Current Therapy in

EXOTIC PET PRACTICE

Current Therapy in

EXOTIC PET PRACTICE

MARK A. MITCHELL, DVM, MS, PHD, DECZM (HERPETOLOGY)
Professor, Zoological Medicine
Department of Veterinary Clinical Medicine
College of Veterinary Medicine
University of Illinois
Urbana, Illinois

THOMAS N. TULLY, JR., DVM, MS, DABVP (Avian), DECZM (Avian)
Professor, Zoological Medicine
Department of Veterinary Clinical Sciences
School of Veterinary Medicine
Louisiana State University
Baton Rouge, Louisiana

ELSEVIER

ELSEVIER

3251 Riverport Lane
St. Louis, Missouri 63043

CURRENT THERAPY IN EXOTIC PET PRACTICE   ISBN: 978-1-4557-4084-0

Library of Congress Cataloging-in-Publication Data

Names: Mitchell, Mark A., 1967- | Tully, Thomas N., Jr., 1959-
Title: Current therapy in exotic pet practice / [edited by] Mark A. Mitchell
  DVM,MS,PhD, Dip. ECZM (Herpetology), Professor, Zoological Medicine.
  Department of Veterinary Clinical Medicine, College of Veterinary
  Medicine, University of Illinois, Urbana, Illinois, Thomas N. Tully, Jr.,
  DVM, MS, Professor, Avian Medicine, Louisiana State University, School of
  Veterinary Medicine, Department of Veterinary Clinical Sciences, Baton
  Rouge, Louisiana.
Description: St. Louis, Missouri : Elsevier, 2015. | "Companion trext to
  Manual of exotic pet practice"—Preface. | Includes index.
Identifiers: LCCN 2015033862
Subjects: LCSH: Exotic animals—Diseases. | Pet medicine. | Wildlife
  diseases. | Wild animals as pets.
Classification: LCC SF997.5.E95 C87 2015 | DDC 636.089—dc23 LC record
  available at http://lccn.loc.gov/2015033862

Director, Content Strategy: Penny S. Rudolph
Content Development Manager: Jolynn Gower
Senior Content Development Specialist: Brian Loehr
Publishing Services Manager: Hemamalini Rajendrababu
Project Manager: Maria Bernard
Design Direction: Ashley Miner

Printed in India

Last digit is the print number: 9   8   7   6   5   4

Working together to grow libraries in developing countries

www.elsevier.com • www.bookaid.org

I dedicate this book to my wife, Lorrie, and children, Mary and RJ. You are the true joys of my life! Because of your love, I feel that I can achieve anything. I would also like to thank my co-editor Tom Tully for being "the big chief." If everybody had the opportunity to have a mentor like Tom, the world would be a much better place.

Mark A. Mitchell

I dedicate this book to Susie, Claudia, and Fiona Tully. Anything I accomplish is a direct result of the love and support I receive from my wife, Susie, and two lovely daughters, Claudia and Fiona. I cannot thank my family enough for their patience and understanding while I am working on projects, such as this book, late at night, early in the mornings, and on weekends. Finally to the lead co-editor of this text, Mark Mitchell, who is an amazing colleague who is always a joy to work with and an inspiration to achieve more than you believe possible—thank you!

Thomas N. Tully, Jr.

Contributors

Hugues Beaufrère, DrMedVet, PhD, DACZM, DABVP (Avian), DECZM (Avian)
Health Sciences Centre
Ontario Veterinary College
University of Guelph
Guelph, Canada

João Brandão, LMV, MS
Assistant Professor, Zoological Medicine
Veterinary Clinical Sciences
Center for Veterinary Health Sciences
Oklahoma State University
Stillwater, Oklahoma

James G. Johnson III, DVM
Resident, Zoological and Aquatic Animal Medicine
Department of Veterinary Clinical Medicine
College of Veterinary Medicine
University of Illinois
Urbana, Illinois

Amber Labelle, DVM, MS, DACVO
Assistant Professor
Department of Veterinary Clinical Medicine
College of Veterinary Medicine
University of Illinois
Urbana, Illinois

Kim Le, BSc(Vet)(Honsl), BVSc
Health Sciences Centre
Ontario Veterinary College
University of Guelph
Guelph, Canada

Jörg Mayer, DrMedVet, MS, DABVP (Exotic Companion Mammal), DACZM, DECZM (Small Mammal)
Associate Professor
Small Animal Medicine and Surgery
University of Georgia
Athens, Georgia

Michael S. McFadden, MS, DVM, DACVS
North Houston Veterinary Specialists
Department of Surgery
Houston, Texas

Mark A. Mitchell, DVM, MS, PhD, DECZM (Herpetology)
Professor, Zoological Medicine
Department of Veterinary Clinical Medicine
College of Veterinary Medicine
University of Illinois
Urbana, Illinois

Romain Pariaut, DrMedVet, DACVIM (Cardiology), DECVIM-CA (Cardiology)
Associate Professor
Department of Clinical Sciences
College of Veterinary Medicine
Cornell University
Ithaca, New York

Sean M. Perry, DVM
Intern, Emergency and Critical Care
Department of Veterinary Clinical Medicine
College of Veterinary Medicine
University of Illinois
Urbana, Illinois

Markus Rick, DrMedVet, PhD
Assistant Professor, Endocrinology
Michigan State University
Lansing, Michigan

Samantha J. Sander, DVM
Intern, Zoological Medicine
Wildlife Health Sciences
Smithsonian's National Zoological Park
Washington, DC

Lionel Schilliger, DECZM (Herpetology) DVM, DECZM (Herpetology), DABVP (Reptile and Amphibian)
Clinique Vétérinaire du Village d'Auteuil
Paris, France

Noemie Summa, DrMedVet, IPSAV
Department of Medicine and Epidemiology
School of Veterinary Medicine
University of California-Davis
Davis, California

Thomas N. Tully, Jr., DVM, MS, DABVP (Avian), DECZM (Avian)
Professor, Zoological Medicine
Department of Veterinary Clinical Sciences
School of Veterinary Medicine
Louisiana State University
Baton Rouge, Louisiana

Megan K. Watson, DVM, MS
Resident, Zoological and Aquatic Animal Medicine
Department of Veterinary Clinical Medicine
College of Veterinary Medicine
University of Illinois
Urbana, Illinois

Kenneth R. Welle, DVM, DABVP (Avian)
Clinical Assistant Professor
Department of Veterinary Clinical Medicine
College of Veterinary Medicine
University of Illinois
Urbana, Illinois

Preface

The coeditors and authors of this text set forth to construct a medical text based on the body systems of the major exotic animal taxa that are treated in veterinary hospitals. The result of this intense effort is the body of information contained within. The challenge of incorporating material from the body systems of invertebrates, fish, amphibians, reptiles, birds, and exotic small mammals into concise, thorough, and, most important, current information is no different from that faced by veterinarians who treat these species on a daily basis. No other book details the body systems of companion exotic animal species as does *Current Therapy in Exotic Pet Practice*.

Each body system comprises a chapter that covers all of the taxa listed above. Each chapter is further delineated into subject areas such as anatomy, physical examination, diagnostic testing, disease conditions, therapeutics, epidemiology of diseases, and zoonoses. Within each of these subsections detailed current clinically relevant information is provided for each taxon. Naturally, depending on body system and subject area, there is more material provided for certain animal groups than others. The primary objective of the authors was to provide the most relevant clinical resource possible. The coeditors feel this objective has been met and will allow veterinarians and veterinary staff to utilize this extensive medical resource on a daily basis to provide quality veterinary care to their patients. This is also an excellent resource for veterinary students who want to learn more about the underlying pathophysiology of disease processes and recommended pathways for diagnosis and treatment options relating to companion exotic animal care.

A picture is worth a thousand words, and this book is filled with color images that are descriptive and emphasize anatomical, physical examination, diagnostic testing, and disease conditions contained within the text. Tables, examination forms, and appendixes are included for easy reference and clinical use by veterinarians who see these animals. When combined, the material contained within provides an indispensable veterinary medical resource.

Current Therapy in Exotic Pet Practice is a completely new book and is in a format different from that of the *Manual of Exotic Pet Practice*. The coeditors wanted a companion text to *Manual of Exotic Pet Practice*, and they feel this goal has been achieved. While the *Manual of Exotic Pet Practice* is relevant and useful as ever, *Current Therapy in Exotic Pet Practice* expands on the description and underlying aspects of disease conditions reported in companion exotic animal species. The complete set of exotic pet texts allows one to find information that will be applicable to both simple and complex case presentations, including those that provide a moderate amount of difficulty in treating.

The advancement of veterinary medical knowledge is increasing at a rapid pace, but not faster than that of companion exotic animal medicine. When treating these animals, to have optimum success requires providing quality veterinary care. Of course there are secondary options that reduce the veterinarian's ability to properly diagnose and treat, but this is an owner's decision. In order to communicate and inform the owner of the recommended course of action, a veterinarian must be knowledgeable of the subject involved. Owners who have confidence in a veterinarian's knowledge and understanding of the patient's condition will be more likely to follow the primary recommendations for disease diagnosis and treatment. This confidence in the veterinarian may begin with the physical examination through handling of the patient and extend to treatment recommendations and prognosis for recovery. *Current Therapy in Exotic Pet Practice* is an excellent resource for veterinarians to use when contemplating recommended diagnostic and treatment options for their patients. As mentioned, this veterinary medical text is different from any previously published in its scope and depth of body system information related to companion exotic animal species. This book alone will not be able to save a patient, but requires the important addition of quality veterinary care; together, they can give the companion exotic animal patient the best chance of living a long, happy, healthy life.

Acknowledgments

This extensive text that details the body systems of the common exotic animal taxa treated by veterinarians posed a significant challenge for the authors. The coeditors would like to thank each of the authors for their perseverance, effort, and contribution to this work. It is impossible to complete the herculean task of publishing a medical text without the help and support of many people. Our colleagues with whom we work on a daily basis provide the support that has allowed us to "multitask" between clinical responsibilities, teaching, research, continuing education, and writing. We are extremely grateful for their presence in our professional lives. This text would not have been possible without the commitment of our publisher, Elsevier, and production staff to this project. Finally, to Ms. Shelly Stringer, Mr. Brian Loehr, and Ms. Penny Rudolph, a big hug and thank you for holding our hands and pushing us when the finish line appeared as a distant mirage. We cannot express enough gratitude for your efforts, understanding, and, most important, patience during the compilation and production of this text.

Contents

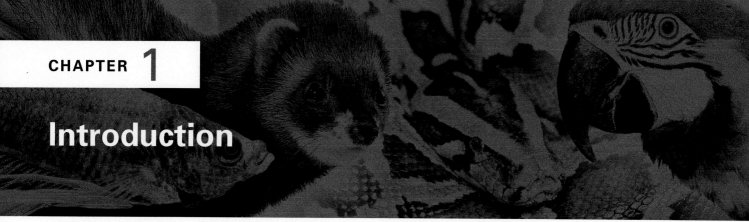

CHAPTER 1

Introduction

Mark A. Mitchell, DVM, MS, PhD, DECZM (Herpetology) •
Thomas N. Tully, Jr., DVM, MS, DABVP (Avian), DECZM (Avian)

Veterinarians working with exotic animals face many challenges. From attempting to interpret how an animal's husbandry may affect its health to determining the most appropriate diagnostic tests required to confirm a specific condition, there are many different questions that veterinarians need to answer to successfully treat their patients. The real challenge for those of us working with exotic animals is that with over 64,000 different species of vertebrates, and another 1,000,000 plus species of invertebrates, developing a knowledge base capable of managing this broad number of species seems impossible. Fortunately, evolution is our friend. Across invertebrates and vertebrates there are patterns in morphology and physiology that have evolved. For example, while a Chilean rose-hair giant spider (*Grammostola rosea*) may have a very different circulatory system (e.g., open system, nonchambered tubular heart) from a bearded dragon (*Pogona vitticeps*; closed system, 3-chambered heart) (Figure 1-1), their basic function is the same: to circulate hemolymph or blood, respectively, and assist with delivering and removing nutrients and gases (see Chapter 5). Using a comparative approach, it is possible to rely on experiences with one species to interpret the needs of another. Of course, there are some limits to this (e.g., hemolymph in spiders and blood in bearded dragons) when dealing with the broad diversity of species; thus the focus of this book, reviewing the similarities and differences among these species using a comparative systems-based approach. By using a systems-based approach, veterinary clinicians can quickly review the differences between phyla or classes of animals and then apply this knowledge to the care of the animals they are managing. For example, clinicians with a strong understanding of the mammalian pulmonary system (e.g., rabbit, ferret) can use their foundation of knowledge with this class of animals to help them to understand the basics of the respiratory system of birds, learn what makes avian respiratory systems unique compared with other vertebrates (see Chapter 3), and apply it to a cockatiel case presenting for respiratory disease (Figure 1-2).

TAKING A PROBLEM-ORIENTED CASE APPROACH: HYPOTHETICAL-DEDUCTIVE REASONING

While exotic animal medicine can seem daunting because of the large number of species that may be presented

to a veterinary hospital, it is important to recognize that veterinarians can manage these many different species if they rely on the hypothetical-deductive reasoning that they use when working with species they are familiar with, such as dogs and cats. This type of approach, regardless of species, directs the veterinarian to identify a problem or problems with the patient, develop a specific hypothesis or hypotheses to solve the problems, perform appropriate diagnostic and therapeutic trials to evaluate each hypothesis or hypotheses, and prove or disprove each hypothesis through critical evaluation of the results. Using a systems-based approach to problem solving will help the veterinarian focus on the fundamentals of medicine, especially when he or she is not familiar with a species. Thus allowing him or her to separate out the physiologic complexity of the patient into its "more digestible" components.

The best method for veterinarians to use when treating an animal species for the first time is to organize the collected data into the standard problem-oriented veterinary record framework. The more we get away from paper-based records, the easier it is for some veterinarians to document more, although some use this as an excuse to document less. In a busy practice, it is essential to document our findings and follow up. This is especially important with new species or species we see infrequently, as it serves as a ready source of knowledge on how we should or should not handle the next case.

Anamnesis (History)

Problem-oriented veterinary medical records are very important for exotic species, because there is often much more information (e.g., husbandry and nutrition) required to determine the underlying cause of the problems identified. To begin with, husbandry-related issues have been and continue to be an important area of concern related to the health of exotic species. When was the last time substrate or perching material had an effect on a dog or cat case? Also, dietary deficiencies are rare in domestic pets but remain a major concern for many exotic species such as reptiles (e.g., insectivores and secondary nutritional hyperparathyroidism), birds (e.g., all-seed diets), and exotic mammals (e.g., hypovitaminosis C in guinea pigs). It is for this reason that the anamnesis (history) is so essential for exotic species. Since husbandry plays such an important role in the well-being of these animals, it is essential that veterinarians take the time to collect

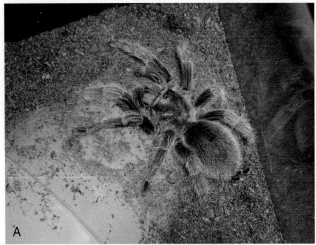

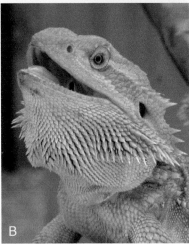

FIGURE 1-1 *A,* Chilean rose-hair giant spider *(Grammostola rosea); B,* bearded dragon *(Pogona vitticeps).* While these animals have evolved to be very different, they share many commonalities regarding the basic "functions" of their different body systems.

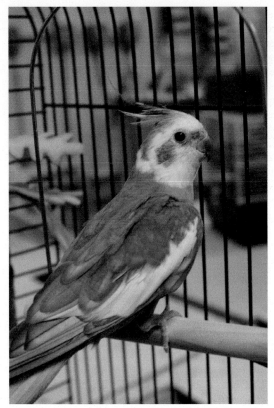

FIGURE 1-2 Birds, like this cockatiel *(Nymphicus hollandicus),* have the most elaborate respiratory system in the animal kingdom. While most veterinarians are comfortable with how the mammalian respiratory system works (e.g., larynx, trachea, and lungs), they may not realize that birds have major morphologic (e.g., air sacs) and physiologic (e.g., air movement through lungs and air sacs) differences compared with their mammalian counterparts. By taking a systems-based approach, a veterinarian can build on their foundation of knowledge with one group of animals to help manage a diverse number of other species.

information that will help them identify disease problems and the hypotheses required for diagnosis and treatment. Figures 1-3 to 1-7 are examples of history collection sheets that may be used by veterinarians or veterinary technicians to identify potential deficiencies in the husbandry of animals presented to their clinic. These "problems" can then be recorded and used in combination with the physical examination findings to direct the case.

An important component of the history to collect for every patient is the signalment; however, this is especially important for exotic animal cases. Knowing the species, age (relative or absolute), and sex will allow the veterinarian to start to organize his or her thoughts on the husbandry needs of the animal, the unique morphologic and physiologic characteristics of the animal, and the potential problems that may exist based on the animal's age (e.g., relative: juvenile, adult, geriatric; absolute: captive born, date of birth known) or sex (e.g., dystocia in a female). Unfortunately, clients may not be able to answer

a veterinarian's questions regarding their pet's signalment. In these cases, it is important for the veterinarian to have a basic knowledge about the different species that they may treat to determine the needs of their patients. As noted earlier, husbandry plays an important role in the welfare of captive exotic animals, therefore it is important to know which species is being examined. When a "turtle" is presented, it may be a species that lives exclusively on land (tortoise), shares a terrestrial and aquatic existence (terrapin), or is exclusively aquatic (turtle). Not being able to differentiate these different "lifestyles" could lead to unreliable information. Fortunately, there are many textbooks available to assist veterinarians with identifying animal species they have not seen before, and the Internet is also a valuable resource for that purpose. However, it is important to recognize that the Internet and some textbooks may provide less than ideal information regarding the care of some animal species. Consequently, veterinarians may want to rely on reference sources to help determine the difference between "valid" and "invalid" information. Ultimately, knowing the signalment allows the veterinarian to determine the husbandry needs of the animal and what may make it unique (morphologically and physiologically). The latter is important when performing a physical examination and determining diagnostic (e.g., where to collect a blood sample from for a complete blood count and biochemistry panel) and therapeutic plans (e.g., using an antibiotic bath for a frog because of its ventral abdominal patch).

Knowing the age of a patient is important because there are certain diseases that are age specific. For example, congenital anomalies are typically identified early in life (juveniles), while reproductive diseases (e.g., dystocia) occur in adult animals. The problem with many exotic species is that it is difficult to accurately age the animal unless a specific date

of birth is known. For these cases, being able to categorize an exotic animal as a juvenile or adult will suffice. However, it may also be possible to further categorize "adult" status by reviewing how long an animal has been under the care of its owner. For example, a ferret (*Mustela putorius furo*) that was adopted as an adult but has been with the same owner for 5 years can be considered geriatric. As veterinarians become more successful providing exotic animals with the husbandry and medical care they need, they are living longer, and as with humans and domestic species, there are new categories (e.g., cardiovascular disease, neoplasia, renal dysfunction) of geriatric diseases that are now being recognized in exotic species.

Determining the sex of an exotic species can be much more difficult than for domestic pets. Species that are sexually dimorphic (e.g., in eclectus parrots *[Eclectus roratus]*, males are

Invertebrate History Form

(form fields)

FIGURE 1-3 Questions to consider when assessing the history of an invertebrate patient.

Fish History Form

Date _____   Clinician _____

Appointment time _____   Client _____

Pet name _____ Species _____ Breed _____

Age _____   Sex _____

Background information

Length of time owned _____   Where acquired (circle) Breeder Pet store Other
location _____

Indoor aquarium or outdoor pond _____

Wild caught or captive bred _____   Previous treatments _____

Any other pets? (circle) Yes No   If yes, specify _____

Any recent additions of fish to aquarium or pond? _____

Husbandry

Size of aquarium/pond (dimension or gallons)_____

Where is pond/aquarium located?_____

Materials (rocks, driftwood, etc.) in aquarium/pond _____

Substrate _____   How often is system/substrate cleaned? _____

What type of disinfection is used to clean aquarium/pond? _____

Type of lighting _____ Photoperiod _____ hours

Water quality

pH _____ Alkalinity _____ Hardness _____ Chlorine _____

Ammonia _____ Nitrite _____ Nitrate _____ Temperature _____

Nutrition

Type of food offered _____

Amount fed/frequency _____ Last feeding _____

Appetite _____

Past medical history/problems

Current presenting problem

Duration of complaint

FIGURE 1-4 Questions to consider when assessing the history of a fish patient.

Reptile and Amphibian History Form

Date _____   Clinician _____

Appointment time _____   Client _____

Pet name _____ Species _____

Sex _____   Age _____

Background information

Length of time owned _____   Where acquired (circle) Breeder Pet store Other
location _____

Wild caught or captive bred _____   Previous treatments _____

How often is animal handled? (circle)   Daily   Occasionally   Never

When did animal last shed? _____   Any trouble shedding? (circle) Yes No

If yes, specify _____

Fecal output (circle) Normal Diarrhea None Urine output (circle) Normal Abnormal

Any other pets? (circle) Yes No   If yes, specify _____

Any other reptiles? (circle) Yes No   If yes, specify _____

Reptile housed singly? (circle) Yes No   If yes, specify _____

Any recent additions of reptiles to the household? _____

Husbandry

Type of enclosure _____   Size of enclosure_____

Where is cage located? _____   Type of cage furniture _____

Cage substrate _____   How often is cage/substrate cleaned? _____

What type of disinfection is used to clean enclosure?_____

Type of lighting _____   Photoperiod _____ hours

Heat source _____   Humidity level _____

Temperature within cage Minimum _____ Maximum_____ Basking spot_____

Nutrition

Type of food offered _____

Amount fed/frequency _____   Last feeding _____

Appetite _____

Water source _____   Frequency changed _____

Past medical history/problems

Current presenting problem

Duration of complaint

FIGURE 1-5 Questions to consider when assessing the history of an amphibian or reptile patient.

Avian History Form

Date _____   Clinician _____

Appointment time _____   Client _____

Pet name _____ Species _____ Breed _____

Age _____   Sex _____

Background information

Length of time owned _____   Where acquired (circle) Breeder Pet store Other
                                      location _____

Housed indoors/outdoors _____   Is animal allowed free roam in house? _____

Wild caught or captive bred _____   Previous treatments _____

How often is animal handled? (circle)   Daily   Occasionally   Never

Fecal output (circle) Normal Diarrhea None Urine output (circle) Normal Abnormal

Any other pets? (circle) Yes   No   If yes, specify _____

Animal housed singly? (circle) Yes   No   If yes, specify _____

Any recent additions of birds to the household? _____

Husbandry

Type of cage _____   Size of cage_____

Where is cage located? _____   Type of cage furniture _____

Cage substrate _____   How often is cage/substrate cleaned? _____

Perch number _____   Perch type _____

What type of disinfection is used to clean enclosure?_____

Type of lighting _____   Photoperiod _____ hours

Nutrition

Type of food offered _____

Amount fed/frequency _____   Last feeding _____

Appetite _____

Water source _____   Frequency changed _____

Past medical history/problems

Current presenting problem

Duration of complaint

FIGURE 1-6 Questions to consider when assessing the history of a bird patient.

Exotic Small Mammal History Form

Date _____   Clinician _____

Appointment time _____   Client _____

Pet name _____ Species _____ Breed _____

Age _____   Sex _____

Background information

Length of time owned _____   Where acquired (circle) Breeder Pet store Other location _____

Housed indoors/outdoors _____   Is the animal allowed free roam in house? _____

Wild caught or captive bred _____   Previous treatments _____

How often is animal handled? (circle)   Daily   Occasionally   Never

Fecal output (circle) Normal Diarrhea None Urine output (circle) Normal Abnormal

Any other pets? (circle) Yes No   If yes, specify _____

Animal housed singly? (circle) Yes No   If yes, specify _____

Any recent additions of exotic mammals to the household? _____

Husbandry

Type of enclosure _____   Size of enclosure _____

Where is cage located? _____   Type of cage furniture _____

Cage substrate _____   How often is cage/substrate cleaned? _____

What type of disinfection is used to clean enclosure? _____

Type of lighting _____ Photoperiod _____ hours

Nutrition

Type of food offered _____

Amount fed/frequency _____ Last feeding _____

Appetite _____

Water source _____ Frequency changed _____

Past medical history/problems

Current presenting problem

Duration of complaint

FIGURE 1-7 Questions to consider when assessing the history of an exotic mammal patient.

green and females are red; in green iguanas *[Iguana iguana]* and bearded dragons, males have large femoral pores and females have small femoral pores (Figure 1-8); in bullfrogs *[Rana catesbeiana]*, the tympanum is larger in males than in females) can be readily sexed; however, the vast majority of captive exotic species are not sexually dimorphic. Even some mammals, such as rabbits *(Oryctolagus cuniculus)*, can be a challenge to sex when young. For species that are not sexually dimorphic, it is important that the veterinarian, at the very least, try to characterize the sex of the animal. In some animals, such as snakes, probing for the reproductive organ can be peformed to confirm sex (Figure 1-9). In others, such as psittacines and reptiles, DNA blood testing or endoscopic sexing (Figure 1-10) is possible. Being able to characterize the sex of

an animal is important as some diseases are specific to one sex (e.g., testicular tumor in bird with intracoelomic testes or dystocia in female bird), and the husbandry needs of some animals may change based on sex (e.g., reproductively active females need more calories than males).

Physical Examination

Once the history and signalment are collected, it is important to perform a thorough examination of the patient. While veterinarians gain a great deal of experience doing this on domestic species, they may have limited experience with exotic pets. In addition, some exotic species may be intimidating, such as macaws or large snakes. However, to be successful with these patients, it is important to thoroughly

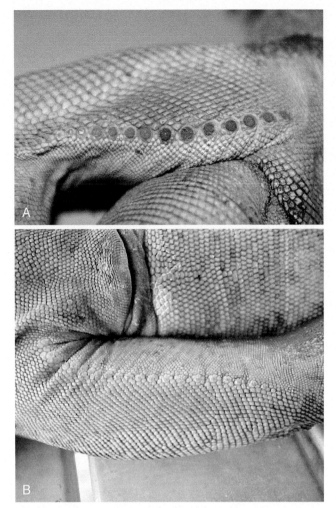

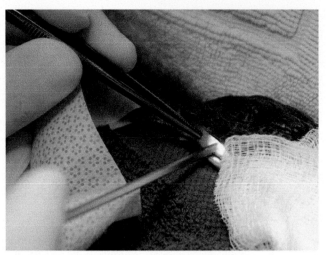

FIGURE 1-10 Endoscopic sexing of a Blanding's turtle *(Emydoidea blandingii).* This procedure was performed in juvenile turtles to determine their sex, as this species does not show sexual dimorphism until they are 5 to 8 years of age.

FIGURE 1-8 Sexual dimorphism in an iguana. Note the larger femoral pores in the male *(A)* than in the female *(B).*

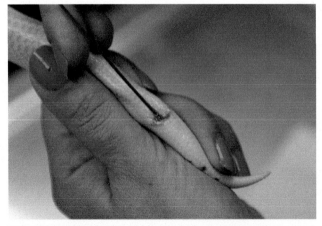

FIGURE 1-9 Snakes can be probed to determine their sex. A lubricated stainless steel probe can be inserted caudo-laterally at the vent. Probe insertion >5 ventral scales is indicative of a male, while probe insertion <5 ventral scales is typical for females.

assess all body systems to develop an idea as to which systems have developed disease problems that need to be addressed. Being hesitant with an examination can result in missing problems and leading a veterinarian toward misdiagnosing the case.

When performing an examination on an exotic species, it is important to divide the procedure into two components: a "hands-off" examination and a "hands-on" examination. All animals have evolved to mask signs of illness. This is a protective measure against being stalked, hunted, and killed. Exotic species, many of which are naturally prey species in the wild, have truly mastered this ability to appear "normal" when ill. Thus, what may appear as an acute presentation to the owner is actually a chronic problem. It is only through a thorough examination that a veterinarian can start to determine the general condition of an exotic pet patient.

The hands-off examination allows veterinarians to evaluate the general mentation, respiratory status, and locomotion of the patient. Exotic species, by their nature, want to appear alert and responsive. An exotic patient that is unable to mask its illness may appear depressed and dull. This finding should alert veterinarians to the severity of the case, providing the basis for a poor to guarded prognosis. When evaluating mentation in exotic species, as with domestic species, it is important to recognize that disease problems that affect different body systems can result in a similar presentation. For example, a reptile that appears dull may have a primary neurologic disease (e.g., larval migrans), hepatic disorder (e.g., hepatic encephalopathy), gastrointestinal disease (e.g., enteritis and secondary sepsis), or excretory problem (e.g., renal failure). Recognizing the correlation between individual body system disease conditions and overt clinical signs is important when developing a hypothesis for an identified physical abnormality to ensure the most appropriate diagnostic tests are selected. Likewise, assessing the respiratory status of the patient becomes important in determining how well the animal is responding to the hands-on examination. Since many exotic species are prey species in their native habitat and obligate nasal breathers, signs of respiratory distress (e.g., open-mouth breathing), are a significant finding. For these cases, it is best to place the patient in a critical care unit with supplemental oxygen to stabilize from the stressful event (i.e., handle the patient like a cat with respiratory distress). Performing a "hands-on" examination on a patient with this type of presentation could further compromise the animal, possibly leading to death. An exception to the recommendation described above is a patient presented with a potential obstruction, such as a tracheal foreign body (e.g., seed in trachea, tracheal *Aspergillus* sp. granuloma). In birds, immediate placement of an air sac tube may alleviate this condition. Further reinforcing the importance of a systems based approach that incorporates different animal groups are locomotion disorders, also important behavior characteristics to assess. A musculoskeletal disease, cardiovascular problem, or sign of discomfort and pain may be considered if an animal is not moving in a normal manner. Noting differences in locomotion and using additional information gained through a physical examination will help guide the veterinarian to develop testable hypotheses that may explain the animal's clinical abnormalities. Finally, the "hands-off" examination can provide some information regarding the function of the gastrointestinal tract and excretory system. Loose diarrhea in birds and no fecal output in rabbits are clinical presentations consistent with disease involving the gastrointestinal tract. Likewise, the overproduction of urine in the droppings of a bird or absence of urine production by a ferret may indicate polyurea (e.g., diabetes insipidus) or blockage of the urethra (e.g., prostatitis in a male ferret with adrenal gland disease), respectively.

Following the "hands-off" examination, a "hands-on" examination that thoroughly and consistently assesses all major body systems should be performed. Examples of physical examination protocols are found in Figures 1-11 to 1-15. Notice how each is divided into body systems, which helps direct the veterinarian by organizing the information collected during the examination. However, when collecting information from the examination, it is important to consider the "quality" of the data. Physical examination data can be classified as subjective or objective. Subjective data, such as mucous membrane color (e.g., pale pink vs. pink), is based on the examiner's interpretation, while objective data are not (e.g., body temperature, heart rate, respiratory rate). Individuals with less experience examining an exotic animal should consider the potential bias that may be introduced when interpreting examination findings. Relying heavily on objective data is recommended and an example relates to body-condition scoring. There are different body-condition scales available for animals (e.g., scoring 1-9, 1-5), and with many cases, there is a degree of subjectivity involved with the assessment. The authors have noted how some veterinarians will score a psittacine differently from a wild bird (e.g., raptor) using the same scale. Most captive psittacines are overweight because their caloric intake is excessive and exercise is limited, whereas wild birds "work for a living." In theory, a wild raptor with a body-condition score of 2.5/5 should be similar to a captive psittacine with a body-condition score of 2.5/5; however, many clinicians have modified their body condition scoring system so that it is relative to the population being assessed. It is rare to find a captive psittacine

with a body-condition score of 3/5 and a wild raptor over 3/5; however, reviews of case reports in the literature show scores outside of these ranges. In these cases, a more objective measurement, such as body weight, is preferred. More objective data are especially useful in cases where follow-up assessment is possible, thus allowing clinicians to use this information (e.g., body weight) to monitor the patient's health.

When performing a physical examination on exotic animals, the veterinarian must consider the morphologic differences between the different classes of exotic animals. For example, as outlined in Chapter 10, amphibians, reptiles, and birds have striated muscles within their irises, hence fundic exams are difficult, if not impossible, in these animals without using an intracameral injection of a muscle paralytic. In cases where assessing the physical condition of the patient is problematic, veterinarians are more reliant on additional testing (e.g., ocular pressures, ultrasound of the globe, performing electroretinograms) to assess ocular function. Using the physical examination sheets provided in Figures 1-10 and 1-11 and reviewing the specific anatomical and physiological differences by system for the different groups of exotic animals will be helpful when evaluating the health status of individual animals. This especially applies to exotic animal species that the veterinarian may have little knowledge of.

Assessing Problems

Once the history is obtained and the physical examination is completed, it is important to document the specific disease problem(s). A systems-based approach can be used to determine the problems that may be linked by body system. For example, an 8-week-old rabbit that is presented with diarrhea may be considered 5% dehydrated during the examination. The list of problems for this rabbit would include problem 1, diarrhea, and problem 2, 5% dehydration. As diarrhea represents an increased volume of water in the feces and a loss of fluids leads to dehydration, the gastrointestinal tract would be the system most likely affected by these two disease conditions. Knowledge regarding the anatomy and physiology of the rabbit gastrointestinal tract (see Chapter 6), including the facts that they are a hindgut fermenter and that alterations to cecal function can lead to colitis and dehydration, can further guide the veterinarian toward, diagnostic testing, a diagnosis, treatment, and hopefully, successful resolution of the presenting problems. By identifying the gastrointestinal system on the problem list, the veterinarian can also develop specific hypotheses (differentials) as to why this rabbit presented with diarrhea and dehydration. Differential disease diagnoses for this case may include endoparasites (e.g., coccidia), bacterial (e.g., *Escherichia coli*) or viral (e.g., rotavirus) enteritis/colitis or a nutritional cause (e.g., diet supplemented with seeds or some carbohydrates that affected intestinal pH and bacterial microflora). For those with less experience with exotic animals, the DAMNIT mnemonic can be used to help guide the clinician with identifying a potential differential disease diagnostic list using a more generic scale. When employing this scheme, it is best to have at least three differential disease diagnoses for a problem, as with the rabbit example. Generic differential disease diagnoses for the DAMNIT scheme can be found in Table 1-1.

Text continued on p. 15

Invertebrate Physical Examination Form

Date _____   Clinician _____

Appointment time _____   Client _____

Pet name _____ Species _____

Sex _____   Age _____   Body weight _____

Hands-off examination

Mentation (circle)   Bright, alert, responsive   Quiet, depressed   Recumbent

Additional comments _____

Respiration (circle)   Normal   Labored   Open mouth

Additional comments _____

Swimming normally? (circle)   Yes   No   Posture _____

Hands-on examination

Sensory systems

Eyes (circle)   Normal   Abnormal   Findings_____

Integument

Skin (circle)   Normal   Abnormal   Findings _____

Ectoparasites? (circle)   Yes   No   Type _____

Gastrointestinal

Oral cavity (circle)   Normal   Abnormal   Findings_____

Abdominal palpation (circle)   Normal   Abnormal   Findings_____

Fecal output? (circle)   Yes   No   Consistency_____

Musculoskeletal system

Body condition (circle)   1   2   3   4   5

Limbs (circle)   Normal   Abnormal   Findings_____

Respiratory system

Respiration rate _____

Cardiovascular system

Heart rate _____

Reproductive system

Active breeding animal? (circle)   Yes   No   Last time bred _____

Last time produced eggs/offspring _____

Nervous system

Awareness of surroundings (circle)   Normal   Abnormal   Findings_____

Proprioception (circle)   Normal   Abnormal   Findings_____

Superficial pain? (circle)   Yes   No   Deep pain? (circle)   Yes   No

List all problems

FIGURE 1-11 Physical examination considerations for an invertebrate patient.

Fish Physical Examination Form

Date _____   Clinician _____

Appointment time _____   Client _____

Pet name _____ Species _____

Sex _____   Age _____   Body weight _____

Hands-off examination

Mentation (circle)   Bright, alert, responsive   Quiet, depressed   Recumbent

Additional comments _____

Respiration (circle)   Normal   Labored   Open mouth

Additional comments _____

Swimming normally? (circle) Yes   No   Posture _____

Hands-on examination

Sensory systems

Eyes Cornea (circle)   Normal   Edema   Ulcer   Findings _____

        Anterior chamber (circle)   Normal   Abnormal   Findings _____

        Posterior chamber (circle)   Normal   Abnormal   Findings _____

Integument

Scales (circle)   Normal   Abnormal   Findings _____

Ectoparasites? (circle) Yes   No   Type _____

Gastrointestinal

Oral cavity (circle)   Normal   Abnormal   Findings _____

Abdominal palpation (circle)   Normal   Abnormal   Findings _____

Fecal output? (circle) Yes   No   Consistency_____

Musculoskeletal system

Body condition (circle)   1   2   3   4   5

Limbs (circle)   Normal   Abnormal   Findings _____

Respiratory system

Gills (circle)   Normal   Abnormal   Findings _____

Respiration rate _____

Cardiovascular system

Heart rate _____

Reproductive system

Active breeding animal? (circle) Yes   No   Last time bred _____

Last time produced eggs/offspring _____

Nervous system

Awareness of surroundings (circle)   Normal   Abnormal   Findings_____

Proprioception (circle)   Normal   Abnormal   Findings_____

Superficial pain? (circle) Yes   No   Deep pain? (circle) Yes   No

List all problems

FIGURE 1-12 Physical examination considerations for a fish patient.

Reptile and Amphibian Physical Examination Form

Date _____ Clinician _____
Appointment time _____ Client _____
Pet name _____ Species _____
Sex _____ Age _____ Body weight _____

Hands-off examination:
Mentation (circle) Bright, alert, responsive   Quiet, depressed   Recumbent
Additional comments _____
Respiration (circle) Normal   Labored   Open mouth
Additional comments _____
Ambulating normally? (circle) Yes   No   Posture _____
Locomotion _____

Hands-on examination:
Sensory systems
Eyes Pupillary light response (circle) Normal   Delayed   Absent
   Cornea (circle) Normal   Edema   Ulcer _____ Findings _____
   Anterior chamber (circle) Normal   Abnormal _____ Findings _____
   Posterior chamber (circle) Normal   Abnormal _____ Findings _____
Ears (circle) Normal   Discharge _____ Findings _____

Integument
Skin (circle) Normal   Abnormal _____ Findings _____
Chelonians
Carapace (circle) Normal   Abnormal _____ Findings _____
Plastron (circle) Normal   Abnormal _____ Findings _____
Abdominal palpation (circle) Normal   Abnormal _____ Findings _____
Ectoparasites? (circle) Yes   No   Type _____
Nails (circle) Normal   Abnormal _____ Findings _____

Gastrointestinal
Teeth or chelonian beak (circle) Normal   Abnormal _____ Findings _____
Mucous membranes (circle) Normal   Abnormal _____ Findings _____
Abdominal palpation (circle) Normal   Abnormal _____ Findings _____
Gut sounds? (circle) Yes   No
Fecal output? (circle) Yes   No   Fecal consistency Normal   Semiformed   Diarrhea

Musculoskeletal system
Body condition (circle) 1   2   3   4   5
Forelimb palpation (circle) Normal   Abnormal _____ Findings _____
Forelimb range of motion (circle) Normal   Abnormal _____ Findings _____
Rear limb palpation (circle) Normal   Abnormal _____ Findings _____
Rear limb range of motion (circle) Normal   Abnormal _____ Findings _____
Pododermatitis? (circle) Yes   No   Findings _____

Urinary system
Urine output? (circle) Yes   No   Urine consistency Normal   Discolored _____

Respiratory system
Nares (circle) Normal   Discharge _____ Findings _____
Auscultation (circle) Normal   Abnormal _____ Findings _____
Respiration rate _____

Cardiovascular system
Hydration status (circle) Normal   Dehydrated _____ % dehydrated _____
Auscultation (circle) Normal   Abnormal _____ Findings _____
Heart rate _____

Reproductive system
Active breeding animal? (circle) Yes   No   Last time bred _____
Last time produced eggs/offspring _____

Nervous system
Awareness of surroundings (circle) Normal   Abnormal _____ Findings _____
Proprioception (circle) Normal   Abnormal _____ Findings _____
Superficial pain? (circle) Yes   No   Deep pain? (circle) Yes   No
List all problems _____

FIGURE 1-13 Physical examination considerations for an amphibian or reptile patient.

Avian Physical Examination Form

Date _____ Clinician _____
Appointment time _____ Client _____
Pet name _____ Species _____
Sex _____ Age _____ Body weight _____

Hands-off examination

Mentation (circle) Bright, alert responsive Quiet, depressed Recumbent
Additional comments
Respiration (circle) Normal Labored Open mouth
Additional comments
Perching normally? (circle) Yes No Posture _____
Locomotion _____

Hands-on examination

Sensory systems

Eyes Pupillary light response (circle) Normal Delayed Absent
  Cornea (circle) Normal Edema Ulcer   Findings
  Anterior chamber (circle) Normal Abnormal   Findings
  Posterior chamber (circle) Normal Abnormal   Findings
Ears (circle) Normal Discharge   Findings

Integument

Feathers contour (circle) Normal Abnormal   Findings
Flight (circle) Normal Abnormal   Findings
Skin (circle) Normal Abnormal   Findings
Ectoparasites? (circle) Yes No   Type
Uropygial gland (circle) Normal Abnormal   Findings
Nails (circle) Normal Abnormal   Findings

Gastrointestinal

Beak (circle) Normal Abnormal   Findings
Oral cavity
  Mucous membranes (circle) Normal Abnormal   Findings
  Choanal papillae (circle) Normal Abnormal   Findings
Crop palpation (circle) Normal Abnormal   Findings
Abdominal palpation (circle) Normal Abnormal   Findings
Cloaca (circle) Normal Abnormal   Findings
Gut sounds? (circle) Yes No
Fecal output? (circle) Yes No   Fecal consistency Normal Semiformed Diarrhea

Musculoskeletal system

Body condition (circle) 1 2 3 4 5
Wing palpation (circle) Normal Abnormal   Findings
Wing range of motion (circle) Normal Abnormal   Findings
Leg palpation (circle) Normal Abnormal   Findings
Leg range of motion (circle) Normal Abnormal   Findings
Pododermatitis? (circle) Yes No   Findings

Urinary system

Urine output? (circle) Yes No   Urine consistency (circle) Normal Discolored

Respiratory system

Nares (circle) Normal Discharge   Rhinolith present? (circle) Yes No   Findings
Glottis (circle) Normal Abnormal   Findings
Auscultation (circle) Normal Abnormal   Findings
Respiration rate

Cardiovascular system

Hydration status (circle) Normal Dehydrated _____ % dehydrated
Auscultation (circle) Normal Abnormal   Findings
Heart rate

Reproductive system

Active breeder? (circle) Yes No   Last time laid eggs

Nervous system

Awareness of surroundings (circle) Normal Abnormal   Findings
Proprioception (circle) Normal Abnormal   Findings
Superficial pain? (circle) Yes No   Deep pain? (circle) Yes No

List all problems

FIGURE 1-14 Physical examination considerations for a bird patient.

Exotic Small Mammal Physical Examination Form

Date _____ Clinician _____

Appointment time _____ Client _____

Pet name _____ Species _____

Sex _____ Age _____ Body weight _____

Hands-off examination

Mentation (circle) Bright, alert responsive Quiet, depressed Recumbent

Additional comments _____

Respiration (circle) Normal Labored Open mouth

Additional comments _____

Ambulating normally? (circle) Yes No Posture _____

Locomotion _____

Hands-on examination

Sensory systems

Eyes Pupillary light response (circle) Normal Delayed Absent

Cornea (circle) Normal Edema Ulcer Findings _____

Anterior chamber (circle) Normal Abnormal Findings _____

Posterior chamber (circle) Normal Abnormal Findings _____

Ears (circle) Normal Discharge Findings _____

Integument

Fur (circle) Normal Abnormal Findings _____

Skin (circle) Normal Abnormal Findings _____

Ectoparasites? (circle) Yes No Type _____

Nails (circle) Normal Abnormal Findings _____

Gastrointestinal

Teeth (circle) Normal Abnormal Findings _____

Mucous membranes (circle) Normal Abnormal Findings _____

Abdominal palpation (circle) Normal Abnormal Findings _____

Gut sounds? (circle) Yes No

Fecal output? (circle) Yes No Fecal consistency (circle) Normal Semiformed Diarrhea

Musculoskeletal system

Body condition (circle) 1 2 3 4 5

Forelimb palpation (circle) Normal Abnormal Findings _____

Forelimb range of motion (circle) Normal Abnormal Findings _____

Rear limb palpation (circle) Normal Abnormal Findings _____

Rear limb range of motion (circle) Normal Abnormal Findings _____

Pododermatitis? (circle) Yes No Findings _____

Urinary system

Urine output? (circle) Yes No Urine consistency Normal Discolored

Kidney palpation (circle) Palpable Nonpalpable Findings _____

Bladder palpation (circle) Palpable Nonpalpable Findings _____

Respiratory system

Nares (circle) Normal Discharge Findings _____

Auscultation (circle) Normal Abnormal Findings _____

Respiration rate _____

Cardiovascular system

Hydration status (circle) Normal Dehydrated _____ % dehydrated

Auscultation (circle) Normal Abnormal Findings _____

Heart rate _____

Reproductive system

Mammary glands (circle) Normal Abnormal Findings _____

Vulva (circle) Normal Abnormal Findings _____

Testicles (circle) Normal Abnormal Findings _____

Penis (circle) Normal Abnormal Findings _____

Nervous system

Awareness of surroundings (circle) Normal Abnormal Findings _____

Proprioception (circle) Normal Abnormal Findings _____

Superficial pain? (circle) Yes No Deep pain? (circle) Yes No

List all problems _____

FIGURE 1-15 Physical examination considerations for an exotic mammal patient.

TABLE 1-1 DAMNIT Mnemonic for Potential Diseases in Exotic Animal Cases

D	Degenerative, developmental
A	Anomalous, autoimmune, atmospheric, allergic
M	Metabolic, mechanical, mental
N	Neoplastic, nutritional
I	Infectious, ischemic, immune mediated, inflammatory, inherited, idiopathic, iatrogenic
T	Toxin, traumatic

Diagnostic Testing

The leading differential disease diagnoses (hypothesis) for a case should be considered the working hypothesis, meaning that the diagnostic plan should follow a logical order to rule in or out this primary differential disease diagnosis. The other differential diseases should represent alternate hypotheses to be ruled in or out based on the diagnostic test results for the working hypothesis. Not following a protocol will increase the likelihood for misdiagnosis. Lack of a diagnostic protocol can be especially problematic for inexperienced clinicians due to a lack of knowledge/experience with an exotic animal species and experienced clinicians who pursue shortcut diagnostics. In the previous case description of the rabbit with diarrhea and dehydration, the top differential disease diagnosis will be determined based on the history and characterization of diarrhea. For example, an animal recently acquired from a breeder is more likely to suffer from an infectious disease than a nutritional disease; however, the difference in the diet (e.g., high-carbohydrate diet or low-carbohydrate diet) could be sufficient enough to result in the disease presentation (and the history should help confirm this). Again, this case description reinforces the need for taking time to obtain a thorough history and why it is so important. In the rabbit example, the diagnostic tests that should be pursued to rule out suspect diseases identified include a fecal flotation, a fecal Gram's stain and bacterial culture, polymerase chain reaction (PCR) assays for various viruses, and a thorough assessment of dietary ingredients. As noted earlier, one of the differential disease diagnoses may rise to the top based on the history and physical examination, thereby improving the selection process regarding which diagnostic test to submit first; however, in some cases there is no obvious top differential disease. In the rabbit case, parasite, virus, and bacterial infections may be considered if the animal came from a large breeding operation or retailer with no quarantine program. In these cases, performing diagnostic tests, based on cost and availability, may determine the order for performing each diagnostic test. For example, a fecal flotation and fecal Gram's stain could be performed in the hospital to rule in or out a coccidial or bacterial infection (e.g., clostridial overgrowth). Results of the diagnostic tests may then be used to guide the initial treatment plan (e.g., ponazuril for coccidia; metronidazole for clostridial organisms) or determine whether additional diagnostic tests are needed (e.g., bacterial culture, viral PCR assays). Of course, it is important to recognize the sensitivity and specificity of diagnostic test assays as well as the potential shortcomings of each when determining their value

in disease diagnostics. For example, a single fecal sample for a fecal flotation or culture may be negative because the parasite or pathogen is shed on an irregular basis. To minimize these risks, the astute clinician may collect and combine several fecal samples to increase the likelihood of identifying an organism that is intermittently shed. Unfortunately, the sensitivity and specificity of many diagnostic tests used for exotic animals are unknown. In these cases, applying the sensitivities and specificities of assays performed in domestic pets may provide some insight. Thorough diagnostic testing is the best way to confirm a diagnosis in an exotic animal; ultimately it will also help guide appropriate therapeutic plans for these patients.

Therapeutic Plans

Therapeutic plans for exotic animals should follow the same basic protocols used for domestic species. However, it is important for veterinarians that treat exotic animal patients to inform pet owners that the drugs used for our patients are off label and that few of the drugs have been thoroughly evaluated with appropriate pharmacokinetic or pharmacodynamic studies. Initially, during the diagnostic workup phase, empirical therapies should be selected that provide appropriate supportive care and stabilize the patient. For example, reptile patients should be immediately transferred to a heated enclosure to maintain their optimal body temperature. Optimal body temperature is important for reptile patients because they are unable to appropriately metabolize and maximize the use of any therapeutic agents (e.g., fluids, antibiotics, analgesics) prescribed, if their body temperature is not appropriate. In the previously described rabbit case, providing fluid therapy to correct its condition of being 5% dehydrated can occur immediately (and before the diagnostic testing) to prevent the condition from becoming worse. Other empirical treatments that are commonly selected for exotic animal patients while diagnostic test results are pending include antimicrobials, anti-inflammatories, and analgesics, among others. However, it is important to recognize that some empirical treatments can cause harm in exotic patients and should not be used, such as oral penicillin in rabbits and rodents that are hindgut fermenters (see Chapter 6). When available, therapeutic agents should be selected using evidence-based criteria (i.e., pharmacokinetic or pharmacodynamic research for that species or class of animal). When evidence based criteria is not available, it is best to use information obtained from similar species or groups of animals to determine the safety, efficacy, and dosage for a particular animal. Regardless, it is important to monitor patients closely and modify the therapeutic plan based on their response to therapy.

Giving a Prognosis

From the time the original history is obtained and physical examination procedure, through the diagnostic testing and treatment of a patient, it is important to provide the pet owner with a realistic prognosis and to explain that the prognosis may change based on diagnostic test results and the patient's response to therapy. In many cases, this information will be used by the owner to determine the best management for the pet's care. For example, if cancer is suspected from the history and physical examination, and confirmation and treatment require expensive testing and surgery, respectively, the client may elect not to pursue the recommended course of action. The authors use the following scale for their exotic pet patients: good, fair, poor, guarded, and grave. When delivering the prognosis to the client, the authors often elect to give a prognosis that is one level below what may be expected. This helps account for the unknown and prepare pet owners for the realties going forward. In addition, some species do not tolerate the stress associated with handling and treatment as well as others. One of the authors (M.A.M.) often states that guinea pigs presented for anything other than a nail trim have a grave prognosis, while the nail trim carries a guarded prognosis. While I (M.A.M.) do not actually believe that guinea pigs are this delicate, they certainly are more likely to suffer from the consequences of stress than other species of rodents (e.g., rats).

Client Education and Follow-Up

Finally, when working with exotic animal patients, much like domestic patients, it is important to provide pet owners with long-term education plans they will need to manage their animal at home. This information is especially important for inexperienced pet owners because they often have to modify their current methods used to care for the animal at home. In addition to husbandry (e.g., providing appropriate environmental temperature for a reptile patient) or nutritional (e.g., weaning parrots off an all-seed diet) recommendations, the client must be properly educated and trained to give any prescribed medications. When and/or if a pet owner is uncomfortable with this, hospitalizing the patient is recommended. Case failure as a result of poor owner compliance can be quite disheartening and often the veterinarian is considered responsible by the client. To limit poor treatment response by the patient due to improper treatment by the owner, regular follow-up (e.g., phone calls or examinations) should be included in the client education handout. The only way to truly determine the success of case management is appropriate follow up on all patients. This is very important for inexperienced clinicians and even experienced clinicians when working on a novel species. The authors commonly follow up with phone calls within 24 to 72 hours and recheck appointments between 7 and 14 days, depending on the diagnosis and therapeutic plan implemented.

CHAPTER 2

Integumentary System

Sean M. Perry, DVM • Samantha J. Sander, DVM • Mark A. Mitchell, DVM, MS, PhD, DECZM (Herpetology)

The thin layer of tissue that covers an animal and represents the largest organ in the body is remarkably variable across taxa. Indeed, even the term for this organ is variable—be it skin, integument, or exoskeleton. Despite the vast differences in structural integrity, the skin plays many of the same roles and has many of the same functions across the animal kingdom. Broadly, the integument acts as an environmental barrier but also has roles in immune regulation, mechanical support, sensory perception, vitamin D production, adnexa production (e.g., hair, claws, spines, scales), glandular secretions, metabolism (and sometimes respiration), and temperature regulation (especially through means of blood flow regulation, sweat excretion, or manipulation of the feathers, fur, or hair that covers it in order to trap or expel heat). Physiologically, each taxon has adapted itself to maximize the functions of this organ in its own unique way. Disorders of the integument can be local or diffuse; affect hair, skin, scale, nail, and beak development; and may even be an indicator of a systemic disease. As with most diseases, a thorough history and physical examination are critical for identifying a specific etiology for a disease problem that involves the integument. Nutritional factors, toxin exposure, stress, and husbandry conditions are important predisposing factors for most disorders of the skin.

ANATOMY & PHYSIOLOGY

Invertebrates

From single-celled organisms to complex arthropods, the integument of invertebrates is as diverse as this grouping. For a thorough review of this system in invertebrates, the reader is referred to *Biology of the Integument, Volume 1*.[1] Coverage in this chapter focuses on some of the most common species presented to veterinarians.

In arthropods, the epidermis takes on a supportive and protective role as the exoskeleton.[2] The exoskeleton is composed of three layers: the epicuticle, procuticle, and epidermal monocellular layer.[3] The epicuticle is typically 1 to 3 μm thick and is a wax depot with waterproofing, pheromone, and antimicrobial roles.[1] The procuticle is 1 to 100 μm thick and contains chitin, which gives the exoskeleton its strength.[3] The phylum Annelida (ringed worms) does not have a chitinous layer.[1] Instead, these invertebrates have a collagenous cuticle that lies external to the epidermis.[1] This cuticle is perforated by sensory and epidermal gland cells.[1] In these animals, the

integument does not prevent water loss or chemical uptake nor is it an avenue for gas exchange.[1] In species where the integument does play a role in gas exchange, such as small-bodied aquatic invertebrates, there is an increased risk of bacterial infections.

The epidermis of a mollusk is quite unique. It can secrete a protective shell that gives the animal its structure and serves as a defense mechanism against predators.[3,4] This shell consists of an outer protein layer (periostratum) with inner calcified layers formed by calcium carbonate.[2,4] The periostracal groove and subepithelial glands form the initial shell membrane, while calcium binding proteins in the space between the mantle and shell allow for mineral deposition.[4] Crustaceans also utilize a calcified cuticle in their exoskeleton.[3] Species with an exoskeleton must molt their shell to allow for growth. The process of molting, or ecdysis, is under endocrine control by the hormone ecdysone.[3] Abnormal molting, or dysecdysis, can result from inappropriate humidity, small enclosure spaces, stress, nutritional deficiencies, or infection (e.g., viral, parasitic). During a molt, the individual is at increased risk for disease and predation.

Different classes of invertebrates handle wound healing in unique ways. For example, higher invertebrates undergo an inflammatory response not observed in lower organisms. Repair of the invertebrate integument after injury can occur remarkably fast. In general, after a traumatic event, there is an escalation in RNA and DNA replication, resulting in increased protein production. This leads to a cascade of events including an elevation in heart rate, improved circulation, and increased hemocyte migration and adhesion, which facilitates wound healing and epithelial regeneration.[3]

Fish

Since fish live in an environment that is either hypotonic (freshwater) or hypertonic (saltwater) to their normal physiologic state, their skin must function as an osmotic barrier to prevent the influx or efflux of water, respectively. Fish skin also functions as a physical barrier and first line of defense against pathogens and physical injury; has sensory roles such as chemoreception, temperature detection, and electroreception; and in certain species can be the source of venom glands and luminescent organs.[5] As in other vertebrates, the fish integument is divided into the epidermis, dermis, and hypodermis. However, the structure (including thickness and composition) of an individual's skin can vary depending on species, life stage, sex, reproductive status, nutritional state, body site, season, water quality, and general health.[6] Despite these apparent differences, many consistencies do exist.

The outermost layer of fish skin is the cuticle or "slime layer." This layer is comprised of mucous and cell debris and is typically 1 µm thick.[6] The primary functions of the slime layer are to reduce friction, prevent abrasions, and function as a part of the innate and acquired immune systems. Immunoglobulin (IgM) antibodies, antimicrobial enzymes, and epidermal lymphocytes and plasma cells in this layer act as an important first line of defense against potential pathogens.[5,6] As such, iatrogenic injuries to this layer through handling or transport can have significant consequences regarding the health of a fish.

Deep to the cuticle is the epidermis.[5,6] This layer is primarily composed of stratified squamous epithelium in two layers: the stratum basale and stratum germinativum.[5,6] Keratinization of the epidermis is species specific and generally limited to the breeding tubercles that form on the pectoral fins and head of male fish during breeding. Numerous goblet cells are scattered throughout the epidermis. These cells produce the mucus that forms the cuticle layer. The number of goblet cells in a fish is inversely proportional to the abundance of scales. Club cells are also located in the epidermis and are responsible for secreting alarm substances and protective exudate in the event of dermal injury.[5,6] These cells are common in certain groups of fish, including members of the families Anguillidae (e.g., eels) and Cyprinidae (e.g., carp and minnows), and the order Siluriformes (e.g., catfish) but absent in others, including the order Gadiformes (e.g., cod, hakes) and the family Petromyzonidae (e.g., lamprey). Some fish can secrete Schreckstoff, a "fear scent" pheromone, to warn individuals from that species of potential danger.[5,6] Some pigment and sensory cells also exist in the epidermis; they assist with chemoreception and tactile recognition.[5,6] In fish, there are no stratum spinosum or stratum corneum layers in the epidermis.[5,6] Epidermal thickness in a fish can vary significantly with age, ranging from 2 cell layers (during larval development) to 10 to 30 cell layers in larvae and adults, respectively.[5,6]

The basement membrane in fish separates the epidermis from the dermis.[5,6] The thickness of the basement membrane varies with both species and location of the fish. The dermis is formed by the stratum spongiosum, which consists of loose and well-vascularized fibrous connective tissue from which the scales develop, and the stratum compactum, which is relatively avascular and provides structural strength.[5,6] Dermal thickness is also species and location dependent but, in general, is minimal over the head, fins, and bony protuberances. Deep to the dermis is the hypodermis, which connects the skin to the underlying muscle and bone and is highly vascular and a common site of infection in many fish.

Scales serve as a protective barrier for fish. Since these animals live in an aquatic medium, they are constantly exposed to potential pathogens.[6] The scales protect against invasion of these pathogens. Consequently veterinarians must use care when handling, examining, and sampling fish to minimize the likelihood of disrupting this component of the innate immune system. Scale types in fish are classified by their size, shape, and structure. The most common scale types, cycloid and ctenoid scales, are thin, translucent, circular discs.[6] Cycloid

scales have a smooth posterior margin and are characteristic of the superorder Malacopterygii (e.g., soft-rayed fishes such as carp, pike, and salmon), whereas ctenoid scales have an irregular toothed posterior margin and are characteristic of some soft-rayed families such as Poeciliidae (e.g., livebearers such as mollies, guppies) and Fundulidae (e.g., killifish). Ctenoid scales are the most evolved scale type. Both cycloid and ctenoid scales can be found concurrently on some fish, such as in *Micropterus* (e.g., black bass), the order Pleuronectiformes (flatfishes), and *Pterophyllum* sp. (freshwater angelfish). These scale types are arranged in an overlapping pattern that reduces friction during swimming. The most primitive scale types are ganoid and placoid, with the latter being the earliest scale type. Ganoid scales have a rhomboid shape with a small peg-like structure on the upper surface that serves as an armor.[6] Placoid scales are also rhomboid shaped but resemble teeth.[6] Fish with placoid scales increase in number, not size, of the scales as they grow.[6] These scales are characteristic of the elasmobranchs (e.g., sharks, skates, rays). Some species of fish lack scales altogether (e.g., order Chimaeriformes), while others have specialized derivatives of scales, including the hard rays in teleosts, spines in stingrays, and bony plates of the seahorses.

Chromatophores are found at the boundaries of the integument between the epidermal, dermal, and hypodermal layers.[5,6] These cells are innervated, contain one or more pigments, and are primarily used for camouflage and communication.[6] Color change can be instigated by adrenergic stimulation (e.g., lightening of color or color loss), cholinergic stimulation (e.g., darkening of the skin color), hormonal stimulation, or environmental changes such as shifts in water quality, temperature, salinity, mechanical pressure, and ultraviolet exposure.[6] Coloration is created by the reflection or refraction of light, with specific cell types being associated with specific color hues.[6] As such, melanophores (dark red, black, and brown hues) contain the pigment melanin, xanthophores (yellow) contain xanthophylls, erythrophores (yellow, orange, and red) contain carotenoids, leucophores (white) contain guanine or purine, and iridophores (iridescent) contain guanine.[6] Some of these pigments, including carotenoids and xanthophylls, are derived from the diet rather than being synthesized directly by the fish.[6]

A number of additional external structures allow fish to thrive in their aquatic environment. The most obvious of these are fins, which vary in size, shape, and position among the different species and serve as a reflection of the niche to which the fish has adapted in its ecosystem. Fins consist of a thin, membranous structure that gains in both support and flexibility with multiple "fin rays."[6] Unpaired fins include the dorsal fin, which is typically large and courses along the dorsal midline; the anal fin, which is located posterior to the vent; the caudal fin (the tail fin); and the adipose fin, which is usually small and located between the dorsal and caudal fins when present.[6] Paired fins include the pectoral and pelvic fins; these fins are associated with the pectoral and pelvic girdles, respectively.[6] The gonopodium is a modified anal fin that is used in live-bearing fish as a copulatory organ; male elasmobranchs have paired claspers that serve the same function but are associated with the pelvic fins.[6] The caudal fin is typically singular but can be paired in some fancy goldfish (*Carassius auratus)*. The shape and size of this fin is directly related to the speed and type of locomotion a fish uses for propulsion during swimming. Additional external structures associated with the integument include barbels, which are paired sensory structures located around the mouth that are used to collect touch and taste sensory input; the nostrils, paired pouches with olfactory receptors; the operculum, a hard bony plate that protects the gills and aids in respiration; and the lateral line, a bilateral sensory structure along the flank that detects sound and changes in pressure.[6]

Amphibians

Amphibian skin is unique among vertebrates because it undergoes significant changes during growth and metamorphosis. A variety of skin cells in amphibians are highly adapted for their unique functions—including hatching and larval adhesion, movement of fluid over the larva, and production of alarm substances. Amphibians are dependent on their skin for respiration, osmoregulation, and excretion of wastes.[7] Veterinarians working with these animals can use this information to their advantage with clinical cases by delivering anesthetics or fluids through the skin and managing apnea during anesthesia by increasing oxygen levels in the water.

In adult amphibians, the epidermis is only a few cell layers thick and is covered with a thin layer of mucus.[7–10] The epidermis is composed of the thin stratum corneum which may or may not be keratinized and is typically shed at regular intervals and eaten, the stratum granulosum, stratum spinosum, and stratum basale.[7,10] Epidermal thickness and keratinocyte distribution vary between species. Amphibian skin is highly vascular and semipermeable, allowing urea, ammonia, and some ions (e.g., sodium and chloride) to diffuse through.[7–10]

The dermis is deep to the epidermis and attaches to the underlying muscle and bone. This layer contains melanophores and chromatophores that provide the many different colors of amphibian species.[7] These pigment cells, as well as smooth muscle, capillaries, nerves, collagen, and elastic fibers, all exist within the stratum spongiosum. Separated from the dermis by the basal lamina are the skin glands, which develop as outgrowths of the epithelium. There are two types of skin glands in amphibians: the mucous and granular (serous) glands.[7] Mucous glands produce a colorless, watery fluid that aids in dermal oxygen permeability and waterproofing. The granular glands produce an irritating and, in some cases, lethal toxin as a defensive mechanism. The composition of the toxin is species specific and may contain peptides, amines, alkaloids, and/or cardiotoxic compounds.[7] The parotid glands are a type of granular gland located on the head just caudal to the tympanum and are prominent in toads (*Bufo* spp.). Modified scales or boney plates (osteoderms) may be observed in the dermis of caecilians and anurans, respectively. The scales in the caecilians form from a combination of collagen and minerals. The small osteoderms found in the anurans are typically located along the body and limbs. In addition, a layer rich in calcium and polysaccharides exists in anurans between the stratum spongiosum and stratum compactum and is thought to play a role in water conservation.

Sexual dimorphism occurs in many amphibians. Sexual dimorphism of amphibian species can be represented by differences in size or skin color but also by a number of modified skin structures. During the breeding season, males of many species develop nuptial pads on their forelimbs that assist in grasping the female during amplexus.[7] Additionally, hairy frog (*Trichobatrachus robustus*) males develop long papillae on their sides, warty toad (*Bufo spinulosus*) males develop granular skin, Rosenberg's treefrog (*Hyla rosenbergi*) males develop "spines" on their forelimbs, and marsupial frog (*Gastrotheca* spp.) females develop a dorsal marsupium.

Reptiles

Reptilian skin evolved to provide physical protection against dehydration, abrasion, and ultraviolet radiation. Less permeable than amphibian skin, it plays a major role in water conservation and allows reptiles to inhabit more arid environments. In some species, the skin can change colors, thereby playing a role in social interactions.

The reptile epidermis consists of three layers and contains the scales.[11] The size, shape, and location of the scales vary between taxonomic groups, as does the anatomic terminology in some cases. In snakes, scales are classified as keeled (ridge down the center) or not keeled. Epidermal thickness is body-site dependent, with dorsal areas thicker than those of the ventrum or near joints. The epidermal layers are divided into the stratum corneum, which is further seperated into the oberhautchen, β-keratin, and α-keratin layers; the intermediate zone; and the stratum germinativum.[11] The stratum corneum is typically 6 to 8 cell layers thick. The scales originate in the stratum germinativum. The β-keratin layer is brittle and forms the scale, whereas the α-keratin layer is pliable and elastic, forming the suture lines between scales. In soft-shell turtles (*Apalone* spp.), the surface of the shell is composed of α- rather than β-keratin.[11] The "horns" of chameleons (Jackson's chameleon, *Chamaeleo jacksonii*) and the "beads" of Gila monsters (*Heloderma* sp.) are formed by thick layers of keratin. The scutes that cover chelonian shells are derived from the stratum corneum.

The dermis is comprised of a mixture of connective tissue, collagen, blood and lymphatic vessels, smooth muscle fibers, nerves, and chromatophores. In chelonians and crocodilians, osteoderms (bony plates) are also found in the dermis. The carapace and plastron of chelonians (upper and lower shells, respectively) are formed by the osteoderms and are fused with the vertebrae, ribs, and sternum. In crocodilians, osteoderms form the thick armor over their dorsum. In the past, some clinicians would suggest that the weight of the shell should be deducted from drug calculations when dosing chelonians; however, osteoderms are metabolically active tissue and the entire weight of a chelonian should be included in dosing calculations.

Coloration of the reptile skin is species dependent and created by a combination of melanocytes (located in the basal layer of the epidermis) and chromatophores (in the outermost layers of the dermis). There are three basic chromatophores: xanthophores (yellow, orange, or red coloration), iridophores (white coloration or reflective), and melanophores (black, brown, or red coloration).[11] The distribution of chromatophores is species dependent, and stacking of these cells is present in species that display color change.

Reptile skin is relatively aglandular; however, there are some site-specific glands to consider. Scent (musk) glands can be found within the vent of both snakes and lizards.[11] A snake's scent glands may be expressed during probing (sexing) or cloacal exams. Some chelonians and lizards (e.g., iguanas) have salt glands within their nares to aid in water conservation. Prefemoral and precloacal glands (represented grossly as pores) are observed in some lizards (e.g., geckos, bearded dragons, and iguanas). These pores are often useful in determining sex in reproductively active animals, with males having larger pores than females. Rathke's (musk) gland is a bilaterally paired gland located at the bridge of the shell of chelonians.[11] Finally, many species of chameleons have temporal glands located at the lateral commissure of their mouth that secrete a malodorous waxy substance that is thought to be used in defensive behavior, territorial marking, or to attract insect prey items.

Ecdysis, or shedding of the skin, is a normal and necessary physiologic process that continues throughout the life of all reptiles. Ecdysis can be broken down into two primary phases (resting and renewal) that can then be further characterized into six stages.[11] The resting phase, or stage 1, is the period between episodes of ecdysis. While the length of this phase is variable, it is shortest in young growing animals and longest in older animals. Environmental temperature, which can affect the growth of reptiles, can also influence this stage. In snakes, the resting phase is maintained by thyroid hormones, whereas thyroid hormones are necessary to induce the renewal phase in lizards. The renewal phase (stages 2 to 6) typically occurs over a two-week period, during which individuals may hide, refuse food, or become aggressive.[11] The skin of reptiles is more fragile during this period; therefore, handling should be minimized to prevent injury. During the renewal phase, the skin becomes characteristically dull and the spectacles (snakes) opaque as the cells of the stratum germinativum proliferate to create a new three-layer epidermis.[11] Lymph then diffuses into the area forming a cleavage zone, enzymatically separating the epidermal generations. Sloughing of the outer epidermal layer then occurs, returning the animal to its natural "shiny" and colorful appearance. While lizards, crocodilians, and chelonians shed their skin in small pieces or flakes, snakes shed their skin *in toto*. Dermatitis, surgical incisions, parasites, hormone imbalances, and trauma can affect normal shedding patterns in reptiles, leading to dysecdysis, or improper shedding. Husbandry deficiencies (e.g., diet, low ambient temperature, humidity, no firm area to rub against to start shedding process) can also lead to dysecdysis.

Birds

As with the lower vertebrates, avian skin is also composed of an epidermis and dermis; however, avian skin is thin when compared to fish, amphibians, and reptiles.[12,13] The outer surface of the skin is covered by a layer of soft keratin, which will typically molt at the same time as the feathers.[13] Additionally, some avian species have scales made of hard keratin on their legs and feet that do not molt.[13] The epidermis itself is divided into the stratum corneum, which forms the hard or soft keratin layer, and the deeper stratum germinativum, which can be further subdivided into the stratum basale, stratum intermedium, and stratum transitivum.[12,13] Deep to these layers is the dermis, which is attached to underlying structures and contains apterial muscles and some fat.[13] Birds have reduced nerve endings and blood vessels in their skin, therefore they are less susceptible to both pain and hemorrhage.

While true glands, including sweat glands, are absent throughout most of the skin, epidermal cells may secrete a lipoid sebaceous material.[13,14] The glands that do exist include the uropygial (preening) gland, located on the dorsum at the base of the tail; pericloacal glands, which secrete mucus; and the glands of the ear canals.[13] The uropygial gland secretes a lipid-rich sebaceous material that is considered important for protecting and waterproofing the feathers and inhibiting bacterial and fungal growth.[13,14] However, despite its absence in some species (e.g., Amazon parrots [*Amazona* spp.], ratites, and members of Columbidae, Picidae, and Otididae), waterproofing of the feathers is not impaired.[13,14]

Avian skin contains several uniquely adapted structures, many of which are genus or species specific. In domestic poultry, the comb, wattle, and snood are present to varying degrees, are rich in blood supply, and, especially in the case of the snood, play an important role in courtship display.[13] The cere is located at the base of the upper beak in some avian orders (Strigiformes, Psittaciformes, and Columbiformes) and is highly innervated by the trigeminal nerve.[13,14] The color of this structure can be used to determine the sex of some species (e.g., budgerigar [*Melopsittacus undulatus*]), while changes in coloration can be a sign of a disease process (e.g., Sertoli cell tumor).[13] The brood patch is a highly vascularized structure over the breast in some male and female birds that aids in egg incubation during brooding.[13] The "nails" (or claws) of birds are similar to the claws of dogs (*Canis lupus familiaris*) and cats (*Felis catus*) and can be present on the feet and the wings of some species (e.g., ratites).[13] The beak (or bill) is a bony core covered by a thin, highly vascularized lamina beneath the rhamphotheca (keratinized horny material).[13,14] The rhamphotheca is further classified as the rhinotheca (maxillary beak) and gnathotheca (mandibular beak); the cutting edge of both is referred to as the tomia.[14] The rhamphotheca contains calcium phosphate and hydroxyapatite to provide strength and, in some species, continuously grows to combat wear from use.[13,14] Innervation of the beak structures is via all three branches of the trigeminal nerve.[13,14] Beak shape and size is dependent on both species feeding and behavior patterns.

Feathers grow from a follicle in the dermis. A dermal papilla projects into the base of the feather, acting as both a blood and nerve supply for the feather.[13,14] Herbst's corpuscles, which detect vibrations, and smooth muscle, which acts to elevate the feather to provide insulation for the bird, are also found at the base of a feather.[13] The feather calamus (quill) attaches to the follicle and contains mesoderm and an axillary artery and vein during feather development.[13] As the feather matures, the calamus becomes hollow. The rachis is the main shaft of the feather and on either side are the vanes. The external and internal vanes are often asymmetric and composed of barbs and barbules that bear hooks (barbicels) that hold the barbs and barbules together. Feathers are arranged in tracts (pterylae) along the body; areas of skin between these tracts (apteria) can be species specific. In some cases, these areas can be utilized to the clinician's advantage, such as using the apteria of the jugular veins to visualize the vessel(s) for venipuncture.

Feather structure and function are dependent on location on the body and age of the individual. Most avian species are covered with natal down feathers at hatching.[13] The natal down feathers are then replaced by juvenile feathers that are smaller and narrower than adult feathers.[13] Adult feathers typically appear at the third molt and are further divided based on structure, function, and location on the body.[13] There are four basic types of feathers: contour, semiplume, bristle, and down. Contour feathers are the outermost layer of feathers that give a bird its shape and coloration. Of these, flight feathers are subdivided into primary, secondary, and tertiary remiges (arising from the manus, antebrachium, and humerus, respectively) and retrices (tail).[14] Remiges and retrices provide surface area to both power and control flight. Contour feathers are covered at their base by covert feathers.[14] Deep to the covert feather is the semiplume feather. Characterized by a large rachis with a fluffy vane, semiplume feathers play an important role in insulation.[14] Filoplume feathers have a long shaft with a tuft of barbs or barbules at the distal end, are highly innervated, and are found near the follicle of each contour feather. Down feathers, or plumules, are fine feathers that lack barbules.[14] Bristle feathers have a stiff rachis, little to no barbs, are typically found near the eyes or the base of the beak, and may serve a tactile function.[14] Powder feathers are those that shed fine granules of keratin, which aids in waterproofing the feathers.[14]

Feather molting occurs in all birds.[13] Some species molt individual feathers gradually and continually over the course of the year (e.g., tropical species); some molt seasonally, with some species molting as infrequently as every 2 years; and others molt as frequently as 3 times per year.[13,14] A molt typically occurs during periods of sexual inactivity and follows a symmetric and distinct pattern in which primary flight feathers are lost first (in a proximal to distal pattern), secondary flight feathers are lost second (in a distal to proximal pattern), and body feathers are lost last.[13] Tail feathers often molt in a pattern that starts at the midline and moves in a lateral direction. Powder feathers are shed continuously and are thus exempt from this molting pattern. While many species will undergo this process slowly to retain flight capabilities during a molt, others will have a catastrophic molt, resulting in a large number of feathers lost at one time and rendering the bird flightless.[13] A molt is triggered by a number of environmental and hormonal cues, including photoperiod, temperature, nutrition, humidity, stress, elevation in thyroid hormone concentrations (T_3 and T_4), and potential alterations in catecholamines and prolactin.[13,14]

Mammals

Mammalian skin is complex, blending with mucous membranes and underlying dermis and having notable differences across mammalian families.[15] As has been discussed for other groups, the thickness of epidermis and dermis are both species and location dependent.[16] The epidermis is formed by several layers of cells, all of which migrate toward the surface where they are later sloughed.[15,16] In this migration, cells are systematically incorporated into each of the four layers (stratum) of the epidermis (basale, spinosum, granulosum, and corneum).[15,16] Approximately 85% of the epidermis is comprised of keratinocytes that are responsible for keratin production.[15,16] Additionally, within the epidermis are melanocytes that contain melanin and are associated with skin and hair coloration, Langerhans cells that process antigens, and Merkel cells, mechanoreceptors that influence skin blood flow and sweat production.[15,16] The thickness of the epidermis is often correlated to the areas that are used the most (e.g., footpads are thicker than the axillary region).[16] The epidermis itself is

devoid of blood and lymphatic vessels.[15,16] Specialized cells within the epidermis will produce hair, glands, digital pads, horn, hoof, and claws.[16]

The dermis is primarily composed of collagen bundles and gives skin its tensile strength.[15] The dermis is divided into the stratum papillare and stratum reticulare, distinguished by the character of collagen fibers located in each region.[15] This region of the skin is highly vascular and innervated, allowing it to supply the overlying epidermis with nutrients via diffusion.[15,16] Additionally, the dermis contains hair follicles, arrector pili muscles, and many glands (e.g., sweat and sebaceous glands).[15,16]

Deep to the dermis is the subcutis or hypodermis, typically the thickest layer of skin.[15,16] The subcutis is composed primarily of loose connective tissue and fat that function to anchor the dermis to the underlying muscle or bone.[15,16] In many species, the subcutis contains white fat, although in rodents, brown fat is located between the scapulae, around the ventral neck, and in the axillary and inguinal regions.[15] In regions where movement is not desirable, such as the lips, eyelids, external ear, and nipple, the subcutis is notably thin or absent, whereas in animals with a scruff over the back of the neck (e.g., small rodents, rabbits [*Oryctolagus cuniculus*], and ferrets [*Mustela putorius*]), this layer is more prominent.[15] The thickness of the subcutis is therefore remarkably variable between species and even when comparing different locations on a single individual.[15]

Hair is a defining characteristic of mammals, providing thermal insulation, sensory perception, and protection of the skin.[15,16] Hairs are characterized as three types: primary or guard (outercoat), secondary or down (undercoat), and tactile (vibrissae).[15] Hair distribution, thickness, and coloration are variable among species and individuals within a given species.[15,16] For example, in rodents, the pinnae are often hairless, with the exception of the gerbil (*Meriones unguiculatus*), while in rabbits, ferrets, dogs, cats, horses (*Equus caballus*), cows (*Bos taurus*), and alpaca (*Vicugna pacos*), the pinnae have hair.[15,16] All hairs develop from follicles and slope caudally and ventrally as a result of the follicle's oblique position in the skin.[15] The number of hairs per follicle varies by species, breed, and age of the individual.[15] Chinchillas (*Chinchilla lanigera*) can have as many as 60 hairs per follicle, the most of any species, creating their naturally dense, soft coat.[15]

Hair is a flexible column of dead epithelial cells that are consolidated and keratinized.[15] The pigment defining hair color is located within the cortex of the hair shaft. Hairs are associated with sebaceous glands, sweat glands, and arrector pili muscles.[15] When the arrector pili muscle is contracted, piloerection causes a thickening of the hair pile, trapping of air, and improved thermal insulation.[15] Hair growth is cyclic and is affected by a number of factors, including photoperiod, ambient temperature, nutritional status, individual health, stress, genetics, and hormonal triggers (especially estrogen, testosterone, adrenal steroids, and thyroid hormone).[15,16] After shaving, hair can take 3 to 18 months to fully regrow, depending on the length of the coat.[16] The three stages of hair growth are classified as, the follicle actively producing hair (anagen), metabolic activity slows as the base of the follicle migrates upward in the skin (catagen), and finally the resting phase, wherein growth stops and dead hair is retained in the follicle until it is eventually shed. (telogen).[15,16]

TABLE 2-1

Number of Teats in Common Mammalian Species

Species	Number of Teats in Males and Females
Ferrets	8
Rabbits	6-8
Guinea pigs	2; reports of up to 4
Chinchillas	6
Mice	10-12
Rats	10-12
Hamsters	12-17
Gerbils	8
Sugar gliders	4
African hedgehogs	2-5 pairs
Prairie dog	8

Meredith A. Structure and function of mammal skin. In: Paterson S, ed. *Skin Diseases of Exotic Pets.* Oxford: Blackwell Science; 2006:175-183.

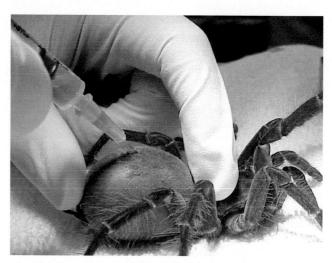

FIGURE 2-1 Bald abdomens are a common finding in captive spiders such as this goliath bird eating spider *(Theraphosa blondi).* The urticating hairs will be replaced after the next molt.

Specialized structures in mammal skin include tactile hairs, footpads, claws, sebaceous scent glands, and mammary glands. Tactile hairs are thicker than primary hairs and are typically located on the upper lip and muzzle, above the eyelid, near the ear, and on the caudal side of the thoracic limbs.[15] These hairs are so named because their follicle extends deep into the subcutis or superficial muscles and is surrounded by a venous sinus; nerve endings in this sinus are responsive to mechanical stimulation.[15] Footpads are areas of thickened epidermis to protect against mechanical trauma, with underlying fat deposits that absorb shock. Claws are dense, thick, cornified epidermis that are retractable in most felids.[15] Sebaceous scent glands are used for scent marking, communication, and territorial behavior. Mammary glands are modified sweat glands that produce milk.[15] The number of mammary glands and teats is variable among species (Table 2-1).[15]

DISEASES OF THE INTEGUMENT

Invertebrates

Husbandry-Related Diseases
The abdomen of a tarantula is covered in urticating hairs that can be shed as a defense mechanism. These hairs are highly irritating and can cause significant hypersensitivity reactions in humans when they contact the skin or conjunctiva. Over time, the abdomen of these spiders will become "bald" (Figure 2-1). Inexperienced caretakers may believe that their pet tarantula has alopecia; however, these hairs will regenerate with the next ecdysis. Spiders that consistently flick their urticating hairs are under some form of stress, so it is important to reevaluate the husbandry of the spider to minimize stressful conditions within their environment.

Traumatic injuries in spiders commonly result in tears to the cuticle. These injuries can lead to a significant loss of hemolymph. Tissue glue can be applied to the injury to minimize hemolymph loss, although these cases carry a grave prognosis. Fluid replacement (e.g., intra-abdomen) can be administered to help control dehydration. Injuries to the legs may be managed by autotomy or by using a pair of hemostats the leg may be removed at a joint. The leg should regenerate with the next ecdysis.

Dysecdysis, or not being able to molt, is a common cause of death for captive spiders. Spiders often lie on their dorsum prior to ecdysis and escape ventrally through the exuvium. Spiders that are dehydrated (e.g., poor husbandry) are most susceptible to dysecdysis. If the spider is completely trapped, the likelihood for survival is low; however, if some pieces of retained shed are found, it may be possible to correct the problem. It is best to minimize handling of a spider immediately after ecdysis because it is more susceptible to injury (e.g., tearing of cuticle). Correcting deficiencies in environmental humidity can prevent dysecdysis. Spiders that retain small parts of the shed on their body or limbs can be anesthetized (e.g., isoflurane anesthetic) several days after the event so that the retained pieces of cuticle can be removed with forceps.

Infectious Diseases
Bacterial and fungal infections of the exoskeleton of spiders are often secondary to husbandry issues. Excessive moisture is a common finding with both bacterial and fungal diseases, although low humidity has also been associated with opportunistic bacterial pathogens. A diagnosis of a bacterial or fungal infection can be made from cytologic evaluation of samples obtained from cotton-tipped swabs rolled over the lesion or direct impression smears. Topical dilute chlorhexidine or Betadine can be applied to the affected area(s) to control the infection. Correcting the environmental humidity and/or altering the substrate can reduce the likelihood of the infection recurring.

Parasitic Diseases
Parasitic mites can be found on giant spiders. The mites are typically found near joints or intersegmental spaces where

they can more easily gain access to feed. Affected spiders may appear irritated or lethargic. A diagnosis can be confirmed by placing mineral oil on a cotton-tipped swab and collecting some of the mites, placing them on a slide, and observing the parasites under light microscopy. Mild infestations may be managed by removing the mites with a cotton swab moistened with mineral oil. One of the editors (M.A.M.) prefers to use predatory mites *(Hypoaspis miles)* to control the spider mites. Correcting environmental humidity issues and quarantining new specimens can help prevent additional infestations.

Fish

Integumentary disease is commonly diagnosed in fish. Due to the role the skin plays in the innate immune system, any defects in the integument can lead to significant disease. Skin diseases in fish can be associated with husbandry deficiencies (e.g., water quality), trauma, infectious diseases (e.g., bacterial, fungal, viral pathogens), parasitism, and cancer.

Husbandry-Related Disease

WATER QUALITY CONCERNS. Testing of water quality should be performed as part of any examination of a fish or group of fish. If water quality issues are, not a primary problem with the case, it is likely that they are, at minimum, a secondary or tertiary issue. The authors cannot overstate the importance that water quality plays in the health of fish, especially as it affects the integumentary system. Many water quality parameters that are tested for fish can adversely affect skin. Ammonia, the end product of protein catabolism in fish, will irritate the skin of fish. Large alterations in pH is also a cause of integument problems. Stabilizing pH in a system is achieved by maintaining appropriate alkalinity levels (>120 part per million [ppm]). Inappropriate salinity levels can also negatively affect skin. The common response of fish to poor water quality conditions is the formation of a protective barrier by increasing mucous production. Often, fish swimming in an aquatic environment of poor quality will appear to have gray or white mucus on their skin and fins. The protective mucus barrier prevents desiccation, irritation, and susceptibility to opportunistic pathogens in the water. As infectious diseases can induce similar clinical signs, it is always important to test the water as part of the fish examination to rule out whether any water quality parameters are associated with the disease process. Commercial test kits are available that can quickly assess water quality parameters. While not all water quality parameters have a direct impact on the skin, the potential for negative effects on other systems (e.g., respiratory) warrants their mention here. The following water parameters should be routinely tested as part of a complete fish examination: ammonia, nitrite, nitrate, alkalinity, pH, hardness, oxygen (ponds), and chlorine. Once the test results are assessed, water changes, the addition of stabilizers (e.g., sodium bicarbonate for pH), alterations to the size and function of the filtration unit, and changes to fish density and feeding habits should be considered.

TRAUMATIC DISEASE. Fish aquariums and ponds are often filled with a diverse number of species and sizes of fish, providing a nice esthetic for the aquarist. However, this diversity can often lead to problems for some fish. Conspecifics will occasionally injure smaller members of the same species, while certain species are just more aggressive to other species.

Fish noted to have scales missing or torn fins are possibly being bullied by others in the system. These fish are often presented for bacterial or fungal dermatitis; however, these lesions are secondary to an underlying problem of conspecific trauma. Certain species of aquarium fish (e.g., arowanas, cichlids) may also develop traumatic injuries secondary to swimming into the sides of the aquarium when startled. These cases often present with rostral abrasions. Traumatic injuries can be avoided by managing stocking densities and sizes of fish, only mixing community fish, and covering the outside walls of the aquarium with colored paper to create a distinct barrier for fish to avoid. Aggressive animals should be removed from an aquarium or pond and affected animals removed and treated for secondary bacterial and water mold infections with rock (aquarium) salt at 3 to 5 g/L.

GAS BUBBLE DISEASE. Gas bubble disease is observed in fish when gas is forced into the water at high pressure. The most common gas associated with this disease is nitrogen. Affected fish have a characteristic appearance of gas bubbles (emboli) under the skin. At first, fish may initially appear to have normal behavior; however, over time, their activity levels decrease. Removing the affected fish from the water is helpful but may not reverse the condition enough to save the fish. Identifying and subsequently correcting the gas leak is important to prevent recurrence.

HEAD AND LATERAL LINE DISEASE. Head and lateral line disease is a skin problem diagnosed in marine tangs, surgeonfish, and angelfish (Figure 2-2); it is also commonly observed in freshwater cichlids (Figure 2-3). There have been several possible etiologies linked to this disease, including hypovitaminosis C, electrical discharges within the aquarium, using activated carbon in the filter, and infectious diseases (protozoal, *Hexamita* spp.; bacterial). In the authors' experience, removing carbon from the system and providing a balanced diet can reduce the incidence of the possible etiologies associated with head and lateral line disease. Submission of skin scrapes and biopsies for diagnostic assessment may aid in ruling out infectious and parasitic diseases.

Infectious Diseases

Ornamental fish are raised in breeding ponds that contain large numbers of fish. These fish continue to be maintained in high densities at commercial retailers. As with other vertebrates, large numbers of fish concentrated in small aquariums can predispose these animals to infectious diseases. In addition, mixing fish from different sources, using a communal filtration unit, and providing no quarantine for fish being moved through retail sources increase the likelihood for the dissemination and exposure to potential pathogens.

BACTERIAL. Bacterial dermatitis is a common finding in aquarium and pond fish; however, this is not surprising as fish are constantly exposed to potential pathogenic organisms circulating in the water. The most common bacteria to adversely affect fish are Gram-negative organisms. Many of these pathogens invade through skin or fin lesions (e.g., trauma, effects of poor water quality). Fish with infectious dermatitis can present with erythema, petechial or ecchymotic hemorrhages, ulcers, erosions, torn and frayed fins, and missing scales. In some cases, infectious dermatitis will develop into a bacterial septicemia. Diagnosis is primarily achieved through cytology, biopsy, and culture. Since many of the bacterial

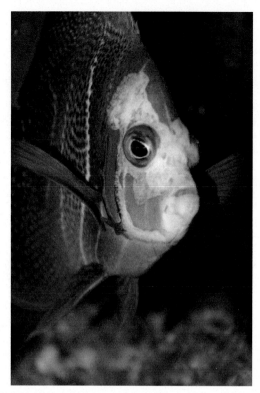

FIGURE 2-2 Head and lateral line disease in a Koran angel-fish *(Pomacanthus semicirculatus).*

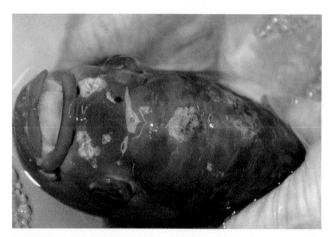

FIGURE 2-3 Head and lateral line disease in an oscar fish *(Astronotus ocellatus).*

pathogens are ubiquitous in the aquarium or pond, it is important to correlate the cytology and/or biopsy diagnostic assessment with the culture results to identify the predominant disease causing organism. Treatment should be based on antimicrobial isolation and sensitivity testing. If this test is not possible, treatment should focus on Gram-negative pathogens. It is also important to ask the aquarist whether she/he has used any over-the-counter medications to treat the fish. The authors prefer to start treatment of freshwater fish with nonantibiotics, such as aquarium or rock salt. Maintaining the fish in a salt solution of 3 to 5 g/L is often sufficient to manage the majority of bacterial infections that affect the integument.

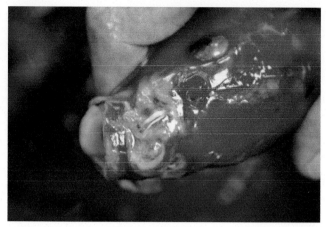

FIGURE 2-4 Ulcerative dermatitis in a koi *(Cyprinus carpio).*

Dipping fish in higher concentrations of the salt solution (10 to 20 mg/L for 10 to 60 sec) is also possible, but the fish must be evaluated closely during this procedure due to the possible toxic effect the saline solution may have on the fish. For marine fish, dipping (10 to 60 sec) in freshwater can have a similar effect.

Koi ulcer disease is a specific type of bacterial dermatitis that is commonly diagnosed in *Cyprinus carpio.* In the authors' experience, koi ulcer disease is diagnosed more often than any other pond fish illness. Affected fish present with erosive ulcers on the body or head (Figure 2-4). Early in the disease process the fish often have normal swimming and eating activity, however the animal's behavioral characteristics degrade through the inevitable development of sepsis. The most common pathogens isolated from koi ulcer disease cases are *Aeromonas salmonicida, Aeromonas hydrophila,* and *Pseudomonas aeruginosa.* Pathogenic bacteria often isolated from fish diagnosed with koi ulcer disease are commonly multidrug resistant and have infectious characteristics similar to that described for "flesh eating bacteria" in humans. It is believed that bacteria in aquatic environments develop multidrug resistance through frequent antibiotic usage during the intensive production process. To minimize losses, breeders and retailers often use antibiotics as prophylactic drugs. In addition, antibiotic medications are often used as the initial treatment for any fish showing signs of illness thus creating multi-drug-resistant bacteria that become ubiquitous in pond water. Frequently, only a single fish within a group will exhibit clinical signs, thereby indicating the importance of an immunocompromised condition (e.g., stress, breeding, bullying) in disease development. Diagnosis of this disease can be made with cytology, biopsy, culture, and antimicrobial sensitivity testing. The treatment of choice for koi ulcer disease is to separate and isolate the affected fish to reduce stress and treat the water with rock salt (5 g/L). In severe disease cases, topical treatment with Betadine and silver sulfadiazine is beneficial; moreover the authors prefer to minimize stress (e.g., no handling), as it appears to exacerbate the condition. Due to the ubiquitous nature of these bacterial pathogens, it is not possible to completely clear all organisms from a pond. Consequently, pond owners are instructed to minimize stress by maintaining good water quality parameters, feeding a proper nutritionally complete diet, and holding stocking densities to appropriate levels.

Columnaris *(Flexibacter columnaris)* disease is commonly diagnosed in freshwater tropical fish. This bacterial pathogen primarily causes dermatitis and fin erosion. Affected fish may develop a characteristic saddle-back lesion, with erosion of the epithelium along the lateral body walls and dorsum. Observation of the characteristic long, narrow rods of *Flexibacter columnaris* microscopically on a wet mount slide preparation will provide enough evidence to tentatively diagnose columnaris disease. Treatment recommendations for columnaris disease include salt (5 g/L) and copper sulfate. Stress reduction and decreasing population densities will help reduce the possibility of disease recurrence.

Mycobacteriosis is a widespread disease in aquarium fish, with *Mycobacterium marinum* and *Mycobacterium fortuitum* the most common organisms isolated. Mycobacteriosis in aquarium fish is a chronic disease. Affected fish present for chronic "poor doing", muscle atrophy, weight loss, and chronic non-healing skin ulcers. In many cases, the fish are eating but losing body condition. A definitive antemortem diagnosis is achieved through microscopic examination of tissue biopsy samples and observing the characteristic acid-fast organisms. Polymerase chain reaction (PCR) testing may be used to confirm mycobacteriosis in aquarium fish. Frequently, postmortem examinations (i.e., granulomas often identified) are performed, allowing one to confirm the diagnosis. *M. marinum* and *M. fortuitum* are potentially zoonotic pathogens, therefore clients should be properly informed of the risk involved. Treatment is not recommended, due to the risk of developing multi-drug-resistant *Mycobacteria* spp. strains. *Mycobactria* spp. are widespread making eradication difficult. As with koi ulcer disease, minimizing stress within an aquarium or pond can reduce the likelihood of individual fish developing a susceptibility to these pathogens.

VIRAL. Viral diseases in tropical and marine fish are not common; however, this may be due to a lack general medical knowledge regarding these infectious organisms. It is important to pursue postmortem and associated histopathologic testing to identify these diseases due to their significant affect on populations of fish in a closed system (e.g., aquarium, pond).

Lymphocystis is a common disease of fish that is caused by an iridovirus and is considered one of the most common viral diseases of tropical fish. Affected fish develop small to large masses that are associated with hypertrophy of fibroblasts. The masses can become so large that they disfigure the fish or affect its ability to swim and eat. Lymphocytosis is self-limiting, therefore treatment is not often required; however, if the lesions affect the ability of a fish to eat or swim, surgical removal is recommended.

Koi herpesvirus (KHV; cyprinid herpesvirus 3) is a highly contagious virus that deserves special attention. This virus can cause devastating losses in koi, with very high mortalities occurring in ponds. Affected fish may be found dead or have mottled gills with necrosis and active hemorrhage. In many cases, opportunistic bacterial infections or parasites are identified at necropsy. When a number of fish die over a short period, the bodies should be submitted for postmortem examination and subsequent histopathological examination of tissues along with full necropsy with histopathology and PCR

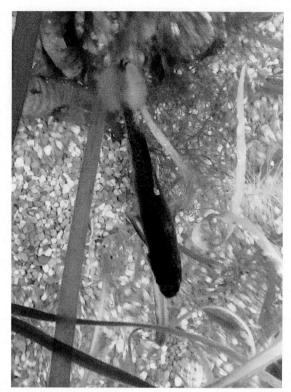

FIGURE 2-5 *Saprolegnia* sp. water mold in a butterfly splitfin *(Ameca splendens).*

testing to possibly diagnose KHV infection. There are no effective treatments for this disease, but there is a commercially available vaccine. Koi herpesvirus requires quarantine (4 to 6 wk preferred) and testing to prevent the introduction of this virus in an established pond.

FUNGI AND WATER MOLDS. There are numerous species of fungi and water molds within aquaria and pond environments. The majority of these organisms function to degrade organic materials within the aquatic system, although some may be identified as opportunistic pathogens. Water molds, such as *Saprolegnia* spp., are most likely to infect freshwater tropical fish. Fish that have epidermal lesions and/or are immunocompromised appear to be predisposed to these infections. Affected animals often present with cotton-like growths on the body and fins (Figure 2-5). A diagnosis can be made through wet mount microscopic examination of the nonseptate hyphae. Recommended treatments for water molds are rock salt (3 to 5 g/L) and increasing the aquarium temperature by 3°C to 5°C.

Parasitic Diseases
Parasites represent an important group of pathogens in freshwater and marine tropical fish. The reason that many pet owners present their fish to veterinarians is over-the-counter antibiotics treatment failure. Thus reinforcing the importance of performing diagnostic tests (e.g., skin scrapes, gill biopsies, and wet mounts) for fish. Dinoflagellates, protozoa, trematodes, and crustaceans are the most common parasites that adversely affect fish skin. Protozoans found to be important pathogens of fish are typically divided into ciliates and

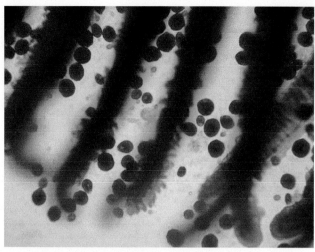

FIGURE 2-6 Gill clip prepared using a wet-mount technique showing evidence of infection with *Amyloodinium*. (Photo courtesy of Shane Boylan.)

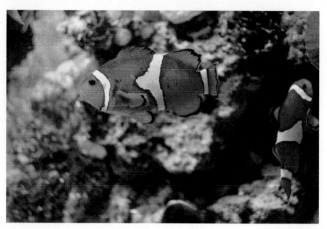

FIGURE 2-7 Marine clown fish (*Amphiprion* spp. and *Premnas* spp.) are the most common species infected with *Brooklynella hostilis.*

flagellates. These organisms can be differentiated by their movement, with ciliates gliding when observed on a microscope slide while flagellates often tumble. The trematodes of importance are monogeneans. These parasites have a direct life cycle and can completely reproduce on fish or within the aquatic system. Crustaceans are macroscopic parasites grossly observed on fish.

MICROSCOPIC PARASITES. *Amyloodinium* spp. and *Piscinoodinium* spp. are dinoflagellates that affect marine and freshwater fish (Figure 2-6). The common names for dinoflagellate diseases are marine and freshwater velvet because the skin of infected fish appears to have a velvet sheen. The life cycle of these parasites is similar to *Ichthyophthirius multifiliis* (see later), with a parasitic trophont feeding stage and an encysted tomont stage. However one difference is the free-swimming, infective stage of dinoflagellates in dinospores rather than theronts. Dinoflagellates can affect both the skin and gills, which results in severe reactions including sudden death. Recommended diagnostic testing to confirm dinoflagellate infections is microscopic examination of slide prepared skin scrape or skin and gill biopsy samples. Treatment can be achieved by increasing the temperature in the aquarium 3° C to 5° C to activate the dinospores and applying copper to the system. Freshwater and saltwater baths can also be used to treat marine and freshwater fish, respectively.

Brooklynella hostilis is a ciliate parasite of marine fish. In the authors' experience, it is most commonly associated with marine clown fish (Figure 2-7). This parasite can be found on the skin and gills. Affected fish often have increased mucus patches (e.g., gray discoloration) on their skin and may be dyspneic or tachypneic. A diagnosis can be made from a wet mount of a skin scrape or gill biopsy. The parasite is circular to oval in shape and has bands of cilia. Formalin is the treatment of choice for this parasite.

Chilodonella piscivorous is a ciliate parasite of freshwater fish; it is similar in appearance and behavior to *B. hostilis*. These parasites can become quite dense in ponds and aquariums. Affected fish may have increased mucus production on their skin, tachypnea, and/or dyspnea. Recommended diagnostic

testing to confirm *Chilodonella pisivorous* infections is microscopic examination of slide prepared skin scrape or skin and gill biopsy samples. The parasite has a round to oval shape with bands of cilia. Salt, formalin, and copper can be used to treat this parasite.

Ichthyobodo necator is a flagellate parasite of freshwater fish that can cause significant morbidity and mortality. In an aquarium or pond, heavy burdens of this parasite on a fish can incite substantial mucus production, leading to generalized mucoid covering of the skin. These parasites can also incite significant hyperplasia of the gills, leading to dyspnea and tachypnea. Diagnosis of this flagellate can be made from wet mounts of skin scrapes and gill biopsies. This parasite has 2 flagella and when curled up takes on a comma-shaped appearance. The recommended treatment for *Ichthyobodo necator* is salt baths (3 to 5 g/L) or formalin.

Ichthyophthirius multifiliis is one of the most common and important pathogens of freshwater fish. This ciliate has a direct life cycle and can overwhelm a population of fish in an aquarium or pond. There are three life stages to this parasite: the trophont, or feeding stage on the fish; the tomont, which encapsulates and adheres to plants or substrates in the aquarium or pond; and the theront or infectious stage, which is derived from binary fission of the tomont. The life cycle of *I. multifiliis* is temperature dependent and clearing an aquatic environment of this organism can be expedited by increasing the temperature by 3° C to 5° C. Increasing the water temperature is most useful when treating an aquarium or pond because it adversely affects the only life stage that can be killed in the water, the free-swimming tomonts. Infected fish present with the classic "ich" clinical signs (i.e., fish appear to be covered in white salt). These small nodules or granulomas contain the trophonts and may be found on the skin or gills. Heavy infestations on the gills may cause the fish to be dyspneic and/or tachypneic. A definitive diagnosis is achieved by performing a skin scrape or gill biopsy and microscopically observing the trophont, which is easy to identify by its holotrichous cilia (covering the organism) and large C-shaped (horseshoe-shaped) macronucleus on a wet mount. Treatment of this parasite should focus on the fish and environment. Salt (3 to 5 g/L), formalin, copper sulfate, and malachite green may be used to treat this parasite in aquariums or ponds. The authors prefer salt because it has the least potential for treatment toxicity. *Cryptocaryon irritans* is the marine version of ich. The life cycle of *C. irritans* is similar to *I. multifiliis*; however, the granulomas on the fish are often smaller in size. Diagnostic test recommendations are similar to that of *I. multifiliis*. The trophonts have a multilobed nucleus instead of a C-shaped nucleus. The recommended treatment for *C. irritans* is to reduce the salinity in the aquatic system; however, this may not be well tolerated by some species of fish. In cases where increased salinity will not be tolerated by the fish, copper sulfate may be used.

Monogenean trematodes are important pathogens of tropical freshwater and marine fish. These parasites have a direct life cycle with two distinct forms of reproduction: oviparity (egg layers) and viviparity (live birth). The monogenean trematodes have a predilection for the skin and gills. In freshwater fish, *Dactylogyrus* spp. and *Gyrodactylus* spp. are most common monogenean trematodes identified, with the former being diagnosed more often on the gills and the latter on the skin; however, they can be found at either site. *Benedenia* spp. and *Neobenedenia* spp. are the marine versions of monogenean trematodes; the latter also have a high predilection for the eye. Low populations of these parasites may not be recognized; however, heavy burdens can result in fish developing generalized mucus over the skin and eyes and hyperplasia of the gills. Microscopic examination of wet mount slide preparations of skin scrapes and gill biopsies will achieve a definitive diagnosis for *Benedenia* spp. and *Neobenedenia* spp. The marine monogenean trematodes have a tube-like body and obvious hooks (opisthohaptor) for attaching themselves to their host (Figure 2-8). Recommended treatment options include praziquantel (preferred); freshwater and saltwater dips for marine and freshwater fish, respectively; copper; and formalin.

Tetrahymena corlissi and *Uronema marinum* are ciliates that affect a variety of freshwater and marine tropical fish, respectively. In the authors' experience, *T. corlissi* is most often associated with livebearers (e.g., guppy killer disease). Ciliate parasites invade the skin, encyst in muscle, and disseminate throughout the body. Affected fish may have integumentary erosions or patches of dermatitis with underlying muscle swelling. A diagnosis is determined through the microscopic evaluation of a skin scrape or muscle biopsy. Ciliate parasites have an oval shape and are holotrichous. Formalin is the treatment of choice for both *Tetrahymena corlissi* and *Uronema marinum*.

Trichodinosis is a ciliate disease that affects both freshwater and marine fish. This group of parasites is often associated with low morbidity but can cause more severe disease in immunocomproprised individuals. These parasites are easy to identify on skin scrapes and gill biopsies because of their round shape and obvious denticular ring of hooks. Salt, formalin, and copper are the recommended aquatic treatments for these parasites.

MACROSCOPIC PARASITES. Fish lice, *Argulus* spp. are commonly diagnosed on koi and goldfish. These crustaceans use a stylet to feed off the fluids and tissues of fish. Affected fish often display abnormal swimming patterns, including rubbing against materials within the aquarium or pond due to the associated irritation caused by the lice infestation. A definitive diagnosis is achieved by observing the parasite moving on the fish. Under light microscopy, one can note the obvious suckers of the lice that attach to fish. Treatment includes manually removing the lice and treating the aquatic system with lufenuron to terminate the life cycle.

Anchor worms (*Lernaea* spp.) are another copepod of importance in pond fish. These parasites have an interesting life cycle. The male and female copepods join together, with the male becoming incorporated into the female and the female being anchored into the fish. Low populations of *Lernaea* spp. typically does not result in significant disease problems but in a closed pond, parasite burdens can become high. Diagnosis is straightforward because the anchor worms are identified when attached to the fish (Figure 2-9). Treatment can be achieved by manually removing the adult anchor worms from the fish using forceps along with pond treatment using lufenuron to inhibit the larval stages from fully developing.

Neoplastic Diseases

Neoplasia presents in fish similar to that of other domestic animal species. Abnormal growths or proliferations may be found at any location on the skin or fins. When a skin mass is identified on a fish, the diagnostic work up should follow

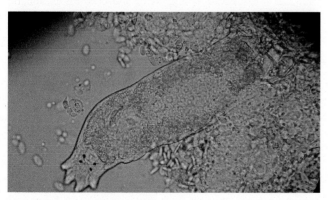

FIGURE 2-8 A monogenean fluke (*Dactylogyrus* sp.) from a koi *(Cyprinus carpio)*. Note the 4 eyespots and the hooks used to attach to the fish.

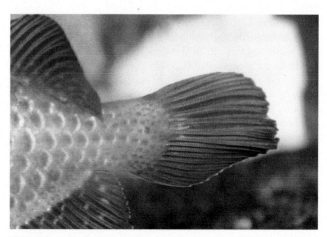

FIGURE 2-9 Anchorworm (*Lernea* sp.) infestation in an Australian arowana *(Scleropages jardini)*.

similar methods described for domestic species, including a fine-needle aspirate and/or biopsy. Surgical excision of the mass is preferred and may be curative depending on type of neoplasm identified and one's ability to obtain clean surgical borders on the removed tissue. Squamous cell carcinomas (SCCs), fibromas, fibrosarcomas, melanomas, and schwannomas have been diagnosed in freshwater and marine tropical fish by one of the authors (M.A.M.).

Amphibians

Husbandry-Related Disease

Hypovitaminosis A is a disease problem diagnosed in captive amphibians as a result of vitamin A–deficient diets. Since adult amphibians are carnivores, captive animals are fed prey species that are commercially available. Many of the invertebrate diets offered to captive animals are deficient in fat-soluble vitamins (e.g., vitamin A). Hypovitaminosis A can lead to the development of squamous metaplasia which results in alterations in the tight junctions between epithelial cells of the skin and linings of the gastrointestinal, excretory, and respiratory systems. Affected animals may present for chronic dermatitis, tears, or erosions in the skin; nasal discharge; tracheitis; pneumonia; and enteritis. A diagnosis of hypovitaminosis A can be made by taking a detailed nutritional history, performing a thorough physical examination, noting systemic changes in the amphibian, and collecting a skin biopsy to identify squamous metaplasia. Measuring vitamin A concentrations in postmortem samples (e.g., liver) may be used to confirm the disease in a population of captive animals. Recommended treatment for hypovitaminosis A is the increased supplementation of the deficient vitamin in the animal's diet. Vitamin A supplementation may be achieved by improving the dietary offerings of prey animals being offered to the amphibians. Parenteral vitamin A can also be administered, but overdosing is possible (hypervitaminosis A). One of the authors (M.A.M.) has observed no complications when using low doses (1000 to 1500 IU/kg) with dosing intervals of at least 10 to 14 days.

Water quality parameters that are important for fish are also important for amphibians. Large fluctuations in pH or ammonia can cause irritation to the skin, effectively disrupting fluid and electrolyte homeostasis. For terrestrial amphibians, alterations of soil pH can also lead to dermatitis and alterations in electrolyte and fluid homeostasis. A diagnosis of poor/inadequate quality of the animal's living environment can be made by testing the water or soil. Water quality measures are determined with commercial kits used for aquarium fish, while soil pH can be measured using commercial meters available for plants.

Rostral abrasions in amphibians, much like reptiles, can occur as a result of the animal chronically running into the sides of an enclosure. Larger anurans (e.g., bullfrogs [*Rana catesbeiana*]), can fracture bones in the jaw as a result of their powerful jumps. Rostral abrasions have the ability of becoming quite severe; in advanced cases, the maxilla and mandible may be exposed, predisposing the animal to osteomyelitis. Rostral trauma and associated lesions can be prevented by providing the amphibian ample space, covering the walls of the enclosure to create a visual barrier, and educating clients on how to remove the animal from its enclosure without pursing it around the terrarium (i.e., dropping a cloth over the amphibian to prevent it from escaping and then picking

it up). Impression smears with Gram and Diff-Quik stains may be used to evaluate the microflora and cell types (e.g., inflammatory cells) associated with the lesion. A uniform population of bacteria may indicate an active infection. These lesions can be managed topically, unless there is boney involvement, and the husbandry improved. For focal disease, topical disinfection with dilute chlorhexidine or Betadine and topical silver sulfadiazine is often sufficient to treat these lesions. For more advanced cases, microbiological culture and antibiotic sensitivity testing is recommended to determine the best course of treatment.

Infectious Diseases

BACTERIAL. Historically, "red leg" has been the descriptive terminology used to describe a specific disease associated with bacterial infections caused by *Aeromonas* spp. and *Pseudomonas* spp. Unfortunately, this has led many clinicians to treat these case presentations with antibiotic medications instead of performing a proper diagnostic evaluation. "Red leg" is best described as a clinical sign of disease. Affected amphibians present for erythema and petechial to ecchymotic hemorrhages on the legs and ventrum (Figure 2-10). These clinical signs are an indication of vasculitis with the animals typically suffering from some form of systemic disease, which may indeed be bacterial in nature but could also be associated with a fungus (e.g., chytrids) or a virus (e.g., ranavirus). *Aeromonas* spp. and *Pseudomonas* spp. are common opportunistic pathogens of amphibians. These bacteria are ubiquitous in nature and are capable of infecting animals suffering from injuries to their integument. Additionally, a number of other genera of Gram-negative bacteria can also cause similar clinical signs. A definitive diagnosis for bacterial dermatitis cases can be obtained by performing skin scrapes or biopsies and antimicrobial culture. The correlation of the diagnostic test results is required to confirm the underlying etiology of the disease process. Other diseases, such as chytrid and ranaviral infections, should also be ruled out in these cases, especially if multiple animals are showing disease signs. Antimicrobial sensitivity testing is recommended to determine the most

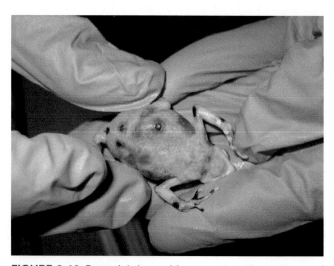

FIGURE 2-10 Bacterial dermatitis present on the ventrum of a Panamanian golden frog *(Atelopus zeteki);* note the petechiations and hemorrhages.

effective medications to treat the pathogenic organisms identified. Amikacin (3 mg/kg, intramuscularly [IM], every 72 h), enrofloxacin (5 mg/kg, orally [per os], every 24 h), and trimethoprim sulfadiazine (25 mg/kg, per os, every 24 h) are antibiotic drugs often administered prior to receiving culture results. Rock salt (3 to 5 g/L) may also be used with aquatic animals to help manage bacterial dermatitis infections.

Mycobacteriosis is not encountered often in amphibians but should be on a differential list for animals presenting with weight loss, especially if associated with a normal appetite, and nonhealing cutaneous lesions (e.g., erosions, ulcers). Mycobacteriosis is an important disease to consider in amphibians because it is considered a zoonotic organism. Exposure to the organism does not only occur through direct contact with the infected animal, but environmental contact is possible. Mycobacteria can lie dormant in aquatic and semiaquatic environments with exposure occurring during water exchanges, wiping down the insides of an aquarium, manipulating the substrate, or cleaning filters. Diagnostic tests commonly used to confirm a diagnosis of mycobacteriosis include cytology and histopathological assessment using acid-fast stains and PCR testing. At this time, treatment is not recommended because of the human health risk. To minimize the risk of zoonotic infection with *Mycobacteria* spp., clients should be educated on the importance of wearing gloves when working with animals with open sores, or when the caretaker has open sores, and hand washing immediately after working in an aquatic environment.

Chlamydia psittaci is a Gram-negative bacterium that is typically associated with disease in birds but has also been associated with infections in amphibians. This infection is most commonly found in captive populations of African clawed frogs. Affected animals may present for "red-leg" syndrome, with erythema, ulcers, and hemorrhages being observed on the ventrum and legs. On postmortem examination, hepatomegaly, splenomegaly, and myositis may be seen. A diagnosis can be made by correlating PCR testing and histopathology results. Doxycycline (5 mg/kg, per os, once a day) or enrofloxacin (5 mg/kg, per os, once a day) are the recommended treatments for amphibian chlamydophilosis; treatment should extend for 45 days and retesting performed to confirm disease status of the patient and therapeutic response.

VIRAL DISEASES. Ranavirus is an important pathogen of amphibians and has been associated with worldwide declines of these animals. In captivity, ranavirus can cause high morbidity and mortality. Frog virus-3 is considered the most common virus isolated from amphibians in captivity and causes widespread systemic disease. The most common skin disease conditions identified in amphibians diagnosed with frog virus-3 include edema, ulcers, erythema, erosions, sloughing of skin, and petechial to ecchymotic hemorrhage. Frog virus-3 is one of the diseases, along with bacteria (e.g., *Aeromonas* spp. and *Pseudomonas* spp.) and fungus (e.g., chytrids), that can present as "red leg." Antemortem diagnosis of this virus is achieved through PCR testing of lesions. Prior to the submission of any diagnostic sample for testing, knowledge of proper sample collection and shipping to the laboratory must be known. Biopsy or postmortem samples can be used to confirm the presence of the intracytoplasmic basophilic inclusion bodies associated with this virus. Currently, there is no effective treatment for frog virus-3 infection;

however, this virus does not tolerate warm temperatures and increasing environmental temperature (>85° C) for amphibian species that can tolerate the elevated warmth may be curative. Quarantine (4 to 6 wk) and PCR testing are the best methods to prevent the introduction of this virus into a collection.

FUNGAL. Chytrid fungi are another pathogen of importance because of their effects on worldwide populations of amphibians. *Batrachochytrium dendrobatidis* and *Batrachochytrium salamandrivorans* are the two species that have been identified as pathogenic organisms to both captive and wild amphibians.[17,18] These fungi have a predilection for keratinized skin. Affected amphibians may present for anorexia, lethargy, weakness, edema, skin sloughing, skin ulcers, and hemorrhage. Morbidity and mortality rates can be high in amphibians infected with these fungi. A definitive diagnosis of chytridiomycosis can be made from a detailed history and physical examination, cytology, histopathology, microbiologic culture, and PCR testing. For antemortem samples, PCR testing is preferred. Collecting swabs from the affected sites on the skin will often yield the best diagnostic test results. Treatment using itraconazole has been found to be effective using both oral (0.1 mg/kg, once daily for 7 to 10 d) and immersion routes (0.01% for 15 min/d for 10 d).[19,20] Avoid compounded itraconazole, as the absence of cyclodextrin appears to reduce the efficacy of the drug.[21] The quarantine of new animals for a minimum of 4 to 6 weeks is strongly recommended. PCR testing animals upon arrival, prior to introduction and immediatly before release from quarantine, is strongly recommended.

There are numerous species of fungi and water molds within aquariums. The majority of these organisms function to degrade organic materials within the aquatic system, although some may cause disease in aquatic amphibians such as African clawed frogs (*Xenopus laevis*) and axolotls (*Ambystoma mexicanum*) as opportunistic pathogens. Water molds (e.g., *Saprolegnia* spp.) represent the group most likely to infect aquatic amphibians. Aquatic amphibians that experience trauma (e.g., thermal injury, bite wounds) or are immunocompromised appear to be predisposed to these infections. Affected animals are often presented for cotton-like growths over the injury. A definitive diagnosis can be made by microscopically examining a cytologic sample on a wet mount slide by visualizing the nonseptate hyphae. Recommended treatments for fungi and water molds are rock salt (3 to 5 g/L) and increasing the aquarium temperature of the amphibian by 3° C to 5° C.

Parasitic Diseases

Protozoal parasites encountered with fish (see Fish, Parasitic Diseases, Microscopic Parasites) can also affect the skin and gills of captive amphibians. Amphibians with excess mucus, erosions, or ulcers on their body or hyperplasia of their gills (larval and neotenic forms) should be examined using the same methods as described for fish, including wet mount examination of skin scrapes and gill biopsies. Recommended treatment protocols are similar, and the parasite should be eliminated from the environment.

Monogenean trematodes are important pathogens of aquatic amphibians. These trematodes have a direct life cycle and a predilection for the skin and gills (larvae and neotenic species). Low burdens of these parasites may not be clinically recognized; however, heavy burdens can result in amphibians developing generalized mucus over the skin and hyperplasia of the gills. Wet mounts of skin scrapes and gill biopsies are diagnostic. These parasites have a tube-like body and obvious hooks (opisthohaptor) for attachment to their host. Successful treatment for monogenean trematoads can be achieved using praziquantel (preferred) or saltwater immersion (5 g/L for axolotls).

Larval migrans is diagnosed in captive and wild amphibians. Since these animals can serve as both intermediate and terminal hosts, it is possible to find larval forms of cestodes or nematodes associated with skin disease. Affected animals present with swellings in skin and subcutaneous space (Figure 2-11). Surgical removal of these parasites is the recommended treatment for the tissue cysts that contain the parasites. For focal lesions, a topical anesthetic can be used. A #15 blade can be used to incise both the surface of the skin and cyst wall, while thumb forceps are inserted through the opening to remove the parasite. Flush the affected area with warmed 0.9% saline then close the skin incision with tissue glue. If the amphibian presents with multiple lesions, general anesthesia (e.g., tricaine methanesulfonate) is preferred during the surgical removal of the multiple parasites.

Different species of ectoparasites may be found on captive amphibians, including mites, ticks, leeches, and crustaceans. These parasites are similar in appearance to those described for other species. Leeches and ticks can be manually removed. The parasite should be grasped near the mouthparts or where it is attached to the skin. Once removed, the site should be disinfected with dilute chlorhexidine or Betadine. For mites,

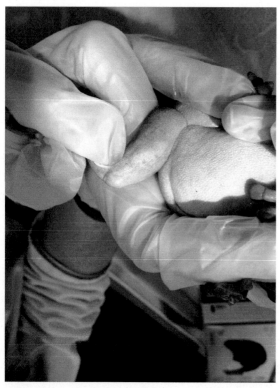

FIGURE 2-11 Subcutaneous parasites in a White's tree frog *(Litoria caerulea)*. A stab incision was made over the white mass and the parasite removed.

ivermectin (0.2 mg/kg, every 14 d, for 3 treatments) may be used to eliminate the ectoparasites. The environment of the amphibian should also be cleaned and disinfected to remove all life stages of the mites. Crustacean parasites, such as *Argulus* spp. (e.g., fish louse), can be manually removed and the aquatic habitat treated with lufenuron.

Neoplastic Diseases

Neoplasia of the integument is not often diagnosed in captive amphibians but does occur. Affected amphibians may present with discoloration of the skin (e.g., melanophoroma), prominent erosion or ulceration of the skin (e.g., SCC), or as a distinct mass (e.g., adenocarcinoma). Biopsy and histopathology are required to confirm a diagnosis. To date, surgical resection of the mass or affected skin appears to be the most effective method of treating cancer in these species. Since some of the neoplasms are malignant, it is important to perform additional diagnostic testing (e.g., radiographs, ultrasound, computed tomography) to determine possible metastasis.

Reptiles

Reptile skin evolved to be less permeable than amphibian skin, decreasing their need for direct contact with an aquatic environment. While this evolutionary advancement reduced the likelihood of certain disease conditions occurring in reptiles (e.g., ammonia toxicity), susceptibility remains to other disease conditions that involve the integument. Skin diseases in reptiles can be associated with husbandry deficiencies (e.g., dysecdysis), trauma (e.g., thermal burns, prey bites), infectious diseases (e.g., bacterial, fungal, and viral pathogens), parasitism (e.g., mites and ticks), and cancer.

Husbandry-Related Disease

DYSECDYSIS. One of the unique features of reptiles is that their outer keratinized layer of skin is periodically shed. Chelonians and crocodilians asynchronously and continuously shed patches of their skin, while snakes and lizards do not have continuously renewing skin. In snakes and lizards, cell replacement in the germinal epidermal layers is cyclic and takes place during a renewal phase. In snakes, skin is shed in a synchronous loss of all keratinized epidermal tissue, which results in the outer skin being lost in one piece (Figures 2-12, 2-13). Lizards often shed their skin in sections. Ecdysis is a complex multifactorial process that is dependent on varied environmental factors (e.g., temperature, humidity, photoperiod) and health status (e.g., hydration). Additionally, thyroid hormones and age play roles in ecydsis. Disease processes such as infection, trauma, malnutrition, crowding, stressors, and parasitism can influence the shedding cycle, leading to dysecdysis (i.e., difficulty shedding) in some cases.

Identifying the underlying cause of dysecdysis is key to formulating a successful treatment plan. Snakes with retained skin patches can be soaked in a shallow warm water bath for 20 minutes to facilitate removal of the shed skin without disturbing the new underlying skin. The container should be deep enough to cover the animal's body with water but kept shallow to prevent interference with the animal's ability to breathe. Reptiles should be monitored when being soaked to decrease the likelihood of drowning. Snakes also can be wrapped or patted down with a warm wet towel to help

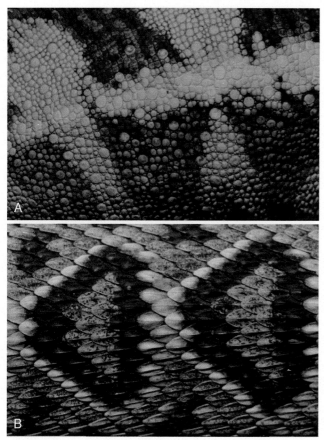

FIGURE 2-12 *(A,B)* Normal chameleon and snake skin in the resting phase before ecydsis.

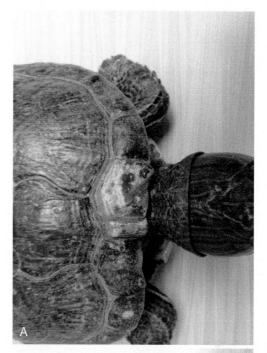

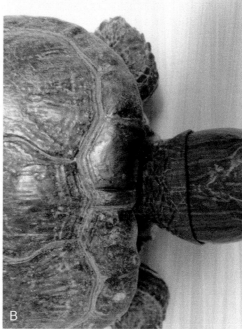

FIGURE 2-13 *(A,B)* Normal chelonian scute before and after ecdysis.

remove retained skin. Veterinarians should aggressively peel back firmly attached shed skin, as this can damage the underlying epidermis. Correcting any husbandry deficiencies (e.g., low temperature and humidity, no cage furniture) will help reduce the likelihood of dysecdysis in the future.

ABRASIONS. Skin abrasions are common in reptiles housed in glass tanks. Skin abrasions can occur anywhere on the reptile's body, although rostral abrasions are the most common. Certain reptile species, such as the Chinese water dragon *(Physignathus cocincinus)*, green iguana *(Iguana iguana)*, and boa constrictor *(Boa constrictor)*, are more prone to develop rostral abrasions because they constantly run into or rub the surfaces of an enclosure in an attempt to escape. These abrasions can progress into ulcers, abscesses, and osteomyelitis if not managed properly. Placing problematic animals into enclosures with solid-colored walls or hanging colored paper over the sides of a glass tank may reduce the incidence of rostral abrasions in captive reptiles that are easily excited.

BITE WOUNDS. Bite wounds from prey or conspecifics (cage mates) are a common reptile disease presentation. In most cases, these wounds are localized, although in severe cases, entire sections of skin and muscle may be traumatized and/or removed. Bite wounds most commonly occur due to mammalian prey (e.g., mice and rats), but crickets can cause severe lesions in small lizards. Bite wounds can be avoided by offering prekilled prey items, separating animals during

feeding times, and rationing food items. For insectivores, juvenile lizards should be fed crickets that are of an appropriate size (i.e., avoid feeding adult crickets to juvenile lizards). It is also important to take into account inter- and intraspecies interactions when housing animals in a communal setting.

THERMAL BURNS. Thermal burns can occur when a reptile is not provided an appropriate heat source. Reptiles typically bask in radiant light to regulate their body temperature. In captivity, "hot rocks," heating pads, exposed incandescent light bulbs, and other unnatural heating elements

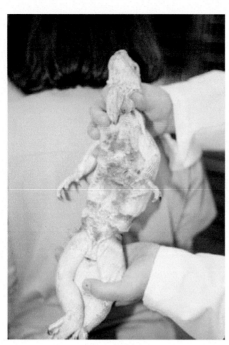

FIGURE 2-14 Severe third-degree thermal burns on the ventrum of a green iguana *(Iguana iguana).*

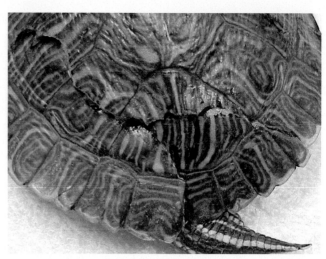

FIGURE 2-15 Carapacial fractures in a turtle. Note that the fractures cross the vertebral, pleural, and marginal scutes. It is important to assess neurologic function in these animals.

have been used to provide "heat". The unnatural heating sources listed above can cause severe burns. Unfortunately, reptiles do not have the same natural reflex to avoid heat found in higher vertebrates, which allows the animal to remain in contact with a heat source while thermal trauma occurs (Figure 2-14).

Thermal burns in reptiles can be classified using the same scale reported for humans and domestic animals. First-degree burns are superficial or partial-thickness injuries that involve only the epidermis, second-degree burns are deeper partial-thickness injuries with full destruction of the epidermis and damage to the underlying dermis, third-degree burns burn through the entire thickness of the skin, and fourth-degree burns affect deeper tissues such as muscle and bone. The clinical signs associated with burns vary; however, erythema, subcutaneous swelling, vesicle formation, blister formation, oozing, discoloration, and scabbing of the skin and deeper tissues are common.

Management of a thermal burn should follow standard protocol. First-degree burns are generally managed using cool compresses and irrigating the wounds with physiologic saline. Second- and third-degree wounds require topical treatment and systemic antimicrobials to prevent opportunistic infections. Fourth-degree burns may require extensive surgical resection and amputation. A broad-spectrum antimicrobial (e.g., fluoroquinolone, third-generation cephalosporin), with activity against *Pseudomonas* spp., should be empirically selected pending culture and sensitivity results.

HYPOVITAMINOSIS A. Hypovitaminosis A is reported in reptiles fed diets that are deficient in vitamin A. Historically, chelonians were the group most often identified as being susceptible to this nutritional deficiency; however, many cases were likely misdiagnosed. Today, hypovitaminosis A is a common problem in reptiles (e.g., chameleons) and amphibians (e.g., frogs) that are insectivores. Hypovitaminosis A leads to squamous metaplasia, which results in epithelial cells undergoing a transitional phase and losing the tight junctions between the cells. Affected animals are often susceptible to infections. Hypovitaminosis A results in systemic disease conditions that affect the respiratory, integumentary, gastrointestinal, and excretory systems.

RENAL DISEASE. Renal disease has been associated with bulla formation due to epidermal or dermal separation in reptiles. Additionally, metastatic mineralization has been observed to lead to dermal vesicle formation.

CONTACT DERMATITIS. Contact dermatitis can occur when a reptile is exposed to novel caustic chemicals within its environment. Erythema and vesicle formation are common sequella associated with contact dermatitis. Removal of the chemical from the environment and aggressive flushing of the wound with warm saline are recommended. Analgesics should also be provided if the reptile appears uncomfortable.

SHELL INJURIES. Shell injuries are a common presentation for both wild and captive chelonians (Figure 2-15). Complete shell fractures should be treated as open fractures. If the shell fracture is greater than 6 hours old, it should be managed as a contaminated injury. Systemic antimicrobial agents are an important component of the treatment plan for these cases, and initial therapy should be directed at treating Gram-positive surface contaminants, ubiquitous opportunistic Gram-negative pathogens, and anaerobes. Microbiological cultures and antimicrobial sensitivity testing should be performed to confirm that the antibiotic medication(s) are appropriate.

Simple, uncontaminated fractures can be reduced using various types of surgical hardware, including metal sutures, cerclage wire, screws, or plates (Figure 2-16). The authors prefer to reduce the shell fractures using screws and cerclage

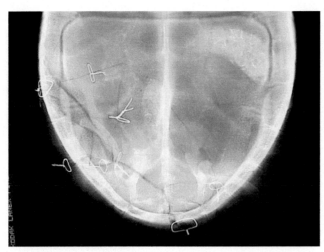

FIGURE 2-16 Radiographic image of a box turtle *(Terrapene carolina)* after surgical correction of a shell fracture with cerclage wire.

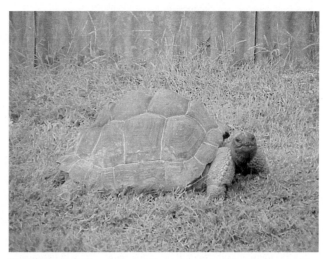

FIGURE 2-17 Shell pyramiding in an Aldabra tortoise *(Aldabrachelys gigantea).*

wire because these products are simple to work with, easy to acquire, and inexpensive. Once fractures have been reduced, they are allowed to resolve by secondary intention healing. The healing process of shell injuries may require 4 to 12 months of convalescence.

The first step in managing contaminated shell fractures is to assess the extent of the injury and remove any devitalized tissue. The injury should be liberally irrigated with warmed, sterile saline. Care is required to avoid introducing a large volume of saline into the coelomic cavity. Wet-to-dry bandages can be applied to the shell surface to facilitate removal of debris. Once the wound is considered decontaminated, it can be closed.

SHELL PYRAMIDING. Shell pyramiding occurs in captive chelonians as a result of receiving a diet that is excessively elevated in protein, nutrients, and calories. The rate of shell growth cannot keep up with the extreme nutritional intake, leading to deviations in the carapace (Figure 2-17). Decreasing caloric consumption can slow the growth of the chelonian and thus its shell. It is best to be preemptive in these cases and grow the chelonian at a slower, more natural pace by providing a proper diet.

Infectious Diseases

BACTERIAL. Abscesses are one of the most common integumentary diseases in reptiles that are presented to veterinary hospitals. Abscesses in reptiles frequently are caseous/inspisated in nature. The inspisated characteristic of reptile abscesses is often attributed to a lack of myeloperoxidase in heterophils. While abscesses can also be associated with fungi, foreign bodies, and parasites, bacteria tend to be the most common cause of these lesions. Abscess formation in reptiles is primarily attributed to skin injuries (e.g., bites, scratches, trauma) that allow opportunistic bacteria to contaminate the wound. Inadequate husbandry also often plays a role in the formation of abscesses, as animals held at low environmental temperatures are often immunocompromised.

Diagnosing an abscess in a reptile is not complicated. A fine-needle aspirate of the abscess often reveals necrotic cells

and debris. Bacteria are rarely identified, as the center of the abscess contains only necrotic material. Abscesses must be surgically opened and debrided. Bacterial cultures should be taken of the abscess body wall interface, because this is the site at which the organism(s) is most likely found.

Bacterial dermatitis is the most common cause of infectious dermatitis in reptiles. Affected animals may develop focal or generalized vesicles, ulcers, crusts, and granulomas. The majority of the infections result from inappropriate husbandry conditions (e.g., chronic low temperatures). Immunosuppression is a common physiologic condition in reptiles maintained at suboptimal environmental temperature, predisposing these animals to chronic infections. The majority of the bacterial dermatitis cases reported in reptiles are associated with Gram-negative bacteria, including *Aeromonas* spp., *Citrobacter* spp., *Escherichia coli*, *Klebsiella* spp., *Proteus* spp., *Pseudomonas* spp., *Salmonella* spp., and *Serratia* spp. Although less common, Gram-positive cocci (*Staphylococcus* spp. and *Streptococcus* spp.), Gram-negative cocci (*Neisseria* spp.), *Dermatophilus congolensis*, *Mycobacterium* spp., and anaerobic bacteria have also been associated with bacterial dermatitis in reptiles.[22] It is important to evaluate the lesion and culture results to determine whether the findings can be attributed to a primary bacterial dermatitis or whether the organisms identified are secondary to some other disease process that must be addressed.

Early signs of bacterial dermatitis include swelling and discoloration of the skin (e.g., erythema). If not identified early in the course of disease, bacterial dermatitis can lead to erosive changes and severe ulcerations. If the skin becomes ulcerated, inflammation can occur in the underlying tissues (e.g., muscle). Alternatively, some cases of bacterial dermatitis can occur secondary to a blood-borne infection by Gram-negative bacteria. Gram-negative bacteremia and septicemia are characterized by petechiation, thrombosis in small vessels, and some degenerative changes to the skin. Some of these bacterial infections lead to abscess/granuloma development. Abscesses in reptiles are caseous/inspisated in nature.

Necrotizing dermatitis or "blister disease" is commonly reported in snakes maintained in enclosures with excess moisture. Affected animals develop coalescing vesicles on their ventral scales. The vesicles are typically sterile but often become infected by an opportunistic microbe as the disease progresses. Placing the snake in an environment with optimal humidity and providing appropriate antimicrobial therapy and supportive care are usually corrective. However, fatal septicemia can occur in severe cases (Figure 2-18).

Septicemic cutaneous ulcerative disease (SCUD) is a common problem in aquatic chelonians living in an enthronement that has poor quality water. *Citrobacter freundii* was the first microbe described as the causative agent of SCUD[23]; however, the authors have isolated other species of Gram-negative microbes (family Enterobacteriaceae) from shell ulcers. It is likely that any opportunistic pathogen producing exotoxins could create similar lesions in the chelonian epidermis. It is also likely that many of SCUD infections are secondary to other disease processes, so it is important for veterinarians to thoroughly assess affected turtles and their environment. Affected animals present with ulcers and erosions on their shell, primarily the plastron. When active,

hemorrhage and ulceration may be noted, although most animals present with chronic, nonhemorrhagic lesions. Diagnosis is often based on clinical signs; however, a definitive diagnosis is possible with more extensive diagnostic testing (e.g., biopsy, histopathology, culture). Treatment often includes decreasing the organic load in the captive system (e.g., more frequent water changes, improved filtration), topical cleaning (e.g., chlorhexidine or Betadine), and/or systemic antibiotic drugs, when bacteria are present.

VIRAL. Viral dermatitis has been reported in chelonians (Figure 2-19), crocodilians, and squamates (Table 2-2). New molecular diagnostic assays (e.g., enzyme-linked immunosorbent assay, PCR) and cell culture lines for isolating viruses have improved the ability to identify viral infections in reptiles.

FUNGAL. Fungal dermatitis has been reported in chelonians, crocodilians, and squamates. *Aspergillosis* spp., *Candida* spp., *Fusarium* spp., *Geotrichum* spp., *Mucor* spp., *Oospora* spp., *Paecilomyces* spp., *Penicillium* spp., *Trichoderma* spp., and *Trichophyton* spp. are the genera of fungi most commonly isolated from skin lesions in reptiles.[29] Most of these fungi have a cosmopolitan distribution and are ubiquitous in the reptile's environment. These fungi are typically considered to be opportunistic invaders and take advantage of a host through

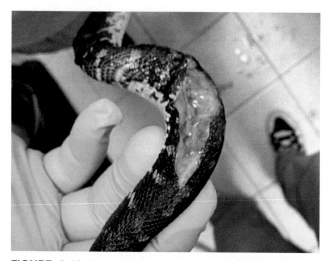

FIGURE 2-18 Neonatal Boelen's python *(Morelia boeleni)* with severe necrotizing dermatitis due to inappropriate husbandry conditions.

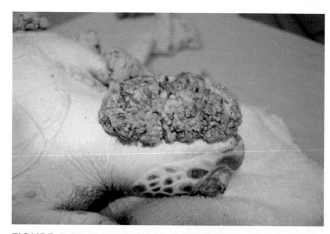

FIGURE 2-19 Green sea turtle *(Chelonia mydas)* with large fibropapillomas diffusely affecting the skin.

TABLE 2-2

Common Causes of Viral Dermatitis in Reptiles

Virus	Reptile Host(s)	Clinical Signs	Diagnosis
Herpesvirus[24]	Green sea turtles *(Chelonia mydas)*	Gray patch disease: gray, coalescing papules	Histopathology: eosinophilic intranuclear inclusion bodies
Iridovirus[25]	Soft-shelled turtles *(Trionyx sinensis)*	Erythematous epidermis in cervical region	Viral culture, PCR
Poxvirus[26]	Crocodilians, squamates	Gray-white epidermal pox lesions	Histopathology
Herpesvirus and/or retrovirus[27,28]	Green sea turtles *(Chelonia mydas)*	Fibropapillomas: large epithelial tumors (Figure 2-19)	Histopathology, PCR

PCR, Polymerase chain reaction.

open lesions. Inappropriate environmental temperature, humidity, and diet; poor sanitation; inadequate ventilation; and inappropriate substrate may predispose reptiles to fungal infections. However, not all cases of fungal infections are associated with poor captive environments, as wild-caught reptiles are also susceptible to fungal infections.[29,30] In addition, some genera of fungi, such as *Chrysosporium* spp., *Nannizziopsis* spp., *Paranannizziopsis* spp., and *Ophidiomyces* spp., are considered to be obligate fungal pathogens and actively infect both captive and wild reptiles.[31]

Fungal infections may be localized or generalized. In severe cases, fungal dermatitis can develop into systemic disease. The clinical signs associated with a fungal dermatitis may be similar to those described for bacterial infections, including erosions/ulcerations, vesicles, granulomas, podo-dermatitis, necrosis, crust formation, and osteomyelitis. *Geotrichum candida* infections are a common problem in farm-raised green iguanas from Central America.[32] Affected iguanas present with generalized black necrotic plaques on their skin. *Chrysosporium* anamorph of *Nannizziopsis vriesii* is a fungus that has been isolated from a variety of reptiles.[31,33] Affected reptiles develop vesicles, black necrotic crusts, and pyogranulomatous lesions (Figures 2-20, 2-21). In bearded dragons, this fungus has been associated with "yellow fungus disease." Since its original identification, this fungus has been reclassified into 4 distinct genera: *Chrysosporium* spp., *Nannizziopsis* spp., *Paranannizziopsis* spp., and *Ophidiomyces* spp.

Diagnosing a fungal infection can be difficult. A cytological sample should be collected from a fresh lesion and evaluated for fungal elements. A cytological evaluation of a skin lesion is often useful in determining the possibility of fungal involvement. Fungi often grow at lower ambient temperatures than bacteria; therefore, the authors prefer to culture samples at both 28°C and 37°C to increase the likelihood of isolating a pathogenic fungus. Certain fungi (e.g., *Chrysosporium* spp., *Nannizziopsis* spp., *Paranannizziopsis* spp., and *Ophidiomyces* spp.) can be difficult to culture using standard methods, therefore the diagnostic laboratory should be informed on the specific media required to isolate the organisms in question. When available, molecular assays can be used to confirm the presence of fungal infections.

Fungal infections are routinely difficult to treat in reptiles and may require long-term therapy. Localized fungal infections can be surgically managed by debulking the lesion or applying a topical antiseptic (e.g., dilute iodine solution) and/or antifungal cream (e.g., miconazole/ketoconazole). Chlorhexidine (2%) has been used topically to successfully treat dermatomycosis in green iguanas.[32] Systemic antifungal agents are not necessary for localized infections; however, generalized infections should be treated with systemic antifungal medication. The literature regarding pharmacokinetic studies for antifungals in reptiles is limited. Ketoconazole, itraconazole, and voriconazole are the antifungal drugs most often used in reptiles. The authors have used itraconazole at 5 to 10 mg/kg once or twice daily (SID-BID) and voriconazole 5 mg/kg SID-BID successfully to manage systemic fungal infections in reptiles. Of the two, voriconazole is preferred, as it appears to be safer and associated with lower mortalities in bearded dragons.[34] Systemic antifungal agents are ineffective for treating against abscesses and granulomas, therefore these masses must be surgically removed.

Parasitic Diseases

ACARIASIS. Captive reptiles are routinely presented to veterinarians infested with a variety of ectoparasites (e.g., ticks, mites). While it is generally considered that wild-caught reptiles have an increased incidence of ectoparasites than captive animals, this unsubstantiated belief is not true. In reality there is often a higher prevalence of ectoparasites in captive reptiles because of high stocking densities and limited quarantine. Reptiles infested with ectoparasites may present for pruritus, discomfort, severe dermatitis, anemia, and a failure to thrive. Several species of ectoparasites are also known to transmit infectious diseases to reptiles. Infestations are serious and must be evaluated and treated immediately to reduce the magnitude of further disease conditions. It can be

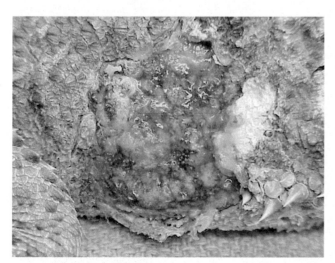

FIGURE 2-20 Pyogranulomatous lesion on the lateral body wall of a bearded dragon *(Pogona vitticeps)* associated with *Paranannizziopsis* sp.

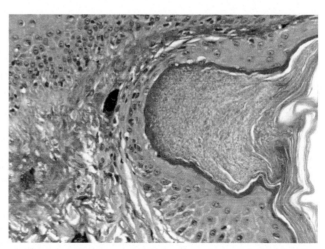

FIGURE 2-21 Histopathology from the bearded dragon *(Pogona vitticeps)* in Figure 2-20. Note how the fungus is "pushing" its way into the skin.

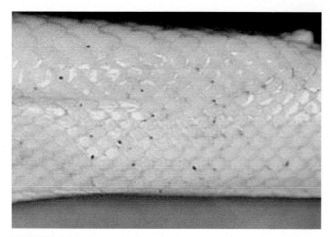

FIGURE 2-22 A heavy *Ophionyssus natricis* infestation on a snake.

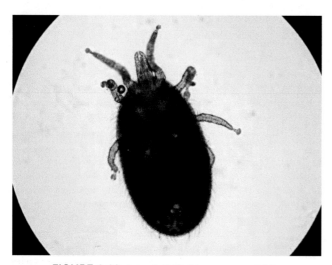

FIGURE 2-23 An adult *Ophionyssus natricis*.

challenging to eliminate ectoparasites, especially in large collections, unless the owners are compliant with treatment and husbandry recommendations. It is important for veterinarians to learn the life cycle of a parasite to ensure complete treatment of both the affected reptiles and their environment.

Snake mites *(Ophionyssus natricis)* can thrive on many different snake and lizard species in captivity (Figure 2-22). Heavy infestations can lead to the dissemination of both bacterial and viral pathogens and cause severe anemia, especially in small reptiles. Captive reptile environments can provide an ideal environment for these mites to thrive through their direct life cycle. After mating and engorgement with blood from their host, adult female mites leave the reptile and search for a site suitable for oviposition (Figure 2-23). The soft larvae hatch and remain in the hatching area. Larvae molt and, once their skin hardens, disperse from the hatching site in search of host animals. Once a host is found, the mites attach themselves and commence feeding. If hosts are not found, the nymphs climb onto objects and await passing reptiles. After engorgement, they leave the host and seek refuge in microhabitats similar to those inhabited by gravid females. During this time, males and females may pair up until mature. After 2 additional molts, they become adults (13 to 19 d total), breed, and once again become more active. The entire mite life cycle is (approximately) 40 days. The newly molted adult mites continue to seek hosts in the environment and feed. After engorgement and falling off the host, the female lays 60 to 80 eggs during the next week or two, feeding several more times. Due to the long mite life cycle (40 d), it is important to treat reptiles and their environment for at least 40 days. Ivermectin (0.2 mg/kg, subcutaneously [SC] or orally q14 d; or 10 mg/L water sprayed topically, q7 d) and Provent-a-mite (Pro Products, Mahopac, NY) have been used to treat the reptiles, while Provent-a-mite and predatory mites (*Hypoaspis* spp.) can be used to eliminate the mites in the reptile's environment. *Ophionyssus natricis* has been shown to be zoonotic, causing intense pruritus in susceptible humans.

Trombiculid mites (*Hirstiella* spp.) are parasitic during their larval stage of development. Adults and nymphs are typically free living within the environment. These mites are six legged and are bright orange to red in color. In the authors' experience, trombiculid mites are most often identified on captive lizards (e.g., iguana). In nonterminal hosts (e.g., humans), these mites can induce an intense pruritic response. Chiggers typically remain on the skin for several days until an "itchy host" actively dislodges them. These parasites do not consume blood from the host but rather use their saliva to inject into the skin, which then digests the cells and lymphatics, resulting in necrotic debris. This necrotic debris is then taken back into the chigger as a meal. These mites can be managed using the same methods described previously for mites.

Hard-bodied ticks that have been documented in reptiles include the following genera: *Ixodes*, *Hyalomma*, *Haemaphysalis*, *Amblyomma*, and *Aponomma*. Soft-body ticks that have been identified on reptile species include *Argasidae* and *Ornithodoros*. Compared with mites, ticks employ different techniques to attach to their hosts. The life stages of a tick consists of an egg, larvae, two or more nymphal stages, and an adult form. Hard ticks usually attach and engorge for several days, while soft ticks attach and engorge for several hours before detaching. Ticks often feed in areas where they do not have to burrow through scales (e.g., conjunctiva, interscalar areas) (Figure 2-24). It is important to remove any ticks that are observed on a reptile to limit the potential for the parasites to cause an anemia or disseminate pathogens to the host. Some species of tick (larval, nymph, and adult stages) can persist within a reptile's captive environment for months, therefore it is important to clean the host's habitat as well.

Leeches are a common finding on aquatic chelonians. In the wild, leech burdens are typically low; however, in captivity, leech burdens can become high in a closed pond system. Leeches attach to the chelonian and feed on blood and tissues. Similar to mites and ticks, leeches can also serve as a mechanical vector and deliver bacterial and viral pathogens to their reptile hosts. Leeches can be removed manually using forceps. Leeches can be zoonotic, consequently it is important to examine the extremities of any human who spends time in a pond with a known infestation.

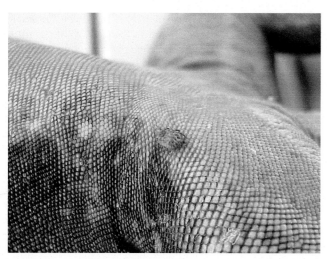

FIGURE 2-24 A tick located on the ventrum of a marine iguana *(Amblyrhynchus cristatus)*.

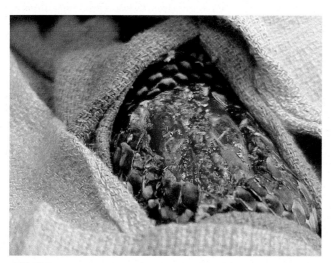

FIGURE 2-25 A squamous cell carcinoma in a king snake. The mass originally looked like an abscess and nonhealing ulcer.

Neoplastic Diseases

The number of reported cases of cutaneous neoplasia in reptiles has been increasing. This finding is likely due to the improved husbandry methods being provided captive reptiles and the resultant increase in age to which these animals are living. However, some forms of cutaneous neoplasia, such as SCC, may actually be the direct consequence of husbandry factors (e.g., exposure to ultraviolet radiation). Any abnormal skin mass on a reptile should be pursued using the same diagnostic methods described for domestic pets. Fine-needle aspirates and tissue biopsies can be performed and submitted to determine a definitive diagnosis.

Squamous cell carcinoma is relatively uncommon in reptiles but may be increasing in incidence. Tumors are often observed in the oral cavity and the skin associated with the head. Cutaneous SCC appears as proliferative, irregular, broad-based masses. In some cases of SCC, the cancer appears as a nonhealing ulcer (Figure 2-25). Overall clinical

observations seem to indicate an increasing rate of SCC in bearded dragons. It has been suggested that this increased incidence may be associated with the high levels of ultraviolet B exposure that these animals receive from full-spectrum lamps in captivity. To date, metastasis has not been documented with these masses; however, they can be locally invasive. Soft tissue sarcomas, such as fibrosarcomas, myxosarcomas, and liposarcomas, have also been documented to affect the skin of reptiles. Many of these tumors appear as swelling involving the skin or underlying tissue structures. Chromatophoromas are also reported in reptiles. These neoplasms are often present in the skin and subcutis and can be aggressive. Tumors may arise from any of the different pigment cells, including melanophores, iridophores, erythrophores, and xanthophores. Typically, tumors involve only one type of pigment cell; however, multiple pigment cells have been reported in some cases. Round cell tumors, including mast cell tumors, lymphoma, lymphosarcoma, plasma cell tumors, and leukemia, have also been described in a variety of reptiles.

Birds

Husbandry-Related Diseases

Feather destructive behavior (FDB) is defined as self-inflicted feather loss, damage, or destruction, regardless of the underlying etiology. Feather destructive behavior can be easily confused with true feather loss or molting; however, once it is identified as self-induced, it is necessary to determine whether the FDB has an underlying medical etiology or is related to husbandry, nutritional, or psychogenic factors.[35] Scant evidence exists in the veterinary literature elucidating the underlying cause of FDB. Medical causes of FDB that have been described include renal disease, hepatic disease, septicemia, endocrinopathies, allergic/inflammatory diseases, viral diseases (e.g., avian bornavirus), bacterial diseases (e.g., *Staphlococcus* spp.), fungal diseases (e.g., *Aspergillius* spp., *Candidia* spp., *Malassezia* spp.), and parasitic diseases (e.g., *Giardia* spp. in mites).[35] Birds with specific FDBs associated with behavior include cockatoos, lovebirds (*Agapornis* spp.), and quaker/monk parrots (*Myiopsitta monachus*).[35] If environmental factors or medical causes are ruled out, psychological factors must be considered. It is important to recognize that birds are a flock animal and removing them from a flock, as we do with pet birds, can lead to stress and the development of negatively reinforced behaviors. Some veterinarians and behaviorists characterize FDB as a stereotypic behavior, similar to trichotillomania in humans and captive primates.[36-38] Feather destructive behavior is only observed in captive birds, which may suggest that living arrangement (singly) and management (environment related) are important contributors to the development of this disease condition.

Chronic ulcerative dermatitis (CUD) is frequently diagnosed in small Psittaciformes (e.g., lovebirds, cockatiels, parakeets).[39,40] The majority of CUD cases appear to be attributed to self-induced trauma. The skin lesions are typically found on the patagium, neck, and back. Chronic ulcerative dermatitis patients often present with a chronic scarified linear lesion or an acutely lacerated hemorrhagic linear lesion. Both polyomavirus and circovirus infections have been implicated in the development of CUD.[41] Diagnosis is based on ruling out other causes of disease. Treatment often includes antimicrobial medications to control secondary bacterial and/or fungal infections in conjunction with using an Elizabethan collar to prevent further mutilation. When lesions of the patagium are healed, scar tissue often restricts movement; this can exacerbate the condition and increases the risk of self-mutilation recurrence.

Xanthomatosis is a condition of proliferative skin lesions of unknown etiology. Xanthomas are nodular lesions that are caused by an accumulation of lipid-containing macrophages.[39,40] These tissue masses are most commonly diagnosed in cockatiels, budgerigars, and smaller psittaciforms. Animals may present with variable-sized yellow masses on the wing, sternopubic area, and keel. It has been hypothesized that these lesions are caused by high-fat diets, trauma, or a disorder in lipid metabolism.[42] To prevent any secondary infection, surgical resection of these masses is necessary when movement or function of the bird is affected or when the lesion becomes traumatized (e.g., hemorrhage). Diagnosis is typically determined through histological evaluation of representative tissue samples. In some species, nutritional therapy (e.g., well-balanced diet with increased vitamin A precursors) may be used to control the growth of these masses.[42]

Allergic skin disease in birds has been reported but is not well documented. Clinical signs associated with cutaneous hypersensitivity in birds include pruritus (possibly seasonal), feather loss, erythema, feather plucking, and skin mutilation.[39,40,43] Definitive diagnosis of allergic skin disease can be difficult. To obtain a diagnosis, it is important to rule out other causes of pruritic skin disease. Food elimination trials (i.e., canine and feline type testing) can be employed and, in some cases, have shown dramatic improvement. Anti-inflammatory medications may be used to treat skin allergies, and resolution of clinical signs with treatment can help with a presumptive diagnosis. Intradermal testing can be performed; however, there is significant difficulty in properly performing this procedure on avian patients.[42] Intradermal skin testing can be difficult to perform due to the need for fresh allergens and accurate injections, the small area of skin available, and difficulty in obtaining positive controls for avian species. Skin biopsies should be used to determine the type and level of inflammation associated with a skin lesion.

Feather follicle cysts may be observed in all avian species. Feather cysts present as an oval or elongated swelling of a feather follicle, that contains an accumulation of keratin. Follicular cysts must be differentiated from folliculitis. Cyst formation can either be inherited or acquired. In canaries, there is a predisposition associated with color and the formation of these cysts.[39,40] The etiology of acquired cysts has not been determined, although infection, trauma, neoplasia, and any other disease abnormalities that can interfere with normal feather growth may lead to cyst formation. Removal of the feather follicle is curative.

Constricted toe syndrome and leg band injuries are common in young, growing psittacines. Fibrous bands of tissue (toe) or identification leg bands can reduce the blood flow to the distal extremity when improperly placed or when there is not enough humidity in the environment.[39,40] Constricted toes are commonly caused by fibrous tissue that are noted as contracting annular rings involving one or more toes; the toe will be swollen distal to the area of compression. Treatment depends on the viability of the tissue distal to the

compression. If the toe is warm and viable, medical management may be sufficient and requires the incision of the tissue "bands" with the bevel of a 22 gauge needle; however, if it is cold and discolored, amputation is recommended. Band injuries can occur in any avian species to which a band (metal or plastic) has been applied. These bands are typically placed on neonatal birds when the foot is small enough to pass through the band. In these cases, the entire foot can swell because of impaired lymphatic and vascular drainage. As with the constricted toe syndrome, medical or surgical management is required and based on tissue viability distal to the compression.

Vitamin A deficiency is a common problem observed in parrots that are fed an exclusive all-seed diet without supplementation. Affected birds often present with hyperkeratosis and scaling of the skin, white plaques in the oral cavity, rhinitis, blepharitis, and sublingual swellings secondary to abscessation of the salivary glands due to squamous metaplasia. Diagnosis of hypovitaminosis A is achieved after collecting a thorough history and evaluating the patient's diet and husbandry in conjunction with clinical signs. Veterinarians treating these cases should use caution when supplementing with vitamin A because it is a fat-soluble vitamin which can result in toxic effects if overdosed.

Gout occurs as a result of the accumulation of monosodium urate crystals in the synovial capsules and the tendon sheaths of joints, leading to the development of swellings around the intertarsal and metatarsal joints. While not in the integument, gout tophi may be confused with skin swellings. Gout lesions are identified most often in small psittacines (e.g., budgerigars, cockatiels). Although unsubstantiated, it is believed if birds have constant access to water and are fed a low protein diet this will reduce the likelihood of gout development. Allopurinol may be used in severe cases to manage hyperuricemia.

Hypothyroidism is a rare disease in psittacines and likely overdiagnosed. Animals with hypothyroidism can have decreased molting events, feather discoloration, hyperkeratosis, and alopecia and may be prone to obesity. To confirm the presence of this disease, it is important to perform the appropriate testing, which can be a challenge. While a thyroid-stimulating hormone (TSH) assay can be performed, there is no avian TSH assay commercially available.[39,40] In the research setting, it has been demonstrated that there is a two- to four-fold increase in circulating T_4 levels when exogenous TSH is administered to the avian patient. Interpretation of baseline T_4 levels has many caveats, as with other domestic species. At this time, a definitive diagnosis of hypothyroidism can only be determined by assessing pathological changes to affected thyroid tissue collected during post mortem examination of the suspect case.

Infectious Diseases

BACTERIAL. Bumblefoot or pododermatitis, a common malady of captive birds of prey, parrots, waterfowl, and poultry, is a degenerative and inflammatory condition that affects the weight-bearing surface of the foot (Figure 2-26). The underlying cause of pododermatitis is multifactorial. Trauma to the plantar surface of the foot or toes can compromise the blood supply to the tissues, leading to tissue necrosis. Lacerations or puncture wounds to the foot may also

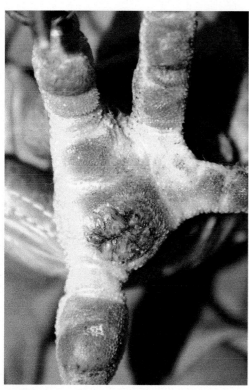

FIGURE 2-26 Pododermatitis in a bald eagle *(Haliaeetus leucocephalus).*

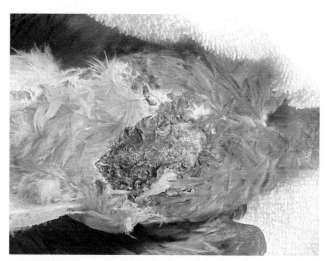

FIGURE 2-27 *Malassezia* spp. dermatitis in an African gray parrot *(Psittacus erithacus).*

predispose the bird to opportunistic bacterial infections. Contributing factors to the development of pododermatitis in captive birds include perches of inappropriate size, shape, and texture; malnutrition; trauma to the foot; and obesity/inactivity. Grading systems have been developed to characterize the severity of disease. Grade I injuries are classified as mild and localized. The epithelium on the plantar surface or toe in these cases is thin and flattended to hypertrophic. Increased swelling and inflammation to the affected area and scabs may be present in these cases. Grade II lesions are associated with infections. Common bacterial pathogens isolated from the foot lesions include *Staphylococcus aureus, E. coli,* and *Pseudomonas aeruginosa.* Increased swelling, heat, and pain are often observed. Grade III lesions are the most severe and carry a guarded prognosis. These are long-standing lesions that are infected and degenerative in nature. Grade III pododermatitis lesions often involve the tendons, joints, and bone. Reommended treatment for birds diagnosed with pododermatitis is focused on correcting the underlying cause, relieving pressure on the affected area, decreasing swelling and inflammation, treating secondary infections, promoting drainage if necessary, and pain management. The overall therapeutic approach is dependent on the severity of the lesions, and a multimodal course of action should be taken; medical and surgical options are further discussed later in this chapter.

Mycobacterial granuloma formation involving the skin of birds is an atypical presentation but can occur. *Mycobacterium tuberculosis* and *M. avium* have both been reported to cause cutaneous lesions in Amazon parrots (*Amazona* spp.) and

macaws (*Ara* spp.).[44] Lesions associated with mycobacterial infections include dermatitis, diffuse nonpruritic skin thickening associated with xanthomatosis, pale soft subcutaneous masses, and tubercle formation within the skin. Mycobacterial granulomas have also been observed around the head or face. In addition to these cutaneous lesions, systemic lesions (e.g., respiratory tract, gastrointestinal tract, and bone) may also be present. Although mycobacterial infections are relatively uncommon, they have important public health implications because *Mycobacterium* spp. are zoonotic. However, at this time there have been no reports of *Mycobacterium* spp. transmission from a bird to a human that resulted in a clinical infection. Diagnosis of *Mycobacterium* spp. is often based on histopathology, microbiology, and PCR testing.

FUNGAL. *Aspergillus fumigatus* skin infections are not common in bird patients; however, these infections can occur secondary to trauma to the skin.[45] Lesions associated with cutaneous *Aspergillus* spp. include blue to dark gray ulcerated epidermal patches. Diagnosis is based on clinical signs, biopsy results, and a positive fungal culture. Impression smears can be initially performed to screen for the fungal organisms; however, appropriate samples should be submitted for histopathology and culture to obtain a definitive diagnosis. Birds with cutaneous aspergillosis should also be screened for a primary fungal respiratory tract infection caused by this fungal pathogen.

Candida albicans is an opportunistic yeast that is rarely considered a primary pathogen. *Candida* spp. infections are typically found in the upper gastrointestinal tract; however, in canaries, they can cause intense head and cervical pruritus that has been associated with feather picking.[35] A diagnosis of a *C. albicans* skin infection are often confirmed based on skin cytology, histopathology, and fungal culture.

Malassezia spp. have been associated with dermatitis and feather picking in birds.[35] (Figure 2-27). Initial cytologic examination of a skin scrape may be used to guide the clinician toward a diagnosis; however, to confirm an infection, both culture and histopathology are required. The role of *Malassezia* spp. as an etiologic agent for feather picking remains controversial, as at least one study reported no difference in *Malassezia* spp. findings between feather-picking and non-feather-picking psittacines.[46]

VIRAL. Psittacine beak and feather disease (PBFD) is caused by the psittacine circovirus. Psittacine beak and feather disease can occur in a wide variety of wild and captive parrots, especially species from Australia, the Pacific islands, and Southeast Asia.[42] Two forms of the disease have been reported: an acute form and a chronic form. The acute form occurs in neonatal birds and is a generalized disease that affects feather growth. Birds with the acute form of PBFD may die within 2 months of showing clinical signs. Alternatively, the chronic form is observed in older birds with clinical signs being observed after the first molt. Clinical signs of the chronic form include feather dystrophy or abnormalities (e.g., clubbing, blunting), feather loss, shiny beak, and deformed beak and nails. Dystrophic feathers ultimately replace normal ones. In cockatoos (*Cacatua* spp.), the powder down feathers are the first affected, thereby reducing the animal's ability to produce "powder". PCR testing and histopathologic examination of biopsy samples can be used in conjunction with clinical signs to confirm a diagnosis of PBFD. Birds that display clinical signs carry a guarded to grave prognosis. Supportive care has prolonged the lives of infected birds for years; however, these birds should be considered contagious. Currently there is no curative treatment nor preventive vaccine available for PBFD.

Polyomavirus is another virus that can cause systemic disease with characteristic skin lesions in birds. Affected birds often develop abnormal feathers (e.g., French molt, budgerigar fledgling disease) and hemorrhages under the skin.[39] Young birds are most susceptible, although adult birds can also become infectious. In addition to the previously noted feather issues, affected birds may be depressed, poor growers, and have delayed gastrointestinal tract emptying (e.g., crop stasis). A PCR assay is available to confirm the disease. There is a vaccine available to protect birds against this virus. Vaccinating animals that may be at risk of exposure (e.g., in aviaries, zoological institutions) is recommended.

Papillomas are thought to be induced by viral disease; however, at this time an etiologic agent for birds has not been confirmed.[39] To date, both a herpesvirus and papillomavirus have been suggested as possible etiologic agents.[39,40] In affected birds, papilloma-like hyperplastic and hyperkeratotic lesions are observed on the palpebrae, beak commissure, and feet. In psittacines, lesions also can be observed on the cloaca or choana. Biopsy and histopathology are required to obtain a definitive diagnosis of papillomatosis. Radiosurgery, cryosurgery, and electrocautery have all been employed to debulk and resect affected tissues.[42]

All avian species appear to be susceptible to poxvirus infections.[42] There are three different forms of disease: dry, wet, and systemic form. The dry form is the most common type of avian pox diagnosed in birds. Hemotogenous exposure through vector blood meals (primary) and open wounds (rare) is the route in which birds become infected with avian pox virus. When draining lesions are observed, a bird is considered contagious to conspecifics in close contact. Birds that have the dry form of avian pox develop small to large nodular lesions on the nonfeathered areas around the face, cere, and feet. The lesions are typically raised and proliferative. Topical disinfection and supportive care should be provided for these

cases until the bird's immune system can control the infection. The wet form, or diphtheritic form, is typically associated with the mucous membranes. The prognosis for cases of wet form avian pox is guarded to grave. Systemic antibiotic and antifungal agents may be required to limit the potential for opportunistic infections (e.g., *Salmonella* spp., *Aspergillus fumigatus*). The systemic form of avian pox carries the most grave prognosis. Affected animals have widespread disease and often die acutely (24 to 48 h) from infection.

Parasitic Diseases

Scaly leg and beak mites (*Cnemidocoptes* spp.) are the most common parasite diagnosed in captive budgerigars. Affected birds present with hyperkeratosis and crusting of the cere, beak, legs, and feet. A definitive diagnosis is achieved by collecting a skin scraping and reviewing the material under light microscopy to positively identify the mites. In addition to *Cnemidocoptes* spp., there are other mites that infest captive passerines and psittacines, including red mites (*Dermanyssus gallinae*), *Ornithonyssus* spp., and quill mites (*Syringophilidae*, *Laminosioptidae*, and *Fainocoptinae*). In all cases, skin scrapings or feather screening can be used as diagnostic options for mite identification.

Giardia psittaci has a cosmopolitan distribution and is known to infect many avian species. In most cases, clinical signs are limited to enteritis; however, in cockatiels, the species most commonly affected, infected individuals have been documented to demonstrate pruritus and a predisposition to feather plucking.[35] However, the clinical belief that there is an association between *Giardia* spp. infections in cockatiels and feather picking has never been scientifically validated. A diagnosis of giardiasis in birds is possible through direct fecal examination or by PCR assay; however, it is important to note that transient shedding of the organism increases the chance of false negative results. To improve one's ability to detect the protozoan parasite on a direct fecal smear it is recommended to warm the slide prior to sample placement and use a warmed dilute Lugol's iodine as contrast solution.

Neoplastic Diseases

Captive avian species are susceptible and often present with integumentary neoplasms. Xanthomas, uropygial adenocarcinomas, lipomas, fibrosarcomas, lymphosarcomas, SCCs, melanomas, hemangiosarcomas, and mucoepidermal carcinomas have all been diagnosed in captive birds.[47] A diagnosis of skin cancer can be made through biopsy collection of suspect tissue and histopathologic evaluation of submitted samples.

MAMMALS: FERRETS

Parasitic Diseases

Ferrets can become infested with the same species of flea that infect dogs and cats (e.g., *Ctenocephalides felis*). Infestation can occur as a result of direct contact with another animal infested with fleas or from exposure within an infested environment. Infested ferrets often present with mild to severe pruritus, scaling, crusting alopecia, and excoriations. Additionally, "flea dirt" or live fleas can be observed on flea combing. Treatments used for cats appear safe for ferrets. One product marketed for control of external parasites, *Advantage Multi®* (Bayer Animal Health), has approval for use on ferrets. It is important to treat both the animal and environment to control the fleas.

Ear mites *(Otodectes cynotis)* are another commonly diagnosed ectoparasite in ferrets. Ear mites are directly transmitted between animals with infestations being subclinical (e.g., dark ceruminous ear wax) or overt (e.g., shaking head, scratching ears). Infestations can be characterized by large amounts of waxy brown otic exudate, although this clinical condition is identified in ferrets that are parasite free. A definitive diagnosis is achieved by swabbing the ears and placing the material, with mineral oil, on a microscope slide with a coverslip and reviewing it under light microscopy to positively identify the mite. The life cycle of *O. cyanotis* is 21 days; therefore, treatment should be administered for at least 4 weeks.[48]

Sarcoptic mange mite *(Sarcoptes scabiei)* infestations are known to cause two types of disease presentations in ferrets, both of which involve intense pruritus. With one clinical condition the infested animal is presented with generalized alopecia (e.g., face, pinna, ventrum), while the other presents as localized disease involving only the paws, which can appear swollen, inflamed, and crusted. Severe infections of the feet can result in deformities of the nails and in more severe cases loss of the nails or toes. The life cycle of *S. scabiei* is 2 to 3 weeks and adults only live a maximum of 10 days; therefore, treatment should be administered until a second skin scrape is negative.[48]

Infectious Diseases
Bacterial
Bacterial pyodermas can present as either a primary skin disease or as a secondary response to an adverse physiologic condition associated with an underlying illness. Bacterial pyodermas can present as a moist dermatitis and diagnosed through procuring a skin scrape and impression smear which are then microscopically evaluated or cultured. Treatment for any bacterial disease should be based on antimicrobial sensitivity testing in order to prevent bacterial resistance. If the bacterial pyoderma is secondary to another disease process, the primary disease should be identified and treated to prevent any further exacerbation of the concurrent bacterial infection.

Fungal
Microsporum canis and *Trichophyton mentagrophytes* have both been diagnosed in ferrets. Exposure to these fungal organisms occurs through direct contact with an infected animal (or human) or contaminated fomites. Overcrowding is thought to be associated with an increased incidence of fungal skin disorders; additionally, the incidence of disease appears to vary according to geographic location.[49] Skin and hair lesions associated with dermatomycosis are similar to those observed in other mammals, including small patches of alopecia, papules that spread to the periphery, crusting, and erythematous pruritus. Excoriations and pyoderma may also be observed secondary to pruritus. Dermatomycosis is more common in younger animals but is generally self-limiting. A definitive diagnosis can be confirmed through dermatophyte (DTM) culture or PCR testing, similar to other domestic species.

Viral
Canine distemper virus (CDV) (paramyxovirus) is a highly fatal disease in ferrets, with reported mortality rates approaching 100%. Canine distemper virus is a preventable disease in ferrets through vaccination. A modified live vaccination should not be used in ferrets since it is believed to induce clinical disease under certain conditions. Although, for the last 30 years, there have been commercially available ferret CDV vaccines. Unfortunately at this time there are no ferret specific CDV products that are regularly available to the practicing veterinarian. Therefore, at this time, the American Ferret Association (AFA) recommends vaccination with Novibac DPv (Merck Animal Health) and provides more information regarding this recommendation on the AFA website. Ferrets infected with canine distemper virus can develop generalized disease involving the central nervous system, respiratory system, and integument, among others. Common dermatologic lesions include brown crusted lesions on the chin, nose, inguinal, and perineal regions. Hyperkeratosis and swelling of the footpads are also common, although relative to the size of the animal. An antemortem diagnosis is based on clinical history (no CDV vaccine), serology, and PCR testing.

Endocrine Disease
Adrenal gland disease (AGD) is common in middle age to geriatric ferrets. One of the first indications of adrenal gland disease is the clinical presentation of bilaterally symmetrical alopecia that is initially observed involving the caudal half of the body (e.g., over pelvis) which then extends to other areas of the body (Figures 2-28, 2-29). Alopecia associated with this disease can begin as a seasonal alopecia that ultimately does not resolve after 2 to 3 seasonal cycles. Pruritus is known to be a clinical disease presentation associated with AGD and often presents as erythema, papules, and excoriations. Other

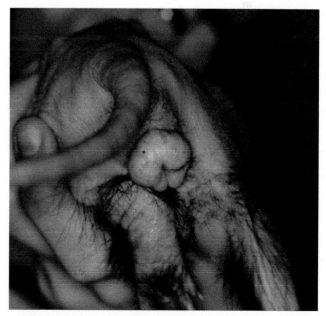

FIGURE 2-28 Adrenal gland disease in a ferret *(Mustela putorius furo)*. Note the generalized alopecia over the hind end and the swollen vulva.

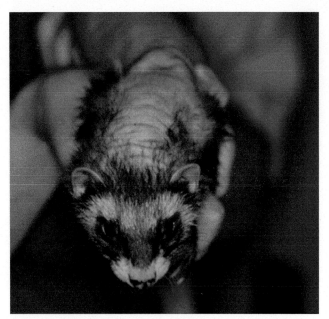

FIGURE 2-29 Adrenal gland disease in a ferret *(Mustela putorius furo)*. Note the generalized alopecia over the dorsum.

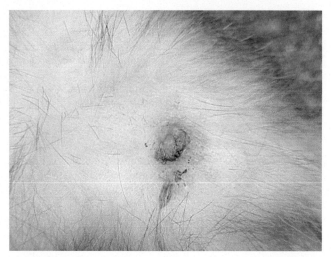

FIGURE 2-30 A sebaceous adenoma in a ferret *(Mustela putorius furo)*.

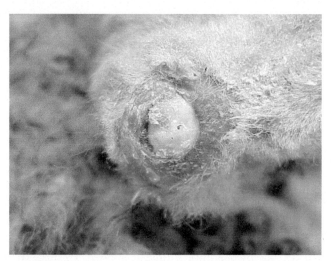

FIGURE 2-31 Pododermatitis in a rabbit *(Oryctolagus cuniculus)*.

clinical signs associated with this disease including prostate enlargement and vulvar enlargement are discussed in the reproductive and endocrinology chapters.

Seasonal alopecia is a common occurrence in ferrets. Typically, the hair is shed and the coat becomes light during the warmer months of the year. Seasonal alopecia can be confused with adrenal gland disease, especially in early cases of the disease when hair loss is light. No treatment is necessary for seasonal alopecia. A proper diagnostic evaluation for adrenal gland disease (e.g., measuring sex steroids and ultrasound) is necessary to determine whether the generalized hair loss is associated with a seasonal event or adrenal gland disease.

Hyperestrogenism in jill ferrets is an uncommon disease presentation because the majority of pet ferrets are spayed as kits. However, veterinarians that see intact breeding ferrets in their practice may encounter this disease; ferrets with remnant ovarian tissue (incomplete surgery) may also present with similar clinical signs as those of hyperestrogenism. Ferrets are seasonally polyestrous-induced ovulators.[50] Female ferrets remain in estrus if they do not ovulate, either through natural or artificial means. Jills diagnosed with hyperestrogenism may present with bilaterally symmetrical nonpruritic alopecia and/or a swollen vulva, which are similar to the clinical signs observed in ferrets with adrenal gland disease. Ferrets affected by hyperestrogenism are typically young animals (1 to 2 yr of age). Concurrent bone marrow suppression (e.g., anemia, leukopenia, pancytopenia) can be observed in individuals that exhibit signs of hyperestrogenism.

Neoplastic Disease

The most common skin tumors diagnosed in ferrets are mast cell tumors, apocrine scent tumors, basal cell tumors, and sebaceous adenomas or epitheliomas (Figure 2-30). These tumors are often focal and benign; metastasis is uncommon. Mast cell tumors in ferrets are often characterized by erythema and hemorrhage, often the result of the animal licking or scratching at the tumor. The tumors may appear as raised growths on the skin and in many cases, regress without treatment. Tumors that involve the ferret integument are often hemorrhagic as a result of self induced trauma due to licking or scratching. Routine diagnostic protocol for tissue masses is required to confirm a diagnosis. Surgical excision of the tissue mass(es) is typically curative.

MAMMALS: RABBITS

Husbandry-Related Disease

Rabbits are unique in that they lack footpads. Rabbit skin is firmly attached to the underlying tissues forming a tarsometatarsal skin pad. Thick fur on the plantar aspect of the metatarsus pads the skin. When walking and/or running, rabbits support most of their weight on their claws, while at rest they distribute most of their weight between their claws and the plantar aspect of the metatarsus.[51] Loss of the fur padding layer on the plantar/palmar surface of the feet can lead to pressure-induced necrosis of the skin or ulcerative dermatitis/pododermatitis (Figure 2-31). Risk factors that predispose rabbits to the development of ulcerative dermatitis/pododermatitis include obesity, inactivity, wet or soiled bedding, and wire flooring. Rex rabbits are commonly affected because they lack protective guard hairs. Improper substrate (e.g., metal screen flooring) can accelerate the development of this disease process. Lesions and associated conditions observed on the feet include alopecia, pain, and erythematous ulcerative dermatitis of the metatarsal and metacarpal regions. *Staphylococcus aureus* and *Pasteurella multocida* are the most common bacteria associated with infectious pododermatitis lesions.[52] As the disease condition continues to progress, there is often a significant loss of structural integrity that involve the surrounding anatomic structures. In severe cases of ulcerative dermatitis/pododermatitis the ligaments of the hock joint are often compromised which can initiate a cascade of associated disease complications. The loss of ligament integrity of the hock joint will allow for medial displacement of the superficial digital flexor tendon. Once the superficial digital flexor tendon is displaced, the rabbit redistributes its weight, disease progression intensifies, and there is a significant decrease in mobility. In severe cases of pododermatitis, it is not unusual to diagnose osteomyelitis in the bone(s) contacting the lesion due to secondary bacterial infections.

Barbering is diagnosed in rabbits and rodents that are maintained in both the laboratory and companion animal environments. Broken hairs and vibrissae, as well as areas of alopecia, may be observed in affected animals. Diagnosis is based on obtaining a thorough history, physical examination, and performing a trichogram (i.e., hair pluck reviewed under light microscopy) to reveal the presence of broken hairs. Barbering is typically the result of one animal displaying dominance over another; however, low-fiber diets have also been associated with barbering. Managing animal densities, providing sufficient cage space to escape from dominant animals, and providing an appropriate coarse-fiber diet will help reduce the incidence of barbering.

Sebaceous adenitis is an immune-mediated disease that targets sebaceous glands. Affected animals develop lesions that include nonpruritic scaling, alopecia, and follicular casting. A diagnosis can be confirmed with biopsy and histopathology testing of identified integumentary lesions. Treatment will depend on the severity of disease, although systemic anti-inflammatory medications are often required to manage the disease.

Telogen defluxion is a condition that affects rabbits in response to systemic stress or illness; but also occurs after parturition. Telogen defluxion is characterized by generalized hair loss over a 4 to 6 week period following systemic stress or illness. Affected rabbits present for nonpruritic patchy alopecia. A detailed history, characterizing the illness or stress, is helpful to diagnose the underlying cause for telogen defluxion.

Cutaneous asthenia is a rare heritable collagen defect that has been documented in rabbits and is characterized by hyperextensible skin.[53] The skin tears easily, which results in lacerations and open wounds. Once healed, the affected tissue remodels into thin atrophic scars. A definitive diagnosis can be achieved through histopathology and electron microscopic evaluation of representative biopsy samples.

A single case of exfoliative dermatitis secondary to the presence of a thymoma in a rabbit has been reported in the literature.[54] Clinical disease signs identified with the

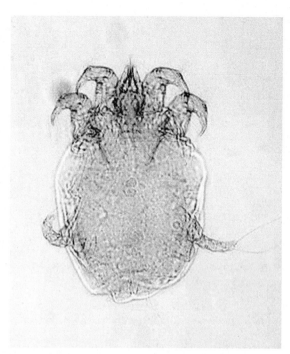

FIGURE 2-32 *Psoroptes cuniculi* from a rabbit *(Oryctolagus cuniculus).*

exfoliative dermatitis rabbit case were generalized scaling and alopecia.

Parasitic Diseases

Sarcoptes scabiei can cause crusty and pruritic lesions over the face, nose, lips, and external genitalia of rabbits. These mites are zoonotic, and owners should be advised to wear gloves when handling or treating infected animals. A confirmative diagnosis is frequently determined by performing a deep skin scrape similar to domestic species.

Psoroptes cuniculi is the common rabbit ear mite and causes severe otitis externa. Affected rabbits often present with excessive crusting and exudate involving the external ear canal and pinna (Figure 2-32). The crusty exudate that develops from the presence of the mites is due to a hypersensitivity reaction to the parasite which causes an intense tissue response in the form of cellular discharge and pruritis. Infestations can be unilateral or bilateral but in most clinical cases, both ears are affected. The mites can also leave the ears, with similar crusting lesions noted on the head, muzzle, and dorsum. Rabbits can be exposed to *P. cuniculi* through direct contact or indirectly via fomites. The life cycle of this mite is 21 days; therefore, treatment should continue for at least 3 to 4 weeks.

Cheyletiella parasitovorax is a skin mite that can cause large white scales on rabbits; these scales may be observed to "move" on the limbs and neck (e.g., "walking dandruff") of affected rabbits. Rabbits with cheyletiellosis present with mild pruritus, large flakes of white scales, alopecia, and oily dermatitis. Infestations can be observed in any animal; however, young, obese, and immunosuppressed individuals appear to be most susceptible to *Cheyletiella parasitovorax*.[55] A definitive diagnosis is determined by reviewing fur and skin tape preparations using light microscopy (Figure 2-33). The life cycle of this parasite is 21 to 28 days, and the adults can live off the host. Thus, it is important to treat the rabbits for at least 4

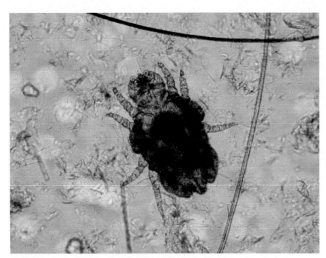

FIGURE 2-33 *Cheyletiella parasitovorax* from a rabbit *(Oryctolagus cuniculus).*

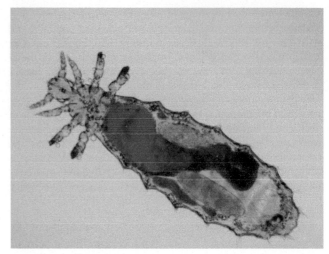

FIGURE 2-34 *Haemodipsus ventricosus* from a rabbit *(Oryctolagus cuniculus).*

weeks (e.g., with ivermectin, 0.2 mg/kg, q10 d, for 3 treatments) and change the bedding regularly during the treatment period. This parasite is zoonotic, therefore it is extremely important to educate owners regarding special precautions one should follow (e.g., wearing gloves) when handling and treating their pet.

The fur-clasping mite *Leporacarus gibbus* is another species of mite that can be found on captive rabbits. Affected animals often present with scaly alopecia, especially over the dorsum and rump. In severe cases, self-mutilation secondary to a hypersensitivity reaction may occur. The fur-clasping mites are ovoid and brown and live their entire life cycle (28 d) on the host. Females attach their eggs to the hair shaft. Thus, diagnosis can be made using tape preparations of fur to identify the attached eggs. Selamectin and ivermectin are both effective for treating *Leporacarus gibbus*.

Dog and cat fleas (*Ctenocephalides canis* and *C. felis*, respectively) are the most common fleas that infest rabbits. The most common location that fleas infest on rabbits is the dorsum from the shoulders to the pelvis. Rabbits, similar to dogs and cats, can develop fleabite hypersensitivities. Flea treatment for rabbits should include both the animal and the environment. Many of the flea treatments used for cats can be used for rabbits and as with ferrets, Advantage-Mutli® (Bayer Animal Health), is effective. It is extremely important for all veterinarians to know that Frontline (Merial, Duluth, GA) should not be used because it has been associated with both morbidity and mortality in rabbits.

Lice can be categorized as either anoplurans (sucking lice) or mallophagans (chewing lice). *Haemodipsus ventricosus*, an anopluran louse, is the clinically relevant species for captive rabbits (Figure 2-34). Adult lice have a head with short antennae and 3 pairs of strong legs with hook-like claws.[55] When eggs are deposited, they adhere to hair. *Haemodipsus ventricosus*, can also serve as a vector for disease such as tularemia in animals and humans. Treatment for this anopluran louse is similar to that for domestic species (ivermectin or selamectin; see treatments for rabbits).

Ticks are most often diagnosed in rabbits that are housed outdoors. In the U.S., rabbits are commonly parasitized by

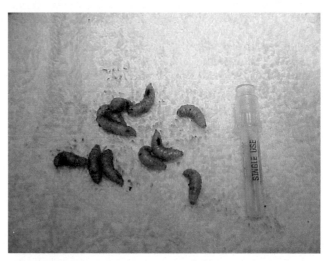

FIGURE 2-35 Fly maggots removed from a rabbit *(Oryctolagus cuniculus).*

Ixodes scapularis, Ixodes dentatus, Haemaphysalis leporispalustris, and *Dermacentor variabilis.*[55] The species of ticks listed above also infest many other species of mammals, consequently it is possible that they may serve as biologic vectors for tick-borne diseases such as *Borrelia burgdorferi, Babesia* spp., and *Anaplasma* spp. At this time, there are no documented cases of *Borrelia burgdorferi, Babesia* spp., and *Anaplasma* spp. in rabbits; however, there has been a single report of antibodies to *B. burgdorferi* in Chinese rabbits.[55]

Myiasis, or fly strike, is commonly observed in rabbits that are housed outdoors during the summer. Unsanitary conditions, dermatitis, and obesity can predispose rabbits to developing myiasis. Diagnosis is straightforward, as the maggots will be found in the wound; however, it is important to define the extent of the wound, as the infested area can be quite deep (Figure 2-35). Removing the maggots, debriding the wounds, and allowing for closure of the wound (delayed primary or secondary) are curative.

Cuterebra larvae, or botflies, will infest both rabbits housed outdoors and those in the wild. Hatched larvae of *Cuterebra*

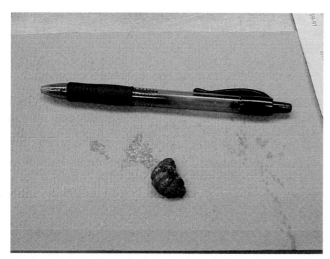

FIGURE 2-36 *Cuterebra* larvae removed from a rabbit *(Oryctolagus cuniculus).*

flies can crawl through the fur and into the subcutis through body openings or injuries of the skin. The larvae are easily diagnosed by the presence of a subcutaneous swelling and the presence of a small breathing hole in the skin. Infected rabbits can have between 1 to 5 botfly larvae under their skin. A rabbit's fur is often matted around the breathing hole as a result of the rabbit licking the wound in reaction to the pain and irritation associated with the larva's presence. Surgical removal of the larvae is necessary for successful treatment (Figure 2-36). A small incision can be made over the larva and the entire larval cyst, which includes the maggot, removed; the area also should be flushed and debrided to prevent secondary bacterial infections. If inappropriately removed (i.e., larvae ruptured), the larvae can induce an anaphylaxis. Rabbits housed outdoors should be protected against flies by appropriate flytraps and cage screening.

Infectious Diseases

Bacterial

Treponematosis *(Treponema cuniculi)*, or rabbit syphilis, is a sexually transmitted disease that is disseminated by direct transmission. Rabbits infected with *T. cuniculi* often present with crusts covering the mucocutaneous junctions of the nose, lips, eyelids, and/or external genitalia. Infected does can abort kits, retain placentas, and potentially develop a fatal metritis. A diagnosis is made through collection of sample material by performing a skin scrape or biopsy of affected tissue. Slides in which the collected sample has been applied should be evaluated with silver stain or under dark-field microscopy to identify the organism. Injectable penicillin (never oral penicillin) can be used to treat affected rabbits.

Subcutaneous abscesses can form anywhere on the body of rabbits but are most often diagnosed secondary to dental disease and bite wounds. Abscesses in rabbits normally contain thick purulent material and do not readily drain (e.g., penrose drains are typically unrewarding). It is best to surgically remove rabbit abscesses in total with the abscess capsule. When this is not possible, the abscess material should be removed and the surrounding tissue void vigorously flushed. Delayed primary or secondary closure is preferred to ensure

that the abscess does not recur. *Pasteurella multocida, Pseudomonas* spp., *Staphylococcus* spp., and *Streptococcus* spp. are common bacterial isolates from rabbit abscesses. Treatment should be based on the results of antimicrobial sensitivity testing, as multidrug resistance is increasing with many of these pathogens.

Fungal

Trichophyton mentagrophytes and *Microsporum canis* are common fungal organisms identified in rabbits that are diagnosed with dermatitis lesions. Lesions observed on rabbits infected with these organisms are similar to those described for domestic animals. Infections with *Trichophyton mentagrophytes* and *Microsporum canis* can occur anywhere on the body and are described as crusty, erythematous alopecia that may be pruritic. These infections are most common in young animals or recent acquisitions where population densities are high and husbandry conditions inadequate. Diagnosis is typically made with a potassium hydroxide (KOH) preparation from a skin scrape or fungal culture. Owners should be asked whether any other animals or people within the household have any similar lesions, because reports of zoonotic transmission and reverse zoonosis are present with rabbits. Owners should be advised to seek medical attention if they or their other animals have lesions typical of fungal dermatitis.

Viral

Myxomatosis is caused by a poxvirus (myxoma virus). In nature, this virus occurs in rabbits and tapeti from Central and South America and forms a mild self-limiting cutaneous fibroma.[56] However, in domestic rabbits, myxomatosis can be a severe, inevitably fatal systemic disease. The virus is transmitted through insect vectors, such as rabbit fleas *(Cediopsylla simplex* and *Odontosyllus multispinous)* and mosquitos *(Aedes* spp., *Anopheles* spp.), although direct transmission has been documented.[56] Clinical signs associated with the nodular form of the myxomatosis include subcutaneous masses and edema of the eyelids and genitals. Purulent ocular discharge, pyrexia, lethargy, depression, and anorexia may also be observed in affected animals. The highly virulent strain of the virus can cause death within 5 to 6 days of infection, with few clinical signs; however, death usually occurs between 10 to 12 days following infection. In rabbits infected with less virulent strains of the virus, the lesions are similar to the virulent form but are less severe. Rabbits can survive the less virulent strain, as the cutaneous lesions eventually scab over and slough.

Shope papilloma virus, a member of the Papovaviridae family, occurs in wild brush rabbits and cottontail rabbits. The Shope papilloma virus is a DNA virus that is typically transmitted by biting arthropods (e.g., ticks). The virus induces oncogenesis, causing multiple hyperkeratotic lesions around the eyes, eyelids, neck, and shoulders. In experimentally infected domestic rabbits, 75% of inoculation sites underwent malignant transformation into SCC.[57] A diagnosis is achieved through biopsy and histopathology of suspect tissue. Surgical removal of the mass can be curative. Vector control is vital to prevent the spread of Shope papilloma virus.

Shope fibroma virus is a leporipoxvirus of wild rabbits in the Americas. The natural host of this virus is the eastern cottontail rabbit *(Sylvilagus flordianus).* This virus is transmitted through arthropod vectors. Domestic rabbits occasionally get infected and develop fibromas that slough at ~30 days postinfection. The fibromas are variable in size and typically occur on the legs, feet, muzzle, and periorbital and perineal regions. Recommended diagnostic tests to confirm disease presence include biopsy, virus isolation, and histopathology. Supportive care and antibiotic therapy for secondary infections is the recommended treatment protocol for Shope fibroma infection.

Rabbit pox is a large DNA virus within the family Poxviridae. Disease outbreaks of rabbit pox infection have been described in the laboratory setting, with clinical signs including pyrexia, lymphadenitis, pox-like lesions on the skin and mucous membranes, keratitis, and orchiditis.[56] Rabbit pox is an extremely uncommon disease presentation in pet rabbits.

Neoplastic Diseases

Many different forms of skin cancer have been reported in rabbits, including trichoblastomas, collagenous hamartomas, Shope fibromas, lipomas, SCCs, myxosarcomas, peripheral nerve sheath tumors, malignant melanomas, fibrosarcomas, carcinomas, squamous papillomas, liposarcomas, leiomyosarcomas, trichoepitheliomas, apocrine carcinomas, and Shope papillomas. Any skin mass encountered in a rabbit patient should be diagnostically evaluated following the same standard practices used for domestic species. A fine-needle aspirate or biopsy with cytology and histopathology, respectively, can be used to confirm the type of neoplasm identified on the patient. For malignant cancers, diagnostic imaging to assess the potential for metastases should be performed. Due to the limited veterinary medical knowledge regarding rabbit neoplasia, surgical resection of a skin tumor remains the primary form of treatment.

MAMMALS: GUINEA PIGS

Husbandry-Related Diseases

Guinea pigs, similar human and nonhuman primates, cannot synthesize vitamin C (ascorbic acid) because they lack L-gulono-δ-lactone oxidase. Subsequently, guinea pigs are predisposed to scurvy if they do not receive sufficient dietary levels of vitamin C. Ascorbic acid plays an important role in collagen synthesis; therefore, a lack of this essential dietary nutrient can result in widespread disruption to collagen structures within the body. Hypovitaminosis C is a common finding in guinea pigs and is frequently underdiagnosed. In mild cases of hypovitaminosis C, the hair coat is in poor condition and scaling may be seen. In severe cases, guinea pigs present with swollen joints, subcutaneous hemorrhages, and active bleeding from wounds or the mucous membranes with pain being apparent upon palpation. When a guinea pig is presented with a history of anorexia, the patient should be treated for hypovitaminosis C. The authors recommend 50 mg/kg once a day during the treatment period or until the animal is eating on its own. Parenteral vitamin C should be used until the guinea pig is eating on its own. Owners should be instructed to provide known daily doses of vitamin C through the form of tablets or vitamin C impregnated "hay tabs" (Oxbow Animal Health).

Pregnancy-associated alopecia is a disease condition that affects guinea pigs. The hair loss associated with pregnancy in guinea pigs is also called effluvium postpartum.[58] Elevated levels of estrogen are responsible for the hair loss. When estrogen concentrations increase, hair follicles enter the telogen phase and stop growing. The alopecia will resolve following the pregnancy period.

Unlike rabbits, guinea pigs have foot pads, and while these padded structures help to protect their feet against some of the disease conditions diagnosed with rabbits, they do not protect the guinea pigs from all potential risk factors (e.g., metal flooring). In most cases, lesions occur secondary to a traumatic event, poor hygiene, or as a result of obesity. Guinea pigs housed in unhygienic conditions or on inadequate flooring may be exposed to a variety of bacterial pathogens (e.g., *Staphylococcus aureus*, *Pseudomonas aeruginosa*) that can invade the footpad. In severe cases, these infections can enter the bone. Obesity often predisposes guinea pigs to pododermatitis, as overconditioned guinea pigs develop abnormal wear patterns on their pads that have an increased susceptibility to puncture wounds and subsequent bacterial invasion. Cytology, culture and antimicrobial sensitivity testing, and diagnostic imaging should be pursued in pododermatitis cases to properly assess the overall extent of the disease process. Treatment often requires long-term topical and systemic antibiotic and analgesic therapy. In severe cases, surgical amputation may be necessary.

Cheilitis, or inflammation of the lips, can occur in guinea pigs and is frequently associated with opportunistic integumentary bacterial infections (e.g., *Staphylococcus aureus* and *Streptococcus* spp.) or yeast (*Candida* spp.). These lesions may arise from cuts or abrasions acquired from the environment. Cytology and culture with antimicrobial sensitivity testing should be performed to identify the pathogen in order to select the appropriate treatment. Reduction of any inciting factors within the animal's living environment (e.g., removing any sharp metal) is also important to ensure a positive treatment response and prevent recurrence.

Barbering has been observed in all age groups of guinea pigs. Guinea pigs presenting with barbering have patchy nonpruritic alopecia and broken hair shafts without inflammation. Lesions on animals that are self-barbering are present on the dorsal lumbar region and flank areas, while barbering of conspecifics typically results in alopecia on the rump, dorsum, ears, vibrissae, and around the eyes. The latter is described as a dominance behavior. It has been hypothesized that barbering may develop due to boredom, stress, a low-fiber diet, and overcrowding. To prevent barbering, it is important to increase dietary roughage by providing high-quality long stem hay, chew toys, weaning animals at an appropriate age, and separating boars.

Anal sac impactions can occur in boars, especially older animals. Anal sac impactions occur as a result of a concentration of cecotropes, the soft nutrient-rich feces that the guinea pigs eat. Warm saline, mineral oil, and a nonirritating soap (Dawn, Procter and Gamble, Cincinnati, OH) can be used to clean the anal sac and remove the mass of cecotropes. To prevent recurrence of an impaction, the anal sac should be cleaned on a regular basis (every 3 to 4 wk); therefore, it is important to educate the guinea pig owner how to perform the procedure. Removing smegma and cleaning the penis should also be accomplished on a regular basis. Warm water or water and a nonirritating soap can be used to clean the

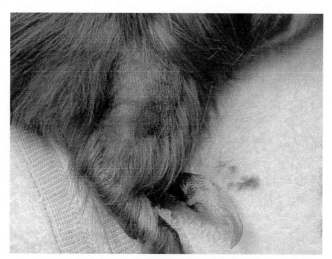

FIGURE 2-37 *Trixacarus caviae* infestation in a guinea pig *(Cavia porcellus)*. Note the alopecia and redness/excoriation on the leg. This animal is recumbent because it was seizuring at the time of the photograph.

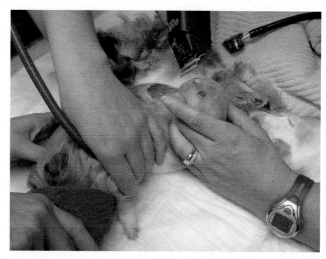

FIGURE 2-38 Trichofolliculoma in a guinea pig *(Cavia porcellus)*. It was surgically removed and the animal had no other complications.

penis and prepuce. Finally, the dorsal scent gland, or grease gland, can also impact as guinea pigs age. The dorsal scent gland can also be cleaned with warm water and soap.

Infectious Diseases

Bacterial

In guinea pigs, the primary etiologic agent associated with cervical lymphadenitis is *Streptococcus zooepidemicus*, although *Yersinia pseudotuberculosis* and *Streptobacillus moniliformis* have been documented in animals that have cervical lymph node swellings.[58] Typically, guinea pigs affected by *S. zooepidemicus* present with severe lymph node swelling in the cervical region. These animals do not typically show any other clinical signs; however, animals may become septic. Septic lesions can be observed in the lungs, kidneys, heart, and skin. Due to the degree of inflammation and caseous nature of the abscesses, these swellings need to be surgically excised in order to obtain full resolution of the condition. In addition, systemic antibiotic therapy, based on culture and antibiotic sensitivity results, and analgesic medication should be prescribed for the patient.

Fungal

Dermatophytosis in guinea pigs is most commonly caused by *Trichophyton mentagrophytes*. Lesions are often associated with patchy hair loss without pruritus and present as circular areas on the face and head. Diagnosis is based on fungal culture. Owners should be aware of the zoonotic potential of this pathogen.

Parasitic Diseases

Guinea pigs can be affected by several different species of mites, including *Trixacarus caviae*, *Sarcoptes scabiei*, *Chirodiscoides caviae*, *Myocoptes musculinus*, *Cheyletiella parasitovorax*, and *Demodex caviae*.[55,58] Fur plucks and deep skin scrapes can be used to identify these mites. One of the mites that deserves special note, and is the most common diagnosed in guinea pigs by the authors, is *T. caviae* (Figure 2-37). This sarcoptic

mite can cause intense pruritus in guinea pigs. The episodes of pruritus associated with this infestation can be so severe that it precipitates seizures in the infested patient. *Trixacarus caviae* is diagnosed more often in young animals processed through commercial pet retailers and is likely exacerbated by stress. Treatment for *Trixacarus caviae* can be accomplished with ivermectin, but high doses may be needed (0.4 to 0.5 mg/kg, every 10 d, for 3 treatments). Advantage-Multi® (Bayer Animal Health) is an effective treatment for guinea pig mites.

Gyropus ovalis and *Gliricola porcelli* are species of lice that commonly affect guinea pigs.[55] These parasites can be distinguished from mites by their long body structure. Most lice infestations in guinea pigs are clinically inapparent; however, pruritus and secondary excoriations may be seen with heavy infestations. Diagnosis can be made from fur plucks and skin scrapes after which the parasite is identified from the collected samples. Ivermectin (0.2 to 0.3 mg/kg, once every 10 d, for 3 treatments) can be used to control these lice. Advantage-Multi® (Bayer Animal Health) is an effective treatment for lice that infest guinea pigs.

Neoplastic Diseases

Trichofolliculomas are a common skin tumor of guinea pigs. These tumors are typically benign and solitary (Figure 2-38). The most common location for trichofolliculomas is over the dorsum and, more specifically, the pelvis. Surgical excision is curative, although additional tumors may occur in the future.

MAMMALS: CHINCHILLAS

Husbandry-Related Disease

Fur chewing is a behavioral dermatopathy that is observed in chinchillas where fur is chewed primarily from the lateral body wall, pelvis, flanks, ventral neck, legs, and paws. The head is not typically affected, which confirms that this is a self-inflicted syndrome rather than barbering by a conspecific. There is no clear evidence that implicates any specific cause for fur chewing in chinchillas; however, it has been hypothesized that dietary deficiencies, endocrine imbalance, dermatophytes, stressors, genetics, and chronic pain may play a role.

Fur slip has been diagnosed in chinchillas as a result of improper handling. Fur slip is considered a natural defense mechanism for these animals. While fur slip does not cause any medical problems, it does affect the aesthetics of the chinchilla's coat. Fur slip occurs during restraint when the fur is grabbed and the animal attempts to flee. Therefore this traumatic condition can be avoided by grasping the chinchilla at the base of the tail and supporting the body, rather than scruffing the fur.

Infectious Diseases

Bacterial

Chinchillas, like other rodents and rabbits, can develop abscesses and moist dermatitis. Abscesses and moist dermatitis lesions typically occur in animals under stress from conspecifics (e.g., bite wounds) or poor hygiene (e.g., high humidity). The management of these cases is similar to that described for other species. Fine-needle aspirates, culture and antibiotic sensitivity testing, and surgical debridement of the abscess are necessary to obtain a diagnosis and direct a therapeutic treatment plan. Similar to rabbits, antibiotic agents with action against cell-wall synthesis (e.g., penicillins and cephalosporins) should be avoided via the oral route. Moist dermatitis is managed in a similar manner as that used for dogs and cats. It is recommended to dry out the wound through the use of an appropriate astringent along with concurrent use of antibiotic medication if a pyoderma is present.

Fungal

Trichophyton mentagrophytes is the most common fungal infection of chinchillas (Figure 2-39). Affected animals may present with alopecia, scaling, and pruritus. Lesions may start on the head around the eyes, nose, and mouth and then spread to the body and legs. Fungal culture is recommended to confirm the fungal infection.

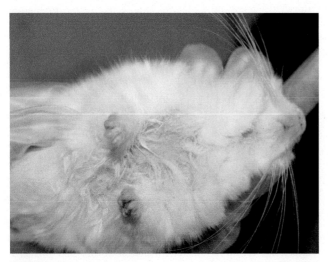

FIGURE 2-39 *Trichophyton mentagrophytes* in a chinchilla (*Chinchilla lanigera*).

MAMMALS: OTHER RODENTS

Husbandry-Related Diseases

Barbering, a common randomly occurring behavior of mice, occurs when they chew, pluck, and remove the whiskers of cage mates. Some individuals manipulate hair after removal and then ingest the hair. The barber mouse often holds down their conspecific when attempting to pluck their hairs, and barbering has even been documented in cage mates of other species. Victims of barbering show nonerythematous pruritic areas of alopecia. Ulcers, scratches, and scabs should not be present in any animal that is suspected of being barbered. Other causes of alopecia should be ruled out prior to making this diagnosis. Several husbandry factors have been suspected to effect barbering, and evidence indicates that higher population densities of mice increase the frequency of barbering secondary to an escalation in the amount of stress to which a mouse is exposed. Additionally, mice are more likely to barber when housed in stainless steel cages and with related individuals. Barbering is not considered to be a dominance behavior. Environmental enrichment is vital in delaying the onset and reducing the prevalence of this unwanted behavior. Some cases of barbering develop secondary to mandibulofacial and maxillofacial abscesses from trapped hair in the gingiva between teeth.

Ringtail is a disease diagnosed in rats, mice, and other rodents. It has traditionally been associated with low environmental humidity and high environmental temperature, although other causes, such as poor diet, genetics, and repeated attempts at tail venipuncture, have been implicated. Affected animals will present with a swollen tail, and in severe cases, the tail can become necrotic. Correcting environmental and dietary deficiencies is often curative. In severe cases, tail amputation is required.

Bald nose is a common finding in small rodents living in wire/bar type cages. The animals develop alopecia over the nose as a result of repeatedly rubbing their nose between the wires or bars. Providing a different housing arrangement and enrichment can reduce the incidence of this behavior.

Tail slip occurs in gerbils as a result of grabbing the tail when attempting to capture or restrain the animal. The entire skin covering the tail can deglove in these instances. Tail slip can be avoided by not restraining or trying to capture gerbils by their tail.

Parasitic Diseases

The most commonly reported fur mite species are *Myocoptes* and *Radfordia* spp. in rats. Infestations with fur mites are characterized by alopecia, excoriations, dermatitis, and a dull haircoat. Lesions can be observed anywhere on the body, especially around the ears and head (*Myobia musculi*) or along the dorsum (*Myocoptes musculinus*).[55] Chronic infestations can lead to significant pathological disease conditions of the skin.

In mice and rats, the most common blood-sucking lice are *Polyplax serrata* and *Polyplax spinulosa*. These mites typically infest young, immunocompromised, and underfed hosts. Affected animals present for alopecia and pruritus, with owners often observing constant scratching behind the ears. Additionally, animals with severe infestations can develop an anemic condition associated with these lice. The lice are long

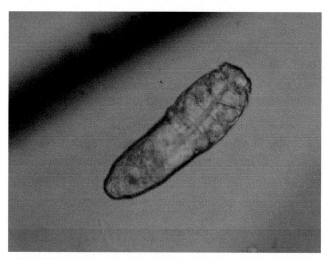

FIGURE 2-40 *Demodex criceti* collected from a Golden Syrian hamster *(Mesocricetus auratus).*

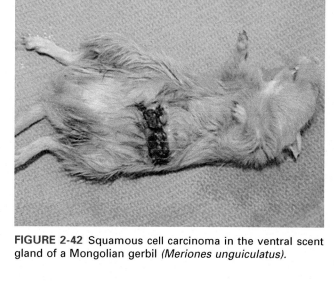

FIGURE 2-42 Squamous cell carcinoma in the ventral scent gland of a Mongolian gerbil *(Meriones unguiculatus).*

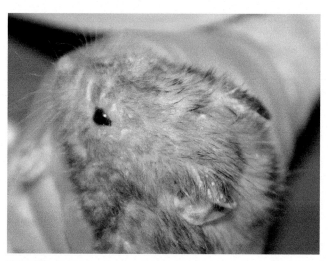

FIGURE 2-41 Generalized alopecia and scaling associated with demodicosis.

and yellow brown in color, with the head lacking eyes and having prominent segmented antenna. Ivermectin (0.2 mg/kg, SC, every 10 d, for 3 treatments) can be used to treat these animals but at this time Advantage-Multi® (Bayer Animal Health) appears to be a much more effective treatment.

Demodicosis is a parasitic disease frequently diagnosed in geriatric hamsters (>1 yr of age). There are two common *Demodex* species found on hamsters: *Demodex aurati* and *Demodex criceti. D. aurati* tends to be more common than *D. criceti.* The *Demodex* species can be differentiated by their body type, with *D. aurati* being cigar shaped and *D. criceti* being short and stumpy (Figure 2-40). Affected animals may present with widespread alopecia, scaling, and pruritus (Figure 2-41). Deep skin scrapes can be used to confirm a diagnosis. Ivermectin (0.2 to 0.4 mg/kg, SC, every 10 d, for 2 to 3 treatments) is curative. However, there appears to be an increasing resistance to ivermectin with small exotic mammal ectoparasites. Therefore Advantage-Multi® (Bayer Animal Health)

may be a better treatment option for *Demodex* spp. infestations in hamsters.

Neoplastic Diseases

The most common skin (subcutaneous, mammary tissue) tumors diagnosed in rats and mice are fibroadenomas and adenocarcinomas, respectively. Fibroadenomas are benign and solitary but can grow to a very large size. Adenocarcinomas are malignant cancers. A fine-needle aspirate or biopsy can be used to confirm the type of tumor. Although surgical excision is temporarily curative for fibroadenomas recurrence is common. More detailed information regarding these tumors is found in Chapter 10.

Cancer of the flank gland in hamsters and scent gland of gerbils may be diagnosed in geriatric animals. Melanomas, adenocarcinomas, and SCCs have been reported to affect these glands. The hamster flank glands are located along the lateral body wall, while in gerbils the scent gland is found on the ventral abdominal wall (Figure 2-42). Hamsters and gerbils with cancer of the scent glands may present for abnormal swellings in the flank and ventrum, respectively. In some cases, blood being lost through the tumor may be found within the cage (i.e., spotting noted on substrate). The diagnosis of scent gland neoplasia can be confirmed through fine-needle aspirate or biopsy suspect tissue mass and subsequent microscopic evaluation of the sample. Surgical resection is the only treatment recommended at this time.

MAMMALS: SUGAR GLIDERS

Self-mutilation can occur with any sugar glider, especially if they are sick or have a surgical incision site. It has been hypothesized that sugar glider self-mutilation is behavioral in origin; however, no validated research has been published documenting the incidence, cause, or potential treatments for this problem. Mutilation of feet, tail, scrotum, and various surgical sites have all been described in the literature.[59] Anecdotally, this problem has been described as being stress related and occurring more often in solitarily housed animals. It has been hypothesized that because most medical conditions can be related back to husbandry and nutrition, this negative behavior in sugar gliders may be similar to the self-injurious behavior observed in nonhuman primates. Alternatively, others have speculated that this behavior may be related to pain or neurasthenia since sugar gliders commonly self-mutilate after surgical procedures.[60] A case report described self-mutilation in sugar glider with a pericloacal mass associated with transitional cell carcinoma, leading to further evidence that self-mutilation may be related to pain or discomfort in this species.[61]

MAMMALS: AFRICAN PYGMY HEDGEHOGS

Husbandry-Related Diseases

In wild African pygmy hedgehogs, pinnal dermatitis is commonly observed. The edges of the ear are often crusty and dry, and skin secretions accumulate at the margins of the ear resulting in a ragged ear edge. Many different factors have been associated with this clinical presentation, including dermatophytosis, acariasis, nutritional deficiency, low humidity, and dry skin.

Infectious Diseases

Fungal

Dermatophytosis is a common clinical disorder in African pygmy hedgehogs. *Trichophyton erinacei*, *Trichophyton mentagrophytes*, and *Microsporum* spp. have all been implicated and isolated as fungal pathogens from African pygmy hedgehogs. Most of the documented fungal organisms have zoonotic potential, consequently it is important to inform your clients about these risks. Clinically, a hedgehog may present with crusting; pruritic dermatitis of the face, pinna, and body; and quill loss. Dermatophyte cultures can be used to confirm a diagnosis.

Parasitic Diseases

Acariasis is a common problem of captive African pygmy hedgehogs. Typically, the mite species that infect hedgehogs are *Caparinia* spp., *Chorioptes* spp., and *Notoedres* spp. In a study of wild hedgehogs, the three mites were found to infect hedgehogs at different rates and with variable pathogenicity.[62] *Notoedres oudesmani* was sporadically observed but usually in infested male hedgehogs resulting in high mortality. *Caparinia erinacei* was the most common mite, but it had a low pathogenicity. *Rodentopus sciuri* was observed on about half of the animals studied, but clinical signs were minimal. In captivity, affected animals often present with scaling, crusting, and spine loss. Diagnosis of the mites can be made with a skin scrape. Ivermectin is commonly used to treat these infestations (0.2 to 0.4 mg/kg, SC, once every 10 d, for 3 treatments).

Ear mites *(Otodectes cynotis)* are occasionally diagnosed in captive African pygmy hedgehogs. Animals may scratch at their ears if infested. Observing mites and eggs on an ear swab confirms the diagnosis. Treatment is similar to that for other mites encountered in hedgehogs.

Tick and mite infestations can predispose hedgehogs to otitis externa which may develop into concurrent bacterial and yeast infections. Clinical signs of infectious otitis externa in hedgehogs include sensitivity to the ears, purulent discharge, and malodor. These cases should be managed using the same methods described for domestic mammals.

Neoplastic Diseases

Neoplasia is one of the most common diseases of African pygmy hedgehogs. Many reports exist within the literature, and ~30% of hedgehogs are diagnosed with neoplasia at necropsy.[63,64] The skin is the most common location for neoplasia in captive hedgehogs. Mast cell tumors, mammary tumors, SCCs, neurofibromas, and fibrous histiocytomas have all been reported as cutaneous neoplasms in African pygmy hedgehogs.[63,64] Diagnosis of skin cancer in these animals is best achieved through biopsy of the suspect tissue mass and subsequent histopathologic evaluation of the sample(s). Surgical management is currently the preferred method of treating African pygmy hedgehogs that have been diagnosed with neoplastic disease.

WORKING UP THE CASE: HISTORY, PHYSICAL EXAMINATION, AND DIAGNOSTIC TESTING

Since skin disease is a very common presenting complaint exotic animal practitioners must become familiar with the methods for evaluating these cases to increase the probability for successful resolution. A systematic diagnostic approach is required to achieve a definitive diagnosis and formulate an effective therapeutic plan. In all exotic species, husbandry is a fundamental contributor to cutaneous disease development and pathogenesis. To elucidate the disease etiology and develop a proper therapeutic plan, one must obtain a thorough history with an extensive understanding of the owner's current husbandry practices. Once a thorough history is obtained, a general physical examination is necessary to systematically evaluate each organ system. Physical examinations should be performed in an identical manner for each patient to ensure one does not miss any overt disease conditions. Diagnostic tests should be selected based on the differential diagnoses. It is best to prioritize the tests based on the differential list; this is especially important for cases where there are financial constraints. The remainder of this section is focused on specific diagnostic methods for skin disease by animal group.

Invertebrates

As with other exotic species, it is important to evaluate the specific husbandry methods used to care for the invertebrate patient, so that it is possible to determine the possible effect of the care provided on it's condition. Since there are a wide variety of invertebrates, ranging from sponges to arthropods, all husbandry inquiries should be tailored to the type of invertebrate evaluated. Their life history traits will also determine how to proceed with a clinical evaluation. The history should focus on the size of the enclosure; temperature, humidity, and methods used to provide them; substrate; filtration for aquatic species; diet; other species of which they are in contact; duration of ownership; and owner's experience with the species (see Chapter 1 for history form). Once the history is completed, a through physical examination of the invertebrate patient should be performed in order to identify all lesions present on the exoskeleton (see Chapter 1 for physical examination form). The initial examination would be an appropriate time to evaluate molts (shedding exoskeletons). Care should be observed when handling invertebrates, as some can sting or bite. Appropriate handling materials (e.g., gloves, forceps, etc.) should always be used to protect both the examiner and the patient.

Water quality is an important component of the physical examination for aquatic invertebrates. Water quality parameters that should be measured include pH, salinity, calcium, alkalinity, hardness, ammonia, nitrate, nitrite, phosphorous, magnesium, strontium, iodine, and temperature. Local aquarium shop personnel may be helpful in deciphering the results of the water quality testing for less experienced individuals. If water parameters are found to be a contributing factor to the skin condition, a plan should be formulated to correct the deficiency (e.g., supplementation, improved biological filtration).

As noted earlier, knowledge regarding invertebrate medicine is limited; therefore, one should utilize the well-known diagnostic methods commonly used in domestic species to guide the management of our invertebrate patients. The following list cites examples of diagnostic tests to consider when evaluating an invertebrate patient with skin disease:

1. Skin (exoskeleton) scrapes, impression smears, and wet mounts can be performed on superficial integumentary wounds to evaluate the bacterial, fungal, and parasitic flora on the skin.
2. Hemolymph can be collected in cases of integumentary disease to assess electrolyte disturbances (e.g., alterations in sodium and chloride concentrations with dehydration) or inflammation.
3. Bacterial and fungal cultures can be collected to specifically isolate potential pathogens from the surface of the skin (exoskeleton).
4. Biopsies of the skin (exoskeleton) can be collected for histopathological assessment.
5. Necropsy can be performed on individual animals to determine a specific disease etiology, which is especially important for invertebrate collections with multiple conspecifics.

Fish

A detailed history regarding the management of a fish is important to confirm a disease diagnosis. The history of the fish or group of fish should focus on the size of the aquarium or pond; water temperature; water quality parameters; plant types; substrate; filtration; diet; other species in the aquarium/pond; duration of ownership; owner's experience with the species; whether any over-the-counter drugs have been used to treat the condition; quarantine protocol used, if any; and the exact lesions and duration of lesions (see Chapter 1 for history form). Once a complete history is obtained, a thorough physical examination should be performed (see Chapter 1 for physical examination form). Most fish require sedation for a good evaluation (examination and diagnostic testing). Tricaine methanesulfonate (MS-222) is the most common anesthetic used for fish. Fish dosages for tricaine methanesulfonate (MS-222) can vary based on species, but the authors recommend 100 to 150 mg/L for induction and 50 to 75 mg/L for maintenance anesthesia. For veterinarians that do not stock MS-222, alfaxalone (Alfaxan, Jurox Limited,

Worcestershire, UK), which is more readily available in small animal practices, can be used.[65] Alfaxalone immersion at 5 to 10 mg/L appears to be well tolerated. When handling fish, it is important to wear examination gloves (preferably nonpowder and nonlatex) to protect the skin of the fish against abrasions and oils from hands and the handler against potential zoonotic diseases (e.g., *Mycobacterium* spp.). Since the focus of this chapter is on the integument, these diagnostic recommendations are centered on that system. The entire skin including the scales and fins should be evaluated. Common abnormalities of the skin and fins that may be observed include discoloration; frayed or irregularly shaped fins; ulcers and erosions; erythema, petechia, and ecchymosis; edema; ectoparasites; papules and nodules; scale loss; and excessive mucus production.

A diagnostic workup for fish presented for dermatologic disease should include direct observation of the fish in its aquarium or pond, a hands-on examination of the fish under anesthesia, and a complete evaluation of the water quality. In addition, skin scrapes, fin biopsies, gill biopsies, microbiologic culture, and PCR testing (e.g., for KHV) may be performed based on the clinical signs and/or lesions identified.

1. Water quality evaluation.
   a. Poor water quality is a common cause of morbidity and mortality for aquarium and pond fish. Every veterinarian that works with fish should have the ability (e.g., a water testing kit) to evaluate the water quality, including the temperature, salinity (marine or brackish systems), pH, alkalinity, hardness, ammonia, nitrite, nitrate, chlorine/chloramines, and dissolved oxygen. If possible, the water testing should be performed tank/pond side or as soon as possible after being presented to the veterinary hospital.
2. Skin scrape, gill biopsy, and fin biopsy.
   a. All of these procedures should be performed under anesthesia (see above) to limit the likelihood of causing unnecessary damage to the skin due to restraint and reduce the pain associated with the procedures (e.g., gill and fin biopsies).
   b. Skin scraping.
      i. In fish, a skin scrape can be performed using a coverslip or the edge of a glass slide. The coverslip or slide should be gently scraped over the lesion on the skin in a cranial to caudal (head to tail) direction (Figure 2-43). This will prevent unnecessary damage to the healthy skin. The collected mucus can be placed on another slide with a drop of water from the aquarium/pond, covered with a new coverslip, and reviewed under light microscopy. Tank or pond water is used to prevent osmotic disruption of any organisms that may be present. In addition, the mucus can be spread over a slide and stained (e.g., Gram stain) to screen for pathogens.
   c. Gill biopsy.
      i. To perform a gill biopsy, lift the operculum with the thumb or finger, insert a pair of small iris scissors, clip the gill at the level of the distal primary lamellae (edge of exposed gill), remove the gill clip, place it on a slide with a drop of water from the pond/aquarium, place a coverslip over the gill biopsy, and review under light microscopy (Figures 2-44, 2-45, 2-46).

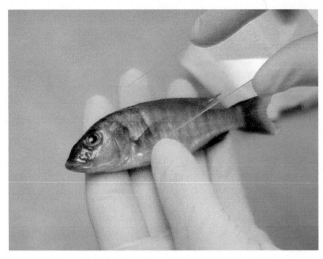

FIGURE 2-43 A skin scrape in a fish.

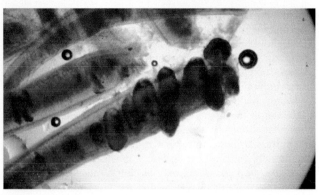

FIGURE 2-46 Wet-mount gill clip at 100× of a gill infected with telangiectasia. (Photo courtesy of Shane Boylan.)

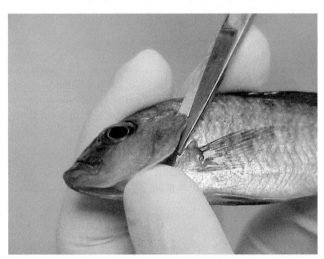

FIGURE 2-44 A gill biopsy in a fish.

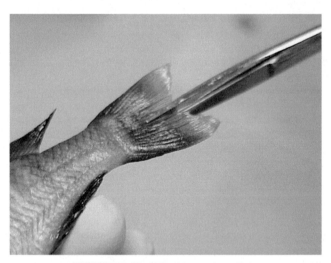

FIGURE 2-47 A fin biopsy in a fish.

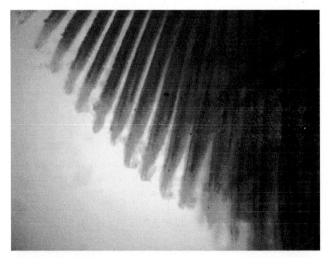

FIGURE 2-45 Normal wet-mount gill clip at 40× prepared using a coverslip and glass slide with a drop of saltwater. (Photo courtesy of Shane Boylan.)

    d. Fin biopsy.
      i. Similar to the gill biopsy described above, iris scissors can be used to remove a lesion from a fin (Figure 2-47). The fin will regrow once the disease process is successfully treated. These samples are prepared as described above for the gill biopsy.
    e. All of these samples should be evaluated with a low power objective (4×, 10×) first and then reevaluated with higher power objectives (40×, 100×). Most parasites can be observed at 4× or 10× magnification; however, some small ciliates and flagellates may need to be evaluated at 40×. Bacteria, fungi, and water molds are best reviewed at 100×. Optimum results can be obtained if the samples are observed when the condenser on the microscope is turned down.
3. Bacterial or fungal culture and antimicrobial sensitivity testing.
    a. A swab or biopsy sample can be collected and submitted for culture; biopsies are preferred. The diagnostic laboratory should be properly informed that the submitted sample was derived from a fish, to ensure the proper incubation temperature of the sample is applied for the aquatic specimen.

4. Complete blood count (CBC) and biochemistry testing.
   a. Underlying systemic disease can manifest as dermatological conditions; therefore, it is important to have a minimum database to help rule in or out a systemic disorder. A CBC and biochemistry analysis can provide insight into the general health of the fish. In fish, blood samples can be collected from the ventral tail vein or heart. A lateral or ventral approach can be used to access the ventral tail vein. The ventral tail vein lies on the ventral aspect of the caudal tail vertebrae. The heart can be approached through the branchial chamber.
5. Viral testing.
   a. Samples can be submitted for evaluation of certain viral diseases, such as KHV. Both serology and PCR diagnostic tests are available to evaluate whether a fish has been infected with KHV. In the future, there will be more viral pathogens identified and more tests to help diagnose these "emerging" diseases as we become more proficient at recognizing viral organisms that cause disease in fish species.
6. Necropsy/histopathology
   a. Necropsy and histopathology are invaluable when trying to identify fish disease. Surgical biopsies can be collected and submitted for antemortem testing. It is important to place the biopsy sample or necropsy samples (e.g., whole fish with belly slit) in formalin as soon as possible to prevent denaturing of the tissues.

Amphibians

Obtaining a thorough history is important when evaluating an amphibian case. An example of the types of questions that should be asked when collecting information regarding the amphibian patient being examined can be found in Chapter 1. Likewise, the systems that should be evaluated during a physical examination of an amphibian are also found in Chapter 1. During an amphibian examination, it is important to always wear gloves (nonlatex and nonpowder preferred) to limit the likelihood of exacerbating any skin conditions on the patient and to prevent the handler from being exposed to any potential zoonotic agents or toxins being produced by the amphibian. When evaluating amphibian skin, it is important to recognize that many diseases can have a similar presentation with skin hyperemia and abnormal coloring, ulceration, hemorrhage, edema, dermal papules, nodules, and excessive mucus production. Excessive mucus production is often one of the most common disease findings that effect amphibian skin.

A diagnostic evaluation for an amphibian presented for dermatologic disease should include direct observation of the amphibian in its terrarium or transport box, a hands-on examination of the amphibian, and a complete water quality evaluation for aquatic species. In addition, skin scrapes or biopsies, microbiologic culture, and PCR testing (e.g., chytrids, ranavirus) may be performed based on the clinical signs/lesions that are identified on the patient.

1. Skin scraping.
   a. In amphibians, a skin scrape can be performed using a coverslip or edge of a glass slide, a procedure similar to that previously described for fish. The collected sample should be placed on a slide and a drop of physiologic saline added to make a wet-mount preparation. These samples should be evaluated immediately to increase the likelihood of pathogen identification. Start with a low power objective and then reevaluate the sample with higher power objectives.
2. Impression swabs or smears, fine-needle aspirates.
   a. Impression smears are often less traumatic than skin scrapes. A slide is typically placed against the surface of the skin, air dried, and then stained. Fine-needle aspirates can be performed by inserting a needle (20 or 22 G) into the affected area (e.g., mass) and aspirating back on the syringe plunger. To increase the probability of collecting a quality sample, the syringe should be removed from the needle, filled with air, reattached to the needle, and the air within the syringe expressed onto a slide. These samples are typically air dried, stained, and evaluated under a light microscope.
3. Bacterial culture.
   a. Bacterial cultures obtained from amphibian skin risk being exposed to normal surface microflora and environmental contamination. For best results, a diagnostic culture should be obtained by irrigating the lesion with sterile physiologic saline and then obtaining a deep sample. Swabs can be pre-moistened with either transport media or sterile saline to maximize the recovery of bacteria and decrease the likelihood of skin damage. The diagnostic laboratory should be informed that the sample was derived from an amphibian, as they may culture the sample at a temperature other than 37°C. Typically, most bacterial isolates from amphibian skin lesions are Gram negative, although Gram positive and mycobacterial infections can also be isolated.
4. Fungal cultures.
   a. Tissue samples can be placed directly onto fungal culture media. Typically, Sabouraud-dextrose agar can be used for most fungal isolates. One advantage of trying to identify fungal organisms is that the sample can be incubated at room temperature.
5. PCR of skin swabs.
   a. PCR is becoming more common as a diagnostic tools for infectious diseases. Several different types of PCR testing are available, including conventional PCR, real-time PCR (RT-PCR), quantitative PCR (q-PCR), and TaqMan PCR. Diagnostic laboratory confirmation is necessary to determine the specific sample collection protocol requirements (e.g., swab type, sample storage conditions, shipping methods) needed for the type of PCR testing methodology used and the pathogen of interest. PCR testing is appropriate to be used on amphibian samples for several different pathogens: *Batrachochytrium dendrobatidis*, ranavirus, chlamydophila, flavobacteria, and mycobacteria.
6. Histopathology.
   a. Excisional or incisional biopsy samples can be harvested from a lesion associated with the skin and placed in a 1:10 ratio of formalin for proper fixation. Samples can be cut and placed on a slide to microscopically evaluate the skin.

Reptiles

Dermatologic disease is a common problem in reptiles. Cutaneous disorders are often multifactorial and frequently associated with husbandry deficiencies, with one report suggesting that as many as 64% of reptile dermatologic lesions can be traced back to husbandry-related issues.[66] Therefore it is imperative to obtain a detailed clinical history of reptile patients that are presented with skin disease. Examples of the types of questions to be asked when obtaining the reptile patient's history can be found in Chapter 1. The types of skin lesions observed in reptiles with dermatological disease include erosions, ulcers, abrasions, wounds, swellings, blisters, vesicles, bullae, dysecydsis, crusts, macroparasites, discoloration, petechiae, ecchymoses, and edema. Reptiles with systemic diseases may also present with dermatologic lesions. Systemic disease lesions that present as integumentary disorders include petechial and ecchymotic hemorrhages in reptiles that are septic and edema associated with renal or liver disease. Approximately 47% of all reptiles with confirmed sepsis had petechial hemorrhages, with chelonians having the highest overall percentage (82%).[66,67]

A diagnostic workup for a reptile presented for dermatologic disease should start with direct observation of the animal in its terrarium or transport box followed by a hands-on examination. In addition, skin scrapes and impression smears, fine-needle aspirates or biopsies, blood work, diagnostic imaging, microbiologic culture, and PCR testing may be performed based on the clinical signs/lesions identified.

1. Skin cytology and impression smears.
   a. Impression smears are often less traumatic than skin scrapes. A slide is typically placed up against the surface of the skin, air dried, and then stained. Once dried the impression smear can be evaluated microscopically for inflammatory cells and infectious agents (e.g., bacteria, fungal elements, viral inclusions).
2. Acetate tape impressions.
   a. Acetate tape is pressed up against the skin and then placed on a microscope slide and evaluated using a light microscope. This technique is useful for diagnosing mites.
3. Skin scrapings
   a. A #15 blade scalpel can be used to collect epidermal samples. The blade is scraped repeatedly over the skin lesion until debris is collected on the blade surface. The debris is then placed on a microscope slide and evaluated. The skin sample can be mixed with mineral oil and reviewed (e.g., mites) or spread on a slide and stained (e.g., bacteria).
4. Microscopic evaluation of shed skin fragments.
   a. Microscopic evaluation of any shed skin will allow one to determine whether there are any organisms (e.g., parasites, fungal) present.
5. Skin biopsies for histopathology.
   a. Punch biopsies or an incisional biopsy can be performed to collect skin samples for histopathologic evaluation. Skin biopsies can be especially valuable in chelonians with shell lesions. These samples should be placed in formalin and fixed.
6. Bacterial and fungal cultures.
   a. Skin cultures can be submitted for diagnostic testing in order to confirm the presence of bacterial or fungal pathogens; however, due to the nature of the sample, there is an increased risk for environmental contamination. Therefore, samples should be collected from deep

within a wound, the abscess wall, or derived from a tissue biopsy. It is best to correlate culture results with histopathology results.
7. Fine-needle aspirates; swellings and growths.
   a. Fine-needle aspirates can be obtained by inserting a needle (20 or 22 G) into the area of concern (e.g., mass) and aspirating back on the syringe plunger. To increase the likelihood of a quality sample, the syringe should be removed from the needle, filled with air, reattached to the needle, and the air within the syringe expressed onto a slide. These samples are typically air dried, stained, and then evaluated under light microscopy.
8. CBC and biochemistry analysis.
   a. A CBC or biochemistry analysis can be used to provide insight into the systemic health of the reptile. This is especially important for those cases where dermatologic lesions are a manifestation of an underlying systemic disease.
9. Diagnostic imaging.
   a. Radiographs or computed tomography imaging can be used to assess damaged osteoderms in chelonians with shell fractures and potential osteomyelitis cases where dermatitis has progressed to a systemic disease.

Birds

Avian species often are presented to veterinary hospitals with disease conditions that involve the integument. Skin and feather disorders in birds are often multifactorial and frequently associated with husbandry (e.g., nutrition, environment). Therefore it is important to obtain a detailed clinical history in birds with skin and feather disease. Examples of the types of questions to be asked when obtaining the history of an avian patient are found in Chapter 1. A dermatologic examination of a bird should be comprehensive and evaluate the feathers, skin, beak and cere, legs and claws, uropygial gland, and vent. Common skin disorders in captive birds include broken or absent feathers, discolored feathers, dystrophic feathers, scaling, crusting, ulcerations, erythema, nodules, and masses.

A diagnostic workup for a bird presented for dermatologic disease should begin with direct observation of the bird in its cage and a hands-on examination. In addition, feather cytologic examination, skin scrapes and impression smears, fine-needle aspirates or biopsies, blood work, heavy metal testing, diagnostic imaging, microbiologic culture, allergy testing, and PCR testing may be performed based on the clinical signs/lesions identified (Figure 2-48).
1. Feather examination.
   a. Gross and microscopic examination of the feathers is necessary in order to evaluate the overall condition of these structures. Ectoparasites, stress bars, and evidence of self-trauma or mutilation may be observed. To increase the likelihood of identifying ectoparasites (e.g., mites) the feather can be further evaluated using potassium hydroxide. The feather's calamus should be placed into 10% potassium hydroxide solution, gently heated, centrifuged, and the sediment removed and evaluated under a light microscope.[13]
2. Feather pulp cytology.
   a. Freshly plucked feathers can be prepared on a slide and microscopically evaluated. The calamus can be

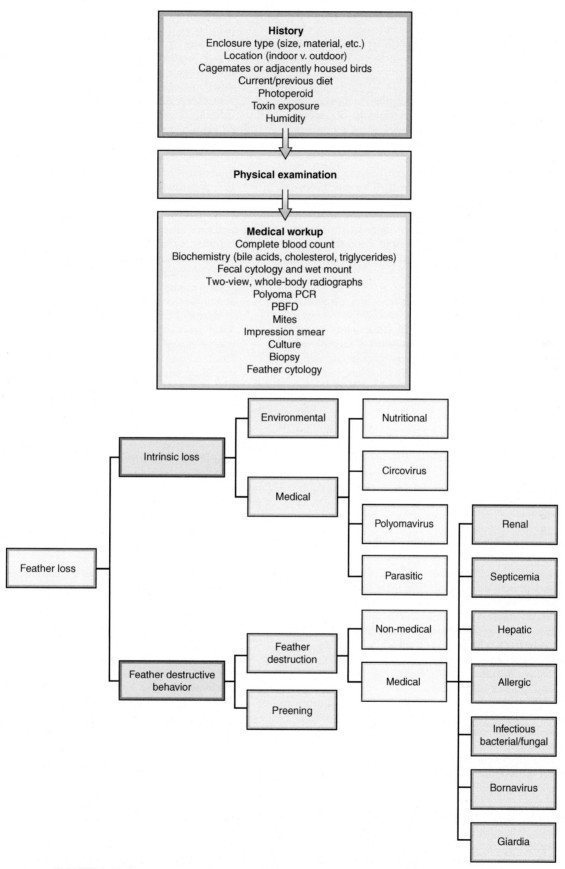

FIGURE 2-48 Flow chart on how to work up a feather-picking bird. *PBFD,* Psittacine beak and feather disease; *PCR,* polymerase chain reaction.

removed from the feather and applied to a slide for cytologic examination. Under the microscope, one can appreciate the presence of folliculitis by observing inflammatory cells, bacteria, viral inclusion bodies, and fungal elements.

3. Acetate tape impression.
   a. Tape preps are primarily used to identify ectoparasites, yeast, and bacterial infections. One must be careful when interpreting tape prep samples, as feather dander and keratin debris can often appear similar to bacteria and yeast.

4. Impression smear.
   a. A direct impression smear can be used for moist, exudative, and crusted lesions. With dry lesions, one can attempt to evaluate impression smears; however, acetate tape preparations may be more diagnostic. If there is difficulty obtaining a sample, a moist cotton-tipped applicator can be rolled over the lesion and then applied to a slide.

5. Skin scraping.
   a. A #15 blade scalpel can be used to collect epidermal samples. The blade is scraped repeatedly over the affected surface of the skin until some debris is collected on the blade surface. The debris is then placed on a microscope slide and microscopically evaluated. The skin sample can be mixed with mineral oil and assessed for (e.g., mites) or spread on a slide and stained (e.g., bacteria).

6. Bacterial and fungal culture.
   a. Several different types of samples can be submitted for bacterial or fungal cultures. Superficial swabs of the skin can be submitted; however, they are subject to false negative results because of environmental contaminants. The feather calamus can also be submitted. Additionally, an aseptically prepared tissue biopsy can be submitted for culture, which is the preferred method.

7. Biopsy.
   a. Skin samples can be submitted for both histopathology and culture. Bird skin is extremely delicate; thus, biopsies should be collected using a scalpel blade rather than a punch biopsy. Placing a piece of acetate tape over the affected skin and incising the tape will ensure complete excision of the skin. The sample, with the tape, can then be placed into formalin; this will prevent the skin from rolling up on itself while providing the pathologist evidence of the skin surface (i.e., the surface next to the attached tape).

8. CBC and biochemistry analysis.
   a. Birds with skin disease, especially feather-based problems, should always have a complete health examination. The CBC and plasma biochemistry analysis can provide important insight into the general health of the bird, including whether skin diseases are having an effect on systemic health.

9. Heavy metal testing.
   a. Exposure to lead and zinc can manifest as skin issues. If heavy metal toxicity is considered a differential disease diagnosis, blood levels should be measured.

10. Diagnostic imaging.
    a. Radiographic evidence of heavy metals in the gastrointestinal tract, or osteomyelitis secondary to pododermatitis, can be used to confirm a diagnosis and plan for specific therapeutic protocols.

11. Crop washes.
    a. A crop wash can be used to diagnose a crop infection (ingluvitis) with *Trichomonas* spp., *Candida* spp., or other microbial pathogen. Feather plucking over the ventral cervical region is considered a sequella to these infections.

12. Fecal examination.
    a. A direct fecal smear may be used to diagnose giardiasis, which has been associated with feather picking in cockatiels. However there is no scientific confirmation regarding the belief that there is a correlation between feather picking and giardiasis infection in cockatiels.

13. Intradermal allergy testing.
    a. Intradermal allergy testing can be used in birds to identify environmental allergens. In small animal medicine, histamine is used as the positive control for this testing method; however, in birds, codeine phosphate at 1 : 100,000 wt/vol is preferred as a positive control.

14. Viral testing (PCR).
    a. Viral pathogens such as polyomavirus and PBFD can be diagnosed using PCR testing methodologies. Contact the diagnostic laboratory for information regarding sample collection and submission.

Mammals

As with the other groups of exotic animals presented in this chapter, a thorough evaluation of husbandry is required to aid in the diagnosis and treatment of mammalian dermatological conditions. See Chapter 1 for an example of the types of questions that should be asked when developing a historical perspective on the patient being examined. After a full physical examination, a thorough dermatological evaluation is required for any animal with skin disease. Integumentary lesions commonly observed in exotic mammals include alopecia, erythema, scaling, crusting, excoriations, erosions, pustules, and ulcers. Due to the small size of many exotic mammals and limited restraint techniques, anesthesia may be required to obtain quality diagnostic samples.

1. Impression smears.
   a. Direct slide impression smears are often used when evaluating moist, exudative, or crusty lesions. For drier lesions, a direct impression smear may be attempted, although results can be variable. With dry lesions, a moistened cotton-tipped applicator can be used to collect the sample; the swab should be rolled onto a slide. If either of these techniques does not work for a dry lesion, an acetate tape impression may be more diagnostic.

2. Skin scrapings.
   a. Traditionally, in small animal medicine, a #10 blade is used to perform a skin scrape; however, because the skin of many exotic mammals is thin and delicate, a #15 blade is preferred.

3. Bacterial and fungal culture and antimicrobial sensitivity testing.
   a. Several different types of samples can be submitted for bacterial or fungal cultures. Superficial swabs of the

skin can be submitted; however, they are subject to false negative results because of environmental contaminants. Deep cultures or cultures derived from biopsied skin are preferred.

4. Wood's lamp.
   a. A Wood's lamp can be used to wave over lesions of which dermtophytosis is suspected. Observations obtained using the Wood's lamp should be compared with fungal culture results.

5. Trichogram.
   a. Trichograms can be used to evaluate hair. Fractured hair shafts are an indication that the hair loss is traumatic rather than a developmental problem (e.g., lost at the hair follicle). Additionally, this allows the practitioner to evaluate the hair for ectoparasites and/or evidence of fungal spores or ectothrix spores.

6. Acetate tape impression
   a. Acetate tape impressions are particularly useful in the collection and identification of surface dwelling ectoparasites such as *Cheyletiella* and *Myobia*.

7. Skin biopsy for histopathology.
   a. Skin biopsy samples can be submitted for histopathology and culture. Skin biopsies are harvested using a scalpel blade or a punch biopsy. If a punch biopsy is employed, additional care must be taken in order to completely appose the skin.

8. Diagnostic imaging,
   a. Radiographic imaging can be used to confirm the presence of osteomyelitis secondary to pododermatitis (e.g., rabbits).

9. CBC and biochemistry analysis.
   a. A complete blood count and plasma biochemistry panel can provide important insight into the general health of an exotic mammal, including if the skin disease(s) is having an affect on the systemic health.

10. Adrenal gland testing in Ferrets
    a. Adrenal gland disease can be diagnosed using ultrasound imaging (enlarged adrenal glands) and androgen testing. See Chapter 6.

TREATMENTS

Since dermatologic diseases can be caused by a variety of different etiologies, Tables 2-3 to 2-8 have been developed by animal group, treatment method, and drug type to guide the veterinarian when managing the various skin disorders listed.

TABLE 2-3

Common Treatments Used to Manage Skin Diseases in Invertebrates

Medication	Route/Type	Dosage
	Topical Therapy: Antimicrobials and Antifungals	
Benzalkonium chloride		0.5 mg/L long term,[68] 10 mg/L for 10 min[69]
Enrofloxacin		2.5 mg/L for 5 h immersion, q12-24 h[70,71]
Nystatin		50 mg/mL[72,73]
Tetracycline		0.01-0.1 ppm as an immersion[74,75]
Trifluralin		100 mL/L for 45 min, q24 h for 7 d as an immersion[76]
	Topical Therapy: Antiparasitics	
Formalin		50-100 µL/L for 4 h, then 25 µL/L indefinitely[76]
Ivermectin		1:1 1% ivermectin:propolene glycol; dilute 1:50 with distilled water prior to topical therapy[69]
Levamisole		8 mg/L immersion for 24 h[75]
Metronidazole		100 mg/L for 16 h[71]
Milbemycin oxime (Interceptor, Novartis)		0.625 mg/L as an immersion[77]
Potassium permanganate		25-30 ppm for 30-60 min[76]
Povidone iodine		25-30 ppm for 30-60 min[69]
	Systemic Therapy: Antimicrobials and Antifungals	
Ceftazidime		20 mg/kg intracardiac, q72 h for 3 wk[69]
Enrofloxacin		5 mg/kg IM, IV[70,71] 10-20 mg/kg PO q24 h[69]
Itraconazole (Sporanox, Janssen)		10 mg/kg IV[78]
Oxytetracycline		50-100 mg/kg PO[79–81]
Sulfamethoxazole/trimethoprim		Bioencapsulated shrimp PO q12 h[82]
Tetracycline		10 mg/kg PO q24 h[71]
Metronidazole		50 mg/kg intracardiac for 1 treatment[69]

IM, Intramuscularly; *IV,* intravenously; *PO,* orally; *ppm,* parts per million; *SC,* subcutaneously.

TABLE 2-4

Common Treatments Used to Manage Skin Diseases in Fish

Medications	Route/Type	Dosage
	Topical Therapy: Antimicrobial and Antifungal Therapeutics	
Benzalkonium chloride		0.5 mg/L long term,[68] 10 mg/L for 10 min[68]
Enrofloxacin		2.5-5 mg/L for 5 h bath q24 h for 5-7 d[83]
Iodine, potentiated (Betadine, Purdue Frederick)		Topical to wound,[82] 20-100 mg/L for 10 min[68]
Malachite green		0.1 mg/L tank water q3 d for 3 treatments[82] 0.25 mg/L for 15 min, q24 h[84]
Methylene blue		2 mg/L tank water q48 h for up to 3 treatments[82]
Oxytetracycline		10-100 mg/L tank water,[82] 10-50 mg/L for 1 h bath[82]
Potassium permanganate		2 mg/L as an indefinite bath[85] 5 mg/L for 30-60 min bath[82]
Trimethoprim/sulfamethoxazole		20 mg/L for 5-12 h bath, q24 for 5-7 d[82]
	Topical Therapy: Antiparasitic Therapeutics	
Formalin/malachite green		(F) 0.025 mL/L + (M) 0.1 mg/L tank water q48 h for 3 treatments[82]
Fresh water		3-25 min bath, repeat q7 d prn[82] for 4-5 min bath[86]
Hydrogen peroxide (3%)		1-1.5 mg/L for 20 min bath[87] 17.5 mL/L for 4-10 min bath once[88]
Levamisole		1 mg/L for 24 h bath[89] 1-2 mg/L for 24 h bath[88] 50 mg/L for 2 h bath[88]
Lufenuron (Program, Novartis)		0.13 mg/L prn[85]
Malachite green		0.1 mg/L tank water q3 d for 3 treatments[82] 1 mg/L for 30-60 min bath[82] 50-60 mg/L for 10-30 sec bath[82] 100 mg/L topical to skin lesions[82]
Mebendazole		1 mg/L 24 or 72 h bath[90] 10-50 mg/L for 2-6 h immersion[91] 100 mg/L for 10 min-2 h baths[88]
Methylene blue		1-3 mg/L tank water[82]
Metronidazole		6.6 mg/L tank water q24 h for 3 d[82] 25 mg/L tank water q48 h for 3 treatments[82]
Praziquantel		5-10 mg/L for 3-6 h bath, repeat in 7 d[86]
Salt (sodium chloride)		1-5 g tank water indefinitely[82] 10-30 g/L up to 30 min bath[82]
Trichlorfon (dimethylphosphonate)		0.25 mg/L tank water 96 h bath[82]
	Systemic Therapy: Antimicrobial and Antifungal Therapeutics	
Amikacin		5 mg/kg ICe q24 h for 3 d, then q48 h for 2 treatments[85]
Amoxicillin		80 mg/kg PO q24 h for 10 d[92] 40-80 mg/kg/d in feed for 10 d[82]
Ampicillin		10 mg/kg q24 h IM, IV[93,94]
Ceftazidime		22 mg/kg IM, ICe q72-96 h for 3-5 treatments[95]
Ciprofloxacin		15 mg/kg IM, IV[96]
Enrofloxacin		5-10 mg/kg PO, IM, ICe q24 h[83] 0.1% feed for 10-14 d
Erythromycin		100-200 mg/kg PO q24 h for 21 d[68]
Florfenicol		40-50 mg/kg PO, IM, ICe[97]
Itraconazole		1-5 mg/kg q24 h in feed q1-7 d[98]
Ketoconazole		2.5-10 mg/kg PO, IM, ICe[98]
Miconazole (Monistat, Janssen)		10-20 mg/kg PO, IM, ICe[98]

TABLE 2-4

Common Treatments Used to Manage Skin Diseases in Fish—cont'd

Medications	Route/Type	Dosage
Nalidixic acid (Neg Gram, Sanofi Winthrop)		5 mg/kg PO, IM, IV q24 h[98] 20 mg/kg PO q24 h[68]
Nifurpirinol		0.45-0.9 mg/kg PO q24 h for 5 d[82] 4-10 mg/kg in feed q12 h for 5 d[99]
Oxolinic acid		5-25 mg/kg PO q24 h[98] 10 mg/kg q24 h PO[68] 25-50 mg/kg PO q24 h[68]
Oxytetracycline		3 mg/kg IV q24 h[100] 7 mg/kg IM q24 h[100] 10 mg/kg IM q24 h[98] 20 mg/kg ICe[68] 20 mg/kg PO q8 h[98] 60 mg/kg IM q7 d[101] 70 mg/kg PO q24 h for 10-14 d[102] 82.8 mg/kg PO for 10[103] d[104] 100 mg/kg IM q24 h[105]
Sarafloxacin (Saraflox, Abbott)		10-14 mg/kg PO q24 h for 10 d[98] 10 mg/kg PO q24 h[68]
Sulfadimethoxine/ormetoprim (Romet, Hoffman-LaRoche)		50 mg/kg/d in feed for 5 d[82]
Thiamphenicol		15 and 30 mg/kg PO[105]
Tobramycin		2.5 mg/kg IM, then 1 mg/kg IM q4 d[106]
Trimethoprim/sulfamethoxazole		30 mg/kg PO q24 h for 10-14 d[82]
	Systemic Therapy: Antiparasitic Therapeutics	
Albendazole		5 mg/kg PO once[107] 10 mg/kg PO once[108]
Chloroquine diphosphate		50 mg/kg PO once[109]
Enamectin (Slice, Schering Plough)		50 µg/kg q24 h for 7 d PO[110]
Fenbendazole		1 mg/kg IV,[111] 5 mg/kg PO for 1 dose[112] 6 mg/kg q24 h PO[113] 50 mg/kg PO q24 h for 2 d, then repeat in 14 d[102] 0.2% in feed q4 d for 2 treatments[87] 40 mg/kg in feed q4 d for 2 treatments[68]
Levamisole (Levasole, Schering Plough)		0.5 mg/kg ICe[114] 10 mg/kg PO q7 d for 3 treatments[88] 11 mg/kg IM q7 d for 2 treatments[88]
Mebendazole		20 mg/kg PO q7 d for 3 treatments[98]
Metronidazole		25 mg/kg q24 h in feed for 5-10 d[82] 50 mg/kg PO q24 for 5 d[88] 100 mg/kg q24 h in feed for 3 d[82]
Piperazine		10 mg/kg q24 h in feed for 3 d[82]
Praziquantel		5 mg/kg PO q24 h for 3 treatments[68] 5 mg/kg PO in feed q7 d for up to 3 treatments[98] 5 mg/kg PO, ICe, repeat in 14-21 d[87]
Pyrantel pamoate		10 mg/kg in feed, once[98]

ICe, Intraceolomically; *IM*, intramuscularly; *IV*, intravenously; *PO*, orally; *prn*, as necessary; *SC*, subcutaneously.

TABLE 2-5

Common Treatments Used to Manage Skin Diseases in Amphibians

Medications	Route/Type	Dosage
	Topical Therapy: Antimicrobial Therapeutics	
Ciprofloxacin		500-750 mg/75 L as 6-8 h bath q24 h[115]
Doxycycline 1% topical gel, compounded		Topical q8-12 h, not to exceed 10 mg/kg/d[116]
Enrofloxacin		500 mg/L as 6-8 h bath q24 h[116]
Gentamicin		1.3 mg/L for 1 h bath q24 h for 7 d[117]
Metronidazole		60 mg/kg topical q24 h for 3 d[115] 50 mg/L for 24 h bath[115]
Silver sulfadiazine cream (Silvadine cream 1%, Marion)		Topical q24 h[118]
Trimethoprim/sulfamethoxazole		20 μg/mL and 80 μg/mL in 0.5% or 0.15% salt solution for 24 h bath[119]
	Topical Therapy: Antifungal Therapeutics	
Florfenicol		30 ppm as continuous bath replaced fresh daily for up to 30 d[116]
Itraconazole		0.01% in 0.6% salt solution as 5 min bath q24 h for 11 d[120]
Ketoconazole		Topical cream[121]
Malachite green		0.15-0.2 mg/L for 1 h bath q24 h[117]
Mercurochrome		4 mg/L for 1 h bath q24 h[122]
Methylene blue		2-4 mg/L bath to effect[123] 4 mg/L for 1 h bath q24 h[122]
Miconazole		Topical[115]
Nystatin 1% cream		Topical[116]
Potassium permanganate		1:5000 water for 5 min bath q24 h[124]
Sodium chlorite (NaOCl₂)		20 mg/L as 6-8 h bath[125]
Temperature elevation		37° C (98.6° C) for 16 h[126]
Tolnaftate (Tinavet cream 1%, Schering)		Topical[117]
	Topical Therapy: Antiparasitic Therapeutics	
Acriflavin		500 mg/L for 30 min bath[127]
Benzalkonium chloride		2 mg/L for 1 h bath q24 h to effect[127]
Copper sulfate		0.1 mg/L as continuous bath to effect[115] 500 mg/L for 2 min bath q24 h to effect[128]
Distilled water		3 h bath[128]
Formalin 10%		1.5 mL/L for 10 min bath q48 h to effect[121] 0.5% for 10 min bath once[128]
Ivermectin		2 mg/kg topical and repeat in 2-3 wk[129] 10 mg/L as 60 min bath, repeat q14 d prn[115]
Malachite green		0.15 mg/L for 1 h bath q24 h to effect[128]
Metronidazole		0.05 mL of 1.008 mg/mL on dorsum q24 h for 3 days[130] 50 mg/L for 24 h bath[131]
Praziquantel		10 mg/L for 3 h bath, repeat q7-21 d[115]
Salt (sodium chloride)		6 g/L for 5-10 min bath q24 h for 3-5 d[127]
Selamectin (Revolution, Pfizer)		6 mg/kg topical[132]

TABLE 2-5

Common Treatments Used to Manage Skin Diseases in Amphibians—cont'd

Medications	Route/Type	Dosage
	Systemic Therapy: Antimicrobial Therapeutics	
Amikacin		5 mg/kg SC, IM, ICe q24-48 h[115]
Ceftazidime		20 mg/kg SC, IM q48-72 h[116]
Ciprofloxacin		10 mg/kg PO q24 h[115]
Doxycycline (Vibramycin, Pfizer)		50 mg/kg IM q7 d[116]
		5-10 mg/kg PO q24 h[133]
Enrofloxacin		5-10 mg/kg PO, SC, IM q24 h[115]
Gentamicin		2.5 mg/kg IM q72 h[134]
Metronidazole		10 mg/kg PO q24 h for 5-10 d[135]
Tetracycline		50 mg/kg PO q12 h[123]
Trimethoprim/sulfa		3 mg/kg PO, SC, IM q24 h[123]
Trimethoprim/sulfadiazine		15-20 mg/kg IM q48 h[136]
Trimethoprim/sulfamethoxazole		15 mg/kg PO q24 h[115]
	Systemic Therapy: Antifungal Therapeutics	
Amphotericin B		1 mg/kg ICe q24 h[115]
Fluconazole		60 mg/kg PO q24 h[115]
Itraconazole		10 mg/kg PO q24 h[115]
Ketoconazole		10 mg/kg PO q24 h[128]
		10-20 mg/kg PO q24 h[115]
Miconazole		5 mg/kg ICe q24 h for 14-28 d[137]
	Systemic Therapy: Antiparasitic Therapeutics	
Febantel		10 mL/kg PO q2-3 wk[138]
Fenbendazole		30-50 mg/kg PO[139]
		50 mg/kg PO q24 h for 3-5 d, repeat in 14-21 d[115]
		50-100 mg/kg PO, repeat in 2-3 wk prn[135]
		100 mg/kg PO, repeat in 2 wk[140]
Ivermectin		0.2-0.4 mg/kg PO, SC, repeat q14 d prn[139]
Levamisole		10 mg/kg IM, ICe, repeat in 2 wk[137]
Moxidectin		200 µg/kg SC q4 mo[141]
Paromomycin		50-75 mg/kg PO q24 h[137]
Ponazuril		30 mg/kg PO q12 h for 3 d, repeat in 3 wk
		30 mg/kg PO q24 h for 30 d[116]
Praziquantel		8-24 mg/kg PO, SC, ICe, topical, repeat in 14 d[115]
Trimethoprim/sulfa		3 mg/kg PO, SC, IM q24 h[127]
	Miscellaneous Therapeutics	
Dexamethasone		1.5 mg/kg SC, IM, IV[116]
Meloxicam		0.4 mg/kg PO, SC ICe q24 h[116]
Prednisolone sodium succinate		5-10 mg/kg IM, IV[115]

ICe, Intracoelomically; *IM*, intramuscularly; *IV*, intravenously; *PO*, orally; *ppm*, parts per million; *prn*, as necessary; *SC*, subcutaneously.

TABLE 2-6

Common Treatments Used to Manage Skin Diseases In Reptiles

Medications	Route/Type	Dosage
	Topical Therapy: Antimicrobial Therapeutics	
Ciprofloxacin ophthalmic ointment or drops		Topical to affected area[142]
Gentamicin ophthalmic ointment or drops		Topical to affected area[143]
Silver sulfadiazine cream		Topical to affected area q24-72 h[144]
	Topical Therapy: Antiviral Therapeutics	
Acyclovir 5% ointment		Apply to lesions q12 h[143]
	Topical Therapy: Antifungal Therapeutics	
Clotrimazole		Topical to affected area[145]
Malachite green		0.15 mg/L water for 1 h bath for 14 d[146]
Miconazole		Topical to affected area[145]
Tolnaftate 1% cream		Topical q12 h prn[147]
	Topical Therapy: Antiparasitic Therapeutics	
Carbaryl powder 5%		Lightly dust animal and environment; rinse after 1 h, repeat in 7 d[148,149]
Fipronil		Spray or wipe on then wash off in 5 min q7-10 d prn[149,150]
Imidocloprid and moxidectin		0.2 mg/kg topical q14 d for 3 treatments[151]
Ivermectin		5-10 mL/L water topical spray q3-5 d for up to 28 d[152]
	Systemic Therapy: Antimicrobial Therapeutics	
Amikacin		5 mg/kg IM, then 2.5 mg/kg q72 h[153,154]
Amoxicillin		10 mg/kg IM q24 h[155] 22 mg/kg PO q12-24 h[143,146]
Azithromycin		10 mg/kg PO q2-7 d[156]
Carbenicillin		200 mg/kg IM q24 h[157] 400 mg/kg SC, IM q24 h[158] 200-400 mg/kg IM q48 h[159]
Ceftazidime		20-40 mg/kg SC, IM q48-72 h[66,149,154] 20 mg/kg SC, IM, IV q48-72 h[153,160]
Ceftiofur sodium		2.2 mg/kg IM q48 h[146] 5 mg/kg SC, IM q24 h[161] 2.2 mg/kg IM q24 h[146] 4 mg/kg IM q24 h[146,162]
Doxycycline		5-10 mg/kg PO q24 h for 10-45 d[131,163]
Enrofloxacin		5-10 mg/kg PO, SC, IM, ICe q24-72 h[131]
Gentamicin		2.5 mg/kg IM q72 h[164,165] 2.5-3 mg/kg IM, then 1.5 mg/kg q96 h[166] 5 mg/kg IM q72 h[159] 6 mg/kg IM q72-96 h[167]
Lincomycin		5 mg/kg IM q12-24[146] 10 mg/kg PO q24 h[146]
Marbofloxacin		10 mg/kg PO q48 h[168]
Oxytetracycline		10 mg/kg IM IV q5 d[169] 5-10 mg/kg IM q24 h[170] 6-10 mg/kg PO, IM, IV q24 h[143,146]
Penicillin, benzathine		10,000-20,000 U/kg IM q48-96 h[149]
Penicillin G		10,000-20,000 U/kg SC, IM, IV, ICe q8-12 h[143]
Piperacillin		50-100 mg/kg IM q24 h[143,146] 50 mg/kg IM, then 25 mg/kg q24 h[131,146] 100 mg/kg IM q48 h[166] 100-200 mg/kg SC, IM q24-48 h[171]

TABLE 2-6

Common Treatments Used to Manage Skin Diseases In Reptiles—cont'd

Medications	Route/Type	Dosage
Streptomycin		10 mg/kg IM q12-24 h[143]
Sulfadiazine		25 mg/kg PO q24 h[131]
Tobramycin		2.5 mg/kg IM q24-72 h[146,162]
		10 mg/kg IM q24-48 h[146]
Trimethoprim/sulfadiazine		15-20 mg/kg PO q24 h[131]
		20-30 mg/kg IM q24-48 h[172]
		30 mg/kg IM q24 for 2 d, then 48 h[143,146,149]
Trimethoprim/sulfamethoxazole		10-30 mg/kg PO q24 h[143]
	Systemic Therapy: Antiviral Therapeutics	
Acyclovir		≥80 mg/kg PO q24 h[173]
		80 mg/kg PO q8 h or 240 mg/kg/d PO[174]
	Systemic Therapy: Antifungal Therapeutics	
Amphotericin B		0.5 mg/kg IV q48-72 h[175]
		0.5-1 mg/kg IV, ICe q24-72 h for 14-28 d[146]
		1 mg/kg q24 h ICe for 2-4 wk[176]
Fluconazole		5 mg/kg PO q24 h[32]
		21 mg/kg SC once, then 10 mg/kg SC 5 d later[177,178]
Griseofulvin		20-40 mg/kg PO q72 h for 5 treatments[145]
Itraconazole		5 mg/kg PO q24 h[179]
		10 mg/kg PO q24 h[180]
		10 mg/kg PO q48 h for 60 d[181]
		23.5 mg/kg PO q24 h[182]
Ketoconazole		15-30 mg/kg PO q24 h for 14-28 d[162]
		25 mg/kg PO q24 h for 21 d[183]
		15 mg/kg PO q72 h[184]
		50 mg/kg PO q24 h for 14-28 d[131]
Thiabendazole		50 mg/kg PO q24 h for 14 d[185]
Voriconazole		10 mg/kg PO[34]
		5 mg/kg SC[186]
	Systemic Therapy: Antiparasitic Therapeutics	
Ivermectin		0.2-0.4 mg/kg PO, SC, repeat q14 d prn (do not use in chelonians, crocodilians, indigo snakes, or skinks)[153,187,188]
Milbemycin		0.25-0.5 mg/kg SC prn[189]
Praziquantel		8 mg/kg PO, SC, IM, repeat in 14 d[131,153,171]
		5-10 mg/kg PO q14 d[190]
		25-50 mg/kg PO q3 h for 3 treatments[191,192]
	Miscellaneous Therapeutics	
Carboplatin		2.5-5 mg/kg IM, intracardiac[193]
Chlorambucil		0.1-0.2 mg/kg PO[193]
Cisplatin		0.5-1 mg/kg IV, IC, or intralesional[193]
Doxorubicin		1 mg/kg IM q7 d for 2 treatments, then q14 d for 2 treatments, then q21 d for 2 treatments[194]
Methimazole		2 mg/kg q24 h for 30 d[195]
Vitamin A		1000-5000 U/kg IM q7-10 d for 4 treatments[162]
Vitamins A, D₃, E		0.15 mL/kg IM, repeat in 21 d[163]
Vitamin D₃		1000 U/kg IM, repeat in 1 wk[196]
Vitamin E/selenium		1 U vitamin E/kg IM[197]

ICe, Intraceolomically; *IM,* intramuscularly; *IV,* intravenously; *PO,* orally; *prn,* as necessary; *SC,* subcutaneously.

TABLE 2-7

Common Treatments Used to Manage Skin Diseases in Birds

Medications	Route/Type	Dosage
	Topical Therapy: Antimicrobial Therapeutics	
Silver sulfadiazine cream (Silvadene, Maron)		Topical to affected area q24-72 h[198,199]
	Topical Therapy: Antiviral Therapeutics	
Imiquimod cream (Aldara, 3M)		Topical 3 ×/wk several hours before morning feeding[200]
	Topical Therapy: Antifungal Therapeutics	
Amphotericin B		Apply 10% solution[201] 3% Cream topical to affected area q12 h[199,202]
Enilconazole emulsion		topical or intratracheal 1:10-1:100 solution[203] 3 topical soakings q3 d[204]
Miconazole		Topical to affected areas q12 h[204,205]
	Topical Therapy: Antiparasitic Therapeutics	
Fipronil (Frontline, Merial)		7.5 mg/kg spray on skin once, repeat in 30 d[206-208]
Ivermectin (Ivomec, Merial)		0.2 mg/kg SC topical on skin, can repeat 1-2 wk for 3-4 applications[207,209,210] 1 drop (0.05 mL) to skin q7 d for 3 treatments[206]
Permethrin (Adams, Pfizer)		Dust plumage lightly[206]
Permethrin/piperonyl butoxide/ methoprene (Avian Insect Liquidator)		Apply to plumage; spray aviaries, bird rooms, surrounding areas.[206]
Selamectin (Revolution, Pfizer)		23 mg/kg topical, repeat in 3-4 wk[211]
	Systemic Therapy: Antimicrobial Therapeutics	
Amikacin		10-20 mg/kg IM, IV q8-12 h[212]
Amoxicillin/clavulanate (Clavamox, Pfizer)		125 mg/kg PO q8 h[213]
Azithromycin		10-20 mg/kg PO q48 h for 5 treatments[214] 40 mg/kg PO q24 h for 30 d[214]
Cefazolin		50-100 mg/kg PO, IM q12 h[215]
Ceftazidime		50-100 mg/kg IM, IV q4-8 h[216,217]
Ceftiofur sodium		10 mg/kg IM q8-12 h[218] 50-100 mg/kg q4-8 h[219-221]
Cephalexin		40-100 mg/kg PO, IM q6-8 h[219-221]
Ciprofloxacin		10-40 mg/kg PO, IV, IM q12 h[199]
Clindamycin		25 mg/kg PO q8 h[222] 100 mg/kg PO q12 h for 7 d[223]
Doxycycline (Vibramycin, Pfizer)		25-100 mg/kg IM q5-7 d for 5-7 treatments[217,224]
Enrofloxacin		5-30 mg/kg PO, SC, IM q12 h[217,219,221] 200-500 mg/L drinking water[225]
Oxytetracycline		50 mg/kg IM q24 h for 5-7 d[201,219] 650-2000 mg/L drinking water for 5-14 d[201] 300 mg/kg soft feed for 5-14 d[201]
Piperacillin		100-200 mg/kg IM, IV q6-12 h[217,219]
Trimethoprim/sulfadiazine		20 mg/kg SC, IM, q12 h[201]
Trimethoprim/sulfamethoxazole		8-50 mg/kg IM, PO q8-12 h[216,219]
	Systemic Therapy: Antiviral Therapeutics	
Acyclovir (Zovirax, Burroughs Wellcome)		20-40 mg/kg IM q12 h[226] ≤400 mg/kg feed[227] 1000 mg/L drinking water[227]

TABLE 2-7

Common Treatments Used to Manage Skin Diseases in Birds—cont'd

Medications	Route/Type	Dosage
	Systemic Therapy: Antifungal Therapeutics	
Amphotericin B		1.5 mg/kg IV q8 h for 3-7 d[204,228,229]
Fluconazole		2-5 mg/kg PO q24 h for 7-10 d[230,231]
		4-6 mg/kg PO q12 h[232]
Itraconazole		2.5-5 mg/kg PO q24 h[233]
		5-10 mg/kg PO q24 h[233]
	Systemic Therapy: Antiparasitic Therapeutics	
Ivermectin		0.2 mg/kg PO, SC, IM once, then repeat in 10-14 d[206,207]
		0.4 mg/kg SC once[234]
Moxidectin		0.2 mg/kg PO, IM once[207,235]
	Psychotropic Drugs	
Amitriptyline		1-5 mg/kg PO q12-24 h[219]
Chlomipramine		1-2 mg/kg PO q24 h[236]
Diphenhydramine		2-4 mg/kg PO q12 h[237]
Fluoxetine (Prozac, Dista)		0.4 mg/kg PO q24 h[203]
Haloperidol		0.1-0.4 mg/kg PO q24 h[236,238]
		1-2 mg/kg IM q14-21 d[221,237]
Nortiptyline (Pamelor, Sandoz)		16 mg/L drinking water[237]
Paroxetine (Paxil, GlaxoSmithKline)		1-2 mg/kg PO q24 h[239]
	Analgesics	
Bupivacaine HCL		2-8 mg/kg SC perineurally[240]
Celecoxib (Celebrex, Pfizer)		10 mg/kg PO q24 h for 6-24 wk[241]
Gabapentin		11 mg/kg PO q12 h[242]
Lidocaine		1-3 mg/kg[243,244]
Meloxicam (Metacam, Boehringer Ingelheim)		0.1-0.2 mg/kg PO, IM q24 h[245,246]
		0.5-1 mg/kg PO, IM, IV q12 h[233]
Piroxicam		0.5 mg/kg PO q12 h[247]
	Miscellaneous Therapeutics	
Acemannan (Carravet, Veterinary Product Labs)		Topical[198]
Desorelin (Suprelorin, Peptech Animal Health)		4.7 mg or 9.4 mg placed SC intrascapularly[248]
Essential fatty acids		0.5 mL/kg PO q24 for 50 d or indefinitely[219]
Fatty acids (omega 3, omega 6)		0.1-0.2 mL/kg of flaxseed oil to corn oil mixed at a ratio of 1:4 PO[249,250]
Prednisolone (prednisone)		0.5-1 mg/kg IM, IV[251]
		2 mg/kg PO q12 h[252]
Vitamin A (Aquasol A Parenteral, Astra)		2000 U/kg, 50,000 U/kg PO, IM[253]
Vitamin D$_3$ (Vital E-A + D, Schering)		6600 U/kg IM once[254]
Vitamin E (Vitamin E$_{20}$, Horse Health Products; BoSe, Schering Plough)		0.06 mg/kg IM q7 d[219]
Vitamin E/γ-linolenic acid, linolenic acid (Derm Caps, DVM Pharmaceuticals)		0.1 mL/kg PO q24 h[202]

ICe, Intraceolomically; *IM*, intramuscularly; *IV*, intravenously; *PO*, orally; *SC*, subcutaneously.

TABLE 2-8		
Common Treatments Used to Manage Skin Diseases in Mammals		
Medications	**Route/Type**	**Dosage**
	Topical Therapy: Antimicrobial Therapeutics	
Mupirocin 2% (Muricin, Dechra)		Topical to cutaneous lesions q12-24 h prn (H)[255]
Neomycin, thiabendazole, dexamethasone solution (Tresaderm, Merial)		Topical to cutaneous lesions or ear canal q12 h prn (H)[255]
Silver sulfadiazine cream (Silvadene, Marion)		Topical q24 h (F, H, Ra, Ro, SG)[256]
	Topical Therapy: Antifungal Therapeutics	
Clotrimazole (Lotrimin, Schering)		Topical (Ra)[257]
Enilconazole (Imaverol, Janssen)		Topical q24 h (H)[258] Dip in a 0.2% solution for 7 d (Ro)[259,260]
Griseofulvin		1.5% in DMSO topical for 5-7 d (Ro)[261]
Lime sulfur		Topical (H)[262] dip q7 d for 4-6 treatments (F, Ra, Ro)[263,264]
Miconazole (Conofite, Schering-Plough)		Topical q24 h for 14-28 d (Ra)[265]
Miconazole/chlorhexidine shampoo		Bathe once daily (Ra)[266]
	Topical Therapy: Antiparasitic Therapeutics	
Amitraz (Mitaban, Pfizer)		0.3% Topical q7 d for 2-3 treatments (H, Ro)[255,267] 1.4 mL/L topical q7-14 d for 3-6 treatments (Ro)[261,263] Topical to affected area q7-14 d for 3-6 treatments (F)[268,269]
Carbaryl powder (5%)		Topical (SG)[270] topical q7 d for 3 treatments (F, Ra, Ro)[271]
Cyromazine 6% (Rear-guard, Novartis)		Topical q6-10 wk (Ra)[266]
Eprinomectin		2 mg/kg topical once (Ra)[272]
Fipronil spray (Frontline, Merial)		Contraindicated in rabbits and rodents, 1 pump topically q60 d (F)[268] 0.2-0.4 mL topical q30 d (F)[273]
Imidacloprid (Advantage, Bayer)		One-half kitten dose topically (Ro)[263] 20 mg/kg topical q30 d (Ro)[274] 10-16 mg/kg as a single application (Ra)[263,275,276] 1 cat dose places along spine topical q30 d (F)[268]
Imidacloprid 10%/moxidectin 1% (Advocate, Bayer)		0.1 mL/animal (Ro)[277] 10 mg/kg (I) + 1 mg/kg (M) topical q4 wk for 3 treatments (Ra)[266]
Imidacloprid 8.8%/permethrin 44% (Advantix, Bayer)		11-16.6 mg/kg topical once (Ra)[278]
Imidacloprid/moxidectin (Advantage Multi, Bayer)		1.9-3.3 µg/kg topical q30 d (F)[279]
Ivermectin		Spray animals or topical drops 4-5 times/yr (Ro)[261,280]
Lime sulfur		Dip q7 d for 4-6 treatments (F, Ra, Ro)[263,264,273,281]
Malathion powder (3%-5%)		Topical 3×/wk for 3 wk (Ro)[281]
Pyrethrins		Topical as directed for puppies and kittens (Ra)[263,282] topical q7 d prn (F)[283]
Selamectin (Revolution, Pfizer)		6-18 mg/kg topical, repeat in 30 d (SG)[284] 6 mg/kg topical q30 d (H, Ro)[285,286] 8-18 mg/kg topical at the base of neck (Ra)[287] 6-10 mg/kg topical (F)[269,288]
	Systemic Therapy: Antimicrobial Therapeutics	
Amikacin		2.5-5 mg/kg IM q8-12 h (H, Ra)[255,265] 5 mg/kg SC, IM q8 h (Ro)[289] 8-16 mg/kg SC, IM, IV divided to q8-24 h (F, Ro)[263,273,290]

TABLE 2-8

Common Treatments Used to Manage Skin Diseases in Mammals—cont'd

Medications	Route/Type	Dosage
Amoxicillin/clavulanate (Clavamox, Pfizer)		12.5 mg/kg PO, SC q12-24 h (F, SG)[271,291,292] 20 mg/kg PO q12 h (Ro)[263]
Ampicillin		20-100 mg/kg PO, SC, IM q8 h (Ro but not hamsters, guinea pigs, or chinchillas)[263,293] 5-30 mg/kg SC, IM, IV q8-12 h (F)[269,294]
Azithromycin		15-30 mg/kg PO q24 h (Ro)[263] 4-5 mg/kg IM q48 h for 7 d (Ra)[295] 5 mg/kg PO q24 h (F)[279]
Cefadroxil		15-20 mg/kg PO q12 h (F)[271]
Ceftazidime		100 mg/kg IM q12 h (Ra)[296]
Cephalexin		30 mg/kg PO, SC q12-24 h (SG)[291,292] 15-25 mg/kg SC q24 h (Ro)[263] 15-30 mg/kg PO q8-12 h (F)[297]
Chloramphenicol		30-50 mg/kg PO q8-12 h (Ro)[263] 50 mg/kg PO, SC, IM, IV q8 h (Ra)[298] 25-50 mg/kg PO q12 h (F)[271]
Ciprofloxacin		5-20 mg/kg PO q12 h (H, Ra, Ro)[261,263] 5-30 mg/kg PO q24 h (F)[271]
Clindamycin		5.5-10 mg/kg PO q12 h (F, H)[255,258,271] 7.5 mg/kg SC q12 h (Ro)[299]
Doxycycline (Vibramycin, Pfizer)		2.5-10 mg/kg PO, SC, IM q12 h (H)[263] 2.5-5 mg/kg PO q12 h (Ro)[261,300] 2.5 mg/kg PO q12 h (Ra)[301] 4 mg/kg PO q24 h (Ra)[302]
Enrofloxacin		5-10 mg/kg PO, SC, M q12 h (F, H)[271] 5-20 mg/kg PO, SC, IM q12 h (Ra, Ro)[261,263]
Penicillin G		22,000 U/kg SC, IM q24 h (Ro but not in guinea pigs and chinchillas)[263] benzathine 42,000-84,000 U/kg IM q7 d for 3 wk (Ra)[303] procaine 40,000 U/kg IM q24 h for 5-7 d[304]
Trimethoprim/sulfa		30 mg/kg PO, SC, IM q12 h (H)[305,306] 15-30 mg/kg PO, SC, IM q12 h (F, Ra, Ro)[261,263,297,307]
	Systemic Therapy: Antifungal Therapeutics	
Amphotericin B		Desoxycholate form: 1 mg/kg IV q24 h (Ra)[308] liposomal form: 5 mg/kg IM q24 h (Ra)[309] 0.4-0.8 mg/kg IV q7 d (F)[310]
Griseofulvin		15-50 mg/kg PO q24 h for 14-28 d (Ro)[261,311] 12.5-25 mg/kg PO q12-24 h for 30-45 d (Ra)[256,264]
Itraconazole		5-10 mg/kg PO q12 h (H, SG)[255,312] 2.5-10 mg/kg PO q24 h (Ro)[259] 20-40 mg/kg PO q24 h (Ra)[313,314]
Nystatin		2,000U/kg PO q12 h (SG)[284] 30,000 U/kg PO q8-24 h (H)[255] 60,000-90,000 U/kg PO q12 h for 7-10 d (Ro)[315]
Terbinafine		10-30 mg/kg PO q24 h for 4-6 wk (Ro)[316] 100 mg/kg PO q12 h for 21 d (Ra)[291,317,318]
	Systemic Therapy: Antiparasitic Therapeutics	
Ivermectin		0.2 mg/kg SC, repeat in 10-14 d (H, SG)[263,319] 0.2-0.4 mg/kg SC q7-14 d (Ro)[320] 0.05-0.3 mg/kg PO q24 h for 1 mo after negative skin scrape (F)[271] 0.5-1 mg/kg in ears and repeat in 14 d (F)[297]
Lufenuron		One-half puppy/kitten dose PO q30 d (H)[321] 30-45 mg/kg PO q30 d (F)[322]

Continued

TABLE 2-8

Common Treatments Used to Manage Skin Diseases in Mammals—cont'd

Medications	Route/Type	Dosage
Nitenpyram (Capstar, Novartis)		1 mg/kg PO once (Ro)[299]
	Analgesics	
Bupivacaine HCL		0.1-1 mg/kg (SG)[312]
		1.1 mg/kg diluted with saline 1:12 (H)[323]
		1-1.5 mg/kg SC locally (F)[324]
Carprofen (Rimadyl, Pfizer)		1-4 mg/kg PO q12-24 h (Ro)[325,326]
		2-4 mg/kg SC, IM q24 h (Ra)[275]
Gabapentin		50 mg/kg PO q24 h (Ro)[327]
		3-5 mg/kg PO q8-24 h (F)[328]
Meloxicam (Metacam, Boehringer Ingelheim)		0.2 mg/kg PO, SC q12-24 h (SG)[329,330]
		0.2 mg/kg PO, SC, IM q24 (F, H)[324,331]
		1-2 mg/kg PO, SC q24 h (Ro)[263]
		0.3 mg/kg PO q24 h (Ra)[332]
	Miscellaneous Therapeutics	
Desorelin (Suprelorin, Peptech Animal Health)		4.7 mg SC intrascapularly (F)[333]
Dexamethasone		0.1-0.6 mg/kg SC, IM, IV (Ra, SG)[291]
		0.1-1.5 mg/kg IM (H)[334]
		0.5-2 mg/kg PO, SC, then taper dose q12 h for 3-12 d (Ro)[261]
		0.5-1 mg/kg IM (F)[271,297]
Diphenhydramine		1-2 mg/kg PO, SC, IM q8-12 h (F, Ro)[263]
Prednisone		0.5-2.2 mg/kg PO, SC, IM (Ro)[263,281]
Thyroxine		0.2-0.4 mg/kg q12 h (F)[335]
Vitamin A		500-5000 U/kg IM (SG)[291]
		400 U/Kg IM q24 h for 10 d (H)[300]
		50-500 U/kg IM (Ro)[326]
		500-1000 U/Kg IM (Ra)[263]
Vitamin C (ascorbic acid)		10-30 mg/kg PO, SC, IM maintenance[259]
		20-200 mg/kg treatment for deficiency (Ro)[300]
Vitamin E		10 U/kg SC (SG)[284]

DSMO, Dimethyl sulfoxide; *F,* ferret; *H,* hedgehog; *IM,* intramuscularly; *IV,* intravenously; *PO,* orally; *prn,* as necessary; *Ra,* rabbit; *Ro,* rodent; *SC,* subcutaneously; *SG,* sugar glider.

REFERENCES

1. Bereiter-Hahn J, Matoltsy AG, Richards KS. *Biology of the Integument 1: Invertebrates.* Berlin, Heidelberg: Springer-Verlag; 1984.
2. Cooper JE. Invertebrate care. *Vet Clin North Am Exot Anim Pract.* 2004;7:473-486.
3. Braun ME, Heatley JJ, Chitty J. Clinical techniques of invertebrates. *Vet Clin North Am Exot Anim Pract.* 2006;9:205-221.
4. Smolowitz R. Gastropods. In: Lewbart GA, ed. *Invertebrate Medicine.* 1st ed. Ames, IA: Blackwell Publishing; 2006:65-78.
5. Fontenot DK, Neiffer DL. Wound management in teleost fish: biology of the healing process, evaluation, and treatment. *Vet Clin North Am Exot Anim Pract.* 2004;7:57-86.
6. Wildgoose W. Structure and function of fish skin. In: Paterson S, ed. *Skin Diseases of Exotic Pets.* Oxford: Blackwell Science; 2006:75-79, 141-145.
7. Wright KM, Whitaker BR. *Amphibian Medicine and Captive Husbandry.* 1st ed. Malabar, FL: Krieger Publishing; 2001.
8. Pessier AP. An overview of amphibian skin disease. *Semin Avian Exot Pet Med.* 2002;11(3):162-174.
9. Poll CP. Wound management in amphibians: etiology and treatment of cutaneous lesions. *J Exot Pet Med.* 2009;18(1):20-35.
10. Voyles J, Rosenblum EB, Berger L. Interactions between *Batrachochytrium dendrobatidis* and its amphibian hosts: a review of pathogenesis and immunity. *Microbes Infect.* 2011;13:25-32.
11. Goodman G. Structure and function of reptile skin. In: Paterson S, ed. *Skin Diseases of Exotic Pets.* Oxford: Blackwell Science; 2006:75-79.
12. Ferrell ST. Avian integumentary surgery. *Semin Avian Exot Pet Med.* 2004;11(3):125-135.
13. Fraser M. Structure and function of bird skin. In: Paterson S, ed. *Skin Diseases of Exotic Pets.* Oxford: Blackwell Science; 2006:3-13.
14. Doneley B. Clinical anatomy and physiology. In: Doneley B, ed. *Avian Medicine & Surgery in Practice: Companion and Aviary Birds.* London: Manson Publishing Ltd.; 2011:7-39.
15. Meredith A. Structure and function of mammal skin. In: Paterson S, ed. *Skin Diseases of Exotic Pets.* Oxford: Blackwell Science; 2006: 175-183.
16. Monteiro-Riviere NA. Integument. In: Eurelle JA, Frappier BL, eds. *Dellmann's Textbook of Veterinary Histology.* 6th ed. Ames, IA: Blackwell Publishing; 2006:320-349.
17. Longcore JE, Pessier AP, Nichols DK. *Batrachochytrium dendrobatidis* gen. et sp. nov., a chytrid pathogenic to amphibians. *Mycologica.* 1999;91:219-227.

18. Martel A, Spitzen-van der Sluijs A, Blooi M, et al. *Batrachochytrium salamandrivorans* sp. nov. causes lethal chytridiomycosis in amphibians. *Proc Natl Acad Sci.* 2013;110:15325-15329. <http://dx.doi.org/10.1073/pnas.1307356110>.

19. Young S, Berger L, Speare R. Amphibian chytridiomycosis: strategies for captive management and conservation. *Int Zoo Yearb.* 2007; 41:1-11.

20. Brannelly LA, Richards-Zawacki CL, Pessier AP. Clinical trials with itraconazole as a treatment for chytrid fungal infections in amphibians. *Dis Aquat Organ.* 2012;101:95-104.

21. Smith JA, Papich MG, Russell G, et al. Effects of compounding on pharmacokinetics of itraconazole in black-footed penguins *(Spheniscus demersus)*. *J Zoo Wildl Med.* 2010;41(3):487-495.

22. Stewart JS. Anaerobic bacterial infections in reptiles. *J Zoo Wildl Med.* 1990;21(2):180-184.

23. Jackson CG, Fulton M. A turtle colony epizootic apparently of microbial origin. *J Wildl Dis.* 1970;6:466-468.

24. Rebell H, Rywlin A, Haines H. A herpesvirus-type agent associated with skin lesions of green sea turtles in aquaculture. *Am J Vet Res.* 1975;36:1221-1224.

25. Chen ZX, Zheng JC, Jiang YL, et al. A new iridovirus isolated from soft-shelled turtles. *Virus Res.* 1999;63:1-2, 147-151.

26. Jacobson ER, Popp JA, Shields RP, et al. Pox-like skin lesions in captive caimans. *J Am Vet Med Assoc.* 1979;175:937-940.

27. Casey RN, Quackenbush SL, Work TM, et al. Evidence for retrovirus infections in green turtles *(Chelonia mydas)* from the Hawaiian islands. *Dis Aquat Organ.* 1997;31:1-7.

28. Herbst LH, Jacobson ER, Klein PA, et al. Comparative pathology and pathogenesis of spontaneous and experimentally induced fibropapilloma of green turtles *(Chelonia mydas)*. *Vet Pathol.* 1999;36: 551-564.

29. Jacobson ER. Diseases of the integumentary system of reptiles. In: Nesbitt GH, Ackerman LJ, eds. *Dermatology for the Small Animal Practitioner.* Lawrenceville, NJ; Veterinary Learning Systems; 1991.

30. Diaz-Figueroa O, Mitchell MA, Ramirez S, et al. *Paecilomyces lilacinus* pneumonia in a free-ranging Louisiana gopher tortoise. *J Herp Med Surg.* 2008;18(2):52-60.

31. Mitchell MA, Walden MR. *Chrysosporium* anamorph *Nannizziopsis vriesii:* An emerging fungal pathogen of captive and wild reptiles. *Vet Clin North Am Exot Anim Pract.* 2013;16(3):659-668.

32. Wissman MA, Parsons B. Dermatophytosis of green iguanas *(Iguana iguana)*. *J Small Exot Anim Med.* 1993;2:133-136.

33. Pare JA, Sigler L, Hunter DB, et al. Cutaneous mycoses in chameleons caused by *Chrysosporium* anamorph of *Nannizziopsis vriesii.* *J Zoo Wildl Med.* 1997;28:443-453.

34. Van Waeyenberghe L, Baert K, Pasmans F, et al. Voriconazole, a safe alternative for treating infections caused by the *Chrysosporium* anamorph of *Nannizziopsis vriesii* in bearded dragons *(Pogona vitticeps)*. *Med Mycol.* 2010;48:880-885.

35. Rubinstein J, Lightfoot T. Feather loss and feather destructive behavior in pet birds. *J Exot Pet Med.* 2012;21:219-234.

36. Zeeland YR, Spruit BM, Rodenburg TD, et al. Feather damaging behavior in parrots: a review with consideration of comparative aspects. *Appl Anim Behav Sci.* 2009;121:75-95.

37. Meehan CL, Garner JP, Mench JA. Environmental enrichment and development of cage stereotypy in orange-winged Amazon parrots *(Amazona amazonica)*. *Dev Psychobiol.* 2004;44:209-218.

38. Seibert LM, Crowell-Davis SL, Wilson GH, et al. Placebo-controlled clomipramine trial for the treatment of feather picking disorder in cockatoos. *J Am Anim Hosp Assoc.* 2004;40:261-269.

39. Girling S. Skin diseases and treatment of caged birds. In: Patterson S, ed. *Skin Disease of Exotic Pets.* Ames, IA: Blackwell; 2006:22-47.

40. Forbes NA. Birds. In: Foster A, Foil C, eds. *BSAVA Manual of Small Animal Dermatology.* Gloucester, UK: British Small Animal Veterinary Association; 2003:256-267.

41. Cornelissen JMM, Gerlach H, Miller H, et al. An investigation into the possible role of circo and avian polyoma virus infections in the etiology of three distinct skin and feather problems (CUD, FLS, PF) in the rose-faced lovebird *(Agapornis roseicollis)*. *Proc Euro Col Avian Med Surg.* 2001;3-5.

42. Schmidt RE, Lightfoot TL. Integument. In: Harrison GJ, Lightfoot TL, eds. *Clinical Avian Medicine, Volume 1.* 1st ed. Palm Beach, FL: Spix Publishing; 2006:395-410.

43. Nett CS, Tully T. Anatomy, clinical presentation and diagnostic approach to feather picking pet bird. *Compend Contin Educ Pract.* 2003;25:206-219.

44. Steinmetz HW, Rutz C, Hoop RK, et al. Possible human–avian transmission of *Mycobacterium tuberculosis* in a green-winged macaw *(Ara chloroptera)*. *Avian Dis.* 2006;50(4):641-645.

45. Ambrams GA, Paul-Murphy J, Ramer JC, et al. *Aspergillus* blepharitis and dermatitis in a peregrine falcon-gyrfalcon hybrid *(Falco peregrinus × Falco rusticolus)*. *J Avian Med Surg.* 2001;15(2): 114-120.

46. Preziosi DVM, Morris DO, Johnston MS, et al. Distribution of *Malassezia* organisms on the skin of unaffected psittacine birds and psittacine birds with feather destructive behavior. *J Am Vet Med Assoc.* 2006;2:216-221.

47. Lightfoot TL. Overview of tumors: Section I: Clinical avian neoplasia and oncology. In: Harrison GJ, Lightfoot TL, eds. *Clinical Avian Medicine, Volume 1.* 1st ed. Palm Beach, FL: Spix Publishing; 2006:560-565.

48. Lewington JH. Parasitic diseases in ferrets. In: Lewington JH, ed. *Ferret Husbandry Medicine and Surgery.* 2nd ed. Philadelphia: Saunders; 2007:224-257.

49. Lewington JH. Viral, bacterial and mycotic disease. In: Lewington JH, ed. *Ferret Husbandry Medicine and Surgery.* 2nd ed. Philadelphia: Saunders; 2007:169-200.

50. Lewington JH. Reproduction and genetics. In: Lewington JH, ed. *Ferret Husbandry Medicine and Surgery.* 2nd ed. Philadelphia: Saunders; 2007:86-121.

51. Harcourt-Brown F. Skin diseases. In: Harcourt-Brown F, ed. *Textbook of Rabbit Medicine.* Oxford: Butterworth-Heinemann; 2002:233-240.

52. Blair J. Bumblefoot: a comparison of clinical presentation and treatment of pododermatitis in rabbits, rodents, and birds. *Vet Clin North Am Exot Anim Pract.* 2013;16(3):715-735.

53. Brown PJ, Young RD, Cripps PJ. Abnormalities of collagen fibrils in a rabbit with a connective tissue defect similar to Ehlers-Danlos syndrome. *Res Vet Sci.* 1993;55:346-350.

54. Florizoone K. Thymoma-associated exfoliative dermatitis in a rabbit. *Vet Dermatol.* 2005;16:281-284.

55. Fehr M, Koestlinger S. Ectoparasites in small exotic mammals. *Vet Clin North Am Exot Anim Pract.* 2013;16:611-657.

56. Meredith AL. Viral skin diseases of the rabbit. *Vet Clin North Am Exot Anim Pract.* 2013;16:705-714.

57. Rous P, Beard JW. The progression to carcinoma of virus-induced rabbit papillomas. *J Exp Med.* 1935;62:523-548.

58. Hawkins MG, Bishop CR. Disease problems of guinea pigs. In: Quesenberry KE, Carpenter JW, eds. *Ferrets, Rabbits, and Rodents: Clinical Medicine and Surgery.* 3rd ed. St. Louis, MO: Saunders; 2012:295-310.

59. Ness RD, Johnson-Delaney CA. Sugar gliders. In: Quesenberry KE, Carpenter JW, eds. *Ferrets, Rabbits, and Rodents: Clinical Medicine and Surgery.* 3rd ed. St. Louis, MO: Saunders; 2012: 393-410.

60. Tynes VV. Behavioral dermatopathies in small mammals. *Vet Clin North Am Exot Anim Pract.* 2013;16:801-820.

61. Marrow JC, Carpenter JW, Lloyd A, et al. A transitional cell carcinoma with squamous differentiation in a pericloacal mass in a sugar glider *(Petaurus breviceps)*. *J Exot Pet Med.* 2010;19:92-95.

62. Rondinini C. Hedgehogs and moonrats. In: MacDonald D, ed. *The Encyclopedia of Mammals.* New York: Facts on File; 2001.

63. Greenacre CB. Spontaneous tumors of small mammals. *Vet Clin North Am Exot Anim Pract.* 2004;7:627-651.

64. Heatley J, Maulden G, Cho D. Neoplasia in the captive African hedgehog (*Atalerix albiventris*). *Semin Avian Exot Pet Med.* 2005;14:182-192.

65. Bauquier SH, Greenwood J, Whittem T. Evaluation of the sedative and anaesthetic effects of five different concentrations of alfaxalone in goldfish (*Carassius auratus*). *Aquaculture.* 2005;396-399, 119-123.

66. White SD, Bourdeau P, Bruet V, et al. Reptiles with dermatological lesions: a retrospective study of 301 cases at two university veterinary teaching hospitals (1992-2008). *Vet Dermatol.* 2011;22:150-161.

67. Palmeiro BS, Roberts H. Clinical approach to dermatologic disease in exotic animals. *Vet Clin North Am Exot Anim Pract.* 2013;16:523-577.

68. Treves-Brown KM. *Applied Fish Pharmacology.* Dordrecht, The Netherlands: Kluwer Academic Publishers; 2000.

69. Pizzi R. Spiders. In: Lewbart GA, ed. *Invertebrate Medicine.* 2nd ed. Ames, IA: Wiley-Blackwell Publishing; 2012:187-221.

70. Gore SR, Harms CA, Kukanich B, et al. Enrofloxacin pharmacokinetics in European cuttlefish, *Sepia officinalis*, after a single i.v. injection and bath administration. *J Vet Pharmacol Ther.* 2005;28:433-439.

71. Scimeca J. Cephalopods. In: Lewbart GA, ed. *Invertebrate Medicine.* 2nd ed. Ames, IA: Wiley-Blackwell Publishing; 2012:113-125.

72. Bodri M. Nematodes. In: Lewbart GA, ed. *Invertebrate Medicine.* 2nd ed. Ames, IA: Wiley-Blackwell Publishing; 2012:335-354.

73. Moens T, Vincx M. On the cultivation of free-living marine and estuarine nematodes. *Helgoländer Meeresunters.* 1998;52:115-139.

74. Hodgson G. Tetracycline reduces sedimentation damage to corals. *Mar Biol.* 1990;104:493-496.

75. Stoskopf MK. Coelenterates. In: Lewbart GA, ed. *Invertebrate Medicine.* 2nd ed. Ames, IA: Wiley-Blackwell Publishing; 2012:21-56.

76. Noga EJ, Hancock A, Bullis R. Crustaceans. In: Lewbart GA, ed. *Invertebrate Medicine.* 2nd ed. Ames, IA: Wiley-Blackwell Publishing; 2012:235-254.

77. Lehmann DW. Reef systems. In: Lewbart GA, ed. *Invertebrate Medicine.* 2nd ed. Ames, IA: Wiley-Blackwell Publishing; 2012:57-75.

78. Allender MC, Schumacher J, Milam J, et al. Pharmacokinetics of intravascular itraconazole in the American horseshoe crab (*Limulus polyphemus*). *J Vet Pharmacol Ther.* 2007;31:83-86.

79. Uno K. Pharmacokinetics of oxolinic acid and oxytetracycline in kuruma shrimp, *Penaeus japonicas*. *Aquaculture.* 2004;230:1-11.

80. Uno K, Aoki T, Kleechaya W, et al. Pharmacokinetics of oxytetracycline in black tiger shrimp, *Penaeus monodon*, and the effect of cooking on the residues. *Aquaculture.* 2006;254:24-31.

81. Reed LA, Siewicki TC, Shah C. The biopharmaceutics and oral bioavailability of two forms of oxytetracycline to white shrimp, *Litopenaeus setiferus*. *Aquaculture.* 2006;258:42-54.

82. Noga EJ. *Fish Disease: Diagnosis and Treatment.* 2nd ed. Ames, IA: Wiley-Blackwell; 2010.

83. Lewbart GA, Vaden S, Deen J, et al. Pharmacokinetics of enrofloxacin in the red pacu (*Colossoma brachypomum*) after intramuscular, oral and bath administration. *J Vet Pharmacol Ther.* 1997;20(2):124-128.

84. Willoughby LG, Roberts RJ. Towards strategic use of fungicides against *Saprolegnia parasitica* in salmonid fish hatcheries. *J Fish Dis.* 1992;15:1-13.

85. Wildgoose WH, Lewbart GA. Therapeutics. In: Wildgoose WH, ed. *BSAVA Manual of Ornamental Fish.* 2nd ed. Gloucester, UK: British Small Animal Veterinary Association; 2001;237-258.

86. Lewbart GA. Emergency and critical care of fish. *Vet Clin North Am Exot Anim Pract.* 1998;1:233-249.

87. Thomasen JM. Hydrogen peroxide as a delousing agent of Atlantic salmon. In: Boxshall GA, Defaye D, eds. *Pathogens of Wild and Farmed Fish: Sea Lice.* Chichester, UK: Ellis Horwood; 1993:290-295.

88. Harms CA. Treatment for parasitic disease of aquarium and ornamental fish. *Semin Avian Exot Pet Med.* 1996;5:54-63.

89. Tarascheewski H, Renner C, Melhorn H. Treatment of fish parasites. 3. Effects of levamisole HCL, metrifonate, fenbendazole, mebendazole, and ivermectin in *Anguillicola crassus* (nematodes) pathogenic in the air bladder of eels. *Parasitol Res.* 1988;74:281-289.

90. Buchmann K, Bjerregaard J. Mebendazole treatment of pseudodactylogyrosis in an intensive eel-culture system. *Aquaculture.* 1990;86:139-153.

91. Schmahl G, Benini J. Treatment of fish parasites. 11. Effects of different benzimidazole derivatives (albendazole, mebendazole, fenbendazole) on *Glugea anomala*, Moniez, 1887 (microsporidia): ultrastructural aspects and efficacy studies. *Parasitol Res.* 1998;60:41-49.

92. della Rocca G, Zaghini A, Zanoni R, et al. Seabream (*Sparus aurata* L.): disposition of amoxicillin after single intravenous injection or oral administration and multiple dose depletion studies. *Aquaculture.* 2004;232:1-10.

93. Brown AG, Grant AN. Use of ampicillin by injection in Atlantic salmon broodstock. *Vet Rec.* 1992;131:237.

94. Plakas SM, DePaola A, Moxey MB. *Bacillus stearothermophilus* disk assay for determining ampicillin residues in fish muscle. *J Assoc Off Anal Chem.* 1991;74:910-912.

95. Roberts HE, Palmerio B, Weber ES III. Bacterial and parasitic diseases of pet fish. *Vet Clin North Am Exot Anim Pract.* 2009;12:609-638.

96. Nouws JFM, Grondel JL, Schutte AR, et al. Pharmacokinetics of ciprofloxacin in carp, African catfish and rainbow trout. *Vet Q.* 1988;211-216.

97. Lewbart GA, Papich MG, Whitt-Smith D. Pharmacokinetics of florfenicol in the red pacu (*Piaractus brachypomus*) after single dose intramuscular administration. *J Vet Pharmacol Ther.* 2005;28:317-319.

98. Stoskopf MK. Fish pharmacotherapeutics. In: Fowler ME, Miller RE, eds. *Zoo and Wild Animal Medicine: Current Therapy 4.* Philadelphia: W.B. Saunders; 1999:182-189.

99. Noga EJ, Wang C, Grindem CB, et al. Comparative clinicopathological response of striped bass and palmetto bass to acute stress. *Trans Am Fish Soc.* 1999;128:680-686.

100. Doi A, Stoskopf MK, Lewbart GA. Pharmacokinetics of oxytetracycline in the red pacu (*Colossoma brachypomus*) following different routes of administration. *J Vet Pharmacol Ther.* 1998;21:364-368.

101. Grondel JL, Nouws JFM, De Jong M, et al. Pharmacokinetics and tissue distribution of oxytetracycline in carp, *Cyprinus carpio* L., following different routes of administration. *J Fish Dis.* 1987;10:153-163.

102. Whitaker BR. Preventive medicine programs for fish. In: Fowler ME, Miller RE, eds. *Zoo and Wild Animal Medicine: Current Therapy 4.* Philadelphia: W.B. Saunders; 1999:163-181.

103. Chen CY, Getchel RG, Wooster GA, et al. Oxytetracycline residues in four species of fish after 10-day oral dosing in feed. *J Aquat Anim Health.* 2004;16:208-219.

104. Reja A, Moreno L, Serrano JM, et al. Concentration-time profiles of oxytetracycline in blood, kidney and liver of tench (*Tinca tinca* L.) after intramuscular administration. *Vet Hum Toxicol.* 1996;38:344-347.

105. Intorre L, Castells G, Cristofol C, et al. Residue depletion of thiamphenicol in the sea-bass. *J Vet Pharmacol Ther.* 2002;25:59-63.

106. Stoskopf MK, Kennedy-Stoskopf S, Arnold J, et al. Therapeutic aminoglycoside antibiotic levels in brown sharks, *Carcharhinus plumbeus* (Nardo). *J Fish Dis.* 1986;9:303-311.

107. Nafstad I, Ingebrigsten K, Langseth W, et al. Benzimidazoles for antiparasitic therapy in salmon. *Acta Vet Scand Suppl.* 1991;87:302-304.

108. Shaikh B, Rummel N, Gieseker C, et al. Metabolism and residue depletion of albendazole in rainbow trout, tilapia, and Atlantic salmon after oral administration. *J Vet Pharmacol Ther.* 2003;26:421-428.

109. Lewis DH, Wenxing W, Ayers A, et al. Preliminary studies on chloroquine as a systemic chemotherapeutic agent for amyloodinosis in red drum (*Sciaenops ocellatus*). *Mar Sci Suppl*. 1988;30:183-189.

110. Schering Plough Animal Health Technical Report 2001; <http://spaqua-culture.com/default. Aspx?pageid=545>; Accessed January 13, 2015.

111. Davis LE, Davis CA, Koritz GD, et al. Comparative studies of pharmacokinetics of fenbendazole in food-producing animals. *Vet Hum Toxicol*. 1988;30(suppl I):9-11.

112. Kitzman JV, Holley JH, Huber WG, et al. Pharmacokinetics and metabolism of fenbandozole in channel catfish. *Vet Res Commun*. 1990;14:217-226.

113. Iosfidou EG, Haagsma N, Tanck MWT, et al. Depletion study of fenbendazole in rainbow trout (*Oncorbynchus mykiss*) after oral and bath treatment. *Aquaculture*. 1997;154:191-199.

114. Kajita Y, Sakai M, Atsuta S, et al. The immunomodulatory effects of levamisole on rainbow trout, *Onciirbynchus mykiss*. *Fish Pathol*. 1990;25:93-98.

115. Wright KM, Whitaker BR. Pharmacotherapeutics. In: Wright KM, Whitaker BR, eds. *Amphibian Medicine and Captive Husbandry*. Malabar, FL: Krieger Publishing; 2001:309-330.

116. Wright KM. Personal observation. 2011.

117. Jacobson E, Kollias GV, Peters LJ. Dosages for antibiotics and parasiticides used in exotic animals. *Compend Contin Educ Pract Vet*. 1983;5:315-324.

118. Fox WF. Treatment and dosages. *Axolotl Newsl*. 1980;9:6.

119. Menard MR. External application of antibiotic to improve survival of adult laboratory frogs (*Rana pipiens*). *Lab Anim Sci*. 1984;34:94-96.

120. Nichols DK, Lamirander EW, Pessier AP, et al. Experimental transmission and treatment of cutaneous chytridiomycosis in poison dart frogs (*Dendrobates auratus* and *Dendrobates tinctorius*). Proc Annu Conf Am Assoc Zoo Vet/Internat Assoc Aquatic Anim Med. 2000;42-44.

121. Crawshaw GJ. Amphibian emergency and critical care. *Vet Clin North Am Exot Anim Pract*. 1998;1:207-231.

122. Williams DL. Amphibians. In: Beynon PH, Cooper JE, eds. *BSAVA Manual of Exotic Pets*. Gloucester, UK: British Small Animal Veterinary Association; 1991:261-271.

123. Crawshaw GJ. Amphibian medicine. In: Kirk RW, Bonagura JD, eds. *Kirk's Current Veterinary Therapy XI: Small Animal Practice*. Philadelphia: W.B. Saunders; 1992:1219-1230.

124. Campbell TW. Amphibian husbandry and medical care. In: Rosenthal KL, ed. *Practical Exotic Animal Medicine (Compendium Collection)*. Trenton, NJ: Veterinary Learning Systems; 1997:65-68.

125. Wright KM. Trauma. In: Wright KM, Whitaker BR, eds. *Amphibian Medicine and Captive Husbandry*. Malabar, FL: Krieger Publishing; 2001:233-238.

126. Woodhams DC, Alford RA, Marantelli G. Emerging disease of amphibians cured by elevated body temperature. *Dis Aquat Organ*. 2003;55:65-67.

127. Willett-Frahm M, Wright KM, Thode BC. Select protozoan disease in amphibians and reptiles. *Bull Assoc Rept Amph Vet*. 1995;5:19-29.

128. Raphael BL. Amphibians. *Vet Clin North Am Small Anim Pract*. 1993;23:1271-1286.

129. Letcher J, Glade M. Efficacy of ivermectin as an anthelmintic in leopard frogs. *J Am Vet Med Assoc*. 1992;200:537-538.

130. Mombarg M, Claessen H, Lambrechts L, et al. Quantification of percutaneous absorption of metronidazole and levamisole in the fire-bellied toad (*Bombina orientalis*). *J Vet Pharmacol Ther*. 1992;15:433-436.

131. Stein G. Reptile and amphibian formulary. In: Mader DR, ed. *Reptile Medicine and Surgery*. Philadelphia: W.B. Saunders; 1996:465-472.

132. D'Agostino JJ, West G, Boothe DM, et al. Plasma pharmacokinetics of selamectin after a single topical administration in the American bullfrog (*Rana catesbeiana*). *J Zoo Wildl Med*. 2007;38:51-54.

133. Wright KM. Chlamydial infections of amphibians. *Bull Assoc Rept Amph Vet*. 1996;6:8-9.

134. Stoskopf MK, Arnold J, Mason M. Aminoglycoside antibiotic levels in the aquatic salamander (*Necturus necturus*). *J Zoo Anim Med*. 1987;18:81-85.

135. Poynton SL, Whitaker BR. Protozoa in poison dart frogs (Dentrobatidae): clinical assessment and identification. *J Zoo Wildl Med*. 1994;25:29-39.

136. Maruska EJ. Procedures for setting up and maintaining a salamander colony. In: Murphy JB, Adler K, Collins JT, eds. *Captive Management and Conservation of Amphibians and Reptiles*. Ithaca, NY: Society for the Study of Amphibians and Reptiles; 1994:229-242.

137. Wright KM. Amphibian formulary. In: Mader DR, ed. *Reptile Medicine and Surgery*. 2nd ed. St. Louis, MO: Saunders/Elsevier; 2006:1140-1146.

138. Pessier AP, Mendelson JR. A Manual for Control of Infectious Diseases in Amphibian Survival Assurance Colonies and Reintroduction Programs. Apple Valley, MN: IUCN/SSC Conservation Breeding Specialist Group. Available at: <www.cbsg.org/cbsg/workshopreports/26/amphibian_disease_manual.pdf>; Accessed December 31, 2010.

139. Crawshaw GJ. Amphibian medicine. In: Fowler ME, ed. *Zoo & Wild Animal Medicine: Current Therapy 3*. Philadelphia: W.B. Saunders; 1993:131-139.

140. Whitaker BR. Developing an effective quarantine program for amphibians. *Proc North Am Vet Conf*. 1997;764-765.

141. Shilton CM, Smith DA, Crawshaw GJ, et al. Corneal lipid deposition in Cuban tree frogs (*Osteopilus septentrionalis*) and its relationship to serum lipids: an experimental study. *J Zoo Wildl Med*. 2001;32:305-319.

142. Mader DR. Antimicrobial therapy in reptiles. Proc South Euro Vet Conf Congresso Nacional. AVEPA; 2007.

143. Frye FL. *Reptile Care. An Atlas of Diseases and Treatments*. Neptune City, NJ: TFH Publications; 1991:1-637.

144. Mader DR. Thermal burns. In: Mader DR, ed. *Reptile Medicine and Surgery*. 2nd ed. St. Louis, MO: Saunders/Elsevier; 2006:916-923.

145. Rossi J. Practical reptile dermatology. Proc North Am Vet Conf. 1995;648-649.

146. Diver SJ. Empirical doses of antimicrobial drugs commonly used in reptiles. *Exotic DVM*. 1998;1:23.

147. Allen DG, Pringle JK, Smith D. *Handbook of Veterinary Drugs*. Philadelphia: Lippincott; 1993:534-567.

148. Fleming GJ. Capture and chemical immobilization of the Nile crocodile (*Crocodylus niloticus*) in South Africa. Proc Annu Conf Assoc Rept Amph Vet. 1996;63-66.

149. Funk RS. A formulary for lizards, snakes, and crocodilians. *Vet Clin North Am Exot Anim Pract*. 2000;3:333-358.

150. Fitzgerald KT, Vera R. Acariasis. In: Mader DR, ed. *Reptile Medicine and Surgery*. 2nd ed. St. Louis, MO: Saunders/Elsevier; 2006:720-738.

151. Groza A, Mederle N, Darabus G. Advocate-therapeutical solution in parasitical infestation in frillneck lizard (*Chlamydosaurus kingii*) and bearded dragon (*Pogona vitticeps*). Lucrari Stiintifice—Universitatea Stiinte Agricole Banatului Timisoara. *Med Vet*. 2009:42:105-108.

152. Klingenberg RJ. *Understanding Reptile Parasites*. Irvine, CA: Advanced Vivarium Systems; 2007:1-200.

153. Barten SL. The medical care of iguanas and other common pet lizards. *Vet Clin North Am Small Anim Pract*. 1993;23:1213-1249.

154. Stahl SJ. Pet lizard conditions and syndromes. *Semin Avian Exot Pet Med*. 2003;12:162-182.

155. Divers SJ. The use of propofol in reptile anesthesia. Proc Annu Conf Assoc Rept Amph Vet. 1996;57-59.

156. Coke RL, Hunter RP, Isaza R, et al. Pharmacokinetics and tissue concentrations of azithromycin in ball pythons (*Python regius*). *Am J Vet Res*. 2003;64:225-228.

157. Holz PH, Burger JP, Baker R, et al. Effect of injection site on carbenicillin pharmacokinetics in the carpet python, *Morelia spilota*. *J Herp Med Surg*. 2002;12:12-16.

158. Lawrence K, Needham JR, Palmer GH, et al. A preliminary study on the use of carbenicillin in snakes. *J Vet Pharmacol Ther*. 1984;7:119-124.

159. Page CD, Mautino M. Clinical management of tortoises. *Compend Contin Educ Pract Vet*. 1990;12:79-85.

160. Lawrence K, Muggleton PW, Needham JR. Preliminary study on the use of ceftazidime, a broad spectrum cephalosporin antibiotic, in snakes. *Res Vet Sci*. 1984;36:16-20.

161. Benson KG, Tell LA, Young LA, et al. Pharmacokinetics of ceftiofur sodium after intramuscular or subcutaneous administration in green iguanas (*Iguana iguana*). *Am J Vet Res*. 2003;64:1278-1282.

162. Gauvin J. Drug therapy in reptiles. *Semin Avian Exot Pet Med*. 1993; 2:48-59.

163. Jenkins JR. Medical management of reptile patients. *Compend Contin Educ Pract Vet*. 1991;13:980-988.

164. Bush M, Smeller JM, Charache PN, et al. Preliminary study of antibiotics in snakes. *Proc Annu Conf Am Assoc Zoo Vet*. 1976; 50-54.

165. Bush M, Smeller JM, Charache P, et al. Biological half-life of gentamicin in gopher snakes. *Am J Vet Res*. 1978;39:171-173.

166. Hilf M, Swanson D, Wagner R, et al. A new dosing schedule for gentamicin in blood pythons (*Python curtus*): a pharmacokinetic study. *Res Vet Sci*. 1991;50:127-130.

167. Raphael B, Clark CH, Hudson R Jr. Plasma concentration of gentamicin in turtles. *J Zoo Anim Med*. 1985;16:136-139.

168. Coke RL, Isaza R, Koch DE, et al. Preliminary single-dose pharmacokinetics of marbofloxacin in ball pythons (*Python regius*). *J Zoo Wildl Med*. 2006;37:6-10.

169. Helmick KE, Papich MG, Vliet KA, et al. Pharmacokinetic disposition of a long-acting oxytetracycline formulation after single-dose intravenous and intramuscular administrations in the American alligator (*Alligator mississippiensis*). *J Zoo Wildl Med*. 2004;35:341-346.

170. Johnson JD, Mangone B, Jarchow JL. A review of mycoplasmosis infections in tortoises and options for treatment. *Proc Annu Conf Assoc Rept Amph Vet*. 1998;89-92.

171. Jenkins JR. Husbandry and diseases of Old World chameleons. *J Small Exot Anim Med*. 1992;1:166-171.

172. Klingenberg RJ. Therapeutics. In: Mader DR, ed. *Reptile Medicine and Surgery*. Philadelphia: W.B. Saunders; 1996:299-321.

173. Gaio C, Rossi T, Villa R, et al. Pharmacokinetics of acyclovir after a single oral administration in marginated tortoises, *Testudo marginata*. *J Herp Med Surg*. 2007;17:8-11.

174. McArthur S. Problem solving approach to common diseases of terrestrial and semi-aquatic chelonians. In: McArthur S, Wilkinson R, Meyer J, eds. *Medicine and Surgery of Tortoises and Turtles*. Oxford: Blackwell Publishing; 2004:309-377.

175. Frye FL. *Reptile Clinician's Handbook*. Malabar, FL: Krieger Publishing; 1994.

176. Lloyd M. Crocodilia. In: Fowler ME, Miller RE, eds. *Zoo and Wild Animal Medicine*. 5th ed. Philadelphia: Saunders/Elsevier; 2003: 59-70.

177. Harms CA, Lewbart GA, Beasley J. Medical management of mixed nocardial and unidentified fungal osteomyelitis in a Kemp's Ridley sea turtle, *Lepidochelys kempii*. *J Herp Med Surg*. 2002;12:21-26.

178. Mallo KM, Harms CA, Lewbart GA, et al. Pharmacokinetics of fluconazole in loggerhead sea turtles (*Caretta caretta*) after single intravenous and subcutaneous injections, and multiple subcutaneous injections. *J Zoo Wildl Med*. 2002;33:29-35.

179. Martel A, Hellebuyck T, Van Waeyenberghe L. Treatment of infections with *Nannizziopsis vriesii*, an emergent reptilian dermatophyte. *Proc Annu Conf Assoc Rept Amph Vet*. 2009;69-70.

180. Mitchell M. Ophidia. In: Fowler ME, Miller RE, eds. *Zoo and Wild Animal Medicine*. 5th ed. Philadelphia: Saunders/Elsevier; 2003:82-91.

181. Bicknese E, Pessier A, Boedeker N. Successful treatment of fungal osteomyelitis in a Parson's chameleon (*Calumma parsonii*) using surgical and anti-fungal treatments. *Proc Annu Conf Assoc Rept Amph Vet*. 2008;86.

182. Gamble KC, Alvarado TP, Bennett CL. Itraconazole plasma and tissue concentrations in the spiny lizard (*Sceloporus* sp.) following once-daily dosing. *J Zoo Wildl Med*. 1997;28:89-93.

183. Jacobson ER. Antimicrobial drug use in reptiles. In: Prescott JF, Baggot JD, eds. *Antimicrobial Therapy in Veterinary Medicine*. Ames, IA: Iowa State University Press; 1993:543-552.

184. Jepson L. Snakes. In: *Exotic Animal Medicine. A Quick Reference Guide*. Philadelphia: Saunders/Elsevier; 2009:315-357.

185. Jacobson E, Kollias GV Jr, Peters LJ. Dosages for antibiotics and parasiticides used in exotic animals. *Compend Contin Educ Pract Vet*. 1983;5:315-324.

186. Innis C, Young D, Wetzlich S, et al. Plasma voriconazole concentrations in four red-eared slider turtles (*Trachemys scripta elegans*) after a single subcutaneous injection. *Proc Annu Conf Assoc Rept Amph Vet*. 2008;72.

187. Flach EJ, Riley J, Mutlow AG, et al. Pentastomiasis in Bosc's monitor lizards (*Varanus exanthematicus*) caused by an undescribed *Sambonia* species. *J Zoo Wildl Med*. 2000;31:91-95.

188. Wilson SC, Carpenter JW. Endoparasitic diseases of reptiles. *Semin Avian Exot Pet Med*. 1996;5:64-74.

189. Bodri MS, Hruba SJ. Safety of milbemycin (A3-A4 oxime) in chelonians. *Proc Joint Conf Am Assoc Zoo Vet/Am Assoc Wildl Vet*. 1992;156-157.

190. Klingenberg RJ. Diagnosing parasites of Old World chameleons. *Exotic DVM*. 2000;1(6):17-21.

191. Adnyana W, Ladds PW, Blair D. Efficacy of praziquantel in the treatment of green sea turtles with spontaneous infection of cardiovascular flukes. *Aust Vet J*. 1997;75:405-407.

192. Jacobson E, Harman G, Laille E, et al. Plasma concentrations of praziquantel in loggerhead sea turtles (*Caretta caretta*) following oral administration of single and multiple doses. *Proc Annu Conf Assoc Rept Amph Vet*. 2002;37-39.

193. Mauldin GN, Done LB. Oncology. In: Mader DR, ed. *Reptile Medicine and Surgery*. 2nd ed. St. Louis, MO: Saunders/Elsevier; 2006: 299-322.

194. Rosenthal K. Chemotherapeutic treatment of a sarcoma in a corn snake. *Proc Joint Conf Am Assoc Zoo Vet/Assoc Rept Amph Vet*. 1994;46.

195. Harkewicz KA. Dermatologic problems of reptiles. *Semin Avian Exot Pet Med*. 2002;11:151-161.

196. Boyer TH. *Essentials of Reptiles. A Guide for Practitioners*. Lakewood, CO: AAHA Press; 1998:1-253.

197. Donoghue S. Nutrition. In: Mader DR, ed. *Reptile Medicine and Surgery*. 2nd ed. St. Louis, MO: Saunders/Elsevier; 2006:251-298.

198. Ferrell ST, Graham JE, Swaim SF. Avian wound healing and management. *Proc Annu Conf Assoc Avian Vet*. 2002;337-347.

199. Ritchie BW, Harrison GJ. Formulary. In: Ritchie BW, Harrison GJ, Harrison LR, eds. *Avian Medicine: Principles and Application. Abridged*. Lake Worth, FL: Wingers Publishing; 1997:227-253.

200. Lennox AM. The use of Aldara™ (imiquimod) for the treatment of cloacal papillomatosis in psittacines. *Exotic DVM*. 2002;4:34-35.

201. Coles BH. Prescribing for exotic birds. In: Bishop Y, ed. *The Veterinary Formulary*. 5th ed. London: Pharmaceutical Press; 2001: 99-105.

202. Johnson-Delaney CA, Harrison LR. *Exotic Companion Medicine Handbook for Veterinarians*. Lake Worth, FL: Wingers Publishing; 1996.

203. Beynon PH, Forbes NA, Lawton MPC. *Manual of Psittacine Birds*. Ames, IA: Iowa State University Press; 1996.

204. Redig P. Infectious diseases; fungal diseases. In: Samour J, ed. *Avian Medicine*. London: Harcourt Publishers; 2000:275-291.

205. Suedmeyer WK, Bermudez A, Fales W. Treatment of epidermal cysts associated with *Aspergillus fumigatus* and an *Alternaria* sp. in a silky bantam chicken *(Gallus gallus)*. Proc Joint Conf Am Assoc Zoo Vet/Internat Assoc Aquatic Anim Med. 2000;307-309.

206. Bailey TA, Apo MM. Pharmaceutics commonly used in avian medicine. In: Samour JH, ed. *Avian Medicine*. 2nd ed. Edinburgh, UK: Mosby Elsevier; 2008:485-509.

207. Chitty J, Lierz M. Formulary. In: Chitty J, Lierz M, eds. *BSAVA Manual of Raptors, Pigeons and Passerine Birds*. Gloucester, UK: British Small Animal Veterinary Association; 2008:384-390.

208. Forbes NA. Raptors. Parasitic diseases. In: Chitty J, Lierz M, eds. *BSAVA Manual of Raptors, Pigeons and Passerine Birds*. Gloucester, UK: British Small Animal Veterinary Association; 2008:202-211.

209. Davies RR. Passerine birds. Going light. In: Chitty J, Lierz M, eds. *BSAVA Manual of Raptors, Pigeons and Passerine Birds*. Gloucester, UK: British Small Animal Veterinary Association; 2008:365-369.

210. Dorrestein GM, Van Der Horst HHA, Cremers HJWM, et al. Quill mite *(Dermoglyphus passerinus)* infestation of canaries *(Serinus canaria):* diagnosis and treatment. *Avian Pathol.* 1997;26:195-199.

211. Bishop CR, Rorabaugh E. Evaluation of the safety and efficacy of selamectin in budgerigars with Knemidokoptes infection. Proc Annu Conf Assoc Avian Vet. 2010;79-84.

212. Gronwall R, Brown MP, Clubb S. Pharmacokinetics of amikacin in African grey parrots. *Am J Vet Res.* 1989;50:250-252.

213. Orosz SE, Jones MP, Cox SK, et al. Pharmacokinetics of amoxicillin plus clavulanic acid in blue-fronted Amazon parrots *(Amazona aestiva aestiva)*. *J Avian Med Surg.* 2000;14:107-112.

214. Carpenter JW, Olsen JH, Randle-Port M, et al. Pharmacokinetics of azithromycin in the blue and gold macaw *(Ara ararauna)* after intravenous and oral administration. *J Zoo Wildl Med.* 2005;36:606-609.

215. Porter SL. Vehicular trauma in owls. Proc Annu Conf Assoc Avian Vet. 1990;164-170.

216. Flammer K. Treatment of bacterial and mycotic diseases of the avian gastrointestinal tract. Proc North Am Vet Conf. 2002;851-852.

217. Rupley AE. Critical care of pet birds. *Vet Clin North Am Exot Anim Pract.* 1998;1:11-41.

218. Tell L, Harrenstien L, Wetzlich S, et al. Pharmacokinetics of ceftiofur sodium in exotic and domestic avian species. *J Vet Pharmacol Ther.* 1998;21:85-91.

219. Dorrestein GM. Passerine and softbill therapeutics. *Vet Clin North Am Exot Anim Pract.* 2000;3:35-57.

220. Samour J. Pharmaceutics commonly used in avian medicine. In: Samour J, ed. *Avian Medicine*. Philadelphia: Mosby; 2000:388-418.

221. Tully TN. Psittacine therapeutics. *Vet Clin North Am Exot Anim Pract.* 2000;3:59-90.

222. Flammer K. Common bacterial infections and antibiotic use in companion birds. *Suppl Comp Cont Edu Pract Vet.* 1998;20(3A):34-48.

223. Phalen DN. Common bacterial and fungal infectious diseases in pet birds. *Suppl Compend Contin Educ Pract Vet.* 2003;25:43-48.

224. Tully TN. Formulary. In: Altman RB, Clubb SL, Dorrestein GM, et al., eds. *Avian Medicine and Surgery*. Philadelphia: W.B. Saunders; 1997:671-688.

225. Flammer K, Whitt-Smith D. Plasma concentrations of enrofloxacin psittacine birds offered water medicated with 200 mg/L of the injectable formulation of enrofloxacin. *J Avian Med Surg.* 2002;16:286-290.

226. Rosskopf WJ, Woerpel RW. Practical avian therapeutics with dosages of commonly used medications. *Proc Basics Avian Med.* 1996;75-81.

227. Cross G. Antiviral therapy. *Semin Avian Exot Pet Med.* 1995;4:96-102.

228. Bauck L, Hillyer E, Hoefer H. Rhinitis: case reports. Proc Annu Conf Assoc Avian Vet. 1992;134-139.

229. Flammer K. An overview of antifungal therapy in birds. Proc Annu Conf Assoc Avian Vet. 1993;1-4.

230. Beynon PH, Forbes NA, Harcourt-Brown NH. *Manual of Raptors, Pigeons and Waterfowl*. Ames, IA: Iowa State University Press; 1996.

231. Orosz SE, Frazier DL. Antifungal agents: a review of their pharmacology and therapeutic indications. *J Avian Med Surg.* 1995;9:8-18.

232. Flammer K. Fluconazole in psittacine birds. Proc Annu Conf Assoc Avian Vet. 1996;203-204.

233. Orosz SE, Schroeder EC, Frazier DL. Pharmacokinetic properties of itraconazole in blue-fronted Amazon parrots *(Amazona aestiva aestiva)*. *J Avian Med Surg.* 1996;10:168-173.

234. Kasper A. Rehabilitation of California towhees. Proc Annu Conf Assoc Avian Vet. 1997;83-90.

235. Samour JH, Naldo J. Serratospiculiasis in captive falcons in the Middle East: a review. *J Avian Med Surg.* 2001;15:2-9.

236. Jenkins JR. Feather picking and self-mutilation in psittacine birds. *Vet Clin North Am Exot Anim Pract.* 2001;4:663-667.

237. Gould WJ. Caring for birds' skin and feathers. *Vet Med.* 1995;6:53-63.

238. Lawton MPC. Anaesthesia. In: Beynon PH, Forbes NA, Lawton MPC, eds. *BSAVA Manual of Psittacine Birds*. Ames, IA: Iowa State University Press; 1996:49-55.

239. Kearns KS. Paroxetine therapy for feather picking and self-mutilation in the waldrapp ibis *(Geronticus eremita)*. Proc Joint Conf Am Assoc Zoo Vet/Am Assoc Wildl Vet/Wildl Dis Assoc. 2004;254-255.

240. Brenner DJ, Larsen RS, Dickinson PJ, et al. Development of an avian brachial plexus nerve block technique for perioperative analgesia in mallard ducks *(Anas platyrhynchos)*. *J Avian Med Surg.* 2010;24:24-34.

241. Dahlhausen B, Aldred S, Colaizzi E. Resolution of clinical proventricular dilatation disease by cyclooxygenase 2 inhibition. Proc Annu Conf Assoc Avian Vet. 2002;9-12.

242. Shaver SL, Robinson NG, Wright BD, et al. A multimodal approach to management of suspected neuropathic pain in a prairie falcon *(Falco mexicanus)*. *J Avian Med Surg.* 2009;23:209-213.

243. Abou-Madi N. Avian anesthesia. *Vet Clin North Am Exot Anim Pract.* 2001;4:147-167.

244. Huckabee JR. Raptor therapeutics. *Vet Clin North Am Exot Anim Pract.* 2000;3:91-116.

245. Cooper JE. Medicines and other agents used in treatment, including emergency anaesthesia kit and avian resuscitation protocol. In: Cooper JE, ed. *Birds of Prey. Health and Disease*. 3rd ed. Ames, IA: Blackwell Publishing, Iowa State Press; 2002:271-277.

246. Stanford M. Cage and aviary birds. In: Meredith A, Redrobe S, eds. *BSAVA Manual of Exotic Pets*. 4th ed. Gloucester, UK: British Small Animal Veterinary Association; 2002:157-167.

247. Edling TM. Anaesthesia and analgesia. In: Chitty J, Harcourt-Brown N, eds. *BSAVA Manual of Psittacine Birds*. Gloucester, UK: British Small Animal Veterinary Association; 2005:87-96.

248. Cook K, Riggs G. Clinical reports: gonadotropic releasing hormones agonist implants. Proc Annu Conf Assoc Avian Vet. 2007;309-315.

249. Baillie JW. Alternative therapy ideas for feather picking. Proc Annu Conf Assoc Avian Vet. 2001;191-196.

250. Echols S, Speer B. Omega-3 fatty acid supplementation: potential uses and limitations. Proc Annu Conf Assoc Avian Vet. 2000;13-16.

251. Ritchie BW, Harrison GJ. Formulary. In: Ritchie BW, Harrison GJ, Harrison LR, eds. *Avian Medicine: Principles and Application*. Lake Worth, FL: Wingers Publishing; 1994:457-478.

252. Axelson RD. Avian dermatology. In: Hoefer HL, ed. *Practical Avian Medicine. The Compendium Collection*. Trenton, NJ: Veterinary Learning Systems; 1997:186-195.

253. Joyner KL. Pediatric therapeutics. Proc Annu Conf Assoc Avian Vet. 1991;188-199.
254. Worell AB. Therapy of noninfectious avian disorders. *Semin Avian Exot Pet Med.* 1993;2:42-47.
255. Lightfoot TL. Therapeutics of African pygmy hedgehogs and prairie dogs. *Vet Clin North Am Exot Anim Pract.* 2000;3:155-172.
256. Jenkins J. *Rabbit Drug Doses.* Lakewood, CO: American Animal Hospital Association; 1995.
257. Harvey C. Rabbit and rodent skin diseases. *Semin Avian Exot Pet Med.* 1995;4:195-204.
258. Stocker L. *Medication for Use in the Treatment of Hedgehogs.* Aylesbury, UK: Marshcliff; 1992.
259. Adamcak A, Otten B. Rodent therapeutics. *Vet Clin North Am Exot Anim Pract.* 2000;3:221-237, viii.
260. Richardson VCG. *Diseases of Small Domestic Rodents.* Malden, MA: Blackwell Scientific Publications; 1997.
261. Harkness JE. *A Practitioner's Guide to Domestic Rodents.* Lakewood, CO: American Animal Hospital Association; 1993.
262. Hoefer HL. Hedgehogs. *Vet Clin North Am Small Anim Pract.* 1994; 24:113-120.
263. Morrisey JK, Carpenter JW. Formulary. In: Quesenberry KE, Carpenter JW, eds. *Ferrets, Rabbits, and Rodents: Clinical Medicine and Surgery.* 3rd ed. St. Louis, MO: Saunders/Elsevier; 2012:566-575.
264. Quesenberry KE. Rabbits. In: Birchard SJ, Sherding RG, eds. *Saunders Manual of Small Animal Practice.* Philadelphia: W.B. Saunders; 1994:1345-1362.
265. Harkness JE, Wagner JE. *The Biology and Medicine of Rabbits and Rodents.* 4th ed. Philadelphia: Williams & Wilkins; 1995.
266. Jepson L. *Exotic Animal Medicine. A Quick Reference Guide.* Philadelphia: Saunders/Elsevier; 2009.
267. Letcher JD. Amitraz as a treatment for acariasis in African hedgehogs *(Atelerix albiventris). J Zoo Anim Med.* 1988;19:24-29.
268. Morrisey JK. Parasites of ferrets, rabbits, and rodents. *Semin Avian Exot Pet Med.* 1996;5:106-114.
269. Morrisey JK. Ferrets. Therapeutics. In: Keeble E, Meredith A, eds. *BSAVA Manual of Rodents and Ferrets.* Gloucester, UK: British Small Animal Veterinary Association; 2009:237-244.
270. Booth RJ. Medicine and husbandry: dasyurids, possums, and bats. Proc 233rd Wildl Post Grad Comm Vet Sci. 1994;423-441.
271. Brown SA. Ferret drug dosages. In: Antinoff N, Bauck L, Boyer TH, et al., eds. *Exotic Formulary.* 2nd ed. Lakewood, CO: American Animal Hospital Association; 1999:43-61.
272. Wen H, Pan B, Wang F, et al. The effect of self-licking behavior on pharmacokinetics of eprinomectin and clinical efficacy against *Psoroptes cuniculi* in topically administered rabbits. *Parasitol Res.* 2010;106:607-613.
273. Williams BH. Therapeutics in ferrets. *Vet Clin North Am Exot Anim Pract.* 2000;3:131-153.
274. Ewringmann A, Glöckner B. *Leitsymptome bei Meerschweinchen, Chinchilla und Degu. Diagnostischer Leitfaden und Therapie.* Stuttgart: Enke Publishing; 2005.
275. Harcourt-Brown F. *Textbook of Rabbit Medicine.* Oxford: Butterworth-Heinemann; 2002.
276. Hutchinson MJ, Jacobs DE, Bell GD, et al. Evaluation of imidacloprid for the treatment and prevention of cat flea *(Ctenocephalides felis felis)* infestations on rabbits. *Vet Rec.* 2001;148:695-696.
277. Jepson L. *Exotic Animal Medicine. A Quick Reference Guide.* New York: W.B. Saunders; 2009:93-173.
278. Birke L, Molina P, Baker D, et al. Comparison of selamectin and imidacloprid plus permethrin in eliminating *Leporacarus gibbus* infestation in laboratory rabbits. *J Am Assoc Lab Anim Sci.* 2009;48: 757-762.
279. Powers LV. Bacterial and parasitic diseases of ferrets. *Vet Clin North Am Exot Anim Pract.* 2009;12:531-561.
280. Baumans V, Havenaar R, Van Herck H, et al. The effectiveness of ivomec and neguvon on the control of murine mites. *Lab Anim.* 1988;22:243-245.
281. Anderson NL. Basic husbandry and medicine of pocket pets. In: Birchard SJ, Sherding RG, eds. *Saunders Manual of Small Animal Practice.* Philadelphia: W.B. Saunders; 1994:1363-1389.
282. Morrisey JK. Ectoparasites of small mammals. Proc North Am Vet Conf. 1998;844-845.
283. Lewington JH. Appendix. In: Lewington JH, ed. *Ferret Husbandry, Medicine and Surgery.* Oxford: Butterworth Heinemann; 2000: 273-282.
284. Brust D. *Sugar Gliders. A Complete Veterinary Care Guide.* Sugarland, TX: Veterinary Interactive Publications; 2009.
285. Carpenter JW. Personal observation. 2011.
286. Beck W, Pantchev N. *Praktische Parasitologie bei Heimtieren.* Hanover, Germany: Schluetersche-Verlagsgesellschaft MBH & Co.; 2006.
287. Kim SH, Lee JY, Jun HK, et al. Efficacy of selamectin in the treatment of cheyletiellosis in pet rabbits. *Vet Dermatol.* 2008;19:26-27.
288. Morrisey JK. Ectoparasites of ferrets and rabbits. Proc North Am Vet Conf. 1998;844-845.
289. Hoefer H. Diagnosis and management of chinchilla diseases. Proc North Am Vet Conf. 1999;833-835.
290. Bishop CR. Reproductive medicine of rabbits and rodents. *Vet Clin North Am Exot Anim Pract.* 2002;5:507-535.
291. Morrisey JK, Carpenter JW. Formulary. In: Quesenberry KE, Carpenter JW, eds. *Ferrets, Rabbits, and Rodents: Clinical Medicine and Surgery.* 2nd ed. St. Louis, MO: Saunders/Elsevier; 2004:436-444.
292. Pye GW, Carpenter JW. A guide to medicine and surgery in sugar gliders. *Vet Med.* 1999;94:891-905.
293. Bistner SI, Ford RB. *Kirk's and Bistner's Handbook of Veterinary Procedures and Emergency Treatment.* 6th ed. Philadelphia: W.B. Saunders; 1994:844-847.
294. Brown SA. Ferrets. In: Jenkins JR, Brown SA, eds. *A Practitioner's Guide to Rabbits and Ferrets.* Lakewood, CO: American Animal Hospital Association; 1993:43-111.
295. Carceles CM, Fernandez-Varon E, Marin P, et al. Tissue disposition of azithromycin after intravenous and intramuscular administration to rabbits. *Vet J.* 2007;174:154-159.
296. Zhou JY, Xu PF, Chen H, et al. Therapeutic effect of ceftazidime in a rabbit model of peritonitis caused by *Escherichia coli* producing CTX-M-14 extended-spectrum beta-lactamase. *Zhonghua Jie He He Hu Xi Za Zhi.* 2005;28:689-693.
297. Hillyer EV, Brown SA. Ferrets. In: Birchard SJ, Sherding RG, eds. *Saunders Manual of Small Animal Practice.* Philadelphia: W.B. Saunders; 1994:1317-1344.
298. Hillyer EV. Pet rabbits. *Vet Clin North Am Small Anim Pract.* 1994; 24:25-64.
299. Ewringmann A, Glöckner B. *Leitsymptome bei Hamster, Ratte, Mause und Rennmaus. Diagnostischer Leitfaden und Therapie.* Stuttgart: Enke Publishing; 2008.
300. Allen DG, Pringle JK, Smith DA. *Handbook of Veterinary Drugs.* Philadelphia: Lippincott; 1993.
301. Carpenter JW, Hawkins MG. Personal communication. 2011.
302. Okerman L, Devriese LA, Gevaert D, et al. In vivo activity of orally administered antibiotics and chemotherapeutics against acute septicaemic pasteurellosis in rabbits. *Lab Anim.* 1990;24:341-344.
303. Gillett CS. Selected drug dosages and clinical reference data. In: Manning PJ, Ringler DH, Newcomer CE, eds. *The Biology of the Laboratory Rabbit.* 2nd ed. San Diego: Academic Press; 1994:467-472.
304. Fish RE, Besch-Williford C. Reproductive disorders in the rabbit and guinea pig. In: Kirk RW, Bonagura JD, eds. *Kirk's Current Veterinary Therapy XI: Small Animal Practice.* Philadelphia: W.B. Saunders; 1992:1175-1179.
305. Hoefer HL. Clinical approach to the African hedgehog. Proc North Am Vet Conf. 1999;836-838.

306. Smith AJ. Husbandry and medicine of African hedgehogs (*Atelerix albiventris*). *J Small Exot Anim Med*. 1992;2:21-28.

307. Burgmann P, Percey DH. Antimicrobial drug use in rodents and rabbits. In: Prescott JF, Baggot JD, eds. *Antimicrobial Therapy in Veterinary Medicine*. Ames, IA: Iowa State University Press; 1993: 524-541.

308. Sanati H, Ramos C, Bayer A, et al. Combination therapy with amphotericin B and fluconazole against invasive candidiasis in neutropenic-mouse and infective-endocarditis rabbit models. *Antimicrob Agents Chemother*. 1997;41:1345-1348.

309. Petraitis V, Petraitiene R, Groll AH, et al. Comparative antifungal activities and plasma pharmacokinetics of micafungin (FK463) against disseminated candidiasis and invasive pulmonary aspergillosis in persistently neutropenic rabbits. *Antimicrob Agents Chemother*. 2002;46:1857-1869.

310. Besch-Williford CL. Biology and medicine of the ferret. *Vet Clin North Am Small Anim Pract*. 1987;17:1155-1183.

311. Quesenberry KE. Guinea pigs. *Vet Clin North Am Small Anim Pract*. 1994;24:67-87.

312. Pye GW. Personal observations. 2010.

313. Walsh TJ, Petraitis V, Petraitiene R, et al. Experimental pulmonary aspergillosis due to *Aspergillus terreus*. Pathogenesis and treatment of an emerging fungal pathogen resistant to amphotericin B. *J Infect Dis*. 2003;188:305-319.

314. Patterson TF, Fothergill AW, Rinaldi MG. Efficacy of itraconazole solution in a rabbit model of invasive aspergillosis. *Antimicrob Agents Chemother*. 1993;37:2307-2310.

315. Harrenstien L. Critical care of ferrets, rabbits, and rodents. *Semin Avian Exot Pet Med*. 1994;3:217-228.

316. Sorensen KN, Sobel RA, Clemons KV, et al. Comparative efficacies of terbinafine and fluconazole in treatment of experimental coccidioidal meningitis in a rabbit model. *Antimicrob Agents Chemother*. 2000;44:3087-3091.

317. Booth RJ. General husbandry and medical care of sugar gliders. In: Bonagura JD, ed. *Kirk's Current Veterinary Therapy XIII: Small Animal Practice*. Philadelphia: W.B. Saunders; 2000:1157-1163.

318. Smith AJ. General husbandry and medical care of hedgehogs. In: Bonagura JD, ed. *Kirk's Current Veterinary Therapy XIII: Small Animal Practice*. Philadelphia: W.B. Saunders; 2000:11.

319. Morrisey JK. Personal communication. 2004.

320. Beaufrere H, Neta M, Smith DA. Demodectic mange associated with lymphoma in a ferret. *J Exot Pet Med*. 2009;18:57-61.

321. Heatley JJ. Hedgehogs. In: Mitchell MA, Tully TN Jr, eds. *Manual of Exotic Pet Practice*. St. Louis, MO: Saunders/Elsevier; 2009: 433-455.

322. Kelleher SA. Skin disease of ferrets. *Semin Avian Exot Pet Med*. 2002;11:136-140.

323. Rhody JL, Schiller CA. Spinal osteosarcoma in a hedgehog with pedal self-mutilation. *Vet Clin North Am Exot Anim Pract*. 2006; 9:625-631.

324. Johnson-Delaney C. Ferrets: anaesthesia and analgesia. In: Keeble E, Meredith A, eds. *BSAVA Manual of Rodents and Ferrets*. Gloucester, UK: British Small Animal Veterinary Association; 2009: 245-253.

325. Eisele PH. Anesthesia for small mammals. Proc North Am Vet Conf. 1997;785-791.

326. Laird KL, Swindle MM, Flecknell PA. *Handbook of Rodent and Rabbit Medicine*. New York: Pergamon; 1996.

327. Granson HJ. Gabapentin for tail trauma in a Syrian hamster (*Mesocricetus auratus*). Proc Annu Conf Assoc Avian Vet/Assoc Exotic Mam Vet. 2010;107-108.

328. Morrisey JK. Personal observation. 2011.

329. Brust DM. What every veterinarian needs to know about sugar gliders. *Exotic DVM*. 2009;11:32-41.

330. Ness RD, Johnson-Delaney C. Sugar gliders. In: Quesenberry KE, Carpenter JW, eds. *Ferrets, Rabbits, and Rodents: Clinical Medicine and Surgery*. 3rd ed. St. Louis, MO: Saunders/Elsevier; 2012:393-410.

331. Hoppes SM. The senior ferret. *Vet Clin North Am Exot Anim Pract*. 2010;13:107-121.

332. Carpenter JW, Pollock CG, Koch DE, et al. Single- and multiple-dose pharmacokinetics of meloxicam after oral administration to the rabbit (*Oryctolagus cuniculus*). *J Zoo Wildl Med*. 2009;40:601-606.

333. Wagner RA, Piche CA, Jöchle W, et al. Clinical and endocrine responses to treatment with deslorelin acetate implants in ferrets with adrenocortical disease. *Am J Vet Res*. 2005;66:910-914.

334. Isenbügel E, Baumgartner RA. Diseases of the hedgehog. In: Fowler ME, ed. *Zoo and Wild Animal Medicine: Current Therapy 3*. Philadelphia: W.B. Saunders; 1993:294-302.

335. Johnson-Delaney C. Ferrets. In: Johnson-Delaney CA, ed. *Exotic Companion Medicine Handbook*. Lake Worth, FL: Zoological Education Network; 2005:1-42.

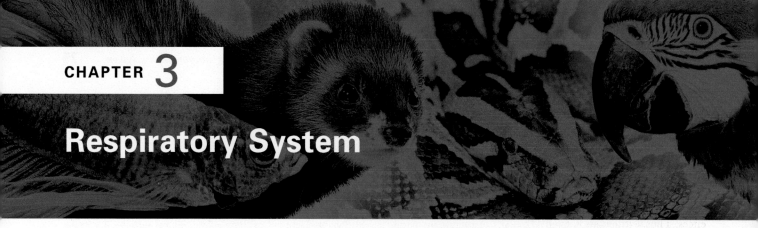

CHAPTER 3

Respiratory System

Hugues Beaufrère, DrMedVet, PhD, DACZM, DABVP (Avian), DECZM (Avian) •
Noemie Summa, DrMedVet, IPSAV • *Kim Le, BSc(Vet)(HonsI), BVSc*

INTRODUCTION

The principal function of the animal respiratory system is to facilitate gas exchange in order to supply the oxygen necessary for aerobic metabolism to individual cells and eliminate the gaseous by-products in the form of carbon dioxide. When the zoological veterinarian is investigating the respiratory system and respiratory diseases of their patients, it should be kept in mind that all living animals are subject to the same constraints. However the respiratory system and its pathologic dysfunction vary with animal groups, metabolic rate, animal size, and environmental factors. As such, all respiratory systems have some characteristics in common including a large capillary network, extended surface area, moist and thin exchange surfaces, and constant renewal of oxygen-rich fluid.[1] As size and metabolism increase, respiratory physiological parameters are optimized to satisfy oxygen demands. Such strategies include maximization of the respiratory surface area to volume ratio, thinner blood/fluid barrier, more efficient ventilation, and increased oxygen extraction through various mechanisms.

Respiratory adaptations usually occur in concert with circulatory adaptations due to the necessity for efficient gas transport (see cardiovascular system: Chapter 4). A panoply of respiratory adaptations have evolved in both aquatic and terrestrial animals to accomplish respiratory functions corresponding to their ecologic and biological needs. Invertebrates show a tremendous variation in respiratory mechanisms from passive diffusion across basic external or internal respiratory surfaces to the more anatomically complex book lungs of Arachnida and tracheal system of Insecta. However, despite this large spectrum of respiratory strategies, invertebrates are limited in size in part due to the metabolic, anatomical, and physiological constraints of their respiratory system. Vertebrates have developed much more sophisticated respiratory systems that maximize respiratory surfaces in a given volume as well as airflow through advanced ventilatory mechanisms. In the aquatic oxygen-poor environment, the cross-current exchange mechanism of the gills, combined with a relatively low poikilothermic metabolism, has allowed fish to thrive. The oxygen-rich terrestrial environment has allowed increased oxygen extraction within the vertebrate lungs, with a high level of complexity culminating in birds where cross-current gas exchange air capillary surfaces power their relatively high metabolism and active biological lifestyle. While homeothermic vertebrates usually rely on a highly specialized pulmonary system for gas exchange, poikilothermic vertebrates frequently combine different systems to meet their overall respiratory needs. This is best exemplified in amphibians, which use gills and skin in their larval life stage and change, as adults, to a combination of cutaneous, oropharyngeal, and pulmonary respiration in response to environmental constraints. Fish may also use an astonishing variety of air-breathing organs to accommodate the low oxygen concentration of tropical water, while reptiles may show extra pulmonary surfaces in various parts of their body (e.g., tracheal lungs in snakes and chameleons, cloacal breathing in aquatic turtles, cutaneous breathing in soft-shell turtles, gular breathing in some reptiles).

Ventilatory mechanisms are also quite diverse in vertebrates and may involve the buccal cavity (e.g., fish, amphibians, reptiles), an internal diaphragm (e.g., mammals), and air sac systems (e.g., some squamates and birds). This ventilation is regulated by various mechanisms triggered by changes in partial pressure of carbon dioxide in arterial blood ($PaCO_2$), partial pressure of oxygen in arterial blood (PaO_2), pH, and intrarespiratory partial pressure of carbon dioxide (PCO_2) and oxygen (PO_2) depending on the species. In the anatomical section of this chapter, primary focus involves the branchial and pulmonary systems with a brief mention of alternate modes of respiration in some poikilothermic taxons. Gas transport and diffusion in the vascular system and cellular respiration are not presented. For obvious reasons, information regarding anatomy and physiology is restricted to that which is general or clinically relavent. Readers are invited to consult specialized texts on respiratory anatomy and physiology for in depth descriptions of this subject area.

The second and third sections of this chapter cover respiratory diseases and their diagnosis in a variety of taxons. Necropsy and pathology are not included in this current therapeutic chapter on the respiratory system of exotic animals. While various vertebrate taxa share similar pathogenic organisms causing respiratory diseases, such as iridoviruses (e.g., fish, amphibians, reptiles), paramyxoviruses (e.g., reptiles, mammals, birds), gram-negative bacteria, mycoplasmas, and fungal species (e.g., reptiles and birds), some are more specific or more prevalent in certain species. Microbial organisms may be opportunistic pathogens (e.g., mycobacteria, saprophytic fungi) or obligate pathogens (e.g., viruses, parasites). The portal of entry into the respiratory system is often directly through the respiratory surfaces. However some pathogens may gain access by other means such as the circulatory system. Husbandry factors and concurrent stress in captivity may contribute to the pathophysiology of most disease processes. This condition is evident with poikilothermic species in which an enclosed and controlled artificial biotope must be recreated. As with many diseases, some species that are phylogenetically closely related may share common disease conditions but may also show marked differences. Thus, extrapolation from one species to another should not only consider taxonomy but also species ecology and physiology. Indeed, vertebrate species with similar ecologic niches may be susceptible to similar diseases regardless of their phylogenetic relationship. Therefore the zoological medicine veterinarian must always extrapolate carefully what is known of a disease for one species to another, regardless of their potential biological relationships. One should always remember that species-specific knowledge is paramount in practicing sound medicine. Since mammalian medicine is more advanced than nonmammalian medicine, the reader may refer to the literature on common domestic mammals for a more in-depth review of some mammalian diseases, diagnostic tests, and therapeutics that may be applicable to zoological companion mammals.

The last section of this chapter introduces therapeutic options for a variety of diseases. Since some diseases discussed in this chapter may affect other body systems, one is encouraged to consult other chapters within this book for further information on corresponding medical and surgical treatments.

ANATOMY AND PHYSIOLOGY

Invertebrates

Invertebrates are rarely treated in veterinary clinical practice but constitute almost 90% of the animal kingdom. As a non-monophyletic group, they are extremely diverse in their natural history, with varying degrees of phylogenetic relationships as a whole; ranging from single-cell organisms to more complex and larger metazoans such as arthropods and mollusks.[2,3] As invertebrates become increasingly popular in zoos, museums, and the pet trade, there is a growing need for veterinarians to be familiar with their care. This expertise is even more important for species conservation, where rare specimens are being reserved for captive maintenance and reproductive security.[2-4] In comparison to vertebrates, the respiratory anatomy of invertebrates is drastically different between species. Nevertheless, the constraints of the respiratory function remain the same depending on the terrestrial or aquatic lifestyle of the species. While terrestrial arthropods breathe by means of book lungs or tracheae, aquatic animals possess gills, and many rely on cutaneous respiration. As the size of invertebrates increases and passive diffusion through surfaces becomes insufficient to power cellular metabolism, specialized respiratory systems have developed in conjunction with the cardiovascular system.

Insects and Arachnids

The process of respiration in spiders is closer in function to that of vertebrates in comparison to insects.[5] The functional unit of respiration, the book lung, is structurally uniform and homologous in all pulmonate spiders and scorpions (members of class Arachnida), although it varies in number among species.[6,7] Anatomically, the book lungs lie ventrally in the anterior opisthosoma (abdomen). The entrance to the lungs communicates with the outside by a small enveloped atrium through the lung slit (or spiracle) and extends into many horizontal air sac pockets with hemolymph-filled lamellae.[8] This series of flattened air-filled cuticular plates is where the process of diffusive gas exchange occurs with hemolymph. Hemocyanin is the most common oxygen-carrying pigment of the arachnid hemolymph. This oxygen-carrying, copper-based pigment has a higher oxygen affinity than hemoglobin, and functions more in oxygen storage than transportation.[3,5,9] It is estimated that the surface area of the two-paired book lungs in a large tarantula such as *Tarantula eurypelma* is ~70 cm^2 for a volume of 10 to 30 mm.[3,8]

The tracheal system is a network of branching tubes of decreasing size that come in direct contact with the tissues in their terminal stages by means of specialized epidermal cells called tracheoblasts (Figure 3-1).[10,11] In insects, tracheae are composed of epithelial cells and an inward spiral cuticular layer called the taenidia.[12] The diameter of tracheae at the spiracles may be several millimeters, but tracheae branch and taper down to 1 to 2 μm, at which point they give rise to tracheoles lined by tracheoblasts that transfer oxygen to cell mitochondria.[12] Direct tracheal systems are mainly found in insects, although they are present and rudimentary in some arachnids. In arachnids that have both a tracheal system and book lungs, it has not been determined which is more efficient in oxygenation, nor why some lineages have such differences.[8]

When present, tracheoles are where gas exchange takes place and supply oxygen faster than book lungs.[5,6,9,13] Gas enters the tracheal system from the environment by way of spiracles found on the thoracic and abdominal segments, which may

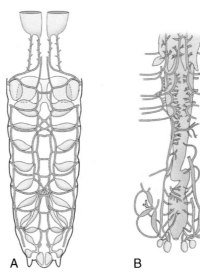

FIGURE 3-1 Views of the locust tracheal system. *A,* Dorsal system in the abdomen; *B,* tracheae associated with the alimentary canal. (From Albrecht FO: The anatomy of the migratory locust, Athlone Press, 1953.)

possess filters or muscular flaps capable of closing the openings and decreasing water loss.[8,12,14] Many insects retain tracheoles between moults.[10,15] Oxygen is transported by passive diffusion. In larger insects, pump mechanisms, such as the flight muscles, thoracic pumping, abdominal pumping, and hemolymph engorgement, may assist with ventilation in order to change tracheal tube volume or work in tandem with tracheal sacs.[12] Insects do not use their circulatory system to transport oxygen, although some species have hemoglobin dissolved in their hemolymph to help with oxygen storage. Aquatic insects have a variety of adaptive respiratory strategies, including submerging air under water (e.g., air bubbles beneath the elytra), passive diffusion through the spiracles, and tracheal gills.[12]

Mollusks

Mollusks are represented by gastropods (e.g., snails and slugs), bivalves (e.g., clams and oysters), and cephalopods (e.g., octopi and squid). The basic respiratory unit of mollusks is generally harmonized, but due to the vast species variations, an exhaustive presentation of mollusk breathing is beyond the scope of this clinical chapter. Most mollusks have true gills or ctenidia, although some have lost these anatomic structures and rely on secondary derived gills for gas exchange across their mantle or general body surface. Cephalopods tend to have a single pair of gills, except the *Nautilus*, which possesses two.[16] In species with absent cilia, the gills are more elongated and highly folded to increase body surface area for efficient gas exchange and for waste excretion.[17,18] The mantle is a secondary constituent of respiration for oxygen storage, although it has other functions in shell deposition, particle collection, retention, and sorting. It has been reported that in gravid unionids (e.g., freshwater mussels), space occupation within the mantle affects oxygen consumption and respiration.[17] In terrestrial species, such as pulmonates, the mantle cavity functions as a primitive lung. Instead of having true gills the pulmonate mantle cavity is modified into a sac-like structure with increased vasculature and an opening called the pneumostome in which a respiratory network of blood sinuses responsible for air exchange is present.[18,19]

Crustaceans

The crustacean class Malacostraca includes crabs, lobsters, shrimps, and krill. Similar to that observed in mollusks, there is a diverse variation of respiratory structure between species. Respiration in conjunction with waste removal generally occurs through the gills, which are composed of vascularized lamellae. The gills of semiterrestrial and terrestrial crabs frequently are fewer in number, have less gill surface area, and have to maintain a reduced respiratory volume compared with aquatic crabs.[20] Some crab gills are enclosed in a branchial chamber, which is formed between the thoracic body wall and the inner surface of the carapace. Respiratory exchange can occur secondarily within the branchial chamber, with variations in function that includes production of negative pressure in burrowing species.[20,21] Due to the significant interaction between the respiratory and cardiovascular systems if ventilation stops there is a subsequent cessation of the heartbeat after which the gill filaments rapidly become deoxygenated, allowing oxygen to diffuse out of the hemolymph into the environment.[21]

Fish

Water Breathing

Fish are the most diverse group of vertebrates, consequently this group of animals has tremendous interspecies differences and adaptations that should be acknowledged by the practicing veterinarian. The aquatic environment contains a lower concentration of oxygen than air because of poor oxygen dissolution in water.[22,23] Compared with air, water is more dense and viscous. Considering the lower oxygen capacity of water, water-oxygen diffusion is about 1/8000th the rate of air-oxygen diffusion.[24] Due to their lower metabolic rate and ectothermic thermoregulation, fish have low oxygen requirements in comparison to terrestrial animals, as it correlates with the oxygen availability in their respective biotopes. Tropical waters have even lower oxygen tension due to the warmer temperatures, and fish in these habitats have been evolutionarily selected for various air-breathing adaptations to enhance their survival in these hypoxic environments.[25] All fish primarily use their gills for gas exchange. There is a wide variety of accessory respiratory organs, including the skin and specialized air-breathing organs, that have evolved in a multitude of families of fish. Some of these accessory respiratory organs are exemplified in several families of ornamental fish commonly kept in private aquaria (see section on Fish: Air Breathing). In addition, gills play important functions in osmoregulation, acid-base balance, and nitrogenous waste excretion, but this chapter only focuses on the respiratory function.[26] Several excellent and comprehensive reviews have been published on the anatomy of the piscine gills and readers are invited to consult these references to gain more detailed information.[27,28] Some scaleless fish, such as catfish in the order Siluriformes, also use their skin for cutaneous respiration. Most fish larvae use passive diffusion in conjunction with cutaneous respiration.

The fish water-breathing respiratory system is composed of the gill arches, the two opercula covering the gills, and the buccal cavity in Actinopterygii (e.g., boney fish) (Figure 3-2). In Chondropterygii (e.g., sharks), which are more primitive, there are no opercula but gill slits (five to seven gill slits in elasmobranchs). In addition, elasmobranchs have a spiracle, which is a small hole caudal to the eyes for the entry of water; it is greatly reduced in some pelagic sharks.[28] Agnatha (e.g., lampreys) have seven gill slits. The general organization of the gills follows the successive subdivision of the gills into gill arches, filaments (or primary lamellae), and secondary lamellae (see Figure 3-2).[24,26-29] Modern fish species have four pairs of respiratory arches and one nonrespiratory pseudobranch on each side of the buccal cavity.

Each gill arch is composed of a skeleton (the hyoid bones) called the gill septum. The gill septum is comprised of connective tissue and bears gill rakers medially that prevent food particles from entering the opercular chamber. Each gill septum supports two hemibranchs, comprised of a series of filaments, that together form a holobranch (see Figure 3-2). The spaces between gill septae are called the gill pouches. Abductor and adductor muscles located on the gill arches regulate the opening of the gill pouches and the spreading of the filaments.[24] The hemibranchs are well differentiated in teleosts but are more fused in elasmobranchs. In elasmobranchs, an additional hemibranch is present on the anterior side of the first branchial slit.[28] The shape of the gills and the

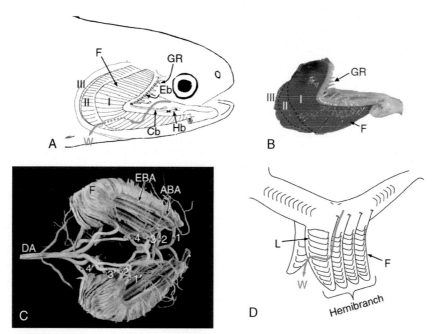

FIGURE 3-2 General orientation of the gills. *(A)* Eight gills line the buccal (mouth) cavity of the fish, four on each side. Three gills, I, II, and III, on the right side of the fish are shown. The gill arch supports the filaments *(F)* and gill rakers *(GR)*. Three bones in the arch, hypobrachial *(Hb)*, ceratobrachial *(Cb)*, and epibrachial *(Eb)*, provide strength and are hinged, permitting the gills to move with the jaw during ventilation. Water flows past the gill rakers, over the arch, and between the filaments *(green arrows, W)*. *(B)* Gills removed from a fish showing three of the four gills (*I, II,* and *III,* separated by *dashed lines*). *Dotted line* indicates plane of cross section through the arch viewed in Figure 3-2a. *(C)* Dorsal view of a vascular corrosion replica of catfish gills, anterior to right. *1-4,* Afferent branchial arteries *(ABA)* deliver blood to corresponding gill arches *(asterisk directly on vessel to left of numbers)*; 19-49 efferent brachial arteries *(EBA)* drain blood from the corresponding gill arches and deliver it to the dorsal aorta *(DA)*. *(D)* Schematic of a single gill arch showing the relationship of the filaments *(F)* of one hemibranch and the direction of water flow *(W; green arrow)* between the filaments of one hemibranch and across the respiratory lamellae *(L)*. GRs on the ventral portion of the arch are not shown. (Reprinted with permission from Olson KR. Design and physiology of arteries and veins I branchial anatomy. In: Farrell AP, ed. *Encyclopedia of Fish Physiology*. Philadelphia, PA: Elsevier; 2011:1095-1103.)

gill filaments vary tremendously among fish species. The number of filaments per hemibranch may differ between 50 to several hundred, providing high surface area for gas exchange.[27] The tips of hemibranchial filaments are in close proximity with one another in teleosts, maximizing the area of water flow across their surface. The filaments are strengthened by a cartilaginous rod providing mechanical support. The secondary lamellae vary in shape, are numerous, and located where the gas exchange occurs. Two arteries, the afferent and efferent, are present and adjacent to the filament nerve. The lamellae are plate-like structures projecting at right angles from the filaments. The direction of lamellar blood flow is counter current to the direction of water, therefore creating a cross-current gas exchange system optimizing function. Seven types of epithelial cells form the lamellae and include pavement cells (barrier), ionocytes (ion transporting cells, also called chloride cells), goblet cells (mucus producing), neuroepithelial cells (chemoreceptor cells), taste cells (absent from filaments and lamellae), undifferentiated cells, and interstitial cells.[24,28]

Two arteries located on the gill arches supply the filamental arterioles and the lamellar capillary network. The afferent branchial artery contains deoxygenated blood, whereas the efferent branchial artery contains oxygenated blood that passes across the lamellar cross-current exchange surface area. These two arteries eventually integrate into the systemic arterial circulation (dorsal aorta).[24,26] Two other vascular networks are present in the gill filaments: the nutrient and interlamellar vascular networks. The nutrient and interlamellar vascular networks perfuse the nonlamellar portion of the branchial filaments. Branchial veins collect blood from nutrient arteries of the nutrient vascular network, which arises from the branchial arteries. Branchial veins flow into the jugular or anterior cardinal veins. The function of the interlamellar vascular network is unknown, although it is believed to be part of a secondary circulatory system of fish.[24]

Ventilation is accomplished in most fish by a pump action of the buccal (buccal pump) and opercular cavities, where the direction of water flow is dependent on which orifice is open or closed. Ventilation is unidirectional in fish and consists of two phases. The first phase consists of increasing the volume of the buccal and opercular cavities, which draws water from the mouth. The second phase involves the closing of the mouth, opening the opercula, and contracting both cavities in order to direct water through the gills and the opercular opening. Water also flows completely or partially through the spiracles in elasmobranchs. In some pelagic species (e.g., tuna, sharks), ventilation is achieved by ram ventilation whereby the water flows through the mouth and gills during forward swimming.[27,29] In lampreys, where anatomically their mouth is fixed on their host, water flows through their branchial slits for both inhalation and exhalation.[28] In comparison to terrestrial mammals, oxygen is the main stimulus in triggering ventilatory changes.[26] Carbon dioxide and pH also have an effect on ventilation, but oxygen demands override acid-base disturbances in fish.[26] Additionally, peripheral chemoreceptors involved in the regulation of ventilation are located in the buccal and branchial cavities.

It is important to note that due to the multifunctional aspect of the fish gill, gill diseases not only lead to respiratory compromise but also impair several osmoregulatory mechanisms.

In cases where environmental oxygen concentrations decrease, the response of fish species may vary. Some fish migrate to more oxygenated areas, while others undergo physiological adaptations such changes in hemoglobin composition and hematocrit level and a decrease in metabolism. Over time, other groups of fish have developed unique and interesting aptitudes regarding adaptation to hypoxic environments by facultative or obligatory air breathing (see the following section).

Fish

Air Breathing

A wide variety of tropical fish have developed air-breathing capabilities. Some of these species, commonly kept as ornamental fish, include bettas, gouramis, and plecos. Aerial respiration has evolved independently over 68 times in fish and there are at least 49 extant fish families with this characteristic; thus, there is a myriad of air-breathing strategies and accessory respiratory organs.[30,31] Due to obvious space limitations to cover such a broad topic, only general features and the most relevant information is presented here. As the swim bladder is not a primary respiratory organ but a hydrostatic organ in most fish, its anatomy, physiology, and diseases are not covered in detail.

Air-breathing organs are extremely varied in form, function, and effectiveness. The air breathing organs in fish can be classified into three groups depending on their body location: organs associated with the skin, structures located on the head or along the digestive tract, and lung and respiratory bladder structures.[25,31] The skin is mainly used by amphibious fish and several species of catfish. The second category of air-breathing organs include the gills (with structural reinforcement to withstand surface tension in air); simple but specialized respiratory epithelia in the buccal, pharyngeal, branchial, and opercular areas; specialized chambers in the roof of the pharynx; specialized structures derived from the gills or opercular chamber (e.g., labyrinth apparatus of the Anabantids such as bettas and gouramis); and intestinal organs such as the esophagus, pneumatic duct, stomach, and intestines.[25,31] The third group comprises fish that have evolved paired primitive lungs from the floor of the alimentary canal with a glottis and proper pulmonary circulation (e.g., lungfish) and fish that use their swim bladder developed from the side or dorsal aspect of the alimentary canal (e.g., gars and bowfins). Lungfish are obligatory air breathers. In fish that use their swim bladder as

an air-breathing organ, the swim bladder is of the physostomous type (with a pneumatic duct connected to the caudal end of the esophagus such as in carp, trout, and salmon) whereas it is of the physoclistous type (no connection) in other fish. In physoclistous fish, oxygen is secreted by the gas gland into the swim bladder and constitutes 80% of the swim bladder gas. Thus, the swim bladder may also act as a storage organ for oxygen in some fish.[22] Certain fish (e.g., Australian gobies), while not having accessory respiratory organs, hold an air bubble within their buccal cavity to increase oxygenation of water immediately before it enters the gills.[25]

Since the vascular system of most fish, except the lungfish, is organized with all organs in serial order, there is a potential for loss of oxygen obtained through the air-breathing organs when this partially oxygenated blood is draining through the gills in poorly oxygenated water. Thus, gill exchange surface area is reduced in most species possessing well-developed air-breathing organs.[25,30]

Ventilation in air-breathing fish is usually achieved by the buccal pump: air is gulped from the surface and forced into the corresponding organ. The inhalation and exhalation process may be complex depending on the individual species' respiratory strategy.[25] Ventilatory control appears to be more complex than the oxygen-driven system of exclusively water-breathing fish, and air breathing itself is periodic.

Amphibians

Physiology and morphology of the respiratory system in amphibians differs significantly among the three different orders (Anura, Caudata, and Gymnophiona) and even within the same order. Knowledge of species variations for respiratory strategy is useful for husbandry, diagnosis, or medical management of amphibians. In this chapter, the respiratory physiology and anatomy of amphibians is presented with emphasis on clinically salient features. As frogs, toads (Anuran), followed by newts, and salamanders (Caudatan) are the most represented animals in captivity, the majority of information focuses on these two orders. Thus, caecilian particularities are rarely described in detail.

Amphibians rely on diverse modes of respiration for gas exchange, including pulmonary, branchial, buccopharyngeal, and cutaneous.[32-45] Each mode involves different vascular adaptations with the respiratory and circulatory systems closely interrelated (see amphibian cardiovascular chapter).[32,46] Depending on species, stage of development, natural history, and oxygen availability, the functional implications of these different respiratory modes may vary.[32-45] In most postmetamorphic terrestrial amphibians, lung or skin is the primary site of respiration, whereas many aquatic species and all premetamorphic stages rely on gills and skin.[32,37,43] Buccopharyngeal respiration is considered a minor site for gas exchange and part of cutaneous respiration by some authors.[35,36,38]

Cutaneous respiration is not discussed in detail in this chapter. However, veterinarians should keep in mind that skin may be the most important site for respiration in some amphibian species such as the aquatic Titicaca water frog (*Telmatobius culeus*) or the lungless salamanders (Plethodontidae).[36,47] Amphibians that predominantly rely on cutaneous respiration usually have an increased cutaneous exchange surface (e.g., skin folds, hair-like structures) and a lower metabolism.[48] Moreover, during hibernation, amphibians may switch to exclusive cutaneous respiration.[48] Skin can also be a major site of excretion of CO_2, even though O_2 may be provided by a different mode of respiration, as described in *Rana catesbeiana*, *Siren lacertina*, and *Amphiuma tridactylum*.[45,49]

Adult Anurans may present three modes of respiration: buccopharyngeal, pulmonic, and cutaneous. Newts and salamanders may rely on four modes of respiration: branchial (retained gills in neotenic species), cutaneous, buccopharyngeal, and pulmonic. Finally, caecilians can have up to three modes of respiration: pulmonic, buccopharyngeal, and cutaneous.[35,36,41]

The respiratory system in amphibians includes external nares, narial ducts, internal nares (choana), buccopharyngeal cavity, glottis, larynx, trachea, bronchi or bronchial tubes, and lungs. When such structures are present, they vary depending on species and the animal's stage of development.[32,35,36,38,50]

Embryonic respiration in both aquatic and terrestrial eggs of salamanders and viviparous caecilians is accomplished by three pairs of external gills.[33] Anuran embryos usually lack gills; however, some species may have two to three pairs of poorly developed gills.[33] In most frog species gill development usually occurs before hatching, except in *Xenopus*, *Discoglossus*, some *Scaphiopus*, and some *Bufo*, which develop these respiratory structures after hatching.[33] Other organs may contribute to embryo respiration such as maternal skin *(Pipa)*, a highly vascularized tail in terrestrial embryos, or a nonvascularized abdominal sac *(Discodeles, Platymantis)*.[33]

Respiratory studies of amphibian larval stages have only been performed in a few species; therefore, extrapolation should carried out with caution.[34] Respiration in most amphibian larvae is branchial and cutaneous.[32,34,38] Tadpoles are the only larval stage amphibian that has internal gills. All Anuran larvae have visible external gills upon hatching that are recovered by an operculum until a pair of branchial spiracles appears and forms the internal gills.[34,36,51] Gills are the major source for gaseous exchange in Anuran larvae.[35] Caudatan larvae have three pairs of plumate external gills, which resorb during metamorphosis in terrestrial forms or remain in neotenic species such as the axolotl *(Ambystoma mexicanum)* and common mudpuppy *(Necturus maculosus)*.[35,36,38] The gills of Caudatan larvae that live in ponds have moderately long fimbriae and a general bushy appearance, whereas the gills of larvae that inhabit streams have shorter and more robust fimbriae.[33,52] Viviparous caecilian larvae strongly resemble adult caecilians, although external gills are present for a few hours after birth.[35,36] Oviparous caecilian larvae have external gills that are also quickly resorbed.[35]

Adult amphibians share some particularities in their respiratory anatomy. The nostrils open to the narial duct, which leads to the buccal cavity via the choana.[32] The nostrils and corresponding narial ducts are intimately associated with the olfactory system. The buccopharyngeal cavity is composed of the mouth and the pharynx, and is covered by a highly vascularized ciliated epithelium.[32,38] The glottis is a longitudinal slit-like structure, on the floor of the pharynx, delineated cranially by the arytenoid cartilages, and is opened and closed by the mm. dilatator laryngis and constrictor laryngis, respectively.[32,50] In aquatic amphibians, the glottis tends to be much smaller than the glottis of a similar-sized terrestrial amphibian.[36] The glottis leads to a triangular chamber, the larynx, which is supported through its length by a series of semicircular cartilages, the lateral cartilages.[32,36] The trachea leads to the bronchi or bronchial tubes depending on species, which end into the lungs, if present.[32] Studies in axolotl *(Ambystoma mexicanum)*, fire

salamander *(Salamandra salamandra)*, red-bellied newt *(Taricha rivularis)*, and African clawed frog *(Xenopus laevi)* suggest that pulmonary surfactant, host defense proteins, and serotonin-positive neuroepithelial endocrine cells in amphibians are similar to those observed in mammals.[53-56]

In Anurans, the nares are closed by an upward swelling of the m. submentalis.[32] The arytenoid cartilages are an integral part of the sound-production system in Anurans and are more developed in males than in females.[32,57] The cricoid cartilage forms a complete ring in most adult amphibians except in pipid frogs *(Xenopus* and *Pipa* spp.).[32] The trachea is extremely short in Anurans and bifurcates within the lungs.[32,35,36,38] Caution should be observed during tracheal intubation and washes in these taxa in order to prevent pulmonary epithelium trauma.[32,35,36] Except in pipid frogs that have bronchi, all Anurans have bronchial tubes.[32] Anurans have simple, highly vascularized, thin, sac-like, paired lungs, which are weakly partitioned by a thin septa composed of connective tissues.[32,35,38,44,57] Positive-pressure ventilation should be carefully performed in Anurans, as pulmonary rupture can occur.[35] Anatomically, the right and the left lungs are approximately the same size, although species variations do exist such as those seen in *Ascaphus*, which are smaller in comparison to aquatic species such as pipid frogs and *Telmatobius*.[32,36] Other anatomical variations have been reported in Anurans, such as the presence of a cartilage in the lungs of pipids and variation in lung compartmentalization across amphibian species.[32,58,59] Compared to Caudatans and Caecilians, Anurans have smaller and more numerous pulmonary compartments.[32]

In Caudata, the nares are closed by smooth muscles.[32] With the exception of some aquatic salamanders *(Amphiumas, Cryptobranchus)*, Caudatans have a very short trachea, which has clinical significance during tracheal intubation, as previously described in Anurans.[35,36,50] The trachea is comprised of cartilaginous rings that also extend into the bronchi of some species.[36] The bronchi are short, wide passages that lead directly to the lungs.[50,60] Most salamanders have simple, well-developed paired lungs, with the exception of some species living in mountain streams *(Salamandrina, Rhyacotriton,* and *Onychodactylus)*, which have smaller lungs.[32,36] Plethodontid salamanders are lungless.[35,36,44] The right and the left lungs of salamanders generally are the same size, with the right side slightly smaller than the left.[36,50] Terrestrial species have sacculated lungs with highly vascularized internal septae, covered by a thin epithelium, while aquatic salamanders (mudpuppies and waterdogs, *Necturus* spp.) have single lobes.[32,35,36] In terrestrial species, each lung has two longitudinal compartments: one containing the pulmonary artery, the other the pulmonary vein.[32,60] Obligate neotenic salamanders and some aquatic salamandrids *(Notophthalmus* spp. and *Triturus* spp.) have few, poorly vascularized septae.[32] Neotenic species *(Siren* spp., *Necturus* spp., *Ambystoma mexicanum, Proteus anguinus, Typhlomolge rathbuni)* possess external gills and rely heavily on branchial respiration.[36] Some of these species *(Siren* spp., *Necturus maculosus)* have both lungs and gills.[36,43] As for Caudatan larvae, gills may present short or as long filaments, depending on their natural environment.[35,36] The hellbender *(Cryptobranchus alleganiensis)* relies almost entirely on cutaneous respiration, although lungs and a singular gill opening are present.[42]

In Caecilians, nares are closed by means of smooth muscles, as in salamanders.[32,36] Compared to Caudatans and Anurans, caecilians have an elongated trachea, which bifurcates into bronchi.[32,36] In Cayenne caecilians (*Typhlonectes compressicauda*) and red caecilians (*Uraeotyphlus oxyurus*), the trachea forms a ventral evagination, which is called the tracheal lung and contributes to gaseous exchange.[32,36] Lungs are extremely elongated paired structures, which are divided in alveoli and are infiltrated with cartilage in most caecilians.[32,36] The left lung is usually shorter in caecilians, although variation may occur with the absence of a left lung in some species.[32,35,36] Aquatic caecilians, especially ill or neonatal animals, should not be placed in an enclosure with relatively deep water, as pulmonic breathing is their most important mode of respiration.[35,36]

Since amphibians lack a diaphragm, all pulmonary and buccopharyngeal ventilation occurs through a buccopharyngeal force-pump mechanism controlled by the cranial nerves.[32,38,52,61] When the nostrils are opened and the buccal floor is depressed by contraction of the throat musculature air enters into the buccal cavity.[32,38] The nostrils then close, the buccal cavity floor is elevated, and the glottis opens, forcing air into the lungs.[32,38] The cycle then reverses: The buccal floor is depressed, the glottis opens while the nares are closed, and air is expulsed from the lungs into the buccal cavity.[32,38] The nares then open while the glottis is closed and the buccal floor is elevated, expelling air out of the mouth.[32,38] In Caudata, expiration is active via muscle contraction, whereas in Anurans and caecilians, it is passive.[52] Expiration and inspiration movements are performed by the nares in *Cryptobranchus*, *Amphiuma*, and *Triturus* and by the mouth in *Sirens*, *Necturus*, pipid frogs, and terrestrials caecilians.[32,36] Respiratory physiology in caecilians is not well described.[36] Similar but faster and oscillatory movements occur in frogs and salamanders corresponding to the ventilation of the olfactory chambers.[38,62]

Reversible adaptations of the respiratory system to the environment, such as change in the preferential mode of respiration or fimbriae development of the gills, may be seen in amphibians. These reversible adaptations of the respiratory system can occur due to oxygen availability, stress, and temperature.[34,39,40,63] Some amphibians may also change their behavior when exposed to low oxygen levels within their aquatic environment. Such behaviors include gulping air behavior in tadpoles or swimming toward the surface in salamanders, newts, and tadpoles.[34]

The respiratory system has a secondary role in amphibians other than gas exchange and includes maintaining hydrostatic, electrolytic, and metabolic homeostasis, waste excretion, and communication through vocalization between conspecifics.[32,36,41,62,63]

Reptiles

Although lungs conserved a similar basic structure and function among the various group of reptiles, major differences with significant clinical implications exist, even within orders. A sound understanding of the respiratory physiology and anatomy of reptiles is a prerequisite for managing respiratory disease, interpreting clinical tests, or monitoring anesthesia in these animals.

Upper Respiratory System

Great variations in the nasal anatomy exist among reptiles, with crocodilians having the most complex nasal cavities of the class Reptilia (clade of Sauropsida).[64] Despite the anatomical variations among reptiles' orders, anatomy of the nasal cavities within an order is very similar.[64] In crocodilians, the nares are slightly raised above the level of the upper jaw, allowing breathing while partially submerged, and adult male gharials have a large nasal excrescence, the ghara, which is supposed to act as a vocal resonator.[65] Crocodilians also maintain the control of the opening of their nares to prevent water aspiration. Moreover this group of reptiles has a large soft tissue valve in the pharynx to prevent aspiration when the oral cavity is filled with water (formed by the velum palati and gular fold).[66] In saurians, the nares are clearly visible in most species and nasal salt glands may be present in others (e.g., green iguana [*Iguana inguana*], desert species).[67] The nasal cavities in reptiles can be divided into five structures, including the vestibulum nasi, the cavum nasi proprium, the ductus nasopharyngeus, the conchae, and the Jacobson's organ.[64]

The vestibulum nasi usually is a short, simple tubular structure, located from the external nares to the cavum nasi proprium, although it may be more complex or longer in some lizards (Varanidae, Chamaelonidae, Iguanidae, and Agamidae), turtles (genera *Caretta*, *Chelonia*, *Dermochelys*, *Eretmochelys*) or snakes (*Laticauda*).[64] In chelonians, the vestibule is divided cranially by a cartilaginous septum into particularly large right and a left nasal chambers.[68,69] In tuatara (*Sphenodon* spp.), many turtles, and squamates, the limit between the vestibulum and the cavum is marked by a ridge in the lateral nasal wall.[64] Erectile tissue may be present around the vestibulum to close off the nares during immersion in some turtles and most species of squamates.[64] Histological structure cannot be generalized, as important variations of the extension of the stratified epithelium occur in lizards.[64]

The cavum nasi proprium is a large and complex chamber, located between the vestibulum and the nasopharyngeal duct, partially covered by a sensory epithelium. The cavum nasi proprium is defined by the presence of a species-dependent number of conchae, which are projections of the lateral wall of the nasal cavity into the former cavity.[64] Anatomy of the cavum nasi is highly variable among reptiles, even within the same order.[64]

The ductus nasopharyngeus is a tubular connection between the *cavum nasi* and the choana. This structure is absent in tuatara, short in most lizards, more developed in snakes and turtles, and reaches its maximum development in crocodilians.[64] The conchae are absent in chelonians but present in other reptiles.[69]

Lower Respiratory System

Reptile lungs are simple sac-like structures, which can be unicameral (snakes and some lizards), paucicameral (transitional, Iguanidae, Chamaelonidae, Agamidae), or multicameral.[69,70] Most chelonians, some squamates (e.g., Varanidae, Helodermatidae), and all crocodilians have complex multichambered lungs, whereas most other reptiles have simple, primary lungs.[69,70] The pulmonary gas exchange sites in reptiles are called ediculi (wider than deep) or faveoli (deeper than wide) and consist of small crypts instead of alveolar sacs.[71] These pulmonary gas exchange sites are much larger than mammalian alveoli and generate much less exchange surface, which is one of the reasons why reptilian lungs are larger and may occupy a large area of the coelomic cavity. Tuataras have a simple single-chambered lung and lack bronchi.[69] In addition, some reptile species may use accessory respiratory surfaces such as the skin (e.g., Trionychidae: soft-shelled turtles), buccopharyngeal (e.g., many lizards), tracheal diverticula (e.g., snakes), and cloacal bursa (e.g., some freshwater turtles).[72]

In chelonians, the air passes from the nares, through the glottis, trachea, and bronchi before entering the lungs.[71] The glottis lies at the base of a muscular fleshy tongue in chelonians.[71,73] Unlike snakes and lizard, the trachea is reinforced by complete cartilage rings and in most chelonians divides after a very short distance into two bronchi.[69,71,73] Therefore, attention should be paid during tracheal intubation to avoid passing the tube too deep into a single bronchus or damage the bronchial bifurcation.[74] The bronchi often enter the lungs dorsally relative to mammalian species.[73] A single cartilage-reinforced intrapulmonary bronchus divides the lungs into a complicated network of bronchioles and faveoli.[70,74] The lungs in chelonians are paired, similar-sized, and large sac-like organs.[68,73] They are divided in many septae and organized in faveoli, with a structure similar to a cross section of a sponge.[68,73] The lungs are located dorsally against the carapace and above the visceral organs.[68] The lungs of chelonians are attached to the ventral carapace and the vertebral column by the pulmonary ligament.[71] All intrapulmonary septae lack perforations and most species possess a complete double capillary network.[70] When the head and limbs are retracted, the lung volume reduces by one-fifth of its initial volume.[74,75] As with all reptile species, chelonians lack a true muscular diaphragm, but many possess thin, membranous, nonmuscular, diaphragm-like structures that separate the lungs from the other viscera. This is called the post-pulmonary septum, the pleuroperitoneal membrane, or the pseudodiaphragm and is absent in seaturtles.[68,71,73,74] A strong vertical membrane separates the left lung from the right.[68]

In ophidians, the glottis opening is composed of two small vertical arytenoid cartilages, is located rostrally on the floor of the oral cavity, and facilitates direct visualization and intubation in conscious snakes.[73,76,77] When swallowing large prey, the larynx can be moved forward between the tips of the mandibles or antero-laterally to the side of the mouth to allow the glottis to open and facilitate ventilation.[76] The trachea in snakes is a long, flexible air duct that goes from the glottis, through the tracheal lung (when present), and ends directly in the right lung at the level of the base of the heart.[73,76] When present, air passes into the left lung via a short left bronchus.[76] The trachea is reinforced by a species-dependent number of incomplete cartilage rings that are separated dorsally by a thin membrane. This tracheal membrane lacks muscle fibers and may expand dorsally to form the tracheal lung or the cardiac lung.[69,73,76] The tracheal lung is usually a single, vascularized, longitudinal organ that is distinguished from the lung by the presence of pulmonary constriction at the level of the heart.[76] In some species, such as marine Hydrophiidae (sea snakes), this constriction is not present and the tracheal lung forms a single structure with the right lung, called the thoraconuchal lung.[76] It is believed the tracheal lung allows gas exchange when the lung is compressed by ingested prey.[73] The cardiac lung is a structure similar to the tracheal lung but is relatively reduced in size and located in the cardiac area.[76] In snakes,

the trachea usually lies ventrally to the esophagus and passes on the left side of the heart. Exceptions exist in Scolecophidia (blind snakes), where the trachea lies on the right of the heart, and in Boidae and most snakes with a well-developed tracheal lung.[76] The lungs in snakes are elongated, membranous, and fusiform in shape with a voluminous tissue-free central axial lumen surrounded by exchange surface.[76] As a general rule, the left lung is absent or vestigial in more advanced snakes (Viperidae), while in primitive snakes (Xenopeltidae, Loxocemidae, Pythonidae, and Boidae), there is a right lung and a small left lung.[70,73,76–79] Pythons usually have two lungs whereas boas' left lung is vestigial or absent. Colubridae, however, have a vestigial left lung.[80] Total length of the lung ranges from 16% (*Uropeltis*) to 94% (*Acrochordus granulatus*) of body length, although most snakes have values between 40% and 80%.[76] All snake lungs are usually arranged in a single longitudinal unit except in Anomalepididae, Typhlopidae, and Acrochordidae, in which the lungs are multichambered.[70,76] The right lung (and the left lung in Boidae) can be divided into two major structural and functional areas.[73,76,81] First, the cranial portion, the alveolar lung, is a thick-walled and highly vascularized structure with major functions in gas exchange and constitutes up to half of the lung mass.[73,76,77] The respiratory tissue is present in this area of the lung and is composed of a honeycomb network of capillary-bearing partitions.[81,82] The second major area of the reptile lung or caudal portion, also known as the membranous lung, is a thin-walled, transparent, nonvascular and nonrespiratory structure, similar to avian air sacs and serves to store air. These two parts are separated by a transitional zone.[76] The cranial portion of the lung usually starts at 20% and ends at ~40% of the snout to cloaca length. The caudal lung extends to the rear of the animal and may reach the cloaca in some species.[73] Aquatic snakes may use this air sac to assist in buoyancy.[80]

Lizards have incomplete tracheal rings similar to those found in snakes.[73] The trachea bifurcates into a left and a right bronchus when it enters the thoracic cavity, near the base of the heart.[73] Intrapulmonary bronchi may be present (Iguanidae and Chamaeleonidae) or absent (Agamidae).[70] Lungs are usually equal in size in lizards, except in Anguimorpha and Amphibaenians.[67] Structurally, the lungs may be very simple, intermediate, air-sac-like organs (Gekkota, Scincomorpha) or a more elaborate reticulated structure with a variable number of faveoli (Varanidae, Helodermatidae).[67,73] In lizards, the lungs represent a significant volume of the coelomic cavity and in some species may extend caudally to the lumbar region during inspiration.[67] As described in snakes, the lungs can be divided into two parts: the cranial respiratory portion of the lungs and the caudal nonrespiratory air-sac-like portion.[73] For example, in skinks (Scincidae), the caudal lungs are organized into an air-sac-like structure as observed in snakes.[83] Chameleons possess large tentacular diverticula projecting from their lungs.[69,73,83] Additionally, some chameleon species have an accessory lung lobe that extends from the anterior trachea cranial to the pectoral girdle (the post-pulmonary septum).[84] Some lizards, such as monitors, possess a membrane that separates the heart and lungs from the rest of the coelomic cavity, similar to a diaphragm in mammals.[73] Two types of pneumocytes have been described in the green lizard.[85] Surfactant quantity is 70 times greater per surface area in the central netted dragon than in mammals.[86]

In Crocodilians, the glottis is caudal to the palatal valve, which seals the glottis while submerged to prevent aspiration.[66] This palatal valve is composed of a dorsal flap from the soft palate, the velum palati, and a ventral flap, the gular fold.[65,66,73] In crocodiles, the trachea passes on the left side into the thorax before bifurcating, avoiding pressure on the trachea while swallowing prey.[70] This anatomic function of the respiratory system is not found in alligators.[70] Crocodilians have complete tracheal rings. The intrapulmonary bronchus is reinforced by cartilage in the cranial half and there is variation among species.[70] In crocodiles, the intrapulmonary bronchus is straight and ends in a terminal sac; in gharials, it lies laterally; in alligators and caimans, it bends medially and terminates against the medial surface of the lung.[70] Similar to chelonians, all crocodilians have tubular, highly vascularized, sac-like multichambered lungs that lie in pleural chambers separated by a complete mediastinum.[70,73,87] The lungs in crocodilians are more complex than those of other reptiles. In crocodiles, the lungs lie loosely in the thoracic cavity, while in the caiman, they are fused to the ventral wall of the thorax.[70] Crocodilians have a pseudodiaphragm that divides the thoracic cavity from the abdomen and is comprised of two membranes: the posthepatic and the postpulmonary membrane.[66,70] The latter separates the lungs from the liver and has a muscular component.[70] The posthepatic membrane is attached to the m. diaphragmaticus, which extends to the pubis.[70] The muscular part of these membranes acts like a diaphragm by pulling the liver in a caudal direction during active inspiration in association with intercostal muscle movement.[70,73]

Microscopic anatomy of the respiratory tract is similar in reptiles.[73] The trachea is lined with a typical pseudostratified columnar epithelium with cilia and goblet cells, which transitions into a squamous epithelium in the bronchi and avascular portion of the snake lung. Pulmonary surfactant is present in faveoli.[88,89] Innervation of the reptile's lung includes cholinergic fibers and adrenergic nerves of sympathetic origin.[90]

Respiratory Physiology

For most reptiles, pulmonary respiration is the main source of oxygen uptake.[70,90] However, some species such as softshelled turtles rely almost entirely on cutaneous respiration in water.[88] One major characteristic of reptile respiratory physiology is their ability to function under anaerobic metabolism utilizing a strong blood buffering system to compensate for lactic acidosis.[73] The ability to function under anaerobic metabolism has an important clinical implication, as it allows reptiles to conceal severe respiratory diseases until the compensatory mechanisms are overwhelmed.[73]

Unlike amphibians and despite the absence of a muscular diaphragm, all reptiles use negative pressure to breathe, except chelonians. Chelonians employ positive-pressure ventilation, allowing these animals to have normal respiration despite shell compromise.[71,74,90] Respiratory cycle patterns vary depending on species.[90,91] However, all reptiles include variable periods of apnea in their respiratory cycle.[90] Lizards and snakes have active expiration and inspiration through the contraction or relaxation of the intercostal muscles, the pulmonary smooth muscles in some species, and dorso-lateral and ventro-lateral muscles.[73,90] One must not restrict ventilation in a lizard patient while holding the animal around the ribs during physical examination.[67] In snakes, the caudal avascular portion of the lung may help ventilate the vascular

portion while ingesting food, as it is cranial to the pylorus in most snakes.[90] In chelonians, respiratory physiology differs between terrestrial and aquatic species.[73,90] On land, expiration is active and inspiration is passive, whereas it is reversed in water because of the effect of gravity and hydrostatic pressure on visceral organs.[73,90] Ventilation is carried out by movements of the inguinal, axial, and shoulder muscles in order to create a pressure change within the coelomic cavity. Thus, movements of the limbs are observed during normal respiration. Some aquatic turtles use other respiratory surfaces, the most notable being the cloacal bursa during periods of underwater hibernation. In crocodilians, expiration and inspiration are both active processes.[90] However, expiration becomes passive when the crocodilians are submerged, as with turtles.[90] The diaphragmaticus muscles in association with the intercostal and abdominal muscles produce coelomic volume variation by pulling on the caudal part of the liver.[65,90]

In reptiles, the stimulus to breathe comes from low blood oxygen concentration.[73] Ventilation is controlled by partial pressures of oxygen (PO_2), and carbon dioxide (PCO_2), acid-base balance, and stretch receptor feedback in the pulmonary parenchyma. Low PO_2 seems to be more important than high PCO_2 in the control of respiration, especially in turtles, although most species are extremely tolerant to hypoxia.[90] Lizards are generally more sensitive to PCO_2 than turtles, depending on species and ecologic behavior (divers, burrowers).[90] In aquatic snakes, hypoxia is the main factor for controlling ventilation.[90] Increase in oxygen demand with higher temperature is not met with an increase in respiratory rate but rather an increase in tidal volume.[73] Hypercapnea causes an increase in tidal volume by suppressing pulmonary stretch receptors. Hypoxia results in an increase in respiratory rate.[71,73]

Some aquatic species have respiratory adaptations related to their diving behavior (e.g., loggerhead sea turtles) where there is reduced airway resistance and muscular contributions toward breathing.[92] The lungs function as a major oxygen store in loggerhead sea turtles and may provide oxygen for up to 20 minutes of submersion.[93] Prolonged submersion (at least 3 h) is possible due to their high anaerobic capacity.[93] This diving reflex may prevent the animal from reaching effective planes of anesthesia.[68]

Gular movements may be observed in some reptiles and are often not related to gas exchange. However gular movements have been associated with communication with conspecifics. This behavior may be displayed with olfaction in turtles and crocodilians, courtship in chameleons by inflation of the gular pouch, or defensive behavior in the chuckwalla.[65,70,90] In snakes, the avascular part of the lung acts as an oxygen store but also cools the testes and plays a role in buoyancy.[90] In chelonians, the lungs play a significant role in buoyancy. Other pulmonary functions found in reptiles are locomotion in snakes, hydrostatic role, behavior and threat display (e.g., lung volume increase in some lizards to prevent them from being extracted from their rock crevice), or vocalization (chameleons, snakes).[67,77,90] In some aquatic and semiaquatic turtles, abnormalities in flotation may be observed with respiratory disease. The abnormal posture of the turtle when floating may be associated with the hydrostatic function of the lungs, although abnormal flotation may also occur with excessive gas in intestines or extrapulmonary ectopic air in the coelomic cavity due to pulmonary trauma.[68]

Mammals

The respiratory system of small mammals is more familiar to veterinarians, as there is a uniform anatomy among all mammalian species with specific adaptations to suit environmental and evolutionary pressures. Detailed descriptions of mammalian anatomy and physiology are beyond the scope of this chapter, in which only a review of comparative differences between the species is outlined.

The primary function of the respiratory system is the gaseous exchange of oxygen and carbon dioxide between the air in the lungs and cells of the body. During the process of respiration, air is moved back and forth through the airways to transport gases and eliminate waste perpetuating gaseous exchange at the level of the respiratory surfaces. Inspired air is a mixture of 79.4% nitrogen, 20.9% oxygen, and 0.03% carbon dioxide. In contrast, expired air in mammals consists of 80% nitrogen, 16% oxygen, and 4% carbon dioxide.[94] In addition to providing gas exchange, the respiratory system has other functions in mammals:[95]

- Facilitation of venous return to the heart
- Participation in bicarbonate buffering system of the blood by regulating the exhalation of CO_2
- Removal of heat and water from the body by warming saturation of inhaled air with water vapor prior to expiration. Respiratory heat loss is due to evaporation.
- Production of sounds and therefore communication
- Homeostatic regulation of other bodily systems such as angiotensin-converting enzyme released from the lung capillaries involved with the renin-angiotensin system in the regulation of systemic blood pressure and fluid homeostasis.

As in other taxons, the mammalian respiratory system anatomically can be divided into the upper and lower respiratory tract. The upper respiratory tract consists of the nares, the paranasal sinuses, pharynx, larynx, and trachea, while the lower respiratory tract consists of the bronchi, lung parenchyma, mediastinum, pleural cavity, and chest wall. Air flows through the nostrils across the alar folds in the nasal cavity. The upper lip, divided by a cleft in rabbits and rodents, is known as the philtrum. The nasal cavity is divided into the left and right septum. In guinea pigs, two recesses are present within the nasal cavity: the rostral and maxillary recess.[96] In rabbits, both dorsal and maxillary recesses are also present. Ventrally, the nasal cavity is separated from the oral cavity, cranially by the hard palate and caudally, the soft palate. Each portion of the nasal cavity has dorsal and ventral nasal conchae that extend into the cavity from the lateral walls.[95] In rabbits and rodents, the nasal conchae also house the vomeronasal organ and olfactory sense organs.[97] Mucosa lines the nasal conchae, which are scrolls of cartilaginous tissue that aim to humidify air as it is inspired and may have olfactory function. The upper respiratory anatomy of the rabbit is outlined in Figure 3-3.

There are extensions into the maxillary, ethmoid paranasal sinuses that open from the nasal conchae. Rabbits and rodents are obligate nasal breathers and any signs of open-mouth breathing are strongly suggestive of primary or secondary respiratory disease.[98,99] The pharynx is located at the caudal ventral area of the oral cavity and continues through the glottis that opens into the larynx. This connection between the pharynx and the trachea also contains paired vocal folds for communication among conspecifics.

Anatomically, the rabbit epiglottis is dorsal to the soft palate, while in rodents, the larynx lies dorsally within the oropharynx in close association with the nasopharynx.[100–103] In rabbits, the epiglottis is large and the glottis small. Rabbits and rodents seem to have a high susceptibility to laryngospasm thus, when associated with their anatomical properties makes these animals difficult to intubate without experience using a blind intubation technique or endoscopic guidance.[97,98,104] There is no laryngeal ventricle in the guinea pigs and the vocal cords are small and poorly developed.[96]

The trachea is divided anatomically into the cervical and thoracic trachea. Rodents possess Clara cells in the bronchial epithelium, which are thought to provide the major component of the distal mucociliary escalator.[105] The trachea bifurcates in the thorax and splits into principal bronchi that ultimately ventilate the pulmonary lobes via first-, second-, and third-order bronchi.[106] Terminal bronchioles anatomically mark the end of the bronchiolar tree and at its termination are the respiratory units consisting of the pulmonary blood vessels to a respiratory bronchiole, alveolar duct, and alveoli.[106] The rabbit lung does not contain respiratory bronchioles but rather terminates into vestibules, which contain alveoli.[107] The guinea pig has very prominent smooth muscle in the distal bronchi.[96]

The lungs consist of several lobes, with number varying between the species of exotic companion mammals commonly treated by veterinarians. Rabbits have three left and three right pulmonary lobes, but the right caudal lung lobe has increased subdivisions, the lateral and medial lobes (Figure 3-4).[103] In most rodents including guinea pigs, hamsters, chinchillas, and degus, the right lung has four lobes (see Figure 3-4).[96,108] In hamsters, the left lung has a single lobe.[109] In rats, the left lung is not subdivided and the right lung has four lobes (see Figure 3-4),[110] while in ferrets, the left lung has two lobes and the right lung four.[111] Generally, the left cranial lobe is smaller than the right due to the presence of the heart. It has been suggested that because there is no septae dividing the lungs into lobules in rabbits and guinea pigs, generalized pneumonia is commonly diagnosed when compared to other small exotic mammalian species.[96,102] The thoracic, as opposed to the abdominal cavity of rabbits and rodents, is relatively small compared to other mammals including the ferret. The pleura is a membrane that lines the visceral and parietal surfaces of the lung. The cavity within the two pleural layers houses a potential space called the pleural cavity. The mediastinum anatomically is the partition between the left and right pleural cavities.

The primary source of oxygenated blood to the respiratory system is via the pulmonary trunk from the conus arteriosus arising from the right ventricle. Blood flow from the respiratory system involves the pulmonary veins that course into the left atrium of the heart after collecting venous blood from the visceral pleura and bronchi. The pulmonary vein of most rodents is thicker.[105] There is a large lymphatic drainage network associated with the respiratory system, where lymph nodes are found within the thoracic cavity including the tracheobronchial lymph nodes. Bronchus-associated lymphoid tissue is common in rabbits and rats, but absent in hamsters.[97] The vagus nerve, sympathetic nerve, and the phrenic nerves contribute to the pulmonary plexus that, in turn, branch away from the lungs. The thymus regresses in adult dogs and cats, although in the rabbit, it persists into adult life and retains

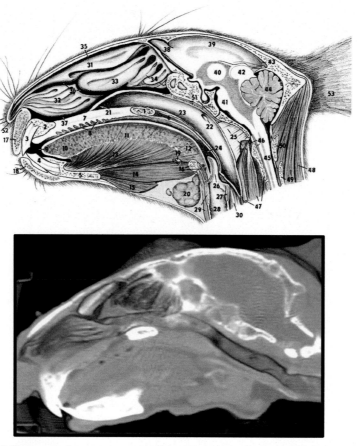

FIGURE 3-3 Upper respiratory system and head anatomy in the rabbit *(top)* with corresponding CT segmentation *(bottom). 1,* Palatin process of maxilla; *2,* incisive bone; *3,* upper incisor; *4,* lower incisor; *5,* body of mandible; *6,* soft palate; *7,* hard palate; *8,* proper oral cavity; *9,* oral cavity; *10,* apex of tongue; *11,* body of tongue; *12,* root of tongue; *13,* genioglossal muscle; *14,* geniohyoid muscle; *15,* mylohyoid muscle; *16,* lingual vein, body of hyoid bone, thyrohyoid muscle; *17,* upper lip; *18,* lower lip; *19,* deep branch of lingual nerve; *20,* mandibular lymph nodes; *21,* choana; *22,* pharyngeal ostium of auditory tube; *23,* nasal part of pharynx; *24,* oral part of pharynx; *25,* pharyngobasilar fascia, medial retropharyngeal lymph nodes; *26,* epiglottis; *27,* cartilaginous cricoid plate; *28,* trachea; *29,* cartilaginous thyroid plate, sternohyoid muscle; *30,* esophagus; *31,* dorsal nasal concha; *32,* ventral nasal concha; *33,* medial nasal concha; *34,* endoturbinate; *35,* dorsal nasal meatus; *36,* medial nasal meatus; *37,* ventral nasal meatus; *38,* olfactory tube; *39,* cerebral hemisphere; *40,* interthalamic adhesion; *41,* pons; *42,* mesencephalic tectum; *43,* dorsal sagittal sinus; *44,* cerebellum; *45,* spinal medulla; *46,* ventral arch of atlas, ventral internal vertebral plexus; *47,* internal jugular vein, long muscle of head, and axis; *48,* trapezius muscle; *49,* spinous process of axis, splenius muscle of head; *50,* dorsal arch of atlas, dorsal straight muscle of head; *51,* nasal venous plexus, sphenopalatine vein; *52,* nostril; *53,* auricle. (Reprinted with permission from Popesko P, et al. *Colour Atlas of Anatomy of Small Laboratory Animals,* Volume 1. London, UK: Saunders, 2003.)

considerable size, lying ventral to the heart and extending forward to the thoracic inlet.[112] Comparatively, only in young ferrets is the thymus prominent, and it can extend up to the cranial mediastinum.[113]

Small mammals often have very high chest wall compliances and low functional residual capacities.[105] Breathing in rabbits is through contraction of the diaphragm and in cases where resuscitation is needed and artificial respiration is required, suspension of the rabbit horizontally in midair with the one hand on each limb rocking head up/head down every 2 seconds can be effective in recovering the patient.[97,112] There

is limited ability for heat exchange in small mammals, particularly in rabbits and rodents that have absence of sweat glands; these animals are unable to pant and rely on heat dissipation primarily through their ears and tail. This is in contrast to canines whose primary form of heat regulation is via the respiratory system and footpads.[114] Additionally, the rabbit glottal and proximal tracheal areas are well vascularized and may be involved with thermoregulation.

The physiology of ventilation in mammals is quite different from other vertebrates in that inspiration is an active process that works using the negative pressure of the pleural

Rabbit

Guinea pig

Rat

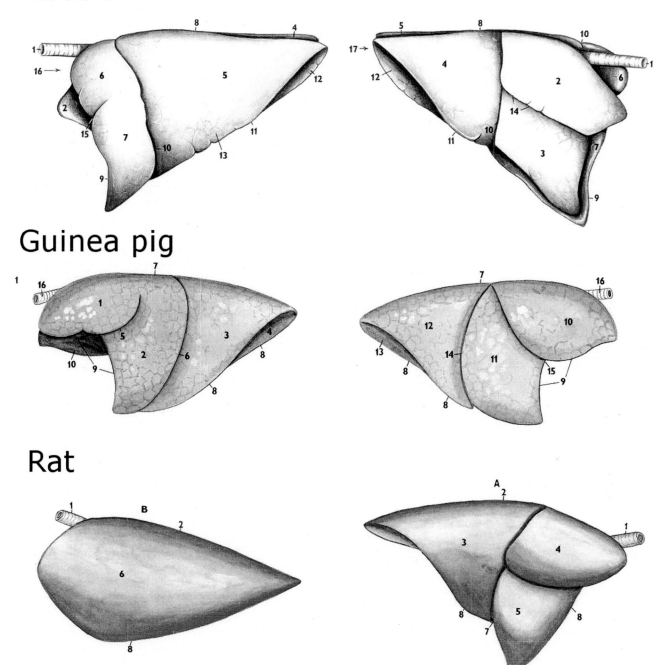

FIGURE 3-4 External anatomy of the left and right surfaces of the lungs in rabbits (*1,* trachea; *2,* right cranial lobe; *3,* right medial lobe; *4,* right caudal lobe; *5,* left caudal lobe; *6,* cranial part of the left cranial lobe; *7,* caudal part of left cranial lobe; *8,* dorsal margin; *9,* ventral margin; *10,* caudal interlobar fissure; *11,* basal margin; *12,* diaphragmatic surface; *13,* costal surface; *14,* cranial interlobar fissure of right lung; *15,* cardiac incisures of left lung; *16,* pulmonary apex; *17,* pulmonary base), guinea pigs (*1,* cranial part of cranial lobe; *2,* caudal part of cranial lobe; *3-4,* caudal lobe; *4,* diaphragmatic surface; *5,* cardiac notch of left lung; *6,* interlobar fissure; *7,* dorsal margin; *8,* acute margin; *9,* ventral margin; *10,* cranial lobe; *11,* medial lobe; *12-13,* caudal lobe; *13,* diaphragmatic surface; *14,* interlobar fissure; *15,* cardiac notch of right lung; *16,* trachea), and rats (*1,* trachea; *2,* dorsal margin; *3,* caudal lobe of right lung; *4,* cranial lobe of right lung; *5,* medial lobe of right lung; *6,* left lung; *7,* interlobar incisures; *8,* ventral margin). (From Popesko P, Rajtová V, Horák J. A *Colour Atlas of the Anatomy of Small Laboratory Animals.* Vol. 1. Wolfe Publishing Ltd; 1992.)

space induced by chest expansion. Expiration is passive. Ventilatory movements are primarily stimulated by dissolved CO_2 in the blood with hypercapnea increasing ventilation, although oxygen and blood pH also contribute.

Birds

The avian respiratory system is probably the most efficient gas exchange system of the animal kingdom and possesses a number of anatomical features unique to birds. When compared with the more familiar respiratory system of domestic mammals, some anatomical and physiological differences are striking and have major clinical implications for anesthesia, diagnostic techniques, and therapeutics (Tables 3-1 and 3-2). An excellent understanding of the complex avian respiratory anatomy is critical to the practice of avian medicine and surgery, as it is found in or around virtually every organ. Therefore, the respiratory system is described in greater detail for birds than for other animal groups.

The Upper Respiratory System

The upper respiratory system of birds is composed of the nasal cavity, the infraorbital sinus, and its diverticula. The external openings to the nasal cavity are the nostrils or nares, which are often located at the base of the beak and may be covered by feathers (e.g., eclectus parrots, some macaws, crows, grouse). There is wide anatomical diversity in the anatomy of the avian nostrils. Avian nares can be perforated (e.g., Gruiformes, Cathartiformes), closed (e.g., some Pelecaniformes), located at the tip of the beak (e.g., kiwis), have a tubular form (e.g., Procellariiformes), and bear a nasal operculum (e.g., Psittaciformes, some Galliformes).[115-117] The left and right nasal cavities are separated by the nasal septum that is perforated in a few species (perforated nares above). The nasal cavity is divided successively into the nasal vestibule with a squamous epithelium that contains the rostral nasal concha, the respiratory region with a mucociliary epithelium and containing the middle nasal concha, and the olfactory chamber

with an olfactory epithelium and caudal nasal concha (absent in African gray parrots).[116,117] In all aquatic birds, a mucosal fold, the nasal valve, arises from the roof of the nasal cavity or the septum. This valve deflects water away from the olfactory chamber.[115-117] The conchae are cartilaginous structures that increase surface areas by scroll formations, which limit heat and water loss during ventilation.[118] The rostral concha is visible through the nostrils in Falconiformes and occludes much of the opening (different from the psittacine nasal

---

TABLE 3-1

Major Anatomical and Physiological Differences in the Respiratory System of Birds Compared to Mammals

Fixed external nares
Larynx: lack of epiglottic and thyroid cartilages
No vocal cords
Complete tracheal rings
Elongated trachea, wider tracheal lumen
Increased tracheal dead space
Sound produced by the syrinx
Single paranasal sinus with many diverticulae
Lungs filled with parabronchi and air capillaries
Presence of large air sacs
Larger tidal volume
No functional diaphragm
Fusion of parietal and visceral pleura
Active exhalation and inspiration
Respiratory system pneumatizes most bones and cavities
Thinner blood-gas barrier
Cross-current gas exchange

TABLE 3-2

Major Clinical Implications of Some Anatomical Peculiarities of the Avian Respiratory System

Medical Area	Implications
Anesthesia	• Use of uncuffed endotracheal tubes • Air sac perfusion anesthesia possible • Increased respiratory depression of inhalants/inhibition of intrapulmonary chemoreceptors • Positive effect of IPPV on cardiac output • Fast induction and recovery • Increased tidal volume and tracheal dead space • Capnography not accurate with breach into the air sac system • Intermittent positive ventilation does not decrease blood pressure
Surgery	• Some surgeries require penetration into the air sac system • Wound irrigation may cause fluid aspiration (e.g., pneumatized bone fracture, abdominal surgery, sinusotomy) • Subcutaneous emphysema is a common minor complication
Disease pathogenesis	• High susceptibility to airborne toxins • Poor drainage of sinusal exudate (dorsal openings into nasal cavity) • Respiratory diseases may spread to organs surrounded by air sac diverticula • Fluid, organomegaly, masses may decrease air sac volumes and thus ventilation
Diagnostics	• Air sac system allows coelioscopy without insufflation • Sinus exudate can be collected via transcutaneous punctures • Decreased ultrasound windows throughout the body • Better delineation of coelomic organs on radiographs than in mammals
Therapeutics	• Nebulized particles should be below 1 to 2 μm to reach air capillaries • Nebulized particles are less likely to be deposited in cranial air sacs • Low drug distribution into air sac membranes

IPPV, Intermittent positive-pressure ventilation.

operculum).[117] The largest concha is the middle, which is lined by a mucociliary epithelium that acts as a primary defense against infections. The rostral and middle conchae communicate with the nasal cavity through a common meatus nasalis, but the caudal concha only connects to the infraorbital sinus. The nasal gland (salt gland in marine birds) discharges salt secretions within the nasal vestibule in marine and some desert birds. The nasolacrimal duct empties into the nasal cavity. The olfactory function is accomplished by the olfactory epithelium lining the nasal surface of the caudal concha within the nasal cavity.[115] Some birds such as kiwis, turkey vultures, petrels, and albatrosses have an exceptional sense of smell. The nasal cavity also participates in air filtration and communicates with the oropharynx through the choana in its roof. The soft palate is absent in birds.

Birds have only one paranasal sinus, the infraorbital sinus, which communicates dorsally with the nasal cavity and the caudal concha and pneumatizes most structures of the head and neck (Figure 3-5).[115,116] It should be noted that the quadrate bone, articular bone, and most bones of the braincase are pneumatized by diverticula arising from the tympanic cavity (whose opening is the infundibular cleft) with no connection to the upper respiratory system.[119] The lateral wall of the infraorbital sinus is made of soft tissues and skin. The sinus is particularly well developed in Psittaciformes where many diverticula are present (see Figure 3-5) but is absent in some cormorants.[116,120-122] In Amazon parrots, one rostral unpaired

diverticulum and six paired diverticula have been described (see Figure 3-5).[121] In macaws, two rostral unpaired diverticula (including the transverse canal) and eight paired diverticula have been identified.[120] However, the terminology and characterization of psittacine paranasal diverticula are not homogeneous and somewhat confusing. Right and left sinuses communicate in psittacine birds through the transverse canal, while this interface is not present in most other birds (e.g., Passeriformes).[116,120,121] The largest diverticulum of the psittacine paranasal sinus is the cervicocephalic diverticulum, which can reach as far as the shoulder and is not connected to the lower respiratory system (see Figure 3-5). The cervicocephalic diverticulum should therefore not be mistaken for an air sac.[116,120]

The Larynx, Trachea, and Syrinx

The avian larynx consists of four cartilages: the cricoid, procricoid, and two arytenoid cartilages.[115,116,123] The cricoid cartilage forms the body of the larynx, the arytenoid cartilages enclose the glottis forming the laryngeal mount, and the procricoid is a small caudal cartilage articulating with the cricoid wings and arytenoids. The epiglottic and thyroid cartilages as well as the vocal cords are lacking in birds. In birds, the larynx does not generate sound but may serve to modulate along with the tongue, as observed in parrots.[123-125] In several species (e.g., pelicans, hornbills, kiwis, penguins, some ducks, etc.) a median crest, the crista ventralis, arises ventrally from the

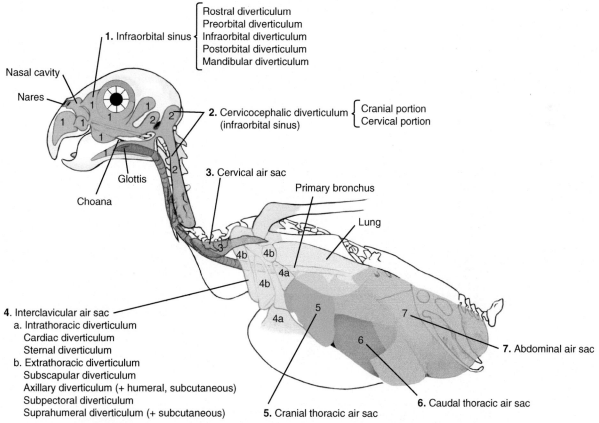

FIGURE 3-5 Respiratory anatomy of the Amazon parrot. (Modified and reprinted with permission from McKibben J, Harrison G. Clinical anatomy, with emphasis on the Amazon parrot. In: Harrison GJ, Harrison LR, eds. *Clinical Avian Medicine and Surgery*. Philadelphia, PA: W.B. Saunders; 1986:31-66.)

cricoid cartilage inside the glottis and should be avoided during endotracheal intubation.[116,123] The dilator and constrictor muscles of the larynx control the glottal opening.[116]

The avian trachea shows a high variability in length and anatomy, which can be extreme and is lined by a ciliated columnar epithelium (see Figure 3-31; see McLelland 1985 for a complete overview).[123] The avian trachea typically starts in the midline and passes slightly to the right side of the neck as it enters the thoracic inlet. In some species, the trachea is particularly elongated and presents as tracheal loops. When present, the loops may be encased into the keel, such as found in trumpeter swans (*Cygnus buccinator*) and whooping cranes (*Grus Americana*) (see Figure 3-31) or located subcutaneously (e.g., helmeted curassows (*Crax pauxi*), magpie geese (*Anseranas semipalmata*), trumpeters (*Psophia* spp.), some birds of paradise). Furthermore, other tracheal adaptations may be encountered including tracheal sacs which are found in the emu (*Dromaius novaehollandiae*) and the male ruddy duck (*Oxyura jamaicensis*). Bulbous expansions of the trachea are also present in the males of certain duck species including the rosy-billed pochard (*Netta peposaca*) and usually occur in the midtrachea (see Figure 3-31). Penguins and petrels have a double trachea formed by a septum extending from the bronchial bifurcation. This septum is particularly pronounced in the black-footed penguin (*Spheniscus demersus*) and *Aptenodytes* penguins but is shortened in most other species of penguins and petrels. Mynahs and toucans have a slight ventral kink to the trachea before it enters the thorax. Tracheal cartilages are complete in birds but asymmetric with a broader half part usually overlapping the narrow parts of the two adjacent rings. The increased tracheal length in birds is compensated by an increased tracheal diameter, resulting in a resistance to tracheal airflow being similar to mammals. However, the tracheal dead space is about four times that of mammals, which is compensated by a larger tidal volume.

The syrinx is a complex structure in voice production unique to birds (Figure 3-6). It is located at the bronchial bifurcation, is surrounded by the interclavicular air sac, and is a particularly advanced structure in Psittaciformes and Passeriformes (songbirds). The syrinx exhibits many variations among species and is typically categorized into tracheobronchial (most common) and bronchial types.[115,116,126] The main structures of the syrinx include the tympanum, the structural body of the organ, the pessulus that divides the airway vertically, and the paired medial and lateral tympaniform membranes, which are the vibrating structures (see Figure 3-6). In addition to these structures, a left dilation of the tympanum, the syringeal bulla, is frequently present in the males of Anatidae.[116] The syrinx of Psittaciformes has been described in detail and lacks the pessulus (see Figures 3-6 and 3-12).[126,127] Sound production is controlled by a number of syringeal muscles. Psittaciformes possess two unique pairs of short syringeal muscles: the superficial and deep syringeal muscles (see Figure 3-6). Passeriformes may have up to five pairs of intrinsic syringeal muscles.[116,126]

The avian airway muscles can be divided into laryngeal, tracheal, and syringeal muscles and a large number of these muscles are encountered with species-specific anatomical variations. The syringeal muscles are the most variable of the avian airway muscles. The reader is invited to consult the *Nomina Anatomica Avium* and the work of King and McLelland for a complete description of the avian airway muscles.[116,123,126]

The Lung-Air Sac System

The avian lungs are located dorsally and do not enclose the heart as in mammals (see cardiology chapter). The lungs are not lobed and are indented dorsally by the vertebral ribs. The caudal border usually reaches to the ilium but may extend as far as the hip joints (e.g., storks, geese).[115,128] The lungs are bordered ventrally by the horizontal septum.

The airways are formed by the two primary bronchi that bifurcate at the level of the syrinx, continue within the pulmonary parenchyma (intrapulmonary primary bronchi),

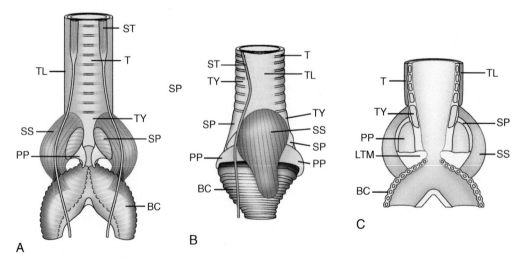

FIGURE 3-6 Diagram of the cockatiel *(Nymphicus hollandicus)* syrinx. *A,* External ventral view; *B,* external left-side view; *C,* horizontal section. *BC,* Bronchial cartilage; *LTM,* lateral tympaniform membrane; *PP,* paired protrusions; *SP,* m. syringealis profundus; *SS,* m. syringealis superficialis; *ST,* m. sternotrachealis; *T,* trachea; *TL,* m. tracheolateralis; *TY,* tympanum (composed of 4 tracheosyringeal cartilages). (Modified and reprinted from Larsen ON, Goller F, 2002. Direct observation of syringeal muscle function in songbirds and a parrot. *J Exp Biol.* 205:25-35, with permission from the Company of Biologists Limited.)

and end caudally into the abdominal air sac (see Figure 3-5). Four groups of secondary bronchi arise from the primary bronchi and are, from cranial to caudal, the medio-ventral, medio-dorsal, latero-ventral, and latero-dorsal secondary bronchi.[115,116,128,129] Multiple parabronchi branch and anatomose off the secondary bronchi. The anastomosed parabronchi carry atria, which lead to infundibula and air capillaries, with the latter constituting the gas exchange structures of the avian lungs. Atria bear atrial muscles forming a network of muscle bundles capable of regulating parabronchial and

atrial diameters. The largest bundles are found at the orifices of the parabronchi.[128] Bronchial muscles are also present in the primary and secondary bronchi. The parabronchial lungs are divided into two structural units: the paleopulmo and the neopulmo (Figure 3-7). The paleopulmo, in which ventilation is unidirectional, is formed by the medioventral-mediodorsal system of bronchi and parabronchi. Located cranially and dorsomedially, the paleopulmo is characterized by layers of hooplike parallel parabronchial connections between the secondary bronchi. The neopulmo, in which ventilation is

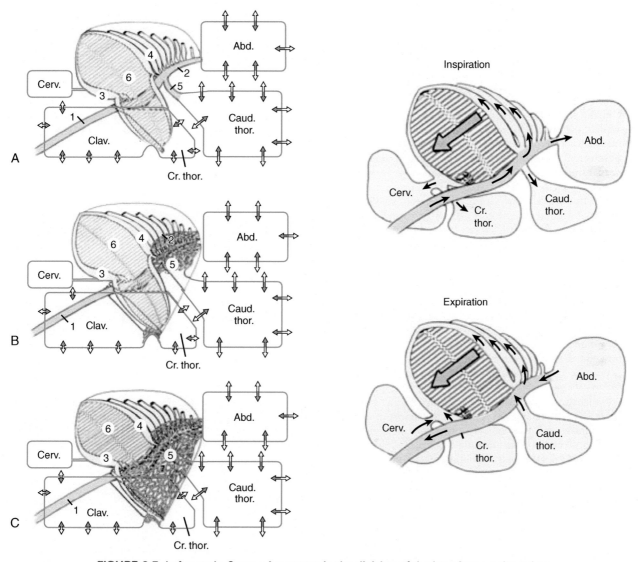

FIGURE 3-7 *Left panels,* Successive stages in the division of the lung into a paleopulmo and neopulmo. *A,* Lungs composed only of the paleopulmo such as observed in Sphenisciformes; *B,* moderate development of the neopulmo forming the caudal part of the lungs such as observed in Anseriformes; *C,* highly developed neopulmo occupying the entire lateroventral aspect of the lungs, such as occuring in Passeriformes. *1,* Trachea; *2,* primary bronchus; *3,* medioventral secondary bronchi; *4,* mediodorsal secondary bronchi; *5,* latero-ventral secondary bronchi; *6,* paleopulmo; *7,* neopulmo. *Right panels,* The length of the *white arrows* indicates the estimated dilatation of the air sacs in inspiration; the length of the *shaded arrows* the estimated compression in expiration. Cerv., cervical air sac; Cr. thor., cranial thoracic air sac; Caud. thor., caudal thoracic air sac; Abd., abdominal air sac, Clv., interclavicular air sac. (Modified and reprinted with permission from McLelland J. Anatomy of the lungs and air sacs. In: King A, McLelland J, eds. *Form and Function in Birds,* Volume 3. London, UK: Academic Press; 1985b:221-280.)

bidirectional, is formed by an anastomosing network of para-bronchi connecting the lateroventral-laterodorsal system of bronchi to each other and to other secondary bronchi. The neopulmo is superficially located caudally and ventrolaterally, constitutes less than a third of the pulmonary parenchyma, absent in Sphenisciformes, and most developed in Passeriformes (see Figure 3-7). In contrast to dead-ending mammalian alveoli, the air capillaries anastomose freely with each other and have a diameter ranging from 3 μm (e.g., passerines) to 10 μm (e.g., penguins, swans). A surfactant covers the exchange surface and prevents collapse.[128–130] Air and blood capillaries are entwined in a cross-current pattern in such a manner that the blood-gas barrier is much thinner than in mammals creating a cross-current system allowing blood to become oxygenated at different degrees along the parabronchus.[115,128,129,131] This arrangement in combination with greater surface exchange areas and thinner blood-gas barrier makes the avian lung a more efficient gas exchange mechanism than other vertebrate lung configurations.

In birds, the lungs communicate with extrapulmonary thin-walled transparent chambers, the air sacs, which are responsible for respiratory ventilation. While six pairs of air sacs develop in the avian embryo, the definitive number is reduced and usually comprises nine air sacs: two cervical air sacs, one interclavicular air sac, two cranial thoracic air sacs, two caudal thoracic air sacs, and two abdominal air sacs (see Figure 3-5). Notable exceptions to this classic configuration include passerines with seven air sacs (cranial thoracic air sacs fused to the interclavicular air sac), chickens with eight (fused cervical air sacs), storks with 11 (caudal thoracic air sacs divided into two), and turkeys with five (caudal thoracic air sacs absent, cervical air sacs fused to two primordial clavicular air sacs, one small pair of clavicular air sacs).[115] Multiple diverticula arise from the air sacs and pneumatize various anatomical structures with important species variations (see Figure 3-5). For a complete description of the air sac topographical anatomy and their different diverticula, the reader is invited to consult the corresponding specific references.[128,129] The cervical air sacs are associated with vertebral and large subcutaneous diverticula depending on species (e.g., gannets, ostriches). The interclavicular air sac is the origin of a large number of intra- and extrathoracic diverticula including two large axillary diverticula; surrounding the heart, and pneumatizing the sternum, coracoids, and humerus. The cranial and caudal thoracic air sacs are located below the lungs and incorporate most of the thoracic space. The walls of the thoracic air sacs are fused medially to the horizontal and oblique septum and laterally and ventrally to the body wall. The abdominal air sacs are the largest air sacs in most species that are commonly presented to veterinary practices, although one of the smallest in penguins. Both the perirenal diverticula, which is dorsal to the kidneys, and femoral diverticula pneumatizing the femurs arise from the abdominal air sacs. The air sac walls are formed of squamous cells and connective tissue with very little vascularization.

The air sacs are connected to the lungs through the ostia, which may network with both primary (termination of bronchi) and secondary (termination of parabronchi). When a large number of parabronchi forms a funnel-like tubular structure, it is termed a saccobronchus (present with the caudal thoracic and abdominal air sacs).[115,128] The cervical,

caudal thoracic, and abdominal air sacs have one ostium and the cranial thoracic and interclavicular air sacs have two (medial and lateral).

Respiratory Mechanics and Regulation

In contrast to mammals, the avian lung does not participate in ventilation. Ventilation in birds is performed by the air sac system, which in turn does not play any direct role in gas exchange. Air sacs act as bellows to ventilate the lungs. Therefore, the avian lungs are practically rigid and vary minimally in volume. Avian lungs are also unique in that ventilation is both tidal as in mammals (bidirectional in neopulmo) and through-flow (unidirectional in paleopulmo). The air sacs are functionally divided into two groups: the cranial group of air sacs composed of the cervical, interclavicular, and cranial thoracic air sacs receiving expiratory air and the caudal group of air sacs that include the caudal thoracic and abdominal air sacs, which receive inspiratory air.[129,131] The inspired air goes directly to the caudal air sacs, bypassing the medioventral secondary bronchi through a process called the inspiratory aerodynamic valving.[129] Expiratory flow from the caudal air sacs is directed through the paleopulmonic lungs through the mediodorsal secondary bronchi by expiratory aerodynamic valving terminating in the cranial air sacs (see Figure 3-7). Air is finally expelled from the cranial air sacs and goes successively through the medioventral secondary bronchi, the intrapulmonary primary bronchi, and the trachea.[129,132] Flow is bidirectional in the neopulmo, which is in series with the caudal air sacs. Two respiratory cycles are necessary for a given volume of inspired air to move through the avian respiratory system.

In birds, both inspiration and expiration are active processes and the relaxed sternal position is at midpoint between end-inspiration and end-expiration. In addition, the thoracic cavity is not at subatmospheric pressure as in mammals and a large number of muscles participate in ventilation. The intercostal and abdominal muscles are the main respiratory muscles but other muscles are also involved (Table 3-3).[128,131] All abdominal muscles are expiratory. In some birds, the furcula and sternum

TABLE 3-3

Ventilatory Muscles in Birds

Inspiratory Muscles	Expiratory Muscles
M. scalenus	Mm. intercostales externi (5th and 6th spaces)
Mm. intercostales externi (except 5th and 6th spaces)	Mm. intercostales interni (3rd to 6th spaces)
M. intercostalis interni (2nd space)	M. costosternalis pars minor
M. costosternalis pars major	M. obliquus externus abdominis
Mm. levatores costarum	M. obliquus internus abdominis
M. serratus profundus	M. transversus abdominis
	M. serratus superficialis pars cranialis and caudalis
	Mm. costoseptalis
	M. rhomboideus profundus
	M. latissimus dorsi
	Mm. iliocostalis and longissimus dorsi
	M. longus colli dorsalis pars thoracica

Adapted from References 128, 131, 136.

are mechanically coupled in such a way that wingbeats assist respiratory ventilation during flight.[133,134] The volume of the air sac system is variable depending on physiological status (intestinal volume, reproductive physiology) and species. Positioning during anesthesia may also influence the air sac and tidal volume and is found to be the lowest in dorsal recumbency.[135,136] While intermittent positive-pressure ventilation usually decreases blood pressure in mammals, no effect or a positive effect has been reported in birds.[137,138]

The basic respiratory rhythm originates from the brainstem but is modulated by reflexes under several well-defined receptors.[131,139,140] Central chemoreceptors are present in birds and initiate an increase in ventilation when $PaCO_2$ increases. Arterial chemoreceptors, located at the carotid bodies near the parathyroid glands, are innervated by the vagus nerve and modulate ventilation in response to changes in PaO_2, $PaCO_2$, and pH. Another group of chemoreceptors, innervated by the vagus nerve and unique to birds and reptiles, is found in the lungs and are known as the intrapulmonary chemoreceptors. These chemoreceptors are stimulated by a decrease in PCO_2. This is in contrast to arterial chemoreceptors, which decrease ventilation. Additionally, air sac mechanoreceptors are also present. In summary, changes in ventilation occur in response to changes in $PaCO_2$, intrapulmonary PCO_2, PaO_2, and pH. The unique anatomy of the lung-air sac system of birds allows anesthetic and respiratory gases through a cannula in the caudal or abdominal air sacs.

RESPIRATORY DISEASES

Invertebrates

Signs of ill health in invertebrates can be nonspecific but are similar to those in other species. Nonspecific clinical signs of invertebrates include weight loss, anorexia, lethargy, color changes, presence of discharge, dysecdysis, behavioral changes, and sudden death.[2] The underlying cause of most respiratory diseases in invertebrates is often secondary to environmental stressors, including poor husbandry (e.g., malnutrition, improper temperature, humidity), inadequate hygiene, and climatic and environmental changes. It is extremely rare that the clinician is specifically presented with an invertebrate suffering from a respiratory problem.[3]

Environmental Diseases

It cannot be stressed enough that poor husbandry and management are the fundamental cause of clinical disease presentations in invertebrate species.[3,21,141,142] Each invertebrate species, whether aquatic or terrestrial, requires the owner to have an in-depth knowledge of ideal environmental conditions and proper diet. Poor hygiene, low ventilation, high stocking densities, and high humidity create ideal environments for bacteria and parasites to thrive and compromise the animal's immune system.[16,142] The health of filtering aquatic organisms such as bivalves is highly correlated to water quality. Gas bubble disease, commonly reported in fish, associated with supersaturation of room air and oxygen or changes in differential pressures of gases in the water, has been described in gastropods and cephalopods.[18] Aquatic invertebrates are more susceptible to high levels of ammonia, nitrites, and nitrates than aquatic vertebrates. Increased release of fine sediments and food may impair respiratory and filtering activities of some invertebrates.

Infectious Diseases

While one can speculate that there are invertebrate diseases with primary underlying etiologies, there is little medical literature to date describing this. Often, the respiratory system is affected secondarily as part of a systemic disease process such as septicemia. Normal external and internal bacterial flora of most invertebrates have not been well investigated, and it is often difficult to determine whether or not bacterial isolates are primary, opportunistic, or nonpathogenic.[4,143] Fungal diseases have been described in insects, although these tend to infect the external cuticular layer.[144] Specific respiratory diseases of invertebrates are rarely reported.

Parasitic Diseases

The oral nematodes of the Panagrolaimidae family are an emerging problem of captive tarantulas and have been reported to be fatal in adult tarantulas through the occlusion of the book lungs.[145] Although infection appears to remain localized to the mouthparts, it is often associated with secondary bacterial infections of the surrounding tissues, with associated necrosis and inflammation.[146] Diagnosis can be made by microscopically examining the oral discharge on low power, whereby numerous small motile nematodes are visible.[147] The nematodes are believed to be transmitted by Phoridae gnats and most often diagnosed in spiderlings, due to their higher humidity requirements. Proper quarantine and prevention of exposure to adult flies appears to be most effective in reducing disease incidence, although flushing mouthparts with saline appears to be as beneficial as antiparasiticides such as ivermectin and fenbendazole, which when administered to spiders can cause toxicosis.[145,146] Parasitic (Prostigmata) and saprophytic (Astigmata and Mesostigmata) mites can cause obstruction to the book lungs.[146,148] Acroceridae flies are true endoparasites of spiders: With the fly larvae being deposited onto the spider's body and entering the book lungs to penetrate the opithosoma. Acroceridae larvae can be present subclinically within the tarantula for months to years with the mature stage larvae consuming the opithosomal tissues before rupturing from the body and pupating.[146]

Microsporidiosis is commonly diagnosed in Crustaceans. These protozoa-like organisms directly attach to the gills, causing destruction and eventually systemic illness which eventually leads to muscle degeneration. The microsporidian organisms have a direct life cycle, and the end of the life cycle is characterized by the production of environmentally resistant spores that disseminate the disease.[21] *Bdelloura candida* is a flatworm found in the gill leaflets of horseshoe crabs with the eggs laid exclusively on gill lamellae.[149] While *Bdelloura candida* are ectosymbionts, they have the potential to be invasive in high numbers.

Insects may also harbor tracheal mites. Among tracheal mites of insects, the most well known and studied is without doubt the honeybee tracheal mite *Acarapis woodi*.[150] It lives in the trachea of bees, sucks hemolymph, and reduces the host life span.

Neoplastic Diseases

Neoplastic diseases are of relatively little clinical importance in invertebrates. Invertebrate, inbreeding and oncogenesis associated with carcinogens have not been well characterized and reported in the literature.[151]

Fish

Environmental Diseases

Low dissolved oxygen (DO) concentration in water leads to environmental hypoxia. Oxygen is poorly soluble in water and solubility decreases with salinity and in warmer water (i.e., aquatic environments for tropical fish and ponds during the summer months). Insufficient water oxygenation may also be promoted by low water-air surface exchange (e.g., ponds, insufficient water circulation, no mechanical aerator, ice coverage in winter), limited quantity of photosynthetic organisms (e.g., plants, algae), high stocking densities, and inadequate water quality (especially regarding nitrogen parameters).[23] In a heavily planted aquarium or a pond with a large algae population, oxygen decreases dramatically at night because of the cessation of photosynthesis and is at its minimum at sunrise.[23] Lack of proper acclimation of new fish or fish introduced to unfamiliar environmental conditions may also precipitate respiratory diseases. Chronic environmental hypoxia is less of a concern in aquaria due to significant mechanical aeration, but acute hypoxia may occur with power outage and equipment failure. A low DO may also lead to decreased numbers of nitrifying bacteria that rely on oxygen to metabolize nitrogen waste (aerobic bacteria), hence increasing ammonia and nitrites in the system. In ponds, low DO may be common in summer often related to increased water temperature, plant growth, and increased metabolism of water organisms. Likewise, in the winter, ice may prevent oxygen diffusion and snow may inhibit plant photosynthesis. Formalin treatment also reduces DO.

Acute hypoxia causes typical signs of fish respiratory disorders (See section on the physical examination on fish). Specific signs of acute environmental hypoxia may include death of non-air-breathing fish and gathering at air-water interface or near water inflow (see Figure 3-18). Chronic hypoxia leads to prolonged stress, which may promote secondary disease conditions.[23] Tolerance to hypoxia varies with fish species (goldfish are particularly resistant).

Ammonia poisoning causes hyperplasia and hypertrophy of the gills and is due to inadequate nitrification. Ammonia poisoning occurs with new tank syndrome (immature biological filtration), overcrowding, overfeeding, improper filter maintenance, and in the presence of toxic substances to nitrifying bacteria such as excessive ammonia, nitrates, chlorine, chloramine, antibiotics, and methylene blue. Ammonia toxicity also causes chronic stress, promotes disease, and induces hyperexcitability and neurologic disorders. Ammonia is present either as NH_3 or NH_4^+ (ammonium), the former being far more toxic. Increased temperature and pH (especially when >8.5) promotes the formation of NH_3. Formalin treatment interferes with the Nessler method, commonly used for measuring ammonium in colorimetric tests, leading to falsely elevated values.

Nitrite poisoning, also due to similar causes as those for ammonia poisoning, specifically targets the respiratory system of fish by inducing methemoglobin formation. Nitrites are actively transported by the gills into the bloodstream. Gills usually appear brown due to the methemoglobin color and is related to the ensuing hypoxia. Nitrite poisoning is affected by several factors, notably the chlorides, which inhibit gill nitrite uptake by the ionocytes.[23,152] Channel catfish are particularly susceptible to the toxic effects of nitrites. Due to the high-chloride water content, marine fish are less susceptible therefore nitrite poisoning is rare in marine aquaria.[23,152]

Nitrate poisoning (old tank syndrome) may also lead to methemoglobin formation. Nitrate is less toxic than nitrite with higher concentrations required to cause clinical disease. Nitrate is the final product of biological filtration and will continue to build up in an enclosed system if not removed by water changes, plant metabolism, or denitrification (anaerobic bacteria in an aquarium and algae). Increasing nitrate concentration may eventually cause death of nitrifying bacteria with an ensuing increase in ammonia. Nitrates may also enter an aquatic system, such as a pond, through agricultural treatment (waste, fertilizer, animal farming).[23] Fish susceptibility varies by species and effects of nitrates are more subtle in an aquatic system due to the lower toxicity and chronic exposure. In a newly established aquarium, ammonia peaks first, followed by nitrites, and finally nitrates.

Acutely low pH may also lead to dyspnea. Fish species vary in their optimum pH range. Most freshwater fish do best in neutral to slightly acidic water (especially South American cichlids) with the exception of African cichlids and brackish water fish, which do best in alkaline water. Marine fish require an alkaline pH and have a narrower range of tolerable pH. A drop in pH may be caused by fish metabolic activity, acid rain in outdoor systems, minerals added to the aquarium (e.g., silicate, stones leaching minerals), environmental contamination, and low alkalinity in water (content of calcium carbonate, buffering capacity of water). pH decreases over time in an enclosed system because of acidic metabolites excreted by living organisms.[23,152] pH also affects the toxicity of many compounds such as ammonium (see above) and metals. Gills are particularly affected by acid stress and low pH which stimulates gill mucus production, ultimately interfering with optimal gas exchange.[23]

Other, less commonly measured parameters that can damage the gill epithelium and/or cause dyspnea include hydrogen sulfide (excessive anaerobic metabolism), dissolved gas hypersaturation (mainly nitrogen that may form bubbles in many organs including the gills and buccal cavity), and toxins.[152] High CO_2 levels may also be encountered in ponds and during bag transportation of fish.

Suboptimal water quality parameters are also major risk factors for numerous gill and integumentary diseases of both freshwater and marine fish.

Infectious and Parasitic Diseases

Low water quality may be a predisposing factor for most infectious and parasitic diseases by lowering fish immunity, increasing fish stress, inducing gill and epithelial changes, and providing potential nutrients to pathogenic organisms. In addition, water temperature influences DO, the fish immune system, and life cycle of common gill parasites and viruses. Many organisms will infect preexisting lesions including bacteria, water molds, and other opportunistic pathogens. Previous gill inflammation may also lead to increased mucus secretion and cuticular substances, which may act as substrates for the growth of pathogenic bacteria.[153]

Bacterial branchial diseases are common and a variety of bacteria may be implicated, primarily gram negative organisms (Table 3-4). Most bacteria infecting the gills are also

TABLE 3-4

Notable Pathogens Responsible for Gill Lesions and Diseases in Fish

BACTERIAL DISEASES	PARASITIC DISEASES
Flavobacterium columnare (FW)*	**Protozoa/Sarcomastigophora/Ciliophora**
Flavobacterium branchiophilum (FW)	*Ichthyophthirius multifiliis* (FW)*
Epitheliocystis (FW, SW)	*Cryptocaryon irritans* (SW)*
Aeromonas hydrophila (FW)*	*Trichodina* (FW, SW)*
Aeromonas salmonicida (FW, SW)*	*Chilodonella* (FW)*
Bacillus cereus (FW)	*Brooklynella* (SW)
Bacillus subtilis (FW)	*Tetrahymena* spp. (FW)
Vibrio spp. (SW)*	Scuticiliatosis (SW)
Mycobacterium spp. (FW, SW)*	*Amyloodinium* (SW)*
	Piscinoodinium (FW)
	Ichthyobodo (FW)*
	Cryptobia (FW, SW)
	Neoparamoeba (FW, SW)
	Ectocommensal ciliates (FW)*
VIRAL DISEASES	
Lymphocystis (FW, SW)*	**Myxozoa**
Channel catfish HV (FW)	*Henneguya ictaluri* (FW)
Viral hemorrhagic septicemia (FW, SW)	*Myxobolus* spp. (FW, SW)
Spring viremia of carp (FW)*	*Sphaerospora molnari* (FW)
Cyprinid HV2 (FW)*	**Crustaceans**
Cyprinid HV3 = KHV (FW)*	Copepods, especially *Lernacea* in goldfish and koi (FW, SW)
Atlantic salmon paramyxovirus (SW)	Isopod (FW, SW)
Grass carp aquareovirus disease (FW)	**Helminths**
Pilchard HV (SW)	Leeches (FW, SW)
Catfish aquareovirus (FW)	Monogenean trematodes (FW, SW)*
Turbot epithelial cell gigantism (SW)	*Centrocestus formosanus* (FW)
	Turbellarian (SW)
FUNGAL DISEASES	
Saprolegniosis (FW)*	
Aphanomyces invadans (FW)	
Branchiomyces spp. (FW)	
Loma salmonae (SW)	

Adapted from References 153-157.
FW, Freshwater; *HV*, herpesvirus; *SW*, saltwater.
*Significant in pet and ornamental fish.

responsible for skin lesions or systemic disease. Depending on the pathogen gill lesions may be associated with the overall clinical picture and observed less often than skin lesions. One should note that gill lesions are usually more serious than skin lesions due to the many physiological functions of fish gills (see the section Anatomy and Physiology at the beginning of this chapter). Columnaris infection caused by *Flavobacterium columnare* is arguably one of the most important bacterial gill/epithelial diseases of aquarium freshwater fish and causes necrotic and erosive lesions, often appearing as cottony fins.[154] Bacterial gill disease, caused by *Flavobacterium branchiophilum*, is mainly a disease of cultured salmonids and produces a proliferative and hyperemic branchitis with no skin lesions.[154] Epitheliocystis is caused by chlamydia-like bacteria and primarily targets gills with minimal skin involvement noted clinically as

small nodules. Other less selective organisms may infect the branchial tissue as part of a systemic syndrome causing septicemic and ulcerative disease due to motile aeromonad bacteria such as *Aeromonas hydrophila*, one of the most common bacterial diseases of freshwater fish, and *Aeromonas salmonicida* in salmons, koi, and goldfish.[155] *Vibrio* spp. cause a common systemic bacterial infection of marine fish.

Viral diseases usually cause branchial lesions as part of a systemic or generalized epithelial process. Lymphocystis is a common sequela to iridovirus infections and is often diagnosed in aquarium fish. The primary clinical condition associated with the disease is the production of highly enlarged dermal fibroblasts macroscopically visible as white nodules, notably in the gills.[153,154] Spring viremia of carp is a rhabdoviral disease that mainly affects the common carp but also is diagnosed in koi and goldfish. Gills are frequently targeted by the rhabdovirus and hemorrhages may be grossly visible. Koi herpesvirus (HV) (cyprinid HV-3) causes pale, swollen, and mottled gills in koi and common carp and may lead to chronic infection.[156]

The main fungal disease that infects the gills of fish is the freshwater mold (saprolegniasis), which causes typical white cottony lesions on the gills and/or skin that may turn brown, green, or red with time, if colonization by algae.[154] Other fungal diseases are also encountered including branchiomycosis (gill rot), which specifically affects gill tissue.[153,154]

Due to an adequate nutrient supply and the relative safety of the opercular cavity, there are a large number of parasites that infest the gills of fish. These parasites belong to various animal phyla such as Arthropoda (e.g., copepods), Annelida (e.g., leeches), Platyhelminthes (e.g., monogenean trematodes), Ciliophora (e.g., ich), Sarcomastigophora (e.g., Ichthyobodo), and Myxozoa (Table 3-4). Some are almost exclusively encountered in wild-caught or pond-raised fish (e.g., copepods, leeches), while others are common in home aquaria (e.g., *Ichthyophthirius* and other protozoan parasites). Life cycles will vary but all protozoan parasites have direct life cycles and most clinically relevant metazoan parasites in home aquaria also have direct cycles. The myxozoan parasite *Henneguya ictaluri* causes proliferative gill disease in channel catfish. Monogenean trematodes (e.g., *Gyrodactylus*) mainly have direct life cycles, while digenean trematodes (e.g., *Centrocestus*) require intermediate hosts such as aquatic mollusks (snails). The monogenean trematodes are external parasites of the gills, while digenean trematodes mainly cause internal infestations and masses. Clinical signs and lesions due to parasitic infestations vary from hyperemic and irritated gills to focal hemorrhages (trematode, copepod) and gill necrosis with associated dyspnea. Parasites may transmit bacterial and viral diseases to their piscine host. Most parasites will also cause disease on the skin and gills, however these disease conditions may be due to secondary complications associated with the infestation. Protozoan parasites are probably the most clinically relevant parasites for aquarium fish. *Ichthyophthirius* (ich) is especially common in freshwater fish and causes white nodules on the skin and gills.[154]

Noninfectious Diseases

Noninfectious diseases of the respiratory system, unrelated to environmental stress are rare in fish. Neoplasms of the gills are very rare but oral tumors may interfere with water movement through the buccal cavity. Papillomas, squamous cell carcinomas, and chondromas have also been documented in fish species.[157] Several cases of branchioblastoma have been reported in koi.[158,159] Tumors of the pseudobranch are described in Atlantic and Pacific cods.[160,161] Environmental contaminants, pollution, and viruses are strongly suspected to promote epithelial oncogenesis in fish.

In addition to inappropriate standard water quality parameters, specific toxins may induce respiratory signs in fish such as copper (environmental contamination, chemicals), iron (environmental contamination, rust), chlorines (tap water), cyanide ("cyanide-collected" marine aquarium fish), manganese, rotenone, detergents, algal biotoxins (wild fish), toxins of zooplankton (jellyfish, siphonophores in wild fish), and mycotoxins.[153,156,157] Overdose of therapeutic agents such as formalin, pesticides, copper, and hydrogen peroxide may also cause gill pathology.

Panthotenic acid and vitamin C deficiencies have been associated with gill lesions.[153] Finally, trauma (e.g., predation attempts) or congenital defects (especially to the opercula) may be observed.[157] Histologic lesions of the various air-breathing organs have also been reported in some fish.[162]

Amphibians

Primary diseases of the respiratory system are uncommon in amphibians.[47] However certain systemic infections, such as mycobacteriosis, may affect amphibians' lungs or gills.[47] These diseases are described elsewhere in this book. Depending on species or environmental conditions, cutaneous disease is likely to affect respiration in amphibians.[47] Cutaneous diseases are also described in Chapter 2 of this book and will not be described here. Very few reports of caecilian disease have been published, and therefore, most reported respiratory diseases concern Anurans and Caudata.[47,163] Systemic diseases of amphibians with respiratory involvement are listed in Table 3-5.

Infectious and Parasitic Diseases

Parasitic infestation of the respiratory system is the most commonly reported respiratory disease of amphibians and includes helminths (e.g., lungworms, flukes), protozoans, and arthropods.[39,63,164,170–179]

Nematodes (*Rhabdias* spp.) are common and represent important pulmonary pathogens in Anurans and possibly in Caudatans.[39,63,164,170,172–176] Animals affected with low worm burdens are generally subclinical, although heavy infestations can easily develop in captivity and are associated with poor hygiene, due to their direct life cycle.[47] Adult nematodes live in amphibian lungs and feed on blood and pulmonary secretions. Larvated eggs and larvae migrate into the oropharynx and are coughed up, swallowed, and deposited in the feces.[47,170] The larvae can be directly infective after being shed by the amphibian or after maturing in the environment. Infective larvae penetrate the skin and migrate to the lungs. Clinical signs in heavy infestations are nonspecific and include lethargy, anorexia, anemia, and dyspnea.[47] Lesions in the respiratory epithelium consist of inflammation and fibrosis secondary to the ventilation-perfusion mismatch and the worms' physical presence.[170] Secondary bacterial infections are common.[170]

Many species of adult trematodes, especially *Haematoloechus* spp., have been reported in the lungs and oropharynx of frogs and toads.[47,63,179] Lung flukes have minor pathologic impacts in the lung, even in heavy infestations.[47,63,179] However the trematode infestation may be fatal if the parasites occlude the bronchial lumen.[63] Lesions such as hyperplasic nodules in the pulmonary epithelium induced by the attachment of flukes may also predispose their host to secondary bacterial and fungal infections and have been mistaken for metastatic adenocarcinomas in the past.[63,177] Other trematodes such as *Clinostomum*, *Diplostomum*, and *Manodistomum* have been

---

TABLE 3-5

Selected Systemic Diseases That Most Commonly Affect the Respiratory System of Amphibians

Type	Disease	Species	Clinical Signs
Viral	Iridoviridae, ranavirus (Bohle iridovirus, frog virus 3)[63,164,165]	Anurans	Hemorrhagic septicemia, multifocal necrosis in liver, spleen, stomach, kidney, and lungs
Bacterial	Chlamydiosis (*Chlamydia pneumoniae*)[39,166]	Anurans	Pneumonia, anemia, pancytopenia, anemia, skin hemorrhage, hepatitis, splenitis, death
	Mycobacteriosis (*Mycobacterium* spp.)[167–169]	All amphibians	Granuloma in visceral organs with systemic disease, rare granuloma in the lungs (6%)
Parasitic	Filariid worms[170]	All amphibians	Heavy infestations may cause capillary clogging in lungs and glomeruli.
Fungal	Chromomycosis (*Cladosporium* spp., *Fonsecaea* spp., *Exophiala* sp., and *Phialophora* spp.)[39,164]	Anurans	Granuloma in lungs and other visceral organs in disseminated infections.
Miscellaneous	Metastatic calcification with hypervitaminosis D, imbalances in dietary calcium and phosphorus, or underlying renal disease[170]	All amphibians	Lungs are a commonly affected site with great vessels, kidney, gut, and skin.
	Melanosis[170]	All amphibians	May be present in liver, spleen, ovary, kidney, lung, heart, skin, brain. Significantly pathologic lesions are only in liver.
	Hypovitaminosis A[170]	All amphibians	Metaplasia of epithelium including the respiratory tract

reported in amphibian lungs.[39,164] Adult flukes of *Sphyranura* spp. are commonly found on the gills of aquatic salamanders, such as the mudpuppy (*Necturus maculosus*).[47,178] *Gyrodactylus* spp., a parasite of fish, are also commonly diagnosed in the gills of tadpoles and may cause death with heavy infestations.[47,164] The trematode *Polystoma* spp. are known to infect gills in larval stages but no specific lesion has been reported.[63]

Ciliated protozoa (*Trichodonella* sp.) or dinoflagellates (*Piscinoodinum pillularis*) may heavily infest the gills of some aquatic amphibians despite being primarily fish parasites.[39,47,164,174] Low-level infestations of ciliated protozoa in ideal husbandry conditions is subclinical; however, clinical signs including dyspnea, anorexia, and lethargy may develop when the animal is immunosuppressed or exposed to inappropriate husbandry conditions.[47] Gray discoloration (*Piscinoodinum pillularis*) or reddening and ulceration (*Trichodonella* sp.) of the gills may be observed along with increased mucus production.[47,164]

Myiasis of the nasal cavity is a common respiratory disease in amphibians, especially in Anurans.[39,47,63] The larvae of two fly species (*Bufolucilia bufonivora* and *Bufolucilia silvarum*) can migrate through the nasal passages of wild amphibians.[47] *B. bufonivora* is a common obligate parasite of Anurans and some salamanders in Europe, Asia, and northern Africa.[47,63] *B. silvarum* is a facultative amphibian parasite and has rarely been reported in Anurans in North America and Europe.[47,63] Adult flies lay eggs on amphibian skin with larval migration moving toward the hosts' nasal passages, which occurs after hatching.[47,63] These parasites cause extensive destruction of the nasal mucosa and surrounding tissues, including nasal bones, and have been reported to migrate to the eyes, tympanic membrane, and brain.[47,63] Infestations are usually severe and fatal in amphibians.[47,63]

Fungal infections may affect the lungs or gills in amphibians. Mycotic pneumonia is rarely reported in amphibians and most reports describe the infestation in Anurans.[180] *Aspergillus* spp., *Geotrichum candidum*, and *Candida* spp. have been cultured from lung tissues in frogs on postmortem examination.[180] Mycotic infections are not common in Giant toads and other *Bufo* spp.[39] One case report describes pulmonary cryptococcosis in a free-living common toad (*Bufo bufo*) confirmed on postmortem examination after being killed by a car.[171] Saprolegniasis gives the appearence of a fungal infection that affects the gills in amphibians, fish, and invertebrates inducing respiratory distress.[47,174] Saprolegniasis infections are commonly associated with poor husbandry or opportunistic development on traumatized gills.[47] Saprolegniasis grossly appears as focal areas of cotton-like material on the skin and gills.[47] *Dermocystidium* spp., a protozoan-like fungus, may grossly appear similar to Saprolegniasis, although it tends to create pinpoint multifocal lesions, with fatalities reported.[164]

Bacterial and viral primary respiratory infections are rarely described in amphibians. Pneumococcal pneumonia has been reported in tadpoles of the Amazon milk frog (*Trachycephalus resinifictrix*).[63] Grossly, pneumococcal pneumonia appears as emphysematous overfilling of the pulmonary parenchyma with gas bubbles, with corresponding ataxia and exercise intolerance.[63]

Two case reports also describe necrotic interstitial pneumonia and death, which were suspected to be secondary to a calicivirus infection in ornate horned frogs (*Ceratophrys ornata*).[63]

Noninfectious Diseases

Due to the highly dependent relationship amphibians have with their environment, any adverse changes to their living conditions are directly associated with immune system compromise and subsequent disease morbidity. As a result, amphibians are often regarded as sentinels of environmental health. The integumentary system of amphibians is well adapted for transcutaneous gas exchange. They have higher requirements for humidity at 70% to 90% and lower preferred optimal temperatures in comparison to most reptiles. Less favorable environmental conditions such as high levels of ammonia, nitrites, and nitrates and low DO levels have direct impacts on respiratory function. The maintenance of excellent water quality is required for those amphibian species that are primarily aquatic in nature. Consequently, the clinician must have a sound knowledge base regarding the husbandry requirements of each species. Hyperplasia of gill epithelial cells has been described in wild and captive salamanders, following prolonged exposure to poor water quality.[47] Just as environmental parameters are vital to understand the possible underlying causes of the presenting disease condition(s), so to is information regarding past medical and treatment history. Developmental stages of amphibians should be properly identified during gross examination as normal physiological changes (e.g., metamorphic degeneration of the gills), which may be mistaken for pathologic conditions.[63] In captivity axolotls, which are usually neotenic, may undergo a metamorphosis and lose their gills with thyroxin supplementation or when living in an inadequate aquatic environment.[181]

Experimental studies have shown that when amphibian larvae were unable to access air, the resultant anatomical changes observed included atrophied or forked lungs, invagination of the posterior body, and abnormal spherical or triangular shaped lungs.[63]

Genetic abnormalities associated with defective gills have been reported in the axolotl.[63]

Environmental toxins may cause respiratory diseases through ecological changes but may also directly affect their highly permeable integument. Rotenone is a pesticide that is known to induce breathing difficulties secondary to respiratory enzyme inhibition in frog larvae.[174,182] Exposure to pesticides will decrease resistance to infection, and has been reported in the larvae of *Rhabdias ranae* (leopard frogs) and is likely to occur in other amphibian species.[183] Tap water that contains chlorine or chloramines may cause gill irritation; hence, it is recommended that water be dechlorinated prior to housing the animal. This irritation and break in local immunity predispose amphibians with gills to infection by opportunistic pathogens.[175]

Other noninfectious diseases to consider are upper airway obstructions, pulmonary rupture due to excessive intermittent positive-pressure ventilation (IPPV) inflation during anesthesia, lesions directly on the trachea, bronchial or pulmonary epithelial trauma from rough handling, thoracic wounds, coelomic masses, and traumatic gill damage from cage mates, especially in neotenic Caudatans.[164] Gastric overload and the presence of a large meal may compress the pulmonary tissue and lead to respiratory compromise in Anurans.

Primary and secondary pulmonary neoplasia is rarely reported in amphibians, although neoplasms in other areas of the respiratory tract, such as the tracheobronchial region, have been described.[177] Reports indicate that axolotls are highly susceptible to nasal cavity neoplasms however the exact tumor classification has yet to be specifically identified. At this time the nasal cavity tumors of axolotls are either an adenocarcinoma of the mucosal epithelium or neuroepithelioma of the neurosensory cells.[177] Gill papilloma can be experimentally induced by injection of perylene in the barred tiger salamander (*Ambystoma tigrinum mavortium*).[177]

Reptiles

General Considerations

Respiratory diseases are one of the most commonly diagnosed disorders of captive and wild reptiles. Reptile respiratory diseases are often multifactorial in origin, and usually are associated with immunosuppression and suboptimal husbandry conditions.[66,73,184] Moreover, viral, bacterial, fungal, and parasitic infections of the respiratory tract may occur as well as disease related to noninfectious causes (e.g., trauma, foreign bodies, toxin inhalation, neoplasia).[184] Respiratory disease may occur due to a primary underlying cause or related to a secondary pathophysiologic condition(s), such as aspiration pneumonia initiated by a generalized neurologic disease condition or or aspiration of necrotic debris due to stomatitis.[66,184] Upper respiratory tract diseases are particularly prevalent in chelonians, while lower respiratory tract diseases are more common in squamates. In this chapter, only primary respiratory disease conditions are covered.

The presence of a poorly ciliated respiratory epithelium and the absence of a true diaphragm make the elimination of foreign body particles or inflammatory exudates from the trachea or lungs difficult in reptiles, especially chelonians and squamates. As a consequence, inflammatory debris tends to accumulate within the respiratory system. In addition, reptiles produce caseous pus that further complicates exudate clearance. Accumulation of cellular and physiologic debris into the caudal extension of both snake and lizards lungs has important clinical implications for medical management, as this area of the lung is poorly vascularized and unaffected by systemic antimicrobials.[73] Debris may also accumulate in the accessory lung of chameleons.[73] The accumulation of inflammatory exudates in association with cellular infiltration and loss of normal tissue elasticity compromise the ability for compensatory increases to tidal volume.[73] In addition, reptiles have an incredible ability to cope with severe respiratory disease by switching to anaerobic metabolism, which may delay the detection of clinical signs by caretakers and lead to more advanced respiratory conditions at presentation.

Due to long incubation periods of some viral diseases and the potential for chronic shedding of organisms from diseased individuals, it is recommended to test species susceptible to particular viruses (e.g., tortoise and mycoplasma/HVs; viperids and paramyxoviruses; boids and inclusion body disease [IBD]) prior to their introduction into a herpetological collection and quarantine for a minimum of 3 to 6 months.

Infectious Diseases

VIRAL DISEASES. Herpes virus infection of the upper respiratory tract is commonly diagnosed in wild tortoises or immunocompromised chelonians that have experienced a stressful event (sudden changes in temperature, nutritional deficiencies, metabolic disease, concurrent diseases, the onset of breeding season) or have been subject to inappropriate husbandry conditions.[74,184] The first case of an upper respiratory tract HV infection was reported in a California desert tortoise (*Gopherus agassizii*) by Harper et al.[185] Since then, HV infections were described in Europe, America, South Africa, and Asia.[186] All tortoises should be considered susceptible to HV infection, although Mediterranean tortoises, especially spur-thighed tortoises (*Testudo graeca*) and Hermann's tortoises (*Testudo hermanni*) both in Europe and in the United States, seem to be the Testudinid species most susceptible to HVs.[73,74,184,187] All characterized reptilian HVs belong to the alphaherpesvirinae, and four different tortoise HV isolates were reported based on genetic characterization: Tortoise HV 1 (TeHV1) primarily identified in Russian (*Agrionemys horsfieldii*) and to a lesser extent in Mediterranean tortoises and is associated with low morbidity and mortality; TeHV2 most often diagnosed in North America and affects desert tortoises (*Gopherus agassizii*); TeHV3 is a European/central Asian virus and is usually reported in Mediterranean tortoises (*Testudo* spp. and Russian tortoise), particularly spur-thighed and Hermann's tortoises with higher mortality than with TeHV1; and finally, TeHV4 has predominantly been reported in Bowsprit tortoises (*Chersina angulata*) and is, at this time, considered a subclinical disease.[186,188–190] TeHVs are suspected to have the ability to switch host species; therefore, mixing of tortoise species should be avoided.[186] In particular, TeHV3 seems to be milder in spur-thighed tortoises but particularly pathogenic in Hermann's tortoises. Hermann's tortoises usually experience high numbers of fatalities to both TeHV1 and TeHV3.[190] As with all HVs, affected individuals should be considered permanently infected and potential chronic shedders of the organism.[191] Latency is thought to occur in the central nervous system and other tissues following primary infection, until recrudescence occurs during a period of stress.[74] Typical presentation of Testudinid HV infection is a glossitis/stomatitis/rhinitis/conjunctivitis complex.[74] Other clinical signs that are commonly observed include nasal discharge, edema of the ventral neck, dehydration, depression, exfoliation of the skin of the head and neck, hypersalivation, dysphagia, dyspnea, nasal discharge, and yellow diphtheritic membrane formation on the tongue, oropharynx, and nasopharynx. Lesions may extend to the trachea, lung, and proximal gastrointestinal system.[74,184,192] Necrotizing hepatitis and neurologic signs (meningoencephalitis) have been reported.[74,184,192,193] Experimental TeHV3 infection provided evidence that the clinical course of the disease may only last 2.5 weeks in spur-thighed tortoises.[194] The virus typically causes necrotizing lesions with characteristic intranuclear inclusion bodies.[192] Shedding mainly occurs through oral and salivary secretions.[192] Lesions may spontaneously regress in spur-thighed (TeHV3) and Russian (TeHV1) tortoises, but death is common in highly sensitive species such as Hermann's tortoises with TeHV1 and 3 and Russian tortoises infected with TeHV3.

In marine turtles, especially Cheloniidae (*Chelonia mydas*), HVs induce several important diseases with respiratory lesions: lung-eye-trachea (LET) disease, fibropapillomatosis associated with the turtle fibropapilloma-associated HV (TFPHV), and loggerhead genital-respiratory HV.[184,191,195] Herpes virus infection was also reported in redheaded agamas (*Agama agama*), with evidence of disease in the liver, lung, and spleen.[196]

Iridovirus of the genus *Ranavirus* induces similar clinical signs to HV and mycoplasma, resulting in upper respiratory tract disease in chelonians including nasal and ocular discharge, conjunctivitis, palpebral edema, caseous plaques in the oral cavity, and pneumonia.[71,74,197,198] Ranavirus has the ability to infect several animal classes such as fish, amphibians, reptiles, and invertebrates.[71,191] Ranaviruses have been reported in a wide variety of tortoises, terrapins, and turtles. Eastern box turtles *(Terrapene carolina carolina)* appear to be frequently infected and chelonian iridovirus infection was first reported in a gopher tortoise *(Gopherus polyphemus)* in North America.[198-200] Chelonians usually become infected following exposure to amphibians in outdoor ponds.[71,74] Necropsy may reveal ulcerative tracheitis, pharyngitis, esophagitis, and pneumonia.[197]

A picornavirus known as virus X has been known to cause rhinitis in Mediterranean tortoises.[191]

Paramyxovirus and reovirus infections are important causes of pneumonia in squamates.[197,201] These viruses are associated with pronounced hyperplasia of respiratory epithelial cells (type-II pneumocytes) and variable diffuse interstitial infiltrates of heterophils, lymphocytes, plasma cells, and macrophages.[201] Paramyxoviruses in snakes include two main agents of respiratory diseases: ferlaviruses (formerly known as ophidian paramyxoviruses) and the emerging Sunshine virus.[202] Ferlavirus has been detected in Colubridae, Elapidae, Viperidae, Crotalidae, Boidae, and Pythonidae but are most commonly found infecting crotalid snakes.[73,77,184,202-204] Pythons seem to be more susceptible to ferlavirus infection than boas.[205] Transmission among snakes occurs by contact, respiratory secretions, fomites, and ectoparasites, especially mites.[77,184,202] No report of vertical transmission has been published at this time.[202] The transmission pathway of this virus is unknown.[202] The disease course of ferlavirus may be acute/peracute death and chronic (wasting syndrome with dysorexia and regurgitations) or subclinical evolution for up to 10 months.[73] Clinical signs may be variable and include stomatitis, open-mouth breathing, and nasal and purulent hemorrhagic tracheal discharge with accumulation of caseous necrotic debris within the lumen of the airways.[73,77,184,197] The lung tissue is often thickened and edematous.[197] Neurologic signs have also been reported in advanced stages of the disease with death occurring within 1 week of the onset of the overt clinical signs.[73,77,184,197,202] Ferlavirus infections are suspected to be immunosuppressive secondary to a potential lymphoid depletion.[202] Sunshine virus causes neurorespiratory disease in Australian snakes.[206] Sunshine virus was reported for the first time in an outbreak of neurorespiratory disease in Australian pythons in 2008. Lethargy, inappetance, and neurologic and respiratory signs were reported.[202] Histologic lesions include hindbrain white matter spongiosis and gliosis and mild bronchointerstitial pneumonia in some snakes.[202,207] At least three genotypes of ferlaviruses have been described. Ferlavirus infections that result in pneumonia have also been reported in lizards and chelonians.[206]

IBD is a viral disease of boid snakes mainly characterized by neurologic lesions. Several snake species can be affected but most reports identify Burmese pythons and boa constrictors. While the disease seems restricted to the neurologic system in pythons, boas suffer from systemic lesions including lesions in the respiratory system. In addition,

secondary bacterial infections including pneumonia are common.[184,208] Retroviruses have historically been implicated, but recently arenaviruses have been strongly associated with the disease.[209-211]

Although adenovirus infection usually affects the liver, intestines, and pancreas, adenoviral pneumonia has been described in crocodilians and snakes.[205,212] Tracheitis caused by an adenovirus was also reported in Jackson's chameleons *(Chamaeleo jacksonii).*[213] Recently, a novel nidovirus has been found to be a major cause of pneumonia in captive ball pythons.[214]

BACTERIAL DISEASES. Bacterial respiratory infections are usually secondary to different primary causes such as suboptimal captive environments or concurrent diseases.[184] In particular, too high or too low humidity seems to promote respiratory infection. Bacterial pneumonias are fairly common in reptiles, especially in ophidians. In snakes, pneumonias may be primary or secondary to bacteremia, bacterial stomatitis, and viral infections (ferlavirus, nidovirus, IBD). Conversely, various bacterial infections such as bacterial endocarditis, stomatitis, abscesses, and dermatitis are frequently associated with pneumonia in snakes.

Bacterial pneumonia can be focal, unilateral, or bilateral and is especially prevalent in captive snakes (Figure 3-8).[73] Aerobic gram-negative bacteria from normal flora of the buccal and respiratory tract or environment are usually implicated in chelonian and ophidian pneumonias, including *Pseudomonas* spp., *Klebsiella* spp., *Proteus* spp., *Aeromonas* spp., *Salmonella* spp., *Morganella* spp., *Providencia* spp., and *Staphylococcus* spp.[73,74,184,197,205,215] In snakes, chronic stomatitis may result in pneumonia due to the snake mite *Ophionyssus natricis* which is capable of transmitting *Aeromonas hydrophila* among snakes.[216] *Pasteurella testudinis* was isolated from desert tortoises *(Gopherus agassizii)* and leopard tortoises *(Geochelone pardalis)* with pneumonia.[184,197,217] In snakes with pneumonia, *Salmonella arizonae* is a common bacterial pathogen.[218] Moreover, for some authors, bacterial infections with *Aeromonas* sp., *Klebsiella* sp., and *Pseudomonas* sp. of the respiratory tract are considered to be common in veiled chameleons.[216] Anaerobic bacteria, such as *Fusobacterium* spp., *Clostridium*

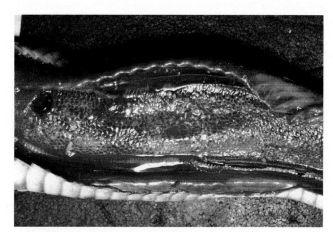

FIGURE 3-8 Pneumonia with gross pulmonary congestion and exudate in a boa constrictor. (Courtesy of Lionel Schilliger.)

spp., *Peptostreptococcus* spp., and *Bacteroides* spp., are not considered part of the normal flora of the respiratory tract; however, these bacteria have been isolated in reptiles with pneumonia.[73,184] Mixed infections with anaerobic and aerobic bacteria have also been described.[184] Snakes with pneumonia have been reported to be susceptible to bacterial valvular endocarditis.[219,220]

Mycoplasmosis is a well-studied upper respiratory tract disease affecting a large variety of captive and free-ranging North American tortoises. This intracellular bacterium is particularly prevalent in desert and gopher tortoises (*Gopherus agassizii* and *G. polyphemus*) with etiological agents being identified as *Mycoplasma agassizii* and *Mycoplasma testudineum*.[73,74,184,197,221–223] Experimental transmission of these organisms has demonstrated their pathogenicity in tortoises.[223–225] *Mycoplasma testudinis* has been cultured from tortoises but does not seem to cause upper respiratory disease in chelonians.[223] All chelonians should be considered susceptible to mycoplasmosis, and additionally, tortoises may be co-infected with TeHV and ranavirus.[74,223] Transmission of the *Mycoplasma* spp. organisms occurs through direct contact with affected tortoises via respiratory secretions and nasal discharges.[73] Mycoplasmosis is often observed in immunocompromised turtles, in the immediate posthibernation period or when suboptimal husbandry conditions are endured.[74] *Mycoplasma agassizii* has been isolated from California desert tortoises (*Gopherus agassizii*), Florida gopher tortoises (*Gopherus polyphemus*), Russian tortoises (*Agrionemys horsfieldii*), Greek tortoises (*Testudo graeca*), marginated tortoises (*Testudo marginata*), and leopard tortoises (*Geochelone pardalis*).[74,184,224,226–228] *Mycoplasma testudineum* has been identified in California desert tortoises (*Gopherus agassizii*) and Florida gopher tortoises (*Gopherus polyphemus*) with upper respiratory tract disease.[229–231] Mycoplasmosis in chelonians has a high morbidity but a low mortality rate, although survival time in the wild is suggested to be lower in affected tortoises compared to unaffected tortoises.[230,232] Typical clinical disease signs include conjunctivitis, serous purulent nasal discharge, increased respiratory sounds, and palpebral edema[73,74,184,197,223] Erosive changes of the nares and pneumonia may be observed in chronic cases.[73,74,184] The incubation period of *Mycoplasma* spp. infections may be as little as 2 weeks, although chronic and subclinical infections are common.[73,222,223,233] Intermittent shedding and clinical signs may occur over several years. With severe infection, tortoises may present with open-mouth dyspnea, lethargy, and anorexia.[184] Aberrant behaviors have been observed in tortoises with mycoplasmosis.[73] Clinical signs may become more apparent in periods of stress caused by shipping, seasonal changes, or suboptimal husbandry.[184] *Mycoplasma agassizii* adheres to the ciliated mucosal epithelium of the tortoise upper respiratory tract. As a result, the infection causes a severe disruption of normal tissue architecture and function, resulting in severe secondary and opportunistic infections, especially gram-negative bacteria.[222,223]

Mycoplasmosis is also a recognized respiratory disease in crocodilians.[66,197] *Mycoplasma alligatoris* has been reported in the American alligator (*Alligator mississippiensis*) and in the broad-nosed caiman (*Caiman latirostris*).[66] Other crocodilians species closely related to alligators may be susceptible to *Mycoplasma alligatoris* infection.[66] *Mycoplasma crocodyli* has been reported in Nile crocodiles.[66,197,212] Clinical signs include

lethargy, weakness, anorexia, white ocular discharge, paresis, and edema (facial, periocular, cervical, limbs).[66,197] Pathologic findings reveal pneumonia, pericarditis, and polyarthritis.[66,197]

A novel *Mycoplasma* sp. was isolated from a Burmese python (*Python molurus bivittatus*) with a proliferative tracheitis and pneumonia.[197,234] *Mycoplasma insons* is considered as part of the normal microbiota of the respiratory tract of the Green iguana (*Iguana iguana*).[235]

Chlamydiosis is a systemic infection that has also been associated with pneumonia in reptiles.[218]

Mycobacteria can cause pneumonia in reptile species, although the respiratory tract is not usually considered the primary site for mycobacterial infection.[73] Pulmonary mycobacteriosis (*Mycobacterium haemophilum* and *Mycobacterium marinum*) was described in a ball python (*Python regius*) while a boa constrictor diagnosed with *Mycobacterium chelonei* developed a pulmonary granuloma along with granulomas in other internal organs.[236,237] *Mycobacterium* spp. were also recovered from a reticulated python (*Python reticulatus*) with pulmonary granulomas.[238] In chelonians, *M. chelonei* caused systemic granulomas including a pulmonary granuloma in a Kemp's Ridley sea turtle (*Lepidochelys kempii*).[239] *Mycobacterium kansasii* caused systemic infection and pulmonary nodules in a Chinese soft-shelled turtle (*Pelodiscus sinensis*).[240] Acid-fast organisms were recovered from pulmonary lesions in a loggerhead sea turtle (*Caretta caretta*) and a Hilaire's side-necked turtle (*Phrynops hilari*).[216] *Mycobacterium szulgai* was the cause of a granulomatous pneumonia in freshwater crocodiles (*Crocodylus johnstoni*).[241]

Pharyngitis has been described in crocodilians secondary to septicemia, with reported cases also involving the tonsils, the dorsal flap of the gular valve, and glottis.[212]

FUNGAL DISEASES. Mycosis of the respiratory tract is commonly diagnosed in reptiles, particularly tortoises, sea turtles, and crocodilians.[73,184,242,243] Most fungi are opportunistic invaders of the respiratory system, integument, and gastrointestinal tract.[66,67,184] Few reports have identified fungal organisms as the primary cause of respiratory disease in reptiles, with most originating as environmental organisms.[184,243] Inappropriate husbandry conditions, especially low environmental temperatures, excessive environmental humidity, chronic stress, excessive fungal spore exposure, and misuse of antibiotics, may promote fungal pneumonia.[66,73,184] Different genera of fungi have been associated with pneumonia in reptiles, including *Aspergillus* spp., *Candida* spp., *Mucor* spp., *Geotrichum* spp., *Penicillium* spp., *Cladosporium* spp., *Rhizopus* spp., *Chrysosporium* spp., *Purpureocillium* spp. (formerly *Paecilomyces*), *Acremonium* spp., and *Beauveria* spp.[73,242–244]

Purpureocillium lilacinum (formerly *Paecilomyces lilacinus*) is the most clinically significant fungus causing respiratory disease in reptiles. *Purpureocillium lilacinum* has been found as the causative agent of pulmonary granulomatous diseases in various species, especially chelonians and crocodilians.[71,242,245,246] Some unspeciated *Penicillium* mycoses may in fact have been due to *Purpureocillium*, which used to be in the *Penicillium* genus and later in the *Paecilomyces* genus.[242] *Aspergillus* spp. have also been isolated several times in association with pulmonary lesions in chelonians and crocodilians.[242] *Aspergillus* pulmonary mycosis has been reported in two green anacondas (*Eunectes murinus*).[247]

Chelonians, especially giant tortoises and sea turtles, appear to be more susceptible overall to fungal pneumonia than any other reptiles with *Candida* spp., *Aspergillus* spp., *Purpureocillium* spp., *Penicillium* spp., and *Beauveria* spp. isolated in animals with respiratory disease.[184,243,246,248-252]

Single cases of pulmonary involvement with *Coccidioides immitis* in a Sonoran gopher snake (*Pituophis melanoleucus*) and *Cryptococcus neoformans* in a captive anaconda (*Eunectes murinus*) have been reported.[73]

In crocodilians, most fungal infections are thought to be of enteric origin and occur in other tissues secondary to an immunocompromised state.[66,212] Fungal pneumonia in crocodilians is usually focal or multifocal, with granulomatous solidification of parts of the pulmonary parenchyma.[212,253] Dilatation of the bronchi and the formation of emphysematous bullae have also been reported.[253] Agents commonly recovered from crocodilian species with fungal infections include *Purpureocillium lilacinum* and *Fusarium* spp.[248] *Beauveria bassiana* was the cause of fatal pneumonia in two American alligators (*Alligator mississippiensis*).[254] *Metarhizium anisopliae* was recovered from a fungal pneumonia in association with pulmonary oxalosis in an American alligator.[255]

Parasitic Diseases

Numerous parasites have been reported in the respiratory system of reptiles.[73,74,77,184,212,253,256] Most respiratory parasites induce localized inflammation and irritation, which often leads to secondary bacterial pneumonia.[73] Therefore, mixed respiratory diseases involving parasitic, bacterial and/or fungal infections are commonly diagnosed in reptiles.[184]

Pentastomids are worm-like, annulated crustacean parasites that affect the lungs, trachea, and nasal passages of wild and captive snakes, lizards, turtles, and crocodilians.[73,184,253,257] Snakes and crocodilians are particularly affected.[184,253] Adult pentastomids feed on tissue fluids and lay embryonated eggs that pass into the oral cavity, are swallowed, and are excreted in the feces.[73] An intermediate host, generally a small mammal or a fish, is necessary to complete the cycle.[73] Genera of clinical importance include *Sebekia*, *Raillietiella*, *Kiricephalus*, *Porocephalus*, and *Armillifer*.[256] *Sebekia* is the main reported pentastomid genus in crocodilians and parasitize the lungs of the final host.[256] Fish serve as the intermediate host of *Sebekia*.[256] The genera *Subtriquetra* sp. and *Leiperia* spp. are found in the nasal passages and in the trachea of crocodilians, respectively and humans may serve as incidental hosts.[73,212,253] *Kiricephalus*, *Porocephalus*, and *Armillifer* spp. parasitize snakes, and several pentastomid species are common lung and air sac parasites of certain wild North American snakes.[256] The genera *Raillietiella* and *Sambonia* have been reported in the lungs of lizards (e.g., geckos, chameleons, monitors).[256,258] Clinical signs of pentastomid infestations in lizards include increased respiratory efforts and open-mouth dyspnea secondary to the obstruction of major airways by the parasites.[73,184,256] If present in the lungs, the parasites may cause inflammation and predispose the animal to secondary bacterial infection.[73,253] Subclinical infestations have also been described in snakes and crocodilians.[77,212]

Lungworms, *Rhabdias* spp. in snakes and lizards, especially *Rhabdias fuscovenosa* in snakes, *Entomelas* sp. in lizards, *Kiricephalus* spp. in snakes, and *Angiostoma carettae* in loggerhead sea turtles (*Caretta caretta*) may also affect the respiratory tract.[73,184,259,260] Infective larvae of *Rhabdias* spp. may directly penetrate the skin or may be ingested through contaminated food or water.[197] Ingested larvae penetrate the oral mucosa, gain access to the circulatory system, and ultimately become distributed to the lungs, where the larvae mature.[197] Heavy infestations may lead to secondary bacterial pneumonia.[73]

Renifers, or lung flukes, are digenetic trematodes of the genera *Dasymetra*, *Lechriochis*, *Zeugorchis*, *Ochestosoma*, and *Stomatrema* that may be found in the buccal cavity, pharynx, esophagus, or occasionally lower respiratory tract of reptiles, especially snakes.[73,77,256] Although most lung fluke infestations are subclinical, a heavy parasite load may predispose the host to secondary bacterial pneumonia.[73] Amphibians have been identified as intermediate hosts.[73,256]

Infection of freshwater and sea turtles with digenetic spirorchiid trematodes of the genera *Spirorchis*, *Henotosoma*, *Unicaecum*, *Vasotrema*, or *Hapalorhynchus* may cause clinical signs suggestive of pneumonia, although the target site for these parasites is the circulatory system.[73,256]

Monogenetic trematodes may inhabit the nasopharynx or urinary bladder of aquatic chelonians and are believed to be nonpathogenic.[74]

Other parasites have been infrequently reported to affect the respiratory system in reptiles, such as the trematode *Hemiuridae* in sea snakes, visceral coccidia in crocodilians and tortoises, *Microsporidium* in an inland bearded dragon (*Pogona vitticeps*), the snake lung mites *Entonyssus* and *Hamertonia* spp., and *Amblyomma exornatum* ticks have been diagnosed in the nasal passages of Nile monitors.[71,73,197,212,256]

Noninfectious Diseases

References to developmental anomalies (congenital disorders) affecting reptile lungs were not found in the literature.

Penetrating injuries to the lungs may be diagnosed in snakes, chelonians, and lizards, secondary to bite wounds from other pets or secondary to car or lawn mower traumas in chelonians.[71,184]

Respiratory foreign bodies are also commonly reported in chelonians and lizards, especially green iguanas (*Iguana iguana*).[184] Foreign bodies, such as plastic objects or fishhooks in free-ranging aquatic turtles, may lodge within the oropharynx and cause acute obstructive dyspnea in reptiles.[184,261]

Trauma, inflammation, or neoplastic proliferation of the surrounding tissue of the respiratory tract may also result in obstructive dyspnea.[71,184] Primary neoplasia of the respiratory tract or pulmonary metastasis has rarely been reported in reptiles (e.g., fibromas, fibroadenoma, fibrosarcoma, adenocarcinoma, oviductal carcinoma, chondrosarcoma, squamous cell carcinoma, lymphosarcoma, plasma cell tumor).[73,262,263] Lymphoma commonly affects oral tissues and lungs in snakes, lizards, and chelonians.[184] Several cases of tracheal chondromas associated with severe dyspnea have been reported in ball pythons (*Python regius*), suggesting a predisposition of this ophidian species to the tracheal neoplasia.[264,265] In sea turtles, fibropapillomas caused by chelonid HV5 may be located in the lungs.

Pulmonary edema from cardiac or hepatic disease may present as respiratory in origin and is uncommon.[73] A single case of pulmonary edema has been reported in a spur-thighed tortoise (*Testudo graeca*).[266]

Respiratory distress, especially on inspiration, due to reduction in tidal volume, may be caused by coelomic distension secondary to organomegaly, ascites, obesity, or pregnancy (see Figure 3-25).[73,184] Loosening of the skin around the nares just before shedding may produce noises during respiration and can be interpreted as respiratory tract disease.[73] A New Caledonia giant gecko (*Rhacodactylus leachianus*) was reported with an intussusception of the proximal left lung into the left bronchus and trachea causing hyperinflation of the right lung, lethargy, abdominal distention, and death.[267] Interstitial pulmonary fibrosis was documented in a leopard tortoise (*Geochelone pardalis*) presented with dyspnea.[268]

Hypovitaminosis A is a common disease in chelonians and results in the degeneration of epithelial surfaces including the lung faveoli.[67,71,74,269] Hypovitaminosis A can cause pathological changes that result in a large variety of clinical signs associated with rhinitis and lower tract diseases in chelonians.[71,73,74] Semiaquatic chelonians with acute hypovitaminosis A commonly present with periocular changes, whereas chronic deficiency in terrestrial chelonians is typically associated with respiratory, hepatic, renal, and/or pancreatic epithelial abnormalities.[74]

Pleural urate deposition has been reported in cases of visceral gout.[270]

Mammals

General Considerations

Upper and lower respiratory diseases are common in small mammals, with respiratory distress a common presenting complaint. Signs of respiratory illness can go unnoticed for a significant period by owners. Therefore, clinicians are often diagnosing and treating animals that have a chronic disease, consequently management of these cases can be challenging. Prompt recognition and appropriate therapeutic intervention are essential, as a delay can result in severe compromise or death of the patient. Rabbits and rodents are obligate nasal breathers, thus any lesion and/or disease affecting the upper respiratory system may present as a respiratory illness.

It must be emphasized that the onset of many diseases is related to physiopathogenic and environmental factors that lead to a compromise in host immunity. Stressors such as poor husbandry, sanitation, diet, high stocking densities, poor diet, and concurrent and underlying illnesses are examples that contribute to this. Consequently it is important to obtain a thorough history regarding the animal's signalment and also understand appropriate husbandry practices in order to gauge the likelihood of environmental contributions to the clinical picture.

Bacterial respiratory diseases are a major cause of morbidity and mortality in rabbits, guinea pigs, and rats, with mixed infections composed of multiple pathogens commonly diagnosed. Ferrets will present with secondary pneumonia due to a primary viral etiology, while hamsters and gerbils, in the context of clinical significance, do not commonly develop primary respiratory diseases.[271–273] African hedgehogs have been reported to present for respiratory disease and have similar etiological bacterial agents as rodents.[274]

Infectious Diseases
BACTERIAL DISEASES
RABBITS. Despite its presence as a commensal, *Pasteurella multocida* is an important bacterial pathogen in rabbits, causing

opportunistic infections.[275–277] Pasteurellaceae are gram-negative bacteria considered part of the normal flora of the rabbit mucous membranes. Pathogenicity is related to the type of strain affecting the animal and is more likely to occur in immunosuppressed animals.[278] Different disease states exist—once an individual is infected, acute disease such as bacteremia and pneumonia may develop after which the animal may become a chronic carrier or develop chronic clinical disease.[102] Studies have shown that there is a lack of passive transfer of antibody in weanlings, and none is actively acquired in adulthood.[276] As a result, adults are often presented with a vast array of clinical signs including rhinitis, sinusitis, conjunctivitis, nasolacrimal duct infection, otitis interna and media, tracheitis, pneumonia, and abscessation.[276,279]

Bordetella bronchiseptica is not considered a primary pathogen in rabbits despite historic reports of pure cultures being isolated from clinically ill animals.[276,277] *Bordetella bronchiseptica* is a common inhabitant of the upper airways in rabbits, but reports suggest that this bacterium could lead to pneumonia in some cases. It has been suggested that *Bordetella bronchiseptica* predisposes individuals to *Pasteurella* spp. infections. However, *Bordetella bronchiseptica* is a pathogen of clinical significance in rodents, and exposure to rabbits may be a predisposing factor to respiratory disease in these species.[102,276]

Treponema cuniculi is a venereal disease that is transmitted horizontally and associated with poorly managed colonies. The bacterium is a spirochete that has an affinity for mucocutaneous junctions.[279] *Treponema cuniculi* infection is more commonly known as rabbit syphilis. Overall, rabbit syphilis is rare in nonbreeding rabbits.[279,280] While it is not a primary respiratory pathogen, the presence of ulcers, vesicles, and discharge around the lips, nares, and eyelids resembles upper respiratory tract involvement.[281,282] Lesions are generally found in the genital region and can cause local lymphadenopathy.[279] Diagnosis is made by confirming the presence of the spiral organisms in lesions using silver stains.[280]

Other isolated bacterial organisms from rabbit respiratory lesions include *Staphylococcus* spp., *Pseudomonas* spp., *Moraxella* spp., *Yersinia pestis*, *Escherichia coli*, *Mycoplasma pulmonis*, *Mycobacterium* spp., *Streptococcus* spp., *Staphylococcus* spp., *Vibrio* spp., *Bacillus* spp., *Chlamydia* spp., and other *Pasteurella* spp.[278,283,284]

RODENTS. Chronic infectious respiratory disease is probably the most common disease of pet rats. Chronic infectious respiratory disease in rats is classically caused by the action of one or several bacterial and viral pathogens (see the section on rat respiratory viruses below under Rodents). The most important rat respiratory bacterial pathogens are *Mycoplasma pulmonis*, *Streptococcus pneumonia*, and *Corynebacterium kutscheri*. Bacteria of lesser importance that may precipitate clinical signs by potentiating the pathogenic actions of the major murine pathogens include cilia-associated respiratory (CAR) *Bacillus* and *Haemophilus* spp.

Mycoplasma pulmonis, an intracellular bacterium that is commonly isolated in rats, is a major respiratory disease of concern in older pet rats. It is a chronic disease to which acquisition occurs at a young age and may persist for life as subclinical disease.[285–287] *Mycoplasma pulmonis* infection varies in clinical presentation due to the complex host, environment, and pathogen relationship. Examples of predisposing history include high levels of ammonia as a result of poor sanitation and hygiene, concurrent viral infections, bacterial virulence, and dietary vitamin A and E deficiency.[288,289] Often, the organism is isolated with other etiological agents, commonly with CAR *Bacillus*.[290] *M. pulmonis* is transmitted horizontally through aerosolization and vertically in utero.[291] The pathophysiology of the disease has been described as a low-level airway inflammation, sustained damage, and remodeling of airway epithelium progression to bronchiectasis.[287] Clinical signs are not only associated with the respiratory tract but can appear as neurologic signs associated with otitis interna. *Mycoplasma pulmonis* infection has also been reported to present as endometritis associated with bacterial dissemination.[287,288,291,292] Elimination of *M. pulmonis* from large populations of rats and mice is impossible without rederivation or depopulation.[105]

Streptococcus pneumoniae is considered a commensal bacterium of the nasal passages and ear of rodents. This grampositive bacteria is pathogenic in rats and guinea pigs but can also cause subclinical disease.[293] The presence of *Streptococcus pneumoniae* can potentiate other diseases such as mycoplasma, as it causes suppurative inflammation of the upper respiratory tract spreading to the lungs, resulting in bronchopneumonia.[286,293] Serotypes III, IV, and XIX cause disease in guinea pigs and may be associated with poor husbandry and hypovitaminosis C.[294,295]

Corynebacterium kutscheri may also be part of the natural microbiota of rodents. Infections are usually subclinical, with development of pulmonary abscesses associated with immunosuppression or concurrent infection with other pathogens, in particular, *M. pulmonis*.[289,293] In mice, the disease is more generalized, and it has been reported to cause mucopurulent visceral disease in the kidneys and liver and septic polyarthritis.[296]

The identification of the CAR *Bacillus* is still pending phylogenetic classification, although has been described as a filamentous rod that adheres to the ciliary respiratory epithelium.[296] The CAR *Bacillus* has been described as a potentiator of other diseases such as mycoplasma and Sendai virus.[290,297] Subclinical infection can occur in rats and mice, with transmission likely associated with direct contact to affected individuals.[293]

Bordetella bronchiseptica is a gram-negative aerobic rod that causes purulent bronchopneumonia and suppurative pleuritis.[295] Bacterial pneumonia is exceedingly common in pet guinea pigs, and other bacteria may be implicated.[295] Guinea pigs are highly susceptible to *B. bronchiseptica*, while mice, hamsters, and rats appear to be more resistant to the disease, which presents as an opportunistic infection.[105] Some individuals can develop immunity and eliminate disease, while others become subclinical carriers.[100,114] Rabbits, dogs, and nonhuman primates are known subclinical carriers of the disease, therefore it is recommended not to house these animals together with guinea pigs.[295]

OTHER SPECIES. Bacterial pneumonia is reported to be uncommon in ferrets, but *Escherichia coli*, *Klebsiella pneumoniae*, *Pseudomonas aeruginosa*, *Streptococcus zooepidemicus*, *Listeria monocytogenes*, and *Bordetella bronchiseptica* have been isolated from ferrets diagnosed with respiratory disease.[298]

Pneumonia is reported in African hedgehogs and sugar gliders but there are few reports pertaining to specific pathogens. There is one article that described *P. multocida* being isolated from a sugar glider that was housed in the same area with rabbits. A sugar glider housed in the same area as rabbits, culturing *P. multocida*.[299,300] A case of *Corynebacterial* bronchopneumonia was documented in an African hedgehog.[301] Other cases of pneumonia have been reported in nonpet species of hedgehogs.

VIRAL DISEASES

FERRETS. Canine distemper virus (CDV) is a single-stranded RNA virus of the genus *Morbillivirus* in the Paramyxoviridae family. It is a highly contagious disease, although because of the above properties, it is a short-lived virus prone to environmental desiccation. Domestic ferrets are highly susceptible to CDV, with reported mortalities close to 100%.[302] Due to the ubiquity of CDV in dogs, young and unvaccinated ferrets are at risk of being exposed to the disease through canine companions.[298,303] The primary mode of transmission of CDV is aerosolization of viral particles onto mucous membranes from respiratory and other bodily secretions. The respiratory system is a preferred site for a virus replication, causing upper respiratory tract signs. The incubation period of CDV is 7 to 10 days, anorexia, pyrexia, and serous nasal discharge are the initial clinical signs observed with the disease in ferrets.[304] Progressive clinical signs include fever, oculonasal discharge, dermatitis from crusting, hyperkeratosis of footpads, secondary bacterial pneumonia, and death.[305,306] Due to routine vaccination in ferrets, CDV is not a common clinical presentation.[306] Antemortem diagnosis of CDV infection in ferrets is achieved by fluorescent antibody of conjunctival swabs or blood smears and postmortem, brain tissue.

Influenza virus, an RNA virus from the Orthomyxoviridae family, is classified into three species: A, B, and C, with A being most medically relevant to ferrets.[307] The ferret is extensively used as a model for human influenza research, as disease progression in ferrets is similar to humans.[304] Influenza virus is a zoonotic and an anthroponotic disease, transmitted primarily by aerosolization of respiratory secretions, and causes primarily upper respiratory disease.[298,306] Ferrets may exhibit high fever that may undulate, heavy bouts of productive sneezing, lethargy, and inappetence.[308] In comparison to distemper, influenza virus has a low mortality rate and clinical signs resolve within a 10- to 14-day period.[309] Similarly, respiratory secretions are often mucoserous rather than mucopurulent.[306] Since the disease is self-resolving, supportive care is recommended, including force-feeding, cough suppressants, antihistamines, antimucolytics, and antibiotics to control secondary bacterial infections.[273] Antiviral medications can be used but their efficacy and therapeutic effect are unknown.[310]

The systemic ferret coronavirus has been documented to cause pulmonary lesions and upper respiratory signs in young ferrets, and Aleutian disease parvovirus is known to induce interstitial pneumonia in minks.[298,311]

RABBITS. Reported viral diseases of pet rabbits are uncommon and some only appear to pose problems with laboratory animals. In Europe, the myxoma virus is highly virulent to *Oryctolagus cuniculus* and can lead to hemorrhagic pneumonia, suppurative bronchopneumonia, fibrinous pleuritis, and nasal disease in the atypical form of myxomatosis (amyxomatous form).[284] An outbreak of HV caused respiratory signs in a commercial rabbit facility in mini-Rex and meat-type rabbits in Alaska.[312,313]

RODENTS. The Sendai virus belongs to the paramyxovirus family. This RNA virus causes acute respiratory disease in rats and is regularly associated with co-infection with organisms such as mycoplasma.[288,291,293] Rodents are natural hosts for this virus, and infections often reduces fertility and fecundity and in young individuals results in retardation of growth.[293,296]

The sialodacryoadenitis virus is a coronavirus and is not considered primary respiratory pathogen in rats. The sialodacryoadenitis virus causes inflammation and edema of the cervical salivary glands, initially causing rhinitis that may appear as an upper respiratory infection. This coronavirus is a highly contagious disease, spread through aerosolization and fomites to which epizootics do occur, and clinical signs include lymphadenomegaly, corneal lesions, conjunctivitis, keratitis, and porphyrin staining.[288,289] The virus has tissue tropism for salivary glands, with chronic focal lesions having been identified in the harderian glands.[293,314] Mortalities associated with the sialodacryoadenitis virus in rats are rare.

Other viruses known to cause respiratory disease in Muridae include the rat respiratory virus (hantavirus) and the pneumonia virus of mice (paramyxovirus).

The guinea pig adenovirus is responsible for bronchopneumonia in this species and has low morbidity but high mortality.[315] Subclinical infections have also been described in guinea pigs diagnosed with adenovirus.

PARASITIC DISEASES. Parasitic respiratory diseases are uncommon in exotic companion mammals. European hedgehogs (*Erinaceus europaeus*) and one species of hedgehogs of the same genus as the African pygmy hedgehogs, the Algerian hedgehog (*Atelerix algirus*), have been reported to have an endemic primary lungworm disease, *Crenosoma striatum*.[316] The life cycle of the lungworm is completed in the hedgehog and acquired through snail ingestion. Clinical signs commonly observed in hedgehogs with lungworm disease are wasting and difficulty breathing associated with larval migration.[317]

FUNGAL DISEASES. As primary respiratory pathogens, fungal diseases appear to be rarely reported in small mammals.

Cryptococcus spp. are a type of capsulated, dimorphic, basidiomycetous fungi that is ubiquitous in the environment. *Cryptococcus* spp. has been isolated in dogs and cats with upper respiratory disease, but in dogs, it has been reported to disseminate to include the eyes and central nervous system.[318] The few reports confirming disease in ferrets have been described all presentations listed above and are commonly associated with immunosuppression.[307] Other fungal pneumonia that has been reported in ferrets includes *Pneumocystis carinii*, *Blastomyces dermatitidis*, and *Coccidioides immitis*.[298] *Aspergillus* pleuritis was diagnosed in a ferret with concurrent lymphosarcoma by one of the above authors.

Fungal sinusitis has been described in rabbits.[278]

Noninfectious Diseases

Perhaps the most common disease in pet rabbits and some rodents is dental disease, with strong correlations to poor diet and congenital conformation. The disease may cause abscessation of periapical tissues and may present as upper respiratory signs, as anatomically, rabbits and most rodents are obligate nasal breathers (see Figures 3-26 and 3-28). In addition, disseminated bacteremia may lead to pneumonia.[99,319,320] Similarly in prairie dogs, pseudo-odontoma is a common presentation and is due to the space-occupying

mass associated with an elongated maxillary incisor tooth root.[98]

Cranial thoracic masses may lead to signs of respiratory disease by compression of lungs and major airways. Rabbits normally have a well-developed thymus into adulthood, and in cases where animals diagnostically have a cranial thoracic mass, this organ is often associated with an abnormal mass. Differential disease diagnoses for cranial thoracic masses include thymic hyperplasia, thymoma, thymic lymphosarcoma, thymic carcinoma, chemodectoma, ectopic thyroid tissue, thyroid carcinoma, thymic branchial cysts, mediastinal granuloma or abscess, hemorrhage, mast cell tumor, and metastatic neoplasia.[99] Thymic lymphoma and lymphepithelial thymomas appear to be the most commonly reported cranial thoracic masses diagnosed in exotic small mammals in the literature.[321] These cases often present acutely for signs of respiratory distress, although they may also be associated with "cranial vena cava" syndrome, where there is exophthalmos due to impedance of venous return to the heart.[289,321,322] Nevertheless in ferrets cranial mediastinal masses are often caused by lymphosarcoma.[273,322] Primary neoplasia is rare, although guinea pigs are known to develop bronchogenic papillary adenomas.[289] Bronchogenic papillary adenomas have been reported as underdiagnosed in guinea pigs and should be a differential in cases where there is no response to conventional treatment for pneumonia. The prevalence of bronchogenic papillary adenomas is approximately 30%, and while the tumor is slow growing, rarely metastasizing, it does reduce the functional volume of the lungs.[100,323] In rabbits, secondary pulmonary metastases due to uterine adenocarcinoma in nonspayed females are common.[292,322] There are few reports of respiratory neoplasia in hedgehogs and sugar gliders (Figure 3-9).

Ferrets have been reported to commonly present for respiratory distress as a result of underlying cardiac disease (see cardiology section). Pleural effusion due to congestive heart failure is common in this species (Figure 3-10).

Small mammals may be presented for predator bites, conspecific confrontation, accidental falls, and motor vehicle accidents. This occurs more often to ferrets due to their curious nature but other species are just as susceptible. Animals may present with fractures, pneumomediastinum, pneumothorax, and hemothorax, for which emergency and critical care is recommended.[104,273,322]

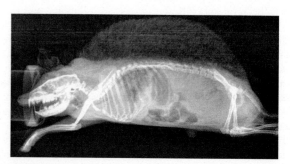

FIGURE 3-9 Lateral thoracic radiograph showing a diffuse thoracic mass in an African hedgehog; the final diagnosis was histiocytic sarcoma. (Courtesy of Isabelle Langlois.)

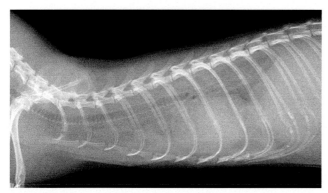

FIGURE 3-10 Lateral thoracic radiograph showing pleural effusion due to congestive heart failure in a ferret.

Vitamin C deficiency in guinea pigs causes nonspecific illnesses including signs of recurrent pneumonia, painful joints, immobility, anorexia, pathologic fractures, weakness, petechiation, and diarrhea.[100] Ascorbic acid is required as a cofactor for the synthesis of collagen and dietary supplementation if recommended for prevention. Supplementation may be administered using commercially available vitamin C tablets and offering dark-leafy greens in the diet, with response being rapid.[324] Supportive care and therapy is recommended in ongoing management of the patient's overall disease conditions.[99]

Intestinal obstruction and gastric stasis in guinea pigs and rabbits can cause reduced thoracic volume and resulting in respiratory distress.[295] Aspiration pneumonia has been reported as well as iatrogenic induced pneumonia due to force-feeding mineral oil to ferrets with suspected foreign body.[298] Endogenous lipid pneumonia has also been reported in ferrets.[325]

Respiratory hypersensitivity or irritation has not been well documented in exotic companion mammals but does appear with some frequency in rabbits. Dusty, moldy, or allergenic hay may be implicated in some cases of respiratory hypersensitivity in rabbits. Nasal foreign bodies are possible and hay is frequently identified as the cause in many cases.[326] Short-nosed rabbits seem also to be affected by a syndrome presenting with clinical similarities to the canine brachiocephalic syndrome, but this disease condition has not been well described. Laryngeal paralysis may be encountered in rabbits as well as laryngeal and tracheal trauma after repeated or difficult intubations.

Birds

Nasal and Sinus Diseases

Rhinitis and sinusitis are common diseases in birds and have the potential to spread to most structures of the head, owing to the extensive pneumatization of the beak, skull, and cervical area. Diseases that cause rhinitis and sinusitis in birds frequently extend to the periorbital region.

Chronic granulomatous rhinitis (or rhinolith) is frequently diagnosed in psittacine birds fed a seed-only diet and is particularly common in cockatiels, African gray parrots, and Amazon parrots. Chronic granulomatous rhinitis appears to be strongly correlated with nutritional deficiencies, notably vitamin A. Concretions of desquamated epithelium, debris, and necrotic and inflammatory materials occupy the nasal cavity and induce progressive tissue destruction, which can be extensive. Upon debridement, permanent damage to the nasal cavities and nasal conchae is often present. Since the normal function of the upper respiratory system is compromised and chronic nasal irritation occurs, rhinoliths periodically recur. Opportunistic organisms frequently involved in the disease process include a variety of gram-negative bacteria (*Escherichia coli*, *Enterobacter* spp., *Pseudomonas* spp., *Klebsiella* spp.) and fungus (*Aspergillus* spp., *Candida* spp., zygomycetes).[327,328] Nasal plugs caused by exudate secondary to chronic rhinitis also occur in falcons.[329] Spiral bacteria have been implicated in upper respiratory disease and infection of the choanal slit and oral cavity in cockatiels.[330]

Infectious rhinitis and sinusitis may be caused by a variety of organisms and frequently manifest as nasal discharge, periorbital swellings, redness, and facial feather loss. Hypovitaminosis A may also cause squamous metaplasia in various locations of the oropharynx.

Chronic sinusitis in macaws is responsible for a so-called sunken-eye syndrome.[327,328] Sinusal exudates do not drain well in birds because of the dorsal location of the sinusal opening into the nasal cavity (see the Anatomy and Physiology section at the beginning of the chapter) and the viscous consistency of avian inflammatory exudates, gram-negative bacteria, *Chlamydia psittaci* (*Chlamydophila psittaci*), and *Mycoplasma* spp. are frequently cited as common etiological agents respiratory disease in various species of birds. Uncomplicated avian chlamydiosis frequently presents as only a mild rhinitis and conjunctivitis in cockatiels and pigeons. Gallinaceous suffer from a high rate of sinusitis for which *Mycoplasma gallisepticum*, *Avibacterium paragallinarum* (infectious coryza of chicken, formerly *Haemophilus*), and *Bordetella avium* (turkey coryza) are common etiological agents.[331] *Mycoplasma gallisepticum* is also a significant disease of house finches in North America and presents with conjunctivitis, sinusitis, and significant morbidity.[332] Mycoplasma infection is also associated with upper respiratory disease in psittacine birds.[333] *Mycoplasma* spp. appear to be commensal organisms in Falconiformes and Accipitriformes.[334,335] *Mycobacterium tuberculosis* and *M. marinum* have been associated with upper respiratory granulomas in psittacine birds.[327,336-339] Viruses with specific nasal and sinusal tropism are uncommon. Rhinotracheitis in turkeys is caused by a pneumovirus. Localized skin diseases around the nostrils, such as cnemidocoptic infestation and poxvirus infection, may constrict the external nasal openings. *Cryptococcus neoformans* has been identified as a cause of a chronic rhinosinusitis in a cockatoo.[340]

Parasitic diseases of the nasal and sinusal system are less common than infections with bacterial organisms. Cnemidocoptic mites may cause hyperkeratosis of the cere with subsequent obstruction of the nares in budgerigars. Trichomoniasis may extend to the choanal area and sinus in raptors and pigeons. *Cryptosporidium baileyi* was the cause of upper respiratory infections in falcons and scops owls.[341-343] Various helminth parasites may be found in the nasal and sinusal tissues in wild water birds, in particular Anseriformes, and include trematodes of the Cyclocoelidae family, *Trichobilharzia* spp. schistosomes, and *Theromyzon* spp. nasal leeches.[344-346]

Plant or seed foreign bodies can be lodged in the nasal cavity or the choanal opening, and chicks may aspirate formula through their choana. Respiratory irritants may also promote nasal inflammation and sneezing. Choanal atresia has been reported in African gray parrots and an Umbrella cockatoo and is characterized by the incomplete development of the choanal region.[327,347]

Hyperinflation or rupture of the cervicocephalic diverticulum of the infraorbital sinus is a relatively common occurrence and manifests as one or multiple large subcutaneous air pockets. This condition has been described in multiple avian species.[327,348–350] In severe cases, it may significantly restrict cervical movement (Figure 3-11). The pathophysiology is poorly understood and the exact location of air leakage in cases of a rupture is difficult if not impossible to determine. This condition may be caused by different diseases of the cervicocephalic diverticulum such as trauma, infection, congenital abnormality, and disruption of normal connection with the infraorbital sinus.

Choanal and sinusal squamous cell carcinoma have been reported in a black-footed penguin and an eclectus parrot.[351,352] Other nasal and sinus neoplasia reported in psittacine birds includes lymphosarcoma, carcinoma, fibrosarcoma, and melanoma.[328]

Tracheal Diseases

Diseases of the avian larynx are uncommon. They include glottal internal papillomatosis (mainly in green-winged macaws) and laryngeal trauma from intubation (damage to the *crista ventralis*).[353–355]

Postintubation tracheal stenosis occurs approximately 1 to 2 weeks after an intubation event and has been reported in blue and gold macaws, geese, bald eagles, red-tailed hawks, a curassow, and other avian species (Figure 3-12).[356–360] The authors have also diagnosed postintubation tracheal stenosis in a sandhill crane, a Jandaya conure, an African gray parrot, and a screech owl. Tracheal stenosis secondary to severe tracheitis or tracheal trauma has also been reported.[361–363] Tracheal foreign bodies are more common in small psittacine birds, particularly cockatiels, in which a millet seed is commonly aspirated.[348,364–366]

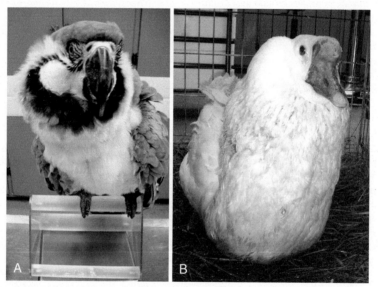

FIGURE 3-11 Cervicocephalic diverticulum rupture in a blue and gold macaw *(A)* and a domestic goose *(B)*.

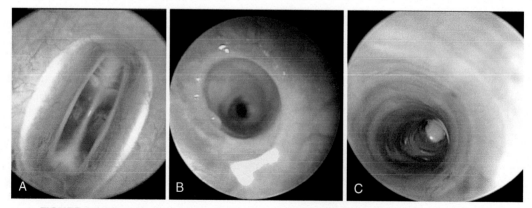

FIGURE 3-12 Tracheoscopy in birds showing the normal syrinx in an eclectus parrot *(A)*, a xanthogranulomatous lesion associated with tracheal stenosis in a blue and gold macaw *(B)*, and a syringeal aspergilloma in an eclectus parrot *(C)*.

Viral diseases of the trachea cause diphtheritic lesions and primarily include HV infections such as the infectious laryngotracheitis virus in chickens (and also pheasants and guinea fowls), the Amazon tracheitis virus in Amazon parrots and other psittacine species (in recently imported birds), cytomegalovirus in Australian finches, psittacid HV3 infection in eclectus parrots and Bourke's parakeets, and poxviruses such as the diphtheric or wet form of poxviruses typically encountered in passerine birds, various parakeets, lovebirds, and mynahs.[327,328,331,353,367-370] Vaccination of galliformes species, other than chickens, with chicken-attenuated infectious laryngotracheitis virus may cause disease.

Various bacterial agents implicated in tracheitis may lead to tracheal stenosis, either by fibrous tissue or granuloma formation. The trachea was found to be the principal replication site for experimental *Chlamydia psittaci* infection in the turkey.[371] *Bordetella avium* primarily infects the trachea in turkeys.[331] *Mycoplasma* spp. are routinely recovered from the trachea of normal birds of prey.[334,335] *Enterococcus faecalis* is associated with chronic tracheitis in canaries.[372,373] A granulomatous tracheitis caused by *Mycobacterium genavense* was diagnosed in an Amazon parrot.[374]

Tracheal and syringeal aspergillosis is the most common fungal infection diagnosed in the avian trachea (see Figure 3-12). Species frequently diagnosed with tracheal aspergillosis include Amazon parrots, African gray parrots, macaws, and falcons. Hypovitaminosis A is frequently cited as a predisposing factor for the formation of tracheal and syringeal aspergilloma.

Several parasites are known to infest the avian trachea and include nematodes such as *Syngamus* spp. (mainly, *Syngamus trachea*) and *Cyathostoma* spp. (mainly *Cyathostoma bronchialis*) and acarids such as *Sternostoma tracheacolum*.[327,331,375] Tracheal worms infest a wide range of species but clinical disease is most frequently encountered in captive birds of prey, poultry, and game birds. The life cycle of *S. trachea* is direct and earthworms may act as paratenic hosts (larvae may remain viable for up to 3 yr in earthworms), which facilitates reexposure in a closed environment with access to the ground. *C. bronchialis* infests mainly Anseriformes and birds of prey and requires earthworms as intermediate hosts.[375] *Sternostoma tracheacolum* (tracheal, air sac mites) infests primarily canaries and Gouldian finches. The mite has a direct life cycle and is passed from parents to chicks.[328,376]

Inhaled toxins and smoke-inhalation injuries may cause severe necrotizing tracheitis (see the next section). Hypovitaminosis A not only predisposes birds to respiratory diseases by altering mucosal defenses but may also promotes epithelial changes, notably in the syrinx. Tracheal neoplasias are uncommon, but tracheal osteochondroma has been reported in parrots.[328]

Diseases of the Lungs and Air Sacs

Lower respiratory diseases are common in birds, and infectious causes tend to predominate. Bacterial pneumonia and airsacculitis have been reported, with a variety of organisms being identified as causative agents, but gram-negative bacteria seem to predominate. Bacteria commonly reported to cause lower respiratory infections in birds include *Pasteurella multocida*, *Ornithobacterium rhinotracheale* (mainly chickens), *Escherichia coli*, *Klebsiella* spp., *Salmonella* spp., *Chlamydia psittaci*, *Riemerella anatipestifer* (mainly waterfowl), *Pseudomonas aeruginosa*, *Staphylococcus* spp., *Streptococcus* spp., *Mycoplasma* spp., and *Mycobacterium* spp.[327,329,331] The importance and pathogenicity of bacterial isolates also depend on the species of bird involved. *Chlamydia psittaci* frequently causes diffuse airsacculitis, and *Mycobacterium* spp. generally produce large granulomatous lesions.[331,377-379] Avian chlamydiosis is an important disease of birds, especially Psittaciformes due to its zoonotic potential. Chlamydial strains are host specific and often produce mild disease in their natural hosts (e.g., cockatiels).[371,380,381] In addition, long-term presence of chlamydial organisms in nonclinical natural hosts is suspected. Large avian wildlife reservoirs have been identified and are sources of exposure to susceptible species. Different avian serotypes are described, and serotype A is predominant in Psittaciformes, but serotype E is associated with more significant clinical disease. Serotype B is the most frequent in pigeons, and serotype D has been characterized as highly virulent in turkeys. Clinical signs are variable in avian chlamydiosis but commonly involve the respiratory system, where mild to severe airsacculitis is a frequent necropsy finding.

Viral diseases of the lungs are less common than other infectious causes but include paramyxovirus I, avian influenza, infectious bronchitis (chickens), avian polyomavirus (nestling cockatoos), and canarypox.[328,331,353]

Aspergillosis is a predominant respiratory fungal infection in birds. Avian species reported to be more susceptible to respiratory aspergillosis include northern raptorial species (e.g., snowy owls, gyrfalcons, rough-legged hawks), juvenile red-tailed hawks, golden eagles, northern goshawks, penguins, flamingos, seabirds (e.g., pelicans, auks, gannets, gulls, petrels, loons), certain parrot species (e.g., African gray parrots, Pionus parrots, blue-fronted Amazon parrots), waterfowl, storks, and mynahs. Large epizootics in wild birds have been reported when gregarious species are exposed simultaneously to large quantities of spores.[382] Wild bird chicks of susceptible species may have a high mortality rate, and the infection appears to be associated with nest materials and dynamics promoting high local spore loads.[382] *Aspergillus fumigatus* is the primary fungal species isolated in birds, but other *Aspergillus* species can be cultured (e.g., *flavus*, *nigricans*, *nidulans*, etc.). Aspergillosis is neither zoonotic nor contagious, but any environmental strain has the potential to be pathogenic. Pathogenesis appears to be associated with exposure to high spore loads, resulting in acute pulmonary aspergillosis or some degree of immunosuppression leading to chronic pulmonary-air sac aspergillosis (Figures 3-13 and 3-14). Tracheal and syringeal aspergillosis constitutes a third form of the disease (see Figure 3-12). Risk factors that have been associated with an increased susceptibility respiratory fungal disease include lead toxicosis (waterfowls, raptors), smoke-inhalation injury, captivity (especially seabirds), stress, steroids, tetracycline (likely due to immunomodulatory effect of long-term use), neoplasia, circovirus infection, hypovitaminosis A, and others.[382-386] In the authors' experience, an air sac cannula maintained for several days, frequently leads to focal aspergillosis lesions. Since the air sac system pneumatizes most of the avian body, aspergillosis lesions may extend to any internal organ by local invasion or distantly by hematogenous dissemination, as *Aspergillus* spp. presents as angiotropism in tissues. Moreover, *Aspergillus* spp. produce a wide

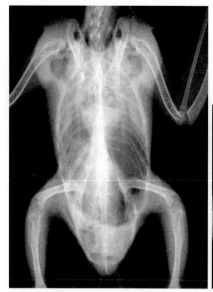
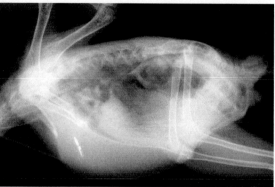

FIGURE 3-13 Whole-body radiographs of an African gray parrot with respiratory aspergillosis. On the ventrodorsal view *(left),* the right part of the air sac system presents some soft tissue opacities, and on the lateral view *(right),* the air sacs are considerably thickened by aspergillosis lesions, which form characteristic "caverns."

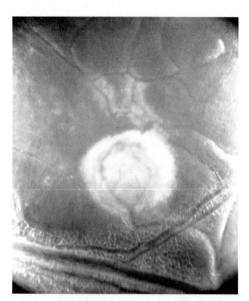

FIGURE 3-14 Close-up view of a focal lesion of aspergillosis on an air sac membrane in a snowy owl. The air sac is displaying mild thickening and hypervascularization, and the small fungal plaque is supplied by a small vessel.

variety of mycotoxins, some with immunosuppressive effects such as the gliotoxin, which may participate in the disease progression and pathogenesis.[387] Various experimental avian models have been developed to further elucidate the pathogenesis and progression of the disease.[388–392]

Several lower respiratory parasitic diseases are of significance in birds. *Sarcocystis falcatula* is a protozoan parasite that has an indirect life cycle, with the Virginia opossum serving as the final host and cockroaches as potential mechanical vectors. *Sarcocystis falcatula* is associated with an acute pulmonary form of the disease in Old World species, such as cockatoos, rather than the classic muscular form.[393,394] Pulmonary lesions are also common, with disseminated visceral coccidiosis in cranes.[395] *Toxoplasma gondii* is a protozoan parasite whose final host is the cat, and that can affect a wide range of avian species. In birds, pulmonary lesions are common with toxoplasmosis. Atoxoplasmosis is caused by the coccidian parasite *Isospora serini* and affects diverse passerine birds from various families, with canaries and finches commonly reported with the disease. Pulmonary lesions are reported with *Isospora serini*, but hepatic and splenic lesions predominate. The air sac mites *Sternostoma tracheacolum* live in the air sacs and lungs but are most often pathogenic in the upper airways (see section on tracheal diseases). Various filarioid nematodes, identified in the lower respiratory system of birds, include the genera *Paronchocerca, Splendidofilaria, Chandlerella, Serratospiculum,* and *Diplotriaena.*[396,397] Most infections of filarioid nematodes in birds do not produce clinical disease. *Serratospiculum seurati* is a common parasite of air sacs in saker and other falcons in the Middle East, and beetle species are the intermediate hosts. Other species of *Serratospiculum* have been reported in birds of prey from various geographical locations. *Serratospiculum* and *Diplotriaena* do not produce microfilariae but rather eggs that developed in insect hosts. These parasites may produce airsacculitis and promote lower respiratory infections. Several genera of air sac flukes (trematodes) have been reported to parasitize wild and captive zoo birds and are associated with mollusks as intermediate hosts.[346,398]

Birds are quite sensitive to smoke-inhalation toxicosis and airborne toxins because of their large and efficient pulmonary exchange surface. Incriminated toxic fumes frequently include polytetrafluoroethylene (PTFE; teflon) from overheated cookware, cigarette smoke, household aerosols (e.g., house perfumes, candles, disinfectants), carbon monoxide, and ammonia. Signs are most often acute, especially in PTFE inhalation and other toxic fumes, with severe pulmonary hemorrhage and congestion observed on postmortem examination (see Figure 3-33). Respiratory signs may develop as long as 3 days after toxin exposure.

Several other noninfectious diseases of clinical significance have been reported in captive birds. Aspiration pneumonia may be encountered in baby birds (chronic poor-doers) and gavage fed hospitalized birds. The "conure bleeding syndrome" frequently manifests as bleeding in the respiratory tract and hemoptysis. Hemoptysis and pulmonary hemorrhage also occur in birds of prey with secondary rodenticide poisoning.[399] Advanced atherosclerosis and cardiac diseases can also cause respiratory signs. Chronic pulmonary interstitial fibrosis has been reported in Amazon parrots and has been associated with right-sided heart failure in some birds.[400,401] A chronic obstructive respiratory disease has been reported in blue and gold macaws (these authors have also seen several affected green-winged macaws) housed with species that produce higher levels of feather powder such as cockatoos, cockatiels, and African gray parrots.[328,402] This syndrome is characterized by polycythemia, pulmonary congestion, and atrial smooth muscle hypertrophy. Severe inspiratory dyspnea with open-mouth breathing is often observed and is intermittent in birds diagnosed with chronic obstructive respiratory disease. Pneumoconiosis (anthracosis, silicosis) results from the accumulation of foreign material (dust) and dust-laden macrophages in the lungs and has been reported in various avian species.[328] Pulmonary fat embolism has been reported in an osprey and pet psittacine birds.[328,403] Air sac cannulation for several days often causes a moderate to marked air sac inflammatory reaction. Subcutaneous emphysema around the body may be caused by air sac trauma such as that resulting from a coeliotomy, coelioscopy, or fracture of a pneumatized bone.

Neoplasias of the lower respiratory tract include pulmonary adenocarcinoma, air sac adenocarcinoma, and metastasis of malignant tumors. Pulmonary and bronchogenic carcinomas have been reported in macaws, a partridge, and a cockatoo and often manifest as hind limb ataxia/paresis due to local invasion of the tumor into the spine.[404-408] These tumors frequently invade the humeral air sac diverticulum. Air sac cystadenocarcinomas have mainly been reported in cockatoos, but an African gray parrot case has also been documented. These tumors usually arise from the proximal humeral and axillary air sac diverticulum.[409-412] Undifferentiated neoplasia of the lungs and air sacs has been recognized in cockatiels and seems to be diagnosed most often in the thoracic inlet occasionally compressing the trachea (Figures 3-15 and 3-16).[328,353] Marek's disease may cause pulmonary tumors in chickens.[331]

Extrarespiratory Diseases: Airflow Occlusion and Air Sac Compression

Due to the extensive nature of the air sac system in birds, especially that of the abdomen and thorax, any extrarespiratory disease resulting in reduction of air sac volume or occlusion of major airways may result in respiratory clinical signs.

In the thoracic inlet, masses of nonrespiratory origin may occlude the trachea, syrinx, and interclavicular air sac, leading to inspiratory dyspnea, aphonia, or voice changes (see Figures 3-15 and 3-16). These masses include thyroid masses (goiter,

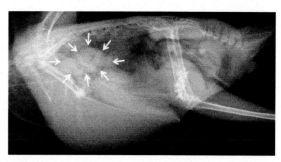

FIGURE 3-15 Cranial lung/air sac mass in a cockatiel with dyspnea and regurgitation. The final diagnosis was lymphoma. *White arrows delineate the mass.*

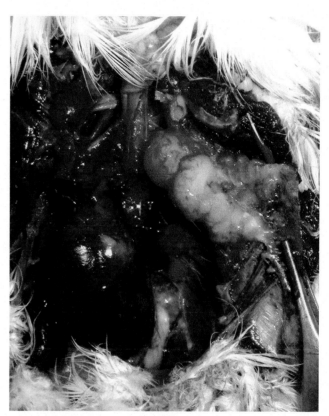

FIGURE 3-16 Soft tissue sarcoma in the interclavicular air sac of a cockatiel that presented with open-mouth breathing and regurgitation.

especially in budgerigars, thyroid neoplasia), bony callus from a coracoid fracture, aneurysm, large granulomas, neoplasia such as undifferentiated sarcoma (see Figure 3-16), hemangiosarcoma, thymoma, and other tumors.[413-416] Typically cardiomegaly does not induce coughing in birds as it does in mammals.

A significant reduction in air space may occur with fluid accumulation in the coelomic cavities of birds, such as ascites resulting from cardiac, hepatic, or neoplastic diseases, and egg-yolk coelomitis. Severe respiratory complications may arise if the fluid/yolk gains access to the respiratory system through a breach in an air sac or coelomic cavity membrane.

Space-occupying masses are also associated with impairment of abdominal ventilation and are encountered with large tumors (e.g., budgerigars), granuloma, eggs, and organomegaly. Obstruction of air sac ostia is rare but may interfere with ventilation. An ostrich was reported with intestinal entrapment in a right pulmonary ostium.[417] Finally, obesity with intracoelomic fat accumulation may impair normal ventilation and induce dyspnea, especially after exercise.

SPECIFIC DIAGNOSTICS

Invertebrates

Physical Examination

A thorough history, including husbandry and control of water quality for aquatic species, is just as important as performing a clinical examination on invertebrates. It is difficult to assess the respiratory rate of invertebrates and determine their effort, especially since most do not have ventilatory movements.[3,9] Diagnosis of diseases in invertebrate species can be frustrating but should nonetheless be pursued to gain a better understanding of the processes involved and their physiological responses.[143,418] The use of magnification through a hand lens, surgical loupes, or an endoscope will facilitate clinical examinations, especially when examining the ospithosomal entrance to the book lungs in arachnids for any evidence of mites or larvae or spiracles in insects and arachnids.[419] Presence of discharge, ulceration, and abnormalities should be noted and properly assessed to develop an appropriate treatment plan.

Judicious use of anesthesia may facilitate a better examination, as it is important not only for the animal's safety but also potentially for the handler.[3] Induction for terrestrial species is carried out with 5% isoflurane that is titrated to effect.[3,148] For immobilization of aquatic patients, tricaine methanesulfanate (MS-222), benzocaine, clove oil, and ethanol have been recommended.[9,148]

Pathology

When establishing a diagnosis in invertebrates, one must consider the potential existence of an ecto- or endosymbiont relationship, given that there is little literature and/or research describing invertebrate pathogens.[145] Routine hemolymph collection submission for culture that may provide evidence of septicemia can be submitted but is nonspecific for the respiratory system.[145] Antemortem wet-mount slides of the integument and aspirated contents allow for cytologic assessment on individual specimens.[3] An example of this diagnostic technique includes identification of the oral nematode Panagrolaimidae under light microscopy on a smear with a drop of saline. Swabs can be taken for microbiology, but it may be challenging to differentiate pathogenic organisms from organisms that are normally part of the invertebrate's environment and microbiota.[141] A fecal sample may also be analyzed as part of the health assessment.

Postmortem examination of an invertebrate patient may be more rewarding than a thorough clinical examination.[419] It may be necessary to sacrifice a number of animals from the collection rather than just obtaining the affected individual in order to establish a diagnosis utilizing a representative sample of the group. Submission of tissues for histopathology after immediate fixation should be interpreted with the help of an experienced invertebrate pathologist to obtain the best results.

Diagnostic Imaging

Radiology, although readily accessible in clinical practice, is not diagnostically useful in most terrestrial invertebrates (e.g., arthropods), as there is no real soft tissue differentiation.[146] Ultrasonography using a 10 MHz phased array curvilinear probe may be a useful diagnostic tool, but the ospithosoma has a water-resistant cuticle that is repellent to ultrasound gel and traps a layer of air on the cuticle; thus, ethanol is preferentially used. Antemortem diagnosis of Acroceridae nematodes may be confirmed by an experienced operator.[148,419] Microcomputer tomography has been reported to be used for imaging invertebrates. Moreover magnetic resonance imaging (MRI) studies have provided excellent images and resolution of ospithosomal anatomy in arachnids.[15,419]

Fish

Water Quality Testing

Taking a thorough history is paramount when practicing fish medicine. Specifically, clients should be questioned on the frequency and water quality testing methods used, quarantine protocols, frequency and amount of water change performed, life support systems present (e.g., filter, protein skimmer, ultraviolet [UV] sterilizer, algae scrubber), general maintenance and feeding, number and type of living organisms in the system (e.g., fish, invertebrates, plants), and a rough idea of morbidity and mortality.

A variety of kits may be used to measure water quality parameters. Continuous monitoring of major parameters such as ammonia, nitrites, and nitrates is also available. Alternatively, semiquantitative commercially available kits, based on color charts and marketed for aquarium hobbyists are perfectly acceptable for use in the clinics for individual patients (Figure 3-17). Quantitative kits and electronic probes are relatively expensive but provide more accurate results than those based on color charts. Test kits that are more accurate are recommended when investigating large culture systems to aid in identifying chronic stressors that may promote diseases or decreased breeding and growth. A minimum database for water quality measurements should include pH, ammonium, nitrites, nitrates, hardness, alkalinity, and salinity in associated species (marine and brackish aquaria, African cichlids). Water samples may be frozen for future analysis of various water quality parameters.

Dissolved oxygen (DO) is defined as the water concentration of oxygen, and this data is measured using a DO meter. Dissolved oxygen should be measured on site relative to the water temperature, as oxygen concentrations will also change in a water sample due to air exposure. Other parameters that may influence respiratory health (e.g., ammonium, nitrites, nitrates) and oxygen dissolution in water (e.g., temperature, pH, salinity) should be measured. Water concentrations of ammonium and nitrites should be near undetectable concentrations using colorimetric kits in a stable aquarium. Fish species vary in their susceptibility to ammonium and nitrite poisoning but the levels of these compounds should remain low within the aquatic environment. Nitrate levels may be higher but keeping levels as low as possible is best, especially when invertebrates are present. Ideal pH depends on the species being maintained within the environment and it influences the amount of toxic unionized ammonia. pH may be measured with a colorimetric test or an electronic pH meter. Water salinity is measured with a conductivity meter or with a refractometer—a cheaper alternative when fish are only occasional patients.

Physical Examination
Signs of respiratory disorders and hypoxia in fish include air piping, deaths of non-air-breathing fish, lethargy, anorexia, gathering at air-water interface (Figure 3-18) or near water inflow, death with opercula and mouth open (agonal response),

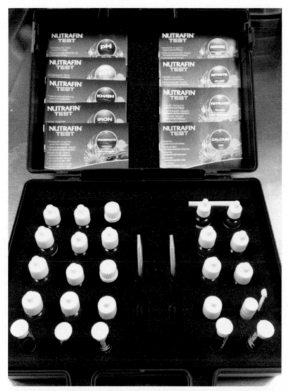

FIGURE 3-17 The Nutrafin Master Test Kit is a commonly used water quality test kit commercially available for private ornamental aquaria.

deaths of larger fish (less tolerant of environmental hypoxia), increased ventilation (more frequent and more important opercular movements), and jumping out of the water.[157]

Close visual inspection of fish can be performed under magnification and can reveal epithelial lesions on the skin and fins. It is common to find small white lesions that are nonspecific to a particular pathogen and warrant further investigation. Examples of the small white lesions include ich, lymphocystis, epitheliocystis, bacterial ulcerative diseases, saprolegniasis, and columnaris infection. Ascites and exophthalmia are common disease syndromes associated with systemic bacterial or viral infections and osmoregulatory failure.

A hands-on physical examination usually requires the use of chemical restraint. A variety of anesthetic agents can be used in fish, with MS-222 and clove oil (isoeugenol) being the most commonly used products. Due to the potential carcinogenicity of MC-222 and clove oil, the use of benzocaine may be a safer alternative when fish anesthesia is a commonly performed procedure (less data are available but this does not require buffering). Sedatives may cause detachment of some surface parasites. As far as the respiratory system is concerned, the buccal cavity, opercula, and gills should be examined.

Gross inspection of the diseased fish patient may reveal lesions, abnormal masses, nodules, discoloration, parasites, and petechiation. Masses may impede water flow through the gill. Pale gills can be associated with anemia, while tanned brown gills suggest methemoglobinemia, and metazoan parasites may be noted as clinically overt lesions. Gill rakers should also be carefully inspected, as many larger parasites may be present in this location.[157] Increased gill mucus production is commonly observed with a variety of branchial diseases.

Clinical Pathology and Laboratory Tests
A gill clip should be performed with the fish under sedation or anesthesia. After grossly examining the gills (mainly color changes), a fine pair of scissors is introduced into the gill chamber. The primary lamellae are lifted with the blade, sectioned at their tips, and immediately transferred to a microscope slide with a drop of aquarium water after which a cover slip is placed over the sample. Bleeding should be minimal. Turning the condenser down on the microscope will enable better contrast for the assessment of gills and aid in identification of parasites. If the wet mount of a gill clip is inconclusive,

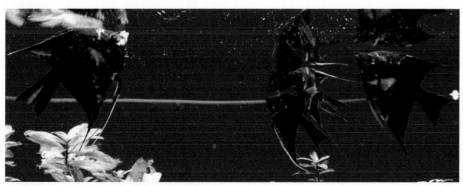

FIGURE 3-18 Angelfish with gill lesions breathing at the water-air interface where dissolved oxygen is the highest.

gill biopsies may be submitted for bacterial culture and histopathological evaluation.

Hyperplasia and fusion of secondary or primary lamellae and increased mucus secretion are commonly associated with gill disease and damage.[153,420] Necrosis of the gills may be detected microscopically after fixing and staining and could be caused by infectious agents. (Table 3-4). In many cases, when gross gill lesions are observed, the gill clip will reveal parasites. A number of parasites can be observed moving, therefore are easier to identify, but nonpathogenic protozoans may also be present. *Ichthyophthirius* and *Cryptocaryon* nodules may be diagnosed on secondary lamella with their encysted trophonts in tropical freshwater and marine fish. *Ichthyophthirius* is easily identified by the presence of its characteristic C-shaped nucleus. Accurate identification of protozoan parasites is not required for most cases, as treatment is similar for all species. The presence of hyphae should raise the suspicion of water mold infection (saprolegniasis). Bacteria may also be identified and specific bacterial shapes in conjunction with macroscopic lesions may point toward specific respiratory pathogens. Long thin rods with flexing or gliding motions in conjunction with epithelial and/or gill lesions are consistent with *Flavobacterium* spp. infections (see Table 3-4).[154] Large fibroblasts visible on the wet mount and concurrent with macroscopic nodular lesions are suggestive of lymphocystis.

Since most gill lesions are frequently associated with skin lesions, skin scrapings and biopsies may also be indicated as part of a thorough diagnostic workup. Skin scraping is performed with the blunt side of a scalpel blade in the direction of the scales. The resulting material is placed on a slide with a drop of aquarium water after which a cover slip is placed over the sample. Skin biopsies are performed using a small punch biopsy using standard surgical methods. The defect is often not closed due to the inelastic nature of the skin. Loosely attached parasites on the skin may be lost during fixation, consequently may not be identified when the sample is histopathologically examined.

Blood samples are generally collected from the caudal tail vein in fish. With respiratory disease, the complete blood cell count (CBC) may show erythrocytosis, polychromasia, or anemia.[157] However, the hematocrit may vary depending on collection sites. Electrolyte changes and increased ammonia may be identified on biochemistry due to disrupted osmoregulatory function or increased environmental ammonia. Elasmobranchs have very different biochemistry profiles and normally maintain a very high blood ammonia concentration.

Bacterial cultures of lesions on live fish are usually complicated by secondary bacterial and fungal invaders. Additionally, bacteria can be fastidious in their growth requirements, therefore specific aquatic animal laboratories may need to be sought for testing. The primary pathogen may also no longer be the most common organism present when the animal is sampled. Nevertheless, secondary pathogens are still part of the overall disease process, therefore most cases should be treated. Molecular testing is commercially available in selected veterinary laboratories for common fish viral diseases (e.g., spring viremia of carp, cyprinid HV3).

When diagnosing disease outbreaks or performing routine health monitoring of commercial stocks, a small percentage of the collection may be sacrificed for postmortem examina-tions, histopathology of internal organs, and culture to determine the potential etiologic cause of the problem.

The vast majority of diseases seen in pet fish may be diagnosed by a combination of water quality testing, physical examination, and diagnostic testing.

Diagnostic Imaging and Endoscopy

While diagnostic imaging modalities are useful in piscine veterinary management, their use is limited to evaluate the fish respiratory system because the gills can be directly evaluated. However, in some species, the gills cannot be directly assessed due to a more enclosed branchial chamber (e.g., puffer fish, elasmobranch). Radiographs are useful when trying to diagnose swim bladder diseases.

A 2.7-mm rigid endoscope can be used in anesthetized fish to evaluate the opercula, gill chamber, gill arches, and their lamellae. The endoscope has a magnification of approximately 20 times with the ability to collect endoscopic biopsies. The gills can be approached through either the opercular opening or the buccal cavity (Figure 3-19).

Amphibians

Physical Examination

As for reptiles, amphibian health is related to the environmental health, thus a complete anamnesis is mandatory.[421] Physical examination should always begin with hands-off observation to evaluate respiratory effort and rates.[164,173] For aquatic species, water quality testing is recommended including DO (only on site), ammonium, nitrites, nitrates, alkalinity, pH, hardness, and bacterial counts (see Fish section). A separate water sample must be supplied by the owner. Water test kits used for fish aquariums can be used for amphibian aquatic environments (see Figure 3-17).

Amphibians with respiratory diseases may present with tachypnea, open-mouth breathing, cyanosis, and changes in behavior, as described earlier.[34,164] A hands-on examination is then accomplished, taking care to handle the amphibian patient carefully with powder-free gloves moistened with chlorine-free water. Chemical restraint using MS-222, clove

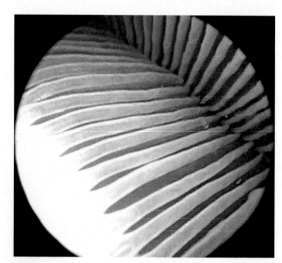

FIGURE 3-19 Gill endoscopy through the opening of the opercular chamber in the mouth of Mbu pufferfish. The gill septa and the hemibranches are clearly visible.

oil, or other anesthetics may be needed to perform a thorough physical evaluation. The nares should be clean, and respiratory disease is suspected if excessive mucus or bubbles are present.[164] If present, gills should be carefully examined, although the internal location of the gills in tadpoles makes external noninvasive examinations difficult.[63] Auscultation of the lungs can be performed accurately only in larger specimens.[164,422]

Clinical Pathology

Tracheal washes may be diagnostic for parasitic, bacterial, or fungal diseases located in the lower respiratory tract amphibians.[164,422,423] Samples may be obtained in anesthetized patients by infusing a small volume of sterile 0.9% saline using a sterile tomcat catheter or intravenous (IV) catheter through the glottis.[164,422] Some clear mucus is physiologically present in the mouth of most animals and contamination with this secretion should be avoided during tracheal washes.[423] As the trachea is very short in most Anurans and Caudatans, extra care is required not to damage the lung epithelial mucosa.[164] A wet mount may be immediately performed after sampling to help in therapeutic decision while the amphibian is still anesthetized.[422] Cytology and culture of the tracheal sample are recommended.[422] A microtip culturette can also be used to swab the trachea.[423]

Confirmation of infestation by *Rhabdias* spp. may also be obtained with fecal examination by observing the typical larval stage of this parasite.[47,164,170] However, *Rhabdias* larvae are indistinguishable from those of relatively common nonpathogenic gastrointestinal nematodes (*Aplectana* spp., *Cosmocerca* spp., and *Cosmocercoides* spp.) therefore proper interpretation of the parasitic larvae is extremely important.[172,173]

Nasal flush may be useful to diagnose myiasis of the nasal cavity by *Bufolucilia* spp. in Anurans and to remove any parasites present.[164]

In amphibian species or larval stages with gills, protoza, helminths (trematodes), or fungus (*Dermocystidium* spp.) may be diagnosed on gill clips, impressions, or scraping.[47,174] Low numbers of protozoa or trematodes are generally not considered a problem in healthy amphibians.[164] The adult trematodes *Gyrodactylus* spp. are small (<1 mm), and microscopic examination of a gill biopsy sample may be required.[47] Histopathology examination of the gill biopsy sample may also be useful.[164] Saprolegniasis may be confirmed by a wet mount of gill lesions and identification of hyphal structures and spores.[47]

CBC and biochemistry may also be helpful for general health assessment, but specific changes related to respiratory disorders may be difficult to interpret in the clinical context such as a high or low packed cell volume (PCV).

Diagnostic Imaging

Radiography is useful for investigating cases of respiratory diseases in amphibians.[172] Most radiographic images can be obtained without chemical restraint, and good patient positioning can be obtained by placing the patient in a moistened sealable plastic bag.[424] For prolonged procedures, small holes can be punched in the bag or the animal should be returned to its environment.[424]

In amphibians of sufficient size, endoscopy can be used to visualize the glottis, trachea, bronchi, and lungs.[173] Biopsies of the respiratory system may also be performed in amphibians during endoscopy or ultrasound.[425] Advanced imaging may be useful in large specimens.

Reptiles

Reptiles with upper or lower respiratory tract diseases generally have initial presentations of subtle, slowly progressive clinical signs, which are often missed by the owner.[73,184] Therefore, most reptiles are presented with chronic respiratory diseases, although acute respiratory distress may occur.[184] Veterinarians should always try to identify the underlying cause to improve their therapeutic plan.[184] The basic diagnostic workup for reptile respiratory diseases usually includes a complete blood cell count, biochemistry panel, tracheal/lung wash with cytology and culture, and diagnostic imaging.[67,74]

Physical Examination

A general physical examination should always be carefully performed, as diseases of other organ systems may be confused with respiratory diseases or may secondarily affect the respiratory tract.[67,73,74,184] The nares, choanae, and glottis should be closely examined for discharge, erythema, edema, masses, debris, and shed skin (Figures 3-20 to 3-23).[71,74,77] Auscultation of lungs in lizards and snakes should reveal only minimal respiratory noise and may be performed using a wet gauze or towel to minimize scratching noises induced by the scales rubbing on the stethoscope's membrane.[73] Transillumination of the coelom can be accomplished in small lizards and may help when assessing the lungs.

Physiological conditions or behaviors, such as vocalization (defensive hissing in lizards and snakes), open-mouth breathing used as a cooling mechanism during overheating in some lizards, gular movements, or a mild increase in respiratory sounds before shedding, may be normal and should not be mistaken for respiratory diseases.[73] Conversely, the inability of a reptile to produce sounds may be noted with consolidated lungs.[73] Increased respiratory sounds, abnormal gurgling, or wheezing on inspiration or especially on expiration should lead to a suspicion of respiratory disorders, such as pneumonia, aspiration, or near drowning.[73] Many reptiles with respiratory diseases become anorexic and lethargic, which may

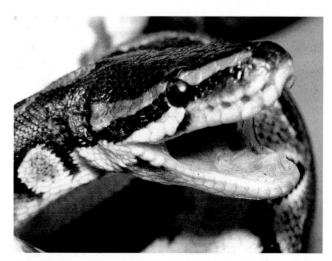

FIGURE 3-20 Open-mouth breathing in a ball python. (Courtesy of Lionel Schilliger.)

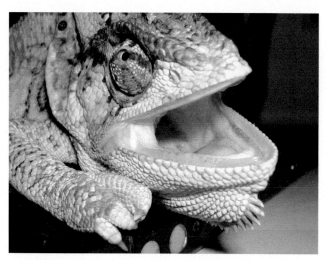

FIGURE 3-21 Veiled chameleon with open-mouth breathing. (Courtesy of Lionel Schilliger.)

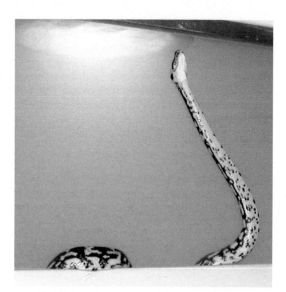

FIGURE 3-22 Carpet python exhibiting a position typical of respiratory disease, in which the head is elevated to facilitate ventilation. (Courtesy of Lionel Schilliger.)

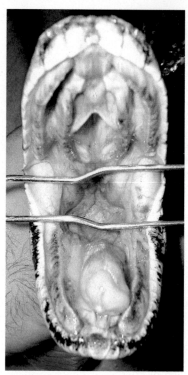

FIGURE 3-23 Glottal exudate in a boa constrictor with pneumonia. (Courtesy of Lionel Schilliger.)

mimic neurologic signs as a result of generalized weakness.[66,73] Monitoring the respiratory frequency is moderately useful in reptiles because in many circumstances, the respiratory response to impaired respiration is through an increased tidal volume.[90]

Respiratory signs in snakes and lizards may include nasal or oral discharge, open-mouth breathing (see Figures 3-20 and 3-21), crusted nares, bubble blowing, sneezing, puffy throat, and increased respiratory sounds.[73] Snakes with respiratory diseases may present in a typical posture, with their head and neck elevated in a 45-degree angle to maximize airflow (orthopnea) (see Figure 3-21).[73,77] In snakes, stomatitis is a common concurrent disease diagnosis with bacterial pneumonia (see Figure 3-23).[216]

Crocodilians with respiratory diseases usually present with nonspecific clinical signs, such as anorexia, lethargy, weakness, or buoyancy disorders. Respiratory clinical signs may also be observed, including dyspnea, tachypnea, nasal discharges, excessive basking, respiratory stridor, and abnormal swimming (either in circles or on one side of the body).[66]

In chelonians, cutaneous erosion, softness, or depigmentation around the nares is often associated with chronic upper respiratory tract diseases.[71,74,223] Clinical signs of dyspnea may include neck stretching, open mouth breathing, increased or abnormal respiratory sounds, abnormal buoyancy in aquatic or semiaquatic species, and increased movements of the head and thoracic limbs during inspiration.[73,74] Movements of the head and limbs are a normal part of respiration cycle in chelonians; however, these movements should not be too pronounced.[71,73] Abnormal respiratory sounds, such as clicks or a slight whistle, are usually suggestive of a lower respiratory tract disease.[73]

Clinical Pathology and Laboratory Tests

A CBC and biochemical panel can help to determine the presence of infectious diseases or concomitant pathologies in reptiles.[67,71,74] Hematologic changes are usually nonspecific and depend on captive environmental factors, although they may reveal an inflammatory leukogram or an erythrocytosis associated with chronic disease. The biochemistry panel may reveal bicarbonate changes from a compensated respiratory acidosis or metabolic acidosis, due to sustained anaerobic metabolism. High lactate levels are also common in dyspneic reptiles due to their ability to switch to anaerobic metabolism for long periods of time. Venous blood gases may be useful in further characterizing other acid-base imbalances but arterial blood gases are typically very challenging to collect in reptile patients. On the other hand, hemoglobin oxygen saturation

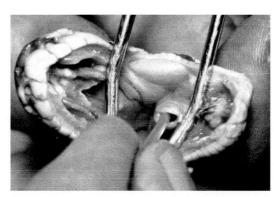

FIGURE 3-24 Tracheal wash in a boa constrictor using a small, long flexible tube. (Courtesy of Lionel Schilliger.)

may be obtained using pulse oximeters. Surprisingly, pulse oximetry using human hemoglobin calibration curve has been found to be accurate in green iguanas (*Iguana iguana*), which is different from other nonmammalian vertebrates such as birds.

Respiratory washes can be very useful and may be collected from reptiles that are presented with respiratory disease. Nasal and sinus washes may be collected for mycoplasma and/ or TeHV testing in tortoises under manual restraint or sedation. Lung or tracheal washes are particularly useful to diagnose the etiologic cause of pneumonia, especially in snakes.[218,426] Lung wash can be performed on most reptiles using manual restraint (snakes, some lizards) or under sedation (chelonians, some lizards). A sterile flexible tube is guided through the glottis into the trachea while the jaws are maintained in an open position (Figure 3-24). In large species, a bronchoscope can be used. The tube should be carefully inserted in the glottis to minimize contamination with commensal bacteria in the oral cavity or bacteria responsible for stomatitis in cases where these lesions are present. Alternatively, a sterile endotracheal tube may be placed first and the collecting tube fed through to minimize oral and glottal contamination.[426] Anatomical particularities of the trachea of the affected species should be known, as the location of the tracheal bifurcation varies greatly among reptiles. Sterile saline (e.g., 0.5 to 1 mL per 100 g in snakes) can be injected and aspirated several times.[426] Suction pumps may be used to improve fluid recovery. In snakes, tilting the body head-down may also help with fluid recovery. In chelonians, a long needle may be inserted dorsocranially in the prefemoral fossa at the level of a lung to perform a unilateral lung wash.[426] The collected fluid may be submitted for cytology, microbiological culture, electron microscopy, or molecular testing. For some authors, bacterial and viral diagnosis of tracheal washes is also a reliable tool in snakes with respiratory signs, having a good sensibility for the detection of ferlavirus infection.[205] Tracheal washes of healthy subadult alligators should be sterile, and cytology is similar to that described in domestic mammals.[427] Lung washes in snakes may also recover embryonated eggs of lung worms (*Rhabdias* spp.) and eggs of pentastomids (e.g., *Armillifer* spp.).[256]

Microbiological cultures are important to identify primary or secondary bacterial or fungal infections and to determine proper antimicrobial therapy.[67,428] Although *Pseudomonas* spp.,

Klebsiella spp., *Proteus* spp., *Aeromonas* spp., *Salmonella* spp., *Morganella* spp., *Providencia* spp., and *Staphylococcus* spp. can be considered normal flora in a healthy reptile, isolation of these bacteria from a tracheal wash of a reptile with respiratory disease is suggestive of pathogenic involvement.[184] Mycoplasma isolation may be difficult, as it requires specific harvesting techniques, transport media, storage, and transportation of submission materials.[428] Mycoplasmas are fastidious and grow slowly over several weeks. A nasal flush is more sensitive and representative than swabbing the nares because typical mycoplasma infections are frequently too deep to be accessible by swabbing.[223] Enrichment with bovine serum albumin is recommended before shipping fluid collected from a nasal flush. As most mesophilic fungal organisms associated with reptile fungal diseases do not usually occur in homeothermic vertebrates, medical laboratories may not be able to isolate, speciate, or correctly identify the causative fungus.[242] Veterinary laboratories with experience in reptile fungal identification or mycology laboratories should be selected (e.g., Microfungus Collection and Herbarium, University of Alberta).

When a viral agent is suspected, samples for electron microscopy, virus isolation, serology, or polymerase chain reaction (PCR) assay may be submitted.[184] Testudinid HV infections may be diagnosed by demonstrating eosinophilic intranuclear inclusion bodies on histopathology, with electron microscopy on nasal flushes, or biopsies from oral lesions in chelonians.[74,184,428] IBD in snakes (especially boa constrictor) with interstitial pneumonia may be confirmed by the presence of typical eosinophilic intracytoplasmic inclusion bodies in epithelial cells.[184] Basophilic cytoplasmic inclusion bodies are compatible with iridovirus infection in chelonians.[74] Inclusion bodies have been reported in snakes infected with ferlaviruses.[202] Virus isolation may be realized on nasal flushes (e.g., chelonians) or tissue samples.[428] HV may be isolated from fresh or rapidly frozen tissue samples or from tissue swabs in chelonians.[74] Oropharyngeal swabs seem to be more accurate than conjunctival or cloacal samples.[74] However, viral organisms may be shed intermittently in oral secretions, either during primary infection or recrudescence, consequently false negatives are possible.[74] Isolation of iridovirus requires proper transport media, transport conditions, and sample collection procedures.[74] Caution should be taken when interpreting viral diagnostic test results. Even though a viral agent may be isolated from a diseased individual, this does not necessarily imply that this virus is the underlying cause of the disease process.[74]

Serology may prove to be helpful in the diagnosis and management of some reptilian infectious diseases.[428] In chelonians, serology for HV, mycoplasma (enzyme-linked immunosorbent assay [ELISA]), and iridovirus (ELISA) are available in selected laboratories.[192,200,428] Since HVs are responsible for permanent infection, a single serology is enough for identifying infected individuals. Rising titers may be needed to confirm clinical disease. Egg-yolk immunoglobulin (IgY) tests may only be positive after the onset of clinical signs, and some animals may not seroconvert. Consequently, two negative tests 8 weeks apart are needed to classify a tortoise as "HV negative."[192] In addition, some TeHV serotypes may not cross react. Serology testing using ELISA for mycoplasma is a sensitive test but does not distinguish past exposure from current infections. Cross reactivity with antibodies to similar bacterial antigens may also lead to false-positive results.[74] Specific anti-mycoplasmal antibodies may only be detected 6 to 8 weeks after infection.[429] Paired antibody titers in combination with compatible clinical signs are needed to confirm a tortoise's mycoplasmosis clinical status. Only *Mycoplasma agassizii* is detected using ELISA, and infections with other mycoplasmas may not cross react with the assay.[223] Serology by hemagglutination inhibition assay is also available to determine exposure of ferlavirus in snakes and lizards.[67,77,184] Paired samples, 8 weeks apart, are required to tentatively an active infection of ferlavirus in snakes and lizards.[77,202] As there is limited agreement among results from different laboratories, caution should be taken when interpreting the results of the hemagglutination inhibition assay test.[77]

PCR assays for HVs, mycoplasma, and intranuclear coccidiosis in chelonians have been developed to test ocular and nasal swabs/flush.[71,223,428,430] Ocular swabs may result in less secondary bacterial contamination and should be considered if ocular lesions are present.[74] Oral, tracheal, and cloacal swabs and nasal flush may also be used to identify pathogenic bacteria depending on the disease presentation of the patient. Pan-herpesviral or nested PCR may be needed to detect all TeHVs in tortoises.[191,192] Negative detection of ferlavirus by PCR using oral and cloacal swabs in infected snakes has also been reported.[202] Consequently, this test should be carefully interpreted, as the shedding patterns of ferlaviruses are unknown in snakes.[202] PCR for mycoplasma disease in tortoises is available in some laboratories but seems less sensitive than serology. This may be due to the difficulties in obtaining a representative sample from the affected area of the chelonian upper respiratory system using a nasal flush.[223]

Diagnostic Imaging

Diagnostic modalities, including radiographs, endoscopy, and advanced imaging, are the most useful tools in the detection of space-occupying masses, such as cartilaginous granuloma, and to guide pulmonary biopsies.[184]

Radiographs may be helpful to diagnose lower respiratory diseases in reptiles.[67,71,218,428,431] The lungs are best evaluated in the craniocaudal and lateral projections in chelonians and on lateral projection in squamates, with reptiles positioned to obtain a horizontal radiograph beam.[73] Left and right lateral views should be taken in chelonians and lizards, with the lateral measurement being greater than 6 cm.[73] As for evaluation of other organs with radiography, the legs and head of chelonians should be extended out of the shell, which usually requires anesthesia or sedation.[73,428] Craniocaudal and lateral views are useful to localize lung lesions in chelonians for microbiological samplings, intrapulmonary therapy, or to ensure the position of intrapulmonary catheters.[428] In snakes, localization of the heart apex can be used as a landmark for the cranial position of the lung. In lizards, the pectoral limbs should be positioned as cranially as possible to minimize superimposition with the lungs.[73] Positioning, positive-pressure ventilation, depth of respiration and digestion, and coelomic contents all have an effect on the radiographic appearance of lung tissue.[73] Anesthesia with endotracheal intubation and positive-pressure ventilation are usually recommended in lizards and snakes, as positive-pressure ventilation decreases pulmonary radiopacity.[73] The standard classification of mammalian pulmonary radiographic patterns

(alveolar, interstitial, bronchial, and pleural patterns) cannot be used in reptiles, as the lung structure differs greatly from mammals.[73,428] The lungs of snakes and most lizards, except the chameleons, present a relatively homogenous tissue density on radiographic images.[73] However, pulmonary vasculature is usually more prominent in the cranial portion of the lungs.[73] In snakes, a diffuse increase in pulmonary radiopacity is generally observed, while focal area of increased pulmonary opacity is more common in chelonians and occasionally in lizards. In chelonians, acute pneumonia is generally visualized as a focal increase of pulmonary radiopacity that is ventrally localized.[428] Such lesions are common in cold-stunned sea turtles.[431] In chelonians, radiographic images of chronic lesions are usually discrete.[428]

Radiography can be also useful to monitor the response to treatment and the resolution of lower respiratory tract diseases.[428] Radiographic evaluation might be necessary to determine involvement of bony structures such as the mandible or maxilla, when severe upper respiratory diseases are diagnosed.[184]

Ultrasonography is a useful adjunct to radiography and aids in the detection or sample collection of pulmonary masses, such as granuloma or neoplasia, which may compress pulmonary spaces.[184]

Advanced imaging offers a much better resolution and is highly sensitive in detecting pulmonary lesions in reptiles. In chelonians, because of the superimposition of the shell in all views, advanced imaging is recommended whenever possible (Figure 3-25). Computed tomography (CT) has extensively been used in reptile pneumonology cases.[71,73,184,255,428,432] Positive-pressure ventilation with anesthesia is recommended to enhance CT details, especially in lizards because of their rapid respiratory rate.[73] CT imaging provides a detailed appearance of the respiratory tract in chelonians.[433] Reference values have been established for the CT lung assessment in some species of snakes, and significant differences in attenuation of the lungs on CT imaging have been reported among species.[78,432] MRI may also provide precise detail of the lower respiratory tract in reptiles, especially chelonians.[71,184,428]

Diagnostic Endoscopy

The usefulness of diagnostic endoscopy in reptile medicine cannot be overemphasized. To investigate respiratory diseases, several approaches may be employed including rhinoscopy, tracheobronchoscopy, pulmonoscopy, coelioscopy, and air sac endoscopy (e.g., snakes and some lizards). Since it is

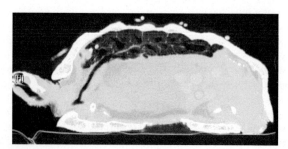

FIGURE 3-25 CT scan of a red-footed tortoise, sagittal section, where the bronchus and lungs are well visualized. This tortoise was in terminal renal failure with coelomic fluid accumulation, reducing the space available for the lungs.

beyond the scope of this chapter to give an exhaustive description of reptilian diagnostic endoscopy, the reader is invited to consult recent descriptions of techniques used in reptile species for this imaging modality.[434,435] Adequate endoscopic approaches depend on many factors in reptiles including species, size of the individuals, and clinical findings. As with other zoological companion animals, a 2.7-mm 30°-angle rigid endoscope is the ideal tool for most reptile endoscopic procedures. However, a flexible endoscope is required for tracheobronchoscopy in larger reptiles. Endoscopy allows targeted pulmonary or gross lesion biopsy samples, video documentation of lesions, topical therapy, treatment, and lesion monitoring. Reptilian airways are smaller than found in mammals and birds of similar sizes, which may restrict the introduction of endoscopes in the trachea and bronchi. General anesthesia is strongly recommended for all endoscopy procedures to minimize instrument damage and harm to the patients.

In chelonians, the buccal cavity, glottis, trachea, and proximal bronchi can be examined with an unsheathed endoscope. Endoscopy of the lungs through the glottis and trachea is generally not possible, as the primary bronchus undergoes an acute deviation before entering the lungs.[428] However, a fine diameter flexible bronchoscope may allow more depth of the instrument into the lungs of giant tortoises and sea turtles.[434] Retrograde endoscopy through an esophagostomy incision is possible in chelonians to visualize the upper respiratory tract via the choana, or a 1-mm or 1.3-mm semirigid scope can be used via the nares in most adult chelonians. A flexible fiberoptic bronchoscopy in large specimens also allows direct visualization of the lower respiratory tract.[197] For access to the lungs, a coelioscopy is performed using a rigid endoscope which is inserted through a prefemoral approach. Entering ventrally into the lungs via the pleuroperitoneum during coelioscopy is generally contraindicated, as it may lead to a pneumocoelom. Due to the presence of the postpulmonary septum, correct visualization of the lungs is hampered in chelonians during the standard coeliotomy procedure. Thus, in chelonians, the postpulmonary septum, which covers the serosal aspect of the lungs, must be incised prior to examination (pulmonoscopy) and biopsy collection. After entering through the skin and coelomic membrane, repeated insufflation of the lungs is performed until the caudolateral lung is visualized. Stay sutures are placed in the caudoventral border of the lung, which is apposed to the skin incision, and entered through a stab incision.[434] Then, a pulmonoscopy is performed using a rigid endoscope. After the examination is complete, the lung is closed to prevent pneumocoelom. An alternative approach has also been described in chelonians through the carapace. A 4-mm temporary osteotomy of the carapace is performed over an affected region of the lungs, the pleuroperitoneal membrane is punctured with the animal at maximum inspiration, and a rigid endoscope is inserted through the osteotomy and incision to examine the lungs.[434] Radiographic or CT images should be obtained prior to the osteotomy to localize the lesions, as the endoscope movements are limited by the hole size in the shell.[428] The hole is then closed by replacing the shell fragment and securing with epoxy or acrylic compound.

In squamates, tracheoscopy and bronchoscopy are relatively easy and usually requires a flexible bronchoscope in

snakes due to their long trachea. The tracheal lung of snakes may also be examined. In snakes, a transcutaneous pulmonoscopy approach has been described and is an effective and safe technique to examine the ophidian lower respiratory tract.[434,436] The skin is incised in the area of the lung, at 90 ventral scales caudal to the head and nine scales lateral on the right side in ball pythons, or 35% to 45% from snout to vent. Since most snake species only have a right lung, the incision should be performed on the right side of the animal. The subcutaneous layer is bluntly dissected and the intercostal muscles are penetrated with mosquito hemostats between two adjacent ribs. The serosal surface of the right lung is then penetrated with mosquito hemostats during inflation of the lungs and a 2.7-mm rigid endoscope is placed into the opening. In large snakes, a rigid endoscope may be inserted into the lungs which allows for good visualization of the distal portion of the trachea, primary bronchus, intrapulmonary bronchus, the cranial lung lobe faveolar, and semisaccular and saccular lung regions in snakes.[436] The lung and skin are closed separately. Iatrogenic lesions secondary to the endoscopy are minimal and complete healing of at least 1 year later has been reported.[436] In lizards, a standard coelioscopic approach through a paramedian or paralumbar entry point allows visualization of the lungs.[434] Since there is no postpulmonary membrane (septum horizontal) in most lizards, the lungs are directly visualized, except in monitors and some tegus. In snakes, coelomic endoscopy is limited by their elongated anatomy and the presence of diffuse fat.[434] Since a better approach to the ophidian lungs has been described, standard coelomic endoscopy is rarely indicated in snakes to examine the lower respiratory system.

The use of bronchoscopy has been described in crocodilians, but coelioscopy has not been well investigated.[427]

Pulmonary Biopsy

Biopsies may also be very useful to reveal a causative agent in upper and lower respiratory diseases and should be considered if cytology is unsuccessful. Pulmonary biopsies may be obtained through a standard coeliotomy or by endoscopy (see previous section on endoscopy). In chelonians, a carapace osteotomy over the affected portion of the lungs (ideally located using advanced imaging) may be necessary for pulmonary biopsy collection. Histopathology with specific stains and microbiological culture should be performed on collected biopsy samples.[428] Most viral respiratory diseases that infect reptiles lead to histologically visible inclusion bodies.

Mammals
Physical Examination
The physical examination of companion exotic mammals is very similar to other mammals. Observation of the animal should comprise the first part of the examination, including evaluation of the respiratory system. Some rabbits and rodents differ in their receptiveness to manual restraint and examination, consequently it is important to be aware of the patient's comfort with being handled and severity of the disease.[437] Clinical signs may include one or a combination of the following disease conditions, sneezing, nasal discharge, coughing, dyspnea, orthopnea, cyanosis, syncope, and ascites. Anatomical localization can be identified to determine whether the upper respiratory tract or the lower respiratory

TABLE 3-6

Normal Respiration Rates of Commonly Seen Small Mammals in Practice

Species	Respiration Rate (bpm)	Reference
Ferrets	33-36	306
Guinea pigs	90-150	324
Hedgehogs	25-50	281
Mice	100-250	287
Rabbits	30-60	438
Rats	70-150	287
Sugar gliders	16-40	299, 439

bpm, Beats per minute.

tract is affected. While upper respiratory signs may be clinically apparent, the signs of lower respiratory disease usually are subtle and there may not be premonitory signs except decreased activity, weight loss, or sudden death.[104,105,273] Additionally, respiratory disease can be further classified as primary or secondary. Primary disease may include infectious bronchitis, while secondary causes of respiratory disease include pulmonary edema or pleural effusion (see Figure 3-9), associated with congestive heart failure or systemic illness such as acidosis or anemia.

Targeting the respiratory system when performing a physical examination should focus on examining the upper and lower respiratory tract through observation and auscultation with minimal stress to the patient. Auscultation of the thorax may produce muffled heart sounds, harsh lung sounds, friction (pleuritis), and fluid sounds (edema), while percussion may reveal increased or decreased resonance (less useful considering the size of most companion exotic mammals). Resting respiratory rates for common small mammals are given in Table 3-6. Auscultation of the nasal cavities is also easily performed in rabbits. In addition, an oral and dental assessment should be performed in every examination. Porphyrin staining can be detected using a Wood's lamp and its presence, although not specific to respiratory tract disease, can be a result of generalized illness.[114] Poor body condition is more likely to be associated with chronic disease and prognosis is generally poor once respiratory distress is evident.

Clinical Pathology and Laboratory Tests

Hematologic changes that may be expected in respiratory diseases are likely to be similar to dogs and cats. In rabbits, however, leukocytosis is not commonly associated with infectious diseases, while leukopenia is often noted with acute infectious cases.[440] Additionally, compared to dogs and cats, paraneoplastic syndromes associated with thymoma, such as hemolytic anemia or immune mediated signs, are less common.[278,441] Arterial blood samples are readily collected in rabbits from the central ear artery and sometimes in ferrets from the tail artery and may be useful in assessing respiratory efficiency.

Serologic tests are available through commercial laboratories for a variety of infectious diseases of exotic companion mammals but turn-around time may be prolonged and classically ~7 days, by which time a presumptive diagnosis has already been made.[296,442,443] Serology also fails to detect subclinical cases and cannot distinguish those that are infected or recently exposed.[276] Serology panels for an impressive number of rabbit and rodent pathogens are being offered by companies specializing in laboratory animal medicine such as Charles Rivers Laboratories as part of preventive screening and specific pathogen-free testing. Likewise, PCR assays for most respiratory pathogens are also available. However, the interpretation of these tests, is dependent on the agent tested, and can be challenging in the clinical context of individualized medicine. Furthermore, many viral infections in small exotic mammals are subclinical unless complicated further by secondary bacterial infections. Frequently the diagnosis of viral infections is based on clinical signs and the in-clinic diagnostic workup rather than on laboratory tests.[437]

A positive serology for canine distemper in an unvaccinated ferret is highly suggestive for this disease.[298] A fluorescent antibody test is also available for various biological samples and useful in the first few days of CDV infection. A PCR assay on blood, urine, feces, pharyngeal swabs, and tissue may also be used to test for CDV in ferrets. For ferret influenzaviral disease, several diagnostic tests are available such as PCR assay and in-clinic antigen detection assays (e.g., Directigen Flu).[298]

Bacterial culture and sensitivity testing is useful for identifying specific pathogens from swabs and/or samples collected from appropriate anatomic locations such as deep nasal swabs (e.g., rabbits), bronchoalveolar lavage, or ultrasound-guided fine-needle aspirates of lung lesions.[278,444,445] Tracheal and nasal secretions often harbor mixed infections.[446] One of the problems faced with culturing potential disease locations in small exotic mammals, especially those associated with *Mycoplasma* species, are the bacteria's fastidious growth requirements, with cultures failing to detect up to 30% of infected animals.[296] When pleural effusion or a pneumothorax is identified, ultrasound-guided collection of the fluid or air may not only be diagnostic for laboratory submission but is likely therapeutic in relieving the intrathoracic pressure related to the disease process. Similarly, ultrasound-guided fine-needle aspirates of intrathoracic masses in rabbits will provide a good indication where the mass originates.[447] The collection and testing of diagnostic samples must be interpreted in conjunction with clinical signs, as many primary pathogens described are also considered commensal bacterial organisms in a normal animal. Anaerobic culture should be submitted in cases of dental abscessation, as anaerobic bacteria are frequently implicated.

Diagnostic Imaging

Radiographic images are efficient for determining disease severity, although the patient must be carefully selected, as individuals in severe respiratory distress may easily decompensate (see Figures 3-9, 3-10, and 3-26). Radiographic quality is of diagnostic importance, therefore sedation and or general anesthetic may need to be administered. Two orthogonal views are necessary to make diagnostic assessments, although multiple projections are required for the upper respiratory tract and the skull.[437]

Thoracic ultrasound examinations may be useful for masses or lesions that are close to the body wall as well as for fine-needle aspiration. Pleural effusion is also readily identified and ultrasound-guided thoracocentesis may be performed.

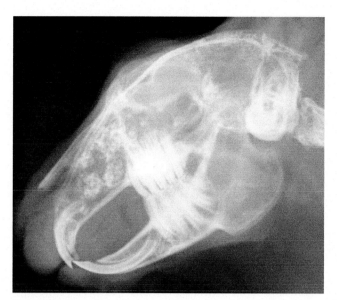

FIGURE 3-26 Lateral radiographic view of the skull of a rabbit exhibiting severe and mineralized rhinitis.

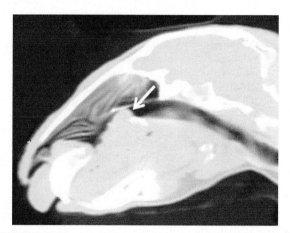

FIGURE 3-27 Sagittal view of a CT scan of the skull of a rabbit diagnosed with a periapical abscess obstructing the upper airways *(arrow)*. The rabbit presented in severe dyspnea with open-mouth breathing. A ventral rhinotomy allowed surgical debridement of the abscess.

CT is now increasingly available and becoming useful in diagnosing, not only subclinical respiratory disease, but also potential underlying dental, nasal, bullae involvement, and intrathoracic neoplasia.[278,288] The use of CT appears to be used more often for rabbits due to the high prevalence of thymoma and dental disease (see Figures 3-3 and 3-27). The evaluation of the structures without superimposition can be complemented with the use of injectable contrast medium to emphasize particular soft tissue regions and highlight vascularized lesions.[448]

MRI is the modality of choice in animals suspected to have soft tissue diseases and has been described in aiding the diagnosis of intrathoracic masses in rabbits.[289,321,448] However, prolonged scanning time associated with extended general anesthesia and limited resolution in small animals are two potential disadvantages of using MRI in small exotic mammals.

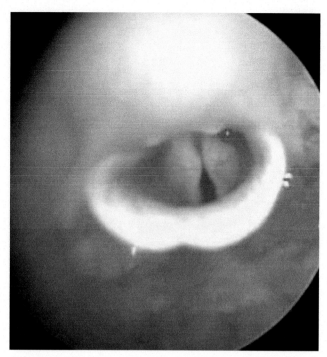

FIGURE 3-28 Endoscopic view of the glottis of a rabbit during over-the-endoscope intubation. Ventrally, the long epiglottis can be seen. At the upper part of the view, the soft palate is visualized, and the arytenoid cartilages are seen within the glottis.

Endoscopy

Various endoscopic approaches useful for assessing the respiratory system have been described in small exotic mammals and include rhinoscopy, tracheoscopy, bronchoscopy, and stomatoscopy.

Rhinoscopy and tracheoscopy using a rigid endoscope or a flexible bronchoscope are readily performed in rabbits. Saline-infusion rhinoscopy using a 2.7- or a 1.9-mm endoscope may be performed in rabbits.[449] The endoscope should be maintained medially to prevent iatrogenic damage to the nasal mucosa. The ventral and middle nasal meati may be explored to examine nasal conchae. Tracheoscopy has been used and is well described for intubation in rabbits, although its use in the smaller exotic mammals is limited to a certain extent by the size of the patient (Figure 3-28).[277,437,448] In the very small species, it may be the only means of visualizing the soft palate and glottis for diagnostic purposes. A small flexible bronchoscope is needed to perform tracheobronchoscopy in medium to large exotic mammal species, and the head should be kept straight during this procedure. A report thoroughly describes flexible bronchoscopy and bronchial morphology in rabbits using a 2.5-mm endoscope.[450] Thoracoscopy has been described for pleural disease or to biopsy intrathoracic masses, but its use appears to be limited because of the small size of exotic mammals.[449]

Birds

Physical Examination

A thorough history may help one determine the source of a respiratory problem. Respiratory diseases in birds may be

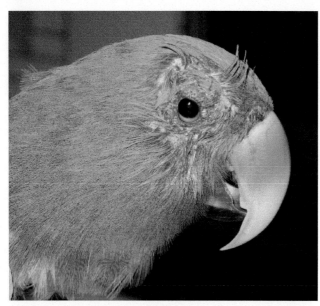

FIGURE 3-29 Periocular feather loss in an eclectus parrot diagnosed with infraorbital sinusitis.

species-specific (e.g., chronic obstructive pulmonary disease in macaws, respiratory neoplasia in cockatiels and cockatoos, goiter in budgerigars) or species susceptibility may vary (e.g., aspergillosis). Knowledge of the bird's sex is important, as female birds may present with reproductive-associated ascites, leading to dyspnea or yolk embolism. Anamnesis questions should particularly focus on housing and environment since birds are particularly susceptible to airborne toxins. Age is associated with chronic exposure to airborne particulate and/ or toxins that may lead to pulmonary silicosis, fibrosis, or neoplasia. Assessment of the diet is also indicated, as nutritional deficiencies may contribute to respiratory diseases (e.g., hypovitaminosis A) and seeds may act as foreign bodies.

The nature of the presenting complaint and chronicity of clinical signs provide valuable information. Acute severe inspiratory dyspnea with open-mouth breathing is usually an indication of upper airway obstruction. Avian clinicians should remain aware that respiratory diseases may lead to nonspecific clinical signs including those that effect the eye (Figure 3-29) and hind limb paresis (e.g., aspergillosis, pulmonary carcinoma). Conversely, diseases that are not specific to the respiratory system may lead to respiratory signs associated with reduction in air sac volumes and occlusion of upper airways. Clinical signs that are frequently observed with respiratory diseases in birds include nasal or ocular discharge, sneezing, coughing, dyspnea, collapse, exercise intolerance, voice changes, voice loss, respiratory noises, tail bobbing, open-mouth breathing, subcutaneous emphysema (see Figure 3-11), ataxia, lethargy, anorexia, and weight loss. Falconry birds may only show a decrease in flight or hunting performance. Birds with severe respiratory signs must be oxygenated prior to handling or not handled at all.

Before a hands-on physical examination is performed, the abnormal respiratory presentation must be characterized, if possible, as inspiratory, expiratory, or mixed, which usually provides clues used to differentiating between upper (inspiratory) and lower (expiratory) airway disease. Increased

respiratory frequencies and efforts should be noted. Increased ventilatory efforts and volume are partially achieved in birds by using additional muscle groups, that include the tail depressor and suprapubic muscles.[451] The amplified activity of these muscles under certain conditions leads to the clinical manifestation of tail bobbing in dyspneic birds. With nasal and sinusal diseases, the periorbital area frequently expands during expiration. Abnormal body posture is also frequent with increased respiratory efforts.

Examination of the head may further identify periorbital swelling or depression, feather staining around the nares or eyes, nasal discharges, nasal granuloma, blunting of choanal papillae, inflamed choana, inflamed glottis, masses on choana or glottis, and upper beak abnormalities (i.e., grooves continuous with nares may indicate weeks or months of rhinitis, sinusitis) (Figure 3-29). Examination of the body may reveal subcutaneous emphysema or abdominal distention. Pulmonary auscultation is not very sensitive in birds, but wheezes, crackles, and other pulmonary noises may be detected. The stethoscope is placed over the dorsum right above the location of the lungs in the coelom or on different areas of the abdomen to auscultate the air sacs. Repeating pulmonary auscultation with manual ventilations is valuable in some cases. Similar to classifying a dyspnic condition, increased inspiratory noises may correlate with upper respiratory diseases and increased expiratory noises with lower respiratory diseases. Cardiac auscultation should also be performed (see cardiology: Chapter 4). Transillumination of the trachea may help identify foreign bodies, mites (canaries), or other tracheal abnormalities. Cyanosis may be evident on periorbital skin and mucous membranes. Weight loss is a nonspecific clinical disease condition but may be associated with chronic respiratory disease. In a healthy bird, normal respiration should return within minutes after restraint or a short period of wing flapping.[327]

Clinical Pathology and Laboratory Tests

Clinical pathologic changes depend on the respiratory disease process. When an infectious or inflammatory process is present, heterophilic leukocytosis and/or monocytosis are classically observed but are nonspecific. Avian chlamydiosis, aspergillosis, mycobacteriosis, sepsis, and other bacterial lower respiratory diseases usually cause marked leukocytosis. However, some avian cases diagnosed with aspergillosis may have a near-normal white blood cell count. Erythrocytosis (polycythemia, increased PCV) may be observed with chronic hypoxemia and this condition occurs with primary and chronic pulmonary parenchymal disease (e.g., pulmonary neoplasia, macaw chronic obstructive disease, and pulmonary interstitial fibrosis).[402,452] Likewise, nonspecific alterations of plasma electrophoresis can be observed but the correlation to specific diseases is unknown. Venous or arterial blood gases may help characterize and grade oxygenation and ventilation problems (e.g., hypoxemia, hypercapnia).

Measurement of arterial blood gases is the gold standard for assessing oxygenation (PaO_2: partial pressure in O_2) and ventilation ($PaCO_2$: partial pressure in CO_2), with interpretation being similar to mammals. The $PaCO_2/FiO_2$ ratio (FiO_2: fraction of inspired O_2) is helpful in determining the severity of hypoxemia, with a ratio <300 indicating lung injuries and respiratory distress. In addition, a PaO_2 <80 mmHg indicates hypoxemia.

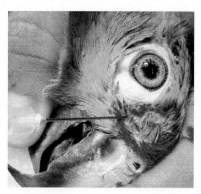

FIGURE 3-30 Aspiration of the infraorbital sinus in a red-lored Amazon parrot. The point of insertion for this approach is located about midway between the eye and the nare in a small depression that can easily be palpated.

Cytology of upper respiratory exudates and nasal granulomas may be helpful. Specific chlamydial stains on conjunctival smears may identify chlamydial elementary bodies. Cytology of tracheal lesions, air sac granulomas, or respiratory washes (sinus, trachea, air sacs) may identify specific organisms such as *Aspergillus* hyphae. Always perform cytology on coelioscopic samples collected from air sac granulomas (e.g., the aspergillosis), since the diagnosis may be confirmed faster than with histopathology.

Swabs or samples may be obtained from the nasal cavity, choanae, sinus, trachea, and biopsy samples. These samples are then submitted for fungal and bacterial culture/isolation. Infraorbital sinus samples can be obtained from different sites. An infraorbital sinus aspirate is performed using a needle that is inserted in a small depression rostral to the eye (Figure 3-30) while the upper beak is extended. Alternatively, with the upper beak flexed, a needle can be inserted underneath the zygomatic arch. A small amount of sterile saline is infused and aspirated. If present, coelomic fluid should always be analyzed. The benefit of a fungal culture for *Aspergillus* is debatable, as the organism is ubiquitous in the environment and a frequent contaminant of culture media. The same holds true for *Aspergillus* PCR. Some bacterial agents may be difficult to identify by culture such as *Mycoplasma* spp. and *Mycobacterium* spp.

Molecular diagnostic and serologic tests are available for a few infectious agents that cause respiratory diseases. In birds, several PCR assays are commercially available including *C. psittaci*, *Mycobacterium genavense/avium/intracellulare*, *Mycoplasma* spp., avian polyomavirus, and atoxoplasma. Serologic diagnostic tests are not widely available except for avian chlamydiosis and some poultry disease causing organisms. Due to the difficulties in diagnosing and screening for avian chlamydiosis, several diagnostics tests should be performed concurrently including serology (elementary agglutination antibody test [IgM], indirect fluorescent antibody, complement fixation, or ELISA tests [IgY]) and PCR on a conjunctival/choanal/cloacal swab. In addition, serologic tests may not have consistent results for all avian species. Serology for aspergillosis is also available but may be of low sensitivity and specificity and is of limited clinical usefulness thus far in diagnosing the disease in most birds. Some avian species also

have high *Aspergillus* seroprevalence and this disease often has an immunosuppressive effect.[383,453] Blood galactomannan (component of the fungal cell wall) assays are not sensitive diagnostic tests,[453] but are considered highly specific, therefore generate false negative results most likely due to a low level of circulating *Aspergillus* antigen in circumscribed or walled-off granulomas. A large study involving various avian species reported a positive predictive value of 63% and a negative predictive value of 76% for blood galactomannan assays, which meant that there is roughly a 1 out of 3 chance that any given positive test is false and a 1 out of 4 chance than any given negative test is false.[453] The use of antifungal medications may further lower the sensitivity of this test. Given the high probability of misdiagnosis, the clinical applications of this promising antigen test seem rather limited for the individual avian patient.

All results should be interpreted in the context of the type of sample collected, species (especially serology; shedding periods and the varying disease susceptibility of individual avian species), sampling site, dynamic of the disease (e.g., shedding of the organism, clinical disease, period of viremia postinfection, shedding routes), and the immune response to the pathogen (e.g., primary cellular immunity in aspergillosis and mycobacteriosis). Knowing the prevalence of the disease is also an important consideration when determining a diagnosis.

Analysis of exhaled breath condensate has been investigated as a possible tool to characterize inflammatory respiratory disease but is limited by availability and useful clinical applications.[454,455]

Respiratory Monitoring

While there is no test currently available to assess the respiratory function in birds, anesthetic monitoring equipment could be used to assess the efficiency of pulmonary gas exchange. Pulse oximetry measures the hemoglobin saturation in oxygen, based on hemoglobin light absorption characteristics. There are differences between avian and human hemoglobin light photometric behavior, consequently most pulse oximeters have not been calibrated for use in birds. Therefore, pulse oximeters frequently underestimate avian hemoglobin saturation, which significantly reduces the benefits of this monitoring device for use as a diagnostic or monitoring tool.[456] Capnometry measures the end-tidal CO_2 in expired air, which is then used to estimate the $PaCO_2$. Capnometry has been determined to be a valuable and accurate monitoring instrument for avian patients. With pulmonary disease, a large difference between the end-tidal CO_2 and the $PaCO_2$ may be evidenced. Normal avian end-tidal CO_2 may be slightly higher than $PaCO_2$, due to the cross-current gaseous exchange in the avian lungs.[457,458]

Radiography

The avian body is "filled" with air and the respiratory system delineates virtually all internal organs. Radiographic images of the avian skull are complex and difficult to interpret, due to superimposition of the many bones that comprise this structure. Nevertheless, the area of the infraorbital sinus is located rostro-ventrally to the eye and the zygomatic bone, as well as pneumatizing most structures of the head. Bone destruction is common in chronic rhinitis and sinusitis.

Contrast media may be used to highlight nasal and sinusal passages. A CT scan is indicated to accurately image upper respiratory disease, as radiographs may only detect a generalized disease process.

The complete rings of the avian trachea are readily identified on radiographic images, and veterinarians must be familiar with species-specific and gender-specific tracheal anatomical peculiarities (see Anatomy and Physiology section at the beginning of the chapter; Figure 3-31). Tracheal diseases are readily diagnosed radiographically, with the diseased section being observed with an increased radiodensity. The syrinx is difficult to identify and evaluate due to summation of surrounding anatomic structures. The tracheal and syringeal cartilages often ossify with age. Masses in the thoracic inlet which may obstruct the syrinx are usually identified through radiographic interpretation (see Figure 3-15).

The avian lungs have a characteristic radiographic pattern: with their honeycomb structure comprised of parabronchi and are best evaluated via a lateral view. Due to anatomical differences, classic division of pulmonary radiographic lesions into interstitial, alveolar, and bronchial patterns is not used for birds. Likewise, due to the altered function of the pleural space, pleural radiographic changes do not occur in birds. Radiographic abnormalities of the avian lung can be diffuse, focal, or multifocal. Bacterial pneumonia frequently causes diffuse patterns, whereas fungal and mycobacterial lesions are often observed as focal or multifocal lesions (see Figure 3-13).[459] In general lung tumors are rare in birds. A "parabronchial" pattern is also recognized radiographically in avian species, in which the parabronchial infiltration leads to prominent ring shadows and an increase in the opaque honeycomb pattern. This is observed with pneumonia, parenchymal disease, and chronic obstructive disease. Pulmonary edema and congestion often cause a more diffuse pattern and are radiographically rarely observed.

The air contained in the air sacs is visible in radiographic images but the air sac membranes are seldom observed in healthy birds. Thickening of the air sac membranes is the most common abnormality and may lead to "cavern" formation (see Figure 3-13). Fat deposition may cause shadowing in the area of the air sac membranes.[459] Focal and more nodular lesions have been identified with granulomatous diseases (e.g., aspergillosis, mycobacteriosis). Overinflation of caudal air sacs may be appreciated with syringeal diseases which cause a valve-like effect, which results in air being trapped at this location. Likewise, overinflation of the interclavicular air sac axillary diverticulum may be present in advanced respiratory diseases when ventilation efforts are increased.[459] When radiographic air sac lesions are present, it is generally acknowledged that the disease process is advanced.

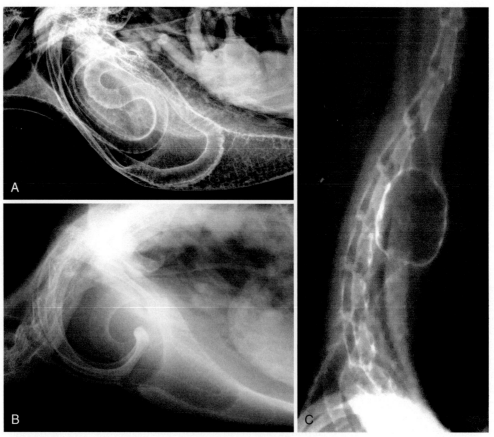

FIGURE 3-31 Radiographic images of tracheal specificities in birds. *A,* Whooping crane *(Grus Americana); B,* trumpeter swan *(Cygnus buccinator); C,* rosy-billed pochard *(Netta peposaca).*

Subcutaneous emphysema occasionally occurs as a result of trauma or fracture of a pneumatized bone.

Endoscopy

Rigid endoscopy is performed within the respiratory system in birds, owing to the extensive volume of the air sacs. Endoscopy is by far the most useful and definitive diagnostic tool to confirm a diagnosis of respiratory disease in birds. Extensive book chapters and review articles have already been published on this topic in birds, and the reader is invited to consult these references for proper endoscopic techniques and approaches.[460,461] A 2.7-mm 30°-angle rigid endoscope is recommended for use when performing most avian endoscopic procedures. The discussion below emphasizes specificities as they relate to the endoscopic assessment of the avian respiratory system.

The upper respiratory system can be investigated by rhinoscopy, oropharyngoscopy, and tracheoscopy. During oropharyngoscopy, the choanal slit is easily identified on the roof of the oropharynx, with the medial concha and nasal septum visualized the oropharyngeal opening. The choanal slit is lined with small papillae, which may appear blunted and short with nutritional deficiencies. The glottis can also be inspected and papillomatous lesions may be identified in green-winged macaws. Tracheoscopy is facilitated by the use of a 0° scope and is easily performed by introducing the unsheathed scope down the trachea through the glottis or an endotracheal tube. The main limitation when performing a tracheoscopy procedure is the length of the trachea when it exceeds the scope length by a significant amount. The syrinx should be evaluated and it should be noted that the pessulus is absent in parrots (see Figure 3-12). Commonly identified tracheal lesions include tracheal worms, tracheal stenosis, foreign bodies, tracheitis, and syringeal aspergilloma (see Figure 3-12).

The respiratory system is classically evaluated using a left or right lateral approach in birds, with an incision in the triangle formed by the last rib cranially, the pubic bone caudally, and the flexor cruris medialis dorsally when the leg is pulled forward (Figure 3-32). The caudal thoracic air sac is penetrated initally, which allows for examination of the air sac membranes cranially (confluent membranes of the cranial thoracic and caudal thoracic air sacs), the air sac membranes caudally (confluent membranes of the caudal thoracic and abdominal air sacs and oblique septum), and the lungs medially perforated with an ostium, for which the exact location is species dependent. Many air passages are visible on the septal surface of the lungs, when observed through the caudal thoracic air sac. Depending on the species, the external visible airways may include the medioventral secondary bronchi, paleopulmo, and neopulmo. The neopulmo is mainly located laterally on the costal aspect of the lungs, but depending on its extent, neopulmonic parabronchi usually cover a large area of the septal surface when examined through the caudal thoracic air sac caudally and ventrally and around the ostia. When examining the caudodorsal coelom of an avian patient, the parietal and visceral pleura may be slightly separated, with extensive fibrous strands often identified. Cranially pleural membranes are completely fused. Upon entering the abdominal air sac caudally, the caudal border of the lungs can be viewed medially deep within the coelom. The ostium of the

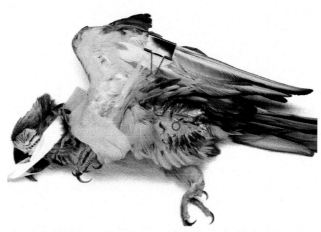

FIGURE 3-32 Blue and gold macaw positioned for a left lateral approach for a coelioscopic examination. The left leg is pulled forward and the wings are secured dorsally. The point of entry is located caudal to the last rib, cranial to the left pubic bone, and ventral to the flexor cruris medialis *(red circle)*.

abdominal air sac may be difficult to access but is typically located dorsally to the lungs. Rotating the scope counterclockwise if one is using the left approach, facilitates visualization of that ostium. Most of the parabronchi observed through the abdominal air sac are neopulmonic. Upon entering the cranial thoracic air sac cranially from the caudal thoracic air sac, areas of the lungs can still be visualized. The ostium of the cranial thoracic air sac may be difficult to localize and is situated deep to the pulmonary veins and arteries. Several ostia may be present depending on the species. Normal air sac membranes should be transparent with minimal to no vessels.

It should acknowledged that endoscopy can only identify pulmonary changes visible from the septal surface of the lungs. Common pulmonary lesions include pulmonary congestion (red patches), hemorrhage (dark red patches), granulomatous lesions (yellow to darkish areas), and pneumoconiosis (small black dots) (Figure 3-33). Iatrogenic mild hemorrhagic pulmonary lesions can easily be induced by the tip of the scope when not being cautious when initially introducing the scope into the caudal thoracic air sac or further manipulations. Common air sac lesions include opacification and hypervascularization, fat deposition, granulomas, and fungal plaques. Early focal lesions can be easily differentiated from fat by the presence of vessels "feeding" the lesion and mild surrounding inflammation (see Figure 3-14).

Pulmonary and Air Sac Biopsy

Pulmonary biopsies are indicated whenever pulmonary abnormalities are identified on radiographic images, CT scans, or coelioscopies. Several biopsies may be collected for histopathology and cultures. The easiest way to obtain a targeted biopsy of a pulmonary lesion is by endoscopy. Within the caudal thoracic air sac, the parietal pleura (thoracic air sac membrane + horizontal septum) and visceral pleura should be incised using endoscopic single-action scissors. Doing so with the fixed blade up facilitates the process. The incision can be enlarged bluntly with the closed biopsy forceps, and the pleura may be partially separated from the lungs. The pulmonary biopsy is then obtained using cup-shaped endoscopic biopsy forceps with the cups partially closed to facilitate penetration into the lung tissue using their cutting edges and to prevent crushing artifacts (Figure 3-34).

Bleeding is usually minimal to moderate and depends on the location and depth from which the biopsy sample was harvested. Another technique has been described using a dorsal intercostal approach and is indicated when lesions are not endoscopically accessible (usually as identified on a CT scan). The intercostal approach is performed by first incising the skin over the second or third intercostal space after which the intercostal space is bluntly dissected. A small section of a

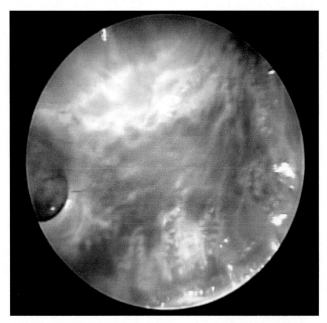

FIGURE 3-33 Pulmonary congestion diagnosed in an African gray parrot with smoke-inhalation injury. The tip of the endoscope is in the left caudal thoracic air sac.

rib may be excised to facilitate exposure of the lung. The biopsy is then harvested using 5-Fr biopsy forceps. A piece of Gelfoam may be placed in the biopsy site to control bleeding, which can be significant.

Air sac biopsies are fairly straightforward. Mildly thickened air sacs are difficult to sample without inducing tissue artifacts.

Ultrasound

Ultrasound does not have direct applications to evaluate the avian respiratory system because of the extensive pneumatization of the avian body. On the other hand, coelomic ultrasound may provide valuable information when investigating abdominal distention caused by fluids or masses that could be the cause of respiratory clinical signs.

Advanced Imaging

Computed tomography has tremendous applications and high sensitivity for assessing the avian respiratory system.[459] The lack of summation of organs and extensive air spaces throughout the avian body makes CT a very powerful and noninvasive diagnostic modality.

Perhaps the main indication for CT imaging that other diagnostic tests, including endoscopy, are of lesser value is upper respiratory disease.[120,462,463] The complex three-dimensional anatomy of the infraorbital sinus and nasal cavity makes the diagnosis of lesions challenging through the use of conventional radiographic imaging and endoscopy. CT has shown to be highly sensitive in detecting upper respiratory lesions, compared with conventional radiographic imaging.[463] Sinusitis may induce a decrease in air volume in the sinus, and in chronic cases cause calcification, and bone destruction that can be detected by CT. The volume of the aerated spaces in the skull of Amazon and African gray parrots has been determined to be about 5% to 6% of the total cranial volume.[463]

CT is also more sensitive in detecting mild to moderate lesions in the lungs and air sacs, compared with traditional radiographic imaging.[464] In addition, the lungs, air sacs, and their diverticula can be thoroughly evaluated using CT, and even the air sac membranes are visible. On average, the

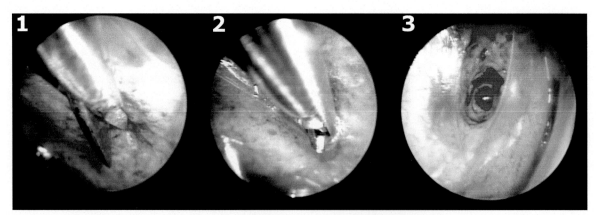

FIGURE 3-34 Endoscopic pulmonary biopsy in a Mississippi kite. *1,* The pleural membranes are incised with the fixed blade of an endoscopic single-action scissor passed through the operating channel of the endoscope; *2,* a small endoscopic biopsy forceps is introduced in the pleural incision and a lung biopsy is harvested; *3,* minimal bleeding is usually encountered but its magnitude depends on the location and depth of the biopsy.

normal lung density values are 600 to 650 HU in medium-sized parrots.[459] When endoscopy is not indicated or possible, a whole-body CT scan is the diagnostic test of choice for evaluating lower respiratory disease. Costal pulmonary lesions and granulomas/obstruction in the primary bronchi may only be diagnosed through CT imaging.

MRI is also an excellent diagnostic tool for diagnosing psittacine sinusitis.[465] However, scanning time is significantly longer than that required for CT imaging.

TREATMENTS

General Concepts in Respiratory Medical Therapy

Principles of Oxygen Therapy

The goal of oxygen supplementation is to increase the oxygen concentration of inspired air (fraction of inspired O_2: FiO_2), improve blood oxygenation, and increase tissue delivery of O_2. General hypoxia may be due to anoxic hypoxia (low FiO_2, hypoventilation, diffusion impairment, ventilation/perfusion mismatching), anemic hypoxia (anemia, methemoglobinemia, CO poisoning), stagnant hypoxia (low blood flow due to cardiac failure or hemorrhage), and histiocytic hypoxia (cyanide poisoning).[466] Common indications of oxygen therapy include severe anemia, hemodynamic compromise, and hypoxemia (decreased blood oxygen concentration) due to pulmonary and obstructive airway diseases.[467]

Oxygen therapy is typically implemented using an oxygen cage for avian and exotic patients because it is low stress and noninvasive (Figure 3-35). Veterinarians are strongly encouraged to measure the FiO_2 which can be achieved in the oxygen cages using an oxygen sensor to confirm performance before administering supplemental oxygen to patients. FiO_2 measured by the authors is 60% in the Lyon Procare Large Exotic Animal Care Unit (see Figure 3-35A) and about 40% in the Lyon Small Animal Care Unit, with oxygen at 6 to 8 L/min.

The former has doors within doors, which allow manipulation of the animal without a massive loss of O_2 from the cage. A fraction of inspired oxygen (FiO_2) of 25% to 45% may be reached through the use of "flow-by" oxygen and 35% to 60% using facemasks.[466,467] It is ideal to monitor the SpO_2 or PaO_2 during oxygen supplementation, but this is rarely practical in most companion exotic patients except rabbits, since a pulse oximeter is easily maintained on an ear.

Response to therapy should also be used for monitoring and to titrate the oxygen flow. The response to oxygen therapy may be poor depending on the disease. As an example, a poor to fair response may be observed in diseases producing a low ventilation/perfusion mismatch (perfusion predominates, with decreased supply in O_2 to the exchange surface) and includes pulmonary edema, pneumonia, asthma, pulmonary neoplasia, and atelectasis. In extreme cases of these diseases (severe pneumonia), oxygen therapy may not be efficacious because blood makes no contact with ventilated lungs. Response is good in diseases with a high ventilation/perfusion mismatch (low perfusion in normally ventilated lungs) such as pulmonary thromboembolism.[466] Improving cardiac function and fluid resuscitation are recommendations to correct stagnant hypoxemia. While the degree of response to oxygen therapy may be variable, regardless of the underlying conditions, any patient with acute respiratory distress and signs of hypoxia (cyanosis, dyspnea, tachypnea, open-mouth breathing) may benefit from supplemental oxygen.

Oxygen therapy seems extremely beneficial to birds, which have a higher metabolic demand for oxygen and which may benefit more by increasing FiO_2, due to their more efficient gas exchange surface. Conversely, oxygen supplementation may provide variable results in reptiles because increased FiO_2 may significantly decrease ventilation (oxygen is the main ventilator stimulus) and movements of inflammatory exudate from the lungs, while promoting right-to-left cardiac shunting, leading to decreased vascularization of pulmonary tissues.[468] For this reason, a slow increase of FiO_2 to 30% to 40% for a short period may be sufficent for reptile species.

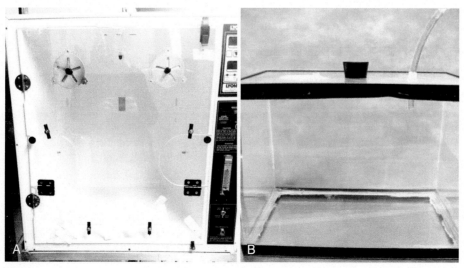

FIGURE 3-35 *A,* Commercial oxygen cage/incubator designed for birds; *B,* glass aquarium converted into a small oxygen cage.

Due to their aquatic environment, oxygen therapy is difficult in aquatic patients (e.g., fish). However, a bubbler connected to an oxygen tank or the addition of hydrogen peroxide may increase water DO, thereby benefiting dyspneic animals.

The most common complication associated with oxygen therapy is oxygen toxicity due to its ability to act as a potent oxidizing agent. The degree of potential toxicity is related to the level of oxygen and duration of therapy, and the organ most vulnerable to oxygen radicals is the lung. General guidelines recommend not to supplement oxygen at 60% to 100% for more than 24 to 48 hours in mammals.[466,467] Depletion of endogenous antioxidant levels may also promote oxygen toxicity at lower oxygen percentages. Oxygen toxicity has been primarily reported in birds. A study demonstrated oxygen toxicity in canaries and budgerigars of 68% to 100% after 3 to 8 days.[469] In another research investigation, budgerigars were found to have pulmonary lesions 3 hours after exposure to 100% oxygen.[470]

Principles of Aerosol Therapy

The goals of aerosol therapy are to deliver airborne therapeutics directly to diseased respiratory tissues and to hydrate airways in order to increase clearance of exudates and necrotic debris.[327] Local therapeutic delivery may be indicated when vascularization is decreased in diseased tissues (e.g., right-to-left shunt in reptiles, inflammatory and infected exudates in airways) or in low-perfused respiratory areas such as reptilian and avian air sacs. Nebulization allows medications to reach high therapeutic concentrations, maximizing its efficacy while minimizing systemic absorption, reducing potential for toxicity, and drug biotransformation. Humidification of the mucociliary escalator may also improve its efficiency.

Depending on particle size and airway diameter, aerosolized therapeutics may only reach the upper respiratory system, larger airways, or lungs and air sacs. Birds' airways have the smallest diameters in vertebrate species, with parabronchi diameters ranging from 0.5 mm (e.g., hummingbirds) to 2 mm (e.g., chicken, penguins) and air capillaries ranging from 3 μm (e.g., passerines) to 10 μm (e.g., swans, coots).[115] In comparison, mammalian alveoli have an approximate diameter of 30 to 150 μm (smallest is in mice) and reptilian faveoli are nearly 100 times larger than mammalian alveoli.[468,471] Likewise, amphibian alveoli are large, at 1 to 2 mm in diameter.[472] Air-breathing invertebrates, due to their size, also have ultrasmall airways; insects' tracheal systems may narrow at 0.1 μm and arachnid book lungs' airways are about 0.5 to 2 μm or less.[6,12,473]

Consequently, depending on the species and the anatomical location of the respiratory tract for drug delivery, nebulizers that can generate the required therapeutic particle sizes should be selected. In mammals, optimal particle size for drug delivery is 2 to 20 μm for the trachea and 0.5 to 5 μm for the distal airways.[474] Moreover these particle sizes are likely optimal for reptiles due to their larger airway diameters (see Figure 3-37). However, birds having smaller airways require smaller particle sizes, and particle diameters of 0.5 to 3 μm are generally recommended.[327,475] During coelioscopy, the authors have observed amphotericin B coating caudal air sacs of birds that have been nebulized, suggesting that nebulized drugs also reach the caudal thoracic and abdominal air sacs in diseased birds.

Aerosol therapy includes humidification, vaporization, and nebulization. The first two methods produce particles that are too large to reach the lower respiratory system but may be adequate for upper respiratory or tracheal diseases. The latter produces particles small enough to be deposited into smaller pulmonary airways. Nebulization can be achieved with a variety of devices that utilize different technologies such as air-jet nebulizers and ultrasonic nebulizers (including vibrating mesh technology).[476] Air-jet nebulizers are noisier and heavier but are less expensive and have a greater ability to nebulize viscous liquid than ultrasonic nebulizers (Figure 3-36). Pressurized metered-dose inhaler aerosols, such as those classically available for albuterol, are a type of air-jet nebulizer and deliver 1 to 2 μm particles.[477] Drugs used for nebulization should ideally be hydrosoluble, of low viscosity, and display adequate nebulization characteristics.[477] Drugs that are commonly nebulized include 0.9% saline, antibiotic, antifungal, antiparasitic, bronchodilation, and mucolytic agents (Table 3-7). Nebulized drugs may induce bronchospasm, and patients should be assessed before and after administration (e.g., N-acetylcysteine [NAC]).

In companion exotic animals, nebulization is mainly used to treat bird and rat lower respiratory diseases and rabbit and tortoise patients that are presented with rhinitis and sinusitis. Nebulization treatment is typically for 15 to 30 minutes, twice a day. In birds, the respiratory surface and functional efficiency of avian lungs may lead to greater systemic absorption of the drugs being nebulized than in other species. This may be advantageous in certain circumstances to obtain drug plasma therapeutic levels without having to restrain the bird. However, plasma concentrations achieved are usually low and of low duration. For instance, the pharmacokinetics of the following nebulized drugs have been performed in birds: terbinafine, voriconazole, oxytetracycline, and ceftriaxone.[478-482]

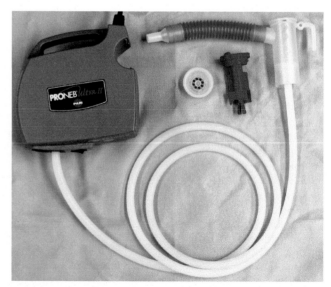

FIGURE 3-36 Air-jet nebulizer commonly used in zoological companion medicine.

TABLE 3-7

Drugs Commonly Used for Nebulization in Companion Zoological Animals

Drug	Dose
ANTIBIOTICS	
Amikacin	5-6 mg/mL sterile water/saline
Cefotaxime	10 mg/mL saline
Gentamicin	3-6 mg/mL sterile water/saline
Tobramycin	1 mg/mL saline
ANTIFUNGALS	
Amphotericin B	0.1-5 mg/mL sterile water
Enilconazol	10 mg/mL sterile water/saline
Terbinafine	1 mg/mL sterile water
Voriconazole	10 mg/mL saline
BRONCHODILATORS	
Aminophylline	3 mg/mL sterile water/saline
Terbutaline	0.01 mg/kg in 5-10 mL saline
OTHER	
N-Acetylcysteine	22 g/mL sterile water

Adapted from References 327, 483, 484.

Principles of Respiratory Pharmacology

Other than antimicrobial and anti-inflammatory agents, the pharmacology of the respiratory system in air-breathing animals includes expectorants, mucolytics, decongestants, bronchodilators, cough suppressors, and respiratory stimulants.[474,485] Most of these drugs have been studied in mammals and their effects may be variable in other vertebrate species, due to different pharmacokinetic properties, different mechanisms of respiratory diseases, and different physiology. Thus, these drugs should be used with caution in nonmammalian animals, as extrapolation from mammals is highly questionable.

The main mucolytic agent used in veterinary medicine is *N*-Acetylcysteine (NAC). *N*-Acetylcysteine breaks the disulfide bonds within mucous molecules, which decreases the viscosity and is mainly used for upper respiratory and tracheal diseases. Another mucolytic drug is bromhexine. Expectorants include potassium iodide and guaifenesin. Expectorants increase mucus production, which aids in airway secretion clearance. The use and efficacy of expectorants and mucolytics are debatable. Moreover, NAC is well known to induce bronchospasm and if used, should be combined with a bronchodilator.[474] Decongestants decrease swelling of the upper respiratory mucous membranes to allow air to freely pass. Sinusitis and rhinitis are frequent indications for the use of decongestants. Decongestants include H1 antihistamines such as diphenhydramine or hydroxyzine and sympathomimetic drugs (e.g., ephedrine, phenylephrine).

Inflammation in noninfectious pulmonary diseases may be treated with various drugs including anti-inflammatory doses of corticosteroids, leukotriene receptor antagonists, cyclosporine, and mast cell stabilizers. Nonsteroidal anti-inflammatory drugs (NSAIDS) have less of a benefit because they have a reduced ability to lower the inhibition of lipooxygenase (involved in the pathogenesis of many antigen-induced pulmonary diseases). If inhibition of cyclooxygenase 1 occurs, NSAIDS have the potential to worsen clinical signs. Corticosteroids should be used with caution in corticosensitive species such as birds, rabbits, and potentially reptiles.

Antitussives are usually opioids and include codeine, hydrocodone, butorphanol, and dextromethorphan. Cough should not be suppressed unless it is nonproductive. Since nonmammalian vertebrates may have different mechanisms and triggers for coughing, antitussive medications may be controversial in these species.

Bronchodilators are beneficial to decrease resistance to airflow but should be used when appropriate. Bronchodilators can increase the ventilation-perfusion mismatch in some diseases, which results in an increase of the hypoxic condition. Most vertebrates have bronchial smooth and airway muscles in the terminal airways such as parabronchial muscles in birds. Different classes of bronchodilators that have different mechanisms of action are available. Parasympatholytic drugs such as atropine and glycopyrrolate induce bronchodilation by competition with acetylcholine at muscarinic receptors in the airways. β_2-sympathomimetic (β-adrenergic) drugs that include albuterol (salbutamol) and terbutaline are the most effective bronchodilators and induce bronchodilation by agonistic effects on adrenergic β_2 receptors in the airways. Side effects are related to residual β_1 effects on the cardiovascular system, potentially leading to tachycardia, and arrhythmias. Methylxanthines (e.g., aminophylline, theophylline) are phosphodiesterase inhibitors that induce bronchodilation and have local anti-inflammatory effects. Adverse effects seen with methylxanthines include nausea, cardiac arrhythmias, and neurologic signs.

Doxapram is a centrally acting respiratory stimulant, but its use is questionable for most respiratory disease cases.

Antibiotic, antiparasitic and antifungal drugs are used when corresponding infections are diagnosed, at doses similar to those used for diseases of other systems.

Invertebrates

Supportive care of individuals, including feeding and fluid therapy, should be considered. Opportunities for pharmacologic intervention are minimal and overall unrewarding. Prevention of diseases and quarantine are most useful in invertebrate diseases.[143] Since invertebrate therapeutics are not specific to the respiratory system and most diseases do not target the respiratory system, readers may consult other chapters in this text for information on drugs that are used to treat commonly kept invertebrates.

Fish

Water Quality Treatments

If an environmental problem is suspected, it is imperative that one locate the origin of the problem, verify life support systems, and identify measures in order to prevent recurrence. Water quality also greatly impacts the susceptibility, occurrence, and course of many fish diseases.

Environmental hypoxia is treated by providing supplemental aeration and correcting underlying causes such as pump dysfunction, lack of mechanical aeration, improper temperature and salinity, overcrowding, or insufficient photosynthetic organisms (drop in algae concentration in ponds). Emergency procedures to increase DO for acute hypoxia in the short term include adding emergency aerators or using hydrogen peroxide (5 mL/gallon).[23,152] Reduction in food offered and lowering the temperature will also reduce a system's organism oxygen consumption. Photosynthetic organisms (e.g., plants, phytoplankton) should be controlled because high numbers may produce large oxygen fluctuations during the day and too few may be associated with low DO.

Ammonia, nitrite, and nitrate levels should be monitored on a regular basis (weekly for aquaria) and sources of nitrogen spikes (dead fish, overcrowding, overfeeding, improper pump maintenance, pump cleaned too vigorously, decreased number of nitrifying bacteria in new tanks, addition of chlorinated water or antibiotics, and anaerobic metabolism in aquarium substrates) corrected. An unstable aquarium with poor water quality may not only directly impact the piscine respiratory system through disease and adverse physiologic response (e.g., brown gill disease, low DO, methemoglobin formation) but also promote stress and secondary gill diseases and provide nutrients for potentially harmful organisms. Furthermore, water parameters are interrelated, therefore an enclosed ecosystem must be approached as a whole.[23,152,486] This interrelationship is noted through a low DO promoting an increase in ammonia and nitrites (nitrifying bacteria need oxygen), temperature and salinity lower the DO, and pH and temperature increasing ammonia toxicity.

Large amounts of ammonia or nitrites require immediate attention. Large water changes (25% to 50%) should be implemented and should be repeated periodically (e.g., daily) until the problem is controlled. Zeolite can be added to the filter to bind ammonia but is ineffective in saltwater. The addition of commercial nitrifying bacteria may help temporarily stabilize the nitrogen cycle by selecting the appropriate bacteria depending on the concentrated metabolites and help repopulate the filter media and aquarium gravels. Biological filtration should be verified and its capacity increased if necessary. Proper aeration should be provided for the biological filtration to be optimal. Feeding should be temporarily stopped to decrease the amount of waste as well as reducing the density of fish within the system. Buffers can be added, as a decrease in pH leads to a decrease in toxic unionized ammonia. Commercial detoxifying and waste control products for aquaria may also be used and usually work by chemical neutralization (AmQuel,® Nutrafin Waste Control®). Temperature may be lowered, which decreases the formation of unionized ammonia and nitrites. Chlorides limit nitrite toxic effects by decreasing gill nitrite absorption and can be added in the form of salt at 0.1 to 0.5 parts per thousand (ppt). The new system may take several weeks/months to establish a stable nitrogen cycle, and until stabilized, fish density and feeding should be minimal. Proper filter maintenance and ensuring that the system does not exceed filter capacity are also paramount.

Lowering nitrate levels is mainly accomplished through water changes, but a biological denitrification system (e.g., algae scrubber filters) may be added. Lava rocks also create anaerobic areas that promote denitrification. As nitrates are an indicator for the increase of other potentially toxic metabolic by-products, it is recommended to perform a water change when nitrate concentration is high.

An acutely acidic pH may require water change along with the addition of commercial buffer agents. The level of ammonia should be known before adjusting the pH, as increasing the pH also increases ammonium toxicity.

A suboptimal temperature should be corrected, as it may decrease fish immunity. Altering the temperature temporarily with some infections/infestations, where pathogens' life cycle/growth may be inhibited, may also be beneficial.

Filtration with granulated activated carbon can be added to the system in case a toxin is suspected and this substance is not already being used.

Water Medications and Bath

Water-borne treatments are the most commonly form of therapeutic administration used for fish and are especially beneficial when applied for external infections and infestations. Medications may be added at low concentration in aquarium water (low concentration and prolonged exposure time), but one should remember that all other fish and live organisms in the tank will also be treated. Thus, water treatments may have unwanted effects on aquarium invertebrates, plants, bacteria, and algae within the enclosed ecosystem and biological filtration. For this reason, many medications cannot be used safely in a reef aquarium. Furthermore, anemones and corals have symbiotic bacteria, algae, and protozoa that may be adversely affected. Scaleless fish, such as catfish and pufferfish) species may also show an increased toxicity to certain drugs (especially nitrofurans) and increased salinity.[487] Juvenile fish also appear more susceptible to the adverse effects of therapeutic agents. Some filters use activated carbon cartridges as part of the chemical filtration and this may have to be temporarily removed to prevent adsorbing the drug, which will decrease treatment efficacy.[488] Likewise, the UV sterilizer and ozonizer may have to be temporarily turned off. Water quality testing should be performed on a regular basis, with specific attention paid to the nitrogen cycle (e.g., ammonium, nitrites, nitrates) to monitor the quality of the biological filtration. Water temperature, salinity, alkalinity, hardness, pH, and other parameters may impact treatment. For example, saltwater may affect the activity of various drugs such as tetracyclines (i.e., chelation of calcium and magnesium), copper, and organophosphates. Marine fish also drink more and may absorb significantly higher drug concentration through the gastrointestinal system than their freshwater counterparts.[487]

Furthermore, pathogens may have different sensitivity to common treatments; even parasites within the same group can express different responses to treatment. Therefore, veterinarians may try different therapies depending on the situation including the fact that protozoan parasites may or may not complete their entire cycle on the host, consequently the system may have to be treated for an extensive period of time to affect the free-living forms. This is typified with the common ich infection (*Ichthyophthirius*), whereby the aquarium may be treated for several days/weeks. In a scenario similar to that used to treat common ich infection, the aquarium temperature should also be increased to accelerate the parasite life cycle so sensitive stages are released more frequently and the overall treatment time is shorter.[154]

Types of drug used depend on the targeted etiological agent. In general, raising the salinity may help one to both prevent and treat multiple infections in freshwater systems, with most freshwater fish tolerating salinity up to 3 ppt. Increasing salinity may also help provide relief from the osmotic stress experienced by fish with damaged gill and cutaneous epithelium as well as limit the uptake of nitrites. Increasing the salinity should be gradual to allow adaptation of the biological filter and fish homeostasis. Likewise, lowering the salinity of the marine aquatic system may be beneficial in some cases. Drugs that are added to the water may also degrade over time into toxic metabolites. Thus repetitive dosing and water changes are likely to be needed (30% to 50% daily) to prevent the buildup of toxic by-products. In general, water-borne treatments are mainly effective for superficial pathogens such as bacteria, fungi, and parasites and are thus well suited for most gill diseases. In addition, gills are highly vascularized and local drug concentration may be able to reach adequate therapeutic concentrations in branchial tissues.

When one does not prefer or cannot treat the whole aquatic system (e.g., because of size, presence of invertebrates, buildup of toxic residues, toxic concentration to nitrifying bacteria, amount of drug used), baths/dips may be employed and higher more precise concentration of the medications can be used for a short period of time (high concentration and short exposure time). It is best to try the treatment on a small number of fish first. Saline baths may be effective in freshwater species and freshwater baths in saltwater species for a variety of pathogens, especially parasites. An AirStone should be placed in the bath during treatment to ensure water oxygenation.

Most drugs used to treat fish in the aquatic environment, including most antibiotics or baths/dips, can be purchased through commercial sources. However, the use of malachite green, nitrofurans, and chloramphenicol should be avoided because of public health concerns and FDA high regulatory priority. Targeted concentrations can easily be calculated by estimating the volume of water to which the drug is to be added either by weighting (1 L = 1 kg) or by approximately calculating its volume (e.g., rectangular cuboid = depth × length × thickness, sphere = $4/3 \pi r^3$, minus estimated volume of aquascaping objects and gravel; note, 1 cm^3 = 0.001 L).

The most common treatments are summarized in Table 3-8. There is no treatment for viral infections other than preventing secondary bacterial and fungal infections (lymphocystis may be self-limiting). Commercial nitrifying bacteria may be added to the tank during treatment to support the biological system (e.g., Nutrafin Cycle). Immunostimulants are widely available for fish (e.g., Melafix®) and may be used in combination with other treatments, but limited data are available regarding their clinical effectiveness.

Other Treatments

Systemic drugs may be warranted for advanced disease cases and depending on the patient's condition (Table 3-9). The fish's weight needs to be known or estimated. Oral medications may be administered in food. Commercial food with added chemicals may be purchased, the drug can be mixed with food using gelatin or by injection in a small food item, or the food may be bioencapsulated in brine shrimp larvae or other crustaceans.[487,490,491] Mazuri® makes various aquatic gel diets that may be combined with medications and possibly improving its palatability and the ease of administration. Doses for oral medications may be calculated on the basis that fish eat an approximate 2% of their body weight daily. However, sick fish are frequently anorexic.

TABLE 3-8	
Common Treatments Used to Treat Fish Respiratory Diseases	
Modality	**Drug**
System water	Enrofloxacin 2.5-5 mg/L q1-2 d (B)
	Furazolidone 1-10 mg/L q1 d (B)
	Kanamycin 50-100 mg/L q3 d (B)
	Neomycin 66 mg/L q3 d (B)
	Nifurpirinol 0.1 mg/L (B)
	Nitrofurazone 2-10 mg/L (B)
	Oxolinic acid 3-10 mg/L q1 d (B)
	Oxytetracycline 10-100 mg/L q1 d (B)
	Chloroquine 10 mg/L q5 d (P)
	Copper 0.15 mg/L
	Formalin 0.015-0.025 mL/L q2 d (P)
	Malachite green 0.1 mg/L (F, P)
	Mebendazole 1 mg/L q1 d (P)
	Trichlorfon 0.25 mg/L q2-3 d (P)
	Praziquantel 2 mg/L (P)
	Salt 2-3 ppt (B, F, P)
Bath/dip	Glacial acetic acid: 1-2 mL/L, 1-10 min (P)
	Flumequine 50-100 mg/L for 3 h (B)
	Nifurpirinol 1-2 mg/L for 5 min-6 h (B)
	Nitrofurazone 100 mg/L for 30 min (B)
	Oxolinic acid 25 mg/L for 15 min (B)
	Oxytetracycline 10-50 mg/L for 1 h (B)
	Bronopol 20 mg/L for 30 min (F)
	Fenbendazole 25 mg/L for 12 h (P)
	Formalin 0.125-0.250 mL/L (P)
	Freshwater for 3-15 min (P)
	Hydrogen peroxide 50-300 mg/L for 10-15 min (B, F, P)
	Malachite green 1-2 mg/L for 30-60 min (F, P)
	Mebendazole 100 mg/L for 10 min (P)
	Potassium permanganate 5-100 mg/L for 5-10 min (B, P)
	Praziquantel 2-10 mg/L for 1-3 h (P)
	Cypermethrin 5 µg/L for 1 h (P)
	Salt 10-30 g/L for 30 min (B, F, P)
	Toltrazuril 5-20 mg/L for 1-4 h (P)

Roberts HE, Smith SA. Disorders of the respiratory system in pet and ornamental fish. *Vet Clin.* 2011;14(2):179-206.[157]
Noga E. Pharmacopoeia. In: Noga E, ed. *Fish Disease: Diagnosis and Treatment.* 2nd ed. Ames, IA: Wiley-Blackwell; 2010:375-420.[489]
B, Bacterial diseases; *F*, fungal diseases; *P*, parasitic diseases; *ppt*, parts per thousand.

Injectable medications (e.g., antibiotics) may be given intramuscularly over the dorsum lateral to the dorsal fin on either side or intracoelomically near the ventral midline. One should remember that few pharmacokinetic studies are published in fish and that fish show tremendous taxonomic and physiological variability, which may affect drug metabolism.

Macroscopic parasites may also be removed manually using surgical magnification and forceps, and focal wounds may be treated topically with ointment.

With most diseases in which zoological species are susceptible, preventive medicine is best. Sterilization systems may be added to an aquatic system including UV and ozone sterilizers which are available for aquaria at pet stores. A 30-day

TABLE 3-9

Common Systemic Treatments* Used to Treat Fish Respiratory Diseases

Route	Drug
Injection	Amikacin 5 mg/kg q12 h
	Amoxicillin 12.5 mg/kg
	Ampicillin 10 mg/kg
	Ceftazidime 5-20 mg/kg q3 d
	Enrofloxacin 5-10 mg/kg q2-3 d
	Flumequine 30 mg/kg (last 10 d)
	Kanamycin 20 mg/kg
	Oxytetracycline 25-50 mg/kg
	Sulfadiazine-trimethoprim 125 mg/kg
	Praziquantel 25 mg/kg once
Oral	Amoxicillin 40-80 mg/kg
	Ampicillin 50-80 mg/kg
	Enrofloxacin 10 mg/kg
	Florfenicol 10-50 mg/kg q1 d
	Flumequine 30 mg/kg
	Kanamycin 50 mg/kg
	Nifurpirinol 4-10 mg/kg
	Oxolinic acid 10 mg/kg
	Oxytetracycline 25-50 mg/kg
	Sulfadiazine-trimethoprim 30-50 mg/kg
	Sulfadimethoxine-ormetoprim 50 mg/kg
	Praziquantel 50 mg/kg once

Roberts HE, Smith SA. Disorders of the respiratory system in pet and ornamental fish. *Vet Clin.* 2011;14(2):179-206.[157]

Noga E. Pharmacopoeia. In: Noga E, ed. *Fish Disease: Diagnosis and Treatment.* 2nd ed. Ames, IA: Wiley-Blackwell; 2010:375-420.[489]

*Frequency of administration may vary; once every 1 to 3 days.

quarantine is recommended before new fish introduction. For fish hobbyists, a quarantine system may just be another smaller tank with its own life support system and cleaning tools. During this period, 2% to 5% of fish may be examined by hands-on physical examination with gill, skin, and blood samples being checked to increase to increase one's odds to find a disease problem. Preventive treatments for ectoparasites, such as formalin, praziquantel, saltwater, or freshwater dips, may also be performed prior to the addition of new fish into an established system. All aquarium supplies and quarantine areas should be thoroughly cleaned with bleach or quaternary ammonium (Rocal®) before use in another aquatic environment. Drying will also kill most aquatic pathogens.

Amphibians

If detected, inappropriate husbandry conditions should be immediately corrected, as these may be directly correlated to the patient condition. Specifically, high humidity and proper water quality should be maintained. An appropriate filtering system should be added to an aquatic enclosure, and maturation of the nitrogen cycle should be verified (see previous section Other Treatments).

Specific treatment should be attempted when necessary and based on the results of diagnostic tests.[164] Animals in critical condition should be placed in an oxygen-rich environment.[172] In cases of infectious diseases, affected amphibians should be isolated and the environment should be cleaned

within 24 hours. Cleaning of the environment with appropriate disinfectants should be frequently repeated during the treatment period.

When parasites are diagnosed in the respiratory system, prophylactic treatment with corticosteroids 3 days before antihelminthics is recommended, especially for heavy infestations.[63,164,172] Dead lung trematodes elicit a significant inflammatory response within lung tissue, and degenerative larvae of *Rhabdias* sp. have been reported to induce bacterial superinfection and toxemia.[63,170] Treatment of *Rhabdias* spp. may be difficult and different protocols have been recommended, including ivermectin (200 to 40 μg/kg, per os [PO], subcutaneous [SC], or topical), levamisole (8 to 10 mg/kg, PO, SC, intramuscular [IM], topical, intratracheal, or intrapneumonic; may be irritant) or fenbendazole (50 to 100 mg/kg PO, repeat in 10 to 14 days).[47,164,173,175,492] Flaccid paralysis may occur with levamisole, especially in aquatic caecilians (*Typhlonectes* spp.), and the Surinam toad (*Pipa pipa*).[492] With prolonged treatment exposure in a medicated bath the paralyzed patient may drown.[492] Any amphibian undergoing treatment with levamisole should be thus monitored regularly, typically every 1 to 8 hours.[492] Infested amphibians should be isolated, as infectious exposure to *Rhabdias* spp. infection is high.[47,173] Fecal monitoring for the presence of the parasite larval stages should be performed frequently and antihelminthic treatments repeated until the fecal examinations test negative.[47] Some authors recommend testing all wild-caught Anurans and salamanders for *Rhabdias* spp. during quarantine or to preemptively treat these animals.[174] Substrate should be changed with each treatment to limit recontamination with infective larvae.[175] Praziquantel (8 to 24 mg/kg, PO, IM, intracoelomic, every 14 days, for three treatments) is usually recommended for treatment of amphibian trematode infestations.[164,492]

Treatment for protozoan infections that infect the respiratory tract of amphibians depends on the organism identified.[47] Husbandry corrections are usually curative for trichodinosis.[47] *Piscinoodinium pillularis* infestations or persistent cases of trichodinosis may be treated with 72-hour immersion in saline (4 to 6 g NaCl/L H₂O) or providing dilute formalin baths (1.5 mL of 10% formalin/L of water, dip for 10 min, every 48 h).[47]

Different therapeutic options may be used to treat saprolegniasis, including formalin or salt baths; dipping briefly in a 1:15,000 solution of malachite green daily for 2 to 3 days; treating the cage water with benzalkonium chloride (0.25 mg/L), methylene blue (4 mg/L), or mercurochrome 3 mg/L; and topical application of dilute benzalkonium chloride, malachite green, or mercurochrome.[47]

Treatment for nasal myiasis, *Dermocystidium* sp. infection, and gill hyperplasia has not been described.[47] Mimicking behavioral fever by elevating temperature has been proposed by some authors as a treatment for *Dermocystidium* spp.[164] Moreover, therapeutic trials for mycotic pneumonia have not been reported, as most cases were diagnosed on postmortem examination.[176]

Reptiles

Medical Therapy

Since most reptiles are presented with advanced chronic respiratory diseases, long-term, multimodal, and aggressive

TABLE 3-10

Selected Drugs Commonly Used to Treat Respiratory Infections in Reptiles

Drug	Dose
MYCOPLASMA INFECTION IN TORTOISES	
Enrofloxacin	5-10 mg/kg IM, PO q24-48 h
Clarithromycin	15 mg/kg PO q48-72 h
Tylosin	5 mg/kg IM q24 h
	50 mg/kg IM, then 25 mg/kg q72 h
ANTIBIOTICS USED IN PNEUMONIA	
Ceftiofur sodium	5 mg/kg SC, IM q24 to 48 h
Ceftazidime	20-40 mg/kg IM q48-72 h (q24 h in chameleons)
Piperacillin	50-100 mg/kg IM q24-48 h
ANTIFUNGALS USED IN MYCOTIC PNEUMONIA	
Itraconazole	5-10 mg/kg PO q24 h
Voriconazole	10 mg/kg PO q24 h
MISCELLANEOUS	
Acyclovir (TeHV infection)	80 mg/kg PO q8 h
Dexamethasone (pharyngeal edema)	0.2 mg/kg IM, IV
Terbutaline	0.01-0.02 mg/kg IM
Vitamin A	1000-5000 U/kg q7-10 d

Adapted from References 184, 223, 500.
IM, Intramuscularly; *IV,* intravenously; *PO,* orally; *SC,* subcutaneously.

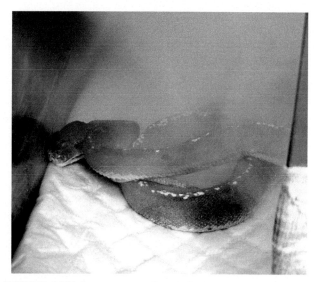

FIGURE 3-37 Green tree python being nebulized. (Courtesy of Lionel Schilliger.)

treatment is generally recommended (Table 3-10).[73,184] Suboptimal husbandry conditions should always be rapidly managed, as they may contribute to the disease process through the subsequent immunosuppression and impaired humidification of airways (low environmental humidity). Moreover, drug metabolism in reptile species depends on environmental temperature.[184] Due to crocodilians having an excessively high gastric pH, oral drugs may not reach plasma therapeutic concentrations in these species. In addition, the increased pulmonary vascular resistance of reptile pulmonary diseases may exacerbate right-to-left shunt. Most reptiles, in particular, aquatic species, have an incredible ability to compensate for the right-to-left shunt through anaerobic metabolism. Consequently, pulmonary concentrations of therapeutic drugs may not be optimal. Oxygen therapy, nebulization, and the use of bronchodilators have been discussed above, and applications to reptile species must take into consideration their unique physiology, as extrapolation from mammals may not always be adequate. As previously discussed, oxygen therapy should be carefully provided to reptile patients. High-oxygen-tension environments often suppress the reptile's spontaneous respiratory rate. Prolonged exposure to an environment of enriched oxygen tension may suppress ventilation in reptiles, which further inhibits the limited excretion of inflammatory exudates from the lungs thereby aggravating clinical conditions such as dyspnea and hypercapnia.[73]

The use of glucocorticoids for severe pharyngeal or laryngeal edema, or bronchodilators for the treatment of obstructive lower respiratory diseases, may be beneficial in selected cases.[184] Supportive care (e.g., fluid therapy, nutritional support), is usually necessary when treating reptile

patients that are presented with severe respiratory disease. Infected reptiles should be isolated from other animals.[74] Until the results of diagnostic tests are received, administration of broad-spectrum antibiotics is generally recommended when treating reptiles diagnosed with upper and lower respiratory disease since the condition is usually chronic and secondary bacterial infections are common (see Table 3-10).[184] The combination of different antibiotic drugs may be required for respiratory disease that is chronic in nature and/or when extremely resistant organisms are identified. In chelonians with pneumonia, an intrapulmonic catheter may be placed within the affected area of the lungs, using the same approach as described for transcarapacial pneumonoscopy, for direct administration of drugs.[184,434] As soon as the etiological agents are determined, specific therapy should be initiated.

For reptile patients diagnosed with upper respiratory disease the combination of systemic antimicrobial administration and local treatments provides the best results.[184] Nasal flushes of diluted antibiotics (i.e., 1:10 solution of enrofloxacin and saline), administered twice daily through a small-gauge catheter inserted into the nares are recommended.[74,184] Debridement of necrotic material should be performed with stomatitis cases.[184] Mycoplasmosis is a chronic infection in chelonians, and complete elimination of the organism may not be possible.[74,184] Treatment of infected tortoises reduces or eliminates overt clinical signs, but infected animals should be considered carriers of the disease, as it is challenging if not impossible to differentiate disease free from subclinical states at this time.[74,184,223] *Mycoplasma* sp. in chelonians may be sensitive to various antibiotics (Table 10).[74,223] Due to the presence of pharmacologic data regarding enrofloxacin and clarithromycin in tortoises, these two antibiotics are the primary drugs of choice.[223,493-496] Ophthalmic ointments and a combination of steroid/antibiotic nasal flushes may also be employed for suspect of confirmed chelonian mycoplasmosis cases.[223] Nebulized antibiotics may be administered using similar doses to those recommended for other exotic animals (see Table 3-7 and Figure 3-37).

Mycoplasma alligatoris usually is susceptible to doxycycline, oxytetracycline, enrofloxacin, sarafloxacin, tilmicosin, or tylosin.[66] The use of an autogenous vaccine for *M. crocodyli* has been described, but its efficacy has not been determined.[66]

Similar to mycoplasma infection, HVs cannot be eliminated in infected chelonians. Therapeutic goals include providing supportive care, address secondary infections, and correct promoting factors until the chelonian's natural defenses are able to suppress the clinical signs. The oral cavity should be rinsed and cleaned under sedation or anesthesia using a cotton tipped applicator soaked with dilute chlorhexidine (0.5%) or povidone-iodine (0.5%), once per day. Acyclovir (45 to 80 mg/kg, PO, every 72 h) and gancyclovir have been reported to be effective in treating HV infections in chelonians, especially if administered early in the course of disease.[74,192,497] Five percent acyclovir ointment may be used topically and has been reported to improve lesions. Acyclovir and gancyclovir have been found to reduce TeHV replication and overall mortality in outbreaks.[192] However, acyclovir has been associated with renal damage in certain chelonian species, therefore this drug should be used with caution and only when there is a strong suspicion of infection or confirmed diagnosis.[73]

Treatment of ranavirus infections in chelonians also includes nursing care, management of secondary bacterial infections, and cleaning of the oral cavity, as previously described for HV.[74] Acyclovir is also a recommended treatment for iridovirus infection in chelonians.[497]

At this time there is no known treatment for snakes infected with ferlavirus.[202] Treatment of clinical signs with broad-spectrum antibiotics has been reported to improve survival time in snakes with ferlavirus infection along with supportive care.[184,202] The use of an antiviral drug, such as ribavin (Virazole®) or BCX 2798, has been advanced, but no in-vitro or in-vivo test have been performed.[202] There are reports of unsuccessful vaccination of snakes with inactivated strains of ferlavirus, while in another study live vaccines were associated with mortality.[202,498,499]

Long-term (at least 2 or 3 months), aggressive, systemic antifungal therapy is the recommended treatment of reptiles diagnosed with pulmonary mycoses (see Table 3-10).[66,184] Aerosol treatments using amphotericin B or F10 may be beneficial in resolving clinical disease signs associated with pulmonary mycoses. Long-term systemic antifungal therapy combined with aerosol therapy offers the best prognosis for respiratory mycotic cases.[184] Surgical removal of fungal granuloma may be required to achieve a successful therapy in chronic disease presentations.[184] However treatment for fungal pneumonia is often unsuccessful in reptiles.[73] In crocodilians, fungal pneumonia is usually diagnosed postmortem.[253] Preventing respiratory fungal disease is achieved by avoiding severe stress and prolonged exposure to poor husbandry conditions.[73,253]

Parasitic infections of the respiratory tract in reptiles should be treated with appropriate antiparasitic agents (see Table 3-10). Praziquantel can be used for trematode and cestode infestations. Nematodes may be treated with ivermectin (do not use in chelonians) or fenbendazole. Precautions against potential zoonotic infections should be considered before initiating treatment.[184] Treatment of pentastomiasis is difficult, but ivermectin, fenbendazole, and other antihelminthics have been somewhat effective in isolated cases.[257] The treatment for pulmonary intranuclear coccidiosis may be challenging, possibly due to the fact that no effective treatment has been reported.[71]

Dietary correction and oral supplementation are recommended in cases of respiratory disorders secondary to hypovitaminosis A.[74]

Prevention of respiratory disorders is based primarily on appropriate quarantine and stress reduction in reptile collections. Quarantine of at least 3 to 6 months for each new reptile specimen is required, including a complete physical examination, hematology, biochemistry, fecal screens, and microbiological testing (e.g., HV and mycoplasma in tortoises, ferlavirus in viperidae) to prevent introduction of sick or subclinical reptiles.[184] Any sick animal should be immediately removed from other specimens and isolated. For parasitic infections, exposure through the intermediate host should be minimized. Crocodilians should be fed with frozen or boiled fish to kill the pentastomid parasite larvae to prevent subsequent infestations.[253]

Surgical Therapy

Surgical treatment of reptilian respiratory diseases has not been well documented.

As in other vertebrates, maintenance of a patent airway is required for life and emergency procedures, such as tracheal intubation, tracheostomy, or tracheal suctioning when fluids are present, are techniques that veterinarians must know to save the critical reptile patient and this includes air sac cannulation in squamates.[184,501] Saccular lung cannulation, similar to bird air sac cannulation, may be performed in snakes with tracheal obstruction (e.g., exudate, tracheal neoplasia, tracheal stenosis) to allow for better ventilation while starting therapeutic management.[501] The approach for a saccular lung cannulation is similar to that described for an ophidian pulmonoscopy. An esophagostomy tube may be placed in chelonians for nutrition support and drug administration.[74,184]

Tracheal resection and anastomosis has been reported in snakes as a treatment of tracheal chondroma, and the technique is similar to that for other species.[264,502] Snakes have C-shaped tracheal rings, and caution must be observed not to damage the dorsal membrane during the procedure.[502]

As there is no effective chemical treatment against pentastomids, surgical removal of worms is recommended.[184] In crocodilians, the parasites can be flushed out of the nasal cavity by injecting saline into the nostrils.[212]

Mammals

Medical Therapy

Treatment of exotic companion mammal respiratory disorders is similar to that used for dogs and cats. Animals that are in severe respiratory distress would benefit from oxygen therapy, mild sedation, and being left along in a dark, quiet environment until further assessment.[289] There are many protocols, published for sedating small exotic mammals, although those commonly used drugs are midazolam and butorphanol. Both midazolam and butorhanol have minimal adverse effects on the cardiovascular and respiratory system and are reliable sedatives in exotic companion mammals.[98]

The antimicrobial treatment response is enhanced with an accurate diagnosis including pathogen identification, ideally derived from culture and sensitivity results, and localization of disease.[278] When culture and sensitivity cannot be performed, antibiotic agents should be selected and used judiciously regarding the organism's potential senstivity to the drug, possible treatment benefits, and potential adverse effects. Rat respiratory disease is frequently caused by *Mycoplasma pulmonis* and *Streptococcus pneumonia*; thus, antibiotics such as doxycycline and azithromycin are particularly useful. A combination of systemic enrofloxacin and doxycycline therapy along with nebulized antimicrobial medication is frequently used to treat chronic respiratory disease in rats. Certain antimicrobial agents, (e.g., penicillin, clindamycin), have adverse treatment effects on rabbit and rodent gastrointestinal microbiota and microfauna when administered orally, although when administered parenterally, this condition is rarely observed.[503] Moreover, doxycycline is readily available in practice, an excellent treatment for intracellular organisms, and known for its anti-inflammatory attributes. Direct delivery of bronchodilators, antimicrobials, acetylcysteine, hypertonic saline, and cortico steroids to the upper respiratory tract through nebulization results in minimal systemic adverse effects therefore can be used in conjunction with other therapeutic protocols (e.g., oral, intramuscular, intravenous). Drug pharmacology and efficacy have not been established for most nebulized agents used to treat, consequently selection is based primarily on empirical or extrapolated data obtained from other mammalian species.[6,291,296] The use of corticosteroids as an anti-inflammatory treatment option is controversial, due to the immunosuppressive effects of this class of drugs, particularly in rabbits, which are a corticosensitive species.[504] Commonly used drugs are presented in Table 3-11.

A vaccination program for ferrets is recommended to protect against canine distemper and rabies viruses is recommended.[298,303,308]

Radiation therapy has been described in rabbits diagnosed with thymomas and is regarded as the treatment of choice for this species. A mean survival time of 313 days was reported in 19 rabbits diagnosed with thymomas and subsequently treated with radiation therapy from which very few therapeutic side effects were noted.[505] Various chemotherapeutic drugs have been used for the treatment of rabbit thymoma and lymphoma, however adverse effects of chemotherapeutic drugs seem to be common in this species.[506] For other classifications of thoracic neoplasms, chemotherapy is an option along with radiation therapy which has been applied to cases where total removal of the tissue mass was in question or the patient was not a suitable surgical candidate. Ferret diagnosed with lymphoma can be treated with a combination chemotherapeutic protocol. Unfortunately, at this time the chemotherapeutic protocol does not significantly prolong nor improve quality of life for the lymphoma patient. Prednisone is a recommended therapeutic treatment for ferrets diagnosed with lymphoma.

Surgical Therapy

In emergency or critical cases in which intubation is not possible a tracheostomy may need to be performed to secure a patent airway. The procedure is similar to that used for dogs and cats, in which a tube is placed approximately two to four rings proximal to the larynx through an incision between the tracheal rings.[507]

TABLE 3-11

Selected Drugs Commonly Used to Treat Respiratory Infections in Exotic Companion Mammals

Drug	Species	Dose
ANTIBIOTICS		
Amoxicillin/ clavulanic acid	Ferrets, hedgehogs	12.5 mg/kg PO q12 h
	Rats	20 mg/kg PO q12 h
Chloramphenicol	All	25-30 mg/kg PO q12 h
Ciprofloxacin	All	5-20 mg/kg PO q12 h
Enrofloxacin	All	5-10 mg/kg IM, IV, PO q12-24 h
Marbofloxacin	All	2 mg/kg IM, IV q24 h 5 mg/kg PO q24 h
Trimethoprim/ sulfamethoxazole	All	15-30 mg/kg PO q12 h
ANTIFUNGALS		
Itraconazole	All	20 mg/kg PO q24 h
Fluconazole	All	5 mg/kg PO q24 h
Terbinafine	All	100 mg/kg PO q12 h
MISCELLANEOUS		
Meloxicam	Rabbits	0.5-1 mg/kg PO q12-24 h
	Guinea pigs	0.5-1 mg/kg PO q12-24 h
	Chinchillas	0.5-1 mg/kg PO q12-24 h
	Rats, mice	1-5 mg/kg PO, SC q24 h
	Ferrets	0.2 mg/kg PO, SC q24 h
Prednisone/ prednisolone	All	0.1-2 mg/kg PO q12-24 h

For rabbits diagnosed with severe or chronic sinusitis, surgical debridement and infusion of topical antimicrobials has been achieved through an indwelling nasal catheter placed during a surgical rhinotomy procedure.[278] The focal administration of antimicrobial therapy through the indwelling catheter provides an aggressive treatment focus in sinusitis cases unresponsive to previous therapeutic protocols. A dorsal rhinotomy and rhinostomy approach has recently been described, which required an osteotomy to gain access to the nasal cavity.[326] One of the authors has successfully performed a ventral rhinotomy using endoscopic-assisted techniques to debride a large periapical abscess that was obstructing the airway in a rabbit (Figure 3-28). This latter approach did not require an osteotomy and was performed on the cranial palate.

Thoracocentesis should be performed in cases of pleural effusion and pneumothorax and is a similar procedure to that used for cats. A thoracotomy procedure used to excise thymoma masses in rabbits has been described but is not well tolerated by the patients.[506] A report with 17 rabbits undergoing thoracotomy and thymoma excision reported that nine died during or within 10 days of the surgery.[508] Thoracotomy surgical procedures have been reported in guinea pigs and chinchillas.[509]

Birds

Medical Therapy

UPPER RESPIRATORY DISEASE. The medical treatment for rhinitis and sinusitis depends on the bacterial or fungal pathogen isolated and the amount of necrotic and caseous debris present in the upper airways. Aerosol therapy, as previously described, may help humidify the nasal passage and aid in the administration of local antimicrobial medication. Flushing the nasal cavity with saline with or without antimicrobial agents may help dislodge nasal debris. The head is typically held down to prevent aspiration of the injected aqueous solution. Nasal flushing may be performed once to twice daily for several days/weeks. A nasal flush formula has been described combining amphotericin B, trypsin, and neomycin (Table 3-12).[510] More drastic debridement is usually required for cases in which rhinoliths have been diagnosed. Increasing the environmental humidity is frequently beneficial to psittacine species, considering their natural tropical range. Improving air quality with high-efficiency particular absorption (HEPA) air filtering and decreasing potential airborne toxins and allergens may be beneficial in some avian cases that exhibit upper respiratory disease signs.

AVIAN CHLAMYDIOSIS. The treatment of avian chlamydiosis relies on using antibiotics such as tetracyclines and macrolides with intracellular distribution. Chloramphenicol and enrofloxacin may also result in clinical improvement and reduced shedding in avian chlamydiosis cases but usually fail to clear the infection. Doxycycline has historically been the drug of choice (see Table 3-12). Doxycycline may be administered orally or with a long-lasting European-formation intramuscular injection every 7 days (Vibramycin IV, formerly Vibravenös). Compounded injectable doxycycline may provide variable results, consequently commercial formulations are always recommended.[511] Injection site irritation usually occurs with single and repeated injections of doxycycline and other tetracyclines. Moreover these intramuscular injections have a tendency to be especially severe with the compounded doxycycline formulations. In addition, tetracyclines may cause hepatic toxicity, while doxycycline decreases immune competence due to its anti-inflammatory properties.[512,513] Regurgitation may occur due to local upper gastrointestinal irritation, particularly in macaws. Gastrointestinal ulceration and cutaneous photosensitivity has been reported with oral doxycycline treatment in penguins.[514] Azithromycin appears to be a safe and effective alternative to doxycycline.[515]

For large colonies of budgerigars, cockatiels, and potentially other psittacine species, tetracyclines may be administered in drinking water or in the feed (see Table 3-12). Doxycycline-medicated food (e.g., seed) reaches adequate therapeutic blood levels to treat avian chlamydiosis.[516-519] Doxycycline-medicated water reaches adequate drug plasma concentrations in several species, but not in budgerigars.[330,517,520,521] Chlortetracycline-medicated feed at 1% may be used but is usually less effective and associated with more toxic side effects than doxycycline. Medication laced water and food consumption should be monitored during the treatment period.

The duration of treatment is recommended to last 45 days because of the potential presence of a latent form. However,

TABLE 3-12

Selected Systemic Dosages for Drugs Used in Common Respiratory Diseases of Birds

Antimicrobials	Dose
AVIAN CHLAMYDIOSIS TREATMENT	
Doxycycline	Food
	• 300 mg mixed with 1 kg hulled seeds and 5-6 mL sunflower oil (budgerigars)
	• 300 mg mixed with 1 kg of pellets (cockatiels)
	• 0.1% corn diet (macaws)
	Water
	• 200-400 mg/L (cockatiels)
	• 400-600 mg/L (Goffin's cockatoos)
	• 800 mg/L (African gray parrots)
	Oral: 25-35 mg/kg q24 h
	Injectable long acting: 75-100 mg/kg q7 d
Chlortetracycline	Food: 1% mash or pelleted diet
Azithromycin	40 mg/kg PO q24-48 h (cockatiels)
ANTIFUNGALS	
Fluconazole	10-20 mg/kg PO q24-48 h
	100 mg/L in drinking water (cockatiels)
Itraconazole	5-10 mg/kg PO q12-24 h
Voriconazole	10-20 mg/kg PO, IV q12-24 h
Amphotericin B	1.5 mg/kg IV q8 h for 3-5 d
	1 mg/kg intratracheal
Terbinafine	10-25 mg/kg PO q12-24 h
	60 mg/kg PO q12 h (Amazon parrot)
ANTIPARASITE DRUGS	
Ivermectin	1-2 mg/kg IM (serratospiculosis)
	0.2-0.4 mg/kg PO or percutaneous q7-10 d × 3 (air sac mites)
Fenbendazole	25-50 mg/kg PO q24 h × 5 d
Praziquantel	5-20 mg/kg PO, SC, IM
Paronomycin	100 mg/kg PO q12 h
Toltrazuril	12.5 mg/kg PO (atoxoplasmosis)
Sulfachloropyridazine	150-300 mg/L drinking water (atoxoplasmosis)
MISCELLANEOUS	
Nasal flush: amphotericin B, neomycin, trypsin	10 mg, 3.5 mg, 124.5 mg in 30 mL diluent; add 0.1-0.4 of base solution to 30 mL diluent

IM, Intramuscularly; *IV,* intravenously; *PO,* orally; *SC,* subcutaneously.

a latent form of *Chlamydia psittaci* has not been confirmed in birds. On another hand, it has been shown that only 30 days treatment with medicated feed was sufficient in budgerigars and that 21 days successfully treated experimental infection in cockatiels, without evidence of a remaining latent form.[515,516] Repeat PCR testing several days/weeks after completion of the treatment is indicated.

ASPERGILLOSIS. The treatment of aspergillosis is complicated, long, and multifaceted. Usually a combination of nebulized, local, and systemic antifungal agents is frequently used, but antifungal monotherapy has resulted in the postive resolution some cases (see Table 3-12).[522] The prognosis should be determined based on radiographic, computed tomographic, and/or coelioscopic evaluation (see Figures 3-13 and 3-14). The treatment is lengthy, with typically 3 to 8 months of oral antifungal medications required. Ideally, the treatment should be based on fungal culture and sensitivity, but laboratories offering fungal sensitivity are few, and minimum inhibitory concentrations of antifungal agents for avian fungal isolates may not be available.

Available antifungal medications include the polyenes (e.g., amphotericin B, nystatin), which bind ergosterol (fungal wall constituent) and permeabilize the fungal cell membrane; the azoles (e.g., ketoconazole, fluconazole, itraconazole, voriconazole, clotrimazole), which inhibit a P450-dependent enzyme of lanosterol 14-α demethylation, thereby decreasing ergosterol synthesis; the allylamines (e.g., terbinafine), which inhibit squalene epoxidase, another enzyme involved in ergosterol synthesis; and echinocandins (e.g., capsofungin), which interfere with glucan synthesis.[523,524] Pharmacokinetic and pharmacodynamics studies have been performed on a few avian species for itraconazole, fluconazole, voriconazole, and terbinafine.[479,522,525-534] Most antifungal agents are fungistatic, but amphotericin B is fungicidal, as are itraconazole, voriconazole, and terbinafine on some fungal isolates, depending on dosages used. Fluconazole is considered to have low therapeutic effectiveness for aspergillosis and other filamentous fungi. Systemic enilconazole and ketoconazole are highly toxic in birds and should not be administered through this route. Using a combination of antifungal drugs with different mechanisms of action may have a synergistic effect and a subsequent reduction in fungal resistance. Voriconazole is the newest antifungal medication used in birds and appears to be particularly effective. Voriconazole has been shown to be effective in treating experimental aspergillosis in pigeons and spontaneous aspergillosis in falcons.[479,522,525] Sensitivity of avian *Aspergillus* isolates to voriconazole and itraconazole has been reported with resistance noted, in particular with itraconazole.[535,536]

Adverse effects also occur when avian patients are administered antifungal therapy. Amphotericin B treatment is associated with nephrotoxicity in mammals, but this has not yet been witnessed in birds. Triazoles may cause hepatotoxicity in cytochrome P450-sensitive species such as African gray parrots, in which the use of voriconazole seems to be safer.

The authors typically favor an aggressive treatment approach in moderate to advanced cases using a combination of antifungal agents for potential synergistic effects consisting of 1 to 3 days of IV amphotericin B or voriconazole combined with nebulized amphotericin B and oral voriconazole occasionally combined with terbinafine. Endoscopic-guided local instillation over fungal plaques or intragranuloma injections of antifungal medications are also advised depending on the case presentation. Intratracheal administration of amphotericine B may also be performed. The use of multiple routes and methods of delivery and antifungal drugs with different mechanisms of action may enhance therapeutic effectiveness and are still well tolerated by most patients. In addition, the slow onset of some triazoles may make early combination therapy advisable. However, no avian research has been performed to identify antifungal synergisms and antagonism in vivo, thus combination therapy is largely empirical. Various results have been obtained in humans, where concentration-dependent synergism or antagonism was observed between antifungal drugs.[537] Synergistic action between triazoles and amphotericin B or triazoles and terbinafine has been observed in human *Aspergillus* isolates in vitro.[538]

RESPIRATORY HELMINTHIASIS, COCCIDIOSIS, AND ACARIASIS. Treatment of respiratory parasites mainly consists of administering parenteral antiparasite medications (see Table 3-12). Intramuscular ivermectin is commonly used for helminthiasis (e.g., falcon serratospiculosis, tracheal worms).[539] Fenbendazole is also effective in treating tracheal worms. Endoscopic removal of tracheal worms may be indicated if tracheal obstruction is an issue. Endoscopic removal of nematodes from air sacs may also be performed but is rarely necessary if an appropriate ivermectin dose is administered. Endoscopic removal of nasal leeches and trematodes is considered a viable treatment option. Although praziquantel has been used to treat birds diagnosed with air sac flukes the effectiveness of this drug varies.[398] Preventive measures should also be implemented by reducing access to an intermediate host of the air sac fluke, such as limiting access to the ground and having appropriate aviary design.[539]

Treatment of respiratory cryptosporidiosis may be attempted using paronomycin or azithromycin but again the therapeutic effect of these drugs varies.[341,342,539] Air sac acariasis in finches is usually treated with oral or percutaneous ivermectin.

The treatment of atoxoplasmosis can be challenging and treatment response is usually highly variable. Drugs, specifically toltrazuril and sulfachloropyridazine, have been used to treat systemic coccidiosis in passerines.[540,541]

NONINFECTIOUS LOWER RESPIRATORY DISEASES. The macaw chronic obstructive pulmonary syndrome is typically treated with short- or long-term bronchodilators (see Principles of Respiratory Pharmacology above). The authors frequently use nebulized terbutaline or albuterol for acute presentations in combination with oxygen therapy and oral theophylline for chronic cases. Theophylline blood levels may also be monitored and correlated with response to therapy. Increasing the relative humidity of ambient air appears to be beneficial when treating macaws. Short-term low-dose corticosteroids may also help to initially decrease pulmonary inflammation (prednisone 0.1 to 0.2 mg/kg PO q12 to 24 h). It appears that advanced disease no longer responds to bronchodilators when chronic histopathological changes in the lung parenchyma are too severe.

Respiratory neoplasias are treated as for other organ systems. Extrarespiratory diseases causing respiratory lesions are treated according to the inciting cause. Coelomic fluid should be drained by abdominocentesis until the respiratory distress has improved.

Surgical Therapy

CHRONIC GRANULOMATOUS RHINITIS. It is recommended to use surgical loupes with a light source to facilitate thorough debridement of the nasal cavities and preserve the psittacine nasal operculum. In addition, the nasal structures of birds are fragile and prone to bleeding. A small dental curette or an equivalent instrument with a narrow extremity should be used to remove the concretion starting at the edges to detach from the nasal wall. The granuloma is either removed in toto or fragmented. Once the bulk of the granuloma is removed, the nasal cavity is thoroughly debrided with a mixture of curettage and flushing with physiological saline (the bird should be intubated to prevent aspiration during nasal irrigation). The nasal deficit left by the granuloma is often extensive. Granulomatous materials should be submitted for bacterial and fungal culture and topical treatment should be pursued. Since the integrity and function of the nasal structures are compromised, this procedure would unfortunately have to be repeated periodically to clean nasal debris that continues to accumulate. A rigid endoscope may be used to explore the nasal cavities after debridement.

SINUSOTOMY/TREPHINATION. The infraorbital sinus is a triangular space located primarily under the eyes, whose topography changes with the position of the upper (prokinesis) and lower beak. Approaches to the infraorbital sinus have been described in large macaws and African gray parrots.

In large macaws, a skin incision is made in the ventral jugal arch, exposing the lateral wall of the sinus (Figure 3-38). The upper beak is flexed and the lower beak extended, which increases the space in this location of the sinus. The wall of the sinus is then incised and the exposed area inspected. A rigid endoscope can also be used to explore the sinus further when the source of the infection is deep. All granulomatous material is debrided. The area is also prone to bleeding. Once debridement is complet, the sinus lateral wall and the skin are sutured. Sinus irrigation may also be performed, but due to the sinus' many connections with diverticula, this is generally not recommended. A sinus swab may also be submitted for bacterial and fungal culture. Other, more cranial sinusotomy approaches are described but are associated with an increased tendency for bleeding.[542] The cranial approaches do not appropriate for African gray parrots, in which a more caudal approach is indicated, but it still provides limited access to the sinusal space.[543]

Sinusal trephination is not commonly performed in avian patients. However in certain cases of infection or neoplasia this surgical technique allows access to the maxillary diverticulum of the infraorbital sinus, after a maxillary trephination in the upper beak, or to the preorbital diverticulum of the infraorbital sinus, after a frontal trephination. A CT scan is recommended before performing trephination procedures to ascertain the location of the lesion. Maxillary trephination is performed by drilling a hole on the side of the upper beak.

Any granulomas are debrided with a curette after which the collected material is submitted for bacterial and fungal cultures. The area is left open for local treatment and can subsequently be closed by application of a resin. For the frontal trephination, the skin is incised about 1/4 to 1/5 of the distance between the orbit and the nostril on one side. A hole is made with the drill bit oriented slightly toward the middle. This procedure is difficult given the size of the ocular structures in birds and interspecific anatomical variations and it is preferable that the approach is based on a CT scan. A drain may be placed for treatment and the skin sutured.

CHOANAL ATRESIA. This surgical approach consists of creating an artificial choanal opening. However, the infraorbital sinus area is highly vascularized and heavy bleeding may be experienced when an inappropriate technique is used. A pin is used to perforate a connection through each nostril to the choanae. The pin is then inserted perpendicularly to the frontal bone into the nostril. A fenestrated (e.g., red rubber catheter) tube is passed through one nostril to the choanae and passed through the contralateral nostril. The tube ends are then tied on the back of the head and the tube is left in place for 4 to 6 weeks until tissue heals around it, which creates a permanent choanal fistula.

CERVICOCEPHALIC DIVERTICULUM RUPTURE. The skin over the inflated area is incised and the subcutaneous tissues are marsupialized to the skin or a Teflon stent is placed. This procedure is only a temporary resolution: The stoma often closes with tissue healing or the lumen of the stent becomes clogged with exudate or granulation tissue. Another approach consists of connecting the inflated cervicocephalic diverticulum to the interclavicular air sac, deep between the clavicles to shunt air into the lower respiratory system.

Finally, a technique of "pleurodesis" or "ablation" of the diverticulum may be attempted. A wide catheter is inserted into the head-neck and directed cranially into the diverticulum. The catheter is sutured in place. A sclerosant drug such as tetradecyl sodium sulfate (2 mg/kg diluted at 5% with sterile water; DSM Guzman, pers. commun.) or doxycycline[544] is then injected into the air space. The neck is massaged to distribute the solution in the entire area. A light bandage is placed with cotton and tape to protect the catheter and maintain pressure between the walls of the diverticulum. A second injection may be performed after several days if

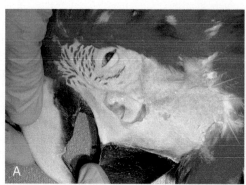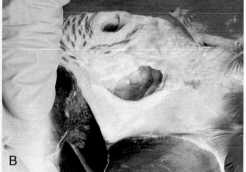

FIGURE 3-38 *A,B,* Sinusotomy in a green-winged macaw. The upper beak is flexed and the lower beak is extended, which opens the infraorbital space. (Courtesy of M. Scott Echols.)

necessary. These drugs induced local inflammation, which may cause adherences of the wall of the diverticulum or obstruct any patent connections with the infraorbital sinus.

TRACHEOTOMY. Prior to the removal of a tracheal foreign body, a tracheoscopy or transillumination of the trachea for small avian species may be required to precisely locate the foreign body and mark the area or insert a needle into the trachea to prevent distal migration. A tube is also placed in the esophagus for identification during surgery and to prevent iatrogenic damage.

The skin is incised over the trachea or for deep access to the syrinx, at the thoracic inlet, cranial to the furcula. For the thoracic inlet approach, the crop should be retracted to access the distal trachea. Tracheal muscles may also be transected. The interclavicular air sac is entered at the level of the clavicles. The syrinx cannot be retracted out of the thorax in most species, however stay sutures may be placed in the trachea to apply a mild cranial traction.

The tracheotomy is performed between the tracheal rings over 50% of its circumference. The foreign body is removed or granulomatous materials debrided using suction or fine forceps. A rigid endoscope may also be used to facilitate the procedure when the syrinx is difficult to visualize. If necessary, the surgical access can be expanded by elevating the superficial pectoral muscle and transecting the clavicle at its central junction. Once the procedure is completed, the tracheostomy is repaired with absorbable suture material using a simple interrupted pattern comprising of at least one ring on each side of the incision, taking care to tie the knots outside the lumen. The preplacement of all sutures before tying the knots is recommended. The clavicles are then apposed and the crop sutured to its original position to close the interclavicular air sac. The skin is sutured routinely.

TRACHEAL RESECTION AND ANASTOMOSIS. This surgical approach is similar to tracheotomy procedures except that it is often performed in a more cranial location, due to the usual area of tracheal stenosis. Five to 10 tracheal rings can usually be removed, and up to 12 to 15 rings have been removed in extreme cases.[357–360,362,363,545] It is essential to remove all of the tracheal tissue affected by fibroproliferation or recurrences may be inevitable. Several methods of anastomosing the tracheal ends are described. The tracheal incision can be made in the center of a ring or between the tracheal rings. Sutures are placed on either side, incorporating at least one tracheal ring proximally and distally. When a large portion of the trachea is excised (>10%), two additional sutures to counteract tension may be placed by incorporating two tracheal rings on both sides without overtightening. The nodes must be located outside of the tracheal lumen. All sutures are usually placed in advance before tying to facilitate tracheal apposition. Even when minimally reactive sutures are used (e.g., polydioxanone), granulomas and exudates around the sutures are not uncommon and it is recommended to monitor the trachea periodically by tracheoscopy during the following months/years. Voice changes may also be encountered due to neurologic and muscular trauma that adversely affect the syringeal muscles and modification of tracheal airflow.

Stenting of the trachea has been described using a custom-made nitinol stent in an eclectus parrot. The stent was deployed in the trachea by tracheoscopy and fluoroscopy.[546]

AIR SAC TUBE PLACEMENT. When tracheal obstruction is suspected, an air sac tube may be placed either in the caudal thoracic or abdominal air sac. The tube is placed between the last two ribs with the leg positioned caudally or behind the last rib with the leg positioned cranially (i.e., the conventional endoscopic approach). A small incision is made and the muscular wall is exposed. The abdominal wall is then punctured with a small hemostat while the respiratory system is distended by the anesthetist to prevent the puncture of the abdominal organs (the proventriculus is frequently distended due to aerophagia during open-mouth breathing). The hemostat is then opened and held in place to guide the insertion of a tube between the open end of the instrument in the body wall. The tube used may be a cut sterile endotracheal tube. The tubes frequently get obstructed therefore it is advisable to fenestrate its extremity. During the placement of the air sac tube, it is recommended to perform a brief endoscopic examination through the tube to both ensure correct placement in regard to the caudal ostia and perform an examination of the air sac, lung, and coelomic organs. The tube is sutured to the skin using a retention disc or tape or directly onto the tube using a Chinese finger-trap suture (Figure 3-39). A cruciate suture is placed over the musculocutaneous incision around the tube. A filtering system should be placed on the tip of the tube to avoid inhalation of dust and feather debris. Several materials may be used as a filter including the material found in surgical or facial masks.

The tube is maintained for a maximum of 5 days, and another tube placed in the contralateral air sac, if needed. When the air sac tube is removed, it is recommended to culture the previously inserted tip and perform a brief endoscopic examination of the area. Air sac tubes induce a

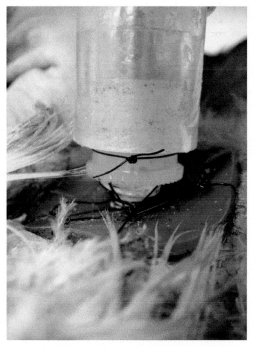

FIGURE 3-39 Air sac cannula placed in a blue and gold macaw and connected to an anesthesia machine. The approach is similar to that depicted in Figure 3-32.

significant amount of inflammatory reaction and it is not uncommon to diagnose focal aspergillosis. If such lesions are observed, topical administration of amphotericin B is recommended. The stoma should remain patent until it heals by secondary intention. Topical ointment may be used to prevent or treat local infections of the incision site.

AIR SAC SURGERY. Air sac surgery is primarily indicated for air sac granulomas induced by aspergillosis. Debridement may be performed using single- or double-entry endoscopic surgery with either biopsy/dissecting forceps or laser/radio-surgical instrumentation.[547]

Targeted endoscopic therapy may be advantageous for a variety of conditions including mass debulking, parasite removal, and local administration of medications.

A more invasive surgical approach may be performed but rarely indicated. Bilateral coeliotomy is typically required to resect or debride all granulomas using microsurgical techniques.

REFERENCES

1. Maina JN. Comparative respiratory morphology: themes and principles in the design and construction of the gas exchangers. *Anat Rec.* 2000;261(1):25-44.
2. Cooper JE. Invertebrate care. *Vet Clin.* 2004;7(2):473-486, viii. doi:10.1016/j.cvex.2004.02.004.
3. Dombrowski D, De Voe R. Emergency care of invertebrates. *Vet Clin.* 2007;10(2):621-645. doi:10.1016/j.cvex.2007.01.005.
4. Pizzi R. Disease management in ex-situ invertebrate conservation programs. In: Fowler ME, Miller RE, eds. *Zoo and Wild Animal Medicine Current Therapy.* 6th ed. St. Louis, MO: Saunders; 2008:88-94.
5. Anderson JF, Prestwich KN. Respiratory gas exchange in spiders. *Physiol Zool.* 1983;55(1):72-90.
6. Schmitz A, Perry SF. Respiratory system of arachnids I: morphology of the respiratory system of *Salticus scenicus* and *Euophrys lanigera* (Arachnida, Araneae, Salticidae). *Arthropod Struct Dev.* 2000;29(1): 3-12.
7. Scholtz G, Kamenz C. The book lungs of scorpiones and tetrapulmonata (Chelicerata, Arachnida): evidence for homology and a single terrestrialisation event of a common arachnid ancestor. *Zoology (Jena).* 2006;109(1):2-13.
8. Foelix RF. *Biology of Spiders.* 2nd ed. USA: Oxford University Press; 1996:61-67.
9. O'Brien M. Invertebrate anesthesia. In: *Anaesthesia of Exotic Pets.* Edinburgh and New York: Elsevier Ltd.; 2008:279-295. doi:10.1016/ B978-0-7020-2888-5.50020-4.
10. Lundgren JG, Jurat-Fuentes JL. Physiology and ecology of host defense against microbial invaders. In: *Insect Pathology.* 2nd ed. Elsevier Inc.; 2012:461-480. doi:10.1016/B978-0-12-384984-7 .00013-0.
11. Harrison R, Hoover K. Baculoviruses and other occluded insect viruses. In: Vega FE, Kaya HK, eds. *Insect Pathology.* 2nd ed. Elsevier Inc.; 2012:73-131. doi:10.1016/B978-0-12-384984-7.00004-X.
12. Klowden M. Respiratory systems. In: Klowden M, ed. *Physiological Systems in Insects.* 2nd ed. Burlington, MA: Academic Press; 2007:433-462.
13. Levi HW. Adaptations of respiratory systems of spiders. *Evolution (NY).* 1967;21(3):571-583.
14. Frye F. Scorpions. In: Lewbart GA, ed. *Invertebrate Medicine.* Wiley-Blackwell; 2012:223-234.
15. Shaha RK, Vogt JR, Han C-S, et al. A micro-CT approach for determination of insect respiratory volume. *Arthropod Struct Dev.* 2013;42(5):437-442. doi:10.1016/j.asd.2013.06.003.
16. Simeca JM. Cephalopods. In: *Invertebrate Medicine.* 2012:113-125.
17. Levine JF, Law M, Corsin F. Bivalves. In: Lewbart GA, ed. *Invertebrate Medicine.* Malaysia: Wiley-Blackwell; 2012:127-152.
18. Smolowitz R. Gastropods. In: Lewbart GA, ed. *Invertebrate Medicine.* USA: Wiley-Blackwell; 2012:95-111.
19. Zachariah T, Mitchell MA. Invertebrates. In: *Manual of Exotic Pet Practice.* 2008:11-38.
20. Mantel LH. Internal anatomy and physiological regulation. In: Bliss DE, ed. *The Biology of Crustacea.* London: Academic Press, Inc.; 1983.
21. Noga EJ, Hancock AL, Bullis RA. Crustaceans. In: *Invertebrate Biology.* 2012;235-254.
22. Kisia S, Onyango D. Adaptation of gas exchange systems in fish living in different environments. In: Fernandes M, Rantin F, Glass M, et al., eds. *Fish Respiration and Environment.* Enfield, NH: Science Publishers; 2007:1-12.
23. Noga E. Problems 1 through 10. In: Noga E, ed. *Fish Disease: Diagnosis and Treatment.* 2nd ed. Ames, IA: Wiley-Blackwell; 2010:83-106.
24. Olson KR. Design and physiology of arteries and veins | branchial anatomy. In: Farrell AP, ed. *Encyclopedia of Fish Physiology.* Philadelphia, PA: Elsevier; 2011:1095-1103.
25. Reid S, Sundin L, Milsom W. The cardiorespiratory system in tropical fishes: structure, function, and control. In: Val A, de Almeida-Val V, Randall D, eds. *Fish physiology: Volume 21, The Physiology of Tropical Fishes.* San Diego, CA: Academic Press; 2006:225-276.
26. Evans DH, Piermarini PM, Choe KP. The multifunctional fish gill: dominant site of gas exchange, osmoregulation, acid-base regulation, and excretion of nitrogenous waste. *Physiol Rev.* 2005;85(1):97-177. doi:10.1152/physrev.00050.2003.
27. Hughes G. General anatomy of the gills. In: Hoar W, Randall D, eds. *Fish Physiology: Volume X.* Orlando, FL: Academic Press; 1984:1-72.
28. Wilson JM, Laurent P. Fish gill morphology: inside out. *J Exp Zool.* 2002;293(3):192-213. doi:10.1002/jez.10124.
29. Strange R. Anatomy and physiology. In: Roberts H, ed. *Fundamentals of Ornamental Fish Health.* Ames, IA: Wiley-Blackwell; 2010:5-24.
30. Brauner C, Val A. Oxygen transfer. In: Val A, de Almeida-Val V, Randall D, eds. *Fish Physiology: Volume 21, The Physiology of Tropical Fishes.* San Diego, CA: Academic Press; 2006:277-306.
31. Graham J. *Air-Breathing Fishes.* San Diego, CA: Academic Press; 1997:299.
32. Duellman WE, Trueb L. Integumentary, sensory, and visceral systems. In: *Biology of Amphibians.* Baltimore, MD: JHU Press; 1994:367-414.
33. Duellman WE, Trueb L. Eggs and development. In: Duellman WE, Trueb L, eds. *Biology of Amphibians.* Baltimore, MD: JHU Press; 1994:109-139.
34. Duellman WE, Trueb L. Larvae. In: Duellman WE, Trueb L, eds. *Biology of Amphibians.* Baltimore, MD: JHU Press; 1994:141-171.
35. Mylniczenko N. Manual of exotic pet practice. In: Mitchell MA, Tully TN, eds. *Manual of Exotic Pet Practice.* St. Louis, MO: Saunders Elsevier; 2009:73-111.
36. Wright KM. Anatomy for the clinician. In: Wright KM, Whitaker BR, eds. *Amphibian Medicine and Captive Husbandry.* Malaba, FL: Krieger Publishing Company; 2001:15-30.
37. Redrobe S, Wilkinson RJ. Reptile and amphibian anatomy and imaging. In: Meredith A, Sharon R, eds. *British Small Animal Veterinary Association Manual of Exotic Pets.* Quedgeley, Gloucester: John Wiley & Sons; 2002:193-207.
38. Zug GR, Vitt LJ, Caldwell JP. Anatomy of amphibians and reptiles. In: Zug GR, Vitt LJ, Caldwell JP, eds. *Herpetology: An Introductory Biology of Amphibians and Reptiles.* Orlando, FL: Academic Press; 2001:33-76.
39. Crawshaw G. Anurans (Anura, Salienta): frogs, toads. In: Fowler M, Miller ER, eds. *Fowler's Zoo and Wild Animal Medicine, Volume 5.* St. Louis, MO: Elsevier Science; 2003.

40. Cooper JE. Urodela (Caudata, Urodela): salamanders, sirens. In: Fowler ME, Miller ER, eds. *Fowler's Zoo and Wild Animal Medicine, Volume 5.* St. Louis, MO: Elsevier Science; 2003:33-40.

41. Mylniczenko ND. Caecilians (Gymniophona, Caecilia). In: Fowler ME, Miller ER, eds. *Fowler's Zoo and Wild Animal Medicine, Volume 5.* St. Louis, MO: Elsevier Science; 2003:41-45.

42. Junge RE. Hellbender medicine. In: Miller ER, Fowler M, eds. *Fowler's Zoo and Wild Animal Medicine Current Therapy, Volume 7.* St. Louis, MO: Elsevier Saunders; 2012:260-264.

43. Lenfant C, Johansen K. Respiratory adaptations in selected amphibians. *Respir Physiol.* 1967;2(3):247-260. doi:10.1016/0034-5687(67)90030-8.

44. Tenney SM, Tenney JB. Quantitative morphology of cold-blooded lungs: amphibia and reptilia. *Respir Physiol.* 1970;9(2):197-215. doi:10.1016/0034-5687(70)90071-X.

45. Burggren WW, West NH. Changing respiratory importance of gills, lungs and skin during metamorphosis in the bullfrog *Rana catesbeiana. Respir Physiol.* 1982;47(2):151-164. doi:10.1016/0034-5687(82)90108-6.

46. Czopek J. Vascularization of respiratory surfaces in some Caudata. *Amer Soc Ichthy Herp.* 1962;3:576-587.

47. Nichols DK. Amphibian respiratory diseases. *Vet Clin North Am Exot Anim Pract.* 2000;3(2):551-554, ix.

48. Helmer P, Whiteside D. Amphibian anatomy and physiology. In: O'Malley B, ed. *Clinical Anatomy and Physiology of Exotic Pets.* London, UK: Elsevier; 2005:3-17.

49. Crawshaw G. Amphibian Viral Diseases. In: Miller RE, Fowler ME, eds. *Fowler's Zoo and Wild Animal Medicine Current Therapy, Volume 7.* St. Louis, MO: Elsevier Saunders; 2012:231-238.

50. Hilton WA. *The Pulmonary Respiratory System of Salamanders.* 2008.

51. Saint-Aubain ML de. Blood flow patterns of the respiratory systems in larval and adult amphibians: Functional morphology and phylogenetic significance. *J Zool Syst Evol Res.* 2009;23(3):229-240. doi:10.1111/j.1439-0469.1985.tb00585.x.

52. Wells KD. Respiration. In: Wells KD, ed. *The Ecology and Behavior of Amphibians.* Chicago, IL: University of Chicago Press; 2007:157-183.

53. Miller LD, Wert SE, Whitsett JA. Surfactant proteins and cell markers in the respiratory epithelium of the amphibian, *Ambystoma mexicanum. Comp Biochem Physiol A Mol Integr Physiol.* 2001;129(1):141-149.

54. Meban C. An electron microscope study of the respiratory epithelium in the lungs of the fire salamander *(Salamandra salamandra). J Anat.* 1979;128(Pt 1):215-224.

55. Meban C. The pneumonocytes in the lung of *Xenopus laevis. J Anat.* 1973;114(Pt 2):235-244.

56. Naruse H, Gomi T, Kimura A, et al. Structure of the respiratory tract of the red-bellied newt *Cynops pyrrhogaster,* with reference to serotonin-positive neuroepithelial endocrine cells. *Anat Sci Int.* 2005;80(2):97-104. doi:10.1111/j.1447-073x.2005.00103.x.

57. Ecker A, Haslam G. *The Anatomy of the Frog.* Oxford, UK: Oxford University Press; 1889:449.

58. Smith DG, Rapson L. Differences in pulmonary microvascular anatomy between *Bufo marinus* and *Xenopus laevis. Cell Tissue Res.* 1977;178(1):1-15. doi:10.1007/BF00232820.

59. Smith DG, Campbell G. The anatomy of the pulmonary vascular bed in the toad *Bufo marinus. Cell Tissue Res.* 1976;165(2):199-213. doi:10.1007/BF00226659.

60. Francis ET. *The Anatomy of the Salamander.* London, UK: Oxford University Press; 1934:381.

61. Wang T, Hedrick MS, Ihmied YM, et al. Control and interaction of the cardiovascular and respiratory systems in Anuran amphibians. *Comp Biochem Physiol Part A Mol Integr Physiol.* 1999;124(4):393-406. doi:10.1016/S1095-6433(99)00131-2.

62. Jørgensen CB. Amphibian respiration and olfaction and their relationships: from Robert Townson (1794) to the present. *Biol Rev.* 2007;75(3):297-345. doi:10.1111/j.1469-185X.2000.tb00047.x.

63. Green DE. Pathology of amphibia. In: Wright KM, Whitaker BR, eds. *Amphibian Medicine and Captive Husbandry.* Malabar, FL: Krieger Publishing Company; 2001:401-467.

64. Parsons TS. The nose and Jacobson's organ. In: Gans C, Dawson WR, eds. *Biology of the Reptilia: Volume 5, Physiology A.* London, UK: Academic Press; 1976:99-191.

65. Huchzermeyer FW. Crocodiles and alligators. In: Huchzermeyer FW, ed. *Crocodiles: Biology, Husbandry and Diseases.* Oxon, UK: CABI Publishing; 2003:1-52.

66. Nevarez JG. Crocodilians. In: Mitchell MA, Tully TN, eds. *Manual of Exotic Pet Practice.* St. Louis, MO: Saunders Elsevier; 2009:112-135.

67. Nevarez J. Lizards. In: Mitchell MA, Tully TN, eds. *Manual of Exotic Pet Practice.* St. Louis, MO: Saunders Elsevier; 2009:164-206.

68. McArthur S, Meyer J, Innis C. Anatomy and physiology. In: McArthur S, Wilkinson R, Meyer J, eds. *Medine and Surgery of Tortoises and Turtles.* Oxford, UK: Blackwell Publishing; 2004:35-72.

69. Jacobson E. Overview of reptile biology, anatomy, and histology. In: Jacobson E, ed. *Infectious Diseases and Pathology of Reptiles.* Boca Raton, FL: CRC Press; 2007:1-130.

70. Perry FS. Lungs: comparative anatomy, functional morphology and evolution. In: Gans C, Dawson WR, eds. *Biology of the Reptilia, Volume 5, Physiology A.* London, UK: Academic Press; 1976:192.

71. Bennett T. The chelonian respiratory system. *Vet Clin.* 2011; 14(2):225-239, v.

72. O'Malley B. General anatomy and physiology of reptiles. In: O'Malley B, ed. *Clinical Anatomy and Physiology of Exotic Pets.* London, UK: Elsevier Saunders; 2005:17-40.

73. Murray MJ. Cardiopulmonary anatomy and physiology. In: Mader DR, ed. *Reptile Medicine and Surgery.* 2nd ed. St. Louis, MO: Elsevier Saunders; 2006:124-134.

74. Kirchgessner M, Mitchell MA. Chelonians. In: Mitchell MA, Tully TN, eds. *Manual of Exotic Pet Practice.* St. Louis, MO: Saunders Elsevier; 2009:207-249.

75. Mans C, Drees R, Sladky KK, et al. Effects of body position and extension of the neck and extremities on lung volume measured via computed tomography in red-eared slider turtles *(Trachemys scripta elegans). J Am Vet Med Assoc.* 2013;243(8):1190-1196. doi:10.2460/javma.243.8.1190.

76. Wallach V. The lungs of snakes. In: Gans C, Dawson WR, eds. *Biology of the Reptilia, Volume 5, Physiology A.* London, UK: Academic Press; 1976:93-295.

77. Mitchell MA. Snakes. In: Mitchell MA, Tully TN, eds. *Manual of Exotic Pet Practice.* St. Louis, MO: Elsevier Saunders; 2009:136-163.

78. Pees M, Kiefer I, Thielebein J, et al. Computed tomography of the lung of healthy snakes of the species *Python regius,* boa constrictor, *Python reticulatus, Morelia viridis, Epicrates cenchria,* and *Morelia spilota. Vet Radiol Ultrasound.* 2009;50(5):487-491.

79. Pees MC, Kiefer I, Ludewig EW, et al. Computed tomography of the lungs of Indian pythons *(Python molurus). Am J Vet Res.* 2007;68(4):428-434. doi:10.2460/ajvr.68.4.428.

80. O'Malley B. Snakes. In: O'Malley B, ed. *Clinical Anatomy and Physiology of Exotic Pets.* London, UK: Elsevier Saunders; 2005:77-93.

81. Maina JN. The morphology of the lung of the black mamba *Dendroaspis polylepis* (Reptilia: Ophidia: Elapidae). A scanning and transmission electron microscopic study. *J Anat.* 1989;167:31-46.

82. Stinner JN. Functional anatomy of the lung of the snake *Pituophis melanoleucus. Am J Physiol Regul Integr Comp Physiol.* 1982;243(3): R251-R257.

83. O'Malley B. Lizards. In: O'Malley B, ed. *Clinical Anatomy and Physiology of Exotic Pets.* London, UK: Elsevier Saunders; 2008:57-75.

84. Barten S. Lizards. In: Mader D, ed. *Reptile Medicine and Surgery.* 2nd ed. St. Louis, MO: Elsevier Saunders; 2006:59-77.

85. Meban C. Functional anatomy of the lungs of the green lizard, *Lacerta viridis. J Anat.* 1978;125(Pt 2):421-431.

86. McGregor LK, Daniels CB, Nicholas TE. Lung ultrastructure and the surfactant-like system of the central netted dragon, *Ctenophorus nuchalis*. *Amer Soc Ichthy Herpetol.* 1993(2):326-333.

87. Perry S. Functional morphology of the lungs of the Nile crocodile, *Crocodylus niloticus*: non-respiratory parameters. *J Exp Biol.* 1988; 134(1):99-117.

88. Wang T, Smits AW, Burggren WW. Pulmonary function in reptiles. In: Gans C, Dawson WR, eds. *Biology of the Reptilia, Volume 5, Physiology A.* London, UK: Academic Press; 1976:297-374.

89. Solomon SE, Purton M. The respiratory epithelium of the lung in the green turtle *(Chelonia mydas* L.). *J Anat.* 1984;139(Pt 2): 353-370.

90. Wood CS, Lenfant CJM. Respiration: mechanics, control and gas exchange. In: Gans C, Dawson WR, eds. *Biology of the Reptilia, Volume 5, Physiology A.* London, UK: Academic Press; 1976: 225-274.

91. Naifeh KH, Huggins SE, Hoff HE, et al. Respiratory patterns in crocodilian reptiles. *Respir Physiol.* 1970;9(1):21-42.

92. Lutcavage ME, Lutz PL, Baier H. Respiratory mechanics of the loggerhead sea turtle, *Caretta caretta*. *Respir Physiol.* 1989;76(1): 13-24.

93. Lutz PL, Bentley TB. Respiratory physiology of diving in the sea turtle. *Amer Soc Ichthy Herpetol.* 1985;3:326-333.

94. Konig HE, Liebich HG. Respiratory system (apparatus respiratorius). In: Konig HE, Liebich HG, eds. *Veterinary Anatomy of Domestic Mammals.* 4th ed. Germany: Schattauer Stuttgart; 2009:369-390.

95. Sjaastad OV, Sand O, Hove K. The respiratory system. In: Sjaastad OV, Sand O, Hove K, eds. *Physiology of Domestic Animals.* Slovenia: Scandinavian Veterinary Press; 2010:426-464.

96. Hargaden M, Singer L. Guinea pigs: anatomy, physiology, and behavior. In: Suckow M, Stevens K, Wilson R, eds. *The Laboratory Rabbit, Guinea Pig, Hamster, and Other Rodents.* San Diego, CA: Academic Press; 2012:575-602.

97. Brewer NR, Cruise LJ. Physiology, Chapter 4. In: Manning PJ, Ringler DH, Newcomer CE, eds. *The Biology of the Laboratory Rabbit.* 2nd ed. USA: Academic Press, Inc.; 1994:63-70.

98. Lichtenberger M, Lennox AM. Critical care of the exotic companion mammal (with a focus on herbivorous species): the first twenty-four hours. *J Exot Pet Med.* 2012;21(4):284-292. doi:10.1053/ j.jepm.2012.09.004.

99. Vella D. Emergency presentations of exotic mammal herbivores. *J Exot Pet Med.* 2012;21(4):293-299. doi:10.1053/j.jepm.2012.09.005.

100. Yarto-Jaramillo E. Respiratory system anatomy, physiology, and disease: guinea pigs and chinchillas. *Vet Clin North Am Exot Anim Pr.* 2011;14(2):339-355.

101. Vennen KM, Mitchell MA. Rabbits. In: *Manual of Exotic Pet Practice.* China: Saunders Elsevier; 2009:375-405.

102. Johnson-Delaney CA, Orosz SE. Rabbit respiratory system: clinical anatomy, physiology and disease. *Vet Clin North Am Exot Anim Pract.* 2011;14(2):257-266, vi. doi:10.1016/j.cvex.2011.03.002.

103. Sohn J, Couto M. Anatomy, physiology, and behavior. In: Suckow M, Stevens K, Wilson R, eds. *The Laboratory Rabbit, Guinea Pig, Hamster, and Other Rodents.* San Diego, CA: Academic Press; 2012:195-215.

104. Hawkins MG, Graham JE. Emergency and critical care of rodents. *Vet Clin North Am Exot Anim Pract.* 2007;10(2):501-531. doi:10.1016/j .cvex.2007.03.001.

105. Kling MA. A review of respiratory system anatomy, physiology, and disease in the mouse, rat, hamster, and gerbil. *Vet Clin North Am Exot Anim Pr.* 2011;14(2):287-337.

106. Hare WCD. General respiratory system. In: Getty R, ed. *Sisson and Grossman's—The Anatomy of the Domestic Animals.* 5th ed. USA: W.B. Saunders; 1975:113-144.

107. Hargaden M, Singer L, Sohn J, et al. Anatomy, physiology, and behavior. In: Suckow M, Stevens K, Wilson R, eds. *The Laboratory Rabbit, Guinea Pig, Hamster, and Other Rodents.* Oxford, UK: Academic Press; 2012:195-215.

108. Alworth L, Harvey S. Chinchillas: anatomy, physiology, and behavior. In: Suckow M, Stevens K, Wilson R, eds. *The Laboratory Rabbit, Guinea Pig, Hamster, and Other Rodents.* San Diego, CA: Academic Press; 2012:955-966.

109. Murray K. Hamsters: anatomy, physiology, and behavior. In: Suckow M, Stevens K, Wilson R, eds. *The Laboratory Rabbit, Guinea Pig, Hamster, and Other Rodents.* San Diego, CA: Academic Press; 2013:222-223.

110. Hofstetter J, Suckow M, Hickman D. Morphophysiology. In: Suckow M, Weisbroth S, Franklin C, eds. *The Laboratory Rat.* 2nd ed. San Diego, CA: Academic Press; 2006:93-125.

111. Johnson-Delaney CA, Orosz SE. Ferret respiratory system: clinical anatomy, physiology, and disease. *Vet Clin North Am Exot Anim Pr.* 2011;14(2):357-367.

112. Vella D, Donnelly TM. Rabbits: basic anatomy, physiology and husbandry. In: Quesenberry K, Carpenter J, eds. *Ferrets, Rabbits and Rodents: Clinical Medicine and Surgery,* 2nd ed. Philadelphia, PA: Elsevier; 2012:157-173.

113. Powers LV, Brown SA. Ferrets: basic anatomy, physiology and husbandry. In: Quesenberry KA, Carpenter JW, eds. *Ferrets, Rabbits and Rodents: Clinical Medicine and Surgery.* 3rd ed. Philadelphia, PA: Saunders; 2012:1-12.

114. Goodman G. Rodents: respiratory and cardiovascular system disorders. In: *BSAVA Manual of Rodents and Ferrets.* British Small Animal Veterinary Association; 2009:142-149.

115. King A, McLelland J. Respiratory system. In: King A, McLelland J, eds. *Birds: Their Structure and Function.* Eastbourne, UK: Bailliere Tindall; 1984:110-144.

116. King A. Apparatus respiratorius. In: Baumel J, King A, Breazile J, et al., eds. *Handbook of Avian Anatomy: Nomina Anatomica Avium.* 2nd ed. Cambridge, MA: The Nuttal Ornithological Club, N 23; 1993:257-300.

117. Bang B, Wenzel B. Nasal cavity and olfactory system. In: King A, McLelland J, eds. *Form and Function in Birds, Volume 3.* London, UK: Academic Press; 1985:195-225.

118. Geist NR. Nasal respiratory turbinate function in birds. *Physiol Biochem Zool.* 2000;73(5):581-589. doi:10.1086/317750.

119. Witmer LM. The craniofacial air sac system of mesozoic birds (aves). *Zool J Linn Soc.* 1990;100(4):327-378.

120. Artmann A, Henninger W. Psittacine paranasal sinus—a new definition of compartments. *J Zoo Wildl Med.* 2001;32(4):447-458.

121. McKibben J, Harrison G. Clinical anatomy, with emphasis on the Amazon parrot. In: Harrison G, Harrison L, eds. *Clinical Avian Medicine and Surgery.* W.B. Saunders; 1986:31-66.

122. Henry RW, Antinoff N, Janick L, et al. E12 technique: an aid to study sinuses of psittacine birds. *Acta Anat (Basel).* 1997;158(1): 54-58.

123. McLelland J. Larynx and trachea. In: King A, McLelland J, eds. *Form and Function in Birds, Volume 3.* London, UK: Academic Press; 1985:69-104.

124. Beckers GJL, Nelson BS, Suthers RA. Vocal-tract filtering by lingual articulation in a parrot. *Curr Biol.* 2004;14(17):1592-1597.

125. Patterson DK, Pepperberg IM, Story BH, et al. How parrots talk: insights based on CT scans, image processing, and mathematical models. In: Hoffman EA, ed. *Medical Imaging 1997.* 1997:14-24 doi:10.1117/12.274039.

126. King A. Functional anatomy of the syrinx. In: King A, McLelland J, eds. *Form and Function in Birds, Volume 3.* London, UK: Academic Press; 1985:105-192.

127. Gaban-Lima R, Hofling E. Comparatice anatomy of the syrinx in the tribe Arini (Aves: Psittacidae). *Braz J Morph Sci.* 2006; 23(3-4):501-512.

128. McLelland J. Anatomy of the lungs and air sacs. In: King A, McLelland J, eds. *Form and Function in Birds, Volume 3.* London, UK: Academic Press; 1985:221-280.

129. Maina J. Qualitative morphology. In: Maina J, ed. *The Lung-Air Sac System of Birds.* Berlin, Heidelberg: Springer; 2005:65-124.

130. Bernhard W, Gebert A, Vieten G, et al. Pulmonary surfactant in birds: coping with surface tension in a tubular lung. *Am J Physiol Regul Integr Comp Physiol.* 2001;281(1):R327-R337.

131. Powell F. Respiration. In: Whittow G, ed. *Sturkie's Avian Physiology.* 5th ed. San Diego, CA: Academic Press; 2000:233-264.

132. Brackenbury J. Ventilation of the lung-air sac system. In: Seller T, ed. *Bird Respiration, Volume 1.* Boca Raton, FL: CRC Press; 1987:39-69.

133. Funk GD, Milsom WK, Steeves JD. Coordination of wingbeat and respiration in the Canada goose. I. Passive wing flapping. *J Appl Physiol.* 1992;73(3):1014-1024.

134. Jenkins FA, Dial KP, Goslow GE. A cineradiographic analysis of bird flight: the wishbone in starlings is a spring. *Science.* 1988; 241(4872):1495-1498.

135. Malka S, Hawkins MG, Jones JH, et al. Effect of body position on respiratory system volumes in anesthetized red-tailed hawks *(Buteo jamaicensis)* as measured via computed tomography. *Am J Vet Res.* 2009;70(9):1155-1160.

136. Fedde M. Respiratory muscles. In: Seller T, ed. *Bird respiration, Volume 1.* Boca Raton, FL: CRC Press; 1987:3-37.

137. Pettifer G, Cornick-Seahorn J, Smith J, et al. The comparative cardiopulmonary effects of spontaneous and controlled ventilation by using the Hallowell EMC anesthesia workstation in Hispaniolan Amazon parrots *(Amazona ventralis)*. *J Avian Med Surg.* 2002; 16(4):268-276.

138. Ludders JW, Rode J, Mitchell GS. Isoflurane anesthesia in sandhill cranes *(Grus canadensis)*: minimal anesthetic concentration and cardiopulmonary dose-response during spontaneous and controlled breathing. *Anesth Analg.* 1989;68(4):511-516.

139. Gleeson M, Molony V. Control of breathing. In: King AS, McLelland JM, eds. *Form and Function in Birds, Volume 4.* London, UK: Academic Press, Inc.; 1989:439-484.

140. Ludders J, Matthews N. Birds. In: Tranquilli W, Thurmon J, Grimm K, eds. *Lumb & Jones' Veterinary Anesthesia and Analgesia.* 4th ed. Ames, IA: Blackwell Publishing; 2007:841-868.

141. Cooper JE. A veterinary approach to spiders. *J Small Anim Pr.* 1987;28(3):229-239. doi:10.1111/j.1748-5827.1987.tb05990.x.

142. Zachariah T. Medicine of common captive invertebrates. In: *AAZV Conference.* Kansas City: 2011.

143. Zachariah T. Bacterial diseases. In: Mayer J, Donnelly TM, eds. *Clinical Veterinary Advisor: Birds and Exotic Pets.* Philadelphia, PA: W.B. Saunders; 2013:4-5.

144. Vega FE, Meyling NV, Luangsa-ard JJ, et al. *Fungal Entomopathogens.* 2nd ed. Elsevier Inc.; 2012:171-220 doi:10.1016/B978-0-12-384984-7.00006-3.

145. Klaphake E. Bacterial and parasitic diseases of selected invertebrates. *Vet Clin.* 2009;12(3):639-648, Table of Contents. doi:10.1016/j.cvex.2009.06.002.

146. Pizzi R. Parasites of tarantulas (Theraphosidae). *J Exot Pet Med.* 2009;18(4):283-288. doi:10.1053/j.jepm.2009.09.006.

147. Pizzi R. Oral nematode: Panagrolaimidae. In: Mayer J, Donnelly TM, eds. *Clinical Veterinary Advisor: Birds and Exotic Pets.* Philadelphia, PA: Saunders; 2013:13-14.

148. Braun ME, Heatley JJ, Chitty J. Clinical techniques of invertebrates. *Vet Clin.* 2006;9(2):205-221, v. doi:10.1016/j.cvex.2006.02.001.

149. Smith SA. Horsehoe crabs. In: Lewbart GA, ed. *Invertebrate Medicine.* USA: Wiley-Blackwell; 2012:173-185.

150. Cooper J. Insects. In: Lewbart G, ed. *Invertebrate Medicine.* 2nd ed. Philadelphia, PA: Wiley; 2012:267-283.

151. Cooper J. Oncology of invertebrates. *Vet Clin.* 2004;7(3):697-703, vii. doi:10.1016/j.cvex.2004.04.003.

152. Stamper M, Semmen K. Basic water quality evaluation for zoo veterinarians. In: Miller R, Fowler M, eds. *Fowler's Zoo and Wild Animal Medicine Current Therapy, Volume 7.* St. Louis, MO: Elsevier Saunders; 2012:177-186.

153. Roberts R, Ellis A. The pathophysiology and systemic pathology of teleosts. In: Roberts R, ed. *Fish Pathology.* 4th ed. Ames, IA: Blackwell Publishing; 2012:62-143.

154. Noga E. Problems 11 through 43. In: Noga E, ed. *Fish Disease: Diagnosis and Treatment.* 2nd ed. Ames, IA: Wiley-Blackwell; 2010: 107-178.

155. Noga E. Problems 45 through 57. In: Noga E, ed. *Fish Disease: Diagnosis and Treatment.* 2nd ed. Ames, IA: Blackwell Publishing; 2010:183-214.

156. Noga E. Problems 77 through 88. In: Noga E, ed. *Fish Disease: Diagnosis and Treatment.* 2nd ed. Ames, IA: Wiley-Blackwell; 2010: 269-304.

157. Roberts HE, Smith SA. Disorders of the respiratory system in pet and ornamental fish. *Vet Clin.* 2011;14(2):179-206.

158. Knüsel R, Brandes K, Lechleiter S, et al. Two independent cases of spontaneously occurring branchioblastomas in koi carp *(Cyprinus carpio)*. *Vet Pathol.* 2007;44(2):237-239. doi:10.1354/vp.44-2-237.

159. Wildgoose W, Bucke D. Spontaneous branchioblastoma in a koi carp *(Cyprinus carpio)*. *Vet Rec.* 1995;136(16):418-419. doi:10.1136/vr.136.16.418.

160. Watermann B, Dethlefsen V. Histology of pseudobranchial tumours in Atlantic cod *(Gadus morhua)* from the North Sea and the Baltic Sea. *Helgoländer Meeresuntersuchungen.* 1982;35(2):231-242. doi:10.1007/BF01997554.

161. Alpers CE, Cain BB, Myers M, et al. Pathologic anatomy of pseudobranch tumors in Pacific cod, *Gadus macrocephalus. J Natl Cancer Inst.* 1977;59(2):377-398. doi:10.1093/jnci/59.2.377.

162. Banerjee TK. Histopathology of respiratory organs of certain air-breathing fishes of India. *Fish Physiol Biochem.* 2007;33(4):441-454. doi:10.1007/s10695-007-9170-5.

163. Mylniczenko ND. A medical health survey of diseases in captive caecilian amphibians. *J Herp Med Surg.* 2006;16(4):120-128.

164. Mylniczenko N. Amphibians. In: Mitchell MA, Tully TN, eds. *Manual of Exotic Pet Practice.* St. Louis, MO: Saunders Elsevier; 2009:73-111.

165. Johnson AJ, Wellehan JFX. Amphibian virology. *Vet Clin.* 2005;8:53-65.

166. Berger L, Volp K, Mathews S, et al. *Chlamydia pneumoniae* in a free-ranging giant barred frog *(Mixophyes iteratus)* from Australia. *J Clin Microbiol.* 1999;37(7):2378-2380.

167. Junge RE. Hellbender medicine. In: Miller ER, Fowler M, eds. *Fowler's Zoo and Wild Animal Medicine Current Therapy, Volume 7.* St. Louis, MO: Elsevier Saunders; 2012:260-264.

168. Chai N. Mycobacteriosis in amphibians. In: Miller RE, Fowler ME, eds. *Fowler's Zoo and Wild Animal Medicine Current Therapy, Volume 7.* St. Louis, MO: Elsevier Saunders; 2012:224-230.

169. Bodetti TJ, Jacobson E, Wan C, et al. Molecular evidence to support the expansion of the hostrange of *Chlamydophila pneumoniae* to include reptiles as well as humans, horses, koalas and amphibians. *Syst Appl Microbiol.* 2002;25(1):146-152.

170. Garner MM. Master class: diseases of amphibians. In: *Proceedings of the Association of Reptilian and Amphibian Veterinarians.* 2009:16-31.

171. Seixas F, Martins Mda L, de Lurdes Pinto M, et al. A case of pulmonary cryptococcosis in a free-living toad *(Bufo bufo)*. *J Wildl Dis.* 2008;44(2):460-463.

172. Hadfield CA, Whitaker BR. Amphibian emergency medicine and care. *Semin Avian Exot Pet Med.* 2005;14(2):79-89.

173. Clayton LA, Gore SR. Amphibian emergency medicine. *Vet Clin.* 2007;10(2):587-620.

174. Densmore CL, Green DE. Diseases of amphibians. *ILAR J.* 2007;48(3):235-254.

175. Baitchman EJ. Amphibian medicine. In: *Proceeding of American Association of Zoo Veterinarians Conference.* 2008.

176. Nichols DK. Amphibian respiratory diseases. *Vet Clin.* 2000;3(2):551-554, ix.

177. Green DE, Harshbarger JC. Spontaneous neoplasia in amphibia. In: Wright KM, Whitaker BR, eds. *Amphibian Medicine and Captive Husbandry.* Malabar, FL: Krieger Publishing Company; 2001: 335-384.

178. McAllister CT, Bursey CR, Steffen MA, et al. *Sphyranura euryceae* (Monogenoidea: Polystomatoinea: Sphyranuridae) from the grotto salamander, *Eurycea spelaea* and Oklahoma salamander, *Eurycea tynerensis* (Caudata: plethodontidae), in Northeastern Oklahoma, U.S.A. *Comp Parasitol*. 2011;78(1):188-192. doi:10.1654/4477.1.
179. Hsu C, Carter DB, Williams D, et al. *Haematoloechus* sp. infection in wild-caught Northern leopard frogs *(Rana pipiens)*. *Contemp Top Lab Anim Sci*. 2004;43(6):14-16, quiz 58.
180. Taylor SK. Mycoses. In: Wright KM, Whitaker BR, eds. *Amphibian Medicine and Captive Husbandry*. Malabar, FL: Krieger Publishing Company; 2001:181-189.
181. Cooper JE. Urodela (Caudata, Urodela): salamanders, sirens. In: Fowler ME, Miller ER, eds. *Fowler's Zoo and Wild Animal Medicine, Volume 5*. St. Louis, MO: Elsevier Science; 2003:33-40.
182. Chandler JH, Marking LL. Toxicity of rotenone to selected aquatic invertebrates and frog larvae. *Progress Fish-Culturist*. 1982;44(2):78-80.
183. Gendron AD, Marcogliese DJ, Barbeau S, et al. Exposure of leopard frogs to a pesticide mixture affects life history characteristics of the lungworm *Rhabdias ranae*. *Oecologia*. 2003;135(3):469-476.
184. Schumacher J. Respiratory medicine of reptiles. *Vet Clin*. 2011;14(2):207-224, v. doi:10.1016/j.cvex.2011.03.010.
185. Harper P, Hammond D, Heuschele W. A herpesvirus-like agent associated with a pharyngeal abscess in a desert tortoise. *J Wildl Dis*. 1982;18:491-494.
186. Stöhr AC, Marschang RE. Detection of a tortoise herpesvirus type 1 in a Hermann's tortoise *(Testudo hermanni boettgeri)* in Germany. *J Herp Med Surg*. 2010;20(2-3):61-63. doi:10.5818/1529-9651-20.2.61.
187. Heckers KO, Rüschoff B, Stöhr A, et al. Detection of a new herpesvirus in European pond turtles *(Emys orbicularis)* in Germany. In: *Proceedings ICARE*. Weisbaden, Germany: 12th European AAV Conference. 2013:137.
188. Bicknese EJ, Childress AL, Wellehan JFX. A novel herpesvirus of the proposed genus *Chelonivirus* from an asymptomatic bowsprit tortoise *(Chersina angulata)*. *J Zoo Wildl Med*. 2010;41(2):353-358.
189. Marschang RE, Gleiser CB, Papp T, et al. Comparison of 11 herpesvirus isolates from tortoises using partial sequences from three conserved genes. *Vet Microbiol*. 2006;117(2-4):258-266. doi:10.1016/j.vetmic.2006.06.009.
190. Origgi FC. Testudinid herpesviruses: a review. *J Herp Med Surg*. 2012;22(1-2):42-54. doi:10.5818/1529-9651-22.1-2.42.
191. Marschang R. Clinical virology. In: Mader D, Divers S, eds. *Current Therapy in Reptile Medicine and Surgery*. 1st ed. St. Louis, MO: Elsevier Saunders; 2014:32-52.
192. Origgi F. Testudinid herpesviruses: a review. *J Herp Med Surg*. 2012;22(1-2):42-54.
193. Hervas J, Sanchez-cordon PJ, De Lara F, et al. Hepatitis associated with herpes viral infection in the tortoise *(Testudo horsfieldii)*. *J Vet Med B*. 2002;49(2):111-114. doi:10.1046/j.1439-0450.2002.00522.x.
194. Origgi FC, Romero CH, Bloom DC, et al. Experimental transmission of a herpesvirus in Greek tortoises *(Testudo graeca)*. *Vet Pathol*. 2004;41(1):50-61.
195. Jacobson ER, Gaskin JM, Roelke M, et al. Conjunctivitis, tracheitis, and pneumonia associated with herpesvirus infection in green sea turtles. *J Am Vet Med Assoc*. 1986;189(9):1020-1023.
196. Watson GL. Herpesvirus in red-headed (common) agamas *(Agama agama)*. *J Vet Diagn Invest*. 1993;5(3):444-445.
197. Jacobson ER. Jacobson ER, ed. *Infectious Diseases and Pathology of Reptiles*. Boca Raton, FL: CRC Press; 2007:716.
198. Westhouse RA, Jacobson ER, Harris RK, et al. Respiratory and pharyngo-esophageal iridovirus infection in a gopher tortoise *(Gopherus polyphemus)*. *J Wildl Dis*. 1996;32(4):682-686.
199. De Voe R, Geissler K, Elmore S, et al. Ranavirus-associated morbidity and mortality in a group of captive Eastern box turtles *(Terrapene carolina carolina)*. *J Zoo Wildl Med*. 2004;35(4):534-543.
200. Johnson AJ, Wendland L, Norton TM, et al. Development and use of an indirect enzyme-linked immunosorbent assay for detection of iridovirus exposure in gopher tortoises *(Gopherus polyphemus)* and Eastern box turtles *(Terrapene carolina carolina)*. *Vet Microbiol*. 2010;142(3-4):160-167. doi:10.1016/j.vetmic.2009.09.059.
201. Stacy BA, Pessier AP. Host response to infectious agents and identification of pathogens in tissue section. In: Jacobson ER, ed. *Infectious Diseases and Pathology of Reptiles*. Boca Raton, FL: CRC Press; 2007:257-267.
202. Hyndman TH, Shilton CM, Marschang RE. Paramyxoviruses in reptiles: a review. *Vet Microbiol*. 2013;165(3-4):200-213. doi:10.1016/j.vetmic.2013.04.002.
203. Potgieter LN, Sigler RE, Russell RG. Pneumonia in ottoman vipers *(Vipera xanthena xanthena)* associated with a parainfluenza 2-like virus. *J Wildl Dis*. 1987;23(3):355-360.
204. Bronson E, Cranfield M. Paramyxoviruses. In: Mader D, ed. *Reptile Medicine and Surgery*. 2nd ed. St. Louis, MO: Saunders Elsevier; 2006:858-861.
205. Schmidt V, Marschang RE, Abbas MD, et al. Detection of pathogens in Boidae and Pythonidae with and without respiratory disease. *Vet Rec*. 2013;172(9):236. doi:10.1136/vr.100972.
206. Hyndman TH, Shilton CM, Marschang RE. Paramyxoviruses in reptiles: a review. *Vet Microbiol*. 2013;165(3-4):200-213. doi:10.1016/j.vetmic.2013.04.002.
207. Hyndman TH, Shilton CM, Doneley RJT, et al. Sunshine virus in Australian pythons. *Vet Microbiol*. 2012;161(1-2):77-87. doi:10.1016/j.vetmic.2012.07.030.
208. Schumacher J. Inclusion body disease virus. In: Mader D, ed. *Reptile Medicine and Surgery*. 2nd ed. St. Louis, MO: Elsevier Saunders; 2006:836-840.
209. Stenglein MD, Sanders C, Kistler AL, et al. Identification, characterization, and in vitro culture of highly divergent arenaviruses from boa constrictors and annulated tree boas: candidate etiological agents for snake inclusion body disease. *MBio*. 2012;3(4):e00180-12. doi:10.1128/mBio.00180-12.
210. Bodewes R, Kik MJL, Raj VS, et al. Detection of novel divergent arenaviruses in boid snakes with inclusion body disease in The Netherlands. *J Gen Virol*. 2013;94(Pt 6):1206-1210. doi:10.1099/vir.0.051995-0.
211. Hetzel U, Sironen T, Laurinmäki P, et al. Isolation, identification, and characterization of novel arenaviruses, the etiological agents of boid inclusion body disease. *J Virol*. 2013;87(20):10918-10935. doi:10.1128/JVI.01123-13.
212. Huchzermeyer FW. Organ diseases and miscellaneous conditions. In: Huchzermeyer FW, ed. *Crocodiles: Biology, Husbandry and Diseases*. Oxon, UK: CABI Publishing; 2003:240-277.
213. Jacobson E. Viruses and viral diseases of reptiles. In: Jacobson E, ed. *Infectious Diseases and Pathology of Reptiles*. Boca Raton, FL: CRC Press; 2007:395-460.
214. Stenglein MD, Jacobson ER, Wozniak EJ, et al. Ball python nidovirus: a candidate etiologic agent for severe respiratory disease in python regius. *MBio*. 2014;5(5):e01484-14.
215. Evans RH. Chronic bacterial pneumonia in free-ranging Eastern box turtles *(Terrapene carolina carolina)*. *J Wildl Dis*. 1983;19(4):349-352.
216. Jacobson E. Bacterial diseases of reptiles. In: Jacobson E, ed. *Infectious Diseases and Pathology of Reptiles*. Boca Raton, FL: CRC Press; 2007:461-526.
217. Henton MM. *Pasteurella testudinis* associated with respiratory disease and septicaemia in leopard *(Geochelone pardalis)* and other tortoises in South Africa. *J South Afr Vet Assoc*. 2003;74(4):135-136.
218. Murray M. Pneumonia and lower respiratory tract disease. In: Mader D, ed. *Reptile Medicine and Surgery*. 2nd ed. St. Louis, MO: Elsevier; 2006:865-877.
219. Schilliger L, Trehiou E, Petit AMP, et al. Double valvular insufficiency in a Burmese python *(Python molurus bivittatus*, Linnaeus,

1758) suffering from concomitant bacterial pneumonia. *J Zoo Wildl Med.* 2010;41(4):742-744.

220. Schroff S, Schmidt V, Kiefer I, et al. Ultrasonographic diagnosis of an endocarditis valvularis in a Burmese python *(Python molurus bivittatus)* with pneumonia. *J Zoo Wildl Med.* 2010;41(4):721-724.

221. Feldman SH, Wimsatt J, Marchang RE, et al. A novel mycoplasma detected in association with upper respiratory disease syndrome in free-ranging Eastern box turtles *(Terrapene carolina carolina)* in Virginia. *J Wildl Dis.* 2006;42(2):279-289.

222. McLaughlin GS, Jacobson ER, Brown DR, et al. Pathology of upper respiratory tract disease of gopher tortoises in Florida. *J Wildl Dis.* 2000;36(2):272-283.

223. Wendland L, Brown D, Klein P, et al. Upper respiratory tract disease (mycoplasmosis) in tortoises. In: Mader D, ed. *Reptile Medicine and Surgery.* 2nd ed. St. Louis, MO: Elsevier Saunders; 2006:931-938.

224. Brown MB, McLaughlin GS, Klein PA, et al. Upper respiratory tract disease in the gopher tortoise is caused by *Mycoplasma agassizii. J Clin Microbiol.* 1999;37(7):2262-2269.

225. Brown MB, Schumacher IM, Klein PA, et al. *Mycoplasma agassizii* causes upper respiratory tract disease in the desert tortoise. *Infect Immun.* 1994;62(10):4580-4586.

226. Lecis R, Paglietti B, Rubino S, et al. Detection and characterization of *Mycoplasma* spp. and *Salmonella* spp. in free-living European tortoises *(Testudo hermanni, Testudo graeca,* and *Testudo marginata). J Wildl Dis.* 2011;47(3):717-724.

227. Dickinson VM, Schumacher IM, Jarchow JL, et al. Mycoplasmosis in free-ranging desert tortoises in Utah and Arizona. *J Wildl Dis.* 2005;41(4):839-842.

228. Brown MB, Brown DR, Klein PA, et al. *Mycoplasma agassizii* sp. nov., isolated from the upper respiratory tract of the desert tortoise *(Gopherus agassizii)* and the gopher tortoise *(Gopherus polyphemus). Int J Syst Evol Microbiol.* 2001;51(Pt 2):413-418.

229. Jacobson ER, Berry KH. *Mycoplasma testudineum* in free-ranging desert tortoises, *Gopherus agassizii. J Wildl Dis.* 2012;48(4):1063-1068. doi:10.7589/2011-09-256.

230. Berish JED, Wendland LD, Kiltie RA, et al. Effects of mycoplasmal upper respiratory tract disease on morbidity and mortality of gopher tortoises in northern and central Florida. *J Wildl Dis.* 2010;46(3):695-705.

231. Brown DR, Merritt JL, Jacobson ER, et al. *Mycoplasma testudineum* sp. nov., from a desert tortoise *(Gopherus agassizii)* with upper respiratory tract disease. *Int J Syst Evol Microbiol.* 2004;54(Pt 5):1527-1529. doi:10.1099/ijs.0.63072-0.

232. Ozgul A, Oli MK, Bolker BM, et al. Upper respiratory tract disease, force of infection, and effects on survival of gopher tortoises. *Ecol Appl.* 2009;19(3):786-798.

233. Brown MB, Berry KH, Schumacher IM, et al. Seroepidemiology of upper respiratory tract disease in the desert tortoise in the western Mojave Desert of California. *J Wildl Dis.* 1999;35(4):716-727.

234. Penner JD, Jacobson ER, Brown DR, et al. A novel *Mycoplasma* sp. associated with proliferative tracheitis and pneumonia in a Burmese python *(Python molurus bivittatus). J Comp Pathol.* 1997;117(3):283-288.

235. Brown DR, Wendland LD, Rotstein DS. Mycoplasmosis in green iguanas *(Iguana iguana). J Zoo Wildl Med.* 2007;38(2):348-351.

236. Hernandez-Divers SJ, Shearer D. Pulmonary mycobacteriosis caused by *Mycobacterium haemophilum* and *M. marinum* in a royal python. *J Am Vet Med Assoc.* 2002;220(11):1661-1663, 1650.

237. Quesenberry K, Jacobson E, Allen J, et al. Ulcerative stomatitis and subcutaneous granulomas caused by *Mycobacterium chelonei* in a boa constrictor. *J Am Vet Med Assoc.* 1986;189:1131-1132.

238. Olson G, Woodard J. Miliary tuberculosis in a reticulated python. *J Am Vet Med Assoc.* 1974;164:733-735.

239. Greer L, Strandberg J, Whitaker B. *Mycobacterium chelonae* osteoarthritis in a Kemp's Ridley sea turtle. *J Wildl Dis.* 2003;39:736-741.

240. Oros J, Acosta B, Gaskin J, et al. *Mycobacterium kansasii* infection in a Chinese soft shell turtle *(Pelodiscus sinensis). Vet Rec.* 2003;152:474-476.

241. Roh Y-S, Park H, Cho A, et al. Granulomatous pneumonia in a captive freshwater crocodile *(Crocodylus johnstoni)* caused by *Mycobacterium szulgai. J Zoo Wildl Med.* 2010;41(3):550-554.

242. Pare J, Jacobson E. Mycotic diseases of reptiles. In: Jacobson E, ed. *Infectious Diseases and Pathology of Reptiles.* Boca Raton, FL: CRC Press; 2007:527-570.

243. Pare J. Update on fungal infections in reptiles. In: Mader D, Divers S, eds. *Current Therapy in Reptile Medicine and Surgery.* St. Louis, MO: Elsevier Saunders; 2013:53-56.

244. Cabo JFG, Serrano JE, Asensio MCB. Mycotic pulmonary disease by *Beauveria bassiana* in a captive tortoise. *Mycoses.* 1995;38(3–4):167-169. doi:10.1111/j.1439-0507.1995.tb00043.x.

245. Maslen M, Whitehead J, Forsyth WM, et al. Systemic mycotic disease of captive crocodile hatchling *(Crocodylus porosus)* caused by *Paecilomyces lilacinus. J Med Vet Mycol.* 1988;26(4):219-225.

246. Heard DJ, Cantor GH, Jacobson ER, et al. Hyalohyphomycosis caused by *Paecilomyces lilacinus* in an Aldabra tortoise. *J Am Vet Med Assoc.* 1986;189(9):1143-1145.

247. Miller DL, Radi ZA, Stiver SL, et al. Cutaneous and pulmonary mycosis in green anacondas *(Euncectes murinus). J Zoo Wildl Med.* 2004;35(4):557-561.

248. Pare J, Jacobson E. Mycotic diseases of reptiles. In: Jacobson E, ed. *Infectious Diseases and Pathology of Reptiles.* Boca Raton, FL: CRC Press; 2007:527-570.

249. Autswick P, Keymer I. Fungi and actinomycetes. In: Cooper J, Jackson O, eds. *Diseases of the Reptilia, Volume I.* New York, NY: Academic Press; 1981:193-231.

250. Hatt J. Raising giant tortoises. In: Fowler M, Miller R, eds. *Zoo and Wild Animal Medicine.* 6th ed. St. Louis, MO: Saunders Elsevier; 2008:144-154.

251. Oros J, Ramirez A, Poveda J, et al. Systemic mycoses caused by *Penicillium brevicompactum* in a Seychelles giant tortoise *(Megalochelys gigantea). Vet Rec.* 1996;139:295-296.

252. Innis C, Nyaoke AC, Williams CR, et al. Pathologic and parasitologic findings of cold-stunned Kemp's Ridley sea turtles *(Lepidochelys kempii)* stranded on Cape Cod, Massachusetts, 2001-2006. *J Wildl Dis.* 2009;45(3):594-610. doi:10.7589/0090-3558-45.3.594.

253. Huchzermeyer FW. Transmissible diseases. In: Huchzermeyer FW, ed. *Crocodiles: Biology, Husbandry and Diseases.* Oxon, UK: CABI Publishing; 2003:139-148.

254. Fromtling R, Jensen J, Robinson B, et al. Fatal mycotic pulmonary disease of captive American alligators. *Vet Pathol.* 1979;16:428-431.

255. Hall N, Conley K, Berry C, et al. Computed tomography of granulomatous pneumonia with oxalosis in an American alligator *(Alligator mississippiensis)* associated with *Metarhizium anisopliae var anisopliae. J Zoo Wildl Med.* 2011;42(4):700-708.

256. Jacobson E. Parasites and parasitic diseases of reptiles. In: Jacobson E, ed. *Infectious Diseases and Pathology of Reptiles.* Boca Raton, FL: CRC Press; 2007:571-665.

257. Paré JA. An overview of pentastomiasis in reptiles and other vertebrates. *J Exot Pet Med.* 2008;17(4):285-294.

258. Flach EJ, Riley J, Mutlow AG, et al. Pentastomiasis in Bosc's monitor lizards *(Varanus exanthematicus)* caused by an undescribed *Sambonia* species. *J Zoo Wildl Med.* 2000;31(1):91-95.

259. Brock AP, Gallagher AE, Walden HDS, et al. *Kiricephalus coarctatus* in an Eastern Indigo snake *(Drymarchon couperi)*; endoscopic removal, identification, and phylogeny. *Vet Q.* 2012;32(2):107-112. doi:10.1080/01652176.2012.709952.

260. Mihalca AD, Miclaus V, Lefkaditis M. Pulmonary lesions caused by the nematode *Rhabdias fuscovenosa* in a grass snake, *Natrix natrix. J Wildl Dis.* 2010;46(2):678-681.

261. Anderson MP. Laryngeal foreign body as a cause of acute respiratory distress in lizards. *Vet Med Small Anim Clin.* 1976;71(7):940.

262. Mauldin G, Done L. Oncology. In: Mader D, ed. *Reptile Medicine and Surgery*. 2nd ed. St. Louis, MO: Elsevier; 2006:299-322.

263. Schmidt R, Reavill D. Metastatic chondrosarcoma in a corn snake *(Pantherophis guttatus). J Herp Med Surg*. 2012;22(3–4):67-69.

264. Diethelm G, Stauber E, Tillson M, et al. Tracheal resection and anastomosis for an intratracheal chondroma in a ball python. *J Am Vet Med Assoc*. 1996;209(4):786-788.

265. Drew ML, Phalen DN, Berridge BR, et al. Partial tracheal obstruction due to chondromas in ball pythons *(Python regius). J Zoo Wildl Med*. 1999;30(1):151-157.

266. Redrobe SP, Scudamore CL. Ultrasonographic diagnosis of pericardial effusion and atrial dilation in a spur-thighed tortoise *(Testudo graeca). Vet Rec*. 2000;146(7):183-185.

267. Hoey S, Keller D, Chamberlin T, et al. Pulmonary-tracheobronchial prolapse in a New Caledonian giant gecko *(Rhacodactylus leachianus). Vet Radiol Ultrasound*. 2013;54(6):630-633.

268. Lim C, Kirberger R, Lane E, et al. Computed tomography imaging of a leopard tortoise *(Geochelone pardalis pardalis)* with confirmed pulmonary fibrosis: a case report. *Acta Vet Scand*. 2013;55:35.

269. Boyer T. Hypovitaminosis A and hypervitaminosis A. In: Mader D, ed. *Reptile Medicine and Surgery*. 2nd ed. St. Louis, MO: Elsevier; 2006:831-835.

270. Mader D. Gout. In: Mader D, ed. *Reptile Medicine and Surgery*. 2nd ed. St. Louis, MO: Elsevier; 2006:793-800.

271. Goodman G. Hamsters. In: Meredith A, Redrobe S, eds. *BSAVA Manual of Exotic Pets*. Barcelona, Spain: British Small Animal Veterinary Association; 2002:26-33.

272. Keeble E. Gerbils. In: Redrobe S, Meredith A, eds. *BSAVA Manual of Exotic Pets*. Barcelona, Spain: British Small Animal Veterinary Association; 2002:34-46.

273. Pollock C. Emergency medicine of the ferret. *Vet Clin North Am Exot Anim Pract*. 2007;10(2):463-500. doi:10.1016/j.cvex.2007.02.002.

274. Johnson-Delaney CA. Other small mammals. In: Meredith A, Redrobe S, eds. *BSAVA Manual of Exotic Pets*. Barcelona, Spain: British Small Animal Veterinary Association; 2002:102-115.

275. Cooper SC, McLellan GJ, Rycroft AN. Conjunctival flora observed in 70 healthy domestic rabbits *(Oryctolagus cuniculus). Vet Rec*. 2001;149(8):232-235.

276. Deeb BJ, DiGiacomo RF, Bernard BL, et al. *Pasteurella multocida* and *Bordetella bronchiseptica* infections in rabbits. *J Clin Microbiol*. 1990;28(1):70-75.

277. Lennox AM, Kelleher S. Bacterial and parasitic diseases of rabbits. *Vet Clin North Am Exot Anim Pract*. 2009;12(3):519-530, Table of Contents. doi:10.1016/j.cvex.2009.06.004.

278. Lennox A. Respiratory disease and pasteurellosis. In: Carpenter J, Quesenberry K, eds. *Ferrets, Rabbits, and Rodents: Clinical Medicine and Surgery*. 3rd ed. Edinburgh and New York: Elsevier; 2012:205-216. doi:10.1016/B978-1-4160-6621-7.00016-6.

279. De Long D, Manning PJ. Bacterial diseases. In: Manning PJ, Ringler DH, Newcomer CE, eds. *The Biology of the Laboratory Rabbit*. 2nd ed. Academic Press; 1994.

280. Suckow M, Brammer D. Biology and diseases of rabbits. In: Fox JG, Anderson LC, Leow FM, et al., eds. *The Laboratory Rabbit, Guinea Pig, Hamster, and Other Rodents*. 2nd ed. Elsevier Inc.; 2002:329-364. doi:10.1016/B978-0-12-263951-7.50012-0.

281. Lennox AM. Emergency and critical care procedures in sugar gliders *(Petaurus breviceps)*, African hedgehogs *(Atelerix albiventris)*, and prairie dogs *(Cynomys* spp.). *Vet Clin North Am Exot Anim Pract*. 2007;10(2):533-555. doi:10.1016/j.cvex.2007.01.001.

282. Kahn CM, Line S, eds. *The Merck Vet Manual*. 9th ed. 2005.

283. Rougier S, Galland D, Boucher S, et al. Epidemiology and susceptibility of pathogenic bacteria responsible for upper respiratory tract infections in pet rabbits. *Vet Microbiol*. 2006;115(1–3):192-198.

284. Marlier D, Mainil J, Linde A, et al. Infectious agents associated with rabbit pneumonia: isolation of amyxomatous myxoma virus strains. *Vet J*. 2000;159(2):171-178.

285. Haines VL. The ancient rat. *Vet Clin North Am Exot Anim Pract*. 2010;13(1):95-105. doi:10.1016/j.cvex.2009.09.001.

286. Monks D, Cowan M. Chronic respiratory disease in rats. In: *Association of Avian Veterinarians, Autralasian Committee and Unusual and Exotic Pets Proceedings*. North Sydney, Australia. 2009.

287. Orr H. Rats and mice. In: Meredith A, Redrobe S, eds. *BSAVA Manual of Exotic Pets*. Barcelona, Spain: British Small Animal Veterinary Association; 2002:13-25.

288. Brown C, Donnelly TM. Disease problems of small rodents. In: Carpenter JW, Quesenberry KE, eds. *Ferrets, Rabbits, and Rodents: Clinical Medicine and Surgery*. 3rd ed. Elsevier; 2012:354-372. doi:10.1016/B978-1-4160-6621-7.00027-0.

289. Meredith A. Respiratory diseases in rabbits, rats and degus. In: *British Small Animal Veterinary Congress*. Birmingham: 2010.

290. Schoeb TR, Dybvig K, Keisling KF, et al. Detection of *Mycoplasma pulmonis* in cilia-associated respiratory *Bacillus* isolates and in respiratory tracts of rats by nested PCR. *J Clin Microbiol*. 1997;35(7).

291. Graham JE, Schoeb TR. *Mycoplasma pulmonis* in rats. *J Exot Pet Med*. 2011;20(4):270-276. doi:10.1053/j.jepm.2011.07.004.

292. Meredith A. Lower respiratory tract disorders. In: Mayer J, Donnelly TM, eds. *Clinical Veterinary Advisor: Birds and Exotic Pets*. 2013:390-391.

293. Kohn DF, Clifford CB. Biology and diseases of rats. In: Fox JG, Anderson LC, Leow FM, et al., eds. *The Laboratory Rabbit, Guinea Pig, Hamster, and Other Rodents*. 2nd ed. San Diego: Elsevier Inc.; 2002:121-165. doi:10.1016/B978-0-12-263951-7.50007-7.

294. Wyre NR, Donnelly TM. Guinea pig respiratory disease. In: Mayer J, Donnelley TM, eds. *Clinical Veterinary Advisor: Birds and Exotic Pets*. 2012:277-278.

295. Hawkins MG, Bishop CR. Disease problems of guinea pigs. In: Carpenter JW, Quesenberry KE, eds. *Ferrets, Rabbits, and Rodents: Clinical Medicine and Surgery*. 3rd ed. Elsevier; 2012:295-310. doi:10.1016/B978-1-4160-6621-7.00023-3.

296. Goodman G. Infectious respiratory disease in rodents. *In Pract*. 2004;26(4):200-205. doi:10.1136/inpract.26.4.200.

297. Griffith JW, White WJ, Danneman PJ, et al. Cilia-associated respiratory (CAR) *Bacillus* infection of obese mice. *Vet Pathol*. 1988;25(1):72-76. doi:10.1177/030098588802500110.

298. Barron HW, Rosenthal K. Respiratory diseases of ferrets. In: *Ferrets, Rabbits, and Rodents: Clinical Medicine and Surgery*. 3rd ed. Elsevier; 2012:78-85. doi:10.1016/B978-1-4160-6621-7.00006-3.

299. Johnson DH. Diagnosing & treating sugar gliders. In: *Western Veterinary Conference*. Las Vegas: 2004.

300. Ness RD, Johnson-Delaney CA. Sugar gliders. In: *Ferrets, Rabbits, and Rodents: Clinical Medicine and Surgery*. 3rd ed. Elsevier; 2012:393-410. doi:10.1016/B978-1-4160-6621-7.00029-4.

301. Raymond JT, Williams C, Wu CC. *Corynebacterial pneumonia* in an African hedgehog. *J Wildl Dis*. 1998;34(2):397-399.

302. Deem SL, Spelman LH, Yates RA, et al. Canine distemper in terrestrial carnivores: a review. *J Zoo Wildl Med*. 2000;31(4):441-451.

303. Graham J. Distemper. In: Mayer J, Donnelly TM, eds. *Clinical Veterinary Advisor: Birds and Exotic Pets*. 2012:444.

304. Fox JG, Pearson RC, Gorham JR. Viral diseases. In: Fox JG, ed. *Biology and Diseases of the Ferret*. 2nd ed. Baltimore, MD: Lippincott Williams and Wilkins; 1998:355-374.

305. Perpiñán D, Ramis A, Tomás A, et al. Outbreak of canine distemper in domestic ferrets *(Mustela putorius furo). Vet Rec*. 2006;163:246-250.

306. Schoemaker NJ. Ferrets. In: Meredith A, Redrobe S, eds. *BSAVA Manual of Exotic Pets*. 4th ed. Barcelona, Spain: British Small Animal Veterinary Association; 2002:93-101.

307. Wyre NR, Michels D, Chen S. Selected emerging diseases in ferrets. *Vet Clin North Am Exot Anim Pract*. 2013;16(2):469-493. doi:10.1016/j.cvex.2013.02.003.

308. Bixler H, Ellis C. Ferret care and husbandry. *Vet Clin North Am Exot Anim Pract*. 2004;7(2):227-255, v. doi:10.1016/j.cvex.2004.02.002.

309. Marini RP, Otto G, Erdman S, et al. Biology and diseases of ferrets. In: Fox JG, Anderson LC, Leow FM, et al., eds. *Laboratory Animal Medicine.* 2nd ed. San Diego, CA: Elsevier Inc.; 2002:483-517. doi:10.1016/B978-0-12-263951-7.50016-8.

310. Graham J. Influenza. In: Donnelly TM, Mayer J, eds. *Clinical Veterinary Advisor: Birds and Exotic Pets.* 2012:468.

311. Murray J, Kiupel M, Maes RK. Ferret coronavirus-associated diseases. *Vet Clin North Am Exot Anim Pract.* 2010;13(3):543-560.

312. Jin L, Valentine BA, Baker RJ, et al. An outbreak of fatal herpesvirus infection in domestic rabbits in Alaska. *Vet Pathol.* 2008;45(3):369-374.

313. Jin L, Löhr CV, Vanarsdall AL, et al. Characterization of a novel alphaherpesvirus associated with fatal infections of domestic rabbits. *Virology.* 2008;378(1):13-20.

314. Fujiwara K. Sialodacryoadenitis virus and rat coronavirus. In: Osterhaus ADME, ed. *Virus Infections of Vertebrates—Virus Infections of Rodents and Lagomorphs.* Utrect: Elsevier Science; 1994:261-264.

315. Brabb T, Newsome D, Burich A, et al. Guinea pigs: infectious diseases. In: Suckow M, Stevens K, Wilson R, eds. *The Laboratory Rabbit, Guinea Pig, Hamster, and Other Rodents.* San Diego, CA: Academic Press; 2012:637-645.

316. Khaldi M. Endoparasites (helminths and coccidians) in the hedgehogs *Atelerix algirus* and *Paraechinus aethiopicus* from Algeria. *African Zool.* 2012;47(1):48.

317. Isenbugel E, Baumgartner RA. Insectivora—diseases of the hedgehog. In: Fowler ME, ed. *Zoo and Wild Animal Medicine Current Therapy.* 3rd ed. Philadelphia, PA: W.B. Saunders; 1993:294-303.

318. Lester SJ, Kowalewich NJ, Bartlett KH, et al. Clinicopathologic features of an unusual outbreak of cryptococcosis in dogs, cats, ferrets, and a bird: 38 cases (January to July 2003). *J Am Vet Med Assoc.* 2004;225(11):1716-1722.

319. Capello V. Diagnosis and treatment of dental disease in pet rodents. *J Exot Pet Med.* 2008;17(2):114-123. doi:10.1053/j.jepm.2008.03.010.

320. Reiter AM. Pathophysiology of dental disease in the rabbit, guinea pig, and chinchilla. *J Exot Pet Med.* 2008;17(2):70-77. doi:10.1053/j.jepm.2008.03.003.

321. Pilny AA, Reavill D. Chylothorax and thymic lymphoma in a pet rabbit *(Oryctolagus cuniculus). J Exot Pet Med.* 2008;17(4):295-299. doi:10.1053/j.jepm.2008.07.006.

322. Antinoff N. Respiratory diseases of ferrets, rabbits, and rodents. In: *International Veterinary Emergency and Critical Care Symposium.* Phoenix, AZ: Veterinary Emergency and Critical Care Society; 2008.

323. Greenacre CB. Spontaneous tumors of small mammals. *Vet Clin North Am Exot Anim Pract.* 2004;7(3):627-651, vi. doi:10.1016/j.cvex.2004.04.009.

324. Flecknell P. Guinea pigs. In: Meredith A, Redrobe S, eds. *BSAVA Manual of Exotic Pets.* 4th ed. Barcelona, Spain: British Small Animal Veterinary Association; 2002:52-64.

325. Perpiñán D, Ramis A. Endogenous lipid pneumonia in a ferret *(Mustela putorius furo). J Exot Pet Med.* 2011;20(1):51-55.

326. Lennox AM. Rhinotomy and rhinostomy for surgical treatment of chronic rhinitis in two rabbits. *J Exot Pet Med.* 2013;22(4):383-392.

327. Tully T, Harrison G. Pneumonology. In: Ritchie B, Harrison G, Harrison L, eds. *Avian Medicine: Principles and Applications.* Palm Beach, FL: Wingers Publishing; 1994:559-581.

328. Schmidt R, Reavill D, Phalen D. Respiratory disease. In: Schmidt R, Reavill D, Phalen D, eds. *Pathology of Pet and Aviary Birds.* Ames, IA: Blackwell Publishing; 2003:17-40.

329. Bailey T. Raptors: respiratory problems. In: Chitty J, Lierz M, eds. *BSAVA Manual of Raptors, Pigeons and Passerine Birds.* Gloucester, UK: The British Small Animal Veterinary Association; 2008:223-234.

330. Evans EE, Wade LL, Flammer K. Administration of doxycycline in drinking water for treatment of spiral bacterial infection in cockatiels. *J Am Vet Med Assoc.* 2008;232(3):389-393. doi:10.2460/javma.232.3.389.

331. Fletcher O, Abdul-Aziz T, Barnes H. Respiratory system. In: Fletcher O, Abdul-Aziz T, eds. *Avian Histopathology.* 3rd ed. Jacksonville, FL: American Association of Avian Pathologists, Inc; 2008:128-163.

332. Luttrell P, Fischer J. Mycoplasmosis. In: Thomas N, Hunter D, Atkinson C, eds. *Infectious Diseases of Wild Birds.* Oxford, UK: Blackwell Publishing; 2007:317-331.

333. Lierz M, Hafez HM. *Mycoplasma* species in psittacine birds with respiratory disease. *Vet Rec.* 2009;164(20):629-630.

334. Lierz M, Hagen N, Lueschow D, et al. Use of polymerase chain reactions to detect *Mycoplasma gallisepticum, Mycoplasma imitans, Mycoplasma iowae, Mycoplasma meleagridis* and *Mycoplasma synoviae* in birds of prey. *Avian Pathol.* 2008;37(5):471-476. doi:10.1080/03079450802272952.

335. Lierz M, Hagen N, Hernadez-Divers SJ, et al. Occurrence of mycoplasmas in free-ranging birds of prey in Germany. *J Wildl Dis.* 2008;44(4):845-850.

336. Woerpel R, Rosskopf W. Retro-orbital *Mycobacterium tuberculosis* infection in a yellow-napped Amazon parrot *(Amazona ochrocephala auropalliata).* In: *Proc Annu Conf Assoc Avian Vet.* 1983:71-76.

337. Washko RM, Hoefer H, Kiehn TE, et al. *Mycobacterium tuberculosis* infection in a green-winged macaw *(Ara chloroptera):* report with public health implications. *J Clin Microbiol.* 1998;36(4):1101-1102.

338. Ackerman LJ, Benbrook SC, Walton BC. *Mycobacterium tuberculosis* infection in a parrot *(Amazona farinosa). Am Rev Resp Dis.* 1974;109(3):388-390.

339. Hannon DE, Bemis DA, Garner MM. *Mycobacterium marinum* infection in a blue-fronted Amazon parrot *(Amazona aestiva). J Avian Med Surg.* 2012;26(4):239-247.

340. Raidal SR, Butler R. Chronic rhinosinusitis and rhamphothecal destruction in a major mitchell's cockatoo *(Cacatua leadbeateri)* due to *Cryptococcus neoformans var gattii. J Avian Med Surg.* 2001;15(2):121-125.

341. van Zeeland YRA, Schoemaker NJ, Kik MJL, et al. Upper respiratory tract infection caused by *Cryptosporidium baileyi* in three mixed-bred falcons *(Falco rusticolus × falco cherrug). Av Dis.* 2008;52(2):357-363.

342. Molina-Lopez RA, Ramis A, Martin-Vazquez S, et al. *Cryptosporidium baileyi* infection associated with an outbreak of ocular and respiratory disease in otus owls *(Otus scops)* in a rehabilitation centre. *Avian Pathol.* 2010;39(3):171-176.

343. Bougiouklis PA, Weissenböck H, Wells A, et al. Otitis media associated with *Cryptosporidium baileyi* in a saker falcon *(Falco cherrug). J Comp Pathol.* 2013;148(4):419-423.

344. Davies R, Govedich F, Moser W. Leech parasites of birds. In: Atkinson C, Thomas N, Hunter D, eds. *Parasitic Diseases of Wild Birds.* Ames, IA: Blackwell Publishing; 2008:501-514.

345. Huffman J, Fried B. Schistosomes. In: Atkinson C, Thomas N, Hunter D, eds. *Parasitic Diseases of Wild Birds.* Ames, IA: Blackwell Publishing; 2008:246-260.

346. Huffman J. Trematodes. In: Atkinson C, Thomas N, Hunter D, eds. *Parasitic Diseases of Wild Birds.* Ames, IA: Blackwell Publishing; 2008:225-245.

347. Greenacre C, Watson E, Ritchie B. Choanal atresia in an African grey parrot *(Psittacus erithacus erithacus)* and an umbrella cockatoo *(Cacatua alba). J Assoc Avian Vet.* 1993;7(1):19-22.

348. Bennett R, Harrison G. Soft tissue surgery. In: Ritchie B, Harrison G, Harrison L, eds. *Avian Medicine: Principles and Applications.* Lake Worth, FL: Wingers Publishing; 1994:1096-1136.

349. Olsen G, Carpenter J, Langenberg J. Medicine and surgery. In: Ellis D, Gee G, Mirande C, eds. *Cranes: Their Biology, Husbandry, and Conservation.* Washington, DC: US Department of the Interior, National Biological Service, and the International Crane Foundation, Baraboo, WI; 1996:137-174.

350. Petevinos H. A method for resolving subcutaneous emphysema in a griffon vulture chick *(Gyps fulvus). J Exot Pet Med.* 2006;15(2):132-137.

351. Ferrell ST, Marlar AB, Garner M, et al. Intralesional cisplatin chemotherapy and topical cyrotherapy for the control of choanal squamous cell carcinoma in an African black footed penguin (*Spheniscus demersus*). *J Zoo Wildl Med*. 2006;37(4):539-541.

352. Diaz-Figueroa O, Tully TN, Williams J, et al. Squamous cell carcinoma of the infraorbital sinus with fungal tracheitis and ingluvitis in an adult Solomon eclectus parrot (*Eclectus roratus solomonensis*). *J Avian Med Surg*. 2006;20(2):113-119.

353. Phalen D. Implications of viruses in clinical disorders. In: Harrison G, Lightfoot T, eds. *Clinical Avian Medicine*. Palm Beach, FL: Spix Publishing; 2006:721-745.

354. Beaufrere H, Aertsens A, Fouquet J, et al. Tracheostomy in a hooded vulture (*Necrosyrtes monachus*). In: *Proc Annu Conf Assoc Avian Vet*. 2007:83-86.

355. Lennox AM, Nemetz LP. Tracheostomy in the avian patient. *Semin Avian Exot Pet Med*. 2005;14(2):131-134.

356. Jankowski G, Nevarez JG, Beaufrere H, et al. Multiple tracheal resections and anastomoses in a blue and gold macaw (*Ara ararauna*). *J Avian Med Surg*. 2010;24(4):322-329.

357. De Matos REC, Morrisey JK, Steffey M. Postintubation tracheal stenosis in a blue and gold macaw (*Ara ararauna*) resolved with tracheal resection and anastomosis. *J Avian Med Surg*. 2006;20(3):167-174. doi:10.1647/2005-012R.1.

358. Evans A, Atkins A, Citino SB. Tracheal stenosis in a blue-billed currasow (*Crax alberti*). *J Zoo Wildl Med*. 2009;40(2):373-377.

359. Clippinger T, Bennett R. Successful treatment of a traumatic tracheal stenosis in a goose by surgical resection and anastomosis. *J Avian Med Surg*. 1998;12(4):243-247.

360. Monks D, Zsivanovits P, Cooper J, et al. Successful treatment of tracheal xanthogranulomatosis in a red-tailed hawk (*Buteo jamaicensis*) by tracheal resection and anastomosis. *J Avian Med Surg*. 2006;20(4):247-252.

361. McClure SR, Taylor TS, Johnson JH, et al. Surgical repair of traumatically induced collapsing trachea in an ostrich. *J Am Vet Med Assoc*. 1995;207(4):479-480.

362. Doneley RJT, Raidal SR. Tracheal resection and anastomosis in a red-tailed black cockatoo (*Calyptorhynchus banksii banksii*). *Aust Vet J*. 2010;88(11):451-454. doi:10.1111/j.1751-0813.2010.00634.x.

363. Guzman DS-M, Mitchell M, Hedlund CS, et al. Tracheal resection and anastomosis in a mallard duck (*Anas platyrhynchos*) with traumatic segmental tracheal collapse. *J Avian Med Surg*. 2007;21(2):150-157.

364. Clayton L, Ritzman T. Endoscopic-assisted removal of a tracheal seed foreign body in a cockatiel (*Nymphicus hollandicus*). *J Av Med Surg*. 2005;19(1):14-18.

365. Dennis P, Bennett R, Newell S, et al. Diagnosis and treatment of tracheal obstruction in a cockatiel (*Nymphicus hollandicus*). *J Av Med Surg*. 1999;13(4):275-278.

366. Ford S. Tracheal foreign body removal in small birds. In: *Proc Annu Conf Assoc Avian Vet*. Providence, RI, USA: Publisher is the Association of Avian Veterinarians; 2007:49-55.

367. Kaleta A, Docherty D. Avian herpesviruses. In: Thomas N, Hunter D, Atkinson C, eds. *Infectious Diseases of Wild Birds*. Ames, IA: Blackwell Publishing; 2007:63-86.

368. Van Riper C, Forrester D. Avian pox. In: Thomas N, Hunter D, Atkinson C, eds. *Infectious Diseases of Wild Birds*. Ames, IA: Blackwell Publishing; 2007:131-176.

369. Wellehan J, Gagea M, Smith D, et al. Characterization of a herpesvirus associated with tracheitis in gouldian finches (*Erythrura [chloebia] gouldiae*). *J Clin Microbiol*. 2003;41(9):4054-4057.

370. Gabor M, Gabor LJ, Peacock L, et al. Psittacid herpesvirus 3 infection in the eclectus parrot (*Eclectus roratus*) in Australia. *Vet Pathol*. 2013;50(6):1053-1057. doi:10.1177/0300985813490753.

371. Andersen A, Vanrompay D. Avian chlamydiosis (psittacosis, ornithosis). In: Saif Y, Fadly A, Glisson J, et al., eds. *Diseases of Poultry*. 12th ed. Ames, IA: Blackwell Publishing; 2008:971-986.

372. Devriese L, Uyttebroek E, Geraert D. Tracheitis due to *Enterococcus faecalis* infection in canaries. *J Assoc Avian Vet*. 1990;2:113-116.

373. Sandmeier P, Coutteel P. Management of canaries, finches and mynahs. In: Harrison G, Lightfoot TL, eds. *Clinical Avian Medicine*. Palm Beach, FL: Spix Publishing; 2006:879-914.

374. Kiehn TE, Hoefer H, Bottger EC, et al. *Mycobacterium genavense* infections in pet animals. *J Clin Microbiol*. 1996;34(7):1840-1842.

375. Fernando M, Barta J. Tracheal worms. In: Atkinson C, Thomas N, Hunter D, eds. *Parasitic Diseases of Wild Birds*. Ames, IA: Blackwell Publishing; 2008:343-354.

376. Best J. Passerine birds: approach to the sick individual. In: Chitty J, Lierz M, eds. *BSAVA Manual of Raptors, Pigeons and Passerine Birds*. Gloucester, UK: British Small Animal Veterinary Association; 2008:356-364.

377. Lanteri G, Marino F, Reale S, et al. *Mycobacterium tuberculosis* in a red-crowned parakeet (*Cyanoramphus novaezelandiae*). *J Avian Med Surg*. 2011;25(1):40-43.

378. Peters M, Prodinger WM, Gümmer H, et al. *Mycobacterium tuberculosis* infection in a blue-fronted Amazon parrot (*Amazona aestiva*). *Vet Microbiol*. 2007;122(3–4):381-383.

379. Hoop RK. *Mycobacterium tuberculosis* infection in a canary (*Serinus canana* L.) and a blue-fronted Amazon parrot (*Amazona amazona aestiva*). *Av Dis*. 2002;46(2):502-504.

380. Andersen A, Franson J. Avian chlamydiosis. In: Thomas N, Hunter D, Atkinson C, eds. *Infectious Diseases of Wild Birds*. Ames, IA: Blackwell Publishing; 2007:303-316.

381. Andersen AA. Serotyping of US isolates of *Chlamydophila psittaci* from domestic and wild birds. *J Vet Diagn Invest*. 2005;17(5):479-482.

382. Converse K. Aspergillosis. In: Thomas N, Hunter D, Atkinson C, eds. *Infectious Diseases of Wild Birds*. Ames, IA: Blackwell Publishing; 2007:360-374.

383. Beernaert LA, Pasmans F, Van Waeyenberghe L, et al. Aspergillus infections in birds: a review. *Avian Pathol*. 2010;39(5):325-331. doi:10.1080/03079457.2010.506210.

384. Redig P. Fungal diseases—aspergillosis. In: Samour J, ed. *Avian Medicine*. 2nd ed. Philadelphia, PA: Mosby Elsevier; 2008:373-387.

385. Bauck L. Mycoses. In: Ritchie B, Harrison G, Harrison L, eds. *Avian Medicine: Principles and Applications*. Lake Worth, FL: Wingers Publishing; 1994:997-1006.

386. Dahlhausen R. Implications of mycoses in clinical disorders. In: Harrison G, Lightfoot T, eds. *Clinical Avian Medicine*. Palm Beach, FL: Spix Publishing; 2006:691-709.

387. Kamei K, Watanabe A. Aspergillus mycotoxins and their effect on the host. *Med Mycol*. 2005;43(suppl 1):S95-S99.

388. Atasever A, Gümüşsoy KS. Pathological, clinical and mycological findings in experimental aspergillosis infections of starlings. *J Vet Med A Physiol Pathol Clin Med*. 2004;51(1):19-22.

389. Femenia F, Fontaine J-J, Lair-Fulleringer S, et al. Clinical, mycological and pathological findings in turkeys experimentally infected by *Aspergillus fumigatus*. *Avian Pathol*. 2007;36(3):213-219.

390. Goetting V, Lee KA, Woods L, et al. Inflammatory marker profiles in an avian experimental model of aspergillosis. *Med Mycol*. 2013;51(7):696-703.

391. Beernaert LA, Pasmans F, Haesebrouck F, et al. Modelling *Aspergillus fumigatus* infections in racing pigeons (*Columba livia domestica*). *Av Pathol*. 2008;37(5):545-549.

392. Van Waeyenberghe L, Fischer D, Coenye T, et al. Susceptibility of adult pigeons and hybrid falcons to experimental aspergillosis. *Avian Pathol*. 2012;41(6):563-567.

393. Clubb S, Frenkel J. *Sarcocystis falcatula* of opossums: transmission by cockroaches with fatal pulmonary disease in psittacine birds. *J Parasitol*. 1992;78(1):116-124.

394. Hillyer E, Anderson M, Greiner E, et al. An outbreak of sarcocystis in a collection of psittacines. *J Zoo Wildl Med*. 1991;22(4):434-445.

395. Spalding M, Carpenter J, Novilla M. Disseminated visceral coccidiosis in cranes. In: Atkinson C, Thomas N, Hunter D, eds. *Parasitic Diseases of Wild Birds*. Ames, IA: Blackwell Publishing; 2008: 181-194.

396. Sterner M, Cole R. *Diplotriaena, Serratospiculum*, and *Serratospiculoides*. In: Atkinson C, Thomas N, Hunter D, eds. *Parasitic Diseases of Wild Birds*. Ames, IA: Blackwell Publishing; 2008:434-438.

397. Bartlett C. Filarioid nematodes. In: Atkinson C, Thomas N, Hunter D, eds. *Parasitic Diseases of Wild Birds*. Ames, IA: Blackwell Publishing; 2008:439-462.

398. Libert C, Jouet D, Ferté H, et al. Air sac fluke *Circumvitellatrema momota* in a captive blue-crowned motmot *(Momotus momota)* in France. *J Zoo Wildl Med*. 2012;43(3):689-692.

399. Murray M. Anticoagulant rodenticide exposure and toxicosis in four species of birds of prey presented to a wildlife clinic in Massachusetts, 2006-2010. *J Zoo Wildl Med*. 2011;42(1):88-97.

400. Amann O, Kik MJL, Passon-Vastenburg MHAC, et al. Chronic pulmonary interstitial fibrosis in a blue-fronted Amazon parrot *(Amazona aestiva aestiva)*. *Avian Dis*. 2007;51(1):150-153.

401. Zandvliet M, Dorrestein G, Van Der Hage M. Chronic pulmonary interstitial fibrosis in Amazon parrots. *Avian Pathol*. 2001;30(5): 517-524.

402. Taylor M, Hunter B. A chronic obstructive pulmonary disease of blue and gold macaws. *J Assoc Avian Vet*. 1991;5(2):71.

403. Dennis P, Heard D, Castleman W. Respiratory distress associated with pulmonary fat embolism in an osprey *(Pandion haliaetus)*. *J Avian Med Surg*. 2000;14(4):264-267.

404. Andre J, Delverdier M. Primary bronchial carcinoma with osseous metastasis in an African grey parrot *(Psittacus erithacus)*. *J Avian Med Surg*. 1999;13(3):180-186.

405. Baumgartner WA, Guzman DS-M, Hollibush S, et al. Bronchogenic adenocarcinoma in a hyacinth macaw *(Anodorhynchus hyacinthinus)*. *J Avian Med Surg*. 2008;22(3):218-225.

406. Jones M, Orosz S, Richman L, et al. Pulmonary carcinoma with metastases in a Moluccan cockatoo *(Cacatua moluccensis)*. *J Avian Med Surg*. 2001;15(2):107-113.

407. Fredholm DV, Carpenter JW, Shumacher LL, et al. Pulmonary adenocarcinoma with osseous metastiasis and secondary paresis in a blue and gold macaw *(Ara ararauna)*. *J Zoo Wildl Med*. 2012; 43(4):909-913.

408. Rettenmund C, Sladky KK, Rodriguez D, et al. Pulmonary carcinoma in a great horned owl *(Bubo virginianus)*. *J Zoo Wildl Med*. 2010;41(1):77-82.

409. Grunkemeyer V, Jones M, Greenacre C, et al. Humeral air sac cystadenocarcinoma in a Moluccan cockatoo *(Cacatua moluccensis)* monitored via serial 18F-fluorodeoxyglucose integrated positron emission tomography-computed tomography scans. In: *Proc Annu Conf Assoc Avian Vet*. 2010:343-344.

410. Marshall K, Daniel G, Patton C, et al. Humeral air sac mucinous adenocarcinoma in a salmon-crested cockatoo *(Cacatua moluccensis)*. *J Avian Med Surg*. 2004;18(3):167-174.

411. Azmanis P, Stenkat J, Hübel J, et al. A complicated, metastatic, humeral air sac cystadenocarcinoma in a Timneh African grey parrot *(Psittacus erithacus timneh)*. *J Avian Med Surg*. 2013;27(1):38-43.

412. Raidal SR, Shearer PL, Butler R, et al. Airsac cystadenocarcinomas in cockatoos. *Aust Vet J*. 2006;84(6):213-216.

413. Bates G, Tucker R, Mattix M. Thyroid adenocarcinoma in a bald eagle *(Haliaeetus leucocephalus)*. *J Zoo Wildl Med*. 1999;30(3): 439-442.

414. Andreasen J, Andreasen C, Latimer K, et al. Thoracoabdominal myelolipomas and carcinoma in a lovebird *(Agapornis* sp.). *J Vet Diagn Invest*. 1995;7:271-272.

415. Rahim MA, Amel OB, Hussein MF. Thyroid hyperplasia in a saker falcon *(Falco cherrug)*. *Comp Clin Path*. 2012;22(1):137-140.

416. Hanley CS, Wilson GH, Latimer KS, et al. Interclavicular hemangiosarcoma in a double yellow-headed Amazon parrot *(Amazona ochrocephala oratrix)*. *J Avian*. 2005;19(2):130-137.

417. Pye GW. Intestinal entrapment in the right pulmonary ostium after castration in a juvenile ostrich *(Struthio camelus)*. *J Avian Med Surg*. 2007;21(4):290-293.

418. Pizzi R. Viral diseases. In: Mayer J, Donnelly TM, eds. *Clinical Veterinary Advisor: Birds and Exotic Pets*. Philadelphia, PA: Saunders; 2013:16-17.

419. Pizzi R. Spiders. In: Lewbart GA, ed. *Invertebrate Medicine*. Phiadelphia, PA: Saunders Elsevier; 2012:187-223.

420. Noga E. The clinical workup. In: Noga E, ed. *Fish Disease: Diagnosis and Treatment*. 2nd ed. Ames, IA: Wiley-Blackwell; 2010:13-48.

421. Whitaker BR, Wright KM, Barnett SL. Basic husbandry and clinical assessment of the amphibian patient. *Vet Clin*. 1999;2(2):265-290, v-vi.

422. Whitaker BR, Wright KM. Clinical technique. In: Wright KM, Whitaker BR, eds. *Amphibian Medicine and Captive Husbandry*. Malabar, FL: Krieger Publishing Company; 2001:89-119.

423. McCampben S. Clinical microbiology of amphibians for the exotic practice. In: Wright KM, Whitaker BR, eds. *Amphibian Medicine and Captive Husbandry*. Malabar, FL: Krieger Publishing Company; 2001:121-128.

424. Stetter MD. Diagnostic imaging of amphibians. In: Wright KM, Whitaker BR, eds. *Amphibian Medicine and Captive Husbandry*. Malabar, FL: Krieger Publishing Company; 2001:253-264.

425. Schumacher J. Selected infectious diseases of wild reptiles and amphibians. *J Exot Pet Med*. 2006;15(1):18-24.

426. Hernandez-Divers S. Diagnostic techniques. In: Mader D, ed. *Reptile Medicine and Surgery*. 2nd ed. St. Louis, MO: Elsevier; 2006: 490-532.

427. Lafortune M, Göbel T, Jacobson E, et al. Respiratory bronchoscopy of subadult American alligators *(Alligator mississippiensis)* and tracheal wash evaluation. *J Zoo Wildl Med*. 2005;36(1):12-20.

428. McArthur S, Meyer J, Innis C. Anatomy and physiology. In: McArthur S, Wilkinson R, Meyer J, eds. *Medicine and Surgery of Tortoises and Turtles*. Oxford, UK: Blackwell Publishing; 2004:35-72.

429. Schumacher IM, Brown MB, Jacobson ER, et al. Detection of antibodies to a pathogenic mycoplasma in desert tortoises *(Gopherus agassizii)* with upper respiratory tract disease. *J Clin Microbiol*. 1993; 31(6):1454-1460.

430. Salinas M, Francino O, Sanchez A, et al. Mycoplasma and herpesvirus PCR detection in tortoises with rhinitis-stomatitis complex in Spain. *J Wildl Dis*. 2011;47(1):195-200.

431. Stockman J, Innis CJ, Solano M, et al. Prevalence, distribution, and progression of radiographic abnormalities in the lungs of cold-stunned Kemp's ridley sea turtles *(Lepidochelys kempii)*: 89 cases (2002-2005). *J Am Vet Med Assoc*. 2013;242(5):675-681. doi:10.2460/javma.242.5.675.

432. Pees MC, Kiefer I, Ludewig EW, et al. Computed tomography of the lungs of Indian pythons *(Python molurus)*. *Am J Vet Res*. 2007;68(4):428-434. doi:10.2460/ajvr.68.4.428.

433. Valente ALS, Cuenca R, Zamora M, et al. Computed tomography of the vertebral column and coelomic structures in the normal loggerhead sea turtle *(Caretta caretta)*. *Vet J*. 2007;174(2):362-370. doi:10.1016/j.tvjl.2006.08.018.

434. Divers S. Diagnostic endoscopy. In: Mader D, Divers S, eds. *Current Therapy in Reptile Medicine and Surgery*. St. Louis, MO: Elsevier; 2013:154-175.

435. Taylor W. Endoscopy. In: Mader D, ed. *Reptile Medicine and Surgery*. 2nd ed. St. Louis, MO: Elsevier; 2006:549-563.

436. Stahl SJ, Hernandez-divers SJ, Cooper TL, et al. Evaluation of transcutaneous pulmonoscopy for examination and biopsy of the lungs of ball pythons and determination of preferred biopsy specimen handling and fixation procedures. *J Am Vet Med Assoc*. 2008;233(3):440-445.

437. Evans EE, Souza MJ. Advanced diagnostic approaches and current management of internal disorders of select species (rodents, sugar gliders, hedgehogs). *Vet Clin North Am Exot Anim Pract*. 2010;13(3):453-469. doi:10.1016/j.cvex.2010.05.003.

438. Meredith A, Crossley DA. Rabbits. In: Meredith A, Redrobe S, eds. *BSAVA Manual of Exotic Pets*. Barcelona, Spain: British Small Animal Veterinary Association; 2002:76-92.

439. Booth R. Sugar gliders. *Semin Avian Exot Pet Med*. 2003;12(4):228-231. doi:10.1053/S1055-937X(03)00039-2.

440. Washington I, Van Hoosier G. Clinical biochemistry and hematology. In: Suckow M, Stevens K, Wilson R, eds. *The Laboratory Rabbit, Guinea Pig, Hamster, and Other Rodents*. San Diego, CA: Academic Press; 2012:57-116.

441. Morrisey J, McEntee M. Therapeutic options for thymoma in the rabbit. *Semin Avian Exot Pet Med*. 2005;14(3):175-181. doi:10.1053/j.saep.2005.06.003.

442. Jaglic Z, Jeklova E, Leva L, et al. Experimental study of pathogenicity of *Pasteurella multocida* serogroup F in rabbits. *Vet Microbiol*. 2008;126(1–3):168-177. doi:10.1016/j.vetmic.2007.06.008.

443. Tamura Y. Current approach to rodents as patients. *J Exot Pet Med*. 2010;19(1):36-55. doi:10.1053/j.jepm.2010.01.014.

444. Melillo A. Rabbit clinical pathology. *J Exot Pet Med*. 2007;16(3):135-145. doi:10.1053/j.jepm.2007.06.002.

445. Kawamoto E, Sawada T, Maruyama T. Evaluation of transport media for *Pasteurella multocida* isolates from rabbit nasal specimens. These include: evaluation of transport media for *Pasteurella multocida* isolates from rabbit nasal specimens. *J Clin Microbiol*. 1997; 35(8)1948-1951.

446. Donnelly TM. Disease problems of small rodents. In: *Ferrets, Rabbits and Rodents: Clinical Medicine and Surgery. 2nd ed*. Saunders; 2004:299-315.

447. Künzel F, Hittmair KM, Hassan J, et al. Thymomas in rabbits: clinical evaluation, diagnosis, and treatment. *J Am Anim Hosp Assoc*. 2012;48(2):97-104. doi:10.5326/JAAHA-MS-5683.

448. Capello V, Lennox AM. Diagnostic imaging of the respiratory system in exotic companion mammals. *Vet Clin North Am Exot Anim Pr*. 2011;14(2):369-389.

449. Divers S. Exotic mammal diagnostic and surgical endoscopy. In: Quesenberry K, Carpenter J, eds. *Ferrets, Rabbits and Rodents: Clinical Medicine and Surgery. 3rd ed*. St. Louis, MO: Elsevier Saunders; 2012:485-501.

450. Johnson LR, Drazenovich TL, Hawkins MG. Endoscopic evaluation of bronchial morphology in rabbits. *Am J Vet Res*. 2007;68(9): 1022-1027.

451. Baumel J, Wilson J, Bergren D. The ventilatory movements of the avian pelvis and tail: function of the muscles of the tail region of the pigeon *(Columba livia)*. *J Exp Biol*. 1990;151(1):263-277.

452. Zandvliet MM, Dorrestein GM, Van Der Hage M. Chronic pulmonary interstitial fibrosis in amazon parrots. *Avian Pathol*. 2001;30(5):517-524.

453. Cray C, Watson T, Rodriguez M, et al. Application of galactomannan analysis and protein electrophoresis in the diagnosis of aspergillosis in avian species. *J Zoo Wildl Dis*. 2009;40(1):64-70.

454. Foldenauer U, Simova-Curd S, Nitzl D, et al. Analysis of exhaled breath condensate in a mixed population of psittacine birds. *J Avian Med Surg*. 2010;24(3):185-191.

455. Hatt J-M, Zollinger E, Boehler A, et al. Collection and analysis of breath and breath condensate exhaled by feral pigeons *(Columba livia)* and chickens *(Gallus domesticus)*. *Vet Rec*. 2009;165(16):469-473.

456. Schmidt P, Gobel P, Trautvetter E. Evaluation of pulse oximetry as a monitoring method in avian anesthesia. *J Avian Med Surg*. 1998;12(2):91-99.

457. Desmarchelier M, Rondenay Y, Fitzgerald G, et al. Monitoring of the ventilatory status of anesthetized birds of prey by using end-tidal carbon dioxide measured with a microstream capnometer. *J Zoo Wildl Dis*. 2007;38(1):1-6.

458. Edling TM, Degernes LA, Flammer K, et al. Capnographic monitoring of anesthetized African grey parrots receiving intermittent positive pressure ventilation. *J Am Vet Med Assoc*. 2001;219(12): 1714-1718.

459. Krautwald-Junghanns M. Respiratory tract. In: Krautwald-Junghanns M, Pees M, Reese S, et al., eds. *Diagnostic Imaging of Exotic Pets*. Hannover, Germany: Schlutersche Verlagsgesellschaft mbH & Co; 2011:92-103.

460. Divers SJ. Avian diagnostic endoscopy. *Vet Clin*. 2010;13(2):1 87-202.

461. Taylor W. Endoscopic examination and biopsy techniques. In: Ritchie B, Harrison G, Harrison L, eds. *Avian Medicine: Principles and Applications*. Lake Worth, FL: Wingers Publishing; 1994: 327-354.

462. Krautwald-Junghanns ME, Valerius KP, Duncker HR, et al. CT-assisted versus silicone rubber cast morphometry of the lower respiratory tract in healthy Amazons (genus *Amazona*) and grey parrots (genus *Psittacus*). *Res Vet Sci*. 1998;65(1):1722.

463. Krautwald-Junghanns M, Kostka V, Dorsch B. Comparative studies on the diagnostic value of conventional radiography and computed tomography in evaluating the heads of psittacine and raptorial birds. *J Avian Med Surg*. 1998;12(3):149-157.

464. Krautwald-Junghanns M-E, Schumacher F, Tellhelm B. Evaluation of the lower respiratory tract in psittacines using radiology and computed tomography. *Vet Radiol Ultrasound*. 1993;34(6):382-390.

465. Pye G, Bennett R, Newell S, et al. Magnetic resonance imaging in psittacine birds with chronic sinusitis. *J Avian Med Surg*. 2000; 14(4):243-256.

466. Manning AM. Oxygen therapy and toxicity. *Vet Clin*. 2002;32(5):1005-1020, v.

467. Hopper K. Oxygen therapy. In: Ettinger S, Feldman E, eds. *Textbook of Veterinary Internal Medicine*. 7th ed. St. Louis, MO: Saunders Elsevier; 2010:516-519.

468. Murray M. Cardiopulmonary anatomy and physiology. In: Mader D, ed. *Reptile Medicine and Surgery*. 2nd ed. St. Louis, MO: Elsevier; 2006:124-144.

469. Stauber E. Effects of increased concentration of inspired oxygen. *Proc Eur Assoc Avian Vet*. 1991;105-114.

470. Jaensch S, Cullen L, Raidal SR. Normobaric hyperoxic stress in budgerigars: enzymic antioxidants and lipid peroxidation. *Comp Biochem Physiol Part C Toxicol Pharmacol*. 2001;128(2):173-180. doi:10.1016/S1532-0456(00)00186-1.

471. Lum H, Mitzner W. A species comparison of alveolar size and surface forces. *J Appl Physiol*. 1987;62(5):1865-1871.

472. Tenney SM, Tenney JB. Quantitative morphology of cold-blooded lungs: amphibia and reptilia. *Respir Physiol*. 1970;9(2):197-215. doi:10.1016/0034-5687(70)90071-X.

473. Schmitz A, Perry SF. Respiratory organs in wolf spiders: morphometric analysis of lungs and tracheae in *Pardosa lugubris* (L.) (Arachnida, Araneae, Lycosidae). *Arthropod Struct Dev*. 2002;31(3): 217-230.

474. Riedesel D. Respiratory pharmacology. In: Hsu W, ed. *Handbook of Veterinary Pharmacology*. Ames, IA: Wiley-Blackwell; 2008:221-233.

475. Quesenberry K, Hillyer E. Supportive care and emergency therapy. In: Ritchie B, Harrison G, Harrison L, eds. *Avian Medicine: Principles and Applications*. Lake Worth, FL: Wingers Publishing; 1994:382-416.

476. Watts AB, McConville JT, Williams RO. Current therapies and technological advances in aqueous aerosol drug delivery. *Drug Dev Ind Pharm*. 2008;34(9):913-922. doi:10.1080/03639040802144211.

477. Taylor RH, Lerman J, Chambers C, et al. Dosing efficiency and particle-size characteristics of pressurized metered-dose inhaler aerosols in narrow catheters. *Chest*. 1993;103(3):920-924.

478. Emery LC, Cox SK, Souza MJ. Pharmacokinetics of nebulized terbinafine in Hispaniolan Amazon parrots *(Amazona ventralis)*. *J Avian Med Surg*. 2012;26(3):161-166.

479. Beernaert LA, Baert K, Marin P, et al. Designing voriconazole treatment for racing pigeons: balancing between hepatic enzyme

auto induction and toxicity. *Med Mycol.* 2009;47(3):276-285. doi:10.1080/13693780802262115.

480. Dyer D, Van Alstine W. Antibiotic aerosolization: tissue and plasma oxytetracycline concentrations in parakeets. *Avian Dis.* 1987;31: 677-679.

481. Junge R, Naeger L, LeBeau M, et al. Pharmacokinetics of intramuscular and nebulized ceftriaxone in chickens. *J Zoo Wildl Med.* 1994;25(2):224-228.

482. Van Alstine WG, Dyer DC. Antibiotic aerosolization: tissue and plasma oxytetracycline concentrations in turkey poults. *Avian Dis.* 1985;29(2):430-436.

483. Hawkins M, Barron H, Speer B, et al. Nebulization agents used in birds. In: Carpenter J, Marion C, eds. *Avian and Exotic Formulary.* 4th ed. St. Louis, MO: Elsevier Saunders; 2013:290-292.

484. Hoppes S. Rat medicine. *Proc Annu Conf Assoc Avian Vet, San Diego, CA.* 2010;265-275.

485. Barrett K. Bronchodilators. In: Ettinger S, Feldman E, eds. *Textbook of Veterinary Internal Medicine.* 7th ed. St. Louis, MO: Saunders Elsevier; 2010:1214-1215.

486. Stamper M, Semmen K. Advanced water quality evaluation for zoo veterinarians. In: Miller RE, Fowler DR, eds. *Fowler's Zoo and Wild Animal Medicine Current Therapy, Volume 7.* St. Louis, MO: Elsevier Saunders; 2012:195-201.

487. Noga E. General concepts in therapy. In: Noga E, ed. *Fish Disease: Diagnosis and Treatment.* 2nd ed. Ames, IA: Wiley-Blackwell; 2010: 347-373.

488. Harms C. Fish. In: Fowler M, Miller R, eds. *Zoo and Wild Animal Medicine.* 5th ed. Philadelphia, PA: Saunders; 2003:2-20.

489. Noga E. Pharmacopoeia. In: Noga E, ed. *Fish Disease: Diagnosis and Treatment.* 2nd ed. Ames, IA: Wiley-Blackwell; 2010:375-420.

490. Allender MC, Kastura M, George R, et al. Bioencapsulation of fenbendazole in adult artemia. *J Exot Pet Med.* 2012;21(3):207-212. doi:10.1053/j.jepm.2012.06.018.

491. Chair M, Nellis H, Leger P, et al. Accumulation of trimethoprim, sulfamethoxazole, and N-acetylsulfamethoxazole in fish and shrimp fed medicated *Artemia franciscana. Antimicrob Agents Chemother.* 1996;40(7):1649-1652.

492. Wright KM, Whitaker BR. Pharmacotherapeutics. In: Wright KM, Whitaker BR, eds. *Amphibian Medicine and Captive Husbandry.* Malabar, FL: Krieger Publishing Company; 2001:309-319.

493. Prezant R, Isaza R, Jacobson E. Plasma concentrations and disposition kinetics of enrofloxacin in gopher tortoises (*Gopherus polyphemus*). *J Zoo Wildl Med.* 1994;25(1):82-87.

494. Raphael B, Papich M, Cook R. Pharmacokinetics of enrofloxacin after a single intramuscular injection in Indian star tortoises (*Geochelone elegans*). *J Zoo Wildl Med.* 1994;25(1):88-94.

495. Wimsatt J, Tothill A, Offermann CF, et al. Long-term and per rectum disposition of clarithromycin in the desert tortoise (*Gopherus agassizii*). *J Am Assoc Lab Anim Sci.* 2008;47(4):41-45.

496. Wimsatt JH, Johnson J, Mangone BA, et al. Clarithromycin pharmacokinetics in the desert tortoise (*Gopherus agassizii*). *J Zoo Wildl Med.* 1999;30(1):36-43.

497. Allender MC, Mitchell MA, Yarborough J, et al. Pharmacokinetics of a single oral dose of acyclovir and valacyclovir in North American box turtles (*Terrapene* sp.). *J Vet Pharmacol Ther.* 2012;36:205-208. doi:10.1111/j.1365-2885.2012.01418.x.

498. Mayr A, Franke J, Ahne W. Adaptation of reptilian paramyxovirus to mammalian cells (vero cells). *J Vet Med Ser B.* 2000;47(2):95-98. doi:10.1046/j.1439-0450.2000.00374.x.

499. Jacobson E, Gaskin J, Flanagan J, et al. Antibody responses of Western diamondback rattlesnakes (*Crotalus atrox*) to inactivated ophidian paramyxovirus vaccines. *J Zoo Wildl Med.* 1991;22(2): 184-190.

500. Carpenter J, Klaphake E, Gibbons P. Reptile formulary and laboratory normals. In: Mader D, Divers S, eds. *Current Therapy in Reptile Medicine and Surgery.* St. Louis, MO: Elsevier; 2013:382-410.

501. Myers DA, Wellehan JFX, Isaza R. Saccular lung cannulation in a ball python (*Python regius*) to treat a tracheal obstruction. *J Zoo Wildl Med.* 2009;40(1):214-216.

502. Mader D, Bennett R, Funk R, et al. Surgery. In: Mader D, ed. *Reptile Medicine and Surgery.* 2nd ed. St. Louis, MO: Elsevier; 2006: 581-630.

503. Klaphake E. Common rodent procedures. *Vet Clin North Am Exot Anim Pract.* 2006;9(2):389-413, vii-viii. doi:10.1016/j.cvex.2006 .01.001.

504. Wyre NR. Respiratory tract disease, chronic. In: Mayer J, Donnelly TM, eds. *Clinical Veterinary Advisor: Birds and Exotic Pets.* Elsevier; 2013:249-250.

505. Andres KM, Kent M, Siedlecki CT, et al. The use of megavoltage radiation therapy in the treatment of thymomas in rabbits: 19 cases. *Vet Comp Oncol.* 2012;10(2):82-94.

506. Huston S, Ming-Show Lee P, Quesenberry K, et al. Cardiovascular disease, lymphoproliferative disorders, and thymomas. In: Quesenberry K, Carpenter J, eds. *Ferrets, Rabbits and Rodents: Clinical Medicine and Surgery.* 3rd ed. St. Louis, MO: Elsevier Saunders; 2012: 257-268.

507. Briscoe JA, Syring R. Techniques for emergency airway and vascular access in special species. *Semin Avian Exot Pet Med.* 2004;13(3):118-131. doi:10.1053/j.saep.2004.03.007.

508. Harcourt-Brown F. Complications and outcome of thymic mass removal in rabbits. *Int Conf Avian, Herpetol Exot Mammal Med Wiesbad.* 2013;183-185.

509. Bennett R. Soft tissue surgery. In: Quesenberry K, Carpenter J, eds. *Ferrets, Rabbits and Rodents: Clinical Medicine and Surgery.* 3rd ed. St. Louis, MO: Elsevier Saunders; 2012:326-338.

510. Kirchgessner M. Sinusitis, chronic. In: Mayer J, Donnelly T, eds. *Clinical Veterinary Advisor: Birds and Exotic Pets.* St. Louis, MO: Elsevier; 2013:230-231.

511. Flammer K, Papich M. Assessment of plasma concentrations and effects of injectable doxycycline in three *Psittacine* species. *J Avian Med Surg.* 2005;19(3):216-224.

512. Lienart F, Morissens M, Jacobs P, et al. Doxycycline and hepatotoxicity. *Acta Clin Belg.* 1992;47(3):205-208.

513. Bahrami F, Morris DL, Pourgholami MH. Tetracyclines: drugs with huge therapeutic potential. *Mini Rev Med Chem.* 2012; 12(1):44-52.

514. Jencek JE, Beaufrère H, Tully TN, et al. An outbreak of *Chlamydophila psittaci* in an outdoor colony of Magellanic penguins (*Spheniscus magellanicus*). *J Avian Med Surg.* 2012;26(4):225-231.

515. Guzman DS-M, Diaz-Figueroa O, Tully T, et al. Evaluating 21-day doxycycline and azithromycin treatments for experimental *Chlamydophila psittaci* infection in cockatiels (*Nymphicus hollandicus*). *J Avian Med Surg.* 2010;24(1):35-45.

516. Smith KA, Campbell CT, Murphy J, et al. Compendium of measures to control *Chlamydophila psittaci* infection among humans (psittacosis) and pet birds (avian chlamydiosis). 2010 National Association of State Public Health Veterinarians (NASPHV). *J Exot Pet Med.* 2011;20(1):32-45. doi:10.1053/j.jepm.2010.11.007.

517. Flammer K, Trogdon MM, Papich M. Assessment of plasma concentrations of doxycycline in budgerigars fed medicated seed or water. *J Am Vet Med Assoc.* 2003;223(7):993-998.

518. Flammer K, Massey JG, Meek CJ, et al. Assessment of plasma concentrations and potential adverse effects of doxycycline in cockatiels (*Nymphicus hollandicus*) fed a medicated pelleted diet. *J Avian Med Surg.* 2013;27(3):187-193.

519. Prus SE, Clubb SL, Flammer K. Doxycycline plasma concentrations in macaws fed a medicate corn diet. *Avian Dis.* 1992;36(2): 480-483.

520. Powers L, Flammer K, Papich M. Preliminary investigation of doxycycline plasma concentration in cockatiels (*Nymphicus hollandicus*) after administration by injection or in water or feed. *J Avian Med Surg.* 2000;14(1):23-30.

521. Flammer K, Whitt-Smith D, Papich M. Plasma concentration of doxycycline in selected psittacine birds when administered in water for potential treatment of *Chlamydophila psittaci* infection. *J Avian Med Surg.* 2001;15(4):176-282.

522. Di Somma A, Bailey T, Silvanose C, et al. The use of voriconazole for the treatment of aspergillosis in falcons (*Falco* species). *J Avian Med Surg.* 2007;21(4):307-316.

523. Odds FC, Brown AJP, Gow NAR. Antifungal agents: mechanisms of action. *Trends Microbiol.* 2003;11(6):272-279. doi:10.1016/S0966-842X(03)00117-3.

524. Flammer K, Orosz S. Avian mycoses: managing these difficult diseases. *Proc Annu Conf Assoc Avian Vet, Savannah.* 2008;153-163.

525. Beernaert LA, Pasmans F, Baert K, et al. Designing a treatment protocol with voriconazole to eliminate *Aspergillus fumigatus* from experimentally inoculated pigeons. *V Microbiol.* 2009;139(3–4):393-397. doi:10.1016/j.vetmic.2009.06.007.

526. Flammer K, Nettifee Osborne JA, Webb DJ, et al. Pharmacokinetics of voriconazole after oral administration of single and multiple doses in African grey parrots (*Psittacus erithacus timneh*). *Am J Vet Res.* 2008;69(1):114-121. doi:10.2460/ajvr.69.1.114.

527. Burhenne J, Haefeli WE, Hess M, et al. Pharmacokinetics, tissue concentrations, and safety of the antifungal agent voriconazole in chickens. *J Avian Med Surg.* 2008;22(3):199-207.

528. Tell LA, Clemons K V, Kline Y, et al. Efficacy of voriconazole in Japanese quail (*Coturnix japonica*) experimentally infected with *Aspergillus fumigatus. Med Mycol.* 2010;48(2):234-244. doi:10.1080/13693780903008821.

529. Kline Y, Clemons KV, Woods L, et al. Pharmacokinetics of voriconazole in adult mallard ducks (*Anas platyrhynchos*). *Med Mycol.* 2011;49(5):500-512. doi:10.3109/13693786.2010.542553.

530. Ratzlaff K, Papich MG, Flammer K. Plasma concentrations of fluconazole after a single oral dose and administration in drinking water in cockatiels (*Nymphicus hollandicus*). *J Avian Med Surg.* 2011;25(1):23-31.

531. Schmidt V, Demiraj F, Di Somma A, et al. Plasma concentrations of voriconazole in falcons. *Vet Rec.* 2007;161(8):265-268.

532. Bechert U, Christensen JM, Poppenga R, et al. Pharmacokinetics of terbinafine after single oral dose administration in red-tailed hawks (*Buteo jamaicensis*). *J Avian Med Surg.* 2010;24(2):122-130.

533. Bechert U, Christensen JM, Poppenga R, et al. Pharmacokinetics of orally administered terbinafine in African penguins (*Spheniscus demersus*) for potential treatment of aspergillosis. *J Zoo Wildl Med.* 2010;41(2):263-274.

534. Evans EE, Emery LC, Cox SK, et al. Pharmacokinetics of terbinafine after oral administration of a single dose to Hispaniolan Amazon parrots (*Amazona ventralis*). *Am J Vet Res.* 2013;74(6):835-838. doi:10.2460/ajvr.74.6.835.

535. Silvanose CD, Bailey TA, Di Somma A. Susceptibility of fungi isolated from the respiratory tract of falcons to amphotericin B, itraconazole and voriconazole. *Vet Rec.* 2006;159(9):282-284.

536. Beernaert LA, Pasmans F, Van Waeyenberghe L, et al. Avian *Aspergillus fumigatus* strains resistant to both itraconazole and voriconazole. *Antimicrob Agents Chemother.* 2009;53(5):2199-2201. doi:10.1128/AAC.01492-08.

537. Meletiadis J, Stergiopoulou T, O'Shaughnessy EM, et al. Concentration-dependent synergy and antagonism within a triple antifungal drug combination against *Aspergillus* species: analysis by a new response surface model. *Antimicrob Agents Chemother.* 2007;51(6):2053-2064. doi:10.1128/AAC.00873-06.

538. Ryder NS, Leitner I. Synergistic interaction of terbinafine with triazoles or amphotericin B against *Aspergillus* species. *Med Mycol.* 2001;39(1):91-95.

539. Forbes N. Raptors: parasitic disease. In: Chitty J, Lierz M, eds. *BSAVA manual of raptors, pigeons and passerine birds.* Gloucester, UK: British Small Animal Veterinary Association; 2008:202-211.

540. Jamriška J, Lavilla LA, Thomasson A, et al. Treatment of atoxoplasmosis in the blue-crowned laughing thrush (*Dryonastes courtoisi*). *Avian Pathol.* 2013;42(6):569-571.

541. Davies R. Passerine birds: going light. In: Chitty J, Lierz M, eds. *BSAVA Manual of Raptors, Pigeons and Passerine Birds.* Gloucester, UK: British Small Animal Veterinary Association; 2008:365-369.

542. Speer B, Echols M. Surgical procedures of the psittacine skull. *Proc Annu Conf Assoc Avian Vet*, Jacksonville. 2013:99-109.

543. Speer B, Echols M, Nielson M. Prokinetic and head anatomy of the grey parrot (*Psittacus erithacus*). *Proc Annu Conf Assoc Avian Vet*, Jacksonville. 2013;261.

544. Antinoff N. Attempted pleurodesis for an air sac rupture in an Amazon parrot. *Proc Annu Conf Assoc Avian Vet.* 2008;437-438.

545. Jankowski G, Nevarez JG, Beaufrere H, et al. Multiple tracheal resections and anastomoses in a blue and gold macaw (*Ara ararauna*). *J Avian Med Surg.* 2010;24(4):322-329.

546. Divers S, Meijia-Fava J. Successful management of extensive tracheal strictures using a custom-made nitinol wire stent in an Eclectus parrot (*Eclectus roratus*). *Proc Eur Assoc Avian Vet.* 2013;285.

547. Hernandez-Divers S. Endosurgical debridement and diode laser ablation of lung and air sac granulomas in psittacine birds. *J Avian Med Surg.* 2002;16(2):138-145.

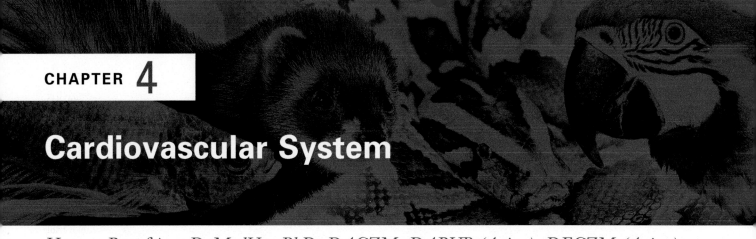

CHAPTER 4

Cardiovascular System

Hugues Beaufrère, DrMedVet, PhD, DACZM, DABVP (Avian), DECZM (Avian)
• Lionel Schilliger, DECZM (Herpetology), DABVP (Reptile and Amphibian) •
Romain Pariaut, DrMedVet, DACVIM (Cardiology), DECVIM-CA (Cardiology)

INTRODUCTION

The primary function of the cardiovascular system is to transport gases, nutrients, waste products, hormones, heat, cells, and molecule transmitters and to broadly participate in homeostasis. The circulatory system is at the interface between the digestive, respiratory, excretory, endocrine, and immune systems. In addition, a plethora of secondary functions has evolved across animal species, such as hydraulic support (e.g., hydroskeleton, locomotion).

Among animals, there is considerable diversity and plasticity to the cardiovascular system. Gas exchange in some phyla with relatively small species is shared between the circulatory system and passive diffusion or other mechanisms (e.g., insects), whereas other phyla of larger species with more active lifestyles greatly rely on an efficient cardiovascular system to allow gas and metabolite exchange for all cells of the organism. This diversity may be approached in terms of increased complexity and improved design as we climb up the evolutionary ladder; however, it may also be viewed as various adaptations to different and specific body plans and ecological niches.[1] For instance, the lack of two ventricles in reptiles should not be misinterpreted for an imperfect heart that fails to avoid mixing oxygenated and deoxygenated blood, but instead as a sophisticated response to group-specific physiological requirements, which is, in fact, favored by evolution in this taxon.[2] Likewise, air-breathing fishes, amphibians, and reptiles breathe air intermittently and are able to match pulmonary perfusion and ventilation using their partially divided circulation and alterations of pulmonary arterial tone or vascular resistance.[3] On the other hand, the evolution of double circulation in birds and mammals allows a higher systemic blood pressure needed for elevated metabolic demands and homeothermy, while keeping a lower pressure in the pulmonary circulation. This permits a thinner air-blood barrier within the pulmonary system and avoids cardiac shunting, which is detrimental in these species. Completely divided circulations have evolved independently in archosaur (crocodilians and birds) and therapsids (mammals), which is a prime example of convergent evolution in cardiovascular physiology

(Figure 4-1).[4] Likewise, the cardiac conduction system has evolved as an adaptation for greater control and coordination of the cardiac cycle and shows the greatest efficiency and specialization in homeothermic species with higher metabolism, while it remains somewhat "rudimentary" or unspecialized in other species.[5] While a slow conducting atrioventricular (AV) canal muscle in combination with the spongy ventricle provides this function in fishes, amphibians, and reptiles, a faster specialized His-Purkinje conduction system develops in mammals and birds.[5,6]

With the basic concepts of evolutionary and ecological anatomy and physiology in mind, the anatomical section of this chapter is organized, aside from invertebrates, which have different body plans, from the most rudimentary system observed in fishes to the most advanced system found in birds. Birds are unrivaled in their cardiovascular abilities to generate high systemic blood pressure and stroke volumes.

The second and third sections of this chapter deal with specific cardiovascular diseases and their diagnoses. These clinical sections do not provide an exhaustive compilation of all cardiovascular diseases diagnosed in exotic companion animals. Instead, they focus on important or unique clinical entities likely to be encountered by veterinarians in each taxon. Considering the substantial diversity found not only in cardiovascular anatomy and physiology but also in disease susceptibility among avian and exotic pets, the authors would like to emphasize that this branch of veterinary cardiology builds on the same foundations as small animal cardiology, and the reader is encouraged to develop a comparative approach to cardiovascular problems in the practice of zoological medicine. While the authors acknowledge that veterinary cardiology is much more advanced in mammals and, to a lesser extent in birds, the same diagnostic and therapeutic principles may be applied across animal taxons and may be adapted depending on the species' anatomical and physiological peculiarities.

Some cardiovascular diseases span the animal kingdom, while others are more species specific. Furthermore, disease prevalence and species susceptibility vary widely across taxons. Overall, cardiovascular diseases are mainly diagnosed in mammals and birds, and, as such, these phyla are covered in

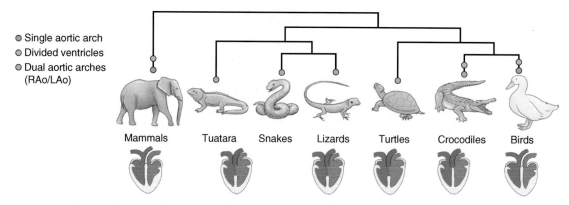

FIGURE 4-1 The evolution of the heart in terrestrial vertebrates. Plotted on the phylogeny are the occurrences of the anatomically divided ventricle *(orange circles)*, single aortic arch *(blue circles)*, and dual aortic arches (RAo/LAo; *green circles*). The relationships suggest the loss of the dual aortic arch system twice independently (mammals and birds) and the independent evolution of the four-chambered heart at least twice (mammals and birds) and possibly three times (mammals, birds, and crocodilians). *RAo*, Right aorta; *LAo*, left aorta. (Reprinted from Hicks J, Wang T. The functional significance of the reptilian heart: new insights into an old question. In: Sedmera D, Wang T, eds. *Ontogeny and Phylogeny of the Vertebrate Heart.* New York, NY: Springer New York; 2012:207-227.)

greater detail in this chapter. Fishes, amphibians, and reptiles do suffer from cardiovascular diseases, but the prevalence and overall clinical significance seem to be low or underreported, except maybe in ophidians. Apart from nonspecific and traumatic fluid loss, cardiovascular conditions seem to be scarce in invertebrates.

Specific diagnostic tests are reviewed in the third section of this chapter. Since mammalian cardiology has been covered extensively in numerous veterinary medical textbooks, the authors restricted the description of mammalian cardiologic diagnostic tests to information specific to exotic companion mammals. Postmortem examination of the cardiovascular system is not covered, and readers are referred to pathology textbooks for necropsy techniques and gross lesion evaluation in avian and exotic pets. While cardiovascular anatomy and physiology are relatively homogeneous in mammals and birds, the veterinary clinician should acknowledge their considerable diversity in other vertebrates and consider how it can impair diagnostic testing interpretation.

Finally, the fourth section deals with the treatment of cardiovascular diseases. Cardiology in zoological companion animals is a nascent field and pharmacologic information is limited in most species. However, clinical information on the treatment of heart failure is available in multiple avian and exotic companion mammal case reports. The scarcity of the scientific literature on invertebrate, piscine, amphibian, and reptilian cardiologic treatment may reflect the combination of the low prevalence of circulatory disorders and the lower pet ownership rates for these species.

ANATOMY AND PHYSIOLOGY

Invertebrates

Invertebrates are not a monophyletic group and make up the vast majority of animal species. Consequently, profound differences are present in the circulatory system within and between invertebrate phyla, and it is beyond the scope of this clinical textbook to review them exhaustively. The authors instead briefly introduce the general circulatory system configurations in the main taxons of invertebrates, with particular focus on important features and design. In addition, some invertebrates are more likely to be presented to veterinarians, such as arachnids kept as pets and cephalopods kept as laboratory animals; thus, a stronger emphasis is placed on these groups.

In small invertebrates, an organized circulatory system does not develop as they can solely rely on diffusion and fluid movements from the gut and body contractions (e.g., most small aquatic invertebrates, small arthropods, and sponges). As size and complexity of multicellular organisms increase, pumping structures and distributional systems develop. They form a circulatory system to transport and exchange gas and metabolites when simple diffusion from the environment and between organs is insufficient to meet all cell requirements. The ancestral vascular system of all animals was likely composed of a ventral and dorsal tubular system with contractile properties, and many invertebrates have a circulatory system composed of a dorsal tubular pumping structure.[5,7] A variety of circulatory systems have evolved from this basic organization in invertebrates to adapt to extreme variability in size and body plans as well as to many environmental and ecological constraints. Furthermore, insects have developed an elaborate tracheal system for oxygen transport, and the circulatory system has little to no respiratory function in these species.[8] Arachnids also have a system of tracheae, but these typically end in the hemolymph, and overall their circulatory system has a greater role in respiration than that in insects.[9] Aside from rudimentary mechanisms, invertebrate circulatory systems are loosely classified into "open" and "closed" systems, although some elaborate open systems can also be viewed as incompletely closed.[7,10-12]

In open circulatory systems, the hemolymph bathes the tissues directly, moves through large sinuses, and is distributed

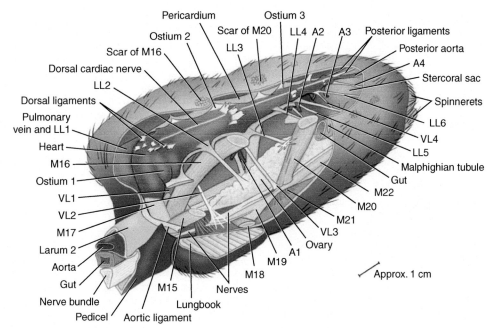

FIGURE 4-2 Example of a complex "open" circulatory system typical of arthropods. Diagram of the abdominal anatomy of a typical large spider showing the heart and open vascular system together with its associated muscles. *A,* Lateral arteries; *LL,* lateral cardiac ligaments; *M,* muscles; *VL,* ventral cardiac ligaments. The heart is located in the pericardial sinus enclosed by the pericardium, which is connected to the exoskeleton by ligaments. Lateral arteries, posterior aorta, and the large anterior aorta that ramifies inside the prosoma are shown. (Modified from Wilson RS. The heart-beat of the spider, *Heteropoda venatoria. J Insect Physiol.* 1967;13(9):1309-1326, with permission from Elsevier.)

through the coelom or pseudocoelom (also called *hemocoelom*) by body musculatures and motions and/or by open-ended muscular vessels or hearts. Ciliated surfaces in water invertebrates such as echinoderms also participate in fluid circulation. Open systems are typical of arthropods and noncephalopod mollusks. For instance, in gastropods a two-chambered heart with a ventricle and an auricle subdivided into two compartments in some species lies in a fluid-filled pericardial cavity. It propels hemolymph in the aorta, which subsequently empties into body sinusoids after dividing into two main vessels.[13–16] In bivalves (e.g., mussels, clams), the heart is composed of two atria and one ventricle and heart function has been thoroughly investigated in oysters.[16,17] In insects the circulatory system is composed of a series of sinuses forming the hemocele (pericardial, perineural, and perivisceral sinuses), a dorsal vessel composed of a caudal heart bearing ostia and an aorta that extends along the length of the body, and accessory pulsatile organs (usually at the bases of appendages).[8,18] In arachnids (e.g., spiders, scorpions), a large tube-like heart is present in the opisthosoma dorsally and is completely surrounded by a pericardium supported by ligaments connected to the exoskeleton and other abdominal structures. The pericardial sinus, delimited by the pericardium, functions as a preliminary cavity for the hemolymph. Hemolymph enters the heart through ostia during a suctioning diastole and is pumped back into the open system of the opisthosoma during systole through lateral arteries and into the prosoma through an anterior aorta, which

subsequently ramifies into smaller arteries (Figure 4-2).[9,19–21] Videos of a spider beating heart captured by magnetic resonance imaging (MRI) are available on the internet for interested readers. In addition, spiders have hydraulic leg extension mechanisms where high pressures (i.e., close to human systemic blood pressure) necessary to extend the legs are generated by prosomal muscles. This may interfere with the circulation during locomotor activity and partially explains spiders' rapid exhaustion after exercise.[9,21]

In closed circulatory systems, the hemolymph is fully enclosed in vascular structures or lined chambers. Large decapod crustaceans have an incomplete closed system with a muscular heart within a pericardium and true arteries lined by an endothelium. However, they lack a complete venous system, and blood/hemolymph returns to large veins through venous sinuses.[7,10] Large annelids have a well-developed vasculature. A contractile vessel is present dorsally and frequently anastomoses to a ventral vessel through connecting lateral vessels that may bear additional hearts.[10] The most advanced circulatory system of invertebrates is found in active cephalopods, which possess two branchial hearts and a multichambered central heart that can generate high pressure in a well-developed cell-lined contractile vascular system (Figure 4-3).[10,22,23] Cephalopods have high metabolic rates but their hemolymph has poor oxygen-carrying capacity. As a consequence, their heart has very high cardiac outputs comparable to mammals of similar size.[22] The tissue structure of

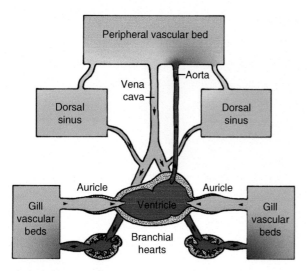

FIGURE 4-3 Example of a "closed" circulatory system typical of cephalopods. *Arrows,* Oxygenated blood; *arrowheads,* deoxygenated blood. (Reprinted and modified from Smith PJS, Boyle PR. The cardiac innervation of *Eledone cirrhosa. Phil Trans R Soc Lond B.* 1983;300:493-511.)

invertebrate blood vessels is different from the vertebrates and varies widely from one species to another.[24]

Invertebrates have various mechanisms of cardiac regulation mainly focused on modulating stroke volume and heart frequencies.[5,7–9,22] Cardiac contractions are either myogenic or neurogenic in invertebrates (myogenic in mammals). In spiders, scorpions, and some insects, heart contractions are neurogenic.[20,25] In peristaltic contractions, electrical impulses are generated in various locations and spread along the tubular hearts. Neural control in advanced arthropods can be accomplished via a pacemaker at the level of the heart or localized in a neural ganglion placed dorsally to the heart.[21,26] Cephalopods have more complex cardiac innervation.[27] Circulatory responses to environmental changes vary in invertebrates. For instance, heartbeat frequency is temperature dependent in cephalopods and bivalves.[17,22]

It is also noteworthy that a large number of parasitic helminth invertebrates inhabit the cardiovascular systems of other animals, which highlights the dual importance of this animal group in comparative cardiology.

Fish

The adult fish heart is composed of the sinus venosus, one atrium, one ventricle, and either an elastic bulbus arteriosus (teleosts) or a contractile conus arteriosus (elasmobranchs) arranged in series (Figure 4-4).[28–31] While the basic body plan for the cardiovascular system is similar for all fish, profound differences may be present in the various families of fish. Major cardiovascular differences are related to branchial circulatory patterns and air-breathing abilities.[32]

The heart, including the outflow tract, is located caudoventrally to the gills in an inelastic pericardial sac. It is separated from the abdominal cavity by the fibrous septum transversum.[33]

The thin-walled sinus venosus receives blood from the ducts of Cuvier (formerly caudal vena cava), the hepatic veins, and the anterior jugular veins.[30] The sinoatrial ostium bears a large sinoatrial valve, and the openings of the hepatic veins are guarded by muscular sphincters, but the Cuverian ducts do not have a valve. The wall of the sinus is mainly composed of connective tissue with a muscular component that widely varies among species. The single atrium has a variable size and shape depending on species, and the atrial myocardium may have trabeculae. The AV region is formed by a distinct ring of myocardium that supports the AV valves.[29,30] The AV valves have two leaflets and lack chordae tendinae; however, ventricular trabecular sheets may help anchor them in the AV muscular ring.[29]

The fish ventricle shows important species variability and does not have a typical shape or tissue organization common to all fishes. Ventricles are usually classified into different types. Morphologically, three ventricular forms are recognized: a saclike ventricle (e.g., elasmobranchs, many marine teleosts), a tubular ventricle (e.g., most fishes with elongate body shape), and a pyramidal ventricle (e.g., active fishes such as salmonids and scombrids).[30,34] The functional significance of these ventricular shapes is still unclear, but they seem to correlate with species lifestyle.[29] Structurally, four ventricular types are also recognized (see Figure 4-4). They are differentiated based on vascularization patterns and on the possession and arrangement of the two histological ventricular layers: the spongiosa (inner layer of trabecular myocardium) and compacta (outer layer of compact myocardium).[28–31,35,36] Metabolism is mainly glycolytic in the spongiosa, whereas it is mainly oxidative in the compacta.[33] Most teleosts (~80%) have a type-I ventricle that lacks a compacta and coronary circulation and is entirely trabeculated. Ventricular types have functional significance. Active species and endothermic sharks have larger ventricles.[30]

The outflow tract in primitive fish is composed of a conus and bulbus arteriosus, the latter containing several conus valves. In modern teleosts, the outflow tract is mainly composed of a prominent bulbus arteriosus, which is an elastic chamber creating even pressure and continuous blood flow to the gills.[29,30] The shape of the bulbus is variable, from pear shaped to elongated and, like arteries, is composed of tunica intima, media, and adventitia and bears a single conus valve made of two leaflets. In elasmobranchs, the outflow tract is composed of the conus arteriosus, which is contractile and prolongs ventricular systole and, like the heart, is composed of epi-, myo-, and endocardium.[30]

Some important physiological differences exist between fish and mammalian hearts that may have some clinical relevance and deserve comment.[30,37] In fish, cardiac output is primarily increased through an increase in stroke volume, and a modest increase in heart rates (HRs) typically occurs, whereas mammals, birds, and reptiles deeply rely on HR increase.[30] In addition, atrial contraction is the sole contributor to ventricular filling in fish, while it accounts for only 25% of ventricular filling in mammalian hearts. Finally, cardiac output in fish varies with environmental temperature, extracellular acidosis, and hypoxia.

Fish lack a specialized conduction system made of Purkinje fibers; however, a sinoatrial node made of specialized

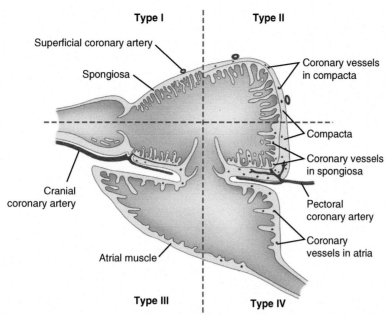

FIGURE 4-4 Anatomical drawing of the heart in fish with the atrium *(bottom)*, ventricle *(middle)*, and bulbus/conus arteriosus *(left)*. Four basic ventricular types have been described in fishes represented by the four quadrants. Type I is characterized by having a single myocardial type (spongiosa) and no capillaries in the ventricular muscle. Most type-I hearts have no coronary vessels whatsoever. Type II is characterized by two muscle layers in the ventricle (inner spongiosa and outer compacta), a coronary circulation, and capillaries only in the outer compacta. Type III is similar to type II, but capillaries are found in both the spongiosa and compacta and, to a limited extent, in the atrium. Type IV has a larger percentage of the ventricle as compacta (>30%) and a more extensive capillarization of the atrium. The coronary circulation, regardless of types, is derived from a cranial supply, as depicted in the *lower left* quadrant, and an additional pectoral supply in some fishes, as depicted in the *lower right* quadrant. (Modified from Farrell AP, Jones D. The heart. In: Hoar WS, Randall DJ, Farrell AP. *Fish Physiology, the Cardiovascular System,* Volume 12, Part A. 1992: 267-304, with permission from Elsevier.)

myocardial pacemaker cells is located in the wall of the sinus venosus, and a functional conduction system made of working cardiomyocytes is present in the ventricle.[28,30,32] The exact location of the sinoatrial node is highly variable in fish.[32] Cardiac regulation is, similarly to other vertebrates, achieved through a combination of sympathetic, parasympathetic, and hormonal pathways.

The arterial system of fish is composed of the ventral aorta, which receives blood from the conus/bulbus arteriosus, and branches into paired afferent branchial arteries.[38] Subsequent efferent branchial arteries form the dorsal aorta, which is paired anteriorly and into a single vessel posteriorly. Since circulation in fish is arranged in sequence, the systemic circulation can be considered an arterial portal system, in which blood flows through two successive capillary beds of comparable resistance that influence each other. Many fish also possess various arterial and venous retia systems with countercurrent exchange (e.g., gills, heat exchangers in muscles, swim bladder, choroid retina of the eye). Major modifications of posterior branchial arteries occur in air-breathing fish. The fish venous system is composed of three subsystems that differ in how they return blood to the heart, their pressure, and their

structure.[39] The first system includes the ducts of Cuvier/ cardinal veins that return blood from the somatic muscular system to the sinus venosus and encompass the renal portal system; the second system is that of the hepatic portal system, which also returns blood from visceral organs directly to the heart; and the third system comprises the veins from the skin, fins, and some mucosal surfaces from which blood is propelled in many fish by a caudal pump or a caudal heart into the caudal vein (most frequent venipuncture site in fish patients). In addition, the renal portal system includes two renal portal veins derived from the caudal vein that drain blood from the somatic muscles into the tubular renal capillary network. The anatomy and importance of the renal portal system vary with species and may have pharmacologic significance. Connections between somatic venous circulation and the hepatic portal venous system are present in some teleosts but do not usually occur.[39] Blood return depends on "pumps," such as swimming and respiratory muscles, but also on auxiliary hearts such as the portal heart of hagfishes (which generates its own electrocardiogram [ECG]) or the caudal heart of some teleosts and elasmobranchs. Fish also possess a secondary vascular system that consists of a separate and parallel

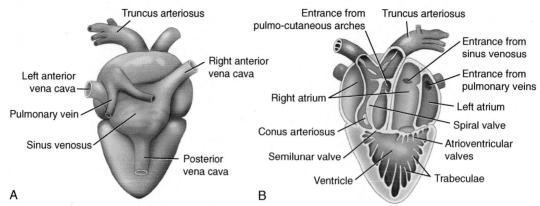

FIGURE 4-5 Anatomical drawing of the heart of the frog (*Anura* spp.), external anatomy, dorsal view *(A)*, and internal anatomy, ventral view *(B)*.

circulatory system. It arises from the main arteries as hundreds of tiny arterioles that re-anastomose into a secondary arterial network with a lower hematocrit and are responsible for supplying blood to the surfaces. This secondary system eventually empties into primary veins.[28,31,40,41] Its function is poorly understood and is sometimes referred to as a lymphatic system, but it is sufficiently different from mammalian lymphatic vessels to be classified in its own category.

A large number of fish have air-breathing capabilities that vary in importance and nature. Since air-breathing has independently evolved in at least 49 different fish families, there is a large diversity in air-breathing organs and location, and consequently, in arrangements among the systemic, branchial, and air-breathing organ's circulation and blood shunting mechanisms between respiratory organs to minimize blood mixing and enhance gas exchange.[28,32,42] The most extreme of these arrangements occurs in the lungfish, which have a different ventricular anatomy with the presence of a partial ventricular septum and extensive trabeculation, such as that observed in amphibians in order to partially separate systemic and respiratory circulations.[32,43] Cardiovascular response to hypoxia, hypercarbia, and other stimuli may vary between water-breathing and air-breathing fishes.[30,42]

Amphibians

The class Amphibia is diverse and, while a similar anatomical plan is conserved, cardiovascular anatomy may vary substantially among the three amphibian orders as well as among species. Most of the anatomy presented here is derived from the order Anura (frogs and toads) and Caudata (salamanders), because detailed anatomical information on the circulatory system is available and frogs and salamanders are more likely to be presented with diseases related to this system than the order Gymnophiona (caecilians). Specifically, amphibian anatomy has been investigated in great depths in the Anuran genus *Rana* and the caudatan genus *Salamandra*.[44-46] In addition, cardiac anatomy has been specifically reported in a few species such as two other caudatans, the hellbender (*Cryptobranchus alleganiensis*) and the greater siren (*Siren lacertina*).[47,48]

The anatomy of the larval cardiovascular system is similar to fish, in which blood flows from an undivided heart to a

truncus arteriosus (ventral aorta), six pairs of arterial branchial arches, and a dorsal aorta.[49] Amphibians acquire an incomplete separation of the systemic and respiratory circulation during metamorphosis through the formation of an arterial anastomosis that eventually takes over the entire branchial blood flow, especially in species in which gills are completely resorbed.[50] This marks an evolutionary or ecological transition from a simple circulation system, such as in fish, to a double circulation system such as in mammals, birds, and crocodilians.

Amphibians have a three-chambered heart with two atria and one ventricle, in which partial mixing of oxygenated arterial and deoxygenated venous blood occurs.[44,45,51,52] The amphibian heart also contains other cavities similar to fishes: a large sinus venosus connected to the right atrium and the combination bulbus cordis/conus arteriosus and truncus arteriosus connected to the ventricle and at the transition between the cardiac and vascular system (Figure 4-5). In frogs, the heart is located on the midline dorsal to the pectoral girdle, ventral to the esophagus, and surrounded caudo-laterally by the liver lobes.[44] The heart lies in the pericardial cavity formed by the pericardium. The pericardium has attachments to the heart vessels and abdominal muscles and is frequently pigmented. In salamanders, the heart is smaller than in frogs, the ventricle is shorter, and the sinus venosus is larger.[45] In salamanders, the dorsal aspect of the ventricle is attached to the pericardium by a large annular ligament. A cardiac ligament attaching the ventricle to the sinus venosus is also described in several sources.[47,48]

The sinus venosus, on the dorsal aspect of the heart (Figure 4-5), is lined by thin walls and joins the right atrium through the ostium venosum sinus, which is guarded by a single flap valve in salamanders and a bicuspid valve in frogs.[44,45] It is much larger in salamanders than in frogs and may be partially divided into two chambers in some species, such as the greater siren or the hellbender.[47,48] The atria are separated by an interatrial septum, which may be incomplete or fenestrated in some species of caecilians and salamanders, such as hellbenders.[47,50,53] The right atrium is larger than the left, except in caecilians. Venous blood from the systemic system enters the sinus venosus and the right atrium through the two anterior and the single posterior venae cavae. The left atrium receives oxygenated blood from the respiratory system (lung + skin in amphibians).[44,45,53] The pulmonary veins do not possess a valve, and regurgitation can only be prevented by contraction of the surrounding muscles. Numerous ridges are present in the atrial walls, forming a multitude of smaller cavities. The largest of these cavities are called *recesses* and a recessus sinister and dextri have notably been identified on the left and right atrium, respectively. The single ventricle possesses extensive trabeculations and compartments (see Figure 4-5). The ventricular cavity is thus divided into a multitude of smaller left and right chambers that minimize the mixing of blood from both circulations.[44,45,47,48,53] These trabeculae are organized in such a way that a partial morphological or functional interventricular septum may be formed in some species. A partial interventricular septum is present in some genera of salamanders and caecilians.[50] The auriculo-ventricular opening is a single large aperture guarded by two valves; these dorsal and ventral valves may be regarded functionally as a single pair, of which the atrial margin is attached to the interatrial septum and the free margin is attached to the ventricular trabeculae by chordae tendineae.[44,45,48] Two pairs of valves may be present in some species. The ventricle pumps blood into the truncus arteriosus, which is separated internally by a spiral valve into two compartments. In most species, a bulbus cordis/conus arteriosus is located before the truncus arteriosus, harbors valves, and is also divided into two compartments that continue into the truncus arteriosus.[45] The conus arteriosus is contractile and is considered a cardiac cavity, whereas the truncus arteriosus is a transitional structure between the heart and the vascular system. In caecilians, the carotid and systemic arches are fused and the heart and the truncus arteriosus are particularly elongated.[50]

The truncus arteriosus is divided into two vessels that each separate into three arterial arches: the carotid, systemic, and pulmo-cutaneous arches. Blood is diverted into each arterial arch depending on the motion of the spiral valve, the contractions of the conus arteriosus, and the differences in arterial arch resistance during the two phases of ventricular contraction.[43,45,53] The results are that most blood from the right atrium is sent to the pulmo-cutaneous arch during the first phase of the ventricular systole and most blood from the left atrium is sent to the carotid and systemic arches during the second phase of the ventricular systole.[53] The amount of cardiac shunting (deoxygenated blood that reenters the systemic circulation) depends on temperature, oxygen availability, activity, and biology of the amphibian species.[53,54] No discernible coronary vascularization is evident in the frog.[46]

There is no histologically discernible specialized conducting system in the amphibian heart; however, evidence exists for a functionally equivalent conducting system, as in higher vertebrates.[5,55] Cardiac innervation has, as in mammals, sympathetic and parasympathetic components and responds to catecholamines and acetylcholine neurotransmitters. Regulation of blood flow is achieved through peripheral and central receptors to arterial pressure and blood-gas composition, and response to oxygen availability is an important cardiovascular stimulus.[54]

Hepatic and renal portal veins are present in amphibians, in which veins from the posterior part of the body connect to the liver (through the ventral abdominal vein) and kidneys (through Jacobson's veins).[45,50,53] Thus, injection of drugs in the caudal half of the amphibian body with hepatic or renal

metabolism should be avoided until more information becomes available.

The lymphatic system is well developed in amphibians. Paired lymph hearts are present, located dorsally and subcutaneously, and can be seen pulsating.[52,53] The contraction rate is independent from the cardiac cycle. The number of lymph hearts varies among species, with the order Gymnophiona having the most (>200), followed by Caudata (~10) and Anura (~4). A central lymph heart associated with the truncus arteriosus is present in some salamander species.[50] Disruption of lymph heart contraction results in edema and weight gain. A terrestrial lifestyle is associated with a lesser dependency on lymphatic circulation due to decreased water cutaneous absorption.[53] Frogs have two pairs of lymph hearts: one anterior pair and one posterior pair.[44] Large lymph sacs and lymph spaces are also present throughout the body and can be extensive, as observed in the frog. Lymphatics empty at different locations along the venous system, including but not limited to the subclavian veins and the renal portal veins.

Reptiles

As observed in amphibians, the cardiac anatomy varies significantly among reptilian taxons, and the internal anatomy of the ventricle can be quite complex (Figures 4-6, 4-7, and 4-8). The basic organization of the heart of reptiles revolves around the presence of two atria and one ventricle, the latter showing various degrees of structural and functional compartmentalization depending on circulatory adaptations to specific ecological and physiological demands.[56,57] Reptilian hearts can be loosely classified as being crocodilian (e.g., crocodiles, alligators, gavials, and caimans) or noncrocodilian (e.g., snakes, lizards, and chelonians). Most published descriptions on specific species (e.g., monitor lizards, pythons, crocodilians, and freshwater turtles) show highly variable designs in anatomy and physiology.[58–65]

The reptilian heart is more or less globoid (e.g., chelonians) or ovoid (e.g., squamates, crocodilians), except in ophidians, in which it is elongated. In most species, the heart is located relatively cranially within the coelom at the level of the pectoral girdle in lizards and crocodilians and immediately past it in chelonians (see Figure 4-6).[57] In some lizards (e.g., varanids, teids, and helodermatids), the heart is more caudally located. In side-necked turtles, the heart is pushed to the right side to accomodate the retracted neck. In snakes, the heart is typically positioned approximately 15% to 35% of the body length from the head, and heart beats can usually be observed ventrally.[66] Some ophidian species, such as aquatic species, the heart can be located much more caudally.[65,67,68] In snakes the heart is mobile within the coelomic cavity; this probably facilitates the movement of large whole prey in the esophagus.[69]

As in other vertebrates, the heart lies in the pericardial cavity. The pericardium is caudally attached to the visceral peritoneum by a ligament, the gubernaculum cordis, except in varanid lizards and snakes.[57,67] The reptilian heart is composed of a sinus venosus, the left and right atria, and one ventricle, except in crocodilians, where two ventricles are present (see Figures 4-7 and 4-8). The ophidian heart is asymmetric, with a large right atrium extending farther back and covering a large surface of the right side of the ventricle.[70]

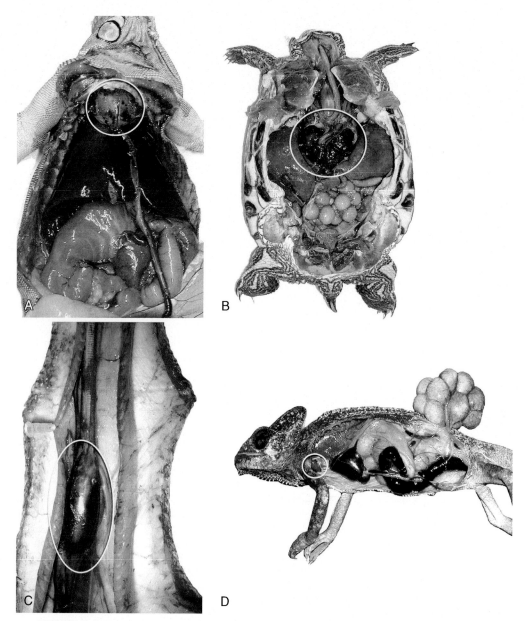

FIGURE 4-6 Topographic anatomy of the heart *(white circles)* in a few species of reptiles. *A,* Green iguana *(Iguana iguana); B,* red-eared slider *(Trachemys scripta elegans); C,* ball python *(Python regius); D,* veiled chameleon *(Chamaeleo calyptratus).*

Three arterial trunks, the left aortic arch, the right aortic arch, and the pulmonary trunk, are visible externally running from the ventricle between the two atria, rotating toward the right and forming an angle of 180°. The two aortic arches merge together caudally to form the common abdominal aorta (dorsal aorta).[56,57,65,69]

The sinus venosus is situated on the dorsal aspect of the heart and attached to the dorsal wall of the ventricle by the dorsal ligament. It receives deoxygenated blood from the two cranial venae cavae and the posterior vena cava and drains into the right atrium through a sinoatrial orifice guarded by a small valve.[56,57,67] In some species, the hepatic vein or jugular vein also drains into the sinus venosus.[61,69] The sinus venosus is much reduced in crocodilians, and harbors a partial septum internally in most squamates and crocodilians.[67] The left atrium tends to be smaller than the right and receives blood from the two pulmonary veins. The atria communicate with the ventricle via the AV funnels guarded by unicuspid AV valves.[56,57,67,71] Chordae tendineae-like fibrous strands attaching the AV valves to the ventricular musculature have been described in some species.[62]

In noncrocodilian reptiles, the ventricle is subdivided into three subchambers: the cavum pulmonale, cavum venosum, and cavum arteriosum (see Figures 4-7 and 4-8).[4,56,57,62,63,65,67,70,71] The ventricle is internally complex, and two-dimensional anatomical drawings may give an incomplete understanding of its structure, depending on the plans and considering the anatomical and topographical diversity among species (see

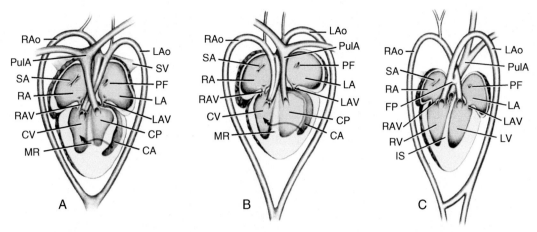

FIGURE 4-7 Anatomical drawing of the different reptilian cardiac configuration. *A*, Chelonian and squamate pattern; *B*, varanid pattern; *C*, crocodilian pattern. *CA*, cavum arteriosum; *CP*, cavum pulmonale; *CV*, cavum venosum; *FP*, foramen of Panizza; *IS*, interventricular septum; *LA*, left atrium; *LAo*, left aorta; *LAV*, left atrioventricular valve; *LV*, left ventricle; *MR*, muscular ridge; *PF*, pulmonary vein foramen; *PulA*, pulmonary artery; *RA*, right atrium; *RAo*, right aorta; *RAV*, right atrioventricular valve; *RV*, right ventricle; *SA*, sinoatrial valve; *SV*, sinus venosus. (Reprinted from Wyneken J. *Vet Clin Exot Anim.* 2009;12:51-63, with permission from Elsevier.)

Figure 4-7). Basically, the cavum venosum and arteriosum (together sometimes referred to as the cavum dorsale) are mostly dorsal and on the left in respect to the cavum pulmonale (also called the cavum ventrale).[65,67,70] Noncrocodilian reptiles have two ventricular septa. One is the muscular ridge (also called the horizontal septum or the "muskelleiste"), which runs from apex to base, is incomplete cranially, and separates the cavum pulmonale from the cavum venosum/cavum arteriosum, especially during the ventricular systole. This muscular ridge is poorly developed in chelonians except in see turtles and giant tortoises.[57,70] The interventricular septum in archosaurs (crocodilians and birds) seems to have evolved from this muscular ridge. An incomplete muscular septum (also called the vertical septum), which is relatively inconstant in structure and position across species (e.g., it is strongly developed in pythons and monitors), divides the cavum dorsale into the cavum arteriosum to the left and the cavum venosum to the right and often joins the muscular ridge at its base. An anterior large interventricular canal, below the AV valves, is the only connection between the cavum arteriosum and the cavum venosum. The AV valves are positioned in such a way that, when pressed medially (open), they partially or completely obstruct the interventricular canal.[71] This system allows a functional separation of the systemic and pulmonary circulation, with the cavum pulmonale being the functional homolog to the mammalian and avian right ventricle and the combined cavum venosum and arteriosum (cavum dorsale) being the functional homolog to the mammalian and avian left ventricle.[4,56,57,65] The cavum venosum is a relatively small cavity that receives both oxygenated and deoxygenated blood at various times during the cardiac cycle. During early ventricular diastole, the cavum venosum and pulmonale receive deoxygenated blood from the right atrium, and the cavum arteriosum receives oxygenated blood from the left atrium.[56,57,72] During late ventricular diastole, blood flow from the atria has ceased and deoxygenated

blood from the cavum venosum flows into the cavum pulmonale; the AV valves then close, which opens the interventricular canal and allows blood flow from the cavum arteriosum into the cavum venosum (see Figure 4-8). During late ventricular systole, the muscular ridge separates the cavum venosum and the cavum pulmonale. Blood from the cavum pulmonale is ejected into the pulmonary artery, and blood from the cavum venosum is ejected into the left and right aortic arches. As in the amphibian heart, sequential ejection into the pulmonary and systemic arterial circuit is partially regulated by pressure gradients between the ventricle and the double arterial circulation. The right but not the left aorta branches off several major arteries, and both aorta later fuse caudally to form the dorsal aorta. Aortic valves are bicuspid. The pulmonary artery later divides into left and right pulmonary arteries. Since the muscular ridge nearly completely divides the ventricular cavity in varanids and pythons, a more pronounced separation of blood flows and higher systemic pressures are seen.[4,62,73] On the other hand, testudines have a larger cavum venosum and more blood mixing occurs.[4,70] Unlike mammals, reptilian atria make an active contribution to ventricular filling.[71]

A different cardiac anatomical pattern is encountered in crocodilians, which possess a four-chambered heart with a complete ventricular septum but still two aortic arches (see Figures 4-7 and 4-8). The left ventricle ejects blood into the right aorta, while the right ventricle ejects blood into the left aorta and the pulmonary artery. The right and left aortic arches anastomose at two locations: first at the foramen of Panizza at the aortic outflow tract and second at the level of the abdomen by the dorsal connecting artery.[4,57] Opening of the foramen of Panizza is actively controlled.

Reptiles have the ability to regulate blood shunting in the ventricle, based on their metabolic needs in a degree that varies across species.[2,4,56,57] While cardiovascular shunting is detrimental in birds and mammals (congenital abnormalities),

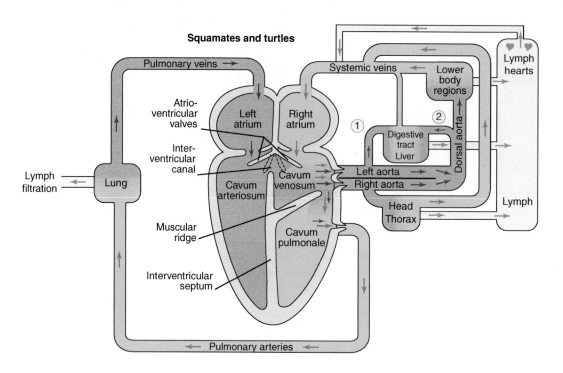

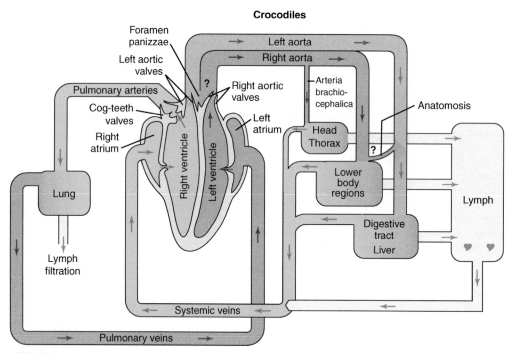

FIGURE 4-8 Schematic illustration of the circulatory and lymphatic systems in squamates/ turtles and crocodiles. *Red,* O_2-rich, CO_2-poor blood; *blue,* O_2-poor, CO_2-rich blood; *shades of violet,* different degrees of mixing; *yellow,* lymph; *arrows,* direction of blood/lymph flow; *top,* illustration of squamates and turtles shows blood supply of the digestive tract via the left aorta in turtles and some varanids; *bottom,* alternative blood supply of the digestive tract via the dorsal aorta in squamates except varanids. (Reprinted from Campen R, Starck M. Cardiovascular circuits and digestive function of intermittent-feeding sauropsids. In: McCue M, ed. *Comparative Physiology of Fasting, Starvation, and Food Limitation.* Berlin, Heidelberg: Springer-Verlag; 2012:133-155.)

it serves important physiological functions in reptiles and is favored by natural selection. The extent of cardiac shunting is determined by the difference between pulmonary and systemic vascular resistance, which is partially regulated by parasympathetic and sympathetic tones. As such, during rest, diving, and apnea (increased parasympathetic tone), a right-to-left shunt may occur, which decreases pulmonary perfusion. When metabolism or activity increases (increased sympathetic tone), a left-to-right shunt may occur, which increases pulmonary perfusion. In most reptiles, breathing is intermittent and long phases of apnea may occur; this system may therefore be optimal to limit ventilation/perfusion mismatching and is advantageous when diving because of increased anaerobic metabolism and bypass of the pulmonary circulation. Other factors may also influence the degree and direction of cardiac shunting in noncrocodilian hearts (e.g., temperature, anesthesia, healing, digestion, vascular sphincters, hibernation (chelonians), and diving reflex in aquatic species), and various investigative approaches have been followed in order to better understand the potential functional and adaptive benefits.[2,4,57,74,75] It is also reasonable to assume that anesthetic drugs, pulmonary ventilation, and the composition of inhaled air may have an effect on cardiac shunting during anesthesia, which varies among species and may impact the duration of anesthetic recovery and isoflurane excretion in reptiles. Interestingly, despite a complete ventricular separation in crocodilians, cardiovascular shunting still occurs through the foramen of Panizza with the two aortae originating from separate ventricles.[2,4,56,57] Crocodilians also have a sphincter at the base of the pulmonary artery that can close down the pulmonary circulation.[3]

As for cardiac shunting, HR, stroke volume, and blood pressure of reptiles greatly depend on environmental and ecological variables such as temperature, oxygen demand, and activity. In addition, different cardiovascular variables are important in reptilian thermoregulation such as HR and cutaneous vasodilation.[56,57] For instance, green iguanas experience tachycardia and about 20% of right-to-left shunting when heated to increase thermal transport.[71] Reptiles may indeed benefit from having two aortas, with the left being the target of cardiac shunting for thermal transport with blood bypassing the lungs while the right (having more branches including carotids) still supplies the brain and major organs with well-oxygenated blood.[71]

An interesting and important physiological feature in intermittent reptile feeders, aside from cardiac shunting, is postprandial hypertrophy of the heart and digestive vascular flow increase, which can be extreme (e.g., ophidians). In postprandial snakes, ventricular mass can increase by up to 40% and blood flow volume to the intestines and portal system up to 30% and 300%, respectively.[75-77] In infrequently feeding Burmese pythons (*Python molurus bivittatus*), heart mass can increase by 40% within 48 to 72 hours after a large meal to support the postprandial increase in metabolism, which seems to be promoted by a plasma-fatty acid mixture.[77]

As in fish, amphibians, and birds, reptiles have a venous renal portal system that exhibits great species variations.

The lymphatic system of reptiles is more developed than the venous system and varies considerably among species. It is made up of anastomosing superficial and deep lymphatic vessels, collecting vessels, sinuses (also called cisterns), and main trunks (see Figure 4-8). The lymphatic vessels form a large network across the body and include perivascular, coelomic, muscular, cutaneous, and vertebral vessels. The collecting vessels drain the superficial and deep lymphatic nets into sinuses and main trunks. The sinuses are dilations of lymphatic vessels, and their anatomical distribution mirrors that of lymph nodes in mammals. These include the precardiac, subpubic, ischiatic, subvesicle, and pelvic sinuses. The main trunks carry the lymph to the venous system. Reptilian lymphatic vessels are also larger, relative to those of mammals.[78-80] Lymphatic vessels contain numerous valves that enable a unidirectional flow. They are particularly numerous in the collecting vessels and in vessels between sinuses and main trunks. In turtles, snakes, and some species of lizards, two lymphatic hearts with contractile activity contribute to propelling lymph through the lymphatic system. In snakes, they are found between the lymphapophysis on either side of the vertebral column at the level of the second or third caudal vertebrae. In turtles, they lie deep under the last vertebral scales of the carapace. In crocodilians, the lymph hearts are found at the base of the tail, between the transverse process of the caudal vertebrae and the caudal border of the ilium.[78]

In reptiles, as observed in amphibians, a specialized cardiac conduction system made of Purkinje cells does not exist, and less specialized cardiac muscle fibers take this function. While no histological evidence for a specialized conduction system has been found, reptiles do have a functional conducting system with the presence of a sinoatrial node or cardiac fibers in the sinus venosus that initiate the electrical impulse, which is then propagated by ventricular electrical channels.[5,57] The heart receives innervations from both parasympathetic and sympathetic fibers. The parasympathetic fibers run in the vagus nerve and provide cholinergic (inhibitory) control. The less well-developed sympathetic fibers cause positive chronotropism via adrenergic innervation.[57,65,69,81]

Mammals

Unlike previously discussed taxons, the mammalian circulatory system can be considered rather uniform from a clinical standpoint. To meet the high metabolic demands associated with the active lifestyle and homeothermy of mammals, the heart has evolved as a particularly efficient pump with a finely tuned regulatory mechanism. The most striking differences from previous vertebrate taxons are that mammalian hearts have two ventricles, with a complete separation of the systemic and pulmonary circulation; only one aorta, the left; and an organized electrical conduction system made of Purkinje fibers (Figure 4-9). The mammalian cardiovascular system is more familiar to veterinarians than that of other vertebrates, and readers are referred to veterinary cardiology and anatomy textbooks for more complete information on the form and function of the cardiovascular system in domestic mammals.[82-86] In addition, more detailed information is available for rodents, rabbits (*Oryctolagus cuniculus*), and ferrets (*Mustela putoriuis furo*) than in other species of companion exotic mammals (Figure 4-10).[87-97]

The mammalian heart is enclosed by a pericardium that blends with the adventitia of the great vessels dorsally and contains a small amount of serous fluid. The pericardium is attached ventrally to the sternum by the sternopericardiac ligament and to the diaphragm by the phrenicopericardiac

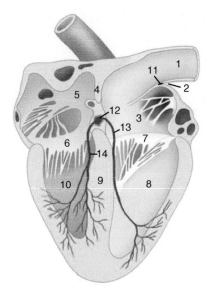

FIGURE 4-9 General internal organization of the mammalian heart. *1,* Cranial vena cava; *2,* terminal sulcus; *3,* right atrium; *4,* interatrial septum; *5,* left atrium; *6,* left AV valve; *7,* right AV valve; *8,* right ventricle; *9,* interventricular septum; *10,* left ventricle; *11,* sinoatrial node; *12,* AV node; *13,14,* right and left branches of AV bundle. (Reprinted and modified from Dyce K, Sack W, Wensing C. *Textbook of Veterinary Anatomy.* 3rd ed. Philadelphia, PA: Saunders; 2002:840, with permission from Elsevier.)

ligament (present in only certain species). The visceral part of the pericardium is the cardiac epicardium. The heart and its pericardium are located in the mediastinum, the partition that separates the pleural cavities in mammals; enclosed by the lungs laterally in the thoracic cavity; and separated from the abdominal cavity by the diaphragm. The cardiac lateral projection within the thoracic cavity is typically between the third and sixth ribs in most mammalian species. In ferrets, which have an elongated thorax, the heart is situated between the sixth and eighth intercostal spaces.[98] Rabbits have small hearts comparatively to other mammals.[97]

The heart of mammals is composed of four chambers: the left and right atria separated by the interatrial septum and the left and right ventricles separated by the interventricular septum (see Figures 4-9 and 4-10). The atria are separated externally from the ventricles by the coronary groove, in which large coronary vessels are found. A fibrous skeleton, also found but less developed in lower vertebrates, separates the atria from the ventricles internally. As in other species, the right atrium receives deoxygenated blood from the caudal vena cava, a single cranial vena cava (two in rabbits, rats *[Rattus norvegicus]*, hamsters, and woodchucks *[Marmota monax]*), and the coronary sinus. The right atrium is divided into the sinus of the venae cavae and a blind sac, the right auricle. The left atrium receives oxygenated blood from the pulmonary veins that enter at different sites. Venous entrances do not bear valves. Each atrium empties into the corresponding ventricle through the AV openings. The right AV valve is usually tricuspid, except in rabbits, in which it is bicuspid.

However, the bicuspid characteristic of this valve is shared by many species (e.g., some dogs, cats, and other exotic mammals), and it often has a bicuspid appearance on echocardiography. The left AV valve is bicuspid and is also known as the mitral valve. Both valves are anchored by the chordae tendineae to the ventricular papillary muscles, which prevent valves from prolapsing into the atrium during ventricular systole. The right ventricle is wrapped around the right and cranial aspects of the left ventricle and is a crescent-shaped cavity with thinner walls than the left ventricle. It pumps blood into the conus arteriosus (anterior part of the single ventricle in lower vertebrates) followed by the pulmonary trunks at a lower pressure than the systemic blood pressure. A pulmonic valve is present at the opening of the pulmonary trunk, which bears three thin cusps thickened in the midportion of their free edge (nodule of Arantius). The left ventricle has a circular cross section, forms the cardiac apex, and has thick walls. It pumps blood into the aorta, which is guarded by a tricuspid aortic valve similar to the pulmonary valve. The widening of the base of the aorta is known as the bulbus aortae. As in other species, the heart is composed of an epicardium, myocardium, and endocardium and the arteries of a tunica intima, media, and adventitia. In marsupials, several morphological differences from placental mammals may be present, such as a larger heart, a monocuspid right AV valve, and a divided right atrium.[92,99,100]

The mammalian heart is well vascularized and receives about 5% to 15% of the cardiac output, depending on the species. The supply is through the left and right coronary arteries. The left coronary artery is usually the largest, but there is an important variation in the pattern or coronary vascularization among mammalian species. The two main coronary veins are the great coronary vein, which returns most of the coronary blood to the right atrium, and the middle coronary vein. In rats, a significant proportion of cardiac arterial vascularization is extracoronary through the mammary and subclavian arteries. Guinea pigs *(Cavia porcellus)* are notable for the important collateral circulation of their coronary arteries, making them particularly resistant to myocardial ischemia. Rabbits, on the other hand, have limited coronary circulation, which may predispose them to myocardial ischemia, especially due to vasoconstriction under anesthesia.

The conduction system of the mammalian heart is composed of specialized myocytes and includes the sinoatrial node located in the right atrial wall, the AV node located at the base of the interatrial septum, the AV bundle (bundle of His), and the subendocardial branches of Purkinje fibers. Most components of this system are capable of spontaneous electrical activity except for the sinoatrial node, which has the highest physiologic rate of depolarization and functions as the primary cardiac pacemaker. The heart is innervated by the sympathetic (cervical cardiac nerves, caudal thoracic nerves) and parasympathetic nervous systems (vagus nerve), which together form the cardiac plexus in the cranial mediastinum. In rabbits, the anatomy of the sinoatrial node region and the conducting tissue is less complex, which makes them the mammal of choice for the laboratory study of Purkinje fibers.

In mammals, the aorta curves to the left of the heart and to the right of the pulmonary trunk (see Figures 4-9 and 4-10) and is commonly divided into ascending and descending

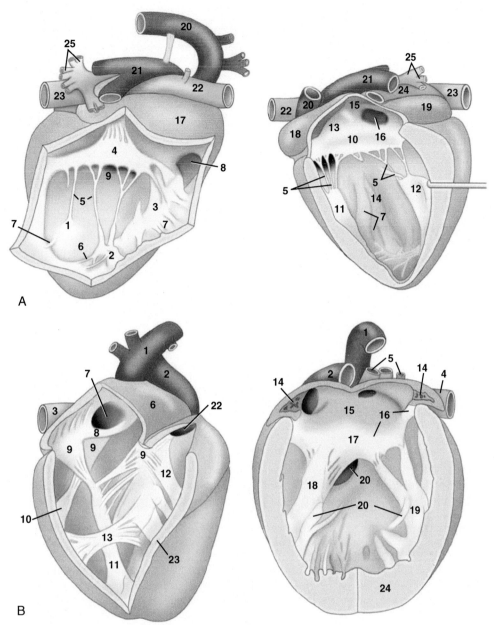

FIGURE 4-10 *A,* Internal anatomy of the heart of the rabbit with the right and left cavities, respectively. *1,* Small papillary muscle; *2,* great papillary muscle; *3,* subarterial papillary muscle; *4,* right AV valve; *5,* chordae tendineae; *6,* septomarginal trabecular; *7,* carneal trabeculae; *8,* opening of the pulmonary trunk; *9,* right AV opening; *10,* left AV valve; *11,* subauricular papillary muscle; *12,* subatrial papillary muscle; *13,* interatrial septum; *14,* interventricular septum; *15,* valve of oval foramen; *16,* ostium of pulmonary vein; *17,* right atrium; *18,* left auricle; *19,* left auricle; *20,* aorta; *21,* pulmonary trunk; *22,* right cranial vena cava; *23,* caudal vena cava; *24,* left cranial vena cava; *25,* pulmonary veins. *B,* Internal anatomy of the heart of the guinea pig of the right and left cavities, respectively. *1,* Aorta; *2,* pulmonary trunk; *3,* cranial vena cava; *4,* caudal vena cava; *5,* pulmonary veins; *6,* right auricle; *7,* sinus venosus; *8,* right AV fibrous ring; *9,* tricuspid valve; *10,* small papillary muscle; *11,* large papillary muscle; *12,* subarterial papillary muscle; *13,* septomarginal trabecula; *14,* left auricle; *15,* left atrium; *16,* left AV fibrous ring; *17,* mitral valve; *18,* subatrial papillary muscle; *19,* subauricular papillary muscle; *20,* septomarginal trabecular; *21,* opening of the aorta; *22,* opening of the pulmonary trunk; *23,* myocardium of right ventricle; *24,* myocardium of left ventricle. (Redrawn from Popesko P, Rajtova V, Horak J. *A Color Atlas of Anatomy of Small Laboratory Animals.* Bratislava: Wolfe Publishing; 1992:255.)

portions. The aorta is connected to the pulmonary trunk by the ligamentum arteriosum, which is the remnant of the ductus arteriosus. The aorta of the rabbit has rhythmic contractions of neurogenic origin.[101] The single brachiocephalic trunk (innominate artery) arising from the ascending aorta usually gives origin to two subclavian arteries and the carotid trunk that supply the pectoral limbs, head, and neck. The descending aorta gives origin to several arteries that supply the trunk, viscera, and posterior limbs. The most prominent branches are the caudal phrenic, lumbar, celiac, cranial mesenteric, renal, gonadal, caudal mesenteric, and external and internal iliac arteries.

The systemic venous system is composed cranially of the unpaired cranial vena cava (except in some species), which receives blood from two large jugular veins, and lymph at its origin from the thoracic duct. The rabbit lacks an anastomosis between the internal and external jugular veins, making it more prone to jugular distension with ensuing exophthalmos. The caudal vena cava receives blood from most posterior veins and is in close association with the right adrenal gland in ferrets. The portal vein drains blood from unpaired organs of the abdominal cavity to the liver, forming the hepatic portal system. The ears of rabbits have a large surface area and a large network of vessels with arteriovenous anastomoses that help with heat exchange.

The mammalian cardiovascular system is regulated through the autonomic nervous system (baroreceptor reflex, chemoreceptor reflex) and hormonal factors including the renin-angiotensin-aldosterone (RAA) system, antidiuretic hormone (ADH), natriuretic peptides, endothelial-derived factors, and inflammatory compounds.

Birds

Like mammals, all birds have a four-chambered heart with complete separation of the pulmonary and systemic circulation. Birds have evolved a highly efficient cardiovascular system that can generate greater cardiac output, stroke volume, and systemic blood pressure than any other animal group to meet the particularly high metabolic requirements of flight. Consequently, the anatomy and physiology of the avian cardiovascular system present some major differences from its mammalian counterparts, as summarized in Table 4-1.[102-106]

Birds have the fastest HR of any animals, but it can actually be lower than mammals of similar body weight. The HR can increase two to four times during flight (see Table 4-13 later).[102,108] The heart is located in the cranial thorax and lies ventrally in a concave indentation of the keel bone, the fascies visceralis sterni pars cardiac.[103] It is partially enclosed laterally and dorsally by the cranial part of the liver and not the lungs as in mammals, which are located dorsally in birds.[102,105] The heart rests dorsally against the bifurcation of the trachea (syrinx), the esophagus, and the horizontal septum on each side. It is surrounded by the cervical air sacs and interclavicular air sac cranially (and ventrally through a diverticulum that raises the pericardium in some species) and the cranial thoracic air sacs laterally.[107]

The heart is located in the pericardial cavity, which is delimited by the pericardium and contains a small volume of serous fluid that acts as a lubricant during the cardiac cycle. The pericardial cavity protrudes into the hepatoperitoneal

TABLE 4-1
Some Avian Cardiovascular Anatomical and Physiological Peculiarities That Differ from Mammals
Muscular unicuspid right AV valve
No chordae tendinae in the right AV valve
Tricuspid (poorly defined) left AV valve
Muscular ring around aortic valve
Ring of Purkinje fibers around aorta and right AV valve
Depolarization of epicardium precedes endocardium
Higher stroke volume, arterial blood pressure, and cardiac output and lower total peripheral resistance
Higher heart/body weight ratio
Smaller cardiac muscle fibers
Absence of T tubules in cardiac myocytes
Absence of M bands connecting myosin filaments
Ascending aorta on the right
Two cranial venae cavae
Brachiocephalic arteries larger than aorta
Cartilage/ossification at base of aorta
Most of myocardial vascularization derived from deep arteries
No cerebral arterial circle of Willis
Renal portal system

Adapted from References 102-104, 107.
AV, Atrioventricular.

cavities. The pericardial sac is attached to the sternum ventrally and laterally; to the hilus of the lungs and the horizontal septum dorsally (to which it is fused); to the oblique septum laterally; and to the liver caudally by the hepatopericardial ligament.[102,109,110] The hepatopericardial ligament is a doubled layer sheet that is continuous to the ventral mesentery caudally.[109] The fibrous layer of the pericardium is also continuous to the adventitia of the large blood vessels cranially.[102,107] The pericardial sac is noncompliant.

The avian cardiac chambers are functionally equivalent to their mammalian counterparts, with two atria and two ventricles composed of the endocardium, myocardium, and epicardium. In some species (e.g., chickens, crows, ostriches, kiwis), a sinus venosus is present as in lower vertebrates, prior to the right atrium. It is not fully incorporated into its wall and presents a thin sinoatrial valve composed of two valvules. It receives blood from the caudal vena cava and the right cranial vena cava and is separated from the opening of the left cranial vena cava by the septum sinus venosi.[103,105] The right atrium is generally larger than the left and possesses a tubular recess (recessus sinister atrii dextri) that extends to the left dorsally to the aortic root.[103,104] The left and right pulmonary veins open into the left atrium, either separately or combined in a common pulmonary vein outside the heart. In the left atrium, the veins coalesce in a single vessel whose opening protrudes into the left atrium (pulmonary chamber) and is guarded by the valve of the pulmonary vein.[105,109] The atrial muscle is composed of muscular bundles. The atria are separated from the ventricles externally by the fat-filled coronary groove and the main coronary arteries. They are separated

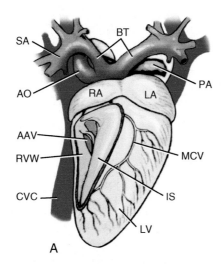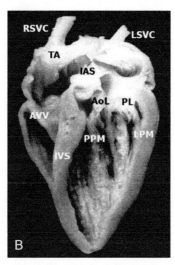

FIGURE 4-11 *A,* Anatomical drawing of the avian heart. The right ventricle is open. *AO,* Aorta; *AAV,* atrioventricular valve; *BT,* brachiocephalic trunks; *CVC,* caudal vena cava; *IS,* interventricular septum; *LA,* left atrium; *LV,* left ventricle; *MCV,* middle cardiac vein; *PA,* pulmonary arteries; *RA,* right atrium; *SA,* subclavian artery; *RVW,* right ventricular wall. *B,* Longitudinal section of the heart of the fowl. *AoL,* aortic leaflet or left atrioventricular valve; *AVV,* right atrioventricular valve; *IAS,* interatrial septum; *IVS,* interventricular septum; *LPM,* left papillary muscle; *LSVC,* left superior vena cava; *PL,* posterior leaflet of left atrioventricular valve; *PPM,* posterior papillary muscle; *RSVC,* right superior vena cava. (**A,** Modified and reprinted from Smith FM, West NH, Jones DR. The cardiovascular system. In: Whittow GC, ed. *Sturkie's Avian Physiology.* London: Academic Press; 2000:141-232, with permission from Elsevier; **B,** From Lu Y, James TN: *Anat Rec* 1993; 235(1):74-86.)

internally by fibrous rings (cardiac skeleton) that are well developed at the origin of the aorta, pulmonary artery, and right AV orifice.[107] A cardiac cartilage, sometimes mineralized, is present in the fibrous rings around the aorta and the pulmonary arteries.[107] The cone-shaped left ventricle extends to the apex of the heart, and its right wall forms the interventricular septum. The right ventricle wraps around the left ventricle (at least one-half of it), forming a crescent-shaped cavity, and does not reach to the apex (Figure 4-11). The wall of the left ventricle is about 2 to 3 times thicker and is able to generate 4 to 5 times higher systolic pressure than the right.[102,105] The right AV valve, unique to birds, is a triangular muscular flap formed of both atrial and ventricular musculature (see Figure 4-11). This valve is also connected to the roof of the right ventricle by a muscle bundle and to the interventricular septum by a small and narrow membrane.[105,107] The mechanisms of the avian right AV valve closure are poorly understood and probably partially active.[102] The left AV valve is a tricuspid valve with poorly defined cusps attached by chordae tendineae to the three left ventricular papillary muscles.[102,107]

The aortic valve located at the root of the ascending aorta also has three cusps and is apparent externally by the bulbus aortae, where in contrast to mammals, a complete sphincter-like ring of muscular tissue is present that may regulate outflow by contraction.[102,105] The pulmonary valve is tricuspid. Avian cardiomyocytes are smaller than those in mammals, lack the T tubules that are invaginations of the sarcolemma, and lack an M band that connects myosin filaments (see Table 4-1).[102] The physiological significance of these differences is poorly understood regarding the conduction velocity and contractile properties of avian cardiomyocytes.

As in mammals, two coronary arteries, the left and right coronary arteries, provide the arterial supply to the heart. They each branch into a superficial and deep ramus near their origin. The superficial branch is located in the coronary groove. Most of the avian cardiac coronary vascularization is provided through the deep rather than the superficial arteries.[102,103,105,107] The right coronary artery is the largest in most species, and the coronary arteries anastomose frequently.[102] Blood is returned to the right ventricle through several cardiac veins, for which the middle cardiac vein and the left circumflex cardiac vein are the largest (see Figure 4-11).

The avian cardiac conduction system is, similarly to mammals, composed of a sinoatrial node, AV node, right AV ring (specific to birds), and Purkinje fibers (bundle of His, bundle branches). The sinoatrial node, or pacemaker, is located between the right cranial vena cava and the caudal vena cava openings into the right atrium.[102,106] The AV node seems to be located at the base of the interatrial septum and serves to transmit electrical activity from the atria to the ventricles and delay ventricular contraction. Right and left ventricular bundle branches composed of Purkinje fibers run the length of the interventricular septum in the subendocardium and penetrate the myocardium along the coronary arteries. In birds, an AV ring of Purkinje fibers is present around the right AV valve and around the aorta in a figure-eight pattern and connected to the AV node.[102] The heart is innervated by both the sympathetic and parasympathetic autonomic nervous systems through the cardiac sympathetic nerve and the vagal nerve, respectively, and is controlled by cathecholamine release.

In birds, the aorta curves to the right and derives from the right fourth aortic arch, which is opposite to mammals, where the left aorta is conserved instead. The coronary arteries are the first to branch off the aorta, followed by two brachiocephalic trunks branching off simultaneously (only one in mammals). These trunks supply the large flight muscles through the subclavian arteries and are consequently larger than the ascending aorta that supplies the rest of the body.[102–104] The common carotid arteries branch from the brachiocephalic trunks as they curve to each side and supply the neck and head. The carotid arteries do not empty distally into a cerebral arterial circle of Willis as in mammals but have instead numerous intercarotid anastomoses with the vertebral arteries.[102] Specific adaptations are present in owls in response to their extreme neck mobility. The ascending aorta supplies the trunk, visceral organs, and pelvic limbs through its successive branches, namely, the celiac, cranial renal, external iliac (femoral artery), ischiatic, caudal mesenteric, and internal iliac arteries for its major arterial trunks.[103] The pulmonary trunk emerges from the right ventricle and divides into the left and right pulmonary arteries.[103] As in other vertebrates, arteries in birds are structurally classified into the elastic arteries composed of the aortic arch, thoracic aorta up to the celiac artery, brachiocephalic trunks, and extrapulmonary portions of the pulmonary arteries, with the muscular arteries comprising the remainder of the arterial system.[102,104] Arteries are also composed of the same three layers (tunica intima, media, and adventitia) as in other vertebrates.

The venous system presents some peculiarities in birds compared to mammals, with notably two cranial venae cavae and a renal portal system. The cranial venae cavae receive blood from the jugular veins and the subclavian veins. The jugular veins anastomose at the base of the head.[102] The renal portal system constitutes a ring ventral to the kidney, with blood supplied from the gut and pelvic region through the vertebral sinus, external iliac vein, ischiatic vein, internal iliac vein, and caudal mesenteric vein. A valve, the renal portal valve, is present in the common iliac vein that is open under sympathetic stimulation, with blood diverting to the caudal vena cava, which increases the blood return directly to the heart. The venous flow can be diverted to the hepatic portal system through the caudal mesenteric vein, where flow can be bidirectional.[104]

As in other vertebrates, the control of peripheral blood flow is achieved by contraction of the muscular fibers modulated by a combination of autoregulatory mechanisms, action of humoral factors, and neural control.

CARDIOVASCULAR DISEASES

Pathophysiology of Congestive Heart Disease

Congestive heart failure is not a disease in itself but the ultimate consequence of a structural or functional problem that affects parts of the cardiovascular and pulmonary systems. The pathophysiology of congestive heart failure has mainly been studied in mammals but is likely to be roughly similar across vertebrate taxons because of shared neuroendocrine

regulatory pathways of circulation and hemodynamic constraints.[111] However, physiological regulation of the cardiovascular system and the relative importance of neural vs. humoral influence may vary across animal taxons. Compared to mammals, which rely mainly on the renal and gastrointestinal systems for volume regulation, other species may have other organs involved in osmoregulation such as salt glands in marine birds, gills in fish, and skin in amphibians. In addition, respiratory physiology, cardiac shunting abilities (e.g., reptiles, amphibians), and reliance on lymphatic circulation (e.g., amphibians and reptiles) may greatly influence mechanisms of heart failure and edema formation across species.

Congestive heart failure occurs when the volume of blood presented to the heart is in excess of what can be pumped into the arterial system, with ensuing organ congestion and decreased cardiac output. Heart failure can be due to abnormalities in the cardiac conduction system, valvular system, cardiac muscle, blood shunting, infection, impaired systolic and diastolic function, and inadequate preload and afterload. Regardless of the inciting cause, each of these events produces a decline in cardiac pump function. All heart diseases do not necessarily lead to congestive heart failure, but it is a frequent clinical end point. Cases of congestive heart failure have mainly been reported in reptiles, birds, and mammals (see sections on Reptiles, Mammals, and Birds).

At the onset of congestive heart failure, decrease in cardiac output and blood pressure is detected by chemoreceptors, baroreceptors, cardiac mechanoreceptors, and the renal juxtaglomerular apparatus. Several compensatory measures similar to those induced by blood loss and dehydration take place to initially preserve cardiac output but may become counterproductive in the long term in the case of congestive heart failure.[112,113] The magnitude, relative importance, and determinants of cardiovascular compensation may vary among animal groups, but the same basic principles and the necessity to maintain cardiac output apply to all. Activation of sympathetic tone causes an increase in HR, contractility, and vasomotor tone as well as the activation of the RAA system (RAAS) and stimulation of arginine vasopressin (arginine vasotocin in nonmammalian vertebrates) release.[112,114] Renin released from the juxtaglomerular complex under stimuli such as hypotension, hypovolemia, decreased plasma sodium, and catecholamines accelerates the conversion of circulating angiotensinogen into angiotensin I, which is itself converted into angiotensin II by the angiotensin-converting enzyme. Angiotensin II promotes thirst, vasomotor tone, and the production of aldosterone, which causes water and sodium retention. Fishes do not produce aldosterone; instead, 11-deoxycorticosterone (precursor of aldosterone in mammals) and/or cortisol are the mineralocorticoid effectors.[111,115] Aldosterone is also a mediator of inflammation and fibrosis. Furthermore, a variety of vasodilatory molecules are released to counteract the excessive vasoconstriction caused by the adrenergic system and RAAS, including the natriuretic peptides, prostaglandins, and nitric oxide.[113] Interestingly, invertebrates also possess a rudimentary renin-angiotensin-like system.[116]

Most clinical signs are the result of these compensatory mechanisms to restore and maintain cardiac output and blood pressure associated with an increase in preload and afterload. Furthermore, the heart undergoes some changes (cardiac remodeling) in response to the hemodynamic challenges (pressure or volume overload), cardiac injury from dilation and hypertrophy, and consequences to neurohormone over-expression.[113,114] The increased preload leads to edema and effusion, and the increased afterload further impairs cardiac output. Low cardiac output and limited cardiovascular adaptive abilities in response to exercise can cause exercise intolerance, syncope, tachycardia, cyanosis, decreased peripheral perfusion, and arrhythmias.

In reptiles and amphibians, considering the physiologic importance of blood shunting mechanisms and the sophistication of differential blood ejection by the single cardiac ventricle, it is reasonable to assume that impaired cardiac function and chamber dilation may have great physiological consequences on blood oxygenation and ventilatory/perfusion mismatch. In addition, global congestive heart failure is to be expected in species possessing only one ventricle.

Invertebrates

Reports of circulatory diseases are scarce in invertebrates despite their wide use in cardiovascular research.[11] Nonspecific circulatory disturbances and lesions of the circulatory system can be encountered as part of systemic infections or with dehydration and hemolymph loss.

Since arthropods have an open circulatory system, insects and arachnids can lose a substantial volume of hemolymph with significant trauma or large wounds. Also, pathogens may easily gain access to the body through the wound and disseminate throughout the open circulatory system. For these reasons, arthropods rely on hemolymph clotting more extensively than vertebrates.[117] Trauma and subsequent hemolymph loss is especially common in spiders, and exsanguination is a frequent cause of death.[20] Wounds over the dorsal opisthosoma where the heart and pericardial sinus reside can lose a large volume of hemolymph quickly, and small wounds on the limbs, depending on their location, may also lead to significant hemolymph loss (hemolymph pressure in the appendages can be high in spiders).[20] Dehydration and hypovolemia are also common occurrences in spiders and impair locomotion that depends on prosomal hydraulic pressure.

Myocarditis has been diagnosed on histopathology in a variety of invertebrates having a central heart, such as mollusks and arthropods, but is generally part of a more systemic condition. Likewise, vasculitis can be encountered in infectious and inflammatory conditions. Five cases of myocarditis were documented in the common cuttlefish associated with *Vibrio* spp. infection, with inflammatory lesions found in the central and two branchial hearts.[118] A significant disease of commercially exploited *Nephrops* lobsters is a microsporidian parasite (*Myospora metanephros*) that causes destruction of heart and skeletal muscles.[119] Vasculitis in brachial arteries has been associated with an automutilation syndrome in nine octopuses from three species.[120]

Changes associated with aging have been reported in the heart of various invertebrates (e.g., honeybee).[121] Neoplasia seems to be quite rare in most invertebrate phyla but are reported more often in bivalves.[17,122] Neoplasias of the circulatory system in bivalves include pericardial tumors in three oysters, a cardiac vesicular cell sarcoma in an Eastern oyster (*Crassostrea virginica*), and a cardiac mesothelioma in an Atlantic surf clam (*Spisula solidissima*).[122–124]

Fish

Piscine Congestive Heart Failure

Specific papers on the pathophysiology of congestive heart failure and edema in fish are scarce, but edema due to cardiac failure is common. The mechanisms of edema formation are incompletely understood and could be due directly to heart failure or failure of the renal and branchial circulations, leading to disruption of normal osmoregulation.[125] Infectious diseases and associated myocardial inflammation and necrosis are the most common causes of piscine heart failure. Peripheral circulatory failure, also reported to be frequent in fish, results from destruction of the skin and loss of fluids through the capillaries.[125]

Infectious and Parasitic Diseases

Reported cardiovascular lesions in fish are mainly infectious, with a wide variety of bacterial, viral, and parasitic agents described (Table 4-2).[33,37] In addition, cardiac infections are usually part of a systemic infection, and infectious agents rarely target specifically the cardiovascular system. A great deal of pathologic information is available in farmed salmonids (e.g., salmon, trout), but cardiovascular literature is minimal in ornamental fish. Pericarditis is common with bacterial

TABLE 4-2

Common Pathogens Affecting the Heart of Fish

Bacteria	*Renibacterium salmoninarum* (salmonids)
	Aeromonas salmonicida
	Pasteurella skyensis
	Flavobacterium psychrophilum (salmonids)
	Vibrio spp.
	Yersinia spp.
	Mycobacteria spp.
	Lactococcus spp.
	Pseudomonas spp.
	Streptococcus spp.
	Nocardia seriolae
Viruses	Viral hemorrhagic septicemia (rhabdovirus)
	Infectious hematopoietic necrosis (rhabdovirus)
	Herpesvirus (trout)
	Alphavirus (pancreatic disease virus of salmons)
	Heart and skeletal muscle inflammation disease
	Cardiomyopathy syndrome of salmon (Totiviridae)
	Infectious salmon anemia virus (Orthomyxoviridae)
Parasites	Digenean trematodes (Metacercariae)
	Cestodes (encapsulated larvae)
	Crustacean *Lernaeocera branchialis*
	Contracaecum spp. nematode larvae
Fungi	*Exophiala* spp.
	Phoma spp.
	Ichthyophonus hoferi

Adapted from References 33, 37, 125.

septicemia, but cardiac lesions may also include epicarditis, myocarditis, and valvular endocarditis (uncommon).[33,125]

Most fish viruses can lead to viremia, generalized disease, and multifocal cardiac lesions, but a few viral diseases have cardiac tropism (see Table 4-2).[33,125] The alphavirus responsible for the salmon pancreas disease induces lesions in the atrium and in the spongy and compact layers of the ventricle.[33] The disease called heart and skeletal muscle inflammation is responsible for myocarditis in salmon but seems to be restricted to farms in Norway and the United Kingdom. Epidemiology of the disease suggests a viral etiology, and a reovirus has been recovered from affected fishes.[33,126] The cardiomyopathy syndrome of Atlantic salmon is associated with myocarditis, thrombosis, and ruptured heart chambers. The cause was unknown until recently when a totivirus was shown to be the causative agent.[33,125,127] The disease affects the atrium and the spongy myocardium and causes death in large adult salmon.

Systemic fungal infections may extend to the heart, and *Ichthyophonus hoferi*, a pathogen of both salmonids and aquarium fish, is a common cause of granulomatous myocarditis and epicarditis.[33,128,129] Encapsulated larvae of cestodes and trematodes are commonly found in myocardium and may block the AV opening.[33] *Contracaecum* spp. nematode larvae seem to preferentially affect the atrium of fishes.[130] *Lernaeocera branchialis*, a crustacean copepod, can feed directly from the ventral aorta and bulbus arteriosus while externally on the host and is a significant parasite in aquaculture.[131]

Developmental Abnormalities
Cardiac anomalies are increasingly diagnosed in farmed salmonids. Aplasia or hypoplasia of the septum transversum causes the heart to herniate into the abdominal cavity.[33,132,133] Affected fish are lethargic, and low mortality may be seen. On necropsy, hearts have an abnormal shape and other concomitant cardiac abnormalities may be seen such as situs invertus and ventricular hypoplasia.[133] Ascites may also be noted. Factors such as genetic selection and high water temperature during egg incubation and larval development may be implicated.[33,125,133,134] Abnormal location of the heart (situs invertus) as a single occurrence is reported to be common in farmed salmon.[33] Hypoplasia of the ventricular myocardium, ventricular aneurysms, and abnormal ventricular shape are also reported.[33]

Miscellaneous Cardiac Diseases
Nutritional cardiomyopathies have been recorded in farmed salmonids and include deficiencies in vitamin E/selenium and excess in linoleic acid.[33,37,125] Another disease with an unknown etiology characterized by posterior paralysis, aortic thrombosis, and intervertebral disk extrusion can affect a large number of fish.[33] Myocardial glycogen storage was described in farmed rainbow trout.[135]

Vascular Diseases
Nonspecific vascular lesions are reported to be common in fish in association with infectious processes.[33] Fish rhabdoviruses (see Table 4-2) have a vascular tropism and induce vasculitis and petechiae.[33,125] Mycotic invasions of vessels occur with *Branchiomyces sanguinis* from branchial vessels and *Saprolegnia* from visceral vessels. Aneurysms and dissecting aneurysms are seen with toxins, trauma, parasites, and bacteria, and lesions appear to be more common in the bulbus arteriosus.[33] Adult flukes of the genus *Sanguinicola* live in branchial and other vessels and may occlude blood vessels.[136]

Arteriosclerosis is a prevalent lesion in wild and farmed salmonids, and lesions typically occur at the main coronary artery, especially at its bifurcation from the bulbus arteriosus ventrally. Lesions consist of smooth muscle proliferation that narrows the arterial lumen, but the lesions seem to have no lipid or calcium, which is very different from the atherosclerotic lesions found in mammals and birds.[33,41,137] Increased cholesterol and low-density lipoprotein (LDL) were reported in association with fish arteriosclerotic lesions as was rapid body growth.[41] However, the clinical significance of coronary arteriosclerosis in fishes is unclear. Lesions are unlikely to lead to acute myocardial ischemia, but chronic ischemia is possible.[41]

Vascular tumors are infrequent in fish, although hemangiomas and hemangioendotheliomas have been reported, especially on the heart.

Amphibians

Edema/Hydrops
Primary cardiovascular diseases seem to be uncommon in amphibians. However, subcutaneous, lymphatic, and abdominal edema (together referred as hydrops) is common (Figure 4-12) and can be due to various causes that disrupt the skin homeostatic function (Table 4-3). Localized edema may also arise. Commonly reported infectious agents causing hydrops include *Mycobacterium* spp., chlamydial agents, *Flavobacterium* spp., systemic fungi, and ranaviruses.[53,138] Edema from sepsis is thought to occur as a result of disruption of capillaries, lymphatics, or epidermis. The tadpole edema virus (ranavirus) is an important emerging disease of amphibians worldwide.[139] Hypocalcemia may impair lymph heart contractions and cause edema.[140] Other diseases of lymph sacs known to cause

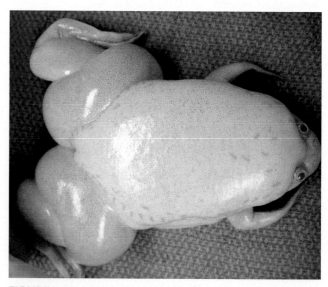

FIGURE 4-12 African clawed frog *(Xenopus laevis)* presented with hydrops.

TABLE 4-3
Differential Diagnosis for Frog Edema
Bacterial septicemia (G–)
Mycobacteriosis
Ranavirus
Parasites
Heart failure
Lymphatic heart disorders
Renal diseases
Hepatic diseases
Skin diseases
Hypoosmolar water
Ovarian hyperstimulation syndrome
Liver diseases
Hypocalcemia
Hypoproteinemia
Neoplastic diseases
Genetic/congenital diseases

Adapted from References 140-142.

hydrops include parasites, toxins, traumatic handling, and outflow obstructions.[140]

Infectious and Parasitic Diseases

Extension of systemic infection to the heart is uncommon in amphibians despite the relatively high prevalence of septicemia.[53,142] With that said, myocarditis, epicarditis, and cardiac granulomas have been diagnosed with *Myobacterium* spp., *Chlamydophila* spp., candidiasis, zygomycosis, geotrichosis, chromomycosis, phaehyphomycosis, and ranaviruses (frog virus 3, tadpole edema virus).[53,142]

Since the skin has important functions in osmoregulation, skin diseases may also cause electrolytic imbalances that have cardiac effects. For instance, it has been demonstrated that chytridiomycosis (caused by the fungus *Batrachochytrium dendrobatidis*) alters epithelial electrolyte transports, resulting in systemic depletion of sodium, potassium, and chloride, subsequently leading to cardiac arrest.[143,144] Electrolyte imbalances altering cardiac conduction may be the main mechanism by which amphibian mortality occurs with chytridiomycosis.[143,144]

A large number of parasites may cause lesions in the myocardium, and their importance depends on the amphibian species and their ecology. Most scientific reports come from wild amphibian populations. Trematode metacercariae of Diplostomidae are found in the pericardial sac of wild-caught African clawed frogs (*Xenopus laevis*), one of its secondary hosts, and cause pericardial effusion and respiratory compromise.[53,145,146] The digenean trematodes *Clinostomum* spp. infect the lymph sacs and pericardial cavity of *Xenopus laevis*.[147] Trypanosomes have been found in the cardiovascular system of Anurans, such as *Trypanosoma inopinatum* in the green frog (*Rana esculante*).[148] Larval migrans from the lungworm *Rhabdias* spp. penetrate the skin of amphibians and can travel through the heart before reaching the lungs.[53,149] In Australasia, the larvae of the dipteran *Batrachomyia* spp. parasitize the dorsal lymph sacs of *Rana* spp. while maintaining breathing holes.[150,151]

Miscellaneous

A variety of congenital and genetic cardiovascular malformations have been described in amphibians.[53,142,152] Laboratory African clawed frogs (*Xenopus laevis*) are sporadically found with nonfunctional lymph hearts, resulting in edema. Newts of the species *Pleurodeles waltl* have been documented with tail edema due to an autosomal recessive trait. A "cardiac nonfunction" mutation is reported in Mexican axolotls (*Ambystoma mexicanum*) that results in a nonbeating heart and edema in homozygous animals. Subcutaneous edema has been observed after metamorphosis in African clawed frogs. In addition, this frog species has been extensively used to study cardiac morphogenesis and congenital defects.

Cuban tree frogs (*Osteopilus septentrionalis*) have been diagnosed with atherosclerosis of the major arteries concomitantly with corneal lipidosis and cutaneous xanthomatosis.[153,154] This lipid disorder was associated with hypercholesterolemia in some but not all cases, and nutritional causes may have been implicated.[153,154] Atherosclerosis and myocarditis were diagnosed in three frogs and a Colombian horned frog (*Ceratophrys* sp.).[155] Cardiovascular neoplasms appear to be extremely rare in amphibians.[142]

Reptiles

Myocardial Diseases

Cardiomyopathy with subsequent congestive heart failure has been reported in a Deckert's rat snake (*Elaphe obsoleta deckertii*) and a mole king snake (*Lampropeltis calligaster rhombomaculata*).[156,157] No underlying etiology was found in either case despite the fact that both animals showed signs of systemic disease. Postmortem examination of the rat snake showed degeneration and necrosis of myocardial fibers and mineralization of blood vessels, with focal aggregates of lymphocytes inside the lamina. The lesions in the king snake were primarily collagen proliferation and osteoid-like material within the myocardium. Cardiomyopathy has also been reported in two pythons, a Children's python (*Liasis childreni*) and a juvenile Burmese python and dilated cardiomyopathy (DCM) was observed post mortem in an adult black king snake (*Lampropeltis niger*) that presented for marked cardiomegaly, dilatation of the ventricle, and congestive heart failure.[158,159]

Vitamin E deficiency has been implicated in myocardial degeneration.[160,161] The lesions resemble those described in mammals; gross examination usually reveals a whitish to gray myocardium, and multifocal losses of myocytes replaced by fibrous stroma are seen on microscopy.

Urate crystals that accumulate during visceral gout have been shown to form within the myocardium.[162] Gout can be of metabolic, nutritional, or iatrogenic origin.[162–164]

Valvular Diseases

The only current valvular diseases described in reptiles are of an infectious etiology: vegetative endocarditis. To the authors' knowledge, degenerative endocardiosis has not been reported in reptiles to date. However, a right AV insufficiency of undetermined origin has been reported in one carpet python (*Morelia spilota variegata*), resulting in bilateral heart failure.[165] Congenital cardiac disease was suspected because of the young age of the reptile patient, clinical signs, and physical examination findings. Due to the lack of septation in Squamata and chelonia, elevated diastolic pressures could be shared across all ventricular compartments, resulting in bilateral heart failure. Valvular regurgitation is usually confirmed on echocardiography, such as in a reported case of sinoatrial and AV insufficiencies in a Burmese python (Figure 4-13).[166]

Pericardial Diseases

Visceral gout can lead to severe pericardial lesions and is easily recognizable on postmortem examination by the thickening of the pericardium, with urate crystal deposition.[162] Primary disease can be metabolic, nutritional, or iatrogenic.[160,162–164]

A Californian desert tortoise (Gopherus agassizii) that presented with cervical fractures was also diagnosed with osteomyelitis and pericardial effusion.[167] Unfortunately, no attempt was made to investigate the importance or underlying cause of the pericardial effusion. An 80-year-old male spur-thighed tortoise (Testudo graeca) with posthibernation anorexia and lethargy was diagnosed on echocardiography with pericardial effusion, atrial dilatation, and liver masses.[168] Radiography showed pneumonia and/or pulmonary edema. Following unsuccessful treatment, the patient was euthanized and postmortem findings confirmed the diagnosis. In another report, pericardial effusion was diagnosed in a 2-year-old male bearded dragon (Pogona vitticeps) that presented with a 3-week history of anorexia and extreme lethargy.[169] The diagnosis was made by ultrasonography and also revealed atherosclerosis in the major arteries at the base of the heart. Another case of pericardial effusion was seen in a bearded dragon by the authors. A female reticulated python (Python reticularis) diagnosed with endocardial fibrosarcoma at the base of the aorta showed concomitant pericardial effusion.[170] Pericardial effusion is typically detected by a combination of radiographs and cardiac ultrasound (Figures 4-14 and 4-15).

Heart venipuncture is the most commonly used site for collecting blood from snakes because it yields a meaningful sample volume, is relatively well tolerated by snakes, and has proven to be safe.[171–173] However, hemopericardium and organized hematoma have been reported.[172,174] Noniatrogenic hemopericardium was also observed in conjunction with a myocardial abscess in a green iguana (Iguana iguana).[175]

Infectious Diseases

In captive reptiles, infectious diseases of the cardiovascular system are usually secondary to systemic infections. West Nile virus has been reported to cause myocardial degeneration and necrosis in farmed American alligators (Alligator mississippiensis).[176–179] Snakes with inclusion body disease (IBD) typically have large eosinophilic intracytoplasmic inclusion bodies in different organs, including the heart.[180–183] Although this disease is thought to be of a viral etiology, the causative agent has not yet been conclusively identified. To date, Koch's postulates have not been fulfilled to conclude on a causal relationship between ferlavirus and IBD.

Cardiovascular lesions caused by Chlamydophila spp. have been reported in various species of reptiles. These included granulomatous pericarditis and myocarditis in a puff adder (Bitis arietans) and necrotizing myocarditis in green sea turtles (Chelonia mydas).[184,185] Histopathological sections from the heart and organs of an emerald tree boa (Corallus caninus) showed histiocytic granulomas and small basophilic organisms.[186] Transmission electron microscopy of an intestinal granuloma demonstrated chlamydial organisms. Other bacterial species have also been implicated in myocardial infections. A granulomatous myocarditis due to Salmonella arizonae was diagnosed in an 8-year-old Dumerili's boa (Acrantophis dumerili) based on positive coelomic effusion culture, ultrasound visualization of abnormal ventricular myocardium, necropsy, and cardiac histological examination.[187] Microscopy demonstrated a granulomatous myocarditis associated with a fibrinous and necrotic pericarditis. Evidence of granulomatous hepatitis, pneumonia, and thyroiditis were also seen with granulomatous infiltration. Bacterial organisms were observed on the histological sections of these organs.

Aerobic gram-negative bacteria are the most common isolates from secondary endocarditis. A mass in the right atrium causing blood flow obstruction in a Burmese python was diagnosed with ultrasonography and angiography. The patient did not survive treatment, and postmortem examination confirmed the mass to be a septic atrial thrombus, from which both Salmonella arizonae and Corynebacterium spp. were isolated.[188] A Vibrio damsela was isolated from a vegetative thrombus attached to the left AV valve and interventricular wall of a stranded leatherback turtle (Dermochelys coriacea).[189] Valvular endocarditis and dilated pulmonary trunk in a Burmese python were diagnosed ante mortem and were associated with a Salmonella enterica sepsis.[190] In a patient from the same species, sinoatrial and AV insufficiencies were diagnosed on echocardiographic examination.[166] In this report, the concomitant finding of a double valvular insufficiency and bacterial pneumonia made the diagnosis of bacterial endocarditis likely, but this could not be confirmed.

Parasitic Diseases

Trematodes have been recorded in the heart chambers and major vessels of chelonians, attached to or freely floating within the lumen.[191] Most cases of fluke infestations occur in saltwater and freshwater turtles, especially in wild and wild-caught animals. Postmortem examination of 96 stranded green sea turtles showed infestation with spirorchid flukes.[192] Cardiovascular lesions speculated to be caused by the infestation included arteritis, endocarditis, thrombosis, and occasional aneurysm formation. A similar necropsy finding in black sea turtles (Chelonia mydas agassizii) noted the presence of spirorchid eggs and adult Learedius learei inside the heart.[59] Sixteen laboratory freshwater turtles (Trachemys scripta elegans and Chrysemys picta) died over a 5-year period. Necropsy revealed, among other lesions, spirorchid eggs in multiple organs including the myocardium, in association with granulomatous lesions.[193]

A study in the United States characterizing the prevalence of the cestode Mesocestoides sp. tetrathyridia in 220 wild whiptail lizards (Cnemidophorus spp.) found a 5% prevalence of encapsulated parasites in the heart, liver, and stomach as well as free coelomic tetrathyridia.[194]

The filarial nematode Macdonaldius oschei has been demonstrated to infest the cardiovascular system of reptiles.[195] Females release large numbers of microfilaria into the circulation, which can be observed on myocardial histology and fresh blood smears.[160] High burdens of adults in the circulatory system can lead to edema, thrombosis, and necrosis.[196] Because M. oschei requires multiple hosts to complete its life cycle, infestation tends to be restricted to wild and wild-caught

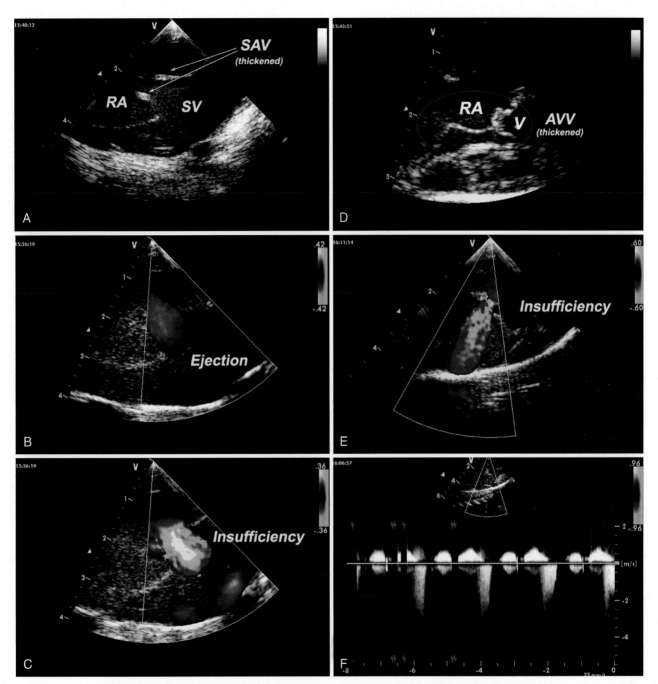

FIGURE 4-13 Double valvular insufficiency diagnosed on echocardiography in a Burmese python *(Python molurus bivittatus);* the insufficiency is evidenced on color Doppler examination of the sinoatrial valves. *A,* Two-dimensional echocardiography (right transatrial short-axis view) showing the abnormal sinoatrial valves during atrial systole; *B,C,* AV insufficiency; *D,* two-dimensional echocardiography (right AV long-axis view) showing the abnormal right AV valvular leaflet; *E,* color Doppler examination of the AV valve showing a marked aliased regurgitation in the right atrium during ventricular systole; *F,* continuous-wave Doppler mode examination confirming a high-velocity regurgitant jet (peak velocity of 4 m/s, *arrows*). *RA,* Right atrium; *SAV,* sinoatrial valve; *SV,* sinus venosus; *V,* ventricle. (Reprinted from Schilliger L, Trehiou E, Petit AMP, et al. Double valvular insufficiency in a Burmese python *(Python molurus bivittatus,* Linnaeus, 1758) suffering from concomitant bacterial pneumonia. *J Zoo Wildl Med.* 2010;41(4):742-744.)

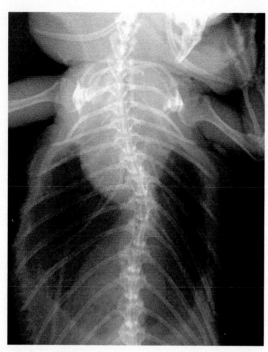

FIGURE 4-14 Enlarged radiographic cardiac silhouette in a bearded dragon *(Pogona vitticeps)* with pericardial effusion and concurrent atherosclerosis. (Reprinted from Schilliger L, Lemberger K, Chai N, et al. Atherosclerosis associated with pericardial effusion in a central bearded dragon [*Pogona vitticeps*, Ahl. 1926]. *J Vet Diagn Invest.* 2010;225:789-792. With permission by the American Association of Veterinary Laboratory Diagnosticians.)

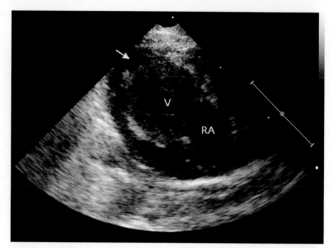

FIGURE 4-15 Pericardial effusion *(arrow)* diagnosed with echocardiography (postpectoral girdle window) in a bearded dragon *(Pogona vitticeps). RA,* right atrium; *V,* ventricle.

animals, because it is possible to break the life cycle in captivity with strategic use of antiparasitic and avoidance of intermediate hosts.

Protozoal infections (besnoitiosis and sarcosporidiosis) are occasionally observed in histological sections of ophidian hearts.[160]

Congenital Defects

It is thought that congenital defects are rare in reptiles. Aortic valvular stenosis with secondary cardiomyopathy was reported in a Children's python, and ventricular mural hypoplasia with plasmacytic pericarditis was reported in a juvenile Burmese python.[159] Aortic stenosis associated with dilatation of the right atrium and the ventricle was found in a green iguana.[197] Histopathological examination revealed atrophy of myocardial fibers and a thickening of the intima of both aortic arches, with consequent narrowing of the lumen. Although the cause was not determined, the authors suggested chronic congenital lesions as a differential. Bilateral subaortic stenosis was described in an alligator.[198] A secundum atrial septal defect was reported in a Komodo dragon *(Varanus komodoensis).*[199] The defect was located on the craniodorsal portion of the interatrial septum. Two cases of bifid ventricles and cardiac malformations were reported in juvenile ball pythons *(Python regius).*[200] In both cases, all cardiac chambers were enlarged and abnormally shaped, with a particularly reduced muscular ridge causing a lack of ventricular pressure separation normally found in pythons.

Vascular Diseases

It is uncommon for vascular diseases to be lethal in reptiles. The low prevalence of atherosclerosis in reptiles is probably related to their comparatively low systemic blood pressure.

A Burmese python was presented with acute respiratory arrest following constriction of a prey. A diagnosis of aortic aneurysm rupture was made on postmortem examination. Multiple organized thrombi were found in the intimal wall and in the heart muscle.[201] Necropsy of a Spanish pond turtle *(Mauremys leprosa)* following sudden death was conclusive of rupture of one of the major arteries of the aortic-pulmonary trunk, causing mediastinal hemorrhage.[202] Histopathology revealed granulomatous arteritis with mural thrombi, lipid deposition, and thickening of the vessel intima, with necrosis and calcification. A dissecting aortic aneurysm was also reported in a sail-tailed lizard *(Hydrosaurus amboinensis),* causing hemorrhage and formation of hematomas in the coelom.[161]

Various forms of medial calcification with or without secondary intimal thickening have been documented in reptiles. In many cases, calcification is thought to be associated with metabolic bone disease.[202] Indeed, animals suffering from secondary nutritional hyperparathyroidism may develop metastatic calcification despite a relative or absolute calcium deficiency.[160,196] Although arteriosclerosis has been documented, mainly in green iguanas, most reported cases consist of subintimal and medial calcifications.[160,161,203,204] Atherosclerosis is poorly documented in reptiles.[169,202,205,206] A few small plaques were found in the abdominal aorta of a two-banded monitor *(Varanus salvator).*[205] In another report, atherosclerosis and pericardial effusion were diagnosed in a 2-year-old male central bearded dragon, based on ultrasound visualization, necropsy, and histological examination.[169]

Neoplasia

Primary neoplasia of the cardiovascular system is uncommon in reptiles. Reported cases include a rhabdomyosarcoma in a boa constrictor *(Boa constrictor),* a cardiac hemangioma of the left atrium in a corn snake *(Pantherophis guttatus),* a fibrosarcoma in a Gaboon viper *(Bitis gabonica),* and a 3 to 4 cm endocardial fibrosarcoma in a reticulated python *(Python reticulatus)*.[170,207-209] In most cases, cardiac tumors in snakes present as a distinct mass that can be visible in the cardiac regions (at ~1/4 of the length of the snake from the rostrum). Tumors of primary or metastatic origin have also been reported, such as lymphoblastic malignant lymphoma.[210,211] A disseminated mast cell tumor diagnosed in an eastern king snake *(Lampropeltis getulus getulus)* involved the heart and numerous other organs.[212] A study of 255 necropsied stranded green turtles suffering from fibropapillomatosis found that 39% had disseminated internal tumors, most of them in the lung, kidney, and heart.[213]

Mammals

Prevalence of Cardiac Diseases in Exotic Mammals
The prevalence of cardiovascular diseases is difficult to estimate with precision in exotic companion mammals because of the lack of epidemiological studies and only a handful of published case reports. Nevertheless, cardiac diseases seem to occur relatively frequently at least in ferrets, rabbits, guinea pigs, chinchillas *(Chinchilla lanigera)*, woodchucks, rats, hamsters, and African hedgehogs *(Atelerix albiventris)* in captivity, based on the few published surveys and personal clinical experience of the authors.[92,98,214-221] In retrospective postmortem surveys, degenerative cardiac diseases were qualified as common in pet ferrets, rabbits, guinea pigs, and hamsters.[220,222-224] A retrospective study of 95 ferrets that had a cardiac evaluation found congestive heart failure in 17 (18%) of them.[225] In a study on 260 chinchillas, 59 (23%) had audible cardiac murmurs on auscultation that translated into echocardiographic abnormalities in 8 (53%) of 15 animals, with valvular disease being the most common finding.[214] A retrospective study found 15% of chinchillas to have degenerative cardiac diseases on postmortem examination.[226] Heart conditions also appear to be prevalent in African hedgehogs. A postmortem study identified cardiomyopathies in 16 (38%) of 42 hedgehogs.[215] Three cases of congestive heart failure have been reported in guinea pigs.[219,227] Laboratory rats suffer from a high prevalence of myocardial degeneration and fibrosis with aging (murine progressive cardiomyopathy) that can reach 70% to 100% by 2 years.[218] Cardiovascular histologic lesions were diagnosed in 14 (5.6%) of 250 hamsters in a postmortem survey.[220] Congestive heart failure is also reported to be frequent in geriatric hamsters.[220] Noninfectious cardiac diseases are not documented in sugar gliders.[226,228]

Dilated Cardiomyopathy
DCM has been described in ferrets, rabbits, guinea pigs, rats, Syrian hamsters *(Mesocricetus auratus)*, and prairie dogs *(Cynomys ludovicianus)*, but it appears to be a common clinical entity only in ferrets and African hedgehogs (see Table 4-21 later).[92,98,215-217,223,227,229-234] The disease is clinically similar to the condition in dogs and cats. The etiology of DCM in ferrets and hedgehogs is unknown, but it results in progressive dilation of the cardiac chambers, decreased contractility, systolic and diastolic dysfunction, and, ultimately, congestive heart failure. DCM is a primary myocardial disease and should be differentiated from other diseases responsible for volume overload and cardiac chamber enlargement. Clinical signs are typical of left or right heart failure in mammals, including pleural effusion, ascites, and pulmonary edema.[98,216,233,235-237]

In ferrets, the disease is thought to account for about 80% of cardiologic cases.[216] A report found a prevalence of 4% (4/95) in ferrets undergoing echocardiographic examinations.[225] Another report from Germany found a 25% prevalence in ferrets.[238] However, the disease seems to have decreased in prevalence in North America, presumably due to improved nutrition.[223] In ferrets and hedgehogs, most cases occur in older animals.[98,230,232] Syrian hamsters are used as an animal model of DCM. In susceptible strains of this species, the disease is due to an inherited genetic defect, resulting in an abnormal sarcoplasmic reticulum.[239] Two spontaneous cases in pet hamsters have also been reported.[233] Several spontaneous DCM cases have been described in rabbits, and giant breeds are thought to be more susceptible.[92,233,240] The chemotherapeutic drug doxorubicin is also known to induce myocardial failure and left ventricular dilation in rabbits, guinea pigs, and mice *(Mus musculus)*.[241,242]

Cardiomegaly secondary to DCM is usually appreciated on thoracic radiographs and echocardiography (Figures 4-16 and 4-17).[98,231] The latter allows the confirmation of the diagnosis; echographic abnormalities are similar to those in dogs and cats, with a reduction of the left ventricular fractional shortening, valvular regurgitations, and dilation of heart chambers. Arrhythmias, when present, may include ventricular and atrial premature contractions, ventricular and atrial tachycardia, and atrial fibrillation. During sinus rhythm, an increase in R-wave amplitude may be present.[98,233,235,243] On necropsy, thinning of the ventricular walls and interventricular septum is usually observed.

Other Myocardial Diseases
Hypertrophic cardiomyopathy appears to be uncommon and results in left ventricular hypertrophy and diastolic failure. The

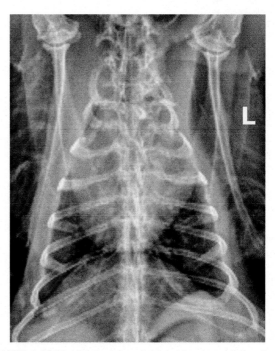

FIGURE 4-16 Ventrodorsal radiographic view of the thorax of a rabbit with cardiomegaly.

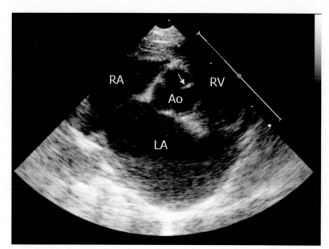

FIGURE 4-17 Rabbit with congestive heart failure and cardiac chamber dilation visible on echocardiography. Right parasternal short-axis view at the level of the aortic valve; *arrow* shows the commissure between the two cusps of the aortic valve. The left atrium and auricle are severely dilated. The interatrial septum bulges toward the right atrium in response to an elevated pressure in the enlarged left atrium. *Ao,* Aorta; *LA,* left atrium; *RA,* right atrium; *RV,* right ventricle.

disease has been documented in ferrets, rabbits, rats, and hamsters, but peer-reviewed case reports are rare or nonexistent in most species, despite the disease being mentioned and documented in multiple textbooks and reviews.[92,98,216,234,239,244,245] Likewise, restrictive cardiomyopathy is rare, but two cases were reported in ferrets.[225] A case of congestive heart failure secondary to hyperthyroidism was diagnosed in a rabbit (J. Brandão, pers. commun.). Hyperthyroidism is not uncommon in guinea pigs, and similar cardiologic conditions may arise in this species as well.[246]

In guinea pigs, rhabdomyomatosis is a disease characterized by excessive glycogen accumulation in myocytes, leading to tan streaks in the myocardium, especially in the left ventricle. However, this disease is of little clinical significance and should not be confused with a neoplasm.[247]

In rats, chronic myocardial degeneration (murine progressive cardiomyopathy) is common and increases in prevalence with age and in males. No clinical signs or histopathologic evidence of congestive heart failure seem to be noted in most cases, but electrocardiographic changes and subclinical cardiac functional changes are reported.[218,248,249] However, it is also cited as a major cause of death in overfed aged male rats.[250] There is a high correlation between the onset and severity of cardiomyopathy and chronic progressive nephropathy in rats.[218] Dietary restriction appears to lower the prevalence of the disease.

In cotton rats (*Sigmodon* spp.), sporadic heart failure cases were described in several laboratory colonies and were associated with exophthalmos due to thrombosis in the orbital venous sinus and skeletal muscle disorders.[251] Cardiomyopathy is reported commonly in woodchucks and frequently results in congestive heart failure.[221]

Myocarditis occurs as a result of infectious diseases or other inflammatory and autoimmune diseases. Myocarditis may cause arrhythmias and an elevation in circulating troponin levels.[98,229] Infectious diseases causing myocarditis in ferrets include *Toxoplasma*-like organisms and Aleutian disease.[252–254] A systemic inflammatory disease, the disseminated idiopathic myofasciitis also causes myocarditis in ferrets.[223,255] In rabbits, myocarditis has been reported with vitamin E deficiency, *Pasteurella multocida, Salmonella* spp., *Clostridium piliforme* (Tyzzer's disease), *Encephalitozoon cuniculi,* and coronavirus.[229,256–258] Ketamine/xylazine myocardial degeneration in this species is attributed to coronary vasoconstriction and myocardial ischemia, with limited collateral myocardial circulation.[256,258] Rabbits also suffer from stress-induced cardiomyopathy supposedly caused by a combination of vasoconstriction and increased cardiac workload associated with catecholamine release.[229,259] Cardiac manifestations of sepsis are reported to be common in sugar gliders.[226]

Valvular Disease
Valvular disease is recognized in ferrets, rabbits, chinchillas, and hedgehogs, although published individual case reports are scant.[98,214,218,220,225,229,260,261] Clinical signs are usually those of congestive heart failure when the valvular leakage is significant enough.

In a retrospective study in ferrets, valvular disease was the most common finding and was identified in 49 (52%) of 95 ferrets, of which 17 (35%) had congestive heart failure.[225] The aortic valve was most commonly affected, followed by the mitral valve. In 4 ferrets, it was concomitant to DCM. Another case described mitral and tricuspid regurgitation concurrently with a ventricular septal defect in a ferret.[260] Using cardiac ultrasound, a rabbit suffering from congestive heart failure was diagnosed with mitral and tricuspid regurgitation.[234] Severe myxomatous valvular degeneration of the AV valve was identified using echocardiography in another rabbit.[233] An aortic insufficiency was documented concomitantly to a ventricular septal defect in a rabbit.[262] A retrospective study in chinchillas identified four animals with mitral regurgitation that was severe in two animals and one other had tricuspid regurgitation.[214] Another case of mitral insufficiency was diagnosed during an echocardiographic study of chinchillas.[263] Congenital anomalies of the aortic valve are common in Syrian hamsters.[220,247] Two cases of valvular disease were diagnosed in African hedgehogs during a cardiac assessment study.[261] Valvular endocardiosis is also seen with some frequency in aging rats but does not seem to be associated with clinical signs.[92,218]

Congenital Defects
Congenital cardiac defects are rare in exotic companion mammals, although they have been reported in ferrets, rabbits, chinchillas, rats, and gerbils.[92,218,250,262,264–266] In rats, ventricular septal defects are most common, but the majority close spontaneously.[264] Two cases of ventricular septal defects have been reported in ferrets.[260,267] In one, the defect was part of a tetralogy of Fallot.[267] A ventricular septal defect was coupled to aortic valve insufficiency and cardiomegaly in a New Zealand white rabbit.[262] A number of other cases of cardiovascular abnormalities have been reported in various breeds of rabbits.[265,268,269]

Vascular Diseases
The rabbit was the first experimental animal model of atherosclerosis, as it was discovered in 1908 that rabbits were extremely

susceptible to dietary cholesterol due to their inability to increase sterol excretion in response to excess intake.[270-272] Spontaneous arteriosclerosis also occurs in all rabbit breeds and has even been observed in wild rabbits. The ascending aorta is the primary site of the blockage. New Zealand white and Flemish giant rabbits appear to be predisposed to this disease, whereas the Dutch and Danish country breeds seem more resistant.[229,273,274] Genetic variants of the New Zealand white, such as the Watanabe strain, are extremely susceptible to atherosclerosis because of genetic abnormalities in lipid metabolism.[272,275] However, spontaneous arteriosclerotic lesions do not contain lipids in rabbits, which differs markedly from atherosclerosis in other species.[273,274] Lesions can be extensively mineralized, resembling Mönckeberg's medial sclerosis in humans. Clinical signs, if present, are usually nonspecific in rabbits, but arterial calcification may be visible on radiographs.[229,257] Most other rodent species have been used as animal models of atherosclerosis, but spontaneous disease is rare without genetic or dietary modifications.[272]

Aortic calcification secondary to renal insufficiency has also been reported in rabbits, which are frequently hypercalcemic with chronic renal disease.[229,276,277] Hamsters also display a high prevalence of calcifying vasculopathy in various arteries, including the aorta.[220] Rats typically exhibit aortic mineralization secondary to chronic nephropathy.[92]

Polyarteritis nodosa is an inflammatory arterial disease of aging laboratory rats primarily affecting mesenteric arteries, although other arteries are also involved.[218,249] The cause is unknown but an autoimmune process is suggested. The tunica media undergoes segmental degenerative and thickening changes with luminal stenosis, thrombosis, and aneurysmal dilations. Polyarteritis nodosa is more common in male rats and those suffering from late-stage chronic nephropathy or hypertension. Depending on the affected arteries the disease may cause unspecific clinic signs or death.[218,249]

Arterial hypertension can be encountered in several species, although there is a high prevalence in aged rats, especially in males, and it is often associated with other age-related diseases in this species.[218] Endometrial aneurysms in rabbits can cause uterine bleeding and are due to episodic rupture of endometrial varices.[278] Affected animals commonly present with frank hemorrhage from the vulva and are anemic.

Dirofilaria immitis has been reported on extensively in ferrets but also occurs infrequently in rabbits.[98,279] Experimental infections have revealed the ferret to be highly susceptible to dirofilariasis, resulting in death in most animals.[280-282] Clinical signs are similar to the infestation in cats, and ferrets can be severely affected by the presence of a single worm (5 to 10 cm in length) that may obstruct blood flow. Worms can be found in the pulmonary arteries, vena cava, and right heart.[98] Clinical and imaging signs in ferrets are consistent with right-sided heart failure and include coughing, dyspnea, and weakness.[98,283]

Aortic rupture is common in woodchucks and results in acute death.[284] Woodchucks also suffer from a high rate of cerebrovascular hemorrhage associated in some cases with atherosclerosis.[284]

Miscellaneous
Arrhythmias are common in exotic companion mammals and their characteristics and causes are similar to other mammals.[98,225,245,285,286] Of interest is the frequency of AV blocks in ferrets.[225,287] Second-degree AV blocks can be normal in ferrets.[98,287] A retrospective study identified AV blocks in 40% (26/65) of ferrets that had a cardiac evaluation, of which 7 had third-degree blocks and 6 congestive heart failure and syncope.[225] Another study found abnormalities in 75% of ferrets that underwent an electrocardiographic examination.[238] A case of third-degree AV block in a ferret was treated with an epicardial pacemaker and was associated with extensive myocardial mineralization.[288] Common arrhythmias in dogs and cats have also been identified in ferrets and seem to share a similar etiology.[225,238,286]

Hamsters exhibit a high prevalence of atrial thrombosis, which occurs subsequently to a consumption coagulopathy.[220,247] The left atrium is most commonly affected. Clinical signs are consistent with heart failure but acute death is common. Atrial thrombosis is also encountered in mice, and intracardiac thrombi occur with age in rats.[218,250]

Endocardial proliferative lesions have been noted in rats on multiple occasions. The fibroproliferative lesions are morphologically similar to Schwann cell tumors.[218]

Two cases of idiopathic pericardial effusion have been reported in guinea pigs (Figure 4-18).[289,290] *Streptococcus pneumoniae* may cause fibrinopurulent pericarditis in guinea pigs.[291]

Primary cardiac neoplasms are rare in exotic companion mammals. In ferret lymphoma, neoplastic lymphocytes may infiltrate the myocardium. Mediastinal lymphoma may also lead to pleural effusion and tracheal elevation in the ferret.[217] Thymoma may cause cranial vena cava occlusion in rabbits. Hemangiosarcoma is uncommon but has been described in rabbits and ferrets, primarily in the liver and spleen.[292-295]

Birds
Avian Congestive Heart Failure
In parrots, the prevalence of cardiovascular diseases has been determined to be between 5.2% and 36% according to various

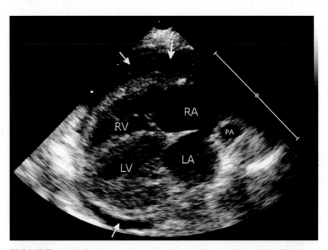

FIGURE 4-18 Guinea pig with idiopathic pericardial effusion. Right parasternal long-axis four-chamber echocardiographic view. The right atrium and ventricle are mildly enlarged. The heart is surrounded by a moderate amount of pericardial fluid. *Arrows,* Pericardial effusion; *LA,* left atrium; *LV,* left ventricle; *PA,* pulmonary artery; *RA,* right atrium; *RV,* right ventricle.

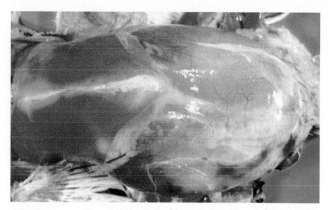

FIGURE 4-19 Ascites syndrome in a broiler chicken; skin was removed. (Courtesy of Dr. John Barnes, North Carolina State University.)

TABLE 4-4

Documented Causes of Congestive Heart Failure in Birds

Causes	References
Valvular insufficiency	300-305
Valvular stenosis	306
Septal defects	307-311
Ischemic cardiomyopathy	312
Dilated cardiomyopathy	311,313-315
Hypertrophic cardiomyopathy	297,309,316
Arrhythmias	317
Nutritional causes	106,315
Pericardial effusion	318,319
Iron storage disease	304,320
Pulmonary arterial hypertension	321,322
Pulmonary fibrosis/aspergillosis	297,323
Cardiac infection	106,309,324,325
Toxic causes	326-328
Atherosclerosis	312,321,329-331

studies that had sample sizes ranging from 107 to 1322 animals.[296-299]

In birds, right-sided congestive heart failure is more common than left-sided failure; this is suspected to be related to the particular anatomy of the right AV valve. In addition, the pathophysiology of avian heart failure has been well studied in the prevalent chicken ascites syndrome, but this disease is mainly related to production systems and rapid growth, so not all findings may translate well to companion avian patients. In chicken ascites syndrome, the increased workload of the heart and oxygen demand brought about by fast growth is coupled with an overall insufficient pulmonary capillary capacity and decreased respiratory efficiency in chickens compared to other birds. This quickly leads to pulmonary hypertension, which in turns leads to right ventricular hypertrophy and ultimately to dilation. Erythrocytosis also develops, which renders the blood more viscous and further increases the cardiac workload. With the dilatory changes affecting the right ventricle, the right AV valve, which extends from its wall, develops insufficiency that in turn increases the preload, leading to systemic congestion and ascites by increased hydrostatic pressure (Figure 4-19). In the turkey, spontaneous DCM, abnormal troponin T structure, and dysregulation of some cardiac enzymatic pathways may participate in the pathogenesis. Documented causes of congestive heart failure in domestic, wild, and companion birds are presented in Table 4-4.

Since right-sided heart failure is more common in birds, signs of fluid retention from the systemic circulation usually prevail, such as ascites, hepatomegaly, pericardial effusion, jugular distension, and dyspnea from air-sac compression. Pulmonary edema and congestion are seen in left-sided heart failure. However, any cardiologic sign can be encountered in bilateral congestive heart failure. Pleural effusion is possible in birds but, if occurring, does not cause dyspnea. Fluid analysis will reveal either a pure or modified transudate. A moderate increase in bile acids due to hepatic congestion is frequently seen.

Electrocardiographic findings may include mean electrical access (MEA) deviations (usually right deviation), tachycardia, widened or tall P waves, atrial fibrillation, widened QRS complexes, prominent R waves, widening of the QT intervals, and AV blocks. These changes are associated with delayed electrical conduction and chamber enlargement. Radiographs usually show a cardiomegaly with ascites and loss of abdominal detail and airspace (Figure 4-20). The axillary diverticula of the interclavicular air sac may appear hyperinflated from volume compensation of the air-sac system and severe dyspnea. Echocardiography is the definitive tool to diagnose congestive heart failure and ascites and some degrees of pericardial effusion, right-side heart dilation, and hepatic congestion are also usually observed (Figure 4-21 and see Figure 4-39 later). In addition, valvular regurgitation and poor contractility may be detected. Angiocardiography will demonstrate an enlarged heart but is seldom indicated when considering other more practical imaging modalities (see Figure 4-40 later).

Arrhythmias

Alterations of the ECG are common but do not always correlate with clinical signs and are rarely primary disease processes in birds. Arrhythmias can be classified into excitability disturbances and conduction disturbances. Reported arrhythmias in birds are summarized in Table 4-5.

Excitability disturbances have various causes and are common with dilated cardiac chambers and organic diseases. AV blocks are associated with disrupted conduction between the sinoatrial and AV node, where the conduction can be delayed (first degree), fail to propagate to the AV node (second degree), or be independent from the AV node (third degree), during which case an AV escape rhythm occurs. Second-degree AV block can be characterized as Mobitz type I (PR [interval] progressively lengthening prior to block), which is usually caused by excessive vagal tone and is atropine responsive, or Mobitz type II (constant PR), which is usually caused by diseases of the His bundle and is not responsive to atropine. AV blocks may be normally found in some avian species (e.g., racing pigeons) and may occur with some frequency during anesthetic events. However, a drop in blood pressure or clinical signs associated with AV blocks are abnormal. Syncope has been reported in a Moluccan cockatoo (*Cacatua moluccensis)* and hypotensive episodes in a Hispaniolan Amazon parrot *(Amazona ventralis)* with second-degree AV blocks.[333,334] Hypotension associated with second-degree AV blocks was observed following dobutamine administration in four Hispaniolan Amazon parrots.[340] A bundle branch block was associated with lead toxicosis in a galah *(Eolophus roseicapilla)*.[331]

In addition, various wave alterations have been associated with cardiac chamber enlargement, toxicities, nutritional imbalances, electrolytic disorders, and infectious agents (see Table 4-5).[106,332]

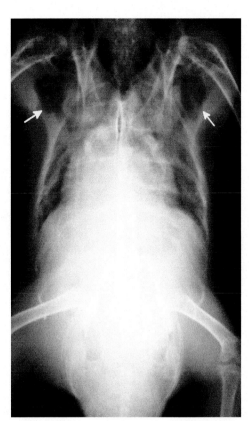

FIGURE 4-20 African grey parrot diagnosed with congestive heart failure. Radiographic findings include cardiomegaly (heart width to thoracic width ratio = 71%), ascites, loss of abdominal details and airspace, and hyperinflation of axillary diverticula *(arrows)*.

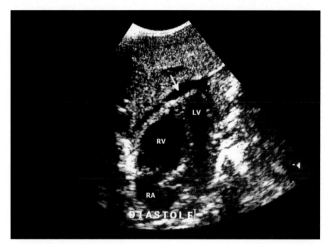

FIGURE 4-21 Four-chamber horizontal view echocardiography in an African grey parrot with congestive heart failure. *Arrow,* Pericardial effusion; *LV,* left ventricle; *RA,* right atrium; *RV,* right ventricle.

TABLE 4-5

Selected Arrhythmias and Some Documented Causes in Birds

Arrhythmias	ECG Changes	Causes
Excitability disturbances		
Respiratory sinus arrhythmia	Slowing of HR during expiration	Physiologic
Sinus bradycardia	Low HR, normal sinus rhythm	Vagal stimulation, atropine, anesthesia, hypokalemia, hyperkalemia, vitamin E deficiency, vitamin B1 deficiency, acetylcholinesterase inhibitors
Sinus tachycardia	High HR, normal sinus rhythm	Sympathetic, catecholamine stimulation
Atrial tachycardia	Series of fast atrial extrasystoles	Atrial distension, ectopic foci
Atrial fibrillation	No normal P waves, irregular SS intervals	Atrial enlargements, cardiac disease
VPCs	Wide, bizarre QRS unrelated to P	Ectopic foci, hypokaliemia, vitamin B1 deficiency, vitamin E deficiency, Paramyxovirus, Avian Influenza, myocardial infarction
Ventricular tachycardia	Series of VPCs	Similar causes as for VPCs
Ventricular fibrillation	Chaotic ventricular depolarization	Myocardial hypoxia, shock, severe disorders
Conduction disturbances		
First-degree AV block	Long PR intervals	Anesthetics, increased vagal tone
Second-degree AV block	Long PR intervals, some P without QRS	Anesthetics, increased vagal tone; occasionally normal in pigeons, parrots, raptors
Third-degree AV block	Escape ventricular rhythm (slow and bizarre QRS), no consistent PR	Severe cardiomegaly
Bundle branch block	Short PR, bizarre and widened QRS	Lead, myopathy, myocarditis; uncommon in birds

Adapted from References 106, 286, 332-340.
AI, Avian influenza; *ECG,* electrocardiogram; *PMV,* Paramyxovirus; *VPCs,* ventricular premature contractions.

Valvular Diseases

Valvular diseases in birds appear to be more prevalent with the right AV valve, frequently resulting in insufficiency. This valve responds to right ventricular dilation by thickening and readily acquires insufficiency because of its fixed position on the ventricular wall.[106,296,297,341,342] A congenital valvular fissure was reported in a blue-fronted Amazon parrot (*Amazona aestiva*) with congestive heart failure.[301] Left AV valve insufficiency with valvular endocardiosis has been reported in an Indian ringneck parakeet (*Psittacula krameri*), an umbrella cockatoo (*Cacatua alba*), an Indian hill mynah (*Gracula religiosa*), and a Pukeko (*Porphyrio melanotus*) (Table 4-4).[300,302,304,343]

Endocardiosis is a noninflammatory nodular thickening of the valves that is more commonly seen on the left AV valve in birds. It is a common lesion of chickens and is a frequent occurrence in the ascites syndrome.[314,344] Valvular stenosis is not common in birds but has been reported in a duck.[305] Idiopathic valvular degeneration may also occur.

Valvular endocarditis, a common manifestation of bacterial cardiac infections, can occur as a result of distant chronic infections and lead to septic emboli.[106,323,324] The left AV valve is most often affected.[308] *Trichomonas* spp. can colonize the AV valves in severe cases in pigeons.[106] A variety of bacterial agents have been isolated (Table 4-6, endocarditis). In cases of significant valvular insufficiency, a systolic murmur may be audible on cardiac auscultation. A complete blood cell count may reveal a leukocytosis, and blood culture can be attempted to isolate a bacterial organism. Cardiomegaly may be evident on radiographs in advanced cases, along with signs of congestive heart failure. Valvular vegetative lesions may be identified on a cardiac ultrasound examination, and signs of congestive heart failure, valvular regurgitation (Doppler echocardiography), and myocardial dysfunction may also be evident.

Myocardial Diseases

Dilated cardiomyopathy refers to primary myocardial disorders leading to a dilated heart. Due to volume overload, the cardiac chambers usually dilate during congestive heart failure, but this should not be confused with spontaneous DCM. Spontaneous DCM is a well-known disorder of 1- to 4-week-old turkeys (*Meleagridis gallopavo*). The exact cause of the disease is unknown, but it is associated with rapid growth and production. Genetic factors, previous myocarditis, hypoxia during incubation, and other environmental and dietary factors have also been proposed to play a role in the etiology.[314,345,346] Gross findings include a large right ventricle with thin walls and signs of congestive heart failure. Histopathologic lesions include degeneration of myofibers with vacuolation, secondary endocardiosis, focal infiltration of lymphocytes, and secondary changes in the liver.[314,344] On the ECG, the following changes, associated with dilation and hypertrophy of the ventricles, can be identified: increased R-wave amplitudes, negative T waves, and rotation of the MEA.[337,347] Chicken round heart disease is characterized by an enlarged heart, hypertrophy of the left ventricle, and myofiber degeneration, but the disease is extremely rare nowadays.[314] In other avian species, the diagnosis of DCM is unclear. A red-tailed hawk (*Buteo jamaicensis*) was reported with primary right-sided DCM and concurrent plasma troponin I elevation. No valvular regurgitation or other potential causes could be identified in that case.[312] A macaw was also

diagnosed with lesions compatible with right-sided DCM.[296] In addition, some cases of left-sided DCM have been diagnosed in pet birds.[308] DCM is best diagnosed by echocardiography and is characterized, apart from chamber enlargement, by poor contractility and systolic dysfunction.

Hypertrophic cardiomyopathy has been poorly documented in birds but is mentioned in several sources.[296,297,308] On echocardiography, hypertrophic cardiomyopathy shows ventricular lumen of diminished dimensions, thickened ventricular walls, and decreased diastolic dysfunction. Restrictive cardiomyopathy does not appear to have been reported in birds. Ischemic cardiomyopathy and myocardial infarction are rare overall but have been documented in several cases in relation to atherosclerosis (see section on atherosclerosis).

Myocarditis can occur with a variety of infectious agents (see Table 4-6). In North American birds of prey, West Nile virus infection seems to be a common cause of myocarditis.[348,349] In psittacines, myocarditis with cell infiltration of Purkinje fibers is encountered with proventricular dilation

TABLE 4-6

Infectious Agents Reported to Cause Cardiovascular Lesions in Birds

Pericarditis/epicarditis	Myocarditis
Listeria monocytogenes	*Escherichia coli*
Riemerella anatipestifer (turkeys, ducks)	*Salmonella* spp.
Chlamydophila psittaci	*Listeria monocytogenes*
Mycoplasma gallisepticum	*Pasteurella multocida*
Salmonella spp.	*Myocabacterium* spp.
Escherichia coli	*Aspergillus* spp.
Myocabacterium spp.	West Nile virus
Aspergillus spp.	Eastern equine encephalitis virus
Trichomonas gallinae (pigeons)	Avian leukosis virus
Reovirus	Parvovirus (geese, Muscovy ducks)
	Avian encephalomyelitis virus
Endocarditis	Reovirus
Enterococcus spp.	Avian paramyxovirus I
Streptococcus spp.	Avian influenza
Staphylococcus spp.	Proventricular dilation disease (ABV)
Pasteurella multocida	*Sarcocystis* spp.
Erysipelothrix rhusopathiae	*Leucocytozoon* spp.
Lactobacillus jensenii	*Toxoplasma gondii*
Escherichia coli	*Atoxoplasma serini* (passerines)
Reovirus	
	Pericardial effusion
Intravascular/intracardiac parasites	Fowl adenovirus (serotype IV)
Trichomonas gallinae (pigeons)	Reovirus
Splendidofilaria spp.	Polyomavirus
Chandlerella spp.	
Cardiofilaria spp.	**Cardiac neoplasias**
Paronchocerca spp.	Marek's disease virus
Sarconema spp. (swans, geese)	Avian leucosis virus
Schistosomes (geese)	Reticuloendotheliosis virus

ABV, Avian bornavirus.

disease, which can be present in up to 79% of the cases.[106,297,350] Iron storage disease can induce myocarditis; however, this disease is only suspected to lead to clinical myocardial disorders in mynahs.[303,319] Electrocardiographic changes usually accompany myocarditis due to increased excitability (see Table 4-5).

Myocardial degeneration is usually the result of nutritional deficiencies (vitamin E/selenium), toxicities, or ischemia.[308] A fatal disease primarily characterized by myocardial degeneration has been reported in great-billed parrot (*Tanygnathus megalorynchos*); skeletal muscle and neural lesions were also found in this animal, and the lesions resembled vitamin E deficiency.[308]

Pericardial Diseases

Pericardial effusion is common with congestive heart disease in birds and can precipitate decompensation if cardiac tamponade occurs.[106,351] Cardiac tamponade first affects the right heart diastolic function because of the lower pressure. Pericardial effusion can also be caused by hypoproteinemia, exudative pericarditis, hemorrhage, atrial rupture, coagulopathy, neoplasia, and idiopathic syndromes. Viral causes of hydropericardium producing transudates have been recorded (see Table 4-6). Avocado toxicity can also induce pericardial effusion.[352] Right auricle rupture leads to hemopericardium and sudden death in poultry.[314,353] Pericardial fluid analysis and culture may be helpful to pinpoint a cause when primary cardiac disease is not suspected. Pericardial fluid can be collected by endoscopy through a midline approach or guided by ultrasound.[317] Pericardial biopsies may also be valuable in some cases. Enlargement of the cardiac silhouette is commonly seen on radiographs, but it may be difficult to differentiate it from true cardiomegaly (Figure 4-22). Echocardiography can be used to readily diagnose pericardial effusion (see Figure 4-21). Electrocardiographic findings may include left axis deviation and low voltage.[106]

Pericarditis has been described with a variety of infectious agents (see Table 4-5). Clinical signs are usually nonspecific, but fibrinous pericarditis can result in constrictive pericarditis. Pericardial filarioids have also been documented in birds (e.g., cockatoos) housed outdoors.[354,355] Uric acid deposits on the pericardium are common with visceral gout and should not be confused with infectious pericarditis. Echocardiography is of low value for pericardial diseases without effusion; however, endoscopy with direct visualization of the pericardium may be more sensitive.

Infectious and Parasitic Diseases

The different bacterial, viral, fungal, and parasitic agents reported to cause cardiovascular disorders are summarized in Table 4-6. Blood culture is the diagnostic test of choice for bacterial cardiopathies. Specific viral diagnostic tests can also be performed depending on the infectious dynamic of the agent. Electrocardiographic changes have been recorded in some instances. Cardiac parasites that can be encountered include myocardial protozoans and filarioid nematodes living in cardiac chambers, vessels, and body cavities.[355-357] These parasites primarily infest birds being housed outside, where they get exposed to final hosts (e.g., cats, opossums) and arthropod hosts or mechanical vectors (e.g., cockroaches, black flies, mosquitoes). Examinations of

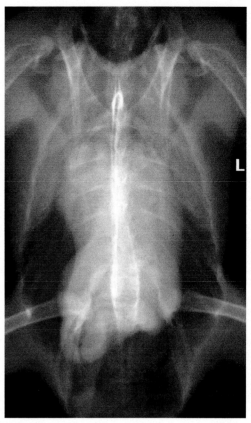

FIGURE 4-22 Ventrodorsal radiographic view of an African grey parrot with pericardial effusion. Note that the cardiac silhouette is enlarged, but no evidence of congestive heart failure is seen (see Figure 4-20). *L,* Left.

blood smears and buffy coats may be helpful in diagnosing these parasites.

Congenital Defects

Congenital diseases are rare and include atrial or ventricular septal defects and valvular stenosis. Some defects may be functionally closed. Among psittacine birds, cockatoos seem to have a higher prevalence of congenital defects than any other species.[306,308] In addition, persistent truncus arteriosus and aortic hypoplasia have been reported, each in combination with septal defects in two cockatoos.[306] In these two cockatoos, an audible murmur and tachycardia were present on cardiac auscultation, and an antemortem diagnosis was reached with a cardiac ultrasound examination. A congenital valvular defect was suspected in a blue-fronted Amazon parrot.[301] Cardiac malformations have also been reported in the chicken and turkey as a result of various chemicals in embryos.[358,359] A ventricular septal defect was reported in a tundra swan (*Cygnus columbianus*), a houbara bustard (*Chlamydotis undulata*), a griffon vulture (*Gyps fulvus*), an ostrich (*Struthio camelus*), and a Chinese goose (*Anser cygnoides*).[307,309,310,360] The ostrich had a defect in the left anterior vena cava in addition to its ventricular septal defect.[360] A duck with an audible heart murmur was diagnosed with congenital mitral stenosis and subvalvular aortic stenosis by echocardiography.[305] Ventricular or atrial septal defects associated with heart murmurs were diagnosed in 7% (8/111) of Mississippi sandhill cranes *(Grus canadensis pulla)* in a mortality survey at the Patuxent Wildlife Research Center.[361] A congenital cardiac aneurysm has been reported in the right ventricle of a pigeon.[362]

Bifid sternum is a congenital defect in which the sternum is split longitudinally, thereby exposing the heart to external trauma. This anomaly has been reported in three African grey parrots *(Psittacus erithacus)* and an orange-winged Amazon parrot *(Amazona amazonica)*.[363,364]

Atherosclerosis

Atherosclerosis is an inflammatory and degenerative disease of the arterial wall characterized by the disorganization of the arterial intima due to the accumulation of inflammatory cells, fat, cholesterol, calcium, and cellular debris, potentially leading to complications such as stenosis, ischemia, thrombosis, hemorrhage, and aneurysm. Atherosclerosis is probably an underlying lesion in the majority of noninfectious cardiovascular diseases diagnosed in pet birds and is undoubtedly the most common lesion of the cardiovascular system found on necropsy in psittacine birds.

The etiology and development of the atherosclerotic lesions can be broadly explained by the response-to-injury hypothesis. While this widely accepted hypothesis has been constantly refined, it postulates that damage to the endothelium lining the artery sets the stage for atherogenesis and is associated with endothelial dysfunction, inflammation, oxidative stress, and entrapment of oxidized lipoproteins in the arterial wall.[365-369]

The histologic lesions have been well described in psittacines and appear similar to humans.[370-374] Psittacine atherosclerotic lesions are classified into seven lesion types. In advanced lesions responsible for clinical signs, there is formation of a lipid core (atheroma; type-IV lesion) covered by a fibrous cap (fibroatheroma; type V), and complications such as fissures, hematomas, and thrombosis (type VI) may occur. In parrots, atherosclerotic lesions are central and most commonly found in the great arteries at the base of the heart, brachiocephalic arteries, ascending aorta, and pulmonary arteries (Figure 4-23).[106,297,351,370,375-379] Lesions in the abdominal aorta and peripheral arteries appear less frequent. However, peripheral lesions have been documented in the abdominal aorta, carotid artery, and coronary arteries in parrot species.[328,330,380-385] Complications and clinical signs are usually due to either severe stenosis from the continuously growing atheromatous plaque or thrombosis and hemorrhage caused by plaque disruption that can decrease or interrupt blood flow or provoke emboli. Atherosclerotic lesions are silent and asymptomatic until such complications arise. Stenosis secondary to atherosclerotic lesions is common in birds, but atherothrombosis and emboli are rare and, in a postmortem study, were found in only 1.9% of atherosclerotic cases.[379]

The prevalence of atherosclerosis in parrots has been documented in multiple sources and ranges from 1.9% to 91.8%.[297,299,371,375,376,380,383,386-389] However, the range of reported prevalence is wide and likely due to reports varying in pathologic inclusion criteria, lesion severity, geographical area, demographics, captive conditions, psittacine species, and the retrospective or prospective nature of the work. A recent large multicenter study including more than 7600 psittacines provided a clearer picture of the epidemiology of atherosclerosis,

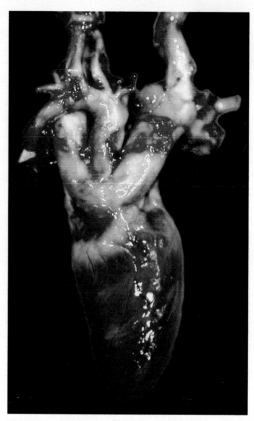

FIGURE 4-23 Atherosclerosis of the main arterial trunks at the base of the heart in a cockatoo. (Courtesy of Dr. Nobuko Wakamatsu, Louisiana State University.)

with the prevalence reported as a function of age, gender, and species.[379] This investigation focused more on the prevalence of clinically important atherosclerotic lesions susceptible to induce disease and interpreted the prevalence in the context of population demographics (Figure 4-24). In nonpsittacine species, atherosclerosis has been described in almost all orders of birds.[298,376,377,384,390] Three large retrospective studies reported the prevalence of atherosclerosis in multiple avian orders.[298,376,384]

Several risk factors have been suggested that may promote the development of atherosclerosis in psittacine birds and include age, gender, species, increased plasma total cholesterol and triglycerides, high-energy and high-fat diets, physical inactivity, thyroid disease, and co-infection with *Chlamydia psittaci*.[371,375,376,378-380,387,388] Female sex and age have been definitely quantified and confirmed as important risk factors.[379] In addition, African grey parrots, Amazon parrots *(Amazona* spp.), and cockatiels *(Nymphicus hollandicus)* are relatively susceptible to the disease, whereas cockatoos *(Cacatua* spp.) and macaws *(Ara* spp.) are relatively resistant.[379] A possible association between *Chlamydia pneumoniae* infection and atherosclerosis has been investigated in multiple studies in humans but remains controversial.[391-393] The association between psittacine atherosclerosis and avian chlamydiosis is equally controversial and is probably not of great clinical significance.[379,387,394,395] Advanced lesions have also been associated with reproductive and hepatic diseases as well

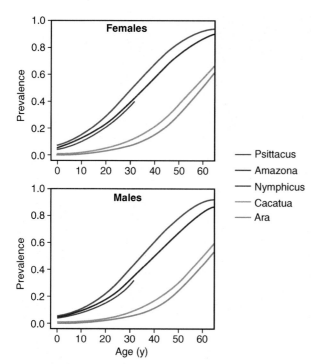

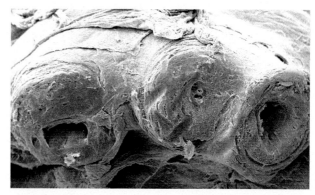

FIGURE 4-25 Scanning electron microscopy of stenotic arteries due to atherosclerosis at the base of the heart in a quaker parrot. Note the severe stenosis, with one artery almost completely obstructed (×60).

FIGURE 4-24 Estimated prevalence of advanced atherosclerosis as a function of age, sex, and genus. (Redrawn from Beaufrere H, Ammersbach M, Reavill D, et al. Prevalence of and risk factors associated with atherosclerosis in psittacine birds. *J Am Vet Med Assoc.* 242(12):1696-1704, 2013)

as myocardial fibrosis.[371,379] Another study identified a correlation between atherosclerosis of the ascending aorta and organ alterations such as myocardial hypertrophy, myocardial fibrosis, pulmonary congestion, and fibrosis.[371]

Dyslipidemic changes with notable hypercholesterolemia are thought to predispose birds to the development of atherosclerotic lesions, as in other animal species. Experimental cholesterol feeding readily induces severe dyslipidemia and advanced atherosclerotic lesions in psittacine birds.[381,396] In a case-controlled study of 22 birds, parrots with atherosclerotic lesions had significantly higher median plasma cholesterol than control birds.[387] A large retrospective study on more than 5600 blood samples showed that the differences observed in atherosclerosis prevalence between psittacine species could partially be explained by differences in their plasma cholesterol levels. Surprisingly, increased high-density lipoprotein (HDL) but not LDL cholesterol was shown to significantly correlate with atherosclerosis prevalence between psittacine species.[397]

The impact of diet on atherosclerosis and dyslipidemia has only been investigated in a few studies. In a feed trial, African grey parrots fed a high-fat diet rich in saturated fatty acids had significantly higher plasma cholesterol than parrots on a low-fat diet or high-fat diet enriched in omega-6 unsaturated fatty acids (linoleic acid).[398] Another feed trial in African grey parrots did not demonstrate a significant difference in cholesterol and lipoprotein plasma concentrations between groups on a pelletized or seed diet.[399] The intake in unsaturated fatty acids, especially in omega-3 fatty acids, seems to protect against atherosclerosis in parrots.[388,400] The severity of atherosclerosis was found to negatively correlate with the muscle and adipose tissue content of α-linolenic acid in parrots.[388] In birds of prey, the common practice of feeding day-old chicks that have a large yolk sac rich in cholesterol may potentiate atherosclerosis in susceptible raptorial species (e.g., insectivorous raptors, falcons).

Clinical signs are uncommonly reported with psittacine atherosclerosis but, when present, consist of sudden death, congestive heart failure, dyspnea, neurologic signs, respiratory signs, exercise intolerance, and ataxia.[106,311,320,328–330,371,375,377,380,383,385,401–403] Most clinical signs reported in parrots are associated with flow-limiting stenosis of the major arteries or the carotid arteries, and clinical signs of thrombosis and thromboemboli are rare (or not diagnosed), unlike in humans (Figure 4-25). The physiologic differences between avian thrombocytes and mammalian platelets may partly explain the clinical differences observed in the nature and prevalence of atherothrombotic diseases.[404] Also, the different pattern of coronary circulation in the avian heart with the predominance of intramyocardial arteries and increased collateral circulation compared with humans may be responsible for the rarity of acute myocardial ischemia. However, it is important to note that ischemic cardiomyopathy and infarction have been reported in a number of birds of prey cases as well as in pigeon and quail models of atherosclerosis.[298,311,405–407]

Intermittent claudication, a clinical manifestation of peripheral arterial disease, was reported in an Amazon parrot and is suspected in a number of other cases with similar clinical presentation.[371,380,385,403,408] Congestive heart failure and valvular insufficiency concurrent to atherosclerosis were also reported in several parrots.[320,328,329] The pathogenesis is unclear, but chronic myocardial ischemia, systemic hypertension, and an increase in the cardiac afterload may contribute to this disease process. Parrots have also been documented to experience ischemic and hemorrhagic stroke events.[401,402,409] Aneurysms secondary to atherosclerosis were reported in a cockatoo and an Alexandrine parakeet (*Psittacula eupatria*).[330,383] Ruptured aneurysms and aorta were also reported in a variety of nonpsittacine birds.[298,383,410] Sudden death or nonspecific clinical signs are generally acknowledged to be the most common presentation of clinical atherosclerosis. These

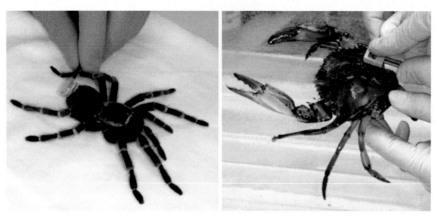

FIGURE 4-26 Heart rate measurement using a Doppler probe in a tarantula *(left)* and a blue crab *(right)*. (Courtesy of Dr. Gregory Lewbart, North Carolina State University.)

may be partially explained by the relative inactivity of some captive parrots, which would allow severe subclinical atherosclerotic lesions to develop without clinical manifestations being detectable by their caretakers. Finally, sudden death from lethal cardiac arrhythmia triggered by myocardial ischemia or undetected cerebral emboli is possible.

Aneurysm and Arterial Rupture

Arterial aneurysm is a focal, blood-filled dilation of the arterial wall communicating with the arterial lumen and may be caused in birds by atherosclerosis, copper deficiency, hypertension, and fungal infection.[330,402,411-415] Nonatherosclerotic aneurysms with aortic dissection and rupture are mainly seen in ostriches and turkeys.[314,411,412,414-416] The exact cause of aortic dissecting aneurysm is not known in these two species. However, systemic hypertension (common in meat-type turkeys, especially young males), genetic factors, connective tissue disorders, peas in the ration (peas' toxin β-aminopropionitrile will cause aortic rupture experimentally by interference with collagen formation), and dietary deficiencies, notably in copper, may contribute to the pathogenesis.[314,342,345,417] A copper-dependent enzyme is needed for connective cross-linking of collagen and elastin in the arterial wall.[308] A spontaneous rupture of the left brachiocephalic artery consecutive to degenerative changes in the tunica media was diagnosed in a whooper swan *(Cygnus cygnus).*[418]

Neoplasia

Cardiovascular neoplasms are rare in birds. Oncogenic viruses can induce various cardiac tumor formations in chickens (see Table 4-6). A vascular hemangiosarcoma arising from the right internal carotid artery was reported in a double yellow-headed Amazon parrot *(Amazona ochrocephala oratrix).*[419] However, in birds, hemangiomas and hemangiosarcomas tend to occur more commonly in a cutaneous location.[378]

SPECIFIC DIAGNOSTICS

Invertebrates

Physical Examination

The information gained from the physical examination as it relates to the circulatory system is limited in invertebrates.

Since most circulatory disorders are associated with generalized disease, trauma, or dehydration, nonspecific clinical signs should be expected.

In terrestrial arthropods that have an open circulatory system, wounds should be examined to ensure that hemolymph loss is stopped. Since spiders are kept as pets by a few hobbyists and in zoological collections, more clinical information on cardiovascular diagnostics is available in arachnids than in most other invertebrate groups. In spiders, joint membranes should be inspected with magnifying glasses for hemolymph leakage.[20]

The heart of large spiders can be seen pulsing in individuals with opisthosoma alopecia.[20] Heart rates may be obtained in some individuals by counting the pulsations of abdominal hairs in a quiet environment.[420] A binocular microscope has been used by some investigators to measure heartbeat frequency.[21] A Doppler ultrasound probe can also be used to noninvasively obtain the HR of arthropods and other invertebrates. In arachnids, the probe should be placed on the top of the opisthosoma (Figure 4-26). In decapod crustaceans, the probe should be placed over the areola region of the cephalothorax, which covers the heart dorsally (see Figure 4-26). Since the spider cuticle is a hydrophobic surface, a small amount of ethanol applied with a cotton tip to the dorsal opisthosoma allows ultrasound gel to adhere better. Ethanol may also contribute to sedating the arachnid patient.[20] Finally, in spiders, the HR may be obtained by transilluminating the opisthosoma from below using a cool laser and observing the heart from the top; normal HRs have been determined in a few species using this technique.[421] Resting HRs of large spiders typically fall ~30 to 70 bpm, but higher values are found in smaller spiders or during exercise.[20,21,422] The normal HR for lobsters is about 5 to 20 bpm.[422] The conditions under which the HR is taken may be of great influence.[420] Octopuses' resting HR is ~8 to 14 bpm.[423] Heart rate monitoring has also been performed in snails and octopuses under anesthesia using a Doppler probe or a pulse oximeter.[422,424] In addition, HRs that are heavily influenced by environmental conditions have been studied in a variety of other species in a large body of scientific literature, ranging from studies of oysters and cephalopods to aquatic and terrestrial arthropods.[8,16,17,22,421,425] However, the clinical interpretation and usefulness of HR measurements may be debatable and more meaningful for anesthetic monitoring.

Hemolymph pressure is generally relatively low in invertebrates, and since the circulatory system is open in most of them, pressure measurement is not practical and would probably have limited clinical usefulness other than in a research setting. Spiders are able to generate considerable prosomal pressure to assist with leg extension during locomotion and jumping. In cephalopods that have a closed circulatory system with true vessels and higher systolic blood pressure than other invertebrates, invasive blood pressure measurements have been obtained by arterial catheterization in laboratory octopuses and other cephalopod species (~30 to 60 mmHg systolic in the aorta).[22,120,423,426]

Clinical Pathology

Abnormalities in clinical pathology parameters are unlikely to be specific to circulatory disorders, which are rare in invertebrates. Instead, they may reflect systemic problems in homeostasis and inflammation.

Electrocardiography

Electrocardiography has been widely studied during experiments on invertebrate physiology, especially in arthropods and mollusks. However, it is frequently accomplished on isolated hearts.[26,427–430] The clinical practicality of this diagnostic is dubious in the light of the rarity of circulatory disorders in invertebrates.

In spiders, the application of pin electrodes on the cranial top of the opisthosoma may allow the recording of an ECG.[21] Electrical activity of a tarantula's heart consists of periodic bursts of ganglionic electrical activity.[26,420] The ECG in most arthropods is of the oscillatory type with a series of rapid potentials, characteristic of neurogenic cardiac contractions.[420] In myogenic contractions, such as in most mollusks, the ECG shows a few simple and slow waves.

Diagnostic Imaging

Radiographs are unrewarding in most invertebrates because of the low definition of body structures and the fact that the heart is not visible without contrast agents. Angiography has been used in a few invertebrate species for anatomical and physiological studies but is not practical.[431,432]

An opisthosomal ultrasound and echocardiography approach has been described in anesthetized spiders and consists of placing the probe over the opisthosoma (Figure 4-27).[20,433] It is recommended to apply a small amount of alcohol to the water-repellent opisthosomal cuticle to induce better adherence of the ultrasound gel. Doppler echocardiography has also been performed.[20,433]

Cardiac ultrasound can also be obtained in cephalopods noninvasively in water through a soft compartment or directly on the anesthetized mollusk. Reports of this technique could be found in the cuttlefish (probe must be placed ventrally because of the cuttlebone) and octopus.[434]

Fish

Physical Examination

As for other organ systems, history taking including husbandry and water quality remains an important aspect of the fish examination. In general, salmonids seem to

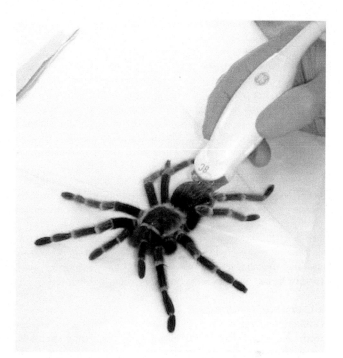

FIGURE 4-27 Opisthosomal and cardiac ultrasound in a tarantula. (Courtesy of Dr. Gregory Lewbart, North Carolina State University.)

have an increased prevalence of infectious and degenerative cardiovascular diseases. Clinical cardiologic information gathered from a remote examination or hands-on examination under anesthesia is limited in fishes. Small ornamental fish can be transilluminated. The heart can be seen beating ventrally in the throat region in some fish. The heart rate can also be obtained using a Doppler probe in the anesthetized patient that can be placed laterally or ventrally on the isthmus and breast area, on the dorsal aspect of the tongue, or inside the operculum underneath the gills.[37,435] A pulse oximeter can also be used to obtain HRs.[37] Heart rates vary widely among species.[30,436]

Fish with cardiovascular diseases usually present with nonspecific signs of decreased appetite and activity. External signs of congestive heart failure in fishes include abdominal distension (dropsy), exophthalmia, softening of the myotomal musculature, and edematous skin.[37,125] The respiratory rate may also be altered and the gill filaments may be hyperemic or pale. Ascites may not only be caused by cardiac diseases but also by gill, skin, liver, and kidney diseases (e.g., kidney microsporidiosis in goldfish).

Blood pressure measurement is unpractical in fish in a clinical setting but has been performed experimentally using arterial catheterization.[37]

Clinical Pathology

Hematologic and biochemical abnormalities are usually nonspecific and associated with generalized conditions and infections. Dyslipidemic changes have been associated with arteriosclerosis in salmonids. Ascitic fluid should be collected and analyzed. Since most cardiovascular diseases in fish are infectious in nature, blood and ascitic fluid microbiologic culture are valuable. In addition, gill clips may help characterize vascular changes in the gill filaments.

Electrocardiography

The ECG, typically used more for anesthetic monitoring than for diagnostic purposes, should be obtained outside of water. Leads are attached using needles inserted subcutaneously (SC). Two needles are placed laterally close to the pectoral fins, and a third one is placed caudally near the anus (Figure 4-28).[436] The piscine ECG is fairly similar to that of mammals, with a few additional waves (Table 4-7).[30] A B wave (usually positive on lead II) occurs during the ST interval in elasmobranchs and corresponds to the contraction of the conus arteriosus. A V wave occurs prior to the P wave in most fishes and represents the contraction of the sinus venosus. The prominence of these extra waves varies with species. Electrocardiography is routinely used in fish anesthesia, but its diagnostic use and the characterization of arrhythmias associated with cardiovascular lesions have not been well documented.

Diagnostic Imaging

Radiographs are not useful to investigate fish cardiovascular diseases because there is a lack of detail regarding their visceral structures. No reports of angiographic techniques could be located in fishes, and angiography seems to be of low practical and clinical value.

Echocardiography can easily be performed directly on the patient in or outside water or through a plastic bag in small individuals. The probe is placed in the midline on the throat region of the immersed fish and the heart appears pyramidal in teleosts. The longitudinal section allows viewing of all four cavities of the heart (sinus venosus, atrium, ventricle, bulbus arteriosus).[437] Echocardiographic measurements have been published for Atlantic salmon and differ between wild and captive animals.[437] The mean ventricular fractional shortening was 17%. Other approaches consist of placing the probe

beneath the gill arches after lifting the operculum or using a transesophageal ultrasound probe, which seems to provide better views in fish with thick scales.[438] Abdominal ultrasound is also an easy method to differentiate ascites from other causes of abdominal enlargements.

Echocardiography has been used in various cardiac conditions.[33,437] Pericardial effusion, loss of definition of the atrium, compression of the ventricle, hepatic congestion, and ascites in salmon affected by the cardiomyopathy syndrome have been identified with this technique.[437] Vascular thrombi may also be identified on the fish echocardiographic examination. Cardiac ultrasound was used to investigate Atlantic salmon with deficient septum transversum and was found to be 100% sensitive and 98% specific in diagnosing the condition.[132] The septum transversum is usually seen as a thin hyperechoic band between the heart and the liver.

Endoscopy

Rigid endoscopic techniques are widely used in fish medicine, but their applications appear to be limited in piscine cardiology. Using a routine approach through a small abdominal incision, the heart is located cranially and is separated from

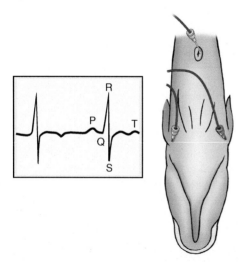

FIGURE 4-28 Needles placement for electrocardiography in a teleost fish with depiction of a typical ECG pattern. (Modified from Stoskopf. *Fish Medicine.* Saunders; 1993:882, with permission from Elsevier.)

TABLE 4-7

Significance of the Different Sections of a Vertebrate ECG during One Cardiac Cycle

ECG Segment	Electrophysiologic Meaning
V or SV wave	Depolarization of sinus venosus in some fishes, amphibians, reptiles
P wave	Depolarization of atria Conduction from SA to AV nodes
F waves	Absent in normal animals Baseline undulations occurring in atrial fibrillation
Ta wave	Present in pigeons, some poultry species Repolarization of atria
PR interval	P wave + delayed conduction at AV node
QRS complex	Ventricular depolarization Q wave absent in most birds Most birds have (Q)rS and mammals have qRs complexes on lead II
R wave	Absent in normal birds Observed in bundle branch block
QT interval	Corresponds to length of ventricular contraction
ST segment	Period between end of ventricular depolarization and beginning of ventricular repolarization
B wave	Conus arteriosus depolarization in elasmobranch fishes Bulbus cordis in amphibians
T wave	Repolarization of the ventricles
U wave	Absent in normal animals Repolarization of papillary muscles or repolarization of conducting system

Sections are in order of appearance.
AV, Atrioventricular; *ECG,* electrocardiogram; *SN,* sinoatrial.

the coelomic cavity by the semitransparent septum transversum; thus, it cannot be directly visualized.[37,439]

Amphibians

Physical Examination

As for other organ systems, a thorough history is important in amphibians, as are water quality and osmolality. The cardiac evaluation is as limited in amphibians as cardiovascular diseases are uncommon. The initial hands-off examination should detect abnormal shape, coelomic distension, localized edema, and cutaneous abnormalities. Most edematous amphibians do not primarily suffer from diseases of the cardiovascular system, but this should remain part of the differential until proven otherwise. The hands-on examination will confirm the presence of edema and coelomic effusion, and an aspirate of the fluid should be collected for analysis. Some frogs may inflate themselves as a defensive measure and this should not be interpreted as abnormal.

The HR can be assessed using a Doppler probe placed on the cranioventral aspect of the animal. By moving the probe, one may be able to differentiate cardiovascular sounds from different vessels.[440] In large frogs, cardiac auscultation is possible, but care should be taken not to damage the fragile skin with the diaphragm or the bell of the stethoscope. In some species, the heart may be seen beating on the ventral aspect of the animal in the area of the xiphoid.[440]

Clinical Pathology

Clinical pathologic changes are nonspecific in amphibians with cardiovascular disease. Changes in plasma/lymph osmolality and electrolytic concentrations may be seen with various causes of hydrops. Hypercholesterolemia was associated with atherosclerosis and lipid disorders in Cuban tree frogs.[154] Effusion fluid should be collected and submitted for fluid analysis, cytology, and bacterial culture. Lymph may be sampled from the lymph hearts caudally. The fluid should be characterized as a transudate or an exudate.

Electrocardiography

Electrocardiography has been extensively used in the frog early on to study cardiac electrophysiology, and it was in frogs that the electrical activity of the heart was first recorded. However, the use of electrocardiography in amphibian medicine has been minimal. It is recommended that amphibians be anesthetized for a proper ECG recording. In addition, Whitaker et al. recommend acclimating the amphibian patient for a minimum of 4 hours to room temperature, inducing anesthesia with tricaine methanesulfonate, and using needle electrodes intramuscularly.[440]

The amphibian ECG is similar to most other vertebrates and is morphologically close to the fish and reptile ECG. SV and B waves are usually present, are of a small magnitude, and denote the depolarization of the sinus venosus and the bulbus cordis, respectively (see Table 4-7).[440,441] A comprehensive study and description of the Anuran ECG was reported by Mullen.[441] Reference intervals have been published with a small sample size (*n* = 3 to 5) on South American common toads *(Bufo margaritifer)*, giant toads *(Bufo marinus)*, Buerger's robber frogs *(Eleuthrodactylus buergeri)*, and mountain water frogs *(Telmatobius montanus)* under pentobarbital anesthesia but are unavailable for most amphibian species.[440,441] Electrocardiographic parameter measurements may vary with temperature. The mean electrical axis (MEA) is usually positive in Anuran but negative MEAs have been recorded in various amphibian species.[441]

Diagnostic Imaging

Radiographs are of limited utility to evaluate amphibian hearts because of a lack of radiographic detail. Echocardiography has been described in Anurans and can be performed by placing the probe directly on the skin on the xyphoid area or through a water-filled plastic container.[438,442] Three views, the parasternal long axis, the subcostal 3 chamber, and the high sternal, were described in two *Xenopus* spp. of different size.[442] In this study on 50 frogs, the intracardiac anatomy, *truncus arteriosus*, and major vascular trunks could be well visualized, Doppler ultrasound could be performed, and two-dimensional and spectral Doppler echocardiographic measurements were reported.[442] Furthermore, lymph heart ultrasound measurements were performed in two Anuran species using a high-frequency sonographic probe.[443] Coelomic effusion can also be differentiated from other causes of abdominal enlargement. Rigid coelomic endoscopy may allow the visualization of the pericardium along other coelomic organs.

Reptiles

Physical Examination

Clinical signs of cardiac disease in reptiles include swelling in the area of the heart (Figure 4-29), cyanosis, peripheral edema, pulmonary edema, ascites, and exercise intolerance. However, nonspecific clinical signs are more frequent, such as lethargy, depression, anorexia, weight loss, weakness, dyspnea, and sudden death. It is important to note that when performing a clinical examination, care should be taken to consider the environmental temperature as this can influence cardiopulmonary parameters and distort the final results.[57,444]

Heart sounds in reptiles are of very low amplitude and hence cannot be consistently auscultated with a standard stethoscope. This problem can be overcome in some species

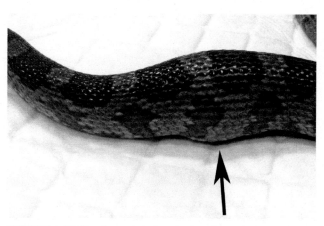

FIGURE 4-29 Cardiomegaly in a ball python *(Python regius)*.

by using a pressure-sensitive acoustic stethoscope (Ultrascope®) that permits diagnosis of heart murmurs. This equipment is, however, only suitable in large species of snakes (e.g., large boids) and species of lizards where the heart lies in the midcoelomic region and is not hidden under the bony pectoral girdle (e.g., monitor lizards, *Varanus* spp.). A Doppler ultrasonic probe can be used for cardiac auscultation in all species of reptiles. The probe is placed with an acoustic gel coating on the epidermal surface at the level of the heart or large efferent arteries. This may enable the clinician to evaluate the HR and rhythm.[57,444,445]

In general, HRs are slower in reptiles compared to mammals or birds. The heart rate is dependent on numerous factors including but not limited to body temperature (increasing during basking and lowering during cooling, myocardial efficiency being optimum when the reptile is within its preferred optimal temperature zone), activity (HR is proportional to metabolic level), respiratory rate (bradycardia is observed during apnea as pulmonary resistance increases and blood flow to the lungs decreases), volemia status, digestion, gravidity, and sensory stimulations such as handling and postural and gravitational stress.[56,69] Heart rates vary with size and species, but the normal reptilian HR can be roughly estimated using allometric formulas such as HR (bpm) $= 20.6 \times W_{(kg)}^{-0.229}$ in ophidians and HR (bpm) $= 33.4 \times W_{(kg)}^{-0.25}$ in general.[68,446]

Blood Pressure Measurement

In indirect arterial blood pressure as measured in small animals with a cuff and Doppler probe is not reliable and therefore not recommended in reptiles. Indeed, no measurement system has been scientifically validated. The thick and highly keratinized skin in the limb and tail regions constitutes a major obstacle to penetration by acoustic waves from the Doppler probe. Oscillometric techniques were assessed in boid snakes and the green iguana and were found to be unreliable or not able to obtain readings.[447,448] In addition, direct blood pressure in reptile species has been obtained experimentally.[449]

Clinical Pathology

In reptiles, hematological and biochemical changes are usually associated with generalized conditions and are nonspecific for heart diseases. Increased plasma creatine kinase (CK) can result from skeletal muscle damage as may occur with traumatic injuries and intramuscular injections (in particular, with certain drugs such as enrofloxacin). CK may also increase with conditions affecting cardiac muscle.[211,450] Dyslipidemias such as hypercholesterolemia have been shown to be associated with atherosclerosis in a bearded dragon.[169] Hypocalcemia, commonly seen with nutritional disorders in reptiles, can affect striated cardiac muscle and be correlated to ECG abnormalities.[445] Because cardiovascular diseases of reptiles are often of an infectious etiology, leukocytosis, lymphocytosis, and heterophilia may be indicative of underlying infections or hematopoietic neoplasia with secondary cardiac effects.

Electrocardiography

Electrocardiography can greatly enhance the diagnosis of cardiac disease in reptiles and is also beneficial for monitoring patients under anesthesia. The main challenge associated with interpreting ECGs in reptiles is the low electric amplitudes (usually <1.0 mV), which do not always provide readings of diagnostic quality. Moreover, standard parameters are not established for many species; thus, interval and segment values may not always be of much use (Table 4-8). Performing routine ECGs on healthy reptile patients can help to build up baseline values for future comparison.[57,444,445,451–453]

Interpretations of ECGs in reptiles are very similar to those in mammals, with P, QRS, and T complexes. An SV wave represented by the depolarization of the sinus venosus (and the postcaval vein) may be measured just before the P wave (see Table 4-7). The SV wave is followed by sinusal contraction, the P wave is followed by atrial contraction, and the R wave is followed by ventricular contraction. The T wave indicates ventricular repolarization.[57,444,445,451–454]

The electrodes used to measure an ECG in a reptile can be self-adhering skin electrodes (designed for human use),

---

TABLE 4-8

ECG Measurement Reference Values (Range) on Lead II in Selected Reptile Species

Species	*Boa Constrictor*[453] Unanesthetized	Metofane	Pentobarbital	Snakes[455]	Lizards[455]	American Alligator[456]
N	6	6	12	101	321	10
HR	11-42	11-37	5-34	22-136	45-230	
SV-P interval		0.24-1.3	0.40-0.60	0.29	0.19	
SV duration		0.04-0.35	0.04-0.18			
P amplitude				Inconsistent	Inconsistent	Inconsistent
P duration	0.06-0.1	0.05-0.2	0.04-0.11	0.02-0.07	0.02-0.06	Inconsistent
PR interval	0.38-0.90	0.40-1.04	0.35-0.56	0.26	0.16	Inconsistent
R amplitude				Inconsistent	Inconsistent	0.03-0.43
QRS duration	0.1-0.24	0.1-0.2	0.11-0.16	0.02-0.12	0.02-0.14	0.064-0.148
T amplitude				Inconsistent	Inconsistent	0.06-0.18
QT interval	0.8-2.0	0.84-1.74	1.16-2.40	0.30-1.36	0.18-1.30	0.93-1.45
MEA				96	95	60-108

Amplitude measured in mV, duration in sec, MEA in degrees. Room temperature was 22°C to 26°C during ECG recording.
ECG, Electrocardiogram; *HR*, heart rate; *MEA*, mean electrical axis; N, sample size; *SN*, supraventricular.

stainless steel hypodermic needles, stainless steel suture material, or alligator clips. Placement of the electrodes varies according to species but is usually inspired from the traditional four limb lead placement. In snakes, they should be placed two heart lengths cranial and caudal to the heart. In lizards, where the heart is encased in the pectoral girdle (e.g., iguanas, bearded dragons, chameleons, water dragons, and skinks), the two cranial electrodes should be placed in the cervical region instead of on the forelimbs. Monitor lizards (*Varanus* spp.), tegus (*Tupinambis* spp.), and crocodilians have a heart positioned caudally to the pectoral girdle and can have the ECG electrodes placed on the limbs or torso. Four limb ECG placement is not appropriate in chelonians due to the low surface voltage generated. In these species, the two cranial electrodes should also be placed in the cervical region, lateral to the neck and medial to the forelimbs.[57,444,445,451–453]

Radiography
The use of diagnostic imaging is an essential part of the examination of the reptile patient (see Figure 4-14). Although conventional radiography has historically been the main imaging tool for reptiles, it remains challenging to deliver images of high diagnostic value, especially for assessing the cardiac silhouette. Radiographs can rarely be used to evaluate the reptilian heart, mainly due to the poor differences in tissue contrast (compared to mammals and birds) and anatomical positioning of organs. Indeed, in chelonians and crocodilians, the heart is superimposed with other visceral organs, and in lizards and chelonians, with the bony pectoral girdle and shell, respectively. Some of these difficulties may be overcome by using corrected settings; however, the use of computed tomography (CT) and digital radiography allows digital enhancement (level and window parameters) and can greatly enhance the diagnostic value of the image.

Nevertheless, radiographs can be used to evaluate heart size in snakes and monitor lizards, because in these species the heart is not located in the vicinity of a radiopaque organ and therefore radiography can be used to confirm the presence of cardiomegaly. Another disadvantage of cardiac radiography is the lack of normal reference parameters; however, this can be overcome by acquiring routine radiographs of healthy patients in order to build up a personal database of standard parameters. When assessing a reptile patient for cardiac enlargement, it is worth noting that cardiomegaly may be normal under some circumstances, such as postprandially in intermittent feeders (see anatomy and physiology section). As with any routine radiographic examination, two orthogonal projections should be taken: a dorso-ventral view and lateral view. In chelonians, a craniocaudal view can be useful but is most useful for visualizing lung fields.[171,445,456,457] Mineralization of the great vessels can sometimes be observed, which may result from hypervitaminosis D or other metabolic disturbances.[444] The shoulder girdles provide good landmarks for increasing image quality in chelonians. The heart is usually just caudal to the level of the acromion processes and cranial to the distal procoracoid process-procoracoid cartilage junction.[57]

Echocardiography
Ultrasound and Doppler examination are diagnostic tools of choice for antemortem evaluation of reptilian heart diseases

(see Figures 4-13, 4-15, and 4-29).[166,187,190,457–462] The size of the patient dictates the transducer probes needed to perform the echocardiographic examination. Smaller animals (e.g., snakes, most lizards, and small chelonians) require the use of a 10- or 15-MHz transducer, while a 5- to 8-MHz transducer can be used for medium to large size patients. A 3.5-MHz probe may be warranted for very large reptiles such as big crocodiles, giant tortoises, large monitors, or sea turtles. A linear array is usually used in snakes and lizards. In chelonians, the use of the biconvex sector scanner is recommended because of the narrow space of the acoustic windows in these reptiles; the linear transducer is too large to fit in the cervical, axillary, or prefemoral areas.

In lizards whose heart is located at the base of the neck, the ultrasonographic window is craniocaudal; the probe must be positioned in front of and above the bony pectoral girdle (this window is relatively narrow and thus restricts a good visualization of the whole organ). In Varanidae and Teiidae, the heart is located more caudally in the coelomic cavity and can be easily accessed via a ventral approach.

In chelonians, placing the transducer in the axillo-cervical (cervico-brachial) fossa will provide access to the heart, which is caudal to the thyroid.[433] It lies immediately above the plastron. The left and right atria are of similar size with thin walls. The ventricle is thick walled and the two AV valves, whose motion is clearly discernible, are very echogenic. They can be seen as highly reflective ribbons.

Since snakes are the group of reptiles most commonly diagnosed with heart disease, a standardization of the two-dimensional echocardiography has been developed in ophidians and is based on approaches used in mammals (Figure 4-30). The ophidian echocardiographic examination has been studied in great detail and is described later; the reader is referred to the original publications for additional information.[458,460] Furthermore, the patterns of blood flow in *Python regius* have been studied using Doppler echocardiography.[72]

In snakes, the position of the heart is indicated by visualization of the ventral precordial tap. As the snake's heart is mobile inside the coelomic cavity, the transducer may be moved by a few centimeters, either cranially or caudally, in relation to the initial position during the ultrasound examination. A thick layer of acoustic coupling gel must be applied ventrally to ensure perfect cohesion between the probe and the snake's scales.

Three approaches to define the ultrasound windows can be used in succession.[445,459,460] Most of the ultrasound examination is carried out by placing the probe ventral to the heart. This ventral approach makes it possible to view the organ from the caudal ventricular apex to the cranial atria and examine the sinus venosus, the AV junctions, and the three arterial trunks. Two other approaches, known as right and left intercostal approaches, are obtained by lateral positioning of the probe. These approaches are used to complete the ventral cranial examination and obtain a lateral visualization of the three arterial trunks and both atria that proceed into the single ventricle.[165,457–463]

By placing the probe ventral to the heart, the operator can scan or "sweep" the organ from the apex to the arterial trunks along its short axis (short-axis views). Thus, two transventricular views can be obtained by a ventral approach:[458,460] on

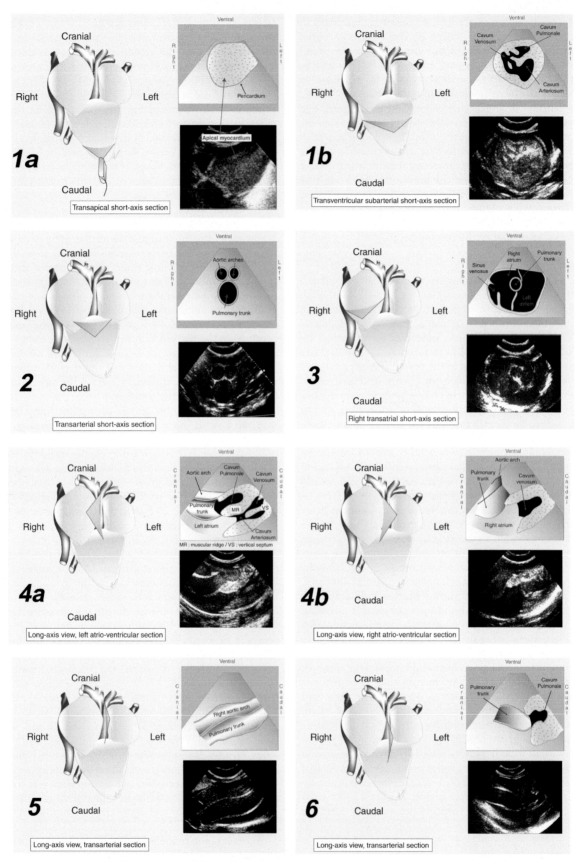

FIGURE 4-30 Standard echocardiographic sections in ophidians. (Reprinted and modified from Schilliger L, Tessier D, Pouchelon JJ, et al. Proposed standardization of the two-dimensional echocardiographic examination in snakes. *J Herp Med Surg.* 2006;16(3):90-102, with permission from the ARAV.)

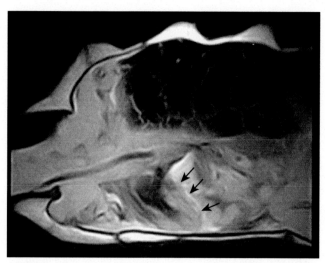

FIGURE 4-31 T2 MRI section of a spur-thighed tortoise *(Testudo graeca)* showing a sagittal view of the heart *(arrows).*

moving the probe caudal to cranial, from the apex toward the base:

The apical or transapical short-axis view shows a transverse view of the apical myocardium and the pericardium from behind, in the form of an echogenic line (Figure 4-30, 1a).

The transventricular subarterial short-axis view shows a transverse view of the three cavae surrounded by the peripheral myocardium (the ventral cavum pulmonale, the right dorsal cavum venosum, the left dorsal cavum arteriosum) (Figure 4-30, 1b). The interventricular (vertical) septum, located in the ventricular cavity between the cavum arteriosum and the cavum venosum, can be partially visualized, as can the muscular ridge (horizontal septum) marking the separation between the cavum venosum and the cavum pulmonale.

By continuing to move the probe cranially, a transarterial short-axis view is obtained, giving a transverse view of the three large arterial trunks: the two aortic arches of equal diameter and the pulmonary trunk of larger diameter (having the shape of a "Mickey Mouse head") (Figure 4-30, 2). By leaving the probe in a ventral position, but by moving it slightly toward the right, the right transatrial short-axis view shows the opening of the sinus venosus into the right atrium and enables the aspect of both sinoatrial valves to be assessed (Figure 4-30, 3).[458,460]

Long-axis views are obtained by turning the probe 90° in relation to the previous projections.[458,460]

Thus, starting from the transventricular or subarterial view, the rotation of the probe enables two long-axis views of the heart to be obtained. These are called AV sections, and they show both atrial cavities opening into the single ventricle. The left AV junction can be observed by orienting the ultrasound plane ventro-dorsally from the right to the left (Figure 4-30, 4a). Similarly, the right AV junction can be observed by orienting the ultrasound plane ventro-dorsally from the left to the right (Figure 4-30, 4b). The AV valves, also known as septal monocuspid valves, can hence be observed.[458,460]

Similarly, starting from the short-axis transarterial view, the probe is rotated 90° to obtain a long-axis transarterial section that reveals the right aortic arch and the pulmonary trunk with parallel paths (Figure 4-30, 5). The path of the pulmonary artery can be located by moving the probe caudally. The path of this artery comes closer to the probe ventrally and then opens out on the right with the cavum pulmonale.[458,460]

Last, starting from the right transatrial short-axis view, the probe is rotated 90° and moved caudally to display the caudal vena cava running parallel to the pulmonary vein: A long-axis transcaval section, starting from the sinus venosus, can thus be obtained (Figure 4-30, 6).[458,460]

When imaging small snakes, the examination may be completed by two intercostal approaches. Thus, the transarterial long-axis section, obtained by the right intercostal approach, provides clear visualization of the left atrium. The probe is placed laterally on the right side so that the cross section is parallel to the animal's body, and the left atrium is removed from the proximal field occupied by the large arterial trunks. Conversely, the left symmetrical intercostal section provides a good approach for observing the right atrium.[458,460]

Advanced Imaging

Computed tomography and MRI are important diagnostic imaging tools in reptile medicine but are not as valuable as echocardiography regarding the investigation of cardiovascular conditions. Moreover, both techniques require that the reptile be immobilized throughout the entire examination. This is usually achieved by general anesthesia, which is contraindicated in case of heart failure.[457] CT is a particularly valuable technique for visualizing lung tissue (e.g., pneumopathy, lung trauma, or road accidents) and bone tissue (e.g., trauma, osteomyelitis, metabolic bone disease). Except for bone tissue, the results obtained with MRI are much more detailed than those obtained with CT (Figure 4-31). In general, MRI is indicated for the examination of soft tissues, particularly the brain, liver, reproductive system, and kidneys.[457] Both CT and MRI are of no help when trying to visualize intracardiac structures and large vessels, except perhaps in cases of marked cardiomegaly, which should be investigated with ultrasound anyway.

Endoscopy

Endoscopy differs from other imaging modalities in that it is an invasive procedure that enables direct inspection of the structures under consideration. Coelioscopy is not an appropriate diagnostic method for investigating cardiac diseases in reptiles. The opaque fibrous pericardium prevents direct visualization of the myocardium with the endoscope, and only gross changes of the pericardium can be appreciated. Endoscopy is mostly used to visualize organs such as the liver, spleen, stomach, lungs, and gonads and can be used to biopsy lesions and masses inside the coelomic cavity. A detailed review of coelioscopy in reptiles has been published.[464]

Mammals

Physical Examination

Patient signalment and clinical history provide important clues to the medical suspicion of cardiovascular diseases.

Some species show higher prevalence than others, and cardiac diseases are more frequent in older animals overall. Geriatric ferrets, rats, and hedgehogs appear particularly susceptible. Some laboratory or pet breeds are reported to have higher susceptibilities (e.g., giant Flemish rabbits). Being a male is also associated with a higher prevalence of a number of degenerative cardiac diseases, particularly in rats. Heartworms should be suspected in ferrets living in endemic areas with access to the outdoors and not on preventive therapy. Clinical signs commonly reported with cardiovascular conditions in exotic mammals include weakness, lethargy, exercise intolerance, anorexia, abdominal distension, cough, cyanosis, dyspnea, posterior limb weakness (ferrets), collapse, and syncope. External examination may reveal the presence of peripheral edema or abdominal distension caused by ascites. Jugular dilation may be present, particularly in rabbits, which are prone to secondary exophthalmia (see Anatomy section of this chapter).

In mammals, cardiopulmonary auscultation is much more rewarding than in all other species of exotic companion animals. However, the HR can be extremely fast in small species, limiting the ability to detect abnormal heart sounds. Physiologic cardiovascular values are provided in Table 4-9 for various species. It is noteworthy that an audible murmur is identified in many cases of congestive heart failure in exotic mammals (see Table 4-20). However, benign and physiologic heart murmurs are also encountered. Murmurs are usually graded on a 1 (very faint, only heard in ideal circumstances) to 6 (very loud, even heard with stethoscope off the chest) scale in mammals.

A study in ferrets found a 28% prevalence of heart murmurs, for which 92.6% were associated with DCM on echocardiography.[238] Another study in chinchillas found a 23% prevalence of heart murmurs, which was considered a normal finding in most animals. However, a murmur of a grade >3 was highly associated with echocardiographic abnormalities.[214] Tachycardia is also frequently noticed in animals with cardiopathies. Bradycardia may be detected in ferrets with second or third AV blocks. Irregular rhythm caused by

premature beats, pauses secondary to periods of sinus arrest, and gallop rhythms can also be identified on auscultation. Pulmonary auscultation may reveal crackles and harsh lung sounds with pulmonary edema. Lungs sounds are muffled in the presence of pleural effusion. Finally, peripheral arterial pulse is easily obtained in ferrets and rabbits (central ear artery) but can be challenging to palpate in smaller mammals.

Blood Pressure Measurement

Indirect over direct arterial blood pressure techniques are typically used in pets. However, while measuring indirect blood pressure is widely advocated in exotic companion mammals, significant limitations exist. Due to the small size of exotic mammals, indirect blood pressure measurements often lack accuracy and only show moderate agreement with direct measurements. Even in larger species such as cats, it was determined that Doppler measurements had poor agreement with direct values.[468] For instance, two studies in ferrets confirmed this lack of agreement and accuracy and showed that Doppler techniques consistently underestimated and oscillometric measurements consistently overestimated systolic blood pressure.[469,470] Underestimation increased with increasing systolic blood pressure.[470] Likewise, a similar trend was observed in rabbits.[471] Tail measurements were found to be more accurate overall in ferrets.[469] For this reason, reference intervals are only provided for direct arterial blood pressure measurements (see Table 4-9). However, rodent-specific equipment has been validated for blood pressure measurement in laboratory rodents and may show adequate accuracy. Indirect arterial pressure is usually obtained from the tail in rats and mice.

Clinical Pathology

As in other species, hematologic and biochemical changes from are not specific to cardiovascular diseases in exotic mammals. Erythrocytosis in response to chronic hypoxia may be noticed and leukocytosis may develop in cases of infectious myocarditis. Myocardial disease may result in an increase in CK (cardiac isoenzyme), lactate dehydrogenase (LDH), and cardiac troponin (cTn)T or I. Troponin assays used in dogs are specific to myocardial injuries and are expected to be applicable to ferrets, rabbits, and guinea pigs because protein sequences are similar at 90% to 95% (basic local alignment search tool [BLAST]; Beaufrère 2013). Cross-species reactivity of laboratory tests is usually considered high in mammals.[472] In experimental cardiotoxicosis, cTnT was an effective biomarker of myocardial injury in ferrets, rats, and mice.[472,473] Normal cTnT values are similar to dogs and humans but not in mice, where normal values are 20-fold higher.[473] For instance, normal ferret values fall within the range of 0.05 to 0.10 ng/mL.[245] Myocardial degeneration in aging rats results in increased cTn.[472]

Fluid recovered by abdominocentesis, thoracocentesis, and pericardiocentesis should be analyzed and is typically a pure or modified transudate. In cases of idiopathic pericardial effusion, fluid can be hemorrhagic.

In ferrets infected with heartworm, microfilariae may be observed on the blood smear (sensitivity of 50%), but heartworm tests should be used to confirm the disease.[98] Antigen enzyme-linked immunosorbent assay (ELISA) (IDEXX's SNAP heartworm rapid treatment [RT] test) tests are most

TABLE 4-9

Heart Rate and Direct Blood Pressure Values in Selected Companion Mammal Species

Species	Heart Rate (bpm)	Systolic (mmHg)	Diastolic (mmHg)
Ferret	200-400	Female 133 Male 161	110-125
Rabbit	200-300	90-130	80-90
Guinea pig	230-380	80-94	55-58
Chinchilla	100-150		
Syrian hamster	280-412	150	100
Rat	300-500	116-145	76-97
Mouse	310-840	133-160	102-110
African hedgehog	180-280		
Sugar glider	200-300		

Adapted from References 465-468.

commonly selected. Sensitivity is 84% and specificity 97% in dogs, but accuracy is unknown in ferrets, especially since only female worms shed antigens and ferrets can develop severe clinical signs from a single worm (www.idexx.com, accessed 01/2013).[98]

Electrocardiography

The mammalian ECG is the most familiar to the veterinary practitioner. In exotic mammals, the leads are placed in a manner similar to that for dogs and cats, and the ECG wave morphology is also similar (see Table 4-7). The ECG is most often obtained on unanesthetized animals restrained in right lateral recumbency. Reference intervals have been published for a few species including three studies in pet ferrets and one in rabbits (Table 4-10). The interpretation of the ECG consists of determining the HR, heart rhythm, MEA, and measurements of wave amplitude and duration. The MEA is positive in most mammals (i.e., a tall R wave is visible in leads II, III, and aVF) (see the section on birds for determination of MEA). ECG recordings are critical to the assessment of arrhythmias and in animals experiencing syncope and may provide clues to chamber enlargement (Figure 4-32). In rabbits, normal rhythm usually does not include sinus arrhythmia but it does in ferrets.[225,245,257] Second-degree AV blocks

TABLE 4-10

ECG Measurement Reference Values on Lead II in Selected Exotic Mammal Species under Anesthesia

	Ferret[476,477]	Ferret[475]	Ferret[239]	Rabbit[478]	Guinea Pig[479]	Hedgehog[262]
N	25-27	80	40	46		13
HR	144-248	250-428	145-354	198-330		104-296
P amplitude	0.108-0.136	0.025-0.200	0.006-0.154	0.04-0.12	0.01	
P duration	0.016-0.032	0.01-0.03	0.008-0.032	0.01-0.05	0.015-0.035	
PR interval	0.040-0.073	0.03-0.06	0.024-0.076	0.04-0.08	0.048-0.060	
R amplitude	0.00-3.05	0.99-2.80	0.482-2.878	0.03-0.039	1.1-1.9	0.00-0.44
QRS duration	0.028-0.060	0.02-0.05	0.012-0.048	0.02-0.06	0.008-0.046	0.03
T amplitude		−0.3-0.1	−0.216-0.516	0.05-0.17	0.062	
QT interval	0.08-0.16	0.06-0.16	0.068-0.132	0.08-0.16	0.106-0.144	
MEA	53.2-101.2	75-100		−43-80	20-80	−36-16

Amplitude measured in mV, duration in sec, MEA in degrees.
Note: To obtain a 95% reference interval, all published results in the form of mean ± SD were reported as mean ± 2SD and in the form of mean ± SEM were reported as mean ± 2SEM√n. When only the range or a 95% reference interval was published, result was reported as is.
ECG, Electrocardiogram; *HR*, heart rate; *MEA*, mean electrical axis; *N*, sample size.

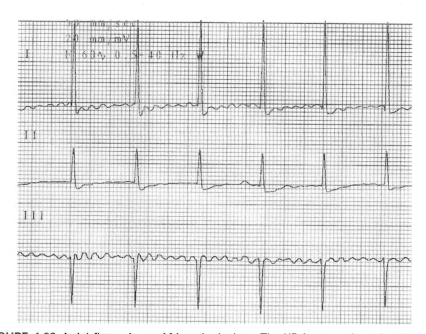

FIGURE 4-32 Atrial flutter in an African hedgehog. The HR is approximately 180 bpm. The rhythm is regular and characterized by tall and narrow R waves in leads I and II, indicating the supraventricular origin of the impulses. There are no P waves; however, the baseline is replaced by rapid flutter waves, visible in leads I and III.

TABLE 4-11

Radiographic Cardiac Sizes in Selected Exotic Companion Mammals

	Ferret*,[†]	Ferret[‡]	Ferret[§]	Rabbit*	Hedgehog[‖]
N	20	18	64	27	13
RL-VHS	4.91-5.91	4.43-6.71	4.20-6.24	6.38-9.16	7.20-9.12
VD-VHS	5.02-6.98	5.34-8.30	4.70-6.01	6.25-9.28	
RL ratio	1.21-1.49				1.31-2.47
VD ratio	1.33-1.69				

Adapted from References 239, 262, 480-482.
RL, right lateral; *VD*, ventro-dorsal; *VHS*, vertebral heart score.
*Starting at cranial edge of T4, [‡]starting at cranial edge of T5, [§]starting at cranial edge of T6; ratios: [†]long axis + short axis/T5-T8 or [‖]long axis/rib 5–rib 7.
Note: To obtain a 95% reference interval, all published results in the form of mean ± SD were reported as mean ± 2SD and in the form of mean ± SEM were reported as mean ± 2SEM√n. When only the range or a 95% reference interval was published, result was reported as is.

can be seen in healthy ferrets. The ferret ECG is reported to be similar to dogs with tall R waves but, otherwise, to small P waves as in cats.[238] A significant effect of body position on electrocardiographic values (P- and R-wave amplitude) has been found in ferrets.[474] The rabbit ECG is reported to be characterized by pointed P waves, peaked T waves, and a relatively long ST segment.[475]

Radiography

Thoracic radiographs, routinely used to assess the presence of cardiomegaly in mammals, must be taken during inspiration. Reference intervals of normal radiographic cardiac dimensions have been determined in ferrets, rabbits, and African hedgehogs using a vertebral scale system, which was calculated differently in each of the published individual studies (Table 4-11).[231,261,479-481]

In ferrets, both vertebral heart scores and vertebral ratios have been described to assess the cardiac silhouette. Three studies investigated the vertebral heart score in ferrets by adding the long- and short-axis length from either the lateral or ventrodorsal view and comparing the measurement obtained to the vertebral length on a right lateral thoracic radiograph starting at the cranial edge of T4, T5, or T6 and estimating to the nearest 0.25 vertebra (see Table 4-11 and Figure 4-33).[238,479,480] A heart/vertebral ratio has also been obtained by adding the heart long- and short-axis length and dividing it by the length of the T5 to T8 segment.[479] Ratios obtained from dividing the long- and short-axis length each by the length of T8 have also been reported.[480] Overall, measurements taken on right lateral radiographic views seemed to be more reliable.[479] A study also showed that the normal ferret's heart usually encompasses 1.7 to 2.9 intercostal spaces.[238] Fat deposition may increase the vertebral heart score.[238] Significant larger radiographic cardiac measurements have been demonstrated in ferrets diagnosed with DCM or other cardiac diseases.[231,238] On mustelid lateral thoracic radiographs, the heart appears globoid and is only slightly in contact with the sternum ventrally. This sternal contact may increase in cases of cardiac diseases.[98]

In rabbits and African hedgehogs, a similar vertebral heart score was determined in terms of vertebral length starting at the cranial edge of T4 (see Table 4-11).[261,481] In addition, in African hedgehogs, a radiographic ratio has been obtained by either dividing the long- or short-axis length by the distance

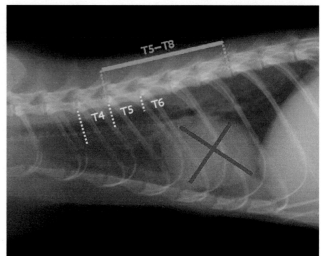

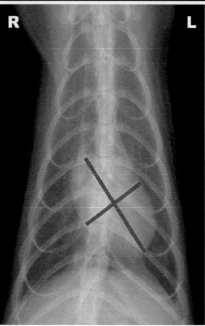

FIGURE 4-33 Radiographic heart size measurement in a ferret. *Red lines* represent the short- and long-axis lengths that should be added. Vertebral heart scores are obtained by comparing this measurement to vertebral length starting at the apical end of T4, T5, or T6. Alternatively, a ratio can be computed with the T5-T8 length.

between the fifth and seventh ribs.[261] Lateral radiographs should be taken in hedgehogs using a clip to hold the dorsal skin and quills dorsally to prevent superimposition with the thorax.[261] It is also interesting to note that the rabbit's chest is small compared to the trunk, which may render radiographic interpretation more challenging in this species.[482]

Other radiographic abnormalities classically seen with cardiac diseases in exotic mammals include pulmonary edema, pulmonary vessel congestion, pleural effusion, tracheal elevation, ascites, hepatomegaly, and arterial mineralization. In rabbits, dorsal elevation of the trachea and soft tissue opacity in the cranial mediastinum should also raise the suspicion of a thymoma.

Echocardiography

The practice of cardiac ultrasound in exotic companion mammals is similar to that in dogs and cats and is the imaging modality of choice for most functional and structural cardiac conditions. Echocardiographic approaches and planes are identical to those used in dogs and cats and can usually be obtained with minimal sedation (Figure 4-34). Readers are referred to cardiologic textbooks for a description of mammalian echocardiography.[483-485] In addition, exotic mammal echocardiography has recently been reviewed in detail in a textbook chapter with the application of standard scanning planes obtained from dogs and cats to exotic species.[486] Reference intervals for echocardiographic measurements have been published in ferrets, rabbits, chinchillas, guinea pigs, rats,

mice, and hamsters (Table 4-12). However, clinicians should be aware that most reference intervals are based on anesthetized patients, laboratory breeds, and single sexes.

Several studies have been reported in ferrets.[238,487,494] However, the rabbit is frequently used in cardiovascular research and therefore there is extensive scientific information on echocardiography available for this species.[256,488,495-500] Differences in echocardiographic measurements have been noted between anesthetized and conscious rabbits.[497] Likewise,

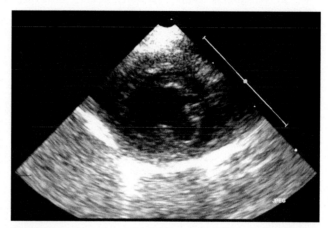

FIGURE 4-34 Echocardiography on a ferret; right parasternal short-axis view at the cardiac apex showing the left ventricle in cross section.

TABLE 4-12

Echocardiographic Reference Intervals in Selected Small Mammal Species

	Ferret[487,488]	Rabbit[489]	Guinea Pig[490]	Chinchilla[264]	Rat[491]	Mouse[492,493]	Hamster[494]	Hedgehog[262]
N	30	52	12	17	44		118	13
IVSd (mm)	2.2-5.0	1.29-2.77	1.13-2.37	1.2-2.4	1.13-1.610	0.64-1.20	0.9-1.1	1.3-1.7
IVSs (mm)	2.6-7.0	2.15-3.95	1.56-2.96			1.18-2.18		1.8-2.6
LVIDd (mm)	5.8-11.8	11.39-17.35	6.13-7.57	5.4-7.4	3.84-7.07	2.38-3.66	3.5-4.7	6.4-8.4
LVIDs (mm)	2.9-8.9	7.61-12.49	4.01-4.69	2.8-4.8	1.20-4.40	0.86-1.62	1.6-3.0	5.2-6.4
LVFWd (mm)	2.0-6.4	1.66-2.66	1.48-3.08	2.2-3.0	1.21-1.77	0.47-1.39	0.9-1.1	1.4-1.8
LVFWs (mm)	3.8-7.8	2.38-4.58	1.64-3.96			0.88-1.88		1.9-2.7
FS (%)	5-61	24.17-36.098	30.38-40.86	30-50	28.2-69.8	34-38	35.3-56.3	16.5-26.5
EF (%)	31-100	51.97-70.61	64.85-76.89		49.89-77.62	62-70		
Ao (mm)	3.3-7.3	6.74-9.78	4.15-5.15	2.6-4.6	2.43-3.91			3.2-4.0
LA (mm)	3.5-10.7	7.38-11.94	4.27-5.63	3.7-6.1	2.36-4.14			4.8-6.4
LA:Ao	7.9-18.7	0.89-1.45		0.98-1.78				1.23-1.87
EPSS (mm)		1.13-2.29		0.0-0.7				0.7-1.5
Ao$_{max}$ (m/s)	0.49-1.29	0.63-1.07		0.26-0.66	0.02-0.06			0.27-0.70
PA$_{max}$ (m/s)	0.82-1.38	0.39-0.79		0.29-0.93	0.00-0.09			0.15-0.52
Mitral E (m/s)	0.5-0.9	0.39-0.79		0.32-0.64	0.45-1.00	0.61-0.69	0.6-0.1	
Mitral A (m/s)	0.30-0.74	0.14-0.42		0.15-0.43	0.16-0.78	0.22-0.30	0.3-0.6	
Mitral E:A	0.74-2.02	1.27-3.11			0.52-2.83	2.1-3.3	1.25-2.87	

Ao, Aorta; *Ao$_{max}$*, aorta maximum velocity; *EF*, ejection fraction; *EPSS*, E-point septal separation; *FS*, fractional shortening; *IVSd*, interventricular septum end diastole; *IVSs*, interventricular septum end systole; *LA*, left atrium; *LVIDd*, left ventricular internal diameter end diastole; *LVIDs*, left ventricular internal diameter end systole; *LVFWd*, left ventricular free wall end diastole; *LVFWs*, left ventricular free wall end systole; *mitral E*, mitral valve E velocity; *mitral A*, mitral valve A velocity; N, sample size; *PA$_{max}$* pulmonary artery maximum velocity.

Note: To obtain a 95% reference interval, all published results in the form of mean ± SD were reported as mean ± 2SD and in the form of mean ± SEM were reported as mean ± 2SEM√n. When only the range or a 95% reference interval was published, result was reported as is.

echocardiography has been extensively performed in laboratory rats and mice since these rodent species are the predominant experimental species in cardiovascular research.[490,491,501–505] However, most murine studies have been conducted using very high-frequency probes that may not be available to veterinary practitioners.

Clinical cases have documented the usefulness of echocardiographic assessment in diagnosing various conditions such as DCM, valvular regurgitation, dirofilariasis, and congestive heart failure (see Table 4-20 later). In addition, several reports demonstrated significant differences in various experimental or spontaneous diseases between normal animals and ferrets, rabbits, hamsters, rats, and mice, such as induction of congestive heart failure or DCM, and showed that echocardiography had a high sensitivity in detecting these abnormalities.[214,225,238,241,263,506]

Ultrasound may also be used to investigate peripheral diseases such as the degree of caudal vena cava occlusion secondary to adrenal gland expansion (e.g., hyperplasia or neoplasia) in ferrets.

Angiography

Clinical applications of angiography have been limited in exotic mammals. Angiographic findings in experimental dirofilariasis have been published in ferrets.[283] In this study, the cranial vena cava, azygous vein, and left caudal lobar pulmonary artery of worms could be visualized.

Computed tomography and MRI angiographies have been used in laboratory animals, especially in species commonly used in cardiovascular research such as rabbits, rats, and mice.

Advanced Imaging

Cerebrovascular diseases are uncommon in companion exotic mammals; therefore, the use of advanced imaging has been restricted. The heart can be imaged using CT and MRI, but echocardiography is much more informative and practical.

Birds

Physical Examination

As for any clinical presentation, a complete history and thorough physical examination should be performed. Species, age, sex, captive lifestyle, and diet may predispose individuals to cardiovascular diseases. Increased age, being female, and certain parrot species (e.g., African grey parrots, Amazon parrots, cockatiels) are at increased risk for atherosclerosis.[379] Parrots are most often diagnosed with congestive heart failure and atherosclerosis, whereas commercial poultry (e.g., broilers, turkeys) suffer more from cardiac diseases related to selection for production.[296,297,342,346,371,379] Specific history of cardiac diseases may include dyspnea, exercise intolerance, falling off the perch, hind limb ataxia, altered mentation, neurological signs, syncope, collapse, and sudden death. Nonspecific signs of disease such as lethargy, weight loss, and anorexia are also frequently present. Coughing does not usually occur in birds due to an enlarged heart, because the aorta curves to the right and cardiac enlargement does not cause bronchial compression.[507] At physical examination, findings observed with cardiovascular diseases often include ascites, cyanosis or hypoperfusion (bluish or pale comb in chicken, bluish periorbital skins in some parrot species [e.g., African grey parrots, macaws], and increased ulnar vein refilling time), and increased

TABLE 4-13

Common Differential Diagnoses for Coelomic Fluids in Birds

Left and right
- Congestive heart failure
- Portal hypertension
- Advanced hepatic disease (fibrosis, amyloidosis, iron storage disease)
- Reproductive-associated ascites (egg yolk coelomitis, ovarian cysts, cystic right oviduct)
- Blockage of lymphatic drainage
- Hypoproteinemia
- Neoplastic ascites (e.g., biliary cystadenoma, ovarian or oviductal neoplasm)
- Viral ascites (avian viral serositis, polyomavirus, eastern equine encephalitis)
- Septic coelomitis (foreign body, ruptured intestine)
- Pancreatitis
- Coelomic hemorrhage

dyspnea when restrained. Ascites, in particular, is frequently present in cases of congestive heart failure but is also commonly seen with other conditions (Table 4-13). Hepatomegaly from liver congestion may be visible under the skin caudal to the keel in some patients. Preoxygenation is indicated to conduct a physical examination in severely distressed patients.

Birds must be handled upright to prevent circulatory collapse.[351] The arterial pulse is difficult to palpate in birds and not practical to procure without anesthesia; it is typically obtained from the ulnar superficial artery at the level of the proximal inner antebrachium. Cardiac auscultation, not sensitive in birds due to their fast HR, can be obtained by placing a pediatric or neonatal stethoscope over the cranial keel bone. The use of a pediatric digital stethoscope may allow the clinician to amplify, record, and slow the recording at a later time for analysis and a more sensitive auscultation examination. In at least one case, a phonocardiogram was used to characterize a cardiac murmur in a bird.[330]

Murmurs and arrhythmias may be detected but are hard to characterize and may be repeated with the patient under anesthesia. However, systolic murmurs have been detected in multiple cardiologic cases in birds.[300–302,305,306,323,330] Muffled heart sounds may indicate pericardial effusion, fluids in the ventral hepatoperitoneal cavities, or hepatomegaly surrounding the heart. In some species (e.g., Pelecaniformes), the presence of air between the heart and the keel from the interclavicular air sac may also muffle the heart sounds. The normal HR of birds is high, scales negatively with body weight, can increase up to four times the resting HR during flying, and can be expected to increase similarly during restraint (Table 4-14). As such, the avian normal HR can vary tremendously in an individual. Pulmonary auscultation is usually of low value to detect pleural effusion or pulmonary edema in birds.

Blood Pressure Measurement

Arterial blood pressure is higher in birds than in any other vertebrate. Direct arterial blood pressure is typically obtained by placing an arterial catheter either in the superficial ulnar artery in the proximal antebrachium or in the deep radial artery in the distal antebrachium. The external carotid artery has also been used. It is then connected to a pressure transducer and measured by an anesthetic monitor (Table 4-15).

Indirect blood pressure can be obtained using a Doppler transducer and a sphygmomanometer placed on the wing or leg with a cuff measured at 30% to 40% of the limb circumference. However, it has been consistently demonstrated that values obtained with this method do not agree with direct systolic blood pressure measurements and may therefore be of low clinical value as a diagnostic tool.[508,511,516] Limits of agreement were wide in a study in Hispaniolan Amazon parrots (*Amazona ventralis*) at −37 to 85 mmHg and −14 to 42 mmHg for wing and leg measurements, respectively.[508] In a study on various species of psittacines, large variation was

seen in repeated indirect blood pressure measurements, with most variability attributable to individual variation and cuff placement.[516] However, this suggested that a monitoring trend in indirect blood pressure measurement may be useful in the same bird during a single cuff placement, such as occurs during an anesthetic event. In an experiment in red-tailed hawks (*Buteo jamaicensis*), indirect blood pressure measurements were found to be in disagreement with direct systolic blood pressure but in acceptable agreement with mean blood pressure, with limits of agreement of −9 to 13.[511] This suggests that accuracy of indirect techniques may be higher in large birds. The oscillometric method of indirect blood pressure measurements has been found unreliable in all studied birds.[508,511]

In general, hypotension is defined as a systolic blood pressure lower than 90 mmHg, with a mean below 60 mmHg.[517] On the other hand, values for hypertension in birds have been poorly defined and are expected to be higher than in mammals owing to their greater blood pressure. Systolic values >200 mmHg have been proposed as hypertensive.[517]

Clinical Pathology

Apart from assessing the general health of the avian patient, clinical pathology tests may reveal specific changes associated with cardiovascular diseases but are of low sensitivity. Erythrocytosis may be caused by chronic hypoxia due to persistent ventilation/perfusion mismatch and increased oxygen demands. Leukocytosis may be seen in bacterial myocarditis and valvular endocarditis. Cardiovascular microfilariae may be observed on the blood smear. Blood samples from patients with severe microfilarial infestation may be positive on canine heartworm antigenic tests.[518] Arterial blood samples and blood-gas analyses may help pinpoint an oxygenation problem. Myocardial damage can lead to a rise in CK (and cardiac CK isoenzyme) and cTnT or cTnI (only 68% and 65% protein sequence homology between chicken and humans, respectively, which may affect diagnostic test accuracy; BLAST, Beaufrère 2013).[312] Electrolyte and mineral disorders (e.g., Ca, Mg, K, Na), hypoproteinemia, and hyperuricemia can also cause arrhythmia and cardiac diseases. Bile acids are

TABLE 4-14

Normal Heart Rates of Birds as a Function of Weight*

Weight (g)	Heart Rate (Resting) (bpm)	Heart Rate (Flight/ Restraint) (bpm)	Factor Increase
25	380	909	2.4
50	329	815	2.5
100	284	731	2.6
200	245	655	2.7
300	226	615	2.7
400	213	588	2.8
500	203	568	2.8
1000	175	509	2.9
2000	152	457	3.0

West N, Langille B, Jones D. Cardiovascular system. In: King A, McLelland J, eds. *Form and Function in Birds*, Volume 2. London: Academic Press; 1981:235-339.

*Function of weight is derived using the following formula: resting HR = $744 \times W^{-0.209}$; flight HR = $1506 \times W^{-0.157}$. The average values likely reflect the approximate range (resting, flight/restraint) of HRs to be expected in most avian species.

TABLE 4-15

Direct Arterial Blood Pressure* in Selected Species of Birds

Species	SAP	MAP	DAP	Reference
Amazon parrot (isoflurane, *n* = 8)	133 (88-177)	117 (76-158)	102 (58-146)	341
Amazon parrot (isoflurane, *n* = 16)	163 (127-199)	155 (119-191)	148 (112-184)	509
Pigeon (isoflurane, *n* = 15)	93 (73-113)	82 (54-110)	72 (46-98)	510
Red-tailed hawk (conscious, *n* = 8)	220 (119-331)	187 (104-271)	160 (70-2500)	511
Red-tailed hawk (sevoflurane, *n* = 6)	178 (124-232)	159 (109-209)	143 (95-191)	512
Great horned owl (conscious, *n* = 6)	231.5 (157-306)	203 (146-260)	178 (128-228)	511
Bald eagle (isoflurane, *n* = 17)	195 (165-225)	171 (142-200)	148 (120-176)	513
Bald eagle (sevoflurane, *n* = 17)	144 (116-172)	139 (111-167)	134.5 (106-163)	513
Chicken (anesthetized, *n* = 40)	141 (118-163)	136 (114-158)	131 (109-153)	514
Turkey (conscious, *n* = 20)	302 (289-315)	253 (242-264)	204 (194-214)	515
Pekin duck (anesthetized, *n* = 72)	165 (138-192)	143 (111-174)	121 (85-157)	516

*Mean (mean ± 2SD reference interval) measured in mmHg.
DAP, Diastolic arterial pressure; *MAP*, mean arterial pressure; *SAP*, systolic arterial pressure.

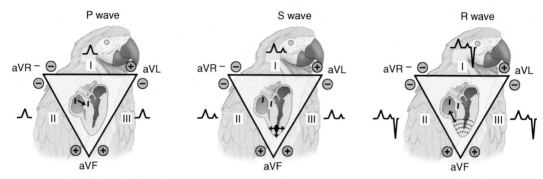

FIGURE 4-35 Schematic representation of the electrical activity of the avian heart with depiction of lead recordings (Einthoven's triangle). Leads I, II, and III are bipolar leads, and leads aVR, aVL, and aVF are augmented unipolar leads. Tracings represent the vectorial projection of the summation of the electrical activity. *P wave,* Atrial depolarization from the SA to the AV node; *R wave,* depolarization at the apex of the left ventricle; *S wave,* ventricular depolarization.

frequently moderately elevated with hepatic congestion secondary to congestive heart failure. Thyroid imbalance may contribute to heart disease but is rare in pet birds. Lipoprotein abnormalities may also be diagnosed in conjunction with some degenerative lesions but have to be interpreted in the context of the egg-laying cycle, and pathologic elevations have been poorly characterized. Experimental cholesterol feeding leads to an increase in total and LDL cholesterol in budgerigars *(Melopsittacus undulatus)* and quaker parrots *(Myiopsitta monachus).*[381,396] In the latter, the plasma cholesterol level was correlated with the severity of atherosclerotic lesions.[396] In addition, psittacine species susceptible to atherosclerosis have higher plasma total cholesterol levels.[375,397]

Finally, ascitic, pericardial, and effusion fluid should always be analyzed and can provide useful information. Cardiac-induced ascitic fluid is a pure or modified transudate; thus, it will have a low protein and cellular content and a low specific gravity. Ascitic fluid should also be submitted for culture. Blood cultures may be valuable to isolate causative agents responsible for cardiac bacterial infections and can be performed with 0.1 to 2 mL only.

Electrocardiography

Most avian cardiovascular diseases are accompanied by changes on the ECG that may also provide clues to chamber enlargement.[106] However, cardiopathies can occur without electrocardiographic changes. The avian ECG is typically obtained in the frontal plane by placing two front electrodes on the propatagia and one (left) or two (earth on right) back electrodes on the knee webs using needle electrodes or flat clips. Each lead evaluates the cardiac electrical activity on a different plane, and a standard examination classically includes three bipolar leads (I, II, and III) and three augmented unipolar leads (aVR, aVL, aVF) (Figure 4-35).

A proper ECG recording is easier to obtain on anesthetized birds, as few will tolerate the procedure or movement and muscle tremors may impair the recordings.[519] However, ECG tracings on conscious birds can still be obtained on pigeons, some raptors, and lethargic birds. Recordings need to be performed at 50 to 100 mm/s, with 100 mm/s being optimal to better assess QRS complex morphology. Electrocardiographic measurements are typically performed on

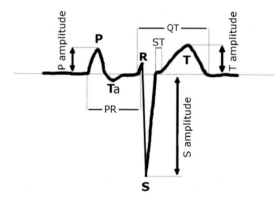

FIGURE 4-36 Typical avian ECG complex with depiction of the different measurement landmarks.

lead-II tracings. Electrical current from heating devices and anesthetic equipment can interfere with ECG tracings, and electrical filters from ECG machines may be used.

The normal avian ECG is usually composed of P, S, T, and a small R wave (see Figure 4-36 and Table 4-7). The Q wave is usually missing and a Ta wave is present in certain birds. The QRS complexes are mainly of the (Q)rS types on lead II, meaning the S wave is the most prominent. This contrasts with mammals, where the QRS complexes are most often of the qRs type. Interpretation of the avian ECG should be methodical, follow the same rules as in mammals, and include determination of the HR, heart rhythm, MEA, and measurements.[106]

In contrast to mammals, the cardiac MEA is negative in birds with a prominent S wave that gives negative QRS complexes on lead II. This is caused by transmission of the depolarization from subepicardially to endocardially.[106] However, some poultry and waterfowl, such as broilers and Pekin ducks, have a positive MEA and QRS complexes. The MEA is affected by changes in heart position and relative dilation of cardiac chambers. The MEA can be calculated using the vector method, the isoelectric method, or the largest net deflection method. The isoelectric method is the most practical and consists of identifying the lead closest to isoelectricity (summation of waves without P and T = 0 mmV) that the

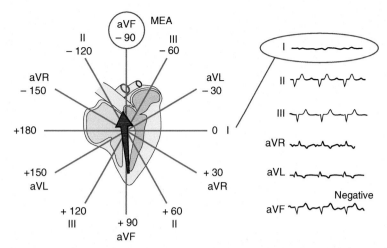

FIGURE 4-37 Determination of the ventricular MEA in birds using the isoelectric method and Bailey's hexaxial system. Example of a tracing where the ventricular depolarization is isoelectric in lead I and negative in the orthogonal aVF lead, resulting in a MEA of –90°.

MEA lies along and has the polarity of the perpendicular lead (Figure 4-36). Changes in ventricular MEA are due to changes in cardiac shape and position and are typically associated with right ventricular enlargement and left ventricular hypertrophy.[106]

Measurements that are usually taken include P amplitude and duration, PR interval, S amplitude, QRS duration, ST segment, T amplitude, QT interval, and MEA (Figure 4-37). The shape of the P wave may indicate left atrial hypertrophy (wide), right atrial hypertrophy (tall), or biatrial hypertrophy (wide and tall). However, the sensitivity and specificity of these ECG criteria are low. Each P wave should precede and be related to a QRS complex. Increase in the PR interval indicates an increased delay in electrical conduction at the AV node (AV block). Morphologic alteration of the QRS complexes may indicate left ventricular hypertrophy (increased S amplitude or QRS complex duration) or right ventricular hypertrophy (prominent R wave). The T wave is always positive in birds in lead II, and a change in polarity indicates myocardial hypoxia.[106] In high HRs, generally >300 to 500 bpm, P and T waves may be fused (atria depolarized before ventricles are completely repolarized) and the P wave indiscernible.[285,332] This P on T phenomenon also seems to be a normal finding in Amazon and African grey parrots.[285,520] ST segment elevation is common in healthy birds and does not indicate cardiac diseases as in mammals.[106,519] The ST segment is often short or absent, with the S wave merged with the T wave (ST slurring).[106,285] With the electrophysiologic specificities of birds in mind, the interpretation of the avian ECG is similar to that of mammals.

Reference intervals have been published for several species (Table 4-16). Anesthesia is suspected to affect the ECG measurements only in HR, QT interval, and the frequency of some arrhythmias (AV blocks).[335,512,520]

Radiography

Radiographic examination is of low sensitivity for cardiovascular diseases, but severe cardiac enlargement and vascular mineralization may be detected.[328,351] Other changes that

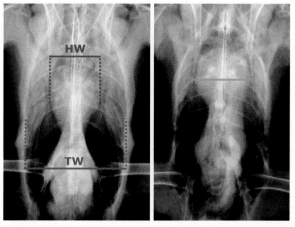

FIGURE 4-38 *Left, (HW)* Heart width and *(TW)* thoracic width landmarks in a macaw *(Ara* spp.). *Right,* Heart width and sternal width landmarks in a peregrine falcon *(Falco peregrinus).*

frequently accompany cardiovascular radiographic signs include loss of abdominal contrast and air-sac space due to ascites, hepatomegaly due to hepatic congestion, and occasionally overinflation of the axillary diverticula of the interclavicular air sac (see Figure 4-20). Several ratios have been determined, but the most practical is the heart width to thoracic width ratio on the ventrodorsal view because these two measurements are highly correlated in birds (Figure 4-38). In medium-sized psittacines, this ratio is 51% to 61%[351,524] and in Harris' hawks *(Parabuteo unicinctus),* it was found to have similar values.[525] This ratio may also vary depending on the respiratory phase, with a variability as high as 10%.[526] In falcons, it is considerably greater, with an upper limit of 70%.[525,526] Rather than using a simple and similar ratio for all individuals, regression-based reference intervals for cardiac radiographic sizes have been determined in peregrine falcons *(Falco peregrinus),* red-tailed hawks *(Buteo jamaicensis),* screech owls *(Otus asio),* and Canada geese *(Branta canadensis).*[526,527]

TABLE 4-16

ECG Measurement Reference Values on Lead II in Selected Avian Species*

Species	Racing Pigeon	Amazon Parrot	Grey Parrot	Macaw	Cockatoo	Red-Tailed Hawk	Bald Eagle	Pekin Duck	Chicken
N	60	37	45	41	31	11	20	50	72
HR	160-300	340-600	340-600	255-555	259-575	80-220	50-160	200-360	180-340
P amplitude	0.4-0.6	0.25-0.60	0.25-0.55	0.03-0.47	0.13-0.53	-0.1-0.175	0.050-0.325		
P duration	0.015-0.020	0.008-0.017	0.012-0.018	0.009-0.021	0.009-0.025	0.020-0.035	0.030-0.060	0.015-0.035	0.035-0.043
PR interval	0.045-0.070	0.042-0.055	0.040-0.055	0.040-0.068	0.039-0.071	0.050-0.090	0.070-0.110	0.04-0.08	0.073-0.089
S amplitude	1.5-2.8	0.7-2.3	0.9-2.2	0.27-1.43	0.27-1.59	0.300-0.900	0.150-1.450	0.35-1.03	0.10-1.0
QRS duration	0.013-0.016	0.010-0.015	0.010-0.016	0.002-0.030	0.014-0.026	0.020-0.030	0.020-0.040	0.028-0.044	0.02-0.028
T amplitude	0.3-0.8	0.3-0.8	0.18-0.6	0.12-0.80	0.17-0.97	0.000-0.300	0.050-0.200	0.04-0.40	0.03-0.28
QT interval	0.060-0.075	0.050-0.095	0.048-0.080	0.053-0.109	0.065-0.125	0.080-0.165	0.110-0.165	0.08-0.12	
MEA	-83 to -99	-90 to -107	-79 to -103	-76 to -87	-73 to -89	-50 to -110	-30 to -150	-160 to 95	-91 to -120

Adapted from References 330, 520-524.

*Amplitude measured in mV, duration in sec, MEA in degrees. To obtain a 95% reference interval, all published results in the form of mean ± SD were reported as mean ± 2SD and in the form of mean ± SEM were reported as mean ± 2SEM√n. When only the range or a 95% reference interval was published, result was reported as is.

ECG, Electrocardiogram; *MEA*, mean electrical axis; N, sample size; *HR*, heart rate.

With this approach, a predictive reference interval is calculated using established regression equations based on either the thoracic or the sternal width on ventrodorsal views and compared with the measured value of the patient (Table 4-17). The sternal width should be measured at the same level as the heart width, but the sternal landmarks may be obscured by an enlarged heart or fluids in diseased birds (see Figure 4-37). In peregrine falcons, the sternal width on the ventrodorsal view was found to be a better predictor of the heart width than the thoracic width, and the sternal and thoracic width were found to be collinear (and thus could not be incorporated into the same equation).[526]

Several authors claim that enlargement and opacification of the arteries can be detected on plain radiographs and are suggestive of atherosclerotic changes. Considering the variability in X-ray exposure, the fast HR of birds, and arterial motion artifacts that are likely present on radiographs in addition to the subjectivity in interpreting such changes, it is doubtful that this approach would have any clinical accuracy.[351,403,528] Severe atherosclerosis may also be present in the absence of vascular radiographic signs, as documented in several case reports.[320,385] Thus, radiographs should be considered an insensitive method of detecting vascular diseases.[529] On the other hand, arterial calcification is fairly specific to advanced atherosclerotic lesions and can be detected on radiographs and CT scans when severe enough (see Figure 4-42, later).[328,528]

Echocardiography
Echocardiography is undoubtedly the single most useful diagnostic tool in avian cardiology, and its clinical application and

TABLE 4-17

Regression-Based Equations for Reference Heart Width* in Selected Avian Species

Species	N	Regression Equation	R Square
Peregrine falcon	60	HW = 0.83 × SW + 0.37 ± 0.16	0.68
		HW = 0.41 × TW + 1.27 ± 0.18	0.33
Red-tailed hawk	50	HW = 0.42 × SW + 0.20 × TW + 3.42 ± 2.02	0.50
Screech owl	50	HW = 0.36 × SW + 0.13 × TW + 7.03 ± 1.40	0.36
Canada goose	50	HW = 0.27 × SW + 0.21 × TW + 15.15 ± 5.00	0.27

Hanley C, Murray H, Torrey S, et al. Establishing cardiac measurement standards in three avian species. *J Avian Med Surg*. 1997;11(1):15-19.

Krautwald-Junghanns M-E, Pees M, Schroff S. Cardiovascular system. In: Krautwald-Junghanns M-E, Pees M, Reese S, et al., eds. *Diagnostic Imaging of Exotic Pets*. Hannover, Germany: Schlutersche Verlagsgesellschaft mbH & Co.; 2011:84-91.

*Reference heart width measured in cm. The higher the R square, the better the precision of the reference limits. These equations are for the 95% confidence interval of the fitted value. The 95% confidence interval of the predictive value is slightly wider, but predictive equations are not practical.

HW, Heart width; N, sample size; *SW*, sternal width; *TW*, thoracic width.

value have been documented in multiple case reports on various species.[300,301,305,306,311,317,320,328-330,341] Echocardiography can detect changes in chamber dimensions, valvular diseases and insufficiency, pericardial diseases, cardiac masses, pulmonary arterial hypertension, wall motion disorders, septal defects, and diastolic disorders. However, cardiac ultrasound examination presents some major limitations in birds due to the location of the heart in an indentation of the keel and the fact that it is surrounded by air sacs (see anatomy section, subsection on birds). Therefore, available acoustic windows and cardiac views are limited.

Two standardized approaches have been described for transcoelomic examination: a ventromedian and a parasternal approach.[351,530-532] A small transducer and high probe frequency and frame rate are recommended. In anesthetized birds, the use of alcohol should be limited to prevent hypothermia. The ventromedian approach consists of placing the probe caudal to the keel and imaging the heart cranially, using the liver as an acoustic window to avoid air sacs laterally and the keel ventrally. This is the most commonly used approach in psittacine and raptorial birds. It can be performed on a conscious, sedated, or anesthetized bird. Birds should be preferentially fasted to limit interference with the gastrointestinal tract. Simultaneous ECG can be performed to better interpret images in relation to the cardiac cycle but is not essential. Only two views can classically be obtained through this approach: the horizontal four-chamber view and the vertical two-chamber view by rotating the probe by 90 degrees (Figure 4-39). All views are longitudinal (long axis); cardiac transverse views (short axis) and M-mode echocardiography have better temporal resolution but cannot be performed in birds by the transcoelomic approach. This precludes the establishment of the same echocardiographic standards in birds as in small

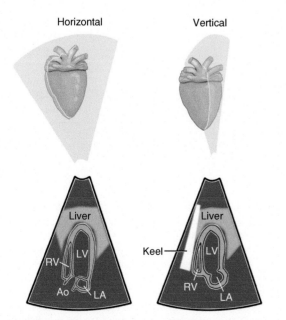

FIGURE 4-39 *Left,* Horizontal four-chamber view and *(right)* vertical two-chamber view in birds as classically obtained through the ventromedian approach. *Ao,* Aorta; *LA,* left atrium; *RA,* right atrium; *LV,* left ventricle; *RV,* right ventricle.

animal cardiology.[483] Therefore, the amount of information gathered from transcoelomic echocardiographic examinations is much more limited in birds, and all morphometric and functional measurements have to be performed on two-dimensional images (B mode). Measurements of several cardiac cycles should be averaged to obtain representative values. Reference intervals have been published for ventricular and atrial dimensions and fractional shortening ([diastole-systole]/diastole %) in several avian species (Table 4-18).[351,530,532] Transcoelomic echocardiography is also thought to underestimate the true fractional shortening of the highly efficient avian heart.[533] Right ventricular measurements are also not routinely taken in mammals due to their complex three-dimensional configuration.[484] Furthermore, recent evidence suggests that taking echocardiographic measurements may not be clinically useful considering avian heart size, HR, current equipment resolution, and the fact that observers can add up to 30% variability.[533] In dogs and cats, in most cases, a good impression of cardiac chamber size and function can be achieved without having made any quantitative measurements.[485] Likewise, an adequate morphologic and functional assessment of the avian heart can be performed qualitatively during the echocardiographic examination. Nevertheless, pathologic changes seen in birds are usually severe when cardiac disease is present, with dramatic chamber dilation (commonly the right heart), pericardial effusion, ascites, and poor contractility, which do not require measurements for confirmation. If measurements are taken for follow-up, it is recommended that the same operator and equipment be used, and changes in measurements should be >20% to be considered genuine. Left ventricular measurements seem to be more reliable overall.[533]

Color Doppler echocardiography can be used for detection of turbulence and reflux, indicative of valvular insufficiency, with right AV insufficiency being most commonly imaged. Spectral Doppler echocardiography can be used to measure inflow and outflow velocities, and reference intervals have been published in a few species (Table 4-19).[351,530,534,535] Fortunately, echocardiographic examinations are easier and more rewarding in birds with cardiac disease, because ascitic fluid, pericardial effusion, hepatomegaly, and cardiac enlargement greatly improve acoustic windows and facilitate the procedure.

The parasternal approach consists of placing the probe laterally (typically on the right to avoid the ventriculus) behind the ribs and above the sternum and imaging the heart craniomedially.[351,532] This can be performed on pigeons and some raptors and is the approach of choice in gallinaceous birds (especially younger chicken). In these birds, the limited caudal extension of the ribs and the larger fenestration of the keel allow a lateral approach to the heart. Typically, more imaging planes can be obtained and transverse views have been described in pigeons and chickens.[532,537]

A transesophageal echocardiographic protocol has been implemented in several species of birds in an attempt to alleviate the limitations associated with the transcoelomic approach. With this technique, a transesophageal ultrasonographic probe is inserted into the upper digestive system with the bird under general anesthesia, and the heart is imaged from inside the proventriculus.[538] Better resolution imaging and better details of cardiac structures are typically obtained, with three positions of the probe (cranial, middle, caudal) giving five

TABLE 4-18

Echocardiographic Reference Intervals* in Selected Avian Species Obtained in the Horizontal Four-Chamber View

Parameter	African Grey Parrots	Amazon Parrots	Cockatoos	Diurnal Raptors[†]	Pigeons (Parasternal)
N	60	10	10	100	50
Left ventricle					
Systole length	18.4-26	16.5-25.7	16.4-21.6	9.1-20.3	15.9-19.9
Systole width	4.8-8.8	4.3-9.1	3.0-9.8	4.1-8.5	4.4-6.0
Diastole length	20.2-27.8	17.7-26.5	16.7-23.1	11.0-21.8	17.3-22.9
Diastole width	6.6-10.6	6.4-10.4	5.3-11.3	5.3-10.1	6.2-8.6
FS (%)	13.8-31.4	14.4-31.2	11.6-39.6		
Right ventricle					
Systole length	6.4-12.0	5.8-13.0	7.9-12.7	7.3-18.1	
Systole width	1.0-4.6	1.7-4.5	7.9-12.7	0.9-3.3	
Diastole length	7.7-15.3	7.7-12.9	6.7-15.9	8.9-18.9	8.3-11.5
Diastole width	2.6-7.0	2.6-7.8	2.5-4.5	0.9-4.1	3.0-5.0
FS (%)	17.0-64.6	26.7-41.5	12.7-53.9		
Aorta					
Systole diameter	2.8-4.4	2.0-4.0		2.0-3.6	2.8-3.2
Diastole diameter	2.8-5.2	2.2-4.6			

Adapted from References 351, 531, 537.

*Reference intervals measured in mm. Echocardiographic measurements may not be reliable or clinically useful. To obtain a 95% reference interval, all published results in the form of mean ± SD were reported as mean ± 2SD and in the form of mean ± SEM were reported as mean ± 2SEM√n. When only the range or a 95% reference interval was published, result was reported as is.

[†]European diurnal raptors included common buzzard, European sparrowhawk, northern goshawk, and black kite.

FS, Fractional shortening; N, sample size.

TABLE 4-19

Spectral Doppler Echocardiographic Reference Intervals* in Selected Avian Species Obtained in the Horizontal Four-Chamber View[351,530,534-536]

Species	N	Left Diastolic Inflow	Right Diastolic Inflow	Aortic Systolic Outflow
Amazon parrots		0.12-0.24	0.12-0.32	0.67-0.99
Cockatoos		0.02-0.62		0.40-1.16
African grey parrots		0.27-0.51		0.63-1.15
Macaws		0.40-0.68		0.55-1.07
Harris' hawks	10	0.13-0.25	0.15-0.27	0.75-1.43
Falcons	15	0.18-0.38	0.17-0.37	1.07-1.43
Common buzzard	10	0.16-0.28	0.13-0.25	1.04-1.68
Barn owls	10	0.14-0.26	0.10-0.34	0.84-1.32

*Reference intervals measured in m/sec. Parrots were anesthetized; raptors were awake. To obtain a 95% reference interval, all published results in the form of mean ± SD were reported as mean ± 2SD and in the form of mean ± SEM were reported as mean ± 2SEM√n. When only the range or a 95% reference interval was published, result was reported as is.

N, Sample size.

consistent echocardiographic views. Furthermore, transverse views and M-mode imaging are possible through the transesophageal approach. However, the equipment is expensive and not widely available, the bird must be anesthetized, and the procedure cannot be performed in small psittacine birds because of a narrow entrance to the thoracic inlet.[538] This procedure has been used to diagnose and monitor a case of DCM in a Harris' hawk at one of the author's (Beaufrere) institutions (Figure 4-40).

Angiography

Since flow-limiting stenosis is the main mechanism leading to clinical signs in psittacine birds, angiography could be useful to assess arterial luminal narrowing. Angiography can be obtained using either fluoroscopy or CT. The circulation of intravenous contrast agents in birds is extremely fast, and image acquisition should be performed during injection or shortly after. The use of angiography in birds has recently been reviewed.[529]

Fluoroscopic angiography can visualize the heart and vascular tree in real time. Under general anesthesia, the bird is initially positioned in left lateral recumbency on a fluoroscopy table. A bolus of nonionic iodinated contrast agent (2 mL/kg IV; iohexol 240 mg/mL; Omnipaque, GE Healthcare Inc., Princeton, NJ) is injected at a rate of 1 to 2 mL/kg/s through a catheter inserted into the basilic or medial

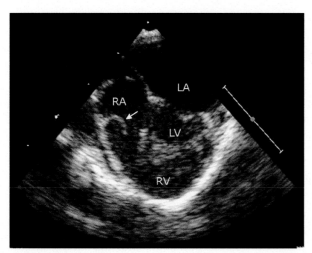

FIGURE 4-40 Transesophageal echocardiography in a Harris' hawk with congestive heart failure. Middle probe position, transverse view at the level of the AV valves. Note the chamber dilations. *Arrow,* Right muscular AV valve; *LA,* left atrium; *LV,* left ventricle; *RA,* right atrium; *RV,* right ventricle.

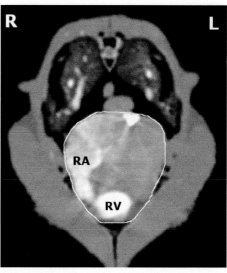

FIGURE 4-41 Computed tomography after injection of contrast in a Harris' hawk with congestive heart failure, bone window. Cross section cranially at the level of the heart. Due to impaired systolic function, incomplete mixing of the contrast agent in the systemic circulation is seen. *RA,* Right atrium; *RV,* right ventricle.

metatarsal vein during video acquisition at a rate of 30 frames/s for the best resolution. The same bolus is repeated to obtain the ventrodorsal view with the bird placed in dorsal recumbency. The brachiocephalic trunks, aorta, pulmonary arteries, pulmonary veins, and caudal vena cava can be seen. The brachiocephalic trunks and aorta can be seen pulsating with the heartbeats. Marked lumen changes can be observed during the cardiac cycle. The procedure is easy and inexpensive and can be recorded for further analysis and measurements. For measurement, to account for different degrees of magnification, a calibrated marker should be kept in the field during fluoroscopic acquisition, although fluoroscopic angiography is likely more useful for qualitative assessment and investigation of aneurysm and stenosis.

In interventional radiology, digital subtraction angiography is a fluoroscopic technique used to clearly visualize blood vessels in a dense soft tissue or bone environment. Images are produced by subtracting a precontrast image from later images once the contrast medium has been introduced into the vascular system, which results in visualizing only the contrast-filled vessels without the background. It considerably increases the outlines of the arteries and the detection of smaller arteries not seen with conventional angiography, specifically for extremities, such as legs, wings, and the head, but images tend to be easily degraded by small motions and noise. A preliminary, nonenhanced fluoroscopic image is recorded before administering a bolus of contrast medium and is digitally subtracted during the angiography procedure. The same bolus technique and a similar dose of contrast medium as used for regular fluoroscopic angiography are used for digital subtraction angiography, except that this option is selected in the machine.

A CT examination provides an excellent assessment of all major arteries and their anatomy in psittacine and raptorial birds.[539,540] The addition of contrast media greatly enhances the visualization of the arteries and veins and their lumens. A CT angiography (CTA) protocol has been standardized and

published for parrots as well as for reference intervals for arterial diameter measurements.[540] As the circulation of contrast is fast in birds and to capture the CT images at the time of greatest intra-arterial contrast concentrations (enhancement peak), it is recommended to start the CTA scanning immediately after administration of contrast. Alternatively, in order to determine the exact time to contrast enhancement peak, a preliminary axial CT scan may be performed.[540]

Reports of angiography applications are still limited in birds. A coronary aneurysm was diagnosed with angiography in an umbrella cockatoo.[330] Angiocardiography has also been used clinically in a racing pigeon, two blue and gold macaws (*Ara ararauna*), and a whooper swan.[106,329]

Advanced Imaging

Computed tomography and MRI are seldom used to image the avian heart, as scans cannot be gated to the fast cardiac cycle in birds to reduce motion artifacts and improve the diagnostic value. However, CT can be used to image the arteries and can readily diagnose cardiomegaly, venous congestion, edema, and arterial calcification associated with advanced atherosclerosis (Figures 4-41 and 4-42). Likewise, cerebral complications such as ischemic and hemorrhagic strokes can be diagnosed using CT or MRI, but concurrent atherosclerosis cannot be detected when calcification of the lesions is not severe enough.[401,402,409] MRI was not found to be of good diagnostic value for the cardiovascular system in pigeons because of the fast circulation of contrast media (gadolinium).[541]

Endoscopy

Coelioscopy allows direct visualization of the heart and major arteries through the standard lateral approaches with the endoscope located in the cranial thoracic air sacs, the

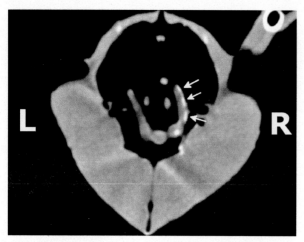

FIGURE 4-42 Computed tomography showing advanced aortic calcification of the ascending aorta in a female African grey parrot *(Psittacus erithacus erithacus)*. Mediastinal window. (Courtesy of Drs. Yvonne van Zeeland and Nico Schoemaker, Utrecht University, The Netherlands.)

interclavicular approach with the endoscope located in the interclavicular air sac, and the ventral midline approach with the endoscope located in the ventral hepatoperitoneal cavities.[529,542] Endoscopy can only detect gross, color, and structural changes to the cardiovascular system such as cardiomegaly, pericardial effusion, pericardial exudate, arterial discoloration, and the presence of granulomas in the area. Pericardial biopsy and pericardiocentesis can be performed via endoscopy. The midline approach is recommended for pericardiocentesis so no fluid leaks into the air sacs. An endoscopic needle is used with its sheath and should only protrude by 1 to 2 mm to prevent puncturing the heart during the procedure. Pericardial fluids should be analzyed cytologically and submitted for cultures.

TREATMENTS

General Therapeutics of Cardiovascular Diseases

Medical treatment is the cornerstone of cardiac disease management and is directed toward the heart, vessels, and volume regulation. The overall treatment goal is to improve quality if life and increase survival time. Since congestive heart failure is not a diagnosis, the correct treatment will also depend on the accurate determination of the cause of heart failure. There is a scarcity of pharmacologic information on cardiovascular agents for zoological companion animals.

Diuretics are used to reduce fluid overload, edema, and effusion. Furosemide, a loop diuretic, is the most commonly used diuretic and inhibits sodium, potassium, and chloride cotransporters in the ascending limb of the loop of Henle in mammals. Furosemide also produces diuresis in vertebrate species lacking looped nephrons (see reptile and fish subsections), suggesting a different mechanism in these species. Furosemide should not be used alone long term as it further activates the RAAS.[543] Electrolytes and renal parameters (e.g.,

BUN, creatinine, and uric acid in some species) should be monitored when using furosemide long term, and hypokalemia is a commonly reported side effect. Cardiac tamponade is a contraindication for the use of furosemide because it decreases cardiac preload, which is necessary in this disease to support ventricular filling and maintain cardiac output. Finally, it should be used with caution in patients with renal disease. Spironolactone is an aldosterone antagonist and classified as a potassium-sparing diuretic. It is also thought to prevent or decrease myocardial fibrosis. It may be used conjointly with furosemide to offset the loss of potassium. However, the real clinical efficacy of spironolactone as a diuretic is uncertain. Therefore, it should not be used as the sole diuretic in animals with pulmonary edema.[543]

Angiotensin-converting enzyme (ACE) inhibitors block the formation of angiotensin II. They promote venous and arterial vasodilation and limit aldosterone production. As a result, they decrease preload and afterload, with a risk of hypotension and hyperkalemia.[544] ACE inhibitors are rarely used alone but rather are combined with diuretics and positive inotropes. Enalapril and benazepril are the most commonly used ACE inhibitors because of their longer half-life.

Positive inotropes are used to enhance cardiac contractility. Disadvantages include an increase in myocardial oxygen consumption and arrhythmias (except [potentially] for pimobendan). They are contraindicated in hypertrophic cardiomyopathy and aortic and pulmonic stenosis. Digoxin, a digitalis glycoside, enhances contractility by directly inhibiting the Na/K ATPase pump, which results in intracellular calcium accumulation through the activation of the Na/Ca exchanger.[545] Beside being a weak positive inotrope, it is also a negative chronotrope and positive lusitrope. However, the use of digoxin is becoming more controversial in small animal and human cardiology because of its failure to reduce overall mortality and its gastrointestinal and proarrhythmic side effects. Recommended therapeutic levels for digoxin are 0.8 to 1.2 ng/mL.[545] Pimobendan is a positive inotrope and arterial vasodilator (inodilator), with its action due to calcium sensitization of myofibrils and phosphodiesterase III inhibition.[545] Pimobendan is commonly used in small animal cardiology and has been shown to increase both survival time and quality of life in canine DCM and in dogs with decompensated mitral valve disease.[546] There have been more clinical trials with pimobendan than with any other drug in veterinary cardiology. Dobutamine is a potent positive inotrope that exerts its activity by selective β_1 adrenergic activity. Since it is short lived, it is used as a constant rate infusion in refractory cases with severe systolic dysfunction and cardiogenic shock.

Beta-blockers (e.g., carvedilol, atenolol, propranolol) and calcium channel blockers (e.g., diltiazem) are negative inotropes. They are mainly used in the treatment of hypertrophic cardiomyopathy and supraventricular tachyarrhythmias. Side effects include bradycardia and hypotension.[547]

The initial treatment of patients with congestive heart failure and severe clinical signs should be aimed at achieving a marked reduction in volemia through the use of diuretics and, on occasion, vasodilators (to trap blood in the venous system, which already contains 70% of total blood volume). Furosemide is the main diuretic for this indication. Oxygen supplementation should be instituted for dyspneic animals, especially if pulmonary edema is present. Injectable inotropes and vasodilators may be indicated in anorexic patients. Administration of intravenous fluids is not indicated in the treatment of congestive heart failure, where the goal is to reduce fluid overload. Acute treatment of congestive heart failure always leads to some degree of dehydration and prerenal azotemia. These abnormalities usually resolve over a few days once the animal resumes normal appetite and water intake. In rare cases of persistent severe azotemia and clinical hypokalemia, small volumes of intravenous fluids can be administered. Fluid accumulation in the thoracic, abdominal, or coelomic cavity should be manually drained by centesis. Long-term management of congestive heart failure is based on the daily administration of furosemide. Once the animal is free of signs of congestion, the dose of diuretics can be tapered to the lowest effective dose. Clinical trials conducted in dogs have shown that the addition of ACE inhibitors to the treatment regimen improves survival. There is also evidence that pimobendan is beneficial to animals already receiving furosemide and an ACE inhibitor.[548] In refractory cases, diuretics may be combined to further decrease the circulatory volume. Data collected from human clinical trials suggest that ACE inhibitors and beta-blockers are the only two types of medications that prevent the progression of cardiac pump dysfunction and prolong survival.[113] This is likely because overstimulation of the adrenergic and RAAS pathways is central in the pathogenesis and progression of congestive heart failure.[113] Finally, moderate dietary sodium restriction is usually recommended.

Invertebrates

Treatments of hemolymph loss in arthropods consist of cleaning and sealing the oozing wound with medical cyanoacrylate glue and replacing fluid loss. Several layers of glue may be needed. In spiders, fluid can be given by placing the ventral prosoma in very shallow water or injecting replacement fluids directly into the pericardial sinus/cardiac cavity dorsally through the opisthosoma using a tuberculin syringe.[20] Overall, hemolymph composition and osmolality vary greatly (200 to 900 mOsm/L) in arthropods, and general recommendations for the type of fluid therapy cannot be given.[549,550] However, normal saline (0.9%) appears to be effective in tarantulas and use of a "spider Ringer's lactate" formula has been published.[20,551] A volume corresponding to 4% to 6% of body weight can be safely administered in spiders. Transfusion of hemolymph from a donor spider may also be performed[552] and may be considered safe in the absence of adaptive immunity in arthropods.

Invertebrate hearts respond to cholinergic and catecholamine compounds, but these drugs are unlikely to be necessary in clinical cases.

Fish

If an antemortem diagnosis can be obtained, treatments are primarily aimed at the cause, which is often infectious in nature. Recommended therapeutics for bacterial diseases can be found in the treatment section, fish subsection of the respiratory chapter. Abdominocentesis to relieve abdominal distension is not efficient in fish, as fluid often reaccumulates quickly. Despite the lack of a loop of Henle in piscine nephrons, furosemide has been found to induce diuresis in fish species.[553]

Amphibians

Treatments for amphibian cardiovascular diseases are aimed at addressing the cause, and no specific treatments have been reported in amphibians other than physiological experiments. Treatments of infectious and cutaneous diseases are considered elsewhere in this book. In addition, fluid therapy is typically managed through altering the composition and osmolality of the fluid in which the amphibian patient is housed (see Chapter 2: Integumentary System, and Chapter 11: Urinary System).

Reptiles

Very little information is available regarding treatment options for cardiac diseases in reptiles, and pharmacokinetic information is unavailable for cardiovascular drugs. Furthermore, reptiles' unique anatomy and physiology makes extrapolation from small animal practice inappropriate.

Furosemide is theoretically ineffective in reptiles because they have loopless nephrons, similar to fish and amphibians. However, administration of furosemide was found to have diuretic effects in chelonians and ophidians.[554-557] One reported treatment involved a carpet python *(Morelia spilota variegata)* that was diagnosed with congestive heart failure causing pulmonary edema and pericardial effusion secondary to AV insufficiency.[165] The authors administered furosemide (5 mg/kg); however, the snake failed to respond to treatment. A spur-thighed tortoise *(Testudo graeca)* with atrial dilatation and pericardial effusion was administered furosemide twice in 3-week intervals at a dose of 5.2 mg/kg. The peripheral edema resolved within 12 hours after each injection.[168] Whether or not other diuretic classes (spirolactone, thiazides) are effective in these species remains unknown. The use of atropine and glycopyrrolate to counter the negative chronotropic effects of vagal stimulation of the heart has been unsuccessful in the green iguana.[558] As reptile medicine continues to evolve, it is hoped that the diagnosis of cardiac diseases will increase and that this will be mirrored by an increase in treatment options.

Mammals

Overall, congestive heart failure in exotic mammals carries a poor long-term prognosis. A review of 13 published clinical cases of congestive heart failure in companion exotic mammals with various conditions and under various treatments showed a median survival time of 21 days, with a maximum survival of 1 year (Table 4-20). There is a paucity of pharmacologic information in these pet species, and no clinical trials could be found. Experimental use of cardiovascular drugs has been performed in laboratory animal models, but the translation of these findings to spontaneous disease in pet animals may be challenging. In the absence of species-specific clinical data, the same approach used for dogs and cats should be followed, as basic therapeutic principles still apply (see section entitled "General Therapeutics of Cardiovascular Diseases"). Recommended drug dosages in exotic mammals are listed in Table 4-21.

Serum drug levels and electrolytes should be monitored in cases where digoxin is used. However, the use of digoxin is falling out of favor, and pimobendan is now considered the inotropic drug of choice for chronic treatment of systolic

TABLE 4-20

Survival Time in Companion Exotic Mammals after Diagnosis of Selected Cases of Spontaneous Congestive Heart Failure with Noninfectious Causes

Species	Diagnosis	CHF	Treatment	Survival Time	Reference
Ferret	DCM	Bilateral	Furosemide Digoxin	7 mo	235
Ferret	DCM	Bilateral	Furosemide Digoxin	3 wk	236
Ferret	DCM Cryptococcosis	Bilateral	Furosemide Digoxin	1 d	237
Ferret	DCM	Bilateral	Furosemide Digoxine Taurine	12 mo	243
Ferret	Ventricular septal defect Valvular disease	Bilateral	Furosemide Benazepril Pimobendan Thoracentesis	At least 5 mo	260
Rabbit	DCM	Left	Furosemide Enalapril Pimobendan Spironolactone	6 wk	233
Rabbit	Valvular disease	Bilateral	Furosemide Enalapril Pimobendan	7 mo	233
Rabbit	HCM	Bilateral	Thoracocentesis	1 d	234
Rabbit	DCM Valvular disease	Right	Furosemide	Few days	234
Rabbit	Cardiomyopathy	Right	Furosemide	3 d	559
Guinea pig	DCM	Bilateral	Furosemide Enalapril	At least 8 wk	227
Syrian hamster	DCM Atrial thrombosis	Bilateral	Furosemide Pimobendan	3 wk	233
Syrian hamster	DCM	Left	Furosemide Pimobendan	2.5 wk	233

CHF, Congestive heart failure; *DCM*, dilated cardiomyopathy; *HCM*, hypertrophic cardiomyopathy.

dysfunction. In a review of four cardiology cases in which treatment with pimobendan was reported, poor survival time was noted except for one rabbit that lived for 7 months.[233] In this rabbit, marked clinical improvement was observed once pimobendan was added to the patient's therapeutic regimen. In hamsters with cardiomyopathy, pimobendan significantly increased survival time in comparison to control animals.[560] Pimobendan dosages reported in rodents are usually much higher than in dogs and cats. A safety trial on the use of pimobendan in ferrets at doses of up to 1.5 mg/kg q12 h for 8 weeks did not report any side effects.[561]

Rats treated with enalapril in an experimental congestive heart failure model had a 95% higher median survival time than controls.[562] Rabbits have plasma atropinase that may interfere with atropine administration. As in domestic carnivores, pleural and pericardial effusion should be tapped to relieved dyspnea and cardiac tamponade.

Preventive treatments for heartworm in ferrets in endemic areas consist of administering monthly macrocyclic lactones (see Table 4-21). The recommended adulticide treatment for ferret dirofilariasis is ivermectin, 0.05 mg/kg SC monthly.[98] Steroids may be added in cases of respiratory signs, and doxycycline may be used to eliminate *Wolbachia* bacteria and decrease inflammation. In addition, heartworm extraction has been documented in a young ferret.[563]

Birds

Once cardiovascular diseases are diagnosed in birds, the long-term prognosis is poor, even with treatment. For instance, a review of 15 published clinical cases of congestive heart failure in birds using various treatments showed a median survival time of 30 days (Table 4-22). The variety of therapeutic treatments, causative conditions, outcomes, and species hampers the formation of any conclusion regarding the association between therapeutic protocols and survival time. In small animals, long-term prognosis for congestive heart failure is also fair to poor, with, for instance, in dogs, median survival times of 27 to 133 days for DCM and 588 days for preclinical mitral valve disease.[579-581] The shorter survival time in birds may be associated with the paucity of pharmacologic information on cardiac drugs, poor standardization of treatment protocols, greater cardiac efficiency and metabolism, late diagnosis, and challenges of chronically medicating birds.

TABLE 4-21

Doses of Selected Cardiac Therapeutic Agents in Small Mammals

Drug	Species	Dose	Basis	Reference
Diuretics				
Furosemide	All	1-4 mg/kg PO, SC, IM, IV q8-12 h	EU	98,257,466,482
Spironolactone	All	1-2 mg/kg q12 h	EU	98,466
Positive inotropes				
Digoxin*	All	0.005-0.01 mg/kg PO q12-24 h	EU	466,482
	Rabbit	0.07 mg/kg PO (Cmax: 5.6-6.0 ng/mL; HL: 20 h)	PK	564
			PK	565
		0.02 mg/kg PO (Cmax: 2.02-2.26 ng/mL; HL: 9.4-11.5 h)	PK	566
	Guinea pigs	0.125 mg/kg IV (concentrations: 0-20 ng/mL; HL: 1.5 h)		
	Rat	1 mg/kg IV (concentrations: 5-32 ng/mL; HL: 2.5 h)	PK	567
Pimobendan	All	0.2-0.5 mg/kg PO q12 h	EU	98,233
	Rabbit	0.1-0.3 mg/kg PO	PD	568
	Hamster	2.8 mg/kg/d PO	PD	560
	Mouse	100 mg/kg q24 h for 30 d (troponin KO mice)	PD	569
Dobutamine	All	5-15 µg/kg/min (CRI)	EU	570
Dopamine	All	5-15 µg/kg/min (CRI)	EU	570
Negative inotropes				
Atenolol	All	3-6.25 mg/kg PO q24 h	EU	466
Diltiazem	All	1.5-7.5 mg/kg PO q12 h	EU	466
Vasodilators				
Enalapril	All	0.25-0.5 mg/kg PO q24-48 h	EU	98,466,482
	Rat	10 mg/kg PO q24 h	PD	571
		17-25 mg/L drinking water	PD	562
Benazepril	Rat	0.3-10 mg/kg PO q24 h	PD	572
Parasympatholytics				
Atropine	All	0.02-0.04 mg/kg SC, IM	EU	466
Glycopyrrolate	All	0.01-0.02 mg/kg SC, IM	EU	466
Antiarrhythmics				
Lidocaine	All	1-2 mg/kg IV	EU	466
Antidirofilaria				
Ivermectin	Ferret	0.05-0.2 mg/kg PO, SC q1 mo larvicide	PD	573–575
		0.05 mg/kg PO, SC q1 mo adulticide	EU	98
Selamectin	Ferret	6-18 mg/kg spot-on q1 mo larvicide	PD	576
Moxidectin	Ferret	0.17-2.0 mg SC once adulticide	EU	577
Moxidectin/imidacloprid	Ferret	1%/10% spot-on 0.4 mL/q1 mo larvicide	PD	578

Cmax, Maximum concentration achieved in a pharmacokinetic study; *EU*, empirical use; *HL*, half-life; *IM*, intramuscular; *IV*, intravenous; *KO*, knockout; *PD*, pharmacodynamics study; *PK*, pharmacokinetic study; *PO*, by mouth; *SC*, subcutaneously.
*Therapeutic levels are 0.8-1.2 ng/mL.

Few pharmacokinetic studies have been performed in birds on cardiovascular therapeutic agents, and no clinical trials have been conducted. This emphasizes the need for therapeutic drug monitoring when treating the individual avian patient whenever possible. Several commercial laboratories offer plasma drug measurements such as for digoxin or carvedilol. Recommended drug dosages in birds are listed in Table 4-23.

In a study of chickens, urine output was measured after administration of several diuretics, namely, furosemide, spironolactone, hydrochlorothiazide, and urotropin.[583] Furosemide was found to have the greatest diuretic effect, especially when given parenterally. Other diuretics did not have a greater effect than controls at the dosage used. Loriidae have been reported to be extremely susceptible to furosemide; therefore, doses used in these species should be much lower.[589] Furosemide is a potent loop diuretic that had good efficiency and

rapid onset of action in birds despite the presence of only 10% to 30% of looped nephrons in the avian kidney.[590]

Among ACE inhibitors, enalapril is the most commonly used in birds. Empirical evidence suggest than enalapril is safe and effective in companion psittacine birds.[587]

For birds, several pharmacokinetic studies on digoxin have been published, and digoxin was used in several cases in which plasma levels were monitored (see Table 4-23).[300,302,304] Only two psittacine cases reported using pimobendan (0.25 to 0.6 mg/kg q12 h in triple therapy), and the results were mixed.[320,582] However, the required pimobendan dose appears to be much higher in parrots, and this may partly explain the poor clinical effect.[586] In Amazon parrots, dopamine and dobutamine significantly increased the blood pressure in a dose-dependent manner.[340] Side effects included arrhythmias and tachycardia.

TABLE 4-22

Survival Time in Birds after Diagnosis of Selected Cases of Congestive Heart Failure with Noninfectious Causes

Species	Diagnosis	CHF	Treatment	Survival Time	Ref
African grey parrot	Atherosclerosis Cor pulmonale	Right	Furosemide Spironolactone Benazepril Pimobendan Coelomocentesis	35 d	320
African grey parrot	Valve regurgitations Hyperechoic aorta	Bilateral	Pimobendan Furosemide Imidapril	30 d	582
Indian ringneck parakeet	Myxomatous degeneration of left AV valve	Bilateral	Furosemide Digoxin	10 mo	300
Amazon parrot	Right AV valve insufficiency	Right	Furosemide Digoxin	8 d	301
Amazon parrot	Right AV valve insufficiency	Right	Enalapril Furosemide	27 mo	341
Blue and gold macaw	Atherosclerosis	Right	Furosemide	70 d	329
Grey-cheeked parakeet	Atherosclerosis	Right	Supportive	3 d	328
Umbrella cockatoo	Atherosclerosis Coronary aneurysm	Right	Supportive	Euthanized at diagnosis	330
Umbrella cockatoo	Myxomatous degeneration of left AV valve	Left	Unspecified	1 d	343
Fischer lovebird	Pericardial effusion Pericarditis Myocarditis	Right	Pericardiocentesis Enalapril Furosemide	11 mo	317
Pukeko	Left AV valve insufficiency	Bilateral	Digoxin	49 d	302
Red-tailed hawk	Dilated cardiomyopathy	Right	Furosemide	Euthanized at diagnosis	312
Mynah	Left AV valve insufficiency	Bilateral	Furosemide Digoxin	10 mo	304
Mynah	Coronary calcification Cause not determined	Right	Abdominocentesis	12 d	303
Duck	Congenital mitral stenosis Subvalvular aortic stenosis	Bilateral	Supportive Furosemide Coelomocentesis	29 d	305

AV, Atrioventricular; CHF, congestive heart failure.

Coelomocentesis is indicated to relieve respiratory signs due to air-sac compression and is an effective means of decreasing volume overload. It can be performed on a regular basis for chronic treatment of right-sided heart failure in birds. Pericardiocentesis (guided by endoscopy or ultrasound) is indicated in severe pericardial effusion and cardiac tamponade.[106,317] Slow aspiration is essential. A permanent surgical window or partial pericardectomy by endoscopy can be performed if necessary.[106]

For the management of atherosclerotic diseases, lifestyle changes that could be implemented include increasing the physical activity of captive parrots by providing more opportunities for locomotion and foraging behaviors and decreasing the stress level in their captive environment. Parrots eat a cholesterol-free diet, as cholesterol is an animal compound for which ergosterol is the vegetal equivalent. Therefore, animal products in the diet should be limited to the strict minimum since they are a source of cholesterol and saturated fat. A well-balanced plant-based diet is primordial. Supplementation with omega-3 fatty acids such as α-linolenic acid that can be found in flaxseed oil has been shown to be beneficial in improving lipid metabolism, minimizing inflammation, and minimizing atherosclerosis in several avian species.[375,388,400] Limiting dietary excess and obesity in captive birds also seems to be a reasonable strategy, but species-specific dietary needs should be considered.

Statins are employed in parrots, but their use is controversial because no pharmacologic information is available, and target levels of blood cholesterol and LDL that would reduce atherosclerosis risks are unknown in psittacine birds.[591,592]

Clinical signs of peripheral arterial disease have been treated with pentoxifylline or isoxsuprine in Amazon parrots.[385,403] Despite the lack of evidence for efficacy in humans, isoxsuprine relieved signs of hind limb weakness in Amazon parrots, but atherosclerotic disease was not confirmed.[403,593] Likewise, the use of antihypertensive medications such as ACE inhibitors and beta-blockers to treat avian hypertension is not yet applicable in birds when there is no accurate and repeatable means of measuring the arterial blood pressure in clinical cases for diagnosis and follow-up.[508,511,516]

TABLE 4-23

Doses of Selected Cardiac Therapeutic Agents in Birds

Drug	Species	Dose	Basis	Ref
Diuretics				
Furosemide	Parrots, raptors	0.15-2 mg/kg PO, IM q12-24 h	EU	351
	Chickens	5 mg/kg PO	PD	583
		2.5 mg/kg IM	PD	583
Spironolactone	Chickens	1 mg/kg PO	PD	583
	Parrots	1 mg/kg PO q12 h	EU	320
Positive inotropes				
Digoxin	Budgerigars	0.02 mg/kg PO q24 h	PK	584
	Sparrows	0.02 mg/kg PO q24 h	PK	584
	Quaker parrots	0.05 mg/kg PO q24 h	PK	585
Pimobendan	Amazon parrots	10 mg/kg PO q12 h	PK	586
	Harris' hawk	0.25 mg/kg PO q12 h	PK, EU	586
	Parrots	0.25 mg/kg PO q12 h	EU	320,333,582
Dobutamine	Amazon parrots	5-15 µg/kg/min (CRI)	PD	340
Dopamine	Amazon parrots	5-10 µg/kg/min (CRI)	PD	340
Negative inotropes				
Propranolol	Most species	0.2 mg/kg IM, 0.04 mg/kg IV	EU	
Atenolol	Most species	5-10 mg/kg PO q12-24 h	EU	
Diltiazem	Most species	1-2 mg/kg PO q8-24 h	EU	
Vasodilators				
Enalapril	Pigeons	1.25 mg/kg PO q8-12 h	PK	587
	Amazons	1.25 mg/kg PO q8-12 h	PK	587
	Parrots	2.5-5 mg/kg PO q12 h	EU	317,341
Benazepril	Parrots	0.5 mg/kg PO q24 h	EU	320
Parasympatholytics				
Atropine	Most species	0.01-0.02 mg/kg IM	EU	
Glycopyrrolate	Most species	0.01-0.02 mg/kg IM	EU	
Antiarrhythmics				
Lidocaine	Amazon parrot	2.5 mg/kg IV	PK	588
Mexiletine	Parrots	4-8 mg/kg PO q12-24 h	EU	
Proprantheline	Parrots	0.1-0.3 mg/kg PO q8 h	EU	333

CRI, Constant rate infusion; *EU,* empirical use; *IM,* intramuscular; *IV,* intravenous; *PD,* pharmacodynamics study; *PK,* pharmacokinetic study; *PO,* by mouth.

REFERENCES

1. Farrell A. Evolution of cardiovascular systems: insights into ontogeny. In: Burggren W, Keller B, eds. *Development of Cardiovascular Systems: Molecules to Organisms.* Cambridge, UK: Cambridge University Press; 1998:101-113.
2. Hicks J. The physiological and evolutionary significance of cardiovascular shunting patterns in reptiles. *News Physiol Sci.* 2002;17:241-245.
3. Farrell AP. Circulation in vertebrates. In: *Encyclopedia of Life Sciences.* London: Nature Publishing Group; 2001:1-15.
4. Hicks J, Wang T. The functional significance of the reptilian heart: new insights into an old question. In: Sedmera D, Wang T, eds. *Ontogeny and Phylogeny of the Vertebrate Heart.* New York, NY: Springer; 2012:207-227.
5. Solc D. The heart and heart conducting system in the kingdom of animals: a comparative approach to its evolution. *Exp Clin Cardiol.* 2007;12(3):113-118.
6. Jensen B, Boukens B, Postma A, et al. Identifying the evolutionary building blocks of the cardiac conduction system. *PLoS ONE.* 2012;7(9):e44231.
7. McMahon B. Comparative evolution and design in non-vertebrate cardiovascular systems. In: Sedmera D, Wang T, eds. *Ontogeny and Phylogeny of the Vertebrate Heart.* New York: Springer Science; 2012:1-33.
8. Klowden M. Circulatory systems. In: Klowden M, ed. *Physiological Systems in Insects.* 2nd ed. San Diego, CA: Academic Press, Inc.; 2007:357-402.
9. Paul R, Bihlmayer S, Colmorgen M, et al. The open circulatory system of spiders (*Eurypelma californicum, Pholcus phalangoides*): a survey of functional morphology and physiology. *Physiol Zool.* 1994;67(6):1360-1382.
10. Reiber C, McGaw I. A review of the "open" and "closed" circulatory systems: new terminology for complex invertebrate circulatory systems in light of current findings. *Int J Zool.* 2009;2009(Article ID 301284):8 pp.
11. Williams D. Cardiac biology and disease in invertebrates. *Vet Clin North Am Exot Anim Pract.* 2009;12(1):1-9, v.
12. Brusca R, Brusca G. *Invertebrates.* 2nd ed. Sunderland, MA: Sinauer Associates, Inc.; 2003:936.
13. Smolowitz R. Gastropods. In: Lewbart G, ed. *Invertebrate Medicine.* 2nd ed. Ames, IA: Blackwell Publishing; 2012:95-111.
14. Civil G, Thompson T. Experiments with the isolated heart of the gastropod *Helix pomatia* in an artificial pericardium. *J Exp Biol.* 1972;56:239-247.

15. Andrews EB, Taylor PM. Fine structure, mechanism of heart function and haemodynamics in the prosobranch gastropod mollusk *Littorina littorea* (L.). *J Comp Physiol [B]*. 1988;158(2):247-262.

16. Jones HD. The circulatory systems of gastropods and bivalves. In: Saleuddin ASM, Wilber KM, eds. *The Mollusca*. Vol 5, Part 2. Orlando, FL: Academic Press; 1983:189-238.

17. Levine J, Law M, Corsin F. Bivalves. In: Lewbart G, ed. *Invertebrate Medicine*. 2nd ed. Ames, IA: Blackwell Publishing; 2012:127-151.

18. Miller T. Structure and physiology of the circulatory system. In: Kerkut G, Gilbert L, eds. *Comprehensive Insect Physiology, Biochemistry, and Pharmacology*. Vol 3. New York, NY: Pergamon Press; 1985:289-353.

19. Klußmann-Fricke B-J, Prendini L, Wirkner CS. Evolutionary morphology of the hemolymph vascular system in scorpions: a character analysis. *Arthropod Struct Dev*. 2012;41(6):545-560.

20. Pizzi R. Spiders. In: Lewbart G, ed. *Invertebrate Medicine*. 2nd ed. Ames, IA: Blackwell Publishing; 2012:187-221.

21. Foelix R. *Biology of Spiders*. 3rd ed. Oxford, UK: Oxford University Press; 2011:419.

22. Wells MJ. The cephalopod heart: the evolution of a high-performance invertebrate pump. *Experientia*. 1992;48(9):800-808.

23. Boyle P. Cephalopods. In: Poole T, ed. *The UFAW Handbook on the Care and Management of Laboratory Animals*. 7th ed. Oxford, UK: Blackwell Publishing; 1999:115-139.

24. Davison I, Wright G, DeMont M. The structure and physical properties of invertebrate and primitive vertebrate arteries. *J Exp Biol*. 1995;198:2185-2196.

25. Krijgsman BJ. Contractile and pacemaker mechanisms of the heart of arthropods. *Biol Rev*. 1952;27(3):320-346.

26. Bursey C, Sherman R. Spider cardiac physiology, I. Structure and function of the cardiac ganglion. *Comp Gen Pharmacol*. 1970; 1(2):160-170.

27. Smith P, Boyle P. The cardiac innervation of *Eledona cirrhosa* (Mollusca: Cephalopoda). *Phil Trans R Soc Lond B Biol Sci*. 1983;300: 493-511.

28. Olson K. The cardiovascular system. In: Evans D, ed. *The Physiology of Fishes*. 2nd ed. Boca Raton, FL: CRC Press; 1998:129-157.

29. Icardo J. The teleost heart: a morphological approach. In: Sedmera D, Wang T, eds. *Ontogeny and Phylogeny of the Vertebrate Heart*. New York: Springer-Verlag; 2012:35-53.

30. Farrell AP, Jones D. The heart. In: Hoar W, Randall D, Farrell A, eds. *Fish Physiology, Volume XII, Part A, The Cardiovascular System*. Vol 12. San Diego, CA: Academic Press, Inc.; 1992:1-88.

31. Olson K. Circulatory system. In: Ostrander G, ed. *The Laboratory Fish*. San Diego, CA: Academic Press; 2000:161-179.

32. Burggren W, Bagatto B. Cardiovascular anatomy and physiology. In: Finn R, Kapoor B, eds. *Fish Larval Physiology*. Enfield, NH: Science Publishers; 2008:119-162.

33. Poppe T, Ferguson H. Cardiovascular system. In: Ferguson H, ed. *Systemic Pathology of Fish*. 2nd ed. Ames, IA: Scotian Press; 2006:141-168.

34. Santer R. Morphology and innervation of the fish heart. *Adv Anat Embryol Cell Biol*. 1985;89:1-102.

35. Tota B, Cimini V, Salvatore G, et al. Comparative study of the arterial and lacunary systems of the ventricular myocardium of elasmobranch and teleost fishes. *Am J Anat*. 1983;167:15-32.

36. Tota B. Myoarchitecture and vascularization of the elasmobranch heart ventricle. *J Exp Zool Suppl*. 1989;2:122-135.

37. Sherrill J, Weber ES, Marty GD, et al. Fish cardiovascular physiology and disease. *Vet Clin North Am Exot Anim Pract*. 2009; 12(1):11-38.

38. Bushnell P, Jones D, Farrell A. The arterial system. In: Hoar W, Randall D, Farrell A, eds. *Fish Physiology, Volume XII, Part A, The Cardiovascular System*. San Diego, CA: Academic Press, Inc.; 1992:89-139.

39. Satchell G. The venous system. In: Hoar W, Randall D, Farrell A, eds. *Fish Physiology, Volume XII, Part A, The Cardiovascular System*. San Diego, CA: Academic Press, Inc.; 1992:141-183.

40. Steffensen J, Lomholt J. The secondary vascular system. In: Hoar W, Randall D, Farrell A, eds. *Fish Physiology, Volume XII, Part A, The Cardiovascular System*. San Diego, CA: Academic Press, Inc.; 1992:185-217.

41. Iwama G, Farrell A. Disorders of the cardiovascular and respiratory systems. In: Leatherland J, Woo P, eds. *Fish Diseases and Disorders*. Vol 2. Non-infectious disorders. New York, NY: CABI Publishing; 2006.

42. Reid S, Sundin L, Milsom W. The cardiorespiratory system in tropical fishes: structure, function, and control. In: Val A, de Almeida-Val V, Randall D, eds. *Fish Physiology*. Vol 21. The Physiology of Tropical Fishes. San Diego, CA: Academic Press, Inc.; 2006:225-275.

43. Johansen K, Hanson D. Functional anatomy of the hearts of lungfishes and amphibians. *Am Zool*. 1968;8(2):191-210.

44. Ecker A, Haslam G. *The Anatomy of the Frog*. Oxford, UK: Oxford University Press; 1889:449.

45. Francis E. *The Anatomy of the Salamander*. Oxford, UK: Oxford University Press; 1934:470.

46. Underhill R. *Laboratory Anatomy of the Frog*. 3rd ed. Dubuque, IA: Wm. C. Brown Company Publishers; 1975:66.

47. Putnam J, Parkerson J. Anatomy of the heart of the Amphibia II. *Cryptobranchus alleganiensis. Herpetologica*. 1985;41(3):287-298.

48. Putnam J. Anatomy of the heart of the Amphibia. I. *Siren lacertina. Copeia*. 1977;3:476-488.

49. De Saint-Aubain M. Blood flow patterns of the respiratory systems in larval and adult amphibians: functional morphology and phylogenetic significance. *J Zool Syst Evol Res*. 1985;23:229-240.

50. Duellman W, Trueb L. Integumentary, sensory, and visceral systems. In: Duellman W, Trueb L, eds. *Biology of Amphibians*. Baltimore, MD: The Johns Hopkins University Press; 1994:367-414.

51. Heinz-Taheny KM. Cardiovascular physiology and diseases of amphibians. *Vet Clin North Am Exot Anim Med*. 2009;12(1):39-50, v-vi.

52. Wright K. Anatomy for the clinician. In: Wright K, Whitaker B, eds. *Amphibian Medicine and Captive Husbandry*. Malabar, FL: Krieger Publishing Company; 2001:15-30.

53. Heinz-Taherny K. Cardiovascular physiology and diseases of amphibian. *Vet Clin North Am Exot Anim Pract*. 2009;12:39-50.

54. Andersen J. Cardio-respiratory responses to reduced oxygen and increased metabolism in amphibians. PhD Dissertation, University of Aarhus, Denmark. 2003:97.

55. Sedmera D, Reckova M, DeAlmeida A, et al. Functional and morphological evidence for a ventricular conduction system in zebrafish and *Xenopus* hearts. *Am J Physiol Heart Circ Physiol*. 2003;284(4): H1152-H1160.

56. Murray M. Cardiopulmonary anatomy and physiology. In: Mader D, ed. *Reptile Medicine and Surgery*. 2nd ed. St. Louis, MO: Elsevier; 2006:124-144.

57. Wyneken J. Normal reptile heart morphology and function. *Vet Clin North Am Exot Anim Pract*. 2009;12(1):51-63.

58. Burgreen W, Johansen K. Ventricular haemodynamics in the monitor lizard *Varanus exanthematicus*: pulmonary and systemic pressure separation. *J Exp Biol*. 1982;96:343-354.

59. Cordero-Tapia A, Gardner SC, Arellano-Blanco J, et al. *Learedius learedi* infection in black turtles (*Chelonia mydas agassizii*), Baja California Sur, Mexico. *J Parasitol*. 2004;90(3):645-647.

60. Jensen B, Nyengaard J, Pedersen M. Anatomy of the python heart. *Anat Sci Int*. 2010;85(4):194-203.

61. Jensen B, Abe A, Andrade D. The heart of the South American rattlesnake, *Crotalus durissus. J Morphol*. 2010;271:1066-1077.

62. Webb G, Heatwole H, De Bavat J. Comparative cardiac anatomy of the Reptilia. I. The chambers and septa of the varanid ventricle. *J Morphol*. 1971;134:335-350.

63. Webb GJ, Heatwole H, De Bavay J. Comparative cardiac anatomy of the Reptilia. II. A critique of the literature on the Squamata and Rhynchocephalia. *J Morphol.* 1974;142(1):1-20.

64. Webb G. Comparative cardiac anatomy of the Reptilia III. The heart of crocodilians and a hypothesis on the completion of the interventricular septum of crocodilians and birds. *J Morphol.* 1979; 161:221-240.

65. White FN. Functional anatomy of the heart of reptiles. *Am Zool.* 1968;8:211-219.

66. McCraken H. Organ location in snakes for diagnostic and surgical evaluation. In: Miller R, ed. *Zoo and Wild Animal Medicine Current Therapy.* 4th ed. Philadelphia, PA: W.B. Saunders; 1999:243-248.

67. Kashyap H. The reptilian heart. *Proc Natl Inst Sci India.* 1959;26(5):234-254.

68. Seymour R. Scaling of cardiovascular physiology in snakes. *Am Zool.* 1987;27:97-109.

69. Farrell A, Gampert A, Francis E. Comparative aspects of heart morphology. In: Gans C, Gaunt A, eds. *Biology of the Reptilia.* Vol 19. Ithaca, NY: Society for the Study of Amphibians and Reptiles; 1998:375-424.

70. Mathur P. The anatomy of the reptilian heart. Part II. Serpentes, Testudinata and Loricata. *Proc Ind Acad Sci Sect B.* 1946;23(3): 129-152.

71. White F. Circulation. In: Gans C, ed. *Biology of the Reptilia.* Vol 5. London, UK: Academic Press; 1976:275-334.

72. Starck JM. Functional morphology and patterns of blood flow in the heart of *Python regius. J Morphol.* 2009;270(6):673-687.

73. Prahlad BY, Mathur N. The anatomy of the reptilian heart. Part I. Varanus monitor. *Proc Ind Acad Sci Sect B.* 1943;20(1):1-29.

74. McArthur S, Meyer J, Innis C. Anatomy and physiology. In: McArthur S, Wilkinson R, Meyer J, eds. *Medicine and Surgery of Tortoises and Turtles.* Ames, IA: Blackwell Publishing; 2004: 35-72.

75. Campen R, Starck M. Cardiovascular circuits and digestive function of intermittent-feeding sauropsids. In: McCue M, ed. *Comparative Physiology of Fasting, Starvation, and Food Limitation.* Berlin, Heidelberg: Springer-Verlag; 2012:133-155.

76. Andersen J, Rourcke B, Caiozzo V, et al. Physiology: postprandial cardiac hypertrophy in pythons. *Nature.* 2005;434:37-38.

77. Riquelme CA, Magida JA, Harrison BC, et al. Fatty acids identified in the Burmese python promote beneficial cardiac growth. *Science.* 2011;334(6055):528-531.

78. Ottavioni G, Tazzi A. The lymphatic system. In: Gans C, Parsons T, eds. *Biology of the Reptilia.* Vol 6. New York, NY: Wiley; 1977:315-462.

79. Aughey E, Frye F. Reptilian lymphatic system. In: *Comparative Veterinary Histology with Clinical Correlates.* London: Mason Publishing Ltd; 2001:259.

80. Origgi F. Reptile immunology. In: Jacobson E, ed. *Infectious Diseases and Pathology of Reptiles.* Boca Raton, FL: CRC Press; 2007:131-166.

81. Wang T, Warburton S, Abe A, et al. Vagal control of heart rate and cardiac shunts in reptiles: relation to metabolic state. *Exp Physiol.* 2001;86(6):777-784.

82. Dyce K, Sack W, Wensing C. *Textbook of Veterinary Anatomy.* 3rd ed. Philadelphia, PA: Saunders; 2002:840.

83. Fox P, Moise N, Evans H, et al. Cardiovascular anatomy. In: Fox P, Sisson D, Moise N, eds. *Textbook of Canine and Feline Cardiology.* 2nd ed. Philadelphia, PA: W.B. Saunders Company; 1999:13-24.

84. Konig H, Ruberte J, Liebich H. Organs of the cardiovascular system. In: Konig H, Liebich H, eds. *Veterinary Anatomy of Domestic Mammals.* Stuttgart, Germany: Schattauer; 2007:441-474.

85. Akers R, Denbow D. Cardiovascular system. In: *Anatomy & Physiology of Domestic Animals.* Ames, IA: Blackwell Publishing; 2008: 345-378.

86. Schummer A, Wilkens H, Volmerhaus B, et al. *The Anatomy of the Domestic Animals.* Vol 3. The Circulatory System, the Skin, and the Cutaneous Organs of the Domestic Mammals. Berlin, Germany: Verlag Paul Parey—Springer Verlag; 1981:610.

87. Breazile J, Brown E. Anatomy. In: Wagner J, Manning P, eds. *The Biology of the Guinea Pig.* London, UK: Academic Press; 1976: 53-62.

88. Chiasson R. *Laboratory Anatomy of the White Rat.* 5th ed. Dubuque, IA: Wm. C. Brown Company Publishers; 1988:129.

89. Cooper G, Schiller A. The cardiovascular system. In: Cooper G, Schiller A, eds. *Anatomy of the Guinea Pig.* Cambridge, MA: Harvard University Press; 1975:147-212.

90. Evans H, Nguyen Q. Anatomy of the ferret. In: Fox J, ed. *Biology and Diseases of the Ferret.* 2nd ed. Baltimore, MD: Lippincott Williams & Wilkins; 1998:19-70.

91. Fox J, Anderson L, Loew F, et al. *Laboratory Animal Medicine.* 2nd ed. San Diego, CA: Academic Press; 2002:1325.

92. Heatley J. Cardiovascular anatomy, physiology, and disease of rodents and small exotic mammals. *Vet Clin North Am Exot Anim Pract.* 2009;12:99-113.

93. Hoyt R, Hawkins J, St Clair M, et al. Mouse physiology. In: Fox J, Barthold S, Davisson M, et al., eds. *The Mouse in Biomedical Research.* 2nd ed. San Diego, CA: Academic Press; 2007:23-90.

94. Kozma C, Macklin W, Cummins L, et al. The anatomy, physiology, and the biochemistry of the rabbit. In: Weisbroth S, Flatt R, Kraus A, eds. *The Biology of the Laboratory Rabbit.* London, UK: Academic Press; 1974:50-73.

95. McLaughlin C, Chiasson R. *Laboratory Anatomy of the Rabbit.* 2nd ed. Dubuque, IA: Wm. C. Brown Company Publishers; 1990:112.

96. Popesko P, Rajtova V, Horak J. *A Colour Atlas of the Anatomy of the Small Laboratory Animals.* Bratislava: Wolfe Publishing; 1992:500.

97. Hargaden M, Singer L, Sohn J, et al. Anatomy, physiology, and behavior. In: Suckow M, Stevens K, Wilson R, eds. *The Laboratory Rabbit, Guinea Pig, Hamster, and other Rodents.* Oxford, UK: Academic Press; 2012:195-215.

98. Morrisey J, Kraus M. Cardiovascular and other diseases. In: Quesenberry K, Carpenter J, eds. *Ferrets, Rabbits, and Rodents. Clinical Medicine and Surgery.* 3rd ed. St. Louis, MO: Elsevier Saunders; 2012:62-77.

99. Dawson TJ, Webster KN, Mifsud B, et al. Functional capacities of marsupial hearts: size and mitochondrial parameters indicate higher aerobic capabilities than generally seen in placental mammals. *J Comp Physiol [B].* 2003;173(7):583-590.

100. Wade O, Neely P. The heart and attached vessels of the opossum, a marsupial. *J Mammal.* 1949;30(2):111-116.

101. Mangel A, Fahim M, Van Breemen C. Rhythmic contractile activity of the in vivo rabbit aorta. *Nature.* 1981;289(5799):692-694.

102. Smith FM, West NH, Jones DR. The cardiovascular system. In: Whittow GC, ed. *Sturkie's Avian Physiology.* London: Academic Press; 2000:141-232.

103. Baumel J. Systema cardiovasculare. In: Baumel J, King A, Breazile J, et al., eds. *Handbook of Avian Anatomy: Nomina Anatomica Avium.* 2nd ed. Cambridge, MA: Nuttall Ornithological Club; 1993: 407-476.

104. West N, Langille B, Jones D. Cardiovascular system. In: King A, McLelland J, eds. *Form and Function in Birds.* Vol 2. London: Academic Press; 1981:235-339.

105. King A, McLelland J. Cardiovascular system. In: King A, MacLelland J, eds. *Birds: Their Structure and Function.* 2nd ed. London: Bailliere Tindall; 1984:214-236.

106. Lumeij J, Ritchie B. Cardiology. In: Ritchie BW, Harrison GJ, Harrison LR, eds. *Avian Medicine: Principles and Applications.* Lake Worth, FL: Wingers Publishing; 1994:695-722.

107. Nickel R, Schummer A, Seiferle E, et al. Circulatory system. In: Nickel R, Schummer A, Seiferle E, et al., eds. *Anatomy of the Domestic Birds.* Berlin: Verlag Paul Parey–Springer Verlag; 1977:85-107.

108. Maina J. Perspectives on the structure and function in birds. In: Rosskopf W, Woerpel R, eds. *Diseases of Cage and Aviary Birds.* 3rd ed. Baltimore, MD: Williams & Wilkins; 1996:163-217.

109. McLelland J. Pericardium, pleura et peritoneum. In: Baumel J, King A, Breazile J, et al., eds. *Handbook of Avian Anatomy: Nomina Anatomica Avium.* 2nd ed. Cambridge, MA: Nuttall Ornithological Club; 1993:251-256.

110. Duncker H. Coelomic cavities. In: King A, McLelland J, eds. *Form and Function in Birds.* Vol 1. London: Academic Press; 1979: 39-68.

111. Fournier D, Luft FC, Bader M, et al. Emergence and evolution of the renin-angiotensin-aldosterone system. *J Mol Med.* 2012;90(5): 495-508.

112. Sisson D. Pathophysiology of heart failure. In: Ettinger S, Feldman E, eds. *Textbook of Veterinary Internal Medicine.* 7th ed. 2010: St. Louis, MO: Saunders Elsevier; 2010:1143-1158.

113. Mann D, Bristow M. Mechanisms and models in heart failure: the biomechanical model and beyond. *Circulation.* 2005;111:2837-2849.

114. Francis GS, Tang WHW. Pathophysiology of congestive heart failure. *Rev Cardiovasc Med.* 2003;4(suppl 2):S14-S20.

115. Takahashi H, Sakamoto T. The role of "mineralocorticoids" in teleost fish: relative importance of glucocorticoid signaling in the osmoregulation and "central" actions of mineralocorticoid receptor. *Gen Comp Endocrinol.* 2013; 181:223-228.

116. Salzet M, Deloffre L, Breton C, et al. The angiotensin system elements in invertebrates. *Brain Res Rev.* 2001;36(1):35-45.

117. Theopold U, Schmidt O, Soderhal K, et al. Coagulation in arthropods: defence, wound closure and healing. *Trends Immunol.* 2004;25(6):289-294.

118. Reimschuessel R, Stoskopf M, Bennett R. Myocarditis in the common cuttlefish *(Sepia oficinalis). J Comp Pathol.* 1990;102(3): 291-297.

119. Stentiford GD, Neil DM. Diseases of *Nephrops* and *Metanephrops:* a review. *J Invert Pathol.* 2011;106(1):92-109.

120. Reimschuessel R, Stoskopf MK. Octopus automutilation syndrome. *J Invert Pathol.* 1990;55(3):394-400.

121. Cruz-Landim C Da. Degenerative changes in heart muscle from senescent honeybee workers *(Apis mellifera adansonii). J Invert Pathol.* 1976;27(1):1-5.

122. Peters E, Smolowitz R, Reynolds T. Neoplasia. In: Lewbart G, ed. *Invertebrate Medicine.* 2nd ed. Ames, IA: Blackwell Publishing; 2012:431-439.

123. Mix MC, Riley RT. A pericardial tumor in a native (Olympia) oyster, *Ostrea lurida,* from Yaquina Bay, Oregon. *J Invert Pathol.* 1977;30(1):104-107.

124. Scharrer B, Lochhead M. Tumors in the invertebrates: a review. *Cancer Res.* 1950;10:403-419.

125. Roberts R, Rodger H. The pathophysiology and systematic pathology of teleosts. In: Roberts R, ed. *Fish Pathology.* 4th ed. Ames, IA: Wiley-Blackwell; 2012:62-143.

126. Palacios G, Lovoll M, Tengs T, et al. Heart and skeletal muscle inflammation of farmed salmon is associated with infection with a novel reovirus. Lindenbach B, ed. *PLoS ONE.* 2010;5(7): e11487.

127. Haugland O, Mikalsen AB, Nilsen P, et al. Cardiomyopathy syndrome of Atlantic salmon *(Salmo salar L.)* is caused by a double-stranded RNA virus of the Totiviridae family. *J Virol.* 2011; 85(11):5275-5286.

128. Prabhuji S, Sinha S. Life cycle (reproductive stages) of *Ichthyophonus hoferi* Plehn & Mulsow, a parasitic fungus causing deep mycoses in fish. *Int J Plant Reprod Biol.* 2009;1(2):93-101.

129. Kocan R, LaPatra S, Gregg J, et al. *Ichthyophonus*-induced cardiac damage: a mechanism for reduced swimming stamina in salmonids. *J Fish Dis.* 2006;29:521-527.

130. Dick TA. The atrium of the fish heart as a site for *Contracaecum* spp. larvae. *J Wildl Dis.* 1987;23(2):328-330.

131. Brooker AJ, Shinn AP, Bron JE. A review of the biology of the parasitic copepod *Lernaeocera branchialis* (L., 1767) (Copepoda: Pennellidae). *Adv Parasitol.* 2007;65:297-341.

132. Poppe TT, Midtlyng P, Sande RD. Examination of abdominal organs and diagnosis of deficient septum transversum in Atlantic salmon, *Salmo salar* L., using diagnostic ultrasound imaging. *J Fish Dis.* 1998;21(1):67-72.

133. Brocklebank J, Raverty S. Sudden mortality caused by cardiac deformities following seining of preharvest farmed Atlantic salmon *(Salmo salar)* and by cardiomyopathy of postintraperitoneally vaccinated Atlantic salmon parr in British Columbia. *Can Vet J.* 2002;43(2):129-130.

134. Poppe T, Taksdal T. Ventricular hypoplasia in farmed Atlantic salmon, *Salmo salar. Dis Aquat Organ.* 2000;42:35-40.

135. Tørud B, Taksdal T, Dale OB, et al. Myocardial glycogen storage disease in farmed rainbow trout, *Oncorhynchus mykiss* (Walbaum). *J Fish Dis.* 2006;29(9):535-540.

136. Kirk RS, Lewis JW. Histopathology of *Sanguinicola inermis* infection in carp, *Cyprinus carpio. J Helminthol.* 1998;72(1):33-38.

137. Moore JF, Mayr W, Hougie C. Number, location and severity of coronary arterial changes in steelhead trout *(Salmo gairdnerii). Atherosclerosis.* 1976;24(3):381-386.

138. Densmore C, Green D. Diseases of amphibians. *ILAR J.* 2007; 48(3):235-254.

139. Daszak P, Berger L, Cunningham A, et al. Emerging infectious diseases and amphibian population declines. *Emerg Infect Dis.* 1999;5(6):735-748.

140. Wright K. Idiopathic syndromes. In: Wright K, Whitaker B, eds. *Amphibian Medicine and Captive Husbandry.* Malabar, FL: Krieger Publishing Company; 2001:239-244.

141. Pessier A. Edematous frogs, urinary tract disease, and disorders of fluid balance in amphibians. *J Exot Pet Med.* 2009;18(1):4-13.

142. Green D. Pathology of Amphibia. In: Wright K, Whitaker B, eds. *Amphibian Medicine and Captive Husbandry.* Malabar, FL: Krieger Publishing Company; 2001:401-485.

143. Voyles J, Young S, Berger L, et al. Pathogenesis of chytridiomycosis, a cause of catastrophic amphibian declines. *Science.* 2009;326(5952):582-585.

144. Campbell CR, Voyles J, Cook DI, et al. Frog skin epithelium: electrolyte transport and chytridiomycosis. *Int J Biochem Cell Biol.* 2012;44(3):431-434.

145. Nigrelli R, Maraventano L. Pericarditis in *Xenopus laevis* caused by *Diplostomulum xenopi* sp. no., a larval strigeid. *J Parasitol.* 1944;30(3): 184-190.

146. King PH, Van As JG. Description of the adult and larval stages of *Tylodelphys xenopi* (Trematoda: Diplostomidae) from southern Africa. *J Parasitol.* 1997;83(2):287-295.

147. Kuperman B, Matey V, Fisher R, et al. Parasites of the African clawed frog, *Xenopus laevis,* in southern California, USA. *Comp Parasitol.* 2004;71(2):229-232.

148. Buttner A, Bourcart N. Some biological particulars of a Trypanosome in the green frog, *Trypanosoma inopinatum* Sergent, 1904. *Ann Parasitol Hum Comp.* 1955;30(5-6):431-445.

149. Pizzatto L, Shilton CM, Shine R. Infection dynamics of the lungworm *Rhabdias pseudosphaerocephala* in its natural host, the cane toad *(Bufo marinus),* and in novel hosts (native Australian frogs). *J Wildl Dis.* 2010;46(4):1152-1164.

150. Lemckert F. Parasitism of the common eastern froglet *Crinia signifera* by flies of the genus *Batrachomyia* (Diptera: Chloropidae): parasitism rates and the influence on frog condition. *Aust Zool.* 2000;31(3):492-495.

151. Kraus F. Fly parasitism in Papuan frogs, with a discussion of ecological factors influencing evolution of life-history differences. *J Nat Hist.* 2007;41(29-32):1863-1874.

152. Murphy T. High incidence of two parasitic infestations and two morphological abnormalities in a population of the frog, *Rana palustris* Le Conte. *Am Midl Natur.* 1965;74(1):233-239.

153. Carpenter J, Bachrach A, Albert D, et al. Xanthomatous keratitis, disseminated xanthomatosis, and atherosclerosis in Cuban tree frogs. *Vet Pathol.* 1986;23:337-339.

154. Russell W, Edwards D, Stair E, et al. Corneal lipidosis, disseminated xanthomatosis, and hypercholesterolemia in Cuban tree frogs *(Osteopilus septentionalis)*. *J Zoo Wildl Med.* 1990;21(1):99-104.

155. Griner L. Amphibians and reptiles—Order Anura. In: Griner L, ed. *Pathology of Zoo Animals.* San Diego, CA: Zoological Society of San Diego; 1983:7-17.

156. Barten S. Cardiomyopathy in a king snake *(Lampropeltis calligaster rhombomaculata)*. *Vet Med Small Anim Clin.* 1980;75:125-129.

157. Jacobson ER, Seely JC, Novilla MN, et al. Heart failure associated with unusual hepatic inclusions in a Deckert's rat snake. *J Wildl Dis.* 1979;15(1):75-81.

158. Wagner R. Clinical challenge. *J Zoo Wildl Med.* 1989;20(2):238.

159. Frye F. Characteristics of cardiomyopathy in two pythons: aortic valvular stenosis and secondary cardiomyopathy in a Children's python, *Liasis childreni*, and ventricular wall hypoplasia, first-degree heart block, and plasmacytic pericarditis in a juvenile Burmese python, *Python bivittatus. Proc IV Int Coll Path Reptiles Amphib.* Bad Nauheim: Germany; 1991.

160. Frye F. Common pathologic lesions & disease processes. In: Frye F, ed. *Reptile Care. An Atlas of Diseases and Treatments.* Vol 2. Neptune City: TFH Publications, Inc.; 1991:533-536.

161. Griner L. Systemic diseases. Sub-order Sauria. In: Griner L, ed. *Pathology of Zoo Animals.* San Diego, CA: Zoological Society of San Diego; 1983:32-35.

162. Mader D. Gout. In: Mader D, ed. *Reptile Medicine and Surgery.* 2nd ed. St. Louis, MO: Elsevier Saunders; 2006:340-343.

163. Jacobson ER. Gentamicin-related visceral gout in two boid snakes. *Vet Med Small Anim Clin.* 1976;71:361-363.

164. Montali RJ, Bush M, Smeller JM. The pathology of nephrotoxicity of gentamicin in snakes. A model for reptilian gout. *Vet Pathol.* 1979;16(1):108-115.

165. Rishniw M, Carmel BP. Atrioventricular valvular insufficiency and congestive heart failure in a carpet python. *Aust Vet J.* 1999;77(9):580-583.

166. Schilliger L, Trehiou E, Petit AMP, et al. Double valvular insufficiency in a Burmese python *(Python molurus bivittatus*, Linnaeus, 1758) suffering from concomitant bacterial pneumonia. *J Zoo Wildl Med.* 2010;41(4):742-744.

167. Penninck DG, Stewart JS, Paul-Murphy J, et al. Ultrasonography of the California desert tortoise *(Zerobates agassizii)*: anatomy and application. *Vet Radiol Ultrasound.* 1991;32(3):112-116.

168. Redrobe SP, Scudamore CL. Ultrasonographic diagnosis of pericardial effusion and atrial dilatation in a spur-thighed tortoise *(Testudo graeca)*. *Vet Rec.* 2000;146(7):183-185.

169. Schilliger L, Lemberger K, Chai N, et al. Atherosclerosis associated with pericardial effusion in a central bearded dragon *(Pogona vitticeps*, Ahl. 1926). *J Vet Diagn Invest.* 2010;22(5):789-792.

170. Gumber S, Nevarez JG, Cho D-Y. Endocardial fibrosarcoma in a reticulated python *(Python reticularis)*. *J Vet Diagn Invest.* 2010;22(6):1013-1016.

171. Hernandez-Divers S. Diagnostic techniques. In: Mader D, ed. *Reptile Medicine and Surgery.* 2nd ed. St. Louis, MO: Saunders Elsevier; 2006:490-532.

172. Isaza R, Andrews G, Coke R, et al. Assessment of multiple cardiocentesis in ball pythons *(Python regius)*. *Contemp Top Lab Anim Sci.* 2004;43(6):35-38.

173. Brown C. Cardiac blood sample collection from snakes. *Lab Anim.* 2010;39(7):208-209.

174. Selleri P, Di Girolamo N. Cardiac tamponade following cardiocentesis in a cardiopathic boa constrictor imperator *(Boa constrictor imperator)*. *J Small Anim Pract.* 2012;53(8):487.

175. Innis C. Myocardial abscess and hemopericardium in a green iguana *(Iguana iguana)*. *Proc 7th Annu Conf Assoc Rept Amph Vet.* 2000;185-188.

176. Jacobson ER, Ginn PPE, Troutman JM, et al. West Nile virus infection in farmed American alligators *(Alligator mississipiensis)* in Florida. *J Wildl Dis.* 2005;41(1):96-106.

177. Ritchie B. Virology. In: Mader D, ed. *Reptile Medicine and Surgery.* 2nd ed. St. Louis, MO: Saunders Elsevier; 2006:391-417.

178. Wellehan JFX, Johnson AJ. Reptile virology. *Vet Clin North Am Exot Anim Pract.* 2005;8(1):27-52, vii.

179. Marschang RE. Viruses infecting reptiles. *Viruses.* 2011;3(11):2087-2126.

180. Schumacher J, Jacobson E, Homer B. Inclusion body disease in boid snakes. *J Zoo Wildl Med.* 1994;25:511-524.

181. Wozniak E, McBride J, DeNardo D, et al. Isolation and characterization of an antigenically distinct 68-kd protein from nonviral intracytoplasmic inclusions in boa constrictors chronically infected with the inclusion body disease virus (IBDV: Retroviridae). *Vet Pathol.* 2000;37(5):449-459.

182. Chang L, Jacobson E. Inclusion body disease, a worldwide infectious disease of boid snakes: a review. *J Exot Pet Med.* 2010;19:216-225.

183. Keilwerth M, Bühler I, Hoffmann R, et al. [Inclusion body disease (IBD of boids)—a haematological, histological and electron microscopical study]. *Berl Munch Tierarztl Wochenschr.* 2012;125(9-10):411-417.

184. Jacobson E, Gaskin J, Mansell J, et al. Chlamydial infection in puff adders *(Bitis arietans)*. *J Zoo Wildl Med.* 1989;20:364-369.

185. Homer B, Jacobson E, Schumacher J, et al. Chlamydiosis in marine culture-reared green sea turtles *(Chelonia mydas)*. *Vet Pathol.* 1994;31:1-7.

186. Jacobson E, Origgi F, Heard D, et al. C. Immunohistochemical staining of chlamydial antigen in emerald tree boas *(Corallus caninus)*. *J Vet Diagn Invest.* 2002;14(6):487-494.

187. Schilliger L, Vanderstylen D, Pietrain J. Granulomatous myocarditis and coelomic effusion due to *Salmonella enterica arizonae* in a Madagascarian Dumeril's boa *(Acrantophis dumerili*, Jan. 1860). *J Vet Cardiol.* 2003;5:43-45.

188. Jacobson E, Homer B, Adams W. Endocarditis and congestive heart failure in a Burmese python *(Python molurus bivittatus)*. *J Zoo Wildl Med.* 1991;22:245-248.

189. Obendorf DL, Carson J, McManus TJ. *Vibrio damsela* infection in a stranded leatherback turtle *(Dermochelys coriacea)*. *J Wildl Dis.* 1987;23(4):666-668.

190. Schroff S, Schmidt V, Kiefer I, et al. Ultrasonographic diagnosis of an endocarditis valvularis in a Burmese python *(Python molurus bivittatus)* with pneumonia. *J Zoo Wildl Med.* 2010;41(4):721-724.

191. Glazebrook J, Campbell R, Blair D. Studies on cardiovascular fluke (Digenea: Spirorchiidae) infections in sea turtles from the Great Barrier Reef, Queensland, Australia. *J Comp Pathol.* 1989;101:231-250.

192. Gordon N, Kelly N, Cribb T. Lesions caused by cardiovascular flukes (Digenea: Spirorchiidae) infections in stranded green turtles *(Chelonia mydas)*. *Vet Pathol.* 1998;35:21-30.

193. Johnson CA, Griffith JW, Tenorio P, et al. Fatal trematodiasis in research turtles. *Lab Anim Sci.* 1998;48(4):340-343.

194. McAllister C, Cordes J, Conn D, et al. Helminth parasites of unisexual and bisexual whiptail lizards (Teiidae) in North America. V. *Mesocestoides* sp. *tetrathyridia* (Cestoidea: Cyclophyllidea) from four species of *Cnemidophorus*. *J Wildl Dis.* 1991;27:494-497.

195. Greiner E, Mader D. Parasitology. In: Mader D, ed. *Reptile Medicine and Surgery.* 2nd ed. St. Louis, MO: Saunders Elsevier; 2006:343-364.

196. Mitchell MA. Reptile cardiology. *Vet Clin North Am Exot Anim Pract.* 2009;12(1):65-79.

197. Clippinger T. Aortic stenosis and atrioventricular dilatation in a green iguana *(Iguana iguana)*. *Proc Am Assoc Zoo Vet.* 1993;342-344.

198. McIntosh HD, Morris JJ, Whalen RE, et al. Bilateral functional subaortic stenosis in the alligator. *Trans Am Clin Climatol Assoc.* 1967;78:119-128.

199. Pizzi R, Pereira YM, Rambaud YF, et al. Secundum atrial septal defect in a Komodo dragon *(Varanus komodoensis)*. *Vet Rec.* 2009;164(15):472-473.

200. Jensen B, Wang T. Hemodynamic consequences of cardiac malformations in two juvenile ball pythons (Python regius). J Zoo Wildl Med. 2009;40(752-756):752-756.
201. Rush E, Donnelly T, Walberg J. What's your diagnosis? Cardiopulmonary arrest in a Burmese python. Aortic aneurysm. Lab Anim Sci. 2001;30:24-27.
202. Finlayson R, Woods S. Arterial disease of reptiles. J Zool Lond. 1977;183:397-410.
203. Schuchman SM, Taylor DO, Schuman S. Arteriosclerosis in an iguana (Iguana iguana). J Am Vet Med Assoc. 1970;157(5):614-616.
204. Griner L. Systemic diseases. Order Testudinata. In: Griner L, ed. Pathology of Zoo Animals. San Diego, CA: Zoological Society of San Diego; 1983:80-85.
205. Vastesaeger M, Delcourt R, Gillot P. Spontaneous atherosclerosis in fishes and reptiles. In: Roberts J, Straus T, eds. Comparative Atherosclerosis: The Morphology of Spontaneous and Induced Atherosclerotic Lesions in Animals and Its Relation to Human Disease. New York, NY: Harper & Row; 1965:129-149.
206. Dangerfield WG, Finlayson R, Myatt G, et al. Serum lipoproteins and atherosclerosis in animals. Atherosclerosis. 1976;25(1):95-106.
207. Elkan E, Cooper JE. Tumours and pseudotumours in some reptiles. J Comp Pathol. 1976;86(3):337-348.
208. Stumpel JBG, Del-Pozo J, French A, et al. Cardiac hemangioma in a corn snake (Pantherophis guttatus). J Zoo Wildl Med. 2012;43(2):360-366.
209. Hruban Z, Vardiman R, Meehan T. Hematopoietic neoplasms in zoo animals. J Comp Pathol. 1992;106:15-24.
210. Orós J, Torrent A, Espinosa de los Monteros A, et al. Multicentric lymphoblastic lymphoma in a loggerhead sea turtle (Caretta caretta). Vet Pathol. 2001;38(4):464-467.
211. Schilliger L, Selleri P, Frye FLF. Lymphoreticular neoplasm and leukemia in a red-tail boa (Boa constrictor constrictor) associated with concurrent inclusion body disease. J Vet Diagn Invest. 2011;23(1):159-162.
212. Schumacher J, Bennett A, Fox LE, et al. Mast cell tumor in an eastern king snake (Lampropeltis getulus getulus). J Vet Diagn Invest. 1998;10(1):101-104.
213. Work TM, Balazs GH, Rameyer RA, et al. Retrospective pathology survey of green turtles Chelonia mydas with fibropapillomatosis in the Hawaiian Islands, 1993-2003. Dis Aquat Organ. 2004;62(1-2):163-176.
214. Pignon C, Sanchez-Migallon Guzman D, Sinclair K, et al. Evaluation of heart murmurs in chinchillas (Chinchilla lanigera): 59 cases (1996-2009). J Am Vet Med Assoc. 2012;241(10):1344-1347.
215. Raymond JT, Garner MM. Cardiomyopathy in captive African hedgehogs (Atelerix albiventris). J Vet Diagn Invest. 2000;12(5):468-472.
216. Lewington J. Diseases of special concern. In: Lewington J, ed. Ferret Husbandry, Medicine and Surgery. 2nd ed. Philadelphia, PA: Saunders Elsevier; 2007:258-288.
217. Fox J. Other systemic diseases. In: Fox J, ed. Biology and Diseases of the Ferret. 2nd ed. 1998: Baltimore: Lippincott Williams & Wilkins; 1998:307-320.
218. King W, Russell S. Metabolic, traumatic, and miscellaneous diseases. In: Suckow M, Weisbroth S, Franklin C, eds. The Laboratory Rat. St. Louis, MO: Academic Press; 2006:513-546.
219. Cox I, Haworth P. Cardiac disease in guinea pigs. Vet Rec. 2000;146(21):620.
220. Schmidt R, Reavill D. Cardiovascular disease in hamsters: review and retrospective study. J Exot Pet Med. 2007;16(1):49-51.
221. Bellezza C, Concannon P, Hornbuckle W, et al. Woodchucks as laboratory animals. In: Fox J, Andersson L, Loew F, et al., eds. Laboratory Animal Medicine. 2nd ed. San Diego, CA: Academic Press; 2002:309-328.
222. Garner M. A review of common diseases in pet rabbits. Proc Annu Conf Assoc Avian Vet. Milwaukee, WI; 2009;207-217.
223. Garner M, Powers L. Diseases of domestic ferrets (Mustela putorius). Proc Annu Conf Assoc Avian Vet. San Diego, CA; 2010;209-219.
224. Garner M, Johnson-Delaney C. Diseases of cavies. Proc Annu Conf Assoc Avian Vet. Savannah, GA; 2008;261-268.
225. Malakoff RL, Laste NJ, Orcutt CJ. Echocardiographic and electrocardiographic findings in client-owned ferrets: 95 cases (1994-2009). J Am Vet Med Assoc. 2012;241(11):1484-1489.
226. Garner M. Diseases of pet hedgehogs, chinchillas, and sugar gliders. Proc Annu Conf Assoc Avian Vet. Seattle, WA; 2011;351-358.
227. Franklin J, Guzman D. Dilated cardiomyopathy and congestive heart failure in a guinea pig. Exotic DVM. 2006;7(6):9-12.
228. Johnson R, Hemsley S. Gliders and possums. In: Vogelnest L, Woods R, eds. Medicine of Australian Mammals. Collingwood, Australia: CSIRO Publishing; 2008:395-438.
229. Orcutt C. Cardiovascular disorders. In: Meredith A, Flecknell P, eds. BSAVA Manual of Rabbit Medicine and Surgery. 2nd ed. Quedgeley, UK: BSAVA; 2006:96-102.
230. Ivey E, Carpenter J. African hedgehogs. In: Quesenberry K, Carpenter J, eds. Ferrets, Rabbits, and Rodents. Clinical Medicine and Surgery. 3rd ed. St. Louis, MO: Elsevier; 2012:411-427.
231. Ono S, Onuma M, Ueki M, et al. Radiographic measurement of cardiac size in ferrets with heart disease. Adv Anim Cardiol. 2008;4(2):37-43.
232. Hoefer H. Heart disease in ferrets. In: Bonagura J, ed. Current Veterinary Therapy XIII Small Animal Practice. Philadelphia, PA: W.B. Saunders Company; 2000:1144-1148.
233. Mitchell E, Zehnder A, Hsu A, et al. Pimobendan: treatment of heart failure in small mammals. Proc Annu Conf Assoc Exot Mammal Vet. Savannah, GA; 2008;71-79.
234. Lord B, Devine C, Smith S. Congestive heart failure in two pet rabbits. J Small Anim Pract. 2010;52(1):46-50.
235. Ensley P, Van Winkle T. Treatment of congestive heart failure in a ferret (Mustela putorius furo). J Zoo Wildl Med. 1982;12:23-25.
236. Lipman N, Murphy J, Fox J. Clinical, functional and pathological changes associated with a case of dilatative cardiomyopathy in a ferret. Lab Anim Sci. 1987;37(2):210-212.
237. Greenlee P, Stephens E. Meningeal cryptococcosis and congestive cardiomyopathy in a ferret. J Am Vet Med Assoc. 1984;184(7):840-841.
238. Boonyapakorn C. Cardiologic examinations in ferrets with and without heart disease. PhD Dissertation, Frelen Universitat, Berlin. 2007;50.
239. Valentine H, Daugherity E, Singh B, et al. The experimental use of Syrian hamsters. In: Suckow M, Stevens K, Wilson R, eds. The Laboratory Rabbit, Guinea Pig, Hamster, and Other Rodents. Oxford, UK: Academic Press; 2012:875-906.
240. Harcourt-Brown F. Cardiorespiratory disease. In: Harcourt-Brown F, ed. Textbook of Rabbit Medicine. Oxford, UK: Butterworth-Heinemann; 1998:324-334.
241. Gava F, Zacche E, Ortiz E, et al. Doxorubicin induced dilated cardiomyopathy in a rabbit model: an update. Res Vet Sci. 2013;94:115-121.
242. Fujita K, Shinpo K, Yamada K, et al. Reduction of adriamycin toxicity by ascorbate in mice and guinea pigs. Cancer Res. 1982;42(1):309-316.
243. Moneva-Jordan A, Moneva-Jordon A. What is your diagnosis? J Small Anim Pract. 1998;39(6):263-303.
244. Goodman G. Rodents: respiratory and cardiovascular system disorders. In: Keeble E, Meredith A, eds. BSAVA Manual of Rodents and Ferrets. Quedgeley, UK: BSAVA; 2009:142-149.
245. Wagner RA. Ferret cardiology. Vet Clin North Am Exot Anim Pract. 2009;12(1):115-134, vii.
246. Brandao J, Vergneau-Grosset C, Mayer J. Hyperthyroidism and hyperparathyroidism in guinea pigs (Cavia porcellus). Vet Clin North Am Exot Anim Pract. 2013;16(2):407-420.
247. Williams B, Karolewski B, Mayer T, et al. Non-infectious diseases. In: Suckow M, Stevens K, Wilson R, eds. The Laboratory Rabbit,

Guinea Pig, Hamster, and Other Rodents. Oxford, UK: Academic Press; 2012:867-873.

248. Ruben Z, Arceo R, Bishop S, et al. Non-proliferative lesions of the heart and vascular in rats. In: *Guides for Toxicologic Pathology*. Washington, DC: STP/ARP/AFIP; 2000:1-10.

249. Percy D, Barthold S. Rat. In: Percy D, Barthold S, eds. *Pathology of Laboratory Rodents and Rabbits*. 3rd ed. Ames, IA: Blackwell Publishing; 2007:125-177.

250. Kohn D, Clifford C, Jacoby R, et al. Biology and diseases of mice. In: Fox J, Andersson L, Loew F, et al., eds. *Laboratory Animal Medicine*. 2nd ed. San Diego, CA: Academic Press; 2002:35-120.

251. Donnelly T, Quimby F. Biology and diseases of other rodents. In: Fox J, Anderson L, Loew F, et al., eds. *Laboratory Animal Medicine*. 2nd ed. San Diego, CA: Academic Press; 2002:247-307.

252. Thornton RN, Cook TG. A congenital *Toxoplasma*-like disease in ferrets (*Mustela putorius furo*). *N Z Vet J*. 1986;34(3):31-33.

253. Daoust PY, Hunter DB. Spontaneous Aleutian disease in ferrets. *Can Vet J*. 1978;19(5):133-135.

254. Welchman Dde B, Oxenham M, Done SH. Aleutian disease in domestic ferrets: diagnostic findings and survey results. *Vet Rec*. 1993;132(19):479-484.

255. Garner MM, Ramsell K, Schoemaker NJ, et al. Myofasciitis in the domestic ferret. *Vet Pathol*. 2007;44(1):25-38.

256. Marini RP, Li X, Harpster NK, et al. Cardiovascular pathology possibly associated with ketamine/xylazine anesthesia in Dutch belted rabbits. *Lab Anim Sci*. 1999;49(2):153-160.

257. Huston S, Lee P, Quesenberry K, et al. Cardiovascular disease, lymphoproliferative disorders, and thymomas. In: Quesenberry K, Carpenter J, eds. *Ferrets, Rabbits, and Rodents. Clinical Medicine and Surgery*. 3rd ed. St. Louis, MO: Elsevier; 2012:257-268.

258. Percy D, Barthold S. Rabbit. In: Percy D, Barthold S, eds. *Pathology of Laboratory Rodents and Rabbits*. 3rd ed. Ames, IA: Blackwell Publishing; 2007:253-307.

259. Jiang JP, Downing SE. Catecholamine cardiomyopathy: review and analysis of pathogenetic mechanisms. *Yale J Biol Med*. 1990;63(6):581-591.

260. Di Girolamo N, Critelli M, Zeyen U, et al. Ventricular septal defect in a ferret (*Mustela putorius furo*). *J Small Anim Pract*. 2012;53(9):549-553.

261. Black PA, Marshall C, Seyfried AW, et al. Cardiac assessment of African hedgehogs (*Atelerix albiventris*). *J Zoo Wildl Med*. 2011;42(1):49-53.

262. Vörös K, Seehusen F, Hungerbühler S, et al. Ventricular septal defect with aortic valve insufficiency in a New Zealand white rabbit. *J Am Anim Hosp Assoc*. 2011;47(4):e42-e49.

263. Linde A, Summerfield NJ, Johnston M, et al. Echocardiography in the chinchilla. *J Vet Intern Med*. 2004;18(5):772-774.

264. Soloman H, Wier PJ, Fish CJ, et al. Spontaneous and induced alterations in the cardiac membranous ventricular septum of fetal, weaning, and adult rats. *Teratology*. 1997;55(3):185-194.

265. Ho S, Michaelsson M. *Congenital Heart Malformations in Mammals*. Hackensack, NJ: World Scientific Publishing Company; 2000:200.

266. Donnelly T. Disease problems of chinchillas. In: Quesenberry K, Carpenter J, eds. *Ferrets, Rabbits, and Rodents. Clinical Medicine and Surgery*. 2nd ed. St. Louis, MO: Elsevier; 2004:255-264.

267. Williams J, Graham J, Laste N, et al. Tetralogy of Fallot in a young ferret (*Mustela putorius furo*). *J Exot Pet Med*. 2011;20(3):232-236.

268. Crary DD, Fox RR. Frequency of congenital abnormalities and of anatomical variations among JAX rabbits. *Teratology*. 1980;21(1):113-121.

269. Crary DD, Fox RR. Hereditary vestigial pulmonary arterial trunk and related defects in rabbits. *J Hered*. 1975;66(2):50-55.

270. Ignatowski AC. Influence of animal food on the organism of rabbits. *St. Peterberg, Izviest Imp Voyenno-Med Akad*. 1908;16:154-173.

271. Yanni AE. The laboratory rabbit: an animal model of atherosclerosis research. *Lab Anim*. 2004;38(3):246-256.

272. Moghadasian MH. Experimental atherosclerosis: a historical overview. *Life Sci*. 2002;70(8):855-865.

273. Gaman EM, Feigenbaum AS, Schenk EA. Spontaneous aortic lesions in rabbits. 3. Incidence and genetic factors. *J Atheroscler Res*. 1967;7(2):131-141.

274. Brock K, Gallaugher L, Bergdall V, et al. Mycoses and non-infectious diseases. In: Suckow M, Stevens K, Wilson R, eds. *The Laboratory Rabbit, Guinea Pig, Hamster, and Other Rodents*. Oxford, UK: Academic Press; 2012:503-528.

275. Watanabe Y. Serial inbreeding of rabbits with hereditary hyperlipidemia (WHHL-rabbit). *Atherosclerosis*. 1980;36(2):261-268.

276. Huynh M, Boyeaux A, Stambouli F, et al. Aortic calcification in a rabbit. *Proc Annu Conf Assoc Avian Vet*. 2012;287.

277. Bas S, Bas A, Estepa JC, et al. Parathyroid gland function in the uremic rabbit. *Domest Anim Endocrinol*. 2004;26(2):99-110.

278. Klaphake E, Paul-Murphy J. Disorders of the reproductive and urinary systems. In: Quesenberry K, Carpenter J, eds. *Ferrets, Rabbits, and Rodents. Clinical Medicine and Surgery*. 3rd ed. St. Louis, MO: Elsevier; 2012:217-231.

279. Pritt S, Cohen K, Sedlacek H. Parasitic diseases. In: Suckow M, Stevens K, Wilson R, eds. *The Laboratory Rabbit, Guinea Pig, Hamster, and Other Rodents*. Oxford, UK: Academic Press; 2012:415-446.

280. McCall JW. Dirofilariasis in the domestic ferret. *Clin Tech Small Anim Pract*. 1998;13(2):109-112.

281. Supakorndej P, McCall J, Jun J. Early migration and development of *Dirofilaria immitis* in the ferret, *Mustela putorius furo*. *J Parasitol*. 1994;80(2):237-244.

282. Campbell W, Blair L. *Dirofilaria immitis*: experimental infections in the ferret (*Mustela putorius furo*). *J Parasitol*. 1978;64(1):119-122.

283. Supakorndej P, Lewis RE, McCall JW, et al. Radiographic and angiographic evaluations of ferrets experimentally infected with *Dirofilaria immitis*. *Vet Radiol Ultrasound*. 1995;36(1):23-29.

284. Snyder RL, Ratcliffe HL. *Marmota monax*: a model for studies of cardiovascular, cerebrovascular and neoplastic disease. *Acta Zool Pathol Antverp*. 1969;48:265-273.

285. Zandvliet M. Electrocardiography in psittacine birds and ferrets. *Sem Avian Exot Pet Pract*. 2005;14(1):34-51.

286. Smith SH, Bishop SP. The electrocardiogram of normal ferrets and ferrets with right ventricular hypertrophy. *Lab Anim Sci*. 1985;35(3):268-271.

287. Malakoff R. Heart disease, AV block. In: Mayer J, Donnelly T, eds. *Clinical Veterinary Advisor: Birds and Exotic Pets*. St. Louis, MO: Elsevier; 2013:458-460.

288. Sanchez-Migallon Guzman D, Mayer J, Melidone R, et al. Pacemaker implantation in a ferret (*Mustela putorius furo*) with third-degree atrioventricular block. *Vet Clin North Am Exot Anim Pract*. 2006;9(3):677-687.

289. Heggem-Perry B, Nevarez J, Tully T. Pericardial effusion, pericardiocentesis, and thoracocentesis in a guinea pig. *Proc Annu Conf Assoc Exot Mammal Vet*. 2012.

290. Dzyban LA, Garrod LA, Besso JG. Pericardial effusion and pericardiocentesis in a guinea pig (*Cavia porcellus*). *J Am Anim Hosp Assoc*. 2001;37(1):21-26.

291. Harkness J, Murray K, Wagner J. Biology and diseases of guinea pigs. In: Fox J, Andersson L, Loew F, et al., eds. *Laboratory Animal Medicine*. 2nd ed. San Diego, CA: Academic Press; 2002:203-246.

292. Li X, Fox J. Neoplastic diseases. In: Fox J, ed. *Biology and Diseases of the Ferret*. 2nd ed. Baltimore, MD: Lippincott Williams & Wilkins; 1998:405-447.

293. Guzman RE, Ehrhart EJ, Wasson K, et al. Primary hepatic hemangiosarcoma with pulmonary metastasis in a New Zealand white rabbit. *J Vet Diagn Invest*. 2000;12(3):284-286.

294. Darby C, Ntavlourou V. Hepatic hemangiosarcoma in two ferrets (*Mustela putorius furo*). *Vet Clin North Am Exot Anim Pract*. 2006;9(3):689-694.

295. Dillberger J, Altman N. Neoplasia in ferrets: eleven cases with a review. *J Comp Pathol.* 1989;100:161-176.
296. Oglesbee BL, Oglesbee MJ. Results of postmortem examination of psittacine birds with cardiac disease: 26 cases (1991-1995). *J Am Vet Med Assoc.* 1998;212(11):1737-1742.
297. Krautwald-Junghanns MEE, Braun S, Pees M, et al. Research on the anatomy and pathology of the psittacine heart. *J Avian Med Surg.* 2004;18(1):2-11.
298. Griner LA. Birds. In: Griner LA, ed. *Pathology of Zoo Animals.* San Diego, CA: Zoological Society of San Diego; 1983:94-267.
299. Kellin N. Auswertung der sektions-und laborbefunde von 1780 vogeln der ordnung Psittaciformes in einem zeitraum von vier jahren (2000 bis 2003). Doctoral thesis. University of Giessen. 2009;252.
300. Oglesbee BL, Lehmkuhl L. Congestive heart failure associated with myxomatous degeneration of the left atrioventricular valve in a parakeet. *J Am Vet Med Assoc.* 2001;218(3):360, 376-380.
301. Pees M, Straub J, Krautwald-Junghanns ME. Insufficiency of the muscular atrioventricular valve in the heart of a blue-fronted Amazon (*Amazona aestiva aestiva*). *Vet Rec.* 2001;148(17):540-543.
302. Beehler B, Montali R, Bush M. Mitral valve insufficiency with congestive heart failure in a Pukeko. *J Am Vet Med Assoc.* 1980;177:934-937.
303. Ensley P, Hatkin J, Silverman S. Congestive heart disease in a greater hill mynah. *J Am Vet Med Assoc.* 1979;175:1010-1013.
304. Rosenthal K, Stamoulis M. Diagnosis of congestive heart failure in an Indian hill mynah bird (*Gracula religiosa*). *J Assoc Avian Vet.* 1993;7(1):27-30.
305. Mitchell EB, Hawkins MG, Orvalho JS, et al. Congenital mitral stenosis, subvalvular aortic stenosis, and congestive heart failure in a duck. *J Vet Cardiol.* 2008;10(1):67-73.
306. Evans D, Tully T, Strickland K, et al. Congenital cardiovascular anomalies, including ventricular septal defects in 2 cockatoos. *J Avian Med Surg.* 2001;15(2):101-106.
307. Bailey T, Kinne J. Ventricular septal defect in a houbara bustard (*Chlamydotis undulata macqueenii*). *Avian Dis.* 2001;45:229-233.
308. Schmidt RE, Reavill DR, Phalen DN. Cardiovascular system. In: Schmidt RE, Reavill DR, Phalen DN, eds. *Pathology of Pet and Aviary Birds.* Ames, IA: Blackwell Publishing; 2003:3-16.
309. Harari J, Miller D. Ventricular septal defect and bacterial endocarditis in a whistling swan. *Avian Pathol.* 1983;183:1296-1297.
310. Risi E, Testault I, Labrut S, et al. A case of congenital atrial communication and dilated cardiomyopathy on a griffon vulture (*Gyps fulvus*). *Proc Annu Conf Eur Assoc Avian Vet.* 2011;244-249.
311. Shrubsole-Cockwill A, Wojnarowicz C, Parker D. Atherosclerosis and ischemic cardiomyopathy in a captive, adult red-tailed hawk (*Buteo jamaicensis*). *Avian Dis.* 2008;52(3):537-539.
312. Knafo SE, Rapoport G, Williams J, et al. Cardiomyopathy and right-sided congestive heart failure in a red-tailed hawk (*Buteo jamaicensis*). *J Avian Med Surg.* 2011;25(1):32-39.
313. Julian RJ. Rapid growth problems: ascites and skeletal deformities in broilers. *Poult Sci.* 1998;77(12):1773-1780.
314. Crespo R, Shivaprasad H. Developmental, metabolic, and other noninfectious disorders. In: Saif Y, Fadly A, Glisson J, et al., eds. *Diseases of Poultry.* 12th ed. Ames, IA: Blackwell Publishing; 2008:1149-1195.
315. Pees M, Krautwald-Junghanns M-E. Cardiovascular physiology and diseases of pet birds. *Vet Clin North Am Exot Anim Pract.* 2009;12(1):81-97, vi.
316. Olkowski AA, Classen HL. Progressive bradycardia, a possible factor in the pathogenesis of ascites in fast growing broiler chickens raised at low altitude. *Br Poult Sci.* 1998;39(1):139-146.
317. Straub J, Pees M, Enders F, et al. Pericardiocentesis and the use of enalapril in a Fischer's lovebird (*Agapornis fischeri*). *Vet Rec.* 2003;152:24-26.
318. Balamurugan V, Kataria JM. The hydropericardium syndrome in poultry—a current scenario. *Vet Res Commun.* 2004;28(2):127-148.
319. Morris P, Avgeris S, Baumgartner RE. Hemochromatosis in a greater Indian hill mynah (*Gracula religiosa*). *J Assoc Avian Vet.* 1989;3(2):87-92.
320. Sedacca CD, Campbell TW, Bright JM, et al. Chronic cor pulmonale secondary to pulmonary atherosclerosis in an African grey parrot. *J Am Vet Med Assoc.* 2009;234(8):1055-1059.
321. Currie RJ. Ascites in poultry: recent investigations. *Avian Pathol.* 1999;28(4):313-326.
322. Zandvliet M, Dorrestein G, Van Der Hage M. Chronic pulmonary interstitial fibrosis in Amazon parrots. *Avian Pathol.* 2001;30(5):517-524.
323. Isaza R, Buergelt C, Kollias GV. Bacteremia and vegetative endocarditis associated with a heart murmur in a blue-and-gold macaw. *Avian Dis.* 1992;36(4):1112-1116.
324. Jessup D. Valvular endocarditis and bacteremia in a bald eagle. *Mod Vet Pract.* 1980;61:49-51.
325. Burger WP, Naudé TW, Van Rensburg IB, et al. Cardiomyopathy in ostriches (*Struthio camelus*) due to avocado (*Persea americana* var. *guatemalensis*) intoxication. *J S Afr Vet Assoc.* 1994;65(3):113-118.
326. Fulton R. Other toxins and poisons. In: Saif Y, Fadly A, Glisson J, et al., eds. *Diseases of Poultry.* 12th ed. Ames, IA: Blackwell Publishing; 2008:1231-1258.
327. Czarnecki CM. Quantitative morphological alterations during the development of furazolidone-induced cardiomyopathy in turkeys. *J Comp Pathol.* 1986;96(1):63-75.
328. Mans C, Brown CJ. Radiographic evidence of atherosclerosis of the descending aorta in a grey-cheeked parakeet (*Brotogeris pyrrhopterus*). *J Avian Med Surg.* 2007;21(1):56-62.
329. Phalen DN, Hays HB, Filippich LJ, et al. Heart failure in a macaw with atherosclerosis of the aorta and brachiocephalic arteries. *J Am Vet Med Assoc.* 1996;209(8):1435-1440.
330. Vink-Nooteboom M, Schoemaker N, Kik M, et al. Clinical diagnosis of aneurysm of the right coronary artery in a white cockatoo (*Cacatua alba*). *J Small Anim Pract.* 1998;39(11):533-537.
331. Westerhof I, Van de Wal M, Lumeij J. Electrocardiographic changes in a galah (*Eolophus roseicapilla*) with lead poisoning. *Proc Annu Conf Europ Assoc Avian Vet.* 2011;59-60.
332. Sturkie P. Heart: contraction, conduction, and electrocardiography. In: Sturkie P, ed. *Avian Physiology.* 3rd ed. New York, NY: Springer Verlag; 1976:103-121.
333. Van Zeeland Y, Schoemaker N, Lumeij J. Syncopes associated with second degree atrioventricular block in a cockatoo. *Proc Annu Conf Assoc Avian Vet.* 2010;345-346.
334. Rembert MS, Smith JA, Strickland KN, et al. Intermittent bradyarrhythmia in a Hispaniolan Amazon parrot (*Amazona ventralis*). *J Avian Med Surg.* 2008;22(1):31-40.
335. Aguilar R, Smith V, Ogburn P, et al. Arrhythmias associated with isoflurane anesthesia in bald eagles (*Haliateeus leucocephalus*). *J Zoo Wildl Med.* 1995;26(4):508-516.
336. Kushner LI. ECG of the month. Atrioventricular block in a Muscovy duck. *J Am Vet Med Assoc.* 1999;214(1):33-36.
337. Martinez L, Jeffrey J, Odom T. Electrocardiographic diagnosis of cardiomyopathies in Aves. *Poul Av Biol Rev.* 1997;8(1):9-20.
338. Odom TW, Hargis BM, Lopez CC, et al. Use of electrocardiographic analysis for investigation of ascites syndrome in broiler chickens. *Avian Dis.* 1991;35(4):738-744.
339. Cote E, Ettinger S. Electrocardiography and cardiac arrhythmias. In: Ettinger S, Feldman E, eds. *Textbook of Veterinary Internal Medicine.* 6th ed. St. Louis, MO: Elsevier Saunders; 2005:1040-1076.
340. Schnellbacher RW, Da Cunha AF, Beaufrère H, et al. Effects of dopamine and dobutamine on isoflurane-induced hypotension in Hispaniolan Amazon parrots (*Amazona ventralis*). *Am J Vet Res.* 2012;73(7):952-958.

341. Pees M, Schmidt V, Coles B, et al. Diagnosis and long-term therapy of right-sided heart failure in a yellow-crowned Amazon (*Amazona ochrocephala*). *Vet Rec*. 2006;158(13):445-447.

342. Julian R. Cardiovascular disease. In: Jordan F, Pattison M, Alexander D, et al., eds. *Poultry Diseases*. 5th ed. London, UK: W.B. Saunders; 2002:484-495.

343. Blaine K. Atypical heart disease in an umbrella cockatoo. *Proc Annu Conf Assoc Avian Vet*. 2012;285.

344. Fletcher O, Abdul-Aziz T. Cardiovascular system. In: Fletcher O, Abdul-Aziz T, eds. *Avian histopathology*. 3rd ed. Madison, WI: American Association of Avian Pathologists, Inc.; 2008:98-129.

345. Charlton B, Bermudez AJ, Boulianne M, et al. Cardiovascular diseases of chickens. In: Charlton B, Bermudez AJ, Boulianne M, et al., eds. *Avian Disease Manual*. 6th ed. Madison, WI: American Association of Avian Pathologists, Inc.; 2006:174-178.

346. Julian RJ. Production and growth related disorders and other metabolic diseases of poultry—a review. *Vet J*. 2005;169(3):350-369.

347. Czarnecki C, Good A. Electrocardiographic technic for identifying developing cardiomyopathies in young turkey poults. *Poult Sci*. 1980;59:1515-1520.

348. Ellis AE, Mead DG, Allison AB, et al. Pathology and epidemiology of natural West Nile viral infection of raptors in Georgia. *J Wildl Dis*. 2007;43(2):214-223.

349. Saito EK, Sileo L, Green DE, et al. Raptor mortality due to West Nile virus in the United States, 2002. *J Wildl Dis*. 2007;43(2):206-213.

350. Gancz A, Clubb S, Shivaprasad H. Advanced diagnostic approaches and current management of proventricular dilation disease. *Vet Clin North Am Exot Anim Pract*. 2012;13(3):471-494.

351. Pees M, Krautwald-Junghanns ME, Straub J. Evaluating and treating the cardiovascular system. In: Harrison GJ, Lightfoot TL, eds. *Clinical Avian Medicine*. Palm Beach, FL: Spix Publishing; 2006:379-394.

352. Hargis A, Stauber E, Casteel S, et al. Avocado (*Persea americana*) intoxication in caged birds. *J Am Vet Med Assoc*. 1989;194(1):64-66.

353. Bougiouklis PA, Brellou G, Georgopoulou I, et al. Rupture of the right auricle in broiler chickens. *Avian Pathol*. 2005;34(5):388-391.

354. Greiner E, Ritchie B. Parasites. In: Ritchie B, Harrison G, Harrison L, eds. *Avian Medicine: Principles and Applications*. Lake Worth, FL: Wingers Publishing; 1994:1007-1029.

355. Greenacre C, Mann K, Latimer K, et al. Adult filarioid nematodes (*Chandlerella* sp.) from the right atrium and major veins of a Ducorps' cockatoo (*Cacatua ducorpsii*). *J Assoc Avian Vet*. 1993;7(3):135-137.

356. Bartlett C. Filarioid nematodes. In: Atkinson C, Thomas N, Hunter D, eds. *Parasitic Diseases of Wild Birds*. Ames, IA: Wiley-Blackwell; 2008:439-462.

357. Latimer KS, Perry RW, Mo IP, et al. Myocardial sarcocystosis in a grand eclectus parrot (*Eclectus roratus*) and a Moluccan cockatoo (*Cacatua moluccensis*). *Avian Dis*. 1990;34(2):501-505.

358. Siller W. Ventricular septal defects in the fowl. *J Pathol Bacteriol*. 1958;76:431-440.

359. Einzig S, Jankus E, Moller J. Ventricular septal defect in turkeys. *Am J Vet Res*. 1972;33:563-566.

360. Murakami T, Uchida K, Naito H, et al. Ventricular septal defects in an ostrich (*Struthio camelus*) and a Chinese goose (*Cygnopsis cygnoid* var. *orientalis*). *Adv Anim Cardiol*. 2000;(1):33-37.

361. Olsen GH, Gee GF. Causes of Mississippi sandhill crane mortality in captivity, 1984-1995. *Proc North Am Crane Workshop*. 1997;7:249-252.

362. Gal A, Tabaran F, Taulescu M, et al. The first description of a congenital right ventricular cardiac aneurysm in a pigeon (*Columba livia domestica*, Cluj blue tumbler pigeon). *Avian Dis*. 2012;56(4):778-780.

363. Buerkle M, Wust E. Bifid sternum in an African grey (*Psittacus erithacus*) and an orange-winged Amazon parrot (*Amazona amazonica*). *Proc Annu Assoc Avian Med*. 2010;331.

364. Bennett RA, Gilson SD. Surgical management of bifid sternum in two African grey parrots. *J Am Vet Med Assoc*. 1999;214(3):372-374, 352.

365. Cullen P, Rauterberg J, Lorkowski S. The pathogenesis of atherosclerosis. In: vonEckardstein A, ed. *Atherosclerosis: Diet and Drugs*. Berlin, Germany: Springer; 2005:3-70.

366. Falk E. Pathogenesis of atherosclerosis. *J Am Coll Cardiol*. 2006;47(8, suppl C):C7-C13.

367. George SJ, Lyon C. Pathogenesis of atherosclerosis. In: George SJ, Johnson J, eds. *Atherosclerosis: Molecular and Cellular Mechanisms*. Weinheim, Germany: Wiley-Vch Gmbh & Co; 2010:3-20.

368. Libby P. Inflammation in atherosclerosis. *Nature*. 2012;420(6917):868-874.

369. Ross R, Glomset J, Harker L. Response to injury and atherogenesis. *Am J Pathol*. 1977;86(3):675-684.

370. Beaufrere H, Nevarez JG, Holder K, et al. Characterization and classification of psittacine atherosclerotic lesions by histopathology, digital image analysis, transmission and scanning electron microscopy. *Avian Pathol*. 2011;40(5):531-544.

371. Fricke C, Schmidt V, Cramer K, et al. Characterization of atherosclerosis by histochemical and immunohistochemical methods in African grey parrots (*Psittacus erithacus*) and Amazon parrots (*Amazona* spp.). *Avian Dis*. 2009;53:466-472.

372. Stary HC, Chandler AB, Glagov S, et al. A definition of initial, fatty streak, and intermediate lesions of atherosclerosis. A report from the Committee on Vascular Lesions of the Council on Arteriosclerosis, American Heart Association. *Arterioscler Thromb Vasc Biol*. 1994;14:840-856.

373. Stary HC, Chandler AB, Dinsmore RE, et al. A definition of advanced types of atherosclerosic lesions and a histological classification of atherosclerosis. A report from the Committee on Vascular Lesions of the Council on Arteriosclerosis, American Heart Association. *Circulation*. 1995;92:1355-1374.

374. Stary HC. Histologic classification of human atherosclerosis lesions. In: Fuster V, Topol E, Nabel E, eds. *Atherothrombosis and Coronary Artery Disease*. 2nd ed. Philadelphia, PA: Lippincott Williams & Wilkins; 2005:441-449.

375. Bavelaar FJ, Beynen AC. Atherosclerosis in parrots. A review. *Vet Q*. 2004;26(2):50-60.

376. Garner MM, Raymond JT. A retrospective study of atherosclerosis in birds. *Proc Annu Conf Assoc Avian Vet*. 2003;59-66.

377. St. Leger J. Avian atherosclerosis. In: Fowler ME, Miller RE, eds. *Zoo and Wild Animal Medicine Current Therapy*. 6th ed. St. Louis, MO: Saunders; 2007:200-205.

378. Reavill DR, Dorrestein GM. Pathology of aging psittacines. *Vet Clin North Am Exot Anim Pract*. 2010;13(1):135-150.

379. Beaufrere H, Ammersbach M, Reavill D, et al. Prevalence of and risk factors associated with atherosclerosis in psittacine birds. *J Am Vet Med Assoc*. 2013;242(12):1696-1704.

380. Johnson JH, Phalen DN, Kondik VH, et al. Atherosclerosis in psittacine birds. *Proc Annu Conf Assoc Avian Vet*. 1992;87-93.

381. Finlayson R, Hirchinson V. Experimental atheroma in budgerigars. *Nature*. 1961;192:369-370.

382. Shivaprasad HL. Diseases of the nervous system in pet birds: a review and report of diseases rarely documented. *Proc Annu Conf Assoc Avian Vet*. 1993;213-222.

383. Finlayson R. Spontaneous arterial disease in exotic animals. *J Zool*. 1965;147:239-343.

384. Finlayson R, Symons C. T-W-Fiennes RN. Atherosclerosis: a comparative study. *BMJ*. 1962;502:501-507.

385. Beaufrere H, Holder KA, Bauer R, et al. Intermittent claudication-like syndrome secondary to atherosclerosis in a yellow-naped Amazon parrot (*Amazona ochrocephala auropalliata*). *J Avian Med Surg*. 2011;25(4):266-276.

386. Pilny AA. Retrospective of atherosclerosis in psittacine birds: clinical and histopathologic findings in 31 cases. *Proc Annu Conf Assoc Avian Vet*. 2004;349-351.

387. Pilny AA, Quesenberry KE, Bartick-Sedrish TE, et al. Evaluation of *Chlamydophila psittaci* infection and other risk factors for atherosclerosis in pet psittacine birds. *J Am Vet Med Assoc.* 2012;240(12):1474-1480.

388. Bavelaar FJ, Beynen AC. Severity of atherosclerosis in parrots in relation to the intake of α-linolenic acid. *Avian Dis.* 2003;47(3):566-577.

389. Grunberg W. Spontaneous arteriosclerosis in birds. *Bull Soc R Zool Anvers.* 1964;43:479-488.

390. Bohorquez F, Stout C. Aortic atherosclerosis in exotic avians. *Exp Mol Pathol.* 1972;17(3):50-60.

391. Dugan JP, Feuge RR, Burgess DS. Review of evidence for a connection between *Chlamydia pneumoniae* and atherosclerotic disease. *Clin Ther.* 2002;24(5):719-735.

392. Sessa R, Nicoletti M, Di Pietro M, et al. *Chlamydia pneumoniae* and atherosclerosis: current state and future perspectives. *Int J Immunol Pharmacol.* 2009;22(1):9-14.

393. Hoymans VY, Bosmans JM, Ieven MM, et al. *Chlamydia pneumoniae*-based atherosclerosis: a smoking gun. *Acta Cardiol.* 2007;62(6):565-571.

394. Beaufrere H. Avian atherosclerosis: parrots and beyond. *J Exot Pet Med.* 2013;22:336-347.

395. Schenker OA, Hoop RK. Chlamydiae and atherosclerosis: can psittacine cases support the link? *Avian Dis.* 2007;51(1):8-13.

396. Beaufrere H, Nevarez J, Clubb S, et al. Diet-induced experimental atherosclerosis in quaker parrots (*Myiopsitta monachus*). *Vet Pathol.* 2013;50:1116-1126.

397. Beaufrere H, Cray C, Ammersbach M, et al. Plasma cholesterol differences mirror interspecies differences in atherosclerosis prevalence in Psittaciformes. *J Avian Med Surg.* 2014;28(3):225-231.

398. Bavelaar FJJ, Beynen ACC. Plasma cholesterol concentrations in African grey parrots fed diets containing psyllium. *Int J Appl Res Vet Med.* 2003;1:1-8.

399. Stanford M. Significance of cholesterol assays in the investigation of hepatic lipidosis and atherosclerosis in psittacine birds. *Exotic DVM.* 2005;7(3):28-34.

400. Petzinger C, Heatley JJ, Cornejo J, et al. Dietary modification of omega-3 fatty acids for birds with atherosclerosis. *J Am Vet Med Assoc.* 2010;236(5):523-528.

401. Beaufrère H, Nevarez J, Gaschen L, et al. Diagnosis of presumed acute ischemic stroke and associated seizure management in a Congo African grey parrot. *J Am Vet Med Assoc.* 2011;239(1):122-128.

402. Grosset C, Guzman DSM, Keating MK, et al. Central vestibular disease in a blue and gold macaw (*Ara ararauna*) with vasculopathy and cerebral infarction and hemorrhage. *Proc Annu Conf Assoc Avian Vet.* 2012;257.

403. Simone-Freilicher E. Use of isoxsuprine for treatment of clinical signs associated with presumptive atherosclerosis in a yellow-naped Amazon parrot (*Amazona ochrocephala auropalliata*). *J Avian Med Surg.* 2007;21(3):215-219.

404. Schmaier AA, Stalker TJ, Runge JJ, et al. Occlusive thrombi arise in mammals but not birds in response to arterial injury: evolutionary insight into human cardiovascular disease. *Blood.* 2011;118(13):3661-3669.

405. Priachard RW, Clarkson TB, Goodman HO. Myocardial infarcts in pigeons. *Am J Pathol.* 1963;43:651-659.

406. Clarkson TB, King JS, Lofland HB, et al. Pathologic characteristics and composition of diet-aggravated atherosclerotic plaques during regression. *Exp Mol Pathol.* 1973;19(3):267-283.

407. Ojerio AD, Pucak GJ, Clarkson TB, et al. Diet-induced atherosclerosis and myocardial infarction in Japanese quail. *Lab Anim Sci.* 1972;22(1):33-39.

408. Bennett RA. Neurology. In: Ritchie BW, Harrison GJ, Harrison LR, eds. *Avian Medicine: Principles and Applications.* Lake Worth, FL: Wingers Publishing; 1994:723-747.

409. Jenkins JR. Use of computed tomography in pet bird practice. *Proc Annu Conf Assoc Avian Vet.* 1991;276-279.

410. St. Leger, J. Acute aortic rupture in Antarctic penguins. *Proc Am Assoc Zoo Vet.* Minneapolis, MN. 2003.

411. Ferreras MC, González J, Pérez V, et al. Proximal aortic dissection (dissecting aortic aneurysm) in a mature ostrich. *Avian Dis.* 2001;45(1):251-256.

412. Baptiste KE, Pyle RL, Robertson JL, et al. Dissecting aortic aneurysm associated with a right ventricular arteriovenous shunt in a mature ostrich (*Struthio camelus*). *J Avian Med Surg.* 1997;11(3):194-200.

413. Courchesne S, Garner M. What is your diagnosis? *J Avian Med Surg.* 2009;23:69-73.

414. Vanhooser SL, Stair E, Edwards WC, et al. Aortic rupture in ostrich associated with copper deficiency. *Vet Hum Toxicol.* 1994;36(3):226-227.

415. Mitchinson MJ, Keymer IF. Aortic rupture in ostriches (*Struthio camelus*)—a comparative study. *J Comp Pathol.* 1977;87(1):27-33.

416. Gresham GA, Howard AN. Aortic rupture in the turkey. *J Atheroscler Res.* 1961;1:75-80.

417. Simpson CF, Kling JM, Palmer RF. β-Aminopropionitrile-induced dissecting aneurysms of turkeys: treatment with propranolol. *Toxicol Appl Pharmacol.* 1970;16(1):143-153.

418. Kashida Y, Seki Y, Machida N, et al. Fatal rupture of the left brachiocephalic artery in a whooper swan (*Cygnus cygnus*). *Adv Anim Cardiol.* 1999;32(1):12-15.

419. Hanley C, Wilson H, Latimer K, et al. Interclavicular hemangiosarcoma in a double yellow-headed Amazon parrot (*Amazona ochrocephala oratrix*). *J Avian Med Surg.* 2005;19(2):130-137.

420. Sherman R, Pax R. The heartbeat of the spider, *Geolycosa missouriensis. Comp Biochem Physiol.* 1968;26(2):529-534.

421. Carrel JE, Heathcote RD. Heart rate in spiders: influence of body size and foraging energetics. *Science.* 1976;193(4248):148-150.

422. Gunkel C, Lewbart G. Invertebrates. In: West G, Heard D, Caulkett N, eds. *Zoo Animal & Wildlife Immobilization and Anesthesia.* Ames, IA: Blackwell Publishing; 2007:147-158.

423. Shadwick RE, Gosline JM, Milson WK. Arterial haemodynamics in the cephalopod mollusc, *Octopus dofleini. J Exp Biol.* 1987;130(1):87-106.

424. Rees Davies R, Chitty J. Cardiovascular monitoring of an *Achatina* snail using a Doppler ultrasound unit. *Proc Br Vet Zool Soc.* London, UK; 2000;101.

425. Spicer JI. Development of cardiac function in crustaceans: patterns and processes. *Integr Comp Biol.* 2001;41(5):1068-1077.

426. Bourne GB. Blood pressure in the squid, *Loligo pealei. Comp Biochem Physiol A.* 1982;72(1):23-27.

427. Jahn TL, Crescitelli F, Taylor AB. The electrocardiogram of the grasshopper (*Melanoplus differentialis*). *J Cell Comp Physiol.* 1937;10(4):439-460.

428. Es'kov EK. Dependence of the structure of electrocardiogram on temperature in the honeybee. *Russ J Ecol.* 2005;36(3):212-215.

429. Brand AR. Heart action of the freshwater bivalve *Anodonta anatina* during activity. *J Exp Biol.* 1976;65(3):685-698.

430. Jakobs PM, Schipp R. The electrocardiogram of *Sepia officinalis* L. (Cephalopoda: Coleoida) and its modulation by neuropeptides of the FMRFamide group. *Comp Biochem Physiol C.* 1992;103(2):399-402.

431. Gribble N, Reynolds K. Use of angiography to outline the cardiovascular anatomy of the sand crab *Portunus pelagicus* Linnaeus. *J Crustacean Biol.* 1993;13(4):627-637.

432. Spotswood T, Smith SA. Cardiovascular and gastrointestinal radiographic contrast studies in the horseshoe crab (*Limulus polyphemus*). *Vet Radiol Ultrasound.* 2007;48(1):14-20.

433. Pereira YM, Pizzi R. Echocardiography of the weird and wonderful: tarantulas, turtles and tigers. *Ultrasound.* 2012;20(2):113-119.

434. King A, Henderson S, Schmidt M, et al. Using ultrasound to understand vascular and mantle contributions to venous return in the cephalopod *Sepia officinalis*. *J Exp Biol*. 2005;208:2071-2082.

435. Neiffer D. Boney fish. In: West G, Heard D, Caulkett N, eds. *Zoo Animal & Wildlife Immobilization and Anesthesia*. Ames, IA: Blackwell Publishing; 2007:159-203.

436. Stoskopf M. Clinical examination and procedures. In: Stoskopf M, ed. *Fish Medicine*. Philadelphia, PA: Saunders; 1993:62-78.

437. Sande R, Poppe T. Diagnostic ultrasound examination and echocardiography in Atlantic salmon *(Salmo salar)*. *Vet Radiol Ultrasound*. 1995;36(6):551-558.

438. Stetter M. Diagnostic imaging of amphibians. In: Wildgoose W, ed. *Amphibian Medicine and Captive Husbandry*. 2nd ed. Malabar, FL: BSAVA; 2001:103-122.

439. Murray M. Endoscopy in fish. In: Murray M, Schildger B, Taylor M, eds. *Endoscopy in Birds, Reptiles, Amphibians, and Fish*. Tuttlingen, Germany: Endo-Press; 1998:57-75.

440. Whitaker B, Wright K. Clinical techniques. In: Wright K, Whitaker B, eds. *Amphibian Medicine and Captive Husbandry*. Malabar, FL: Krieger Publishing Company; 2001:89-110.

441. Mullen RK. Electrocardiographic characteristics of four Anuran amphibia. *Comp Biochem Physiol A*. 1974;49(4):647-654.

442. Bartlett H, Escalera R, Patel S, et al. Echocardiographic assessment of cardiac morphology and function in *Xenopus*. *Comp Med*. 2010; 60(2):107-113.

443. Crossley DA, Hillman SS. Posterior lymph heart function in two species of Anurans: analysis based on both in vivo pressure-volume relationships by conductance manometry and ultrasound. *J Exp Biol*. 2010;213(Pt 21):3710-3716.

444. Kik M, Mitchell MA. A review of anatomy and physiology, diagnostic approaches, and clinical diseases. *Sem Avian Exot Pet Pract*. 2005;14(1):52-60.

445. Murray M. Cardiology. In: Mader D, ed. *Reptile Medicine and Surgery*. 2nd ed. Philadelphia, PA: Elsevier Saunders; 2006: 181-195.

446. Sedwick C. Allometrically scaling the data base for vital sign assessment used in general anesthesia of zoological species. *Proc Am Assoc Zoo Vet*. 1991;360-369.

447. Chinnadurai SK, Wrenn A, DeVoe RS. Evaluation of noninvasive oscillometric blood pressure monitoring in anesthetized boid snakes. *J Am Vet Med Assoc*. 2009;234(5):625-630.

448. Chinnadurai SK, DeVoe R, Koenig A, et al. Comparison of an implantable telemetry device and an oscillometric monitor for measurement of blood pressure in anaesthetized and unrestrained green iguanas *(Iguana iguana)*. *Vet Anaesth Analg*. 2010;37(5):434-439.

449. Wang T, Altimiras J, Klein W, et al. Ventricular haemodynamics in *Python molurus*: separation of pulmonary and systemic pressures. *J Exp Biol*. 2003;206(Pt 23):4241-4245.

450. Campbell T. Clinical pathology of reptiles. In: Mader D, ed. *Reptile Medicine and Surgery*. 2nd ed. St. Louis, MO: Saunders Elsevier; 2006:453-470.

451. Valentinuzzi ME, Hoff HE, Geddes LA. Electrocardiogram of the snake: effect of vagal stimulation on the Q-T duration. *J Electrocardiol*. 1970;3(1):21-27.

452. Valentinuzzi ME, Hoff HE, Geddes LA. Electrocardiogram of the snake: intervals and durations. *J Electrocardiol*. 1969;2(4):343-352.

453. Valentinuzzi ME, Hoff HE, Geddes LA. Observations on the electrical activity of the snake heart. *J Electrocardiol*. 1969;2(1):39-50.

454. Mullen R. Comparative electrocardiography of the Squamata. *Physiol Zool*. 1967;40(2):114-126.

455. Heaton-Jones T, King R. Characterization of the electrocardiogram of the American alligator *(Alligator mississippiensis)*. *J Zoo Wildl Med*. 1994;25(1):40-47.

456. Rubel A, Kuoni W. Radiology and imaging. In: Frye F, ed. *Reptile Care. An Atlas of Diseases and Treatments*. Vol 1. Neptune City: TFH Publications, Inc.; 1991:185-208.

457. Silverman S. Diagnostic imaging. In: Mader D, ed. *Reptile Medicine and Surgery*. 2nd ed. St. Louis, MO: Saunders Elsevier; 2006: 471-489.

458. Chetboul V, Schilliger L, Tessier D. Specific features of echocardiographic examination in ophidians. *Schweiz Arch Tierheilkd*. 2004;146:327-334.

459. Isaza R, Ackerman N, Jacbson E. Ultrasound imaging of the coelomic structures in the boa constrictor *(Boa constrictor)*. *Vet Radiol Ultrasound*. 1993;34:445-450.

460. Schilliger L, Tessier D, Pouchelon JJ, et al. Proposed standardization of the two-dimensional echocardiographic examination in snakes. *J Herpetol Med Surg*. 2006;16(3):90-102.

461. Schildger B, Tenhu H, Kramer M. Ultraschalluntersuchung bei reptilien. *Berl Munch Tierarztl Wochenschr*. 1996;109:136-141.

462. Stetter M. Ultrasonography. In: Mader D, ed. *Reptile Medicine and Surgery*. 2nd ed. St. Louis, MO: Saunders Elsevier; 2006:665-674.

463. Snyder PS, Shaw NG, Heard DJ. Two-dimensional echocardiographic anatomy of the snake heart *(Python molurus bivittatus)*. *Vet Radiol Ultrasound*. 1999;40(1):66-72.

464. Hernandez-Divers S, Hernandez-Divers S, Wilson H. A review of reptile diagnostic coelioscopy. *J Herp Med Surg*. 2005;15(3):16-31.

465. Fox J. Normal clinical and biologic parameters. In: Fox J, ed. *Biology and Diseases of the Ferret*. 2nd ed. Baltimore, MD: Lippincott Williams & Wilkins; 1998:183-210.

466. Carpenter J, Marion C. *Exotic Animal Formulary*. 4th ed. St. Louis, MO: Saunders; 2012:744.

467. Wilson J, Gaertner D, Marx J, et al. Normative values. In: Suckow M, Stevens K, Wilson R, eds. *The Laboratory Rabbit, Guinea Pig, Hamster, and Other Rodents*. Oxford, UK: Academic Press; 2012: 1231-1245.

468. da Cunha A, Saile K, Beaufrère H, et al. Measuring level of agreement between values obtained by directly measured blood pressure and ultrasonic Doppler flow detector in cats. *J Vet Emerg Crit Care (San Antonio)*. 2014;24(3):272-278.

469. Schoemaker N, Bosman I. Intra-arterial blood pressure in ferrets compared to peripheral blood pressure. *Proc Annu Conf Assoc Exot Mammal Vet*. Milwaukee, WI; 2009;59-60.

470. Olin JM, Smith TJ, Talcott MR. Evaluation of noninvasive monitoring techniques in domestic ferrets *(Mustela putorius furo)*. *Am J Vet Res*. 1997;58(10):1065-1069.

471. Nelson M, Mayer J. A comparison of direct and indirect blood pressure monitoring techniques in rabbits. *Proc Annu Conf Assoc Exot Mammal Vet*. Milwaukee, WI; 2009;61.

472. O'Brien PJ. Cardiac troponin is the most effective translational safety biomarker for myocardial injury in cardiotoxicity. *Toxicology*. 2008;245(3):206-218.

473. O'Brien P, Dameron G, Beck M, et al. Cardiac troponin T is a sensitive, specific biomarker of cardiac injury in laboratory animals. *Comp Med*. 1997;47(5):486-495.

474. Bublot I, Wayne Randolph R, Chalvet-Monfray K, et al. The surface electrocardiogram in domestic ferrets. *J Vet Cardiol*. 2006;8(2):87-93.

475. Schnellbacher R, Olson E, Mayer J. Emergency presentations associated with cardiovascular disease in exotic herbivores. *J Exot Pet Med*. 2012;21:316-327.

476. Bone L, Battles AH, Goldfarb RD, et al. Electrocardiographic values from clinically normal, anesthetized ferrets *(Mustela putorius furo)*. *Am J Vet Res*. 1988;49(11):1884-1887.

477. Lord B, Boswood A, Petrie A. Electrocardiography of the normal domestic pet rabbit. *Vet Rec*. 2010;167(25):961-965.

478. Sisk D. Physiology. In: Wagner J, Manning P, eds. *The Biology of the Guinea Pig*. San Diego, CA: Academic Press; 1976:63-92.

479. Stepien RL, Benson KG, Forrest LJ. Radiographic measurement of cardiac size in normal ferrets. *Vet Radiol Ultrasound*. 1999;40(6): 606-610.

480. Onuma M, Kondo H, Ono S, et al. Radiographic measurement of cardiac size in 64 ferrets. *J Vet Med Sci*. 2009;71(3):355-358.

481. Onuma M, Ono S, Ishida T, et al. Radiographic measurement of cardiac size in 27 rabbits. *J Vet Med Sci*. 2010;72(4):529-531.

482. Pariaut R. Cardiovascular physiology and diseases of the rabbit. *Vet Clin North Am Exot Anim Pract*. 2009;12(1):135-144, vii.

483. Thomas WP, Gaber CE, Jacobs GJ, et al. Recommendations for standards in transthoracic two-dimensional echocardiography in the dog and cat. Echocardiography Committee of the Specialty of Cardiology, American College of Veterinary Internal Medicine. *J Vet Intern Med*. 1993;7(4):247-252.

484. Bélanger MC. Echocardiography. In: Ettinger SJ, Feldman EC, eds. *Textbook of Veterinary Internal Medicine*. St. Louis, MO: Elsevier Saunders; 2005:311-326.

485. Boon J. Evaluation of size, function, and hemodynamics. In: Boon J, ed. *Veterinary Echocardiography*. 2nd ed. Oxford, UK: Wiley-Blackwell; 2011:153-266.

486. Poulsen Nautrup C. Thorax: echocardiography. In: Krautwald-Junghanns M-E, Pees M, Reese S, et al., eds. *Diagnostic Imaging of Exotic Pets*. Hannover, Germany: Schlutersche Verlagsgesellschaft mbH & Co.; 2011:188-223.

487. Stepien RL, Benson KG, Wenholz LJ. M-mode and Doppler echocardiographic findings in normal ferrets sedated with ketamine hydrochloride and midazolam. *Vet Radiol Ultrasound*. 2000;41(5):452-456.

488. Fontes-Sousa APN, Brás-Silva C, Moura C, et al. M-mode and Doppler echocardiographic reference values for male New Zealand white rabbits. *Am J Vet Res*. 2006;67(10):1725-1729.

489. Cetin N, Cetin E, Toker M. Echocardiographic variables in healthy guinea pigs anaesthetized with ketamine-xylazine. *Lab Anim*. 2005;39(1):100-106.

490. Watson LE, Sheth M, Denyer RF, et al. Baseline echocardiographic values for adult male rats. *J Am Soc Echocardiog*. 2004;17(2):161-167.

491. Stypmann J, Engelen MA, Troatz C, et al. Echocardiographic assessment of global left ventricular function in mice. *Lab Anim*. 2009;43(2):127-137.

492. Rottman JN, Ni G, Brown M. Echocardiographic evaluation of ventricular function in mice. *Echocardiography*. 2007;24(1):83-89.

493. Salemi VMC, Bilate AMB, Ramires FJA, et al. Reference values from M-mode and Doppler echocardiography for normal Syrian hamsters. *Eur J Echocardiog*. 2005;6(1):41-46.

494. Vastenburg MHAC, Boroffka SAEB, Schoemaker NJ. Echocardiographic measurements in clinically healthy ferrets anesthetized with isoflurane. *Vet Radiol Ultrasound*. 2004;45(3):228-232.

495. Pelosi A, St John L, Gaymer J, et al. Cardiac tissue Doppler and tissue velocity imaging in anesthetized New Zealand white rabbits. *J Am Assoc Lab Anim Sci*. 2011;50(3):317-321.

496. Plehn JF, Foster E, Grice WN, et al. Echocardiographic assessment of LV mass in rabbits: models of pressure and volume overload hypertrophy. *Am J Physiol Heart Circ Physiol*. 1993;265(6):H2066-H2072.

497. Stypmann J, Engelen MA, Breithardt A-K, et al. Doppler echocardiography and tissue Doppler imaging in the healthy rabbit: differences of cardiac function during awake and anaesthetised examination. *Int J Cardiol*. 2007;115(2):164-170.

498. Tello de Meneses R, Mesa MD, Gonzalez V. Echocardiographic assessment of cardiac function in the rabbit: a preliminary study. *Ann Rech Vet*. 1989;20(2):175-185.

499. Bartusevich EV, Roshchevskaia IM. [The echocardiographic study of the rabbit heart left ventricle morpho-functional parameters]. *Ross Fiziol Zh Im I M Sechenova*. 2005;91(7):752-757.

500. Fontes-Sousa AP, Moura C, Carneiro CS, et al. Echocardiographic evaluation including tissue Doppler imaging in New Zealand white rabbits sedated with ketamine and midazolam. *Vet J*. 2009;181(3):326-331.

501. Liu J, Rigel DF. Echocardiographic examination in rats and mice. *Methods Mol Biol*. 2009;573:139-155.

502. Gardin JM, Siri FM, Kitsis RN, et al. Echocardiographic assessment of left ventricular mass and systolic function in mice. *Circ Res*. 1995;76(5):907-914.

503. Stypmann J. Doppler ultrasound in mice. *Echocardiography*. 2007;24(1):97-112.

504. Syed F, Diwan A, Hahn HS. Murine echocardiography: a practical approach for phenotyping genetically manipulated and surgically modeled mice. *J Am Soc Echocardiog*. 2005;18(9):982-990.

505. Scherrer-Crosbie M. Role of echocardiography in studies of murine models of cardiac diseases. *Arch Mal Coeur Vaiss*. 2006;99(3):237-241.

506. Ryoke T, Gu Y, Mao L, et al. Progressive cardiac dysfunction and fibrosis in the cardiomyopathic hamster and effects of growth hormone and angiotensin-converting enzyme inhibition. *Circulation*. 1999;100(16):1734-1743.

507. Rosenthal K, Miller M. Cardiac disease. In: Altman R, Clubb S, Dorrestein G, et al., eds. *Avian Medicine and Surgery*. Philadelphia, PA: W.B. Saunders Company; 1997:491-500.

508. Acierno MJ, Da Cunha A, Smith J, et al. Agreement between direct and indirect blood pressure measurements obtained from anesthetized Hispaniolan Amazon parrots. *J Am Vet Med Assoc*. 2008;233(10):1587-1590.

509. Touzot-Jourde G, Hernandez-Divers SJ, Trim CM. Cardiopulmonary effects of controlled versus spontaneous ventilation in pigeons anesthetized for coelioscopy. *J Am Vet Med Assoc*. 2005;227(9):1424-1428.

510. Hawkins MG, Wright BD, Pascoe PJ, et al. Pharmacokinetics and anesthetic and cardiopulmonary effects of propofol in red-tailed hawks (*Buteo jamaicensis*) and great horned owls (*Bubo virginianus*). *Am J Vet Res*. 2003;64(6):677-683.

511. Zehnder AM, Hawkins MG, Pascoe PJ, et al. Evaluation of indirect blood pressure monitoring in awake and anesthetized red-tailed hawks (*Buteo jamaicensis*): effects of cuff size, cuff placement, and monitoring equipment. *Vet Anaesth Analg*. 2009;36(5):464-479.

512. Joyner PH, Jones MP, Ward D, et al. Induction and recovery characteristics and cardiopulmonary effects of sevoflurane and isoflurane in bald eagles. *Am J Vet Res*. 2008;69(1):13-22.

513. Koch J, Buss EG, Lobaugh B, et al. Blood pressure of chickens selected for leanness or obesity. *Poult Sci*. 1983;62(5):904-907.

514. Speckmann EW, Ringer RK. The cardiac output and carotic and tibial blood pressure of the turkey. *Can J Biochem Physiol*. 1963;41(11):2337-2341.

515. Langille BL, Jones DR. Central cardiovascular dynamics of ducks. *Am J Physiol*. 1975;228(6):1856-1861.

516. Johnston MS, Davidowski LA, Rao S, et al. Precision of repeated, Doppler-derived indirect blood pressure measurements in conscious psittacine birds. *J Avian Med Surg*. 2011;25(2):83-90.

517. Lichtenberger M, Ko J. Critical care monitoring. *Vet Clin North Am Exot Anim Pract*. 2007;10(2):317-344.

518. Echols MS, Craig TM, Speer BL. Heartworm (*Paronchocerca ciconarum*) infection in 2 saddle-billed storks (*Ephippiorhynchus senegalensis*). *J Avian Med Surg*. 2000;14(1):42-47.

519. Oglesbee BL, Avian A, Hamlindvm RL, et al. Electrocardiographic reference values for macaws (*Ara* species) and cockatoos (*Cacatua* species). *J Avian Med Surg*. 2001;15(1):17-22.

520. Nap AM, Lumeij JT, Stokhof AA. Electrocardiogram of the African grey (*Psittacus erithacus*) and Amazon (*Amazona* spp.) parrot. *Avian Pathol*. 1992;21(1):45-53.

521. Lumeij JT, Stokhof AA. Electrocardiogram of the racing pigeon (*Columba livia domestica*). *Res Vet Sci*. 1985;38(3):275-278.

522. Burtnick N, Degernes L. Electrocardiography on fifty-nine anesthetized convalescing raptors. In: Redig P, Cooper J, Remple J, et al., eds. *Raptor Biomedicine*. Minneapolis, MN: University of Minnesota Press; 1993:111-121.

523. Cinar A, Bagci C, Belge F, et al. The electrocardiogram of the Pekin duck. *Avian Dis*. 1996;40(4):919-923.

524. Straub J, Pees M, Krautwald-Junghanns ME. Measurement of the cardiac silhouette in psittacines. *J Am Vet Med Assoc*. 2002;221(1):76-79.

525. Barbon AR, Smith S, Forbes N. Radiographic evaluation of cardiac size in four Falconiform species. *J Avian Med Surg*. 2010;24(3):222-226.

526. Lumeij JT, Shaik MAS, Ali M. Radiographic reference limits for cardiac width in peregrine falcons *(Falco peregrinus)*. *J Am Vet Med Assoc*. 2011;238(11):1459-1463.

527. Hanley C, Murray H, Torrey S, et al. Establishing cardiac measurement standards in three avian species. *J Avian Med Surg*. 1997;11(1):15-19.

528. Krautwald-Junghanns M-E, Pees M, Schroff S. Cardiovascular system. In: Krautwald-Junghanns M-E, Pees M, Reese S, et al., eds. *Diagnostic Imaging of Exotic Pets*. Hannover, Germany: Schlutersche Verlagsgesellschaft mbH & Co.; 2011:84-91.

529. Beaufrere H, Pariaut R, Rodriguez D. Avian vascular imaging: a review. *J Avian Med Surg*. 2010;24(3):174-184.

530. Pees M, Straub J, Krautwald-Junghanns M-E. Echocardiographic examinations of 60 African grey parrots and 30 other psittacine birds. *Vet Rec*. 2004;155(3):73-76.

531. Pees M, Krautwald-Junghanns M. Avian echocardiography. *Sem Avian Exot Pet Pract*. 2005;14(1):14-21.

532. Krautwald-Junghanns M-E, Schulz M, Hagner D, et al. Transcoelomic two-dimensional echocardiography in the avian patient. *J Avian Med Surg*. 1995;9:19-31.

533. Beaufrere H, Pariaut R, Rodriguez D, et al. Comparison of transcoelomic, contrast, and transesophageal echocardiography in anesthetized red-tailed hawk *(Buteo jamaicensis)*. *Am J Vet Res*. 2012;73(10):1560-1568.

534. Straub J, Forbes NA, Pees M, et al. Pulsed-wave Doppler-derived velocity of diastolic ventricular inflow and systolic aortic outflow in raptors. *Vet Rec*. 2004;154(5):145-147.

535. Straub J. Effect of handling-induced stress on the results of spectral Doppler echocardiography in falcons. *Res Vet Sci*. 2003;74(2):119-122.

536. Boskovic M, Krautwald-Junghanns M, Failing K, et al. Moglichkeiten und grenzen echokardiographischer untersuchungen bei tag-und nachgreivogeln (Accipitriformes, Falconiformes, Strigiformes). *Tierarztl Prax*. 1995;27:334-341.

537. Martinez-Lemus LA, Miller MW, Jeffrey JS, et al. Echocardiography evaluation of cardiac structure and function in broiler and leghorn chickens. *Poult Sci*. 1998;77(7):1045-1050.

538. Beaufrere H, Pariaut R, Nevarez JG, et al. Feasibility of transesophageal echocardiography in birds without cardiac disease. *J Am Vet Med Assoc*. 2010;236(5):540-547.

539. Krautwald-Junghanns M-E, Schloemer J, Pees M. Iodine-based contrast media in avian medicine. *J Exot Pet Med*. 2008;17(3):189.

540. Beaufrère H, Rodriguez D, Pariaut R, et al. Estimation of intrathoracic arterial diameter by means of computed tomographic angiography in Hispaniolan Amazon parrots. *Am J Vet Res*. 2011;72(2):210-218.

541. Romagnano A, Shiroma JT, Heard DJ, et al. Magnetic resonance imaging of the brain and coelomic cavity of the domestic pigeon. *Vet Radiol Ultrasound*. 1996;37(6):431-440.

542. Taylor M. Endoscopic examination and biopsy techniques. In: Ritchie B, Harrison GJ, Harrison LR, eds. *Avian Medicine: Principles and Applications*. Lake Worth, FL: Wingers Publishing; 1994:327-354.

543. Schroeder N. Diuretics. In: Ettinger S, Feldman E, eds. *Textbook of Veterinary Internal Medicine*. 7th ed. St. Louis, MO: Saunders Elsevier; 2010:1212-1214.

544. Bulmer B. Angiotensin converting enzyme inhibitors and vasodilators. In: Ettinger S, Feldman E, eds. *Textbook of Veterinary Internal Medicine*. 7th ed. St. Louis, MO: Saunders Elsevier; 2010:1216-1223.

545. Fuentes V. Inotropes: inodilators. In: Ettinger S, Feldman E, eds. *Textbook of Veterinary Internal Medicine*. 7th ed. St. Louis, MO: Saunders Elsevier; 2010:1202-1207.

546. Summerfield NJ, Boswood A, O'Grady MR, et al. Efficacy of pimobendan in the prevention of congestive heart failure or sudden death in Doberman Pinschers with preclinical dilated cardiomyopathy (The PROTECT Study). *J Vet Intern Med*. 2012;26(6):1337-1349.

547. Gordon S. Beta blocking agents. In: Ettinger S, Feldman E, eds. *Textbook of Veterinary Internal Medicine*. 7th ed. St. Louis, MO: Saunders Elsevier; 2010:1207-1212.

548. Keene B, Atkins C, Bonagura J, et al. Guidelines for the diagnosis and treatment of canine chronic valvular heart disease. In: Ettinger S, Feldman E, eds. *Textbook of Veterinary Internal Medicine*. 7th ed. St. Louis, MO: Saunders Elsevier; 2010:1196-1202.

549. Sinclair B, Chown S. Haemolymph osmolality and thermal hysteresis activity in 17 species of arthropods from sub-Antarctic Marion Island. *Polar Biol*. 2002;25(12):928-933.

550. Schartau W, Leidescher T. Composition of the hemolymph of the tarantula, *Eurypelma californicum*. *J Comp Physiol [B]*. 1983;152(1):73-77.

551. Zachariah T, Mitchell M. Invertebrates. In: Mitchell M, Tully T, eds. *Manual of Exotic Pet Practice*. St. Louis, MO: Elsevier; 2009:11-38.

552. Visigalli D. Guide to hemolymph transfusion in giant spiders. *Exotic DVM*. 2004;5:42-43.

553. Nishimura H. Renal responses to diuretic drugs in freshwater catfish, *Ictalurus punctatus*. *Am J Physiol*. 1977;232(3):F278-F285.

554. Cipolle MD, Zehr JE. Renin release in turtles: effects of volume depletion and furosemide administration. *Am J Physiol Regul Integr Comp Physiol*. 1985;249(1):R100-R105.

555. Uva B, Vallarino M. Renin-angiotensin system and osmoregulation in the terrestrial chelonian *Testudo hermanni* Gmelin. *Comp Biochem Physiol A*. 1982;71(3):449-451.

556. Stephens GA, Robertson FM. Renal responses to diuretics in the turtle. *J Comp Physiol [B]*. 1985;155(3):387-393.

557. LeBrie SJ, Boelskevy BD. The effect of furosemide on renal function and renin in water snakes. *Comp Biochem Physiol C*. 1979;63(2):223-228.

558. Pace L, Mader D. Atropine and glycopyrrolate, route of administration and response in the green iguana *(Iguana iguana)*. *Proc Assoc Rept Amph Vet*. 2002;79.

559. Martin M, Darke P, Else R. Congestive heart failure with atrial fibrillation in a rabbit. *Vet Rec*. 1987;121:570-571.

560. Van Meel JC, Mauz AB, Wienen W, et al. Pimobendan increases survival of cardiomyopathic hamsters. *J Cardiovasc Pharmacol*. 1989;13(3):508-509.

561. Hermans K, Geerts T, Cauwerts K, et al. Tolerability of pimobendan in the ferret *(Mustela putorius furo)*. *Vlaam Diergen Tijdschr*. 2008;78:53-56.

562. Sweet C, Emmert S, Inez I, et al. Increased survival in rats with congestive heart failure treated with enalapril. *J Cardiovasc Pharmacol*. 1987;10(6):636-642.

563. Bradbury C, Saunders AB, Heatley JJ, et al. Transvenous heartworm extraction in a ferret with caval syndrome. *J Am Anim Hosp Assoc*. 2010;46(1):31-35.

564. He Z, Li Y, Zhang T, et al. Effects of 2-hydroxypropyl-β-cyclodextrin on pharmacokinetics of digoxin in rabbits and humans. *Pharmacie*. 2004;59(3):200-202.

565. Harrison LI, Gibaldi M. Pharmacokinetics of digoxin in the rat. *Drug Metab Dispos*. 1976;4(1):88-93.

566. Nishihara K, Hibino J, Kotaki H, et al. Effect of itraconazole on the pharmacokinetics of digoxin in guinea pigs. *Biopharm Drug Dispos*. 1999;20(3):145-149.

567. Wójcicki M, Drozdzik M, Sulikowski T, et al. Pharmacokinetics of intragastrically administered digoxin in rabbits with experimental bile duct obstruction. *J Pharm Pharmacol*. 1997;49(11):1082-1085.

568. Van Meel JC, Diederen W. Hemodynamic profile of the cardiotonic agent pimobendan. *J Cardiovasc Pharmacol*. 1989;14(suppl 2): S1-S6.

569. Du C-K, Morimoto S, Nishii K, et al. Knock-in mouse model of dilated cardiomyopathy caused by troponin mutation. *Circ Res*. 2007;101(2):185-194.

570. Haskins S. Monitoring anesthetized patients. In: Tranquilli W, Thurmon J, Grimm K, eds. *Lumb & Jones' Veterinary Anesthesia and Analgesia*. 4th ed. Ames, IA: Blackwell Publishing; 2007:533-558.

571. Pahor M, Bernabei R, Sgadari A, et al. Enalapril prevents cardiac fibrosis and arrhythmias in hypertensive rats. *Hypertension*. 1991;18(2):148-157.

572. Webb RL, Miller D, Traina V, et al. Benazepril. *Cardiovasc Drug Rev*. 1990;8(2):89-104.

573. Blair LS, Williams E, Ewanciw DV. Efficacy of ivermectin against third-stage *Dirofilaria immitis* larvae in ferrets and dogs. *Res Vet Sci*. 1982;33(3):386-387.

574. Blair LS, Campbell WC. Trial of avermectin B1a, mebendazole and melarsoprol against pre-cardiac *Dirofilaria immitis* in the ferret *(Mustela putorius furo)*. *J Parasitol*. 1978;64(6):1032-1034.

575. Blair LS, Campbell WC. Suppression of maturation of *Dirofilaria immitis* in *Mustela putorius furo* by single dose of ivermectin. *J Parasitol*. 1980;66(4):691-692.

576. Fisher M, Beck W, Hutchinson M. Efficacy and safety of selamectin (Stronghold/Revolution) used off-label in exotic pets. *Int J Appl Res Vet Med*. 2007;5(3):87-96.

577. Cottrell D. Use of moxidectin as a heartworm adulticide in four ferrets. *Exotic DVM*. 2004;6:9-12.

578. Schaper R, Heine J, Arther R, et al. Imidacloprid plus moxidectin to prevent heartworm infection *(Dirofilaria immitis)* in ferrets. *Parasitol Res*. 2007;101(1):6.

579. Tidholm A, Svensson H, Sylvén C. Survival and prognostic factors in 189 dogs with dilated cardiomyopathy. *J Am An Hosp Assoc*. 1997;33(4):364-368.

580. Borgarelli M, Crosara S, Lamb K, et al. Survival characteristics and prognostic variables of dogs with preclinical chronic degenerative mitral valve disease attributable to myxomatous degeneration. *J Vet Intern Med*. 2012;26(1):69-75.

581. Martin MWS, Stafford Johnson MJ, et al. Canine dilated cardiomyopathy: a retrospective study of signalment, presentation and clinical findings in 369 cases. *J Small Anim Pract*. 2009;50(1): 23-29.

582. Beaufrere H, Aertsens A, Fouquet J. Un cas d'insuffisance cardiaque congestive chez un perroquet gris. *L'Hebdo Veterinaire*. 2007;200: 8-10.

583. Esfandiary A, Rajaian H, Asasi K, et al. Diuretic effects of several chemical and herbal compounds in adult laying hens. *Int J Poult Sci*. 2010;9(3):247-253.

584. Hamlin R, Stalnaker P. Basis for use of digoxin in small birds. *J Vet Pharmacol Ther*. 1987;10(4):354-356.

585. Wilson R, Zenoble R, Horton C, et al. Single dose digoxin pharmacokinetics in the quaker conure *(Myiopsitta monachus)*. *J Zoo Wildl Med*. 1989;20(4):432-434.

586. Guzman D, Beaufrere H, Kukanich B, et al. Pharmacokinetics of a single oral dose of pimobendan in Hispaniolan Amazon parrot *(Amazona ventralis)*. *J Avian Med Surg*. 2014;28:95-101.

587. Pees M, Kuhring K, Demiraij F, et al. Bioavailability and compatibility of enalapril in birds. *Proc Annu Assoc Avian Med*. 2006;7-11.

588. Da Cunha A, Stout R, Tully T, et al. Pharmacokinetics/pharmacodynamics of bupivacaine and lidocaine in chickens. *Proc Annu Conf Assoc Avian Vet*. 2011;313.

589. Hawkins M, Barron H, Speer B, et al. Birds. In: Carpenter J, Marion C, eds. *Exotic Animal Formulary*. 4th ed. St. Louis, MO: Elsevier; 2013:184-438.

590. Goldstein D, Skadhauge E. Renal and extrarenal regulation of body fluid composition. In: Whittow G, ed. *Sturkie's Avian Physiology*. 5th ed. San Diego, CA: Academic Press; 2000:265-297.

591. Paoletti R, Bolego C, Cignerella A. Lipid and non-lipid effects of statins. In: von Eckarstein A, ed. *Atherosclerosis: Diet and Drugs*. Berlin, Germany: Springer Verlag; 2005:365-388.

592. White C. A review of the pharmacologic and pharmacokinetic aspects of rosuvastatin. *J Clin Pharmacol*. 2002;42(9): 963-970.

593. Hirsch AT, Haskal ZJ, Hertzer NR, et al. ACC/AHA 2005 guidelines for the management of patients with peripheral arterial disease (lower extremity, renal, mesenteric, and abdominal aortic): executive summary a collaborative report from the American Association for Vascular Surgery/Society for Vas. *J Am Coll Cardiol*. 2006; 47(6):1239-1312.

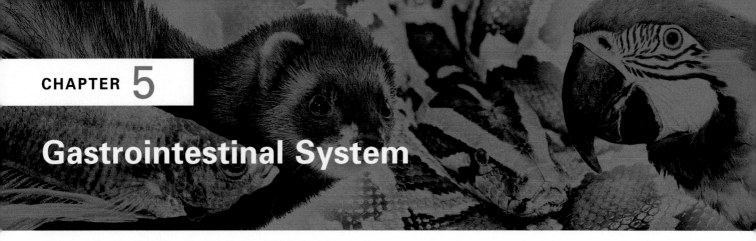

CHAPTER 5

Gastrointestinal System

Kenneth R. Welle, DVM, DABVP (Avian)

INTRODUCTION

The digestive or gastrointestinal (GI) system is one of the primary interfaces an organism has with the environment. The GI tract provides a means for collection of energy, fluids, and other nutrients, while eliminating unnecessary or harmful components. Due to the adaptations for absorbing these nutrients, this body system can also be an entryway for pathogens, toxins, and other diseases. Gastrointestinal disorders are common occurrences in veterinary practice for this reason. A strong knowledge of anatomy, physiology, and diseases of the GI tract is critical to clinical veterinary medicine.

ANATOMY AND PHYSIOLOGY

The digestive system functions in the collection and digestion of food items from the environment. In all but the most primitive of invertebrates, the GI tract is a modified tube. The modifications are dependent on the methods used by the animal to prehend and digest food. To assist in digestion, there are glandular structures both within the digestive tract (gastric and intestinal glands) or connected to it via ducts (e.g., liver, pancreas). A result of the close interface with the environment, the immune system has numerous connections into the GI tract, such as tonsils, Peyer's patches, and GI-associated lymphatic tissue (GALT). There are both commonalities and tremendous variation in the anatomic layout of the GI system. The wide variety of diets that animals eat and the habitats from which they obtain food has led to a number of adaptations in the GI system to allow for efficient extration of nutrients.

Invertebrates

Invertebrates are an incredibly diverse group of animals. Many aquatic invertebrates are commonly sold through the pet trade. These range from simple corals to complex arthropods their digestive anatomy varies greatly among the groups. The most primative of invertebrates simply absorb nutrients from the aquatic medium in which they live. Others will have a mouth but not a "one way" digestive tract. The more complex species have a tubular system similar to vertebrates with an enormous variety of modifications.

Fish

The piscine class is extremely large, consisting of an estimated 25,000 species. As such, there is tremendous variation in the anatomy and physiology of the GI tract.[1] The mouth has four basic positions in fish: inferior, subterminal, terminal, and superior, depending on their feeding biology.[1] Barbels may be present in some species, and serve a sensory function. The presence and location of teeth are also variable.[1] As water passes through the pharynx, food items are trapped by the gill rakers and swallowed. There is little or no processing of food in the mouth area. In most fishes, the mouth is devoid of distinct consolidated salivary glands, although considerable mucus is produced by the buccal glands.[2]

The esophagus is usually short, extremely distensible, has multiple folds, and in general, very muscular. In some fish species, the esophagus is lined with caudally directed papillae to help facilitate the passage of food.

The swim bladder originates as an outpouching of the esophagus. In physostomous species, the connection to the esophagus is retained via the pneumatic duct.[1,2] In other fish, the connection is functionally closed by a sphincter muscle at the pneumatic duct. Physoclistic species have no connection between the esophagus and the swim bladder in adulthood. While the swim bladder primarily functions for buoyancy, in various species of fish it may be involved with gas exchange, sound and pressure detection, or even sound production.[1]

Stomach anatomy in fish is highly variable, from being barely distinguishable from the esophagus to highly muscular. Some surgeonfish have a thick-walled gizzard-like stomach.[1] Some fishes, approximately 10% to 15% of species including the goldfish and carp, do not have a defined stomach. In fish that do have a stomach, it can be straight, U shaped, or J shaped or have gastric diverticula that pouch off of U-shaped stomachs.[1,2] In several species, a widely variable number of blind pouches, called pyloric cecae, project from the pyloric region of the stomach. These appear to function in food absorption.[1]

The intestines of fish also vary significantly between orders and species. As in other vertebrates, the carnivorous species have shorter GI tracts (as little as 20% of body length) while herbivorous species have longer tracts (up to 2000% of body length).[1] The intestines may be a straight tube or loop into numerous coils. In most cases there is no distinction between the large and small intestines, although elasmobranchs do have enlarged spiral colons. The intestines may exit through an anus or into a cloaca that shares an exit with the urinary and reproductive tracts.[1]

The pancreas of fish may be separate (e.g., sharks, lung fishes, some catfishes), diffuse, or part of the liver creating a hepatopancreas.[1,2] The pancreas has both endocrine and

221

exocrine functions. The liver usually does not have one distinct color between species and is large with an accompanying gallbladder.[1] The liver can be very pigmented due to the presence of melanomacrophage centers and are occasionally considered to be an indication of inflammation. Conversely, some fish livers are very pale, almost white, especially in captive-raised fish.[2]

Amphibians

All adult amphibians are carnivorous or insectivorous and have a relatively short and simple GI tract. The oral cavity of adult amphibians is large and wide with poorly developed lips.[3] Some mastication occurs in the oral cavity, but prey are usually swallowed whole. Amphibia have pediceled teeth, with the crown attached to the pedicel (base) that attaches to the jaw. The teeth are shed and replaced throughout life. However bufid toads lack teeth while ranid frogs lack mandibular teeth.[4] The tongues of most amphibians (caecilians with fixed tongues and pipid frogs with no tongues are the exceptions) extend well beyond (up to 80%) the mouth for prehension of food.[3,4] Retraction of the eyes is required for swallowing.[4] Larval Anurans (tadpoles) generally feed by filtering particles from the water, using the branchial sieve, mucus-covered filter plates in the pharynx, located just cranial to the gills.[3] Tadpoles also feed on larger material in their environment by using a keratin beak on the margin of the mouth.

In larval Anurans, food is transported through the esophagus by cilia rather than peristaltic movement.[3] The stomach is a small dilation at the end of the esophagus and produces no enzymes, functioning primarily as a food storage site.[3] The stomach in larval urodeles is similar to that found in adults.

In adult amphibians, there is a strong sphincter between the oral cavity and the esophagus and between the esophagus and stomach.[5] There is also a pyloric sphincter. Some Anurans can evert their stomach and use their forelimbs to wipe ingesta from the mucosal surface, an adaptation allowing removal of toxic substances or indigestible material. Some frogs brood their tadpoles in their stomach.[4] The rest of the GI tract is relatively short and follows typical vertebrate anatomic structure. The delineation between intestinal sections of amphibian species are not obvious although the GI tract does terminate at the cloaca.

The liver and gallbladder have a close association and the pancreas is present in amphibian species. The liver does not have a significant influence in processing nitrogen for excretion in aquatic amphibians, as ammonia is freely defused into the surrounding environment through the skin and via excretion by the kidneys. In terrestrial amphibians, the liver converts ammonia to the less toxic, water-soluble nitrogenous compound urea. In a few terrestrial species, urea is converted to uric acid to conserve water. The amphibian liver serves as an important erythropoietic center, in addition to synthesis and metabolism of nitrogenous compounds, proteins, glucose, lipids, and iron.

Reptiles

There are four main groups of reptiles: the Chelonia (e.g., turtles, tortoises, terrapins), crocodilians, squamates (e.g., lizards, snakes), and tuataras. There is tremendous variation in anatomy and physiology among the reptiles, so it is more difficult to make generalizations for this group. Figures 5-1, 5-2, and 5-3 show the general GI anatomic layout of snake, lizard, and chelonian, respectively.

Reptiles have variable dentition. Agamid lizards and chameleons have acrodont teeth which attach to the crest of the maxillary and mandibular bones. Pleurodont teeth, found in iguanid lizards and snakes, have an eroded lingual side and are attached to a higher sided labial wall. Crocodilians have

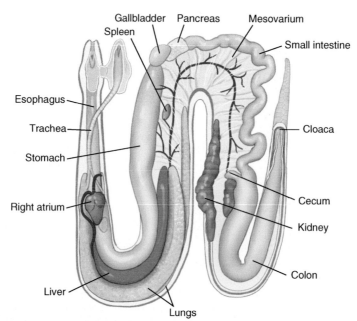

FIGURE 5-1 Gross anatomy of a snake. Most snakes have the same basic anatomical layout. The gastrointestinal system is relatively short, only slightly longer than the length of the snake. (Redrawn from Mader DR, ed. *Reptile Medicine and Surgery*. 2nd ed. St. Louis, MO: Elsevier: 2006.)

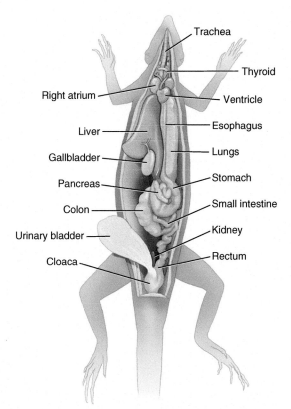

Trachea

Thyroid

Right atrium

Ventricle

Liver

Esophagus

Gallbladder

Lungs

Pancreas

Stomach

Colon

Small intestine

Urinary bladder

Kidney

Cloaca

Rectum

FIGURE 5-2 Gross anatomy of an iguana. Lizards vary somewhat more than snakes in their anatomy, but the basic components remain the same. (Redrawn from Mader DR, ed. *Reptile Medicine and Surgery*. 2nd ed. St. Louis, MO: Elsevier: 2006.)

the codont teeth which are embedded in deep bony socket and have no periodontal membranes.[6] Snakes have two rows of upper teeth (maxillary and pterygoid) and one row of lower teeth (mandibular). Generally, teeth are lost or resorbed and replaced throughout life (polyphyodonty). However, many acrodont reptiles will cease producing new teeth at some point and will use the remaining teeth and jaw margins thereafter. Chelonians lack teeth and are unable to chew. Similar to birds, chelonians have a horny beak with sharp edges. Most herbivorous species have a row of hard ridges on the palate to allow more precise prehension of food.[7]

Salivary glands primarily produce mucus which helps to lubricate food items. Venom glands are modified labial salivary glands, producing collagenases, phospholipases, and proteases. The injection of venom into prey is under voluntary control. Venomous snakes may have rear fangs (opithsoglyphous), fixed front fangs (proteroglyphous), or folding front fangs (solenoglyphous).[8]

The tongue of chameleons is used extensively for food prehension. The sticky tip can protrude over half of the body length to capture prey. Geckos use their tongues to clean their eyes.[9] Snakes, varanids, and tegu lizards all have thin, forked, and mobile tongues which lies in a sheath below the glottis and can be extended through the lingual fossa with the mouth closed. The tongue functions in collecting chemical signals (olfaction and taste).[8,9] The chelonian tongue is short and fleshy.[7]

In most reptiles, the esophagus is a non muscular, thin-walled, highly distensible anatomic structure. The skeletal musculature aids in passage of food.[8] Reptile stomachs are simple and spindle shaped, and the transition from the esophagus is often indistinct.[6] The snake stomach is indistinct, fusiform, and glandular.[8] The stomach secretes hydrochloric acid, which prevents putrefaction, kills live prey, and helps digest food.

Chitin is digested by insectivores by chitinolytic enzymes. Chitinase hydrolyzes chitin into chitobiose and chototriose. Chitobiose is degraded into acetylglucosamine through interaction with chitobiase.[6] Fiber is digested by mibrobial fermentation which requires a large and complex digestive system. The cecum is prominent in herbivorous reptiles (e.g., tortoises) but absent in most snakes. In herbivores, the large intestine is very voluminous, but the cecum is not large. Transit time for ingesta may be 2 to 4 weeks to allow for maxim nutritional absorption.[7] Only 3% of lizards are herbivores and these species depend on high environmental temperatures to facilitate bacterial fermentation of their food.[9]

The colon terminates at the cloaca. The cloaca is the final section of the GI, urinary, and reproductive tracts. The cloaca is comprised of a coprodeum, which receives the colon, the urodeum, where the ureters and genital ducts enter, and the proctodeum, which exits the cloacal orifice. The cloaca of reptiles has substantial activity in fluid and electrolyte homeostasis. In reptile species the majority of fluid reabsorption occurs within the cloaca rather than in the kidneys.[10] The hemipenes of squamates lie in a sulcus caudal to the cloacal orifice. In chelonians and crocodilians, the single phallus lies in the proctodeum.[6]

The reptile liver is large and, in snakes, very elongated. There is no biliverdin reductase, therefore bilirubin is not produced. Alternatively, biliverdin, a very green pigment, is the end product. Liver function is similar to higher vertebrates.

The pancreas may be associated with the stomach or duodenum or intermixed with the spleen, forming a splenopancreas (e.g., boids).[10] The reptile pancreas has both endocrine and exocrine functions, as in mammals. The exocrine tissue secretes digestive enzymes including chitinase and amylolytic, proteolytic, and lipolytic enzymes. Amylolytic enzymes are produced in higher quantities by herbivorous reptile species than found carnivorous species.[10]

Birds

With the varied niches that avian species occupy in nature, many different diets, methods of food prehension, and digestion occur. However, birds conserve anatomical similarity over the various orders more than any of the other vertebrate orders, and enough similarities exist that some generalizations can be made. Many of the commonly kept companion birds have similar digestive tracts (Figure 5-4).

None of the existing species of birds have teeth. In most cases the beak is the organ used for food prehension, although the feet are also used extensively in raptors and psittacine birds to grab prey and food items. The structure of the beak varies with the function. Seedeaters generally have short, stout beaks while psittacine species have strong, hooked bills for both climbing and cracking the hard shell of nuts. Carnivores have narrower, hooked bills for tearing flesh and waterfowl have broad bills for straining their food from water. The

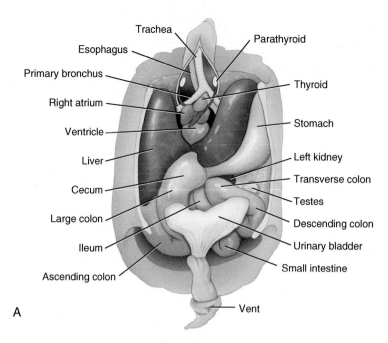

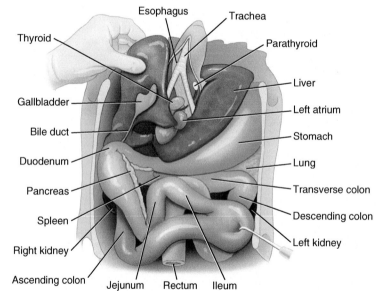

FIGURE 5-3 *A,B,* Gross anatomy of a tortoise. The liver is reflected cranially and the bladder is removed. (Redrawn from Mader DR, ed. *Reptile Medicine and Surgery.* 2nd ed. St. Louis, MO: Elsevier: 2006.)

oral cavity has fewer variations, although psittacine birds are unusual in having a fleshy, sensitive tongue with intrinsic musculature that is used for manipulation of food and other objects.[11] In lories and lorikeets, the tongue has erectile bristles for the collection of pollen and nectar. The lateral edges of ducks' tongues have bristles for filtering food particles.[12] Several other avian species have tongues modified for use when eating their specific diet. Most other birds have a flat, heavily keratinized tongue with no intrinsic musculature. The salivary glands produce small quantities of saliva for lubrication of food and have minimal digestive function.[11] A few species have oral diverticula. In some (e.g., bustards), these

are used for display, while in others (e.g., nutcrackers), they carry food.[11] The entire floor of the pelican mouth stretches for catching fish.[11]

The esophagus is similar to that of mammals, however it may be more distensible, and, in many species, it has an evagination called a crop, or ingluvies, at the coelomic inlet. The presence of the crop is variable. Psittaciformes, Columbiformes, Galliformes, and many Passeriformes possess a crop. Other passerines (canaries), owls, many wading birds, and some others do not have a distinct crop.[11] In Columbiformes, the lining of the crop, under the influence of prolactin, produces a secretion of protein-rich material, called crop milk,

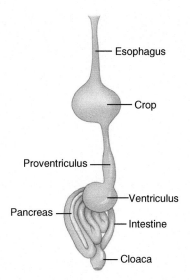

FIGURE 5-4 Basic in situ anatomy of the psittacine digestive tract.

which is regurgitated to the offspring (squabs) as a primary food source.

The stomach of birds is divided into the secretory portion (proventriculus) and a muscular portion (ventriculus or gizzard). Stomach size varies with species, often being quite large and sac-like in fish-eating birds such as penguins and herons[11] where as other orders of birds have a more muscular stomach. Chemical digestion of ingesta begins in the proventriculus. As in the mammalian stomach, hydrochloric acid is produced in the proventriculus. A narrowed isthmus separates the proventriculus from the ventriculus and the mucosa from both these gastrointestinal organs are present and the ventriculus, or gizzard, is lined by the cuticle, a thick layer of koilin that is a tough, carbohydrate-protein material secreted by glands located within the ventricular mucosa.[11] The koilin is composed of interconnecting vertical rods in a horizontal matrix. This substance protects the lining of the ventriculus while food is ground into fine particles. In hornbills, the cuticle is shed and regurgitated as a seed-filled sac that the male feeds to the female in the nest.[11] The ventricular musculature varies depending on the bird's diet, with the most developed musculature being found in granivorous species. In species that primarily eat liquid foods (e.g., nectar), the ventriculus is often not as muscular as in other birds. Release from the ventriculus is particle-size dependent, which explains the fact that foreign objects often settle here. Gastric reflux (egestion or casting) occurs in carnivores (Strigiformes and Falconiformes) to void indigestible portions of their diet from the ventriculus. Egestion or casting involves synchronized contractions of the proventriculus, ventriculus, and duodenum, usually about 12 hours post feeding. The pellet is expelled by antiperistaltic contractions of the esophagus. Owls have both bone and roughage in pellets, while Falconiformes tear up food and digest longer (due to the crop being present), therefore only roughage is present in these casts.[12]

The ventriculus empties into the duodenum, along with the liver and pancreas via the bile and pancreatic ducts at the level of the distal ascending duodenum.[11] The jejunum and ileum follow the duodenum. The presence of ceca is variable. Ceca are absent in psittacines and diurnal raptors, rudimentary in passerines and pigeons, and most developed in ground-feeding birds.[12] Many companion birds do not possess ceca. In these birds, the colon is nearly indistinguishable from the small intestine. When ceca are present, they are paired and also vary in size. Ceca may function in water conservation along with aiding digestion of fibrous material. In the ostrich, the ceca are large and sacculated and appear to aid in digestion of fiber by bacterial fermentation. The colon empties into the coprodeum, the cranial-most portion of the cloaca. The cloaca is the common termius for the digestive, urinary, and reproductive tracts. It consists of the coprodeum, the urodeum, and the proctodeum. The ureters and reproductive tracts (ductus deferens or oviduct) enter the urodeum. The proctodeum has a lymphatic bursa on the dorsal margin. In species that have a phallus, this anatomic structure lies on the ventral floor of the proctodeum. Droppings of birds consist of urine, urates (the insoluble portions of the urine), and feces. Feces, urine, and urates will be retained in the cloaca or retropulsed into the colon for further modification. Much of the water reabsorption from the urine occurs in the GI tract rather than in the kidneys.

The pancreas lies in close association with the duodenum. The pancreas has both endocrine and exocrine functions, very similar to those in mammals. In granivorous birds, glucagon appears to be more important in the regulation of blood glucose than insulin.

The normal avian liver is dark red and composed of a right and left lobe, with the right being slightly larger.[13] The liver lobes may be subdivided in some species. Ventrally, the liver is in contact with the sternum and in most species does not extend past the caudal aspect of sternal margin.[13] The presence of gallbladders varies with species and even between individuals of the same species. Psittacine birds, except the cockatoos, lack a gallbladder. The avian liver is physiologically similar to the mammalian liver. However, similar to reptiles, birds lack biliverdin reductase and cannot produce bilirubin. Therefore, avian feces are usually green in color. Failure of the liver to conjugate and excrete biliverdin into the intestine results in excess biliverdin excretion into the urine.

Mammals

Mammalian digestive anatomy varies significantly, depending on the animal's diet. The digestive anatomy of carnivorous and insectivorous species are often less complex than that of herbivorous animals. Ferrets, hedgehogs, and sugar gliders are the primary exotic pet species that fit this category. The digestive anatomy follows the basic model with which most veterinarians are familiar. Ferrets, in particular, have a very simple digestive tract. They have simple stomachs, no cecum, and little distinction between the large and small intestine. Their teeth are simple, brachydontic teeth, very much like dogs and cats. The dental formulae for common pet species are listed in Table 5-1.

Herbivores require more specialized digestive anatomy. Rabbits and rodents have very specialized teeth. The incisors of all are aradicular (elodont) hypsodont, meaning there is no anatomical root and grow continuously throughout life. In rabbits and hystricomorph rodents, the cheek teeth are also aradicular and hypsodont, while in other rodents, the cheek

TABLE 5-1

Dental Formulae for Various Mammal Species

Species	Incisors	Canines	Premolars	Molars
Sugar gliders	3/1	1/0	3/3	4/4
Hedgehogs	3/2	1/1	3/2	3/3
Ferrets	3/3	1/1	3/3	1/2
Rabbits	1/1	0/0	3/2	3/3
Hystricognathi	1/1	0/0	1/1	3/3
Sciuridae	1/1	0/0	1-2/1	3/3
Muridae	1/1	0/0	0/0	3/3

teeth are radicular (anelodont) and brachydont, similar to carnivores and insectivores.

Dietary fiber requires the assistance of bacterial fermentation for digestion. Therefore, many herbivores have modifications of their stomach or hindgut. Ruminants have four-chambered stomachs that represent the highest degree of specialization. Some primates, in particular those that primarily eat leaves, have modified forestomachs. Rabbits and rodents are herbivorous and omnivorous animals that are commonly maintained as pets. These species are monogastric, and generally are unable to vomit or release gas from the stomach predisposing these species to gastric bloat. Rabbits and hystricomorph rodents (e.g., guinea pigs, chinchillas, and degus) are hindgut fermenters. Part of the digestive process in these species involves coprophagy and with rabbits, distinct cecotrophs are formed and consumed. Cecotrophs provide volatile fatty acids (for energy), microbial proteins, B vitamins, sodium, potassium, and water.[14]

Specific Features of Common Pet Mammal Species

Sugar Gliders

Sugar gliders are diprotodonts, which have only one pair of lower incisors that project rostrally. The dental formula is 2(I3/1 C1/0 P3/3 M4/4).[15] The lower incisors, while they appear similar to rodent teeth, do not grow continually and should never be trimmed. The basic anatomic structure of the sugar glider digestive system follows that of a typical carnivore/omnivore. Marsupials' GI tract, like that in reptiles and birds, ends in a cloaca, a common exit for the urogenital and digestive tracts.[16]

Hedgehogs

Hedgehogs have anelodont brachydont teeth similar to carnivores. The dental formula is 2(I3/2 C1/1 P3/2 M3/3).[17] The upper first incisors are widely separated, project rostrally, and are slightly larger than the next tooth, giving the appearance of canine teeth.[18] The lower first incisors fit in the gap between the uppers when the mouth is closed. Otherwise, the digestive system is similar to other carnivores/insectivores. Hedgehogs do not have a cecum.

Ferrets

Ferrets have typical anelodont brachydont carnivore teeth. The dental formula is 2(I3/3 C1/1 P3/3 M1/2).[19] There are five pairs of salivary glands: parotid, mandibular, sublingual, molar, and zygomatic.[19] Although vomiting is uncommon in ferrets, they are anatomically capable of vomiting.[19] The stomach is a simple, J-shaped organ capable of substantial distension. The small intestine is relatively short, being about 500% of the body length.[20] There is no cecum and the large intestine is not distinguishable from the small intestine on gross examination. The large intestine is about 10 cm long and is comprised of 3 sections; ascending, transverse, and descending.[19] The liver is large and consists of six lobes, the left lateral, quadrate, right medial, right lateral, and caudate. There is a gallbladder between the quadrate and right medial lobes. The cystic duct joins the right and central hepatic ducts to form the common bile duct.[19] The V-shaped pancreas has a section along the duodenum and one adjacent to the stomach and spleen. Ducts from each lobe come together to form the common pancreatic duct, which joins the common bile duct and enters the duodenum approximately 3 cm caudal to the cranial duodenal flexure.[19]

Rabbits

Rabbits have a unique and complex digestive system with continuously growing teeth, simple stomach, large cecum, and a mechanism for sorting food particles by size. It is a two-pass system requiring cecotrophy.

Rabbit dentition is adapted to an herbivorous diet. All rabbit teeth are aradicular hypsodont and grow continuously throughout life.[21] The teeth have no true anatomical root, and are divided into the clinical crown and the reserve crown. The dental formula for rabbit teeth is 2(I2/1 C0/0 P3/2 M3/3).[22] In contrast to rodents, rabbits have two sets of maxillary incisors, with the second tooth directly behind the first and diminished in size. This smaller incisor is referred to as the peg tooth and serves as a stop for the mandibular incisor. The incisors' purpose is to cut pieces of food small enough for the rabbit to eat. There is no true anatomic distinction between the molars and premolars, so they are often referred to collectively as "cheek teeth." During mastication, the jaw moves up to 120 times per minute in both vertical and horizontal directions.[23] Rabbits eat small amounts of food about 30 times a day.[23] Hunger is stimulated by a number of variables, including dry mouth, gastric contractions, or decreased blood levels of metabolites (e.g., glucose, amino acids, volatile fatty acids, lactic acid).[23]

The gastric pH in the rabbit varies from 1.0 to 3.0, with the low occurring after eating. This low pH essentially sterilizes ingesta. Before weaning, the gastric pH is higher (5.0 to 6.5), which allows for the establishment of microbial flora within the large intestine.[23] Before weaning, rabbit kits produce milk oil through a reaction with the doe's milk. This oil is antimicrobial and helps prevent GI infections. Kits receiving milk replacer or milk from other species do not produce this fatty acid, therefore are predisposed to GI infections.[23] The rabbit stomach is rarely void of ingesta, with hair, food, and fluid being found even after 24 hours without eating.

Many nutrients, such as amino acids, lipids, monosaccharides, and electrolytes, are absorbed in the small intestine. However, the natural diet of the rabbit has very little of these nutrients in a form suitable for absorption. However, cecotrophs contain these nutrients in an easy-to-absorb form.[23] Bicarbonate is secreted into the proximal small intestine and neutralizes gastric acid. Pancreatic amylase is not a important component of digestive physiology in the rabbit. The small intestine has significant immune function through extensive lymphoid aggregates called Peyer's patches and the sacculus rotundus, primarily lymphoid tissue, located at the terminal ilium. The sacculus rotundus is unique to rabbits.[23]

The large intestine consists of three functional parts: cecum, proximal colon, and distal colon. The cecum is the largest organ in the abdominal cavity, having 10 times the capacity of the stomach. The rabbit cecum is thin walled, coiled, and ends in the vermiform appendix. The cecum is a long and voluminous structure consisting of three gyri, is heavily sacculated, occupies about one-third of the abdominal cavity and terminates in an appendix, which is similar to the human appendix.[21] The appendix has both lymphoid and secretory functions.[23] Microbial fermentation primarily takes part in the cecum. A wide variety of microorganisms are present in the cecum to assist in fermentation, including anaerobes, facultative anaerobes, protozoa, and a rabbit-specific yeast (*Cyniclomyces guttulatus*). Some nutrients are absorbed through the cecal wall, while others are expelled and reingested as cecotrophs.[23] Cecotrophs are formed when material is expelled from the cecum, enveloped in mucus from the colon, and excreted by rapid peristaltic motility after which they are consumed directly from the anus. Cecotrophs are rich in amino acids, volatile fatty acids, vitamins, enzymes, and microorganisms. Fermentation continues within the cecotrophs for up to 8 hours until the stomach acid dissolves the mucous coating.[23]

Fiber is sorted into digestible fiber, which goes into the cecum, and indigestible fiber, which has a high lignin content and passes into the colon.[21] The digestible fiber is fermented in the cecum by *Bacteroides* spp. and other microorganisms into volatile fatty acids, which are absorbed by the cecal wall and provide energy for the rabbit.[21] The proximal colon is easily recognized by the presence of haustra (sacculations). This is the site where ingesta are separated into digestible and indigestible components. The smaller, digestible particles settle near the mucosa and are propelled back to the cecum by a series of contractions. The larger, indigestible particles stay in the center of the colon and will eventually form hard fecal pellets. While the indigestible particles contribute little nutritionally, they are essential for maintaining normal GI motility. At the junction of the proximal and distal colon is the fusus coli, a thickened ring of muscle with a dense blood and nerve supply, unique to lagomorphs. This structure acts as an intestinal "pacemaker," controlling segmental,

peristaltic, and colonic motility, and is influenced by hormones such as aldosterone and prostaglandins.[23]

The distal colon is smaller in diameter and a simple tubular structure. Here, reabsorption of water and dissolved substances occurs prior to expulsion of the hard feces. Excretion of feces follows a circadian rhythm, with a hard-feces phase usually during feeding activity and a cecotroph phase during resting or nonfeeding periods.[23] The large intestine has GALT, accounting for >50% of the total lymphoid tissue in the rabbit.[23] Intestinal motility is under the influence of the autonomic nervous system, hormones, and fiber levels of the diet. Motilin, one of the hormones that enhances motility, is stimulated by fats but inhibited by carbohydrates.[23]

Rodents

Rodents represent the largest order of mammals, accounting for 40% of all species and are occasionally classified into suborders by the structure of the jaw as either Sciurognathi (squirrel-like) or Hystricognathi (porcupine-like).[24] There are numerous families in each of these suborders.[24] Hystricognathi commonly kept as pets include guinea pigs, chinchillas, and degus. Sciurognathi commonly kept as pets include rats, mice, hamsters, gerbils, and prairie dogs.

As in rabbits, the incisors of all rodents are aradicular hypsodont teeth. With aradicular hypsodont teeth, the part of the tooth embedded in the bone is not a root because there is no anatomical distinction from the exposed crown. The term "reserve crown" is appropriate when referring to this area.[25] The incisors have a chiseled edge caused by more rapid wear on the oral surface.[25] In most rodents, the incisors have an orange coloration on their surface. This is lacking in guinea pigs. Hystricognathi are similar to rabbits in that the cheek teeth are also aradicular hypsodont teeth. Sciurognathi have cheek teeth that are anelodont brachydont teeth, with true roots that do not continuously grow.[22] The Hystricognathi are more specialized for the consumption of fibrous, low-energy diets, while Sciurognathi are more adapted to a grain-based diet. However, within each group there is a degree of both convergence and divergence, with some Sciurognathi (e.g., prairie dogs), being adapted to a fibrous, low-energy diet. The Hystricognathi have greater need for appropriate use of the cheek teeth because of their continuous growth. Wear of the teeth is mainly accomplished by the abrasive nature of the natural diet, another component is the tooth-on-tooth grinding action.[25] The gape of all rodents is very small, and both guinea pigs and chinchillas have a soft palate that is continuous with the base of the tongue. Food passes through the pharynx through the palatal ostium, a hole in the soft palate.[26] Rodents are not capable of vomiting because of a strong esophageal sphincter and a limiting ridge in the stomach.[27] Although rodents are monogastric, many species have a forestomach that has a limiting ridge separating it from the glandular stomach.[27] Hystricognathi have a hindgut fermenting digestive tract similar to rabbits. In guinea pigs, stomach emptying time is about 2 hours, and the entire GI transit time is approximately 20 hours.[26,28] The transit time in chinchillas is 12 to 15 hours. The guinea pig cecum is large and sacculated, while the chinchilla's is somewhat smaller and coiled.[26] Chinchillas produce both nitrogen-rich feces, which are consumed, and nitrogen-poor feces, which are not. However, guinea pigs, while they are coprophagic, do not produce cecotrophs and as a result require more preformed vitamins in their diets.[26] Nonetheless, guinea pigs digest fiber more efficiently than rabbits.[28] Many other rodents are largely herbivorous, but their diet is based on grains which requires significantly less modification of the intestinal tract. Even these rodent species engage in a degree of coprophagy, which may provide them with nutrients (e.g., B vitamins).[27]

DISEASES OF THE GASTROINTESTINAL SYSTEM

Disease of the GI tract may occur by itself or as a part of a systemic process. Selected infectious diseases affecting the digestive tract of several categories of exotic companion species are listed in Table 5-2.

Invertebrates

Invertebrates are uncommon veterinary patients, often presenting for trauma or problems visible from the surface. As such, there are limited data available on the diseases of the digestive system. Giant spiders (e.g., tarantulas) are one of the more frequent pet species of invertebrates presented to veterinarians, and a few conditions are recognized that have at least some GI effects.

Bacterial Diseases

Bacillus spp. appear to be normal digestive tract flora that can act as opportunistic pathogens, especially under poor husbandry conditions. Mortality can occur when humidity is insufficient. Generally, the problem will resolve when the humidity is corrected.[29] *Proteus* spp. infections have been found concurrently with Panagrolaimidae nematode infestations, but the significance of the parasite with this disease condition is not clear.[29]

Parasitic Diseases

Nematodes of the genus *Panagrolaimidae* can cause oral infestations in tarantulas. The infection initially manifests with anorexia and a gradually increasing lethargy that progresses to a huddled posture. Death occurs after several weeks or occasionally months. White discharge around the mouth and chelicerae may be noted during the late stages of infection. The minute motile nematodes may be seen microscopically in a saline prep. Treatments, to date, have been ineffective or in some cases toxic to the host.[29]

Fish

In many cases, GI diseases of fishes occur as part of a systemic disease process. Often the clinical signs are vague and may not be specific to the digestive system. In this chapter, those disease conditions that have prominent GI clinical signs or pathology are discussed. Clinical signs associated with fish GI disease may include visible changes in either the oral or vent regions, anorexia, abnormal feces, coelomic swelling, or dysphagia.

Viral Diseases

Some viral diseases can affect the fish GI tract. The GI disease conditions associated with viral infections in fish are usually related to systemic illness and result in nonspecific clinical signs. Generally, the definative diagnosis is obtained through necropsy. The golden shiner virus may affect the intestinal

tract as part of a more involved systemic process. In spring viremia of carp, a mucoid cast may trail from the inflamed vent.[30] Infectious pancreatic necrosis is caused by a bornavirus and is widely distributed. This bornavirus has commercial significance because it affects salmonids, but several other species are susceptible. Infectious pancreatic necrosis causes catarrhal enteritis and high mortality in young fish.[1] Diagnosis is achieved through immunofluorescent antibody testing, serum enzyme-linked immunosorbent assay (ELISA) testing, or virus isolation.[1,31] A virus similar to infectious pancreatic necrosis virus of salmonids has been isolated from several tropical Caribbean reef fish. In these fish, acute death is frequently observed without the classic pancreatic necrosis however epithelial sloughing in the intestinal tract is often present.[32]

Bacterial Diseases

ENTERIC REDMOUTH. This disease, caused by *Yersinia ruckeri*, is a septicemic disease that has clinical signs associated with the digestive tract. Clinical disease signs associated with enteric redmouth include hyperemia and petechiae of the mouth and a yellow discharge in the vent area.[33] Other signs are typical of septicemia. Diagnosis of enteric redmouth is based on identification of the organism from the kidney.[33] A variety of drugs, including tetracyclines, sulfonamides, tiamulin, and oxalinic acid, have been effective in treatment. Treatment should be continued for at least 14 days.

RED PEST. This disease, caused by *Vibrio anguillarum*, appears similar to enteric redmouth, resulting in erythema of the mouth, vent, and base of fins. Affected fish may have distended intestines, filled with clear mucoid fluid.[34]

MYCOBACTERIOSIS. Mycobacteriosis is a systemic disease that can affect multiple systems, including the digestive tract. It is characterized by multifocal granulomas, consequently the clinical course of this disease is variable, depending on the location of the granulomas.[1] Diagnosis is often tentative until acid-fast bacteria are identified within the lesions through the use of special cytologic stains.[1] This disease is zoonotic, and treatment of affected fish is difficult. Mycobacteriosis is best prevented by appropriate quarantine methods.[1]

ENTERIC SEPTICEMIA OF CATFISH. Enteric septicemia of catfish is a systemic bacterial disease caused by *Edwardsiella ictaluri* that typically enters the body through the intestinal tract, invades the bloodstream, and colonizes various organs. The disease primarily occurs when water temperatures are between 24°C and 28°C (75°F to 82°F), the temperature at which the bacterium optimally grows. Affected fish may "hang" in the water with their head up, show abnormal swimming behaviors, or exhibit abdominal distension, exophthalmos, or pale gills. Skin petechiae may also occur. Histologically, are enteritis and hepatitis is often identified, in addition to lesions in non-GI organs. Diagnosis is determined through culture of the lesions.[1,31] Various antibiotics may be effective, but treatment selection is best attained through antimicrobial sensitivity reports.

SWIM BLADDER DISEASE. Swim bladder abnormalities in koi and goldfish occur periodically. Koi and goldfish have physostomous swim bladders; they are connected to the esophagus by a pneumatic duct. This may serve as an entry site for bacteria. Affected fish may have either positive or negative buoyancy effects when the swim bladders become

TABLE 5-2

Infectious Diseases by Etiology

Etiology	Species	Disease	Etiology	Species	Disease
Viruses	Invertebrates		Fungi	Invertebrates	
	Fish	Golden shiner virus		Fish	Phycomycosis
		Spring viremia of carp		Amphibians	Chromomycosis
		Infectious pancreatic necrosis			Mucormycosis
	Amphibians	Ranavirus			*Candida* spp.
	Reptiles	Inclusion body disease of boids			*Penicillium* spp.
		Herpesvirus		Reptiles	
		Adenovirus		Birds	*Candida* spp.
		Ranavirus			*Macrorhabdus ornithogaster*
	Birds	Pox (avipox)		Mammals	
		Papillomatosis (herpes)	Parasites	Invertebrates	Panagrolaimidae nematodes
		Proventricular dilatation disease (bornavirus)		Fish	Coccidiosis
					Microsporidiosis
		Pacheco's disease (herpesvirus)			Hexamita
		Adenovirus			Cestodes
		Reovirus			Nematodes
		Polyomavirus		Amphibians	Amoeba
		Coronavirus			Pentastomids
		Avian serositis virus		Reptiles	Coccidiosis
	Mammals	Epizootic catarrhal enteritis (coronavirus)			Cryptosporidiosis
					Entamoeba invadens
		Rotavirus			Nematodes
		Rabbit hemorrhagic disease		Birds	Trichomoniasis
		Sialodacryoadenitis virus			Coccidiosis
Bacteria	Invertebrates	Proteus			Cryptosporidiosis
		Bacillus			*Giardia psittaci*
	Fish	Enteric redmouth			*Hexamita* spp.
		Red pest			*Cochlosoma* spp.
		Mycobacteriosis			*Encephalitozoon hellum*
		Enteric septicemia of catfish			Nematodes
		Swim bladder infections			Cestodes
	Amphibians	*Aeromonas hydrophila*		Mammals	Coccidiosis
		Salmonella			Cryptosporidiosis
		Mycobacteria			Protozoa
	Reptiles	Bacterial stomatitis, gastritis, enteritis, cloacitis, hepatitis			*Hymenolepis nana*
					Spironucleus muris
		Aeromonas spp., *Pseudomonas* spp.			*Giardia muris*
		Enterobacteriaciae			
		Mycobacterium spp.			
	Birds	*Chlamydophia psittaci*			
		Mycobacterium spp.			
		Gram-negative bacteria (opportunistic infections)			
		Yersinia pseudotuberculosis			
		Helicobacter spp.			
		Clostridium spp.			
		Campylobacter			
	Mammals	*Helicobacter mustelae*			
		Proliferative bowel disease			
		Dysbiosis			
		Tyzzer's disease			
		Yersinia pseudotuberculosis			

fluid filled or overdistended. A diagnosis is based on imaging (e.g., radiology, ultrasound) and aspirates of the swim bladder for cytology or culture. Removal of fluid or excess air may be included as part of the treatment plan for swim bladder disease.

Fungal Disease

PHOMAMYCOSIS. Chinook salmon are susceptible to phomamycosis which is caused by the fungus *Phoma herbarum*. The infection affects the swim bladder and stomach. Clinical disease signs include the development of swollen vents and abnormal or upside-down swimming. Some affected fish may have a pinched appearance cranial to the vent, fluid present in the swim bladder or stomach, and mycelial tufts in the swim bladder, while others may rest on their side.[35] Necropsy samples or swim bladder aspirates may be used to obtain a fungal culture which is required to confirm the diagnosis. A similar disease condition may be caused by *Paecilomyces farinosus* in Atlantic salmon.

Parasitic Diseases

COCCIDIOSIS. Coccidiosis, caused by *Eimeria* spp., is occasionally diagnosed in pond or aquarium fish that exhibit clinical signs of enteritis. Affected fish present for emaciation, with sunken eyes and having a depressed attitude. The intestines are often filled with yellowish colored fluids.[36,37] Intestinal mucosa infected with coccidia show varying degrees of epithelial necrosis and sloughing. The parasites may be observed on microscopic examination of the feces or intestinal scrapings. Coccidiosis is a potential cause of peritonitis in elasmobranchs and sygnathids.[1] Weight loss, anorexia, blackened feces, and coelomic swelling are characteristic of the disease. Wet-mount preparations of feces or intestinal contents is the recommended diagnostic test to identify the organism in diseased fish. Oocysts can be found in feces or coelomic aspirates, although if in feces, the significance cannot be determined.[1] Treatment with diclazuril, toltrazuril, and sulfadimidine may be effective to treat infected fish.[1]

MICROSPORIDIOSIS. Microsporidiosis can be fatal to fish and is a highly contagious disease. *Pleistophora hyphessobryconis* is a common species found in neon tetras *(Paracheirodon innesi)*. The parasites (primitive fungus) are found in the intestines, pyloric ceca, bile ducts, liver, and other tissues. Oral ingestion is the mode of transmission, but some microsporidian parasites require intermediate hosts. The parasites cause no cellular degeneration but stimulate hypertrophy that results in almost total occlusion of the intestinal lumen. There are no effective treatments for fish diagnosed with microsporidiosis.[37] Cryptosporidiosis has been found in angelfish exhibiting anorexia, regurgitation, and undigested feces.[38]

HEXAMITIASIS. *Hexamita* infections can be found in a variety of fish species. In some infected fish, no clinical signs will be noted. In others, particularly angelfish, discus, and gouramis, hexamitiasis may result in poor condition, weight loss, poor appetite, catarrhal enteritis, and death.[1] Diagnosis of hexamitiasis in fish is achieved by finding the trophozoites in fecal wet-mount preparations. Metronidazole baths can be effective for treatment.[38]

CESTODES. Numerous species of cestodes can affect fish. One of particular importance is the Asian tapeworm *(Bothriocephalus acheilognathi)*. This parasite was introduced from China in imported grass carp *(Ctenopharyngodon idellus)*.[1] It poses a particular risk because it can infect a wide variety of hosts including koi, carp, baitfish, and freshwater aquarium species.[1] The proglottids may be identified in feces with praziquantel being recommended as a treatment option.[1]

NEMATODES. Various nematode species can be found in the fish GI tract. Nematodes appear to be most common in bottom-feeding species.[1] *Capillaria* are frequently found in tropical fishes, but their clinical significance is difficult to determine. Diagnosis of nematodes through identification of

eggs in the feces by flotation or wet-mount preparation. Treatment with fenbendazole or levamisole can be effective.[1,38] Ivermectin has a very low margin of safety in fishes and used with caution.[1]

Noninfectious Diseases

HEPATIC LIPIDOSIS. Hepatic lipidosis may occur in various aquarium or pond fish and usually accompanies obesity resulting from overfeeding or being fed a high-fat diet (>15% in koi).[39] Other initiating causes of hepatic lipidosis in fish include biotin deficiency, choline deficiency, or toxemia. Diagnosis may be made based on biopsy and the liver may appear yellow and mottled. The cut surface of the liver may exude oil while histologically, intracellular fat droplets may be observed.[40] Treatment is primarily dietary improvement and controlling the quantity fed.

NEOPLASIA. A variety of tumors have been reported in fish species. Tumors of the GI tract in koi and goldfish include pancreatic carcinoma and hepatocellular tumors.[41,42] Gastrointestinal tumors reported in freshwater tropical fish all involve the liver, which include cholangioma cholangiocarcinoma and hepatocellular adenoma.[43]

In fish that are large enough, an excisional biopsy can provide the diagnosis but also can be considered part, if not all, of the treatment plan. Neoplasms in fish are often less aggressive and more differentiated than in mammals, and metastasis is uncommon. Removal of the tumor may be curative or at least palliative for the fish.[39]

Foreign Body Ingestion

Fish in private or public aquaria are prone to ingestion of foreign bodies. Such items include balls, decorative items, air stones, lead weights, or even tank mates.[1] If noted in time, the object can be removed nonsurgically with forceps, either blindly or through endoscopy.

Amphibians

Clinical signs of GI disease in amphibians may include anorexia, mouth abnormalities, coelomic swelling or palpable masses, diarrhea or lack of fecal production, and cloacal prolapse.[3]

Viral Diseases

Ranavirus is a major disease threat in wild amphibian populations and may be significant for captive collections as well. Although ranavirus infection is a systemic disease in amphibian species, the liver and intestinal tract may be affected. Diagnosis may be made based on pathologic findings as well as molecular-based diagnostic tests.[1,44]

Bacterial Diseases

Although bacterial disease is common, generally it presents as a systemic septicemia rather than a localized GI problem. Although, *Aeromonas hydrophila* is often implicated in amphibian bacterial GI infections many species may be involved.[1] *Salmonella* spp. can be a normal inhabitant of the amphibian digestive tract.[45] *Mycobacterium* spp. may cause granulomatous disease similar to the fungal diseases. *Mycobacterium marinum, Mycobacterium fortuitum,* and *Mycobacterium xenopi* are common pathogens found in amphibian GI granulomatous disease cases. Usually there is a chronic syndrome, and affected animals may show weight loss despite having a good appetite.[1]

Fungal Diseases

Like bacterial diseases, fungal diseases in amphibians are often systemic but may involve the GI tract. These GI diseases often involve ubiquitous fungal species such as Dematiaceae (chromomycosis) or *Mucor* spp. (mucormycosis).[1] Although fungi tend to be opportunistic pathogens, *Mucor amphibiorum* may behave as a primary pathogen in some species.[1] *Candida* spp. and *Penicillium* spp. have been isolated from liver granulomas in toads.[46] Intestinal fungal infections have also been found in amphibians.[46]

Parasitic Diseases

Although ciliated protozoa are common in amphibians, they appear to be nonpathogenic. A wide variety of flagellates also inhabit the amphibian digestive tract. Generally, these protozoa are considered to be commensal, but if the infestation is heavy and there are clinical signs such as diarrhea, treatment with metronidazole should be considered.[47] Some species of amoeba will cause anorexia and weight loss. Both monogenean and digenean trematodes occur in amphibians but are not usually found in the digestive tract. Likewise, most nematodes are outside of the digestive tract. Pentastomid parasites can affect the respiratory tract or the upper GI tract.[47] Treatment of parasites with metronidazole, fenbendazole, or praziquantel appears to be reasonably safe in amphibians. Ivermectin should be used with caution.[1]

Noninfectious Diseases

PROLAPSES. The underlying causes for the prolapse of rectal, gastric, or cloacal tissues in amphibians often go undiagnosed; however, in some cases it may be associated with GI disease.[1] Underlying causes of prolapse in amphibians include nematodiasis, metabolic disease, gastric overload, intoxication, hypocalcemia, impaction, or obstruction.[48,49] Gastric prolapse is usually terminal, although it may be occur secondary to parasites or toxin exposure.[1] A prolapse is readily recognized on visual examination of the patient as protruding tissue from the vent or mouth (Figure 5-5). Treatment involves surgical reduction of the prolapse, placement

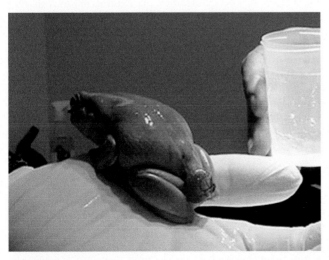

FIGURE 5-5 This White's tree frog was presented for a cloacal prolapse. On close examination, it was discovered that an intestinal loop was herniated through a rent in the muscle and skin of the pelvic area.

of securing sutures, and treatment of any identified underlying conditions.

FOREIGN BODY INGESTION. Consumption of foreign material is a common occurrence in some amphibian species. The distensible esophagus of amphibians often allows the removal of ingested foreign bodies through the mouth. If the object has moved beyond the stomach, surgical removal may be required. Some species will overeat normal food items, resulting in an impaction which can result in severe gastric distension and shock. Diagnosis can be made using radiographs and ultrasound. Treatment for shock and removal of the foreign objects and/or impacted food material are required for successful resolution of these cases.[1]

NEOPLASIA. Five types of spontaneous primary neoplasms of the liver have been reported in amphibians, including hepatoma, hepatocellular carcinoma, hepatoblastoma, cholangioma, and cholangiocarcinoma.[50] Pancreatic tumors primarily involve the islet cells, rarely exocrine cells.[50] Neuroepithelioma of the mouth originates from the olfactory epithelium and have primarily been diagnosed in captive axolotls (*Ambystoma mexicanum*). Additional tumors, characterized as adenocarcinomas, were also detected in axolotls.[50] One gastric adenocarcinoma with metastatic disease has been reported in a captive African clawed frog (*Xenopus laevis*).[50] Four neoplasms, all malignant, have been reported in the intestines of amphibians; an African clawed frog, the giant toad (*Bufo marinus*), a leopard frog (*Rana pipiens*), and an oriental firebelly toad (*Bombina orientalis*). The origin of 3 of the intestinal tumors was questionable, however one (in the giant toad) was clearly an adenocarcinoma.[50]

Reptiles

Reptiles will often present with distinct GI disease or with systemic processes involving the digestive system. It is helpful to localize the disease problem based on the clinical signs. This allows a narrower differential diagnosis list and an appropriate selection of diagnostic tests. Table 5-3 describes the clinical disease signs, diagnostic tests, and differential diagnoses for the various sections of the reptile digestive tract.

Oral disorders are commonly encountered in reptile practice. Due to the visible location of the mouth and the obvious clinical effect of these disorders (anorexia, dysphagia), oral abnormalities may be recognized more easily than those at other sites. Clinical signs of oral disease may include anorexia, dysphagia, exudate adhered to the mucosa or lip margins, or other visible lesions in the mouth. Differential diagnoses for oral disease include infectious stomatitis, oral granulomas, herpesviral or ranaviral stomatitis, proliferative gingivitis, oral neoplasia, and tissue mineralization.[51]

Esophageal and gastric conditions may also present as anorexia along with weight loss and dehydration. Additionally, vomiting or regurgitation may be seen in some cases, although this is not consistent. A midbody swelling may be noted with diseases that involve the stomach (e.g., cryptosporidiosis or foreign body ingestion). Differential diagnoses for esophageal and gastric conditions include nonspecific gastritis, adenovirus, inclusion body disease (IBD), bacterial or fungal gastritis, cryptosporidiosis, nematodes, protozoa, and neoplasia.[51]

Intestinal disease will cause similar clinical signs as described for the stomach, anorexia, weight loss, and dehydration but

TABLE 5-3

Clinical Signs, Diagnostics, and Differential Disease Diagnoses by Anatomic Site in Reptiles

Site	Clinical Signs	Diagnostics	Differentials
Oropharynx	Anorexia Dysphagia Visible lesions, exudates Hypersalivation Halitosis	Visual examination Oral swabs (cytology, microbiology, PCR, etc.) Radiography Biopsy	Infectious stomatitis Herpesvirus Proliferative gingivitis Trauma Neoplasia
Esophagus	Regurgitation Hypersalivation	Esophageal swab Endoscopy Radiography Contrast radiography	Trauma Foreign body Neoplasia
Stomach	Vomiting Anorexia	Gastroscopy Radiography Contrast radiography	Foreign body Gastritis Neoplasia
Intestine/Cecum	Diarrhea	Radiography Contrast radiography	Enteritis (parasitic, bacterial, etc.) Intussusception Foreign body
Cloaca	Tenesmus Protruding tissue	Cloacoscopy Radiography Contrast radiography	Prolapse Cloacalith
Liver	Vague signs Swollen abdomen Enlarged liver	AST Bile acids Radiography Contrast radiography Coelioscopy Coeliotomy Biopsy	Hepatitis (viral, bacterial, etc.) Hepatic lipidosis Toxic
Pancreas	Vague signs	Coelioscopy Coeliotomy Biopsy	Neoplasia

AST, Aspartate transaminase; *PCR*, polymerase chain reaction.

may also include diarrhea. Differential diagnoses for the intestinal tract include cryptosporidiosis, nonspecific enteritis, coccidiosis, adenovirus, trematodes, cestodes, nematodes, and neoplasia.[51]

Since there is an association with the urogenital systems, cloacal disease may or may not be related to the digestive tract. Common clinical signs noted with cloacal disease include bleeding, tenesmus, or tissue protruding from the vent. Common disease conditions of the cloaca in reptile species are constipation, cloacoliths, prolapse, and cloacitis.

Viral Diseases

INCLUSION BODY DISEASE. Regurgitation is a problem that boas and pythons will occasionally present with as a consequence of inclusion body disease (IBD). An arenavirus appears to be the etiologic agent of IBD.[52] Regurgitation and weight loss are common in affected snakes. Neurologic signs are more prominent in affected pythons, but there is great variation in the susceptibility, duration, and clinical signs among snakes. Boa constrictors (*Boa constrictor*) may be more resistant to disease but may also serve as a reservoir of this virus. A complete blood count (CBC) may reveal a leukocytosis or leukopenia, depending on the stage of the disease at the time of presentation. Inclusions within lymphocytes or other cells may occasionally be seen in the peripheral blood smears, although this is not a sensitive indicator of infection. A definitive diagnosis is usually obtained at necropsy; however,

polymerase chain reaction (PCR) assay testing and biopsy of the liver, esophageal tonsils, or pancreas may provide an antemortem diagnosis.[52,53] Histologically, there are eosinophilic intracytoplasmic inclusions in various major organs and tissue necrosis may be evident. Interestingly, in *Python* spp., the inclusions are more abundant in central nervous system (CNS) tissue.[52] No treatment for IBD is available and control involves preventing exposure. Snakes of different species should not be housed together. Boas, in particular, have a slow course of the disease, and a quarantine period of up to 6 months or more is recommended.

HERPESVIRAL STOMATITIS. Herpesviruses have surfaced as important pathogens of the oral cavity and respiratory tract in captive Hermann's tortoises (*Testudo hermanii*), spur-thighed tortoises (*Testudo graeca*), and other tortoises in Europe and the United States.[54] Infections are often associated with high mortality rates. Herpesvirus may be detected by light microscopic observation of intranuclear inclusion bodies in various tissues and/or by PCR.[55] There appears to be several types (four) of herpesviruses that affect tortoises.[55] Concurrent infections with *Mycoplasma* spp. may enhance the disease conditions associated with herpesvirus infection in reptiles. Different species of tortoises with in the same collection may have varied clinical responses to the viral disease.[56] Herpesvirus infection in tortoises is largely characterized by the development of respiratory and oral clinical signs. Systemic lesions in organs such as the liver and spleen are also commonly observed.

Rarely, viral hepatitis with no clinical signs or lesions in the respiratory system, oral cavity, or other organs may occur.[57] An ELISA diagnostic test has been developed for the detection of antibodies to a chelonian herpesvirus.[58] This ELISA test could be used as an important diagnostic tool for screening wild populations and private and zoo collections of tortoises. Alternately, PCR techniques may be used as a screening test.[59] Acyclovir may be effective in the management of this disease, but it is important to recognize that the drug only limits viral replication and would not be curative.[60]

ADENOVIRUS. Numerous adenoviruses have been identified in reptiles. The adenovirus that affects bearded dragons *(Pogona vitticeps)* is of the greatest concern to the reptile practitioner. This disease appears to partly depend on co-infection with coccidian parasites and primarily affects hatchling bearded dragons.[61] Epizootic outbreaks in hatchling bearded dragons may occur. Affected lizards may be found dead after a short period of weakness and lethargy. Neurologic signs are common, including head tilt and circling. Pathologically, hepatocellular necrosis with large basophilic intranuclear inclusion bodies in numerous hepatocytes may be found. Coccidial protozoa *(Isospora amphiboluri)* and basophilic intranuclear inclusion bodies may be found in the small-intestinal enterocytes. Diagnosis of adenovirus in bearded dragons is generally made through post mortem examination. There is no successful treatment for the adenovirus infection in reptile species; however, treating for coccidiosis may reduce mortalities. Likewise, co-infection with dependovirus may precipitate rapid neonatal mortality.[62] In older bearded dragons, adenoviral infection may follow a more chronic, low-grade course of disease, showing poor growth or weight loss and anorexia. Pathology may reveal nonsuppurative hepatitis and nephritis, with large, amphophilic, intranuclear inclusion bodies.[63]

RANAVIRUS. Ranavirus is an uncommon disease of pet reptiles, but is considered an emerging disease of wild reptiles. Ranaviruses have been attributed to worldwide disease epidemics in free-ranging amphibian, turtle, and tortoise populations. Infection is usually fatal in turtles, and the potential impact on endangered populations could be devastating.[64] Diseased turtles primarily exhibit ocular and respiratory signs in the form of conjunctivitis, ocular discharge, nasal discharge, and respiratory distress. However, oral ulcers, plaques, or abscesses are also observed.[64,65] Death generally occurs within days of disease onset.[66] This disease should be considered as a differential diagnosis in turtles that exhibit typical clinical signs, and affected animals should be isolated to avoid transmission to other turtles. Although not commercially available, diagnosis can be made via PCR diagnostic testing.[64] No treatment is currently available for reptile species diagnosed with ranavirus.

Bacterial Diseases

Infectious stomatitis is a commonly encountered digestive tract disorder of reptiles. This is a multifactorial disease and the affected animal can be presented in various stages of infection. While stomatitis can be diagnosed in any reptile, snakes are commonly and severely affected. Stress, trauma (e.g., prey bites), poor temperature regulation, and other factors can suppress the oral defense mechanisms. This allows opportunistic bacteria to invade and cause infection. The bacterial

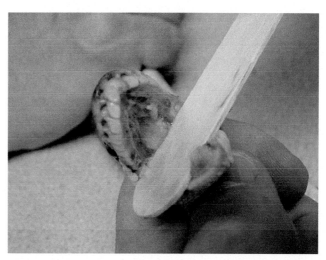

FIGURE 5-6 Ball python with moderate infectious stomatitis. Note the caseous debris, the excessive foamy mucus, and the gingival erosions.

isolates from lesions of snakes with infectious stomatitis predominantly yield Gram-negative bacteria. Common bacterial isolates include *Pseudomonas aeruginosa, Aeromonas hydrophila, Providencia rettgeri,* and *Stenotrophomonas maltophilia.* In contrast, healthy snakes have a predominantly Gram-positive oral flora, with *Corynebacterium* spp. and coagulase-negative *Staphylococcus* spp. being the most frequently isolated organisms.[67] Since cloacal swabbing of healthy snakes also resulted in the isolation of predominantly Gram-negative organisms, it is likely these bacteria are not exogenous pathogens but opportunistic invaders.[67] Initially, small petechiae, excessive salivation, hyperemia, or edema will be observed. In more advanced cases, the development of caseous debris, necrosis, or hemorrhage occurs (Figure 5-6). In very advanced cases, osteomyelitis, necrosis, and deformities are sequela to the disease process. At any point, the infection can proceed to a septicemia and become life threatening. While mildly affected animals may continue to feed, most will become anorectic. The predisposing factors should be identified and eliminated. In mild cases, this may result in the recovery of the patient. The animal's environmental temperature should be kept at the upper end of the preferred optimum temperature zone (POTZ) for the affected species. A deep culture of the affected tissues should be obtained along with a thorough curettage of necrotic tissue. The infected area should be lavaged daily with chlorhexidine or dilute povidone iodine solutions. Topical antibiotic preparations are occasionally prescribed for treating the oral lesions. Finally, systemic antibiotics, based on antibiotic sensitivity results, should be administered.

In lizards, particularly iguanas, gingival proliferation commonly occurs. The proliferative gingival tissue may become so enlarged that it is easily traumatized. Affected lizards often have mild malocclusion, which leads to chronic trauma to the gingiva by the opposing teeth. Histopathology of gingival tissue generally reveals chronic, proliferative, heterophilic inflammation with bacterial colonization. A variety of bacterial isolates may be through culture of the suspect area. Treatment of the acute oral infection involves topical and systemic antimicrobial therapy. Long-term usage of oral antiseptic rinses such as chlorhexidine or zinc ascorbate may be useful in treating lizard infectious stomatitis cases. In some patients, electrosurgical or laser resection of the proliferative tissue is required. Chameleons sometimes develop a syndrome similar to that in snakes.

Opportunistic bacterial infections can occur in the stomach, liver, intestines, and cloaca. The patient will have clinical signs associated with the site of infection, therefore determining a definitive diagnosis become more difficult. However, treatment using systemic antimicrobial therapy is indicated when there is evidence of a generalized systemic infection.

Parasitic Diseases

Intestinal parasitism remains a very common problem in reptiles. While most parasite infestations are subclinical, occasionally diarrhea, anemia, or other clinical signs are encountered. *Entamoeba invadens* is one of the more serious parasites of lizards and snakes while chelonians are occasionally subclinical carriers. From time to time this disease can take on enzootic properties. Treatment with metronidazole is usually effective. *Strongyloides* parasites are commonly found but usually are incidental. Severe infestations can cause weight loss, unthriftiness, and immunosuppression. Treatment with fenbendazole or ivermectin is usually effective; however, ivermectin should not be used in chelonians (turtles, tortoises, or terrapins) because of potentially fatal side effects.

COCCIDIOSIS. Coccidia may be present in a variety of reptile species. However, coccidia (*Isospora amphiboluri*) are very common and persistent parasites in bearded dragons. The presence of disease is variable, but when present, diarrhea, weight loss, and dehydration represent the major clinical signs observed. Rarely, systemic disease will develop from an a primary coccidia infection.[68,69] The oocysts are readily identified on fecal flotation. Treatment using sulfonamides (trimethoprim sulfamethoxazole: 25 mg/kg, orally [PO], once daily for 5 d) or ponazuril (20 mg/kg, PO, once daily for 5 d) is indicated if clinical signs of coccidiosis are present. Ponazuril is preferred because it is coccidiocidal, while the sulfonamides are coccidiostatic.

CRYPTOSPORIDIOSIS. *Cryptosporidium* represents a genus of coccidians that have been found to cause significant disease in a wide range of both wild and captive reptile species. Although avian and mammalian prey species for the reptiles may have *Cryptosporidium* spp. parasites, it does not appear that snakes (or other reptiles) are infected through prey consumption. The mammalian and avian parasite oocysts, however, do pass through into the reptile feces.[70] Cryptosporidiosis (*Cryptosporidium serpentis*) in snakes frequently causes a specific disease condition of gastric hypertrophic inflammation.[71] Weight loss, regurgitation, and a midbody lump characterize the classic form of cryptosporidiosis. Enteritis may be a part of the clinical disease process and can occasionally occur without the gastritis.[72] In some cases, the parasites may enter the biliary tree.[73]

In lizards, proliferative enteritis is the prevalent pathology, although gastritis may occur as well.[74,75] The disease (*Cryptosporidium varanii, Cryptosporidium saurophilum*) is very common in leopard geckos (*Eublepharis macularius*) and savannah monitor lizards (*Varanus exanthematicus*), with affected animals presenting for weight loss, anorexia, lethargy, and diarrhea. Affected lizard collections will have a high

oocyst shedding rate.[76] In severe cases, cloacal or rectal prolapses can occur.[77] An unusual syndrome of aural-pharyngeal polyps associated with *Cryptosporidium* spp. has been reported in green iguanas.[78]

Although less susceptible than squamates, chelonians can also be affected by *Cryptosporidium* spp. Gastrointestinal pathology appears similar to that found in lizards and snakes.[79] Diagnosis of the disease is based on identification of the parasite. The organisms can be found in gastric lavages or feces but are difficult to recognize. Acid-fast staining of the sample will highlight the organisms, as they will stain bright red. While the finding of the acid-fast organisms should be considered supportive evidence of infection, a negative test will not rule out the disease.[80] Alternatively, PCR testing may be used to detect the organism in fecal or tissue samples.[81]

Although considered a zoonotic disease, there is evidence that reptilian isolates are not highly infective to mammals and vice versa.[82,83] Treatment of infected animals is often considered ineffective, but therapeutic responses have been reported with the use of trimethoprim sulfa, paromomycin, nitazoxanide, and spiramycin.[84] It is important to note that in many cases, these drugs appear to suppress rather than eliminate the parasite. A wide variety of other drugs and biologic treatments such as hyperimmune bovine colostrum have been reported to have some degree of success as well.[71,85,86] Unfortunately, some of the novel treatment options are not commercially available and provide inconsistent results.

Noninfectious Diseases

FOREIGN BODIES. Impactions of the GI tract are common in reptiles maintained on particulate substrates. These animals will exhibit signs of obstruction including anorexia, abdominal pain, vomiting, or weight loss. Radiography with or without contrast media will usually provide a diagnosis. Occasionally small undigestible particles will pass through the digestive tract after the administration of psyllium or mineral oil laxatives. Complete obstructions or large foreign bodies will require surgery for removal.

GASTRIC NEUROENDOCRINE CARCINOMA. Gastric neuroendocrine carcinoma is an emerging disease syndrome of bearded dragons.[87] The disease typically affects young adult bearded dragons and is rapidly progressive and is usually metastatic at the time of diagnosis. Affected lizards exhibit anorexia and weight loss. Pale mucus membranes may be identified in affected animals which is usually an indication of an anemic condition. A plasma chemistry panel may reveal severe hyperglycemia, possibly due to somatostatin release by the tumor cells.[88] Radiographic images will often be unrewarding in contributing to a diagnosis. Ultrasound may show the primary or metastatic tumors. Gastric endoscopy will provide a means to identify a tissue mass in the stomach (Figure 5-7); however, mucosal biopsies may not be adequate for a definative diagnosis. Histopathology of a deep section of the tumor is required for diagnosis. At present, no successful treatment of this disease has been reported.

Birds

Birds with localized GI disease frequently will display clinical signs before the onset of generalized GI or systemic disease. Additionally, if there is close contact between the bird and owner, there is an increased chance for earlier disease

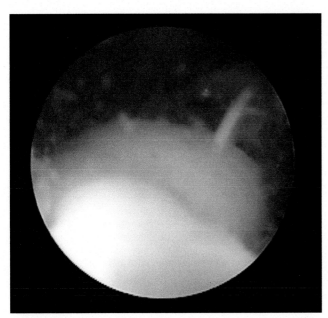

FIGURE 5-7 Endoscopic view of the stomach of a bearded dragon with a gastric neuroendocrine carcinoma. Note the soft tissue mound in the foreground. There is debris floating in the saline medium used to insufflate the stomach. Endoscopic biopsy showed only lymphocytic inflammation, but necropsy confirmed diagnosis.

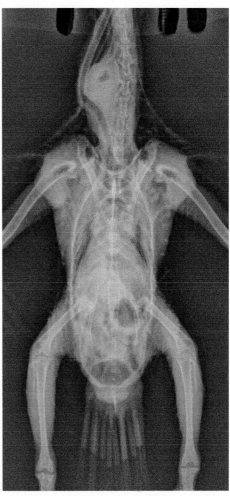

FIGURE 5-8 Radiograph of a young cockatoo with a periesophageal granuloma. The breeder had apparently punctured the esophagus and deposited food under the skin. Note the gas-distended proventriculus, ventriculus, and cloaca. Severe leukocytosis and monocytosis were found on the CBC. The bird responded well to surgical debridement, antimicrobials, and supportive care.

recognition. Consequently, the disease process may exhibit distinct clinical signs attributable to the site that is affected. A thorough history and physical examination may allow the disease to be localized. Table 5-4 lists clinical signs, diagnostics, and differential diagnoses for various areas of the digestive system in birds.

Disorders of the oral cavity are commonly encountered in pet bird practice and wildlife rehabilitation facilities. Lesions are often observed in the oral cavity during physical examination. Hyperemia, increased mucus production, caseous plaques, swollen salivary glands, and other lesions are commonly observed when disease is affecting the oral cavity of a bird. Other clinical disease signs attributable to the avian oral cavity include dysphagia, yawning, head shaking, food adhering to the oral mucosa, or exudate at the corners of the mouth. The head may be extended during swallowing as a result of pain. The differential diagnoses for diseases of the oral cavity include candidiasis, trichomoniasis, *Capillaria*, pox, Gram-negative infections, *Helicobacter*, hypovitaminosis A, trauma, oral papillomas, and neoplasia.

The crop and esophagus are affected by many of the same conditions as the oral cavity. When these areas are diseased, several clinical signs may result: regurgitation, fluctuant crop, matted head feathers (referred to by breeders as head sweating), sour breath odor (sour crop), stasis of the crop, decreased contractions, or fistulas at the thoracic inlet. The crop and esophageal disease conditions that may cause clinical signs include Gram-negative bacterial infections, candidiasis, trichomoniasis, papillomatosis, thermal burns, trauma, foreign bodies, extraluminal obstruction (e.g., goiter, neoplasia), functional ileus, and ingluvioliths (Figure 5-8). Occasionally, the

clinical signs observed may originate from disease farther down the digestive tract.

The two parts of the stomach, the proventriculus and ventriculus, is where significant digestion of the ingested food commences. When the avian stomach not function properly, the consequences are very serious. The clinical signs that may be noted with gastric disease are true vomiting (pH < 5), regurgitation, crop stasis, weight loss, passage of whole grains, diarrhea, and melena. Disorders that affect the proventriculus and/or the ventriculus include proventricular dilatation disease (PDD), neoplasia, *Macrorhabdus ornithogaster*, mycobacteriosis, candidiasis, papillomatosis, foreign bodies, functional ileus (e.g., sepsis, lead toxicosis), Gram-negative infections, and parasites (e.g., *Capillaria*).

Diarrhea is the primary clinical sign associated with intestinal disease. It should be noted that what an owner refers to as diarrhea may be polyuria. Diarrhea is much less common than polyuria and involves increased water content and a

TABLE 5-4

Clinical Signs, Diagnostics, and Differential Disease Diagnoses by Anatomic Site in Birds

Site	Clinical Signs	Diagnostics	Differentials
Oropharynx	Mouth pain (neck stretching, head shaking, yawning, dysphagia, anorexia) Visible lesions (exudates, plaques, swollen salivary glands, hyperemia) Hypersalivation Halitosis	Visual examination Oral swabs (cytology, microbiology, PCR, etc.) Endoscopy Biopsy	Candidiasis Trichomoniasis Pox *Helicobacter* Gram-negative infection Hypovitaminosis A Papillomatosis Capillariasis
Esophagus	Regurgitation Sour breath odor	Esophageal swab Esophagoscopy Radiography Contrast radiography Endoscopy	Gram-negative infection Candidiasis Trichomoniasis Capillariasis Esophageal burns Ingluviolith
Crop	Regurgitation Fluctuant crop Matted head feathers Sour breath odor Crop stasis Reduced contractions Fistulae	Crop wash Crop swab Crop aspirate Radiography Contrast radiography Ingluvioscopy	Gram-negative infections Candidiasis Trichomoniasis Capillariasis Crop burns Crop fistulas Ingluviolith
Proventriculus/ventriculus	Vomiting (pH <5) Regurgitation Crop stasis Weight loss Passing whole grains Diarrhea Melena Proventricular enlargement	Radiography Contrast radiography Feces Proventricular washes Endoscopic samples Crop biopsy Proventricular biopsy Ventricular biopsy	Proventricular dilatation disease Impaction/foreign bodies Candidiasis *Macrorhabdus* Neoplasia Capillariasis, ascariasis Mycobacteria Heavy metal intoxication
Intestine/ceca	Diarrhea Pasting of the vent Mucus in stool Melena Hematochezia Abdominal pain Fecal odor	Feces Radiography Contrast radiography	Gram-negative infections Candidiasis Mycobacteriosis Giardiasis Ascariasis *Campylobacter* Clostridial enteritis Coccidiosis Intussusception
Cloaca	Tenesmus Hematochezia Protruding tissue Fecal odor	Feces Cloacal swab Cloacoscopy Radiography	Papillomatosis Prolapse Cloacalith Gram-negative infection *Clostridium*
Liver	Vague signs Biliverdinuria Abdominal distension Diarrhea Weight loss	AST, GGT, GLDH Bile acids Radiography Ultrasound CT Hepatic biopsy	Hepatitis (*Chlamydophila, Mycobacterium*, viral, opportunistic, etc.) Hepatic lipidosis Hemochromatosis Aflatoxicosis
Pancreas	Shock Diarrhea Abdominal pain Vomiting Polyuria Lipemia Amylorrhea Sudden death	Amylase Fecal iodine test Hematology Biopsy	Pancreatitis Pacheco's disease Neoplasia Exocrine insufficiency

AST, Aspartate transaminase; *CT*, computed tomography; *GGT*, gamma-glutamyltransferase; *GLDH*, glutamyl dehydrogenase; *PCR*, polymerase chain reaction.

lack of form to the fecal portion of the dropping. Other clinical signs associated with intestinal disease are "pasting of the vent," mucus-laden stools, melena, hematochezia (frank blood), or abdominal pain. There are many diseases that can affect the intestinal tract of birds, including Gram-negative bacterial infections (e.g., *Salmonella*), *Clostridium*, *Campylobacter*, *Chlamydophila*, *Giardia*, *Hexamita*, coccidia, candidiasis, mycobacteriosis, intussusception, and ileus.

The ceca are not present in most of the birds that are presented to a pet bird practice; however, chickens and other fowl are being treated with increasing regularity and cecal disease may be seen in these species. Any disease that affects the intestine can also affect the ceca. Additionally, lesions may be identified with cecal coccidia, *Heterakis gallinarum* (cecal worm), or other diseases.

The cloaca is the common terminus of the interstinal, urinary, and reproductive tracts for three systems and can be affected by problems associated with anyone of these body systems. Cloacal disease is often associated with clinical signs of tenesmus, frank blood in (or on) the droppings, a strong fecal odor, tissue protruding from the cloacal orifice, or infertility. Subclinical cloacal disease may be detected during physical examination when the cloaca is everted and the mucosa is examined. The normal cloacal mucosa should be smooth, although there are longitudinal folds around the orifice known as columns. Cloacal diseases include cloacal papillomas, cloacal prolapse, cloacalithiasis, cloacitis (Gram-negative, anaerobes), or paresis (neurologic).

Disease conditions of the liver are a relatively common occurrence in pet birds. Signs of liver disease (hepatosis) often predominate in multisystemic disease because the liver has so many important functions. There are many types of liver disease in birds, but most can be placed into five categories: infectious, metabolic, toxic, neoplastic, and congenital. The signs associated with liver disease can be varied. The liver serves an important function as a digestive organ and is very important in the breakdown of certain nutrients, most notably, fats. If these fats remain undigested, diarrhea and steatorrhea may result. Affected birds are deprived of this high caloric nutrient and may become cachexic. The liver is also responsible for detoxifying and excreting many endogenous and exogenous toxins and waste products. Liver failure can lead to the systemic increase of these toxic substances. One of the endogenous waste products that can increase in the face of liver dysfunction is biliverdin, a green pigment formed through the degradation of red blood cells. Unlike mammals, birds and reptiles lack biliverdin reductase and cannot form bilirubin. When biliverdin levels increase within the body, renal excretion of the pigment through the urine, results in green, watery urine that is often observed in patients with liver disease. Many blood proteins are manufactured in the liver, and hypoproteinemia may occur with liver failure. Since the blood proteins are responsible for maintaining vascular osmotic pressure, excessively low protein levels may lead to fluid leakage into the body cavity (e.g., ascites). This, along with the large size of the diseased liver, may give the appearance of a "potbelly". Some of the proteins in the blood are also responsible for hemostasis consequently low protein levels may cause delayed blood clotting, although this appears to be rare. A pathophysiologic explanation for some of the signs of liver disease have not been identified. For instance, some birds with liver disease will develop overgrown beaks. The beak may be discolored and have keratin defects as well. Very often, birds are presented with "sick bird syndrome" but with no specific clinical signs to indicate the nature of the disease. The clinician depends on a thorough history, physical examination, and diagnostic workup to discover and identify the problem. Diseases that affect the avian liver include Pacheco's disease, *Chlamydia psittaci*, mycobacteriosis, other forms of hepatitis, toxins, hepatic lipidosis, hemochromatosis, neoplasia, and chronic fibrosis.

Pancreatic disease usually results in nonspecific clinical signs of malaise, anorexia, and weight loss. However, occasionally more specific signs including vomiting and amylorrhea may be encountered. In pancreatic exocrine insufficiency, polyphagia, weight loss, and amylorrhea evidenced by pale, bulky droppings may be encountered.[89] Diseases affecting the pancreas include acute or chronic pancreatitis, pancreatic necrosis, pancreatic exocrine insufficiency, or pancreatic neoplasia.

Viral Diseases

AVIAN POX. There are nearly as many poxviruses as there are bird orders, but most are similar in the disease processes that they produce. Small papules that progress to plaques which are deeply rooted in the mucosa and submucosa develop in the oral cavity and upper respiratory tract. When these lesions are scraped, significant bleeding may occur. In some cases the lesions may be localized to the skin. Over time, the affected areas progress to scabs and then scars, which may disfigure the area and predispose the bird to repeated infections. A septicemic form of the disease can occur and seems to be particularly common in canaries. In many cases avian pox can be diagnosed through cytologic examination of samples collected from lesions. Proliferation of epithelial cells with ballooning degeneration and large eosinophilic, intracytoplasmic inclusions called Bollinger bodies is diagnostic for avian pox.[90] Biopsy may be more definitive if typical cells are not identified through cytological evaluation. Treatment is supportive and vitamin. A supplementation may be beneficial in supporting the health and recovery of the infected oral epithelium. Antibiotic therapy may be useful in preventing secondary infections. Survivors often gain a lifetime immunity to avian pox. There are commercial vaccines available, and they are generally effective across different bird orders. Since the virus cannot penetrate intact skin or mucous membranes, controlling biting insects and preventing trauma can significantly reduce disease exposure.

PAPILLOMATOSIS. Papillomatosis or internal papillomatous disease is a common disorder in companion avian practice. The disease is characterized by proliferative tissue on the surfaces of the oral cavity, esophagus, crop, proventriculus, or cloaca.[91] The lesions may appear as a mass with a roughened surface or simply a granular appearance to the mucosa. The application of 5% acetic acid to the mucosa enhances visualization of the papillomatous tissue.[92] Papillomas of the cloaca are most common, but other areas of the digestive tract, including the oral cavity, should be examined. There is also an association between papillomas and neoplasias of the liver and pancreas, particularly in *Amazona* spp.[93] In some cases, cloacal carcinoma may result from a malignant transformation of these lesions.[94] Papillomatosis has only been reported in

New World psittacines. There are some definite species predilections for avian papillomatosis with the most common pet birds diagnosed being the macaws (especially green wings), hawk-headed parrots, and Amazon parrots.[92] The etiologic agent has been proposed to be a herpesvirus and the disease appears to be transmissible.[95] Frequently *Escherichia coli* or other Gram-negative bacteria are cultured from the affected site as secondary pathogens.[92] The clinical disease signs depend on the anatomic site affected. Dyspnea or wheezing may occur with papillomas on the glottis or within the choanal slit, while tenesmus and possible infertility can occur with cloacal papillomas, which are often subclinical. Treatment involves various techniques for surgical removal including electrosurgery, cryosurgery, laser surgery, or chemical cautery (silver nitrate sticks). The proliferative tissue is carefully "shaved" off the mucosa with the selected surgical technique.[92] Vinegar may be applied to help distinguish the diseased from the normal tissue. The resection may have to be performed in stages with severe cases. Significant bleeding may occur and can be minimized by the application of barium suspension to the mucosa. Mucosal stripping has been used for severe lesions but may be associated with increased morbidity.[96] With chemical cautery, silver nitrate sticks are rolled over the affected tissue after which the affected area is rinsed thoroughly with saline. The chemical cautery technique may have to be repeated several times at weekly intervals but has the advantage of being the least likely to cause strictures. The size of the papilloma and associated inflammation can be reduced by the application of a commercial hemorrhoid cream for a few days prior to surgery. If the papilloma is in the oral cavity, the patient should be intubated to prevent aspiration of blood (barium should not be used in the mouth). Recurrence of the papilloma is common following surgery. Antibiotics should be used to control secondary infections. Some clinicians feel that autogenous vaccines prepared from samples of tissue from the papilloma will reduce the recurrence of this problem, while others claim that improving husbandry, nutrition, and treating secondary infections may obviate the need for surgery.[92] Most recommend that surgery should be performed only on cases where clinical signs are present or with that have small lesions that can be completely excised.[92]

PROVENTRICULAR DILATATION DISEASE. Originally called macaw wasting disease, PDD was initially recognized only in macaws, but from there, the list of affected species expanded to include most psittacine species and many non-psittacine birds.[97] Interestingly, it has not been reported in the budgerigar.[97] It usually affects young adults in multiple bird households but can be seen in babies, older adults, and even in single pets (due to the very long incubation). In an aviary, it can occur as sporadic cases or involve many birds. At its most basic level, the disease involves inflammation of certain nerves (splanchnic ganglion neuropathy). The nerves most commonly affected are those supplying the proventriculus (glandular stomach) and ventriculus (gizzard or muscular stomach). The effect is a general neuromuscular dysfunction of part are the majority of the GI tract. The end result is that the proventriculus dilates and becomes very enlarged. Once food starts to accumulate in these dysfunctional organs, that is when clinical signs develop and include weight loss, regurgitation, and passage of undigested seeds or other food. Occasionally, other nerves become affected and cause a variety of

neurological signs (e.g., incoordination, head tilt) develop. Ocular lesions, such as choroiditis and optic neuritis, have also been described in birds diagnosed with PDD.[98]

An avian bornavirus,[97,98] appears to be involved in the disease process associated with PDD and is considered a very unstable virus within the environment. The incubation period can be extremely long, and affected birds may shed virus for years before succumbing to the disease. Many clinically normal birds test positive for bornavirus, so it is thought that other factors may be involved in the development of disease. There is some evidence that in addition to the bornavirus infection, autoimmune responses may play a role in the development of some PDD cases.[98]

Diagnosis of the disease is based on clinical signs, characteristic appearance of GI changes on radiographs, and biopsy of affected areas. Most other clinical data are of little value. Occasionally, a mild anemia, hypoproteinemia, or elevated creatine kinase (CK) will occur with PDD. The radiographic appearance of the proventriculus varies with species, age, and feeding but is normally spindle shaped in adult, fasted psittacine birds. On ventro-dorsal views, the left border is roughly even with the left lateral border of the liver (if the liver is of normal size). On lateral views, the proventriculus curves smoothly into the ventriculus. Gas is never present in normal birds with the exception of dyspneic or extremely fractious individuals in which aerophagia may occur. The presence of gas, enlargement of the proventriculus, or changes in shape or position are common radiographic signs diagnosed with PDD (Figure 5-9). Barium administration is recommended to better delineate the proventriculus and to detect masses, foreign bodies, or other luminal defects that can mimic PDD. Confirmation of PDD can be accomplished only through biopsy of affected GI organs. Biopsy samples of the proventriculus, ventriculus, crop, adrenal gland, or even cloaca can be submitted for histopathologic examination. Mucosal biopsies obtained by endoscopy are nondiagnostic since the lesions are in the muscular tunic. Full-thickness proventricular biopsies are recommended in most of the older references, but collection of these samples is associated with very high

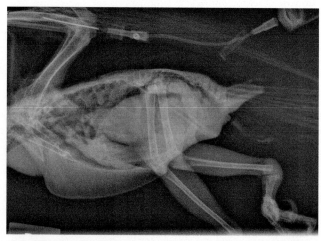

FIGURE 5-9 Lateral view of a macaw with proventricular dilatation disease. This bird presented in critical condition and has an intraosseous catheter in place.

complication and mortality rates. Ventricular biopsies provide only a slightly reduced risk to the patient when collected. Crop biopsies are very low-risk procedures, making this a preferred diagnostic procedure. Approximately 70% to 90% of affected birds have crop lesions. The biopsies must include ganglia, therefore full-thickness samples are required. The nerves follow the vasculature consequently collected samples should include visible vessels. Proventricular dilatation disease is a segmental disease, therefore random biopsy samples may provide false-negative results. Proper selection of the surgical site and the collection of multiple biopsy sections can improve the sensitivity of crop biopsies.[97]

There is no cure for PDD. However, the length and quality of the patient's life expectancy can be improved by supportive and dietary management. Initial treatment often involves removal of accumulated food using careful gastric lavage and prescribing easily digested foods. The care for birds diagnosed with PDD is time consuming and expensive. The use of celecoxib, a cyclooxygenase-2 (COX-2) selective nonsteroidal anti-inflammatory drug (NSAID) (and possibly other COX-2 selective NSAIDs), has been reported to suppress clinical signs and reduce pathologic changes associated with the disease.[99] The status of viral shedding and contagion is assumed to be unchanged. Tepoxalin, a combined COX-1, COX-2, and 5-lipoxygenase (LOX) inhibitor, may have improved effects when compared to celecoxib.[97] It is important to note that clinical response to NSAID treatment in birds diagnosed with PDD is extremely inconsistent. The addition of amantadine hydrochloride may improve therapeutic success for PDD, especially when neurologic involvement occurs.[97] Metoclopramide can be a useful adjunct therapy in severe cases of PDD.[97]

Prevention of PDD in the individual bird or aviary is difficult. Since much is not know about the epidemiology of PDD, only general management guidelines recommended. First, maintain flocks of birds in complete isolation from other birds. Second, follow strict sanitation procedures. Third, control pests. Last, seek rapid veterinary care for any bird showing signs of illness to obtain a rapid diagnosis so that affected birds can be identified and isolated.

PACHECO'S DISEASE. Pacheco's disease is a severe, acute, systemic disease of psittacine birds caused by a herpesvirus.[100] The liver is among the most severely affected organs. In most cases, the affected birds are found dead with no prior clinical signs. In the rare cases in which infected birds are presented alive, severe depression, yellowish or greenish urates, and physiologic shock are typically observed. Heterophilia or heteropenia are hematologic abnormalities associated with Pacheco's disease. However many of these birds usually die within a matter of hours. Gross necropsy findings often include an enlarged, congested liver and spleen. Histopathology is required for definitive diagnosis. Pacheco's disease is generally diagnosed in aviaries, often following the introduction of new birds. While conures are frequently implicated as carriers, any psittacine can be a potential carrier. During an outbreak, acyclovir can be administered to exposed birds to prevent the onset of disease.[100] In rare cases, even birds with early clinical signs can be saved by treating with acyclovir and supportive care; however, it is important to recognize that the acyclovir may only limit viral replication and not be virucidal.[101]

Other Viral Liver Diseases

Most viral hepatitides are sporadically diagnosed post mortem. Adenovirus, reovirus, polyomavirus, coronavirus, and avian serositis virus can all cause liver lesions. The liver lesions may be disease specific or develop as part of a systemic process.

Bacterial Diseases

AVIAN MYCOBACTERIOSIS. Avian mycobarterioisis is caused by a bacterium in the genus *Mycobacterium*. Several species may be involved, including *Mycobacterium genavense* and *Mycobacterium avium*.[102] These organisms are similar to the organism that causes human tuberculosis, *Mycobacterium tuberculosis*. In fact, the avian isolates can cause disease in humans under optimum circumstances (e.g., immune suppression), and birds can become infected with *M. tuberculosis* from infected humans. Mycobacteria are different and may be considered more pathogenic than other bacterial infections because of their ability to avoid the body's defenses. When infected with mycobacteria, the body's immune system is stimulated, often causing extremely high white blood cell counts. Unfortunately, the bacteria hide inside the host cells and cannot be readily destroyed by the white blood cells. Consequently, the body attempts to "wall off" the infection, resulting in a granuloma. Hundreds or thousands of these granulomas may form resulting in tremendous stress to the body. To complicate the disease process, the granulomas in birds are primarily in the intestines and the liver (unlike in humans, where it is a lung disease), resulting in poor absorption of nutrients. Birds become very emaciated with this disease. Weight loss despite a good appetite, chronic diarrhea, lethargy, and a poor appearance are the typical clinical signs observed in birds infected with avian mycobacteriosis. Skin lesions are occasionally seen as well. Mycobacteriosis is most often diagnosed in birds with access to soil. The organism is ubiquitous in the soil and is resistant to many disinfectants. As a result, a majority of avian mycobacteriosis cases are diagnosed in wild-caught birds, although this disease can be seen in any avian species, wild caught or captive born. Immune suppression is thought to occur in many cases. Psittacine birds appear quite susceptible and therefore should not be housed with ground-feeding birds or in aviaries with dirt floors. Although not as highly contagious as human tuberculosis, avian mycobacteriosis is easily propagated under these conditions. Infected birds shed *Mycobacterium* spp. primarily in the feces. The bird may be exposed by eating something contaminated with the organism. Aerosol transmission does not seem to be an important method of infection. Since this is a very chronic disease, clinical signs may take months to years to develop.

Diagnosis of avian mycobacteriosis may involve blood testing (e.g., CBC, biochemistries, protein electrophoresis), plain or contrast radiographs, fecal acid-fast stains, molecular testing (e.g., PCR), or even biopsies (especially liver biopsies). Birds infected with *Mycobacterium* often have extremely high white blood cell counts (>100,000 cells/μL), with a mature heterophilia and monocytosis. Reactive lymphocytosis may occur in some cases.[103] An individual avian patient's response to an avian mycobacteriosis infection is extremely variable, consequently, the absence of such findings cannot rule out the disease. Signs of liver disease, such as elevated aspartate transaminase (AST) or bile acids, may also occur.[103] Radiographs

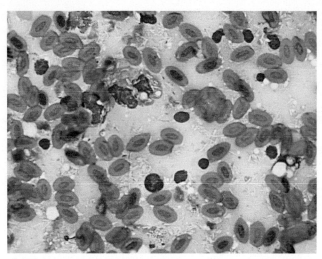

FIGURE 5-10 Impression smear of a mycobacterial granuloma. The mycobacteria resist stain uptake with Wright's stains and appear as clear "ghost-like" rods. Staining with an acid-fast stain confirmed these as acid-fast bacteria.

may reveal dilated or thickened bowel loops, hepatomegaly, splenomegaly, granulomas in the lungs, or GI filling defects (barium study). Lytic bony lesions may also be seen.[103] Diagnosis of mycobacteriosis requires demonstration of acid-fast rods and PCR-positive test results. The pathogenic bacterial organisms may be observed in fecal samples, cytologic specimens, biopsies (liver, skin, intestine), or at necropsy. The initial identification of nonstaining, clear, ghost-like rods on routine cytologic staining (Figure 5-10) may provide evidence of a tentative diagnosis of avian mycobacteriosis. Skin reaction tests and serologic tests are not reliable in birds. The probability for identification of mycobacteria in blood, feces, or tissue samples can be improved using PCR amplification of genus- or species-specific DNA segments.[103] However, since organisms are shed intermittently and have multifocal distribution, there are currently no tests that can definitively determine if a bird is free of the disease or not. Pooling fecal samples over 1 week is recommended to increase the overall sensitivity of testing.

Treatment of infected birds is not usually recommended because of the difficulty of treatment compliance and the real but minimal human health risk. For larger bird collections, quarantine of all exposed birds and complete disinfection of premises are often the only options for controlling the disease. Frequently, only sporadic disease is present when mycobacteriosis is diagnosed within an aviary. Occasionally, an individual bird can be treated with antibiotic cocktail over the course of months to years. Owners must be aware of the potential zoonotic risk and be prepared for a long course of treatment with extensive follow-up. Clinical, hematologic, and microbiologic data are used to determine when treatment can be discontinued. Ethambutol, cycloserine, clofazimine, clarithromycin, rifabutin, aminoglycosides, and fluoroquinolones are among the drugs used to treat avian mycobacteriosis. The costs, duration, and public health risks of treatment must be carefully weighed against the financial and emotional attachment to the bird.[104]

Control of this disease in aviculture is accomplished by following strict sanitation, not combining different avian species (particularly, ground birds with psittacines), prevent bird contact with the ground in aviaries, and having medical workups performed on all birds entering the facility. Since the immune status of the bird may play a role in the course of the disease, quality nutrition and stress reduction are important management recommendations for prevention.

GRAM-NEGATIVE PHARYNGITIS, INGLUVITIS, AND ENTERITIS. Gram-negative infections are usually considered opportunistic infections caused by ubiquitous environmental bacteria. Poor sanitation or stressors that suppress immune function are the usual predisposing factors to avian Gram-negative GI infections. Although these organisms may not be primary pathogens, many of these Gram-negative bacteria cause extremely purulent or erosive disease, while others (e.g. *Salmonella* spp.) are associated with granulomatous lesions. The clinical signs observed in birds will depend on the location of the infection within the GI tract but may include erythema in the oral cavity, regurgitation, crop stasis, and diarrhea. The proventriculus and ventriculus appear to be more resistant to infection from Gram-negative bacteria due to the low pH within the lumen of these organs.

Diagnosis can be difficult to confirm, and in many cases, a response to therapy is the only indication of a GI tract bacterial infection. Suspicion of a GI tract Gram-negative bacterial infection is often first considered based on finding a high number of Gram-negative bacteria identified in a cytologic sample (e.g., Gram stain) collected from a bird with clinical signs. Cytologic evidence (e.g., Diff-Quik stain) of inflammation (e.g., heterophils, lymphocytes, and monocytes) can add supportive evidence that the avian patient has a GI tract bacterial infection. A bacterial culture and antibiotic sensitivity profile can be used to identify the pathogenic organism and to help select an appropriate treatment protocol. PCR diagnostic testing is also available to identify certain pathogenic bacteria, such as *Salmonella* spp. Treatment for bacterial gastroenteritis includes the use of appropriate antibiotics and supportive care. Probiotics may be administered as an adjunct therapy. Sanitation should be addressed to avoid reinfection. Treatment of subclinical Gram-negative infections is controversial. Antibiotics should be avoided unless the level of organisms present is very high or the organism has a high potential for causing disease. Sanitation, probiotics, stress management, and other measures may be used successfully in these cases.

BACTERIAL HEPATITIS. Nearly any bacteria can cause hepatitis if the liver is exposed. Gram-negative bacteria predominate in these cases. The bacteria can come from the intestinal tract via the biliary ducts or the portal vein. Therefore any bacterial enteritis can potentially lead to hepatitis. Moreover hepatitis is often a significant part of septicemic conditions. The clinical course for bacterial hepatitis can vary. In acute cases, the signs can be very severe, while milder signs may predominate in chronic cases. Bacterial hepatitis may induce a moderate to high elevation of the white blood count, with a heterophilia, as well as hepatomegaly, elevated AST, and elevated bile acids. A diagnosis can be confirmed with a liver biopsy and subsequent histopathological evaluation of the collected sample, bacterial culture, and an antibiotic sensitivity profile. Treatment with antibiotics is usually effective.

Enrofloxacin is the drug of choice when culture results are not available because of the bacterial susceptibly to this drug and its excellent tissue penetration into the hepatic tissue. Duration of therapy will be based on the resolution of clinical signs, radiographic changes, and hematologic abnormalities.

PSEUDOTUBERCULOSIS. Although not common in the United States, infections with *Yersinia pseudotuberculosis* are common causes of morbidity and mortality in small psittacines and passerines from Europe and Australia.[105] Infected rodents and wild birds can serve as the source of infection for pet birds. Diarrhea, general malaise, and pneumonia are present in infected birds and the mortality rate is high in diseased birds. Pathologic findings in affected birds include granulomas throughout the GI tract, liver, and body. Bacterial cultures are required to identify the organism. Treatment with disinfectants (e.g., chlorhexidine), in the drinking water may slow transmission within a flock.[105] Rodent control and restricting contact with wild birds are also necessary to control and prevent this disease.

HELICOBACTER *PHARYNGITIS.* Pharyngitis caused by spiral-shaped bacteria, now classified as *Helicobacter* spp., has been diagnosed in small psittacines. Early references described a spiral-shaped bacterium, sometimes associated with upper respiratory signs.[106,107] The organism appears to reside in the palatine salivary glands.[108] Most cases involve cockatiels (*Nymphicus hollandicus*) and lovebirds (*Agapornis* spp.), although (rarely) other psittacines may also be affected. Hyperemia of the pharyngeal mucosa is the most prevalent sign in affected birds, with the pharynx exhibiting a bright, scarlet red color. Increased mucus in the pharynx may also be observed. Signs of oral pain, including head shaking, excessive yawning, dysphagia, and retching, may be observed in diseased animals.[109] Occasionally, infected birds will also have nasal discharge. Unrelated concurrent abnormal physical examination findings are common, possibly suggesting that immune compromise may be a part of this disease condition. Diagnosis is made based on finding spiral-shaped Gram-negative bacterial organisms on Gram-stained pharyngeal swabs (Figure 5-11).

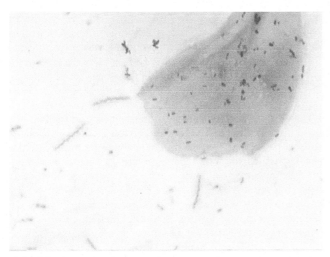

FIGURE 5-11 *Helicobacter* spp. in the choanal swab of a cockatiel. This organism inhabits the salivary glands and causes mild to moderate pathology and discomfort.

PCR testing may be performed to further confirm the presence of this organism. There are generally no hematologic changes observed in birds infected with *Helicobacter* spp.The disease, while apparently uncomfortable, is not usually life threatening. Treatment with oral doxycycline or enrofloxacin is generally successful.

Clostridium spp. Clostridial organisms can cause severe necrotizing enteritis or cloacitis. Alternatively, a mild enteritis or cloacitis may be present. There is often a very strong odor to the feces noted in birds with clostridial gastroenteritis. *Clostridium perfringens* type C or *Clostridium tertium* have been implicated in most cases where anaerobic culture has been performed. Clostridial organisms produce severe toxins, often leading to shock and death. Megacolon or megacloaca may occur secondary to clostridial infections. The sporulated bacteria may be identified on fecal Gram stains. Occasionally, clostridial enteritis may occur without the typical sporulated organisms. Anaerobic cultures can be used to confirm the presence of *Clostridium* spp. With most clostridial species, the feces may be tested for the presence of toxins, but *C. tertium* produces no toxins and acts by colonization of the intestine or cloaca. This disease is unusual in psittacines, but large outbreaks have been reported. Penicillins, especially potentiated products such as amoxicillin/clavulanic acid combinations, macrolides, and metronidazole, are all possible treatment options for avian gastrointestinal clostridial infections.

CAMPYLOBACTER. *Campylobacter* spp. infections are rarely diagnosed in pet bird practice but can occasionally cause chronic diarrhea. The disease is generally mild and not life threatening, although young birds (fledglings) may succumb. Most often, finches are affected. Clinical signs often include diarrhea and amylorrhea, with high mortalities in young birds.[110] The *Campylobacter* spp. organisms are often identified on wet-mount or cytologic preparations (e.g., Gram or differential stains) of the feces. *Campylobacter* spp. have been isolated from clinically normal birds, so it is important to consider the animal's condition (i.e., no clinical signs vs. clinical signs) when interpreting the results. As this disease is contagious and potentially zoonotic, treatment is indicated in affected flocks. Treatment with macrolides or fluoroquinolones may be effective and should continue for a minimum of 3 weeks. Strict sanitation is essential to prevent reoccurrence.

AVIAN CHLAMYDIOSIS. Avian chlamydiosis is a contagious, zoonotic, systemic disease of birds. *Chlamydia psittaci* is the organism responsible for this disease. The course of chlamydophilosis depends of the strain of organism, host defenses, and species of bird, among other factors. *Chlamydia psittaci* organisms can be found and shed through fecal, urine, and respiratory secretions.[111] Humans generally contract *C. psittaci* through inhalation. Although this disease is systemic, respiratory and hepatic signs predominate.[112] The respiratory disease signs observed in birds may include serous oculonasal discharge, conjunctivitis, pneumonia, and air sacculitis. The classical description of psittacosis includes weight loss; green, watery urine (signs of liver disease); and diarrhea. The hemogram of affected birds can vary; however, many birds have an extremely high white blood cell count (>70,000 cells/μL), heterophilia, monocytosis, and mild anemia. Elevations in AST and bile acids are also common. There is considerable species variation in presentation. Neotropical psittacines often have classical signs with respiratory disease, pea green urine, and severe leukocytosis with heterophilia and monocytosis. Australian, Pacific, and Asian psittacines may develop a more chronic form of the disease. African psittacines, especially lovebirds, appear to have the most resistance and may develop a very low-grade disease from months to years without exhibiting clinical signs.

Several tests are available for chlamydia detection. The "gold standard" test is culture of the organism. Since chlamydia are obligate intracellular pathogens, isolation requires the use of tissue culture, chicken embryos, or mouse inoculation.[113] While these methods are very sensitive, only birds shedding viable chlamydia will be positive. Additionally, since shedding is intermittent and the bacteria need to survive transport to the laboratory, false negatives can occur. Fortunately, DNA-based diagnostics are available for detection of chlamydia in avian patients.[114] These tests are extremely sensitive and specific for chlamydia; however, they do require that the patient is shedding organisms at the time the swab is collected. The time delay for results (3 to 7 d) might also be a disadvantage to the clinician. When a quick diagnostic test is required, there are a number of ELISA kits that can be used to detect chlamydia-group-specific antigen. These tests were developed for detecting human venereal chlamydiosis (*Chlamydia trachomatis*), although they do cross react with *C. psittaci*. While greater amounts of the chlamydial antigen are required to produce positive test results, these tests do not require the organisms to be viable. As with other testing techniques, intermittent shedding can give false-negative results. Chlamydial organisms can also be detected by electron microscopy, immunofluorescent antibody staining, staining with Gimenez and Machiavelli, or other special staining of cytologic or histologic samples. Several serologic tests for avian chlamydiosis are available, including latex agglutination (LA), complement fixation (CF), and elementary body agglutination (EBA).[111] Serologic results provide information regarding the host's exposure to the chlamydial organism only. Latex agglutination and EBA are arguably the most useful tests for diagnostic purposes to detect infected subclinical carriers, as the titers drop more rapidly with recovery than do CF titers because they screen for the immunoglobulin M (IgM) antibodies that are produced in the acute stages of infection. These qualities allow the LA and EBA tests to be used for for monitoring a patient during treatment. Paired or multiple sera provide helpful information regarding the disease status of a patient. When screening for avian chlamydiosis in a group of birds, two or more methods should be used on a representative number of birds.

Birds identified as *C. psittaci* positive should be administered a 45-day treatment with a tetracycline antibiotic; doxycyline is the preferred drug.[111] Secondary infections with yeast (*Candida* spp.) or Gram-negative bacteria may occur with long-term tetracycline use. Biweekly rechecks of the avian patient are recommended to evaluate the animal for any potential complications with the disease or treatment. All birds in contact with the affected animal must be treated as well. Larger groups of birds can be treated with medicated (chlortetracycline or doxycycline) feed. Psittacosis is a reportable disease in many states.

Fungal Diseases

CANDIDIASIS. *Candida* yeasts (*Candida albicans*) may be present in low numbers in normal avian GI tracts. Under certain circumstances, the yeast may proliferate beyond the normal state and cause disease. Young birds, particularly before weaning, are more prone to candidiasis, most likely due to their immunocompromised state. Cockatiels appear to be particularly susceptible, and the disease develops characteristics of a primary disease in this species.[115] The consumption of sugary diets may promote yeast growth as well. Antibiotic therapy, especially if prolonged, can provide *Candida* yeasts with a competitive advantage in the gut. Whenever long-term antibiotic therapy is used, the patient should be monitored for candidiasis. In preweaned neonates, antifungal therapy should always accompany antibiotic treatment.

Candida spp. can affect the entire GI tract, with the organisms colonizing the mucosa. The yeast can interfere with normal digestion and absorption of ingesta. Typically, thick caseous lesions will occur on the mucosa of affected areas. In the oral cavity, yeast lesions frequently can be scraped off the epithelium without hemorrhage. Clinical signs associated with candidiasis in an avian patient include a thickened crop wall delayed crop emptying and/or regurgitation. If the stomach or intestine is affected, diarrhea, fecal color changes and foul-smelling droppings may be observed. Weight loss may occur from poor nutrient absorption. Diagnosis can be made by preparing a Gram stain from a swab of the lesion, crop wash, or fecal smear, depending on the affected site. The characteristic budding yeast are easily identified. There is often little or no inflammatory response associated with candidiasis lesions. Hematology is often unremarkable. An effort should be made to establish whether underlying medical conditions exist.[115]

Most of the azole antifungals are usually effective in treatment of a bird diagnosed with candidiasis. Nystatin can be administered prophylactically when antibiotics are prescribed for neonatal birds. One should remember that nystatin only works topically when contacting the organism on the mucosal surface and will not be effective if deeper invasion of tissues has occurred. Therapy may be as short as 10 days or may last months. Clinical signs and monitoring of the crop contents, mouth, and feces for yeasts should be used to determine an end point for therapy. Control of this disease revolves around sanitation, good hand feeding practices, and control of predisposing disease conditions.

AVIAN GASTRIC YEAST. This disease is caused by large, fastidious, recently characterized yeast now known as *Macrorhabdus ornithogaster* or simply as avian gastric yeast (AGY).[116] Originally called megabacteria, the organism, which had not been isolated but could be identified cytologically, was thought to be a bacterium. The infections seem to be limited to the proventriculus but other parts of the gastrointestinal tract may be infected. Globular mucinous cysts form with this pathogen, usually at the isthmus between the proventriculus and ventriculus. Clinically, weight loss and regurgitation are the most prominent feature. Vomiting, melena, or passage of whole seeds may also be observed in affected birds. The disease is commonly diagnosed, especially in smaller bird species, such as budgerigars and finches.

Diagnosis depends on finding the organisms in the feces or from samples taken directly from the crop and/or

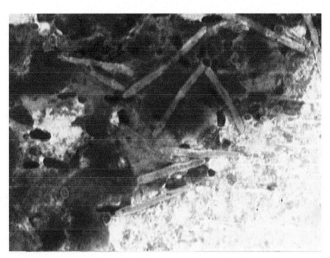

FIGURE 5-12 Proventricular impression smear from the necropsy of a budgerigar. Both *Macrorhabdus ornithogaster* and *Candida* spp. were present, along with ulceration at the isthmus.

proventriculus. On slides that have been Gram stained, these yeasts are Gram positive, while on standard differential stains, they appear "ghost-like" (Figure 5-12). *Macrorhabdus ornithogaster* can also be identified on fecal wet mounts. Avian gastric yeasts are extremely large, measuring 10 μm in width and up to 200 μm in length. The organisms can be found in some clinically "normal" birds, therefore host factors are apparently important in the formation of disease. PCR tests for *Macrorhabdus* DNA are also available. Finding typical proventricular filling defects, using contrast radiography, in commonly affected species may give a presumptive diagnosis, although gastric neoplasia must also be considered in these cases. Affected birds have elevated proventricular pH. Acidification of the drinking water has been suggested as a means of improving survival rates.[117] In one study, the administration of a bolus of *Lactobacillus* was successful in eliminating shedding of AGY.[118] The disease has been described as having high morbidity but low mortality. Oral amphotericin B is currently the most successful treatment. It appears that while amphotericin B may alleviate clinical signs and reduce shedding, it may not eliminate yeast from the stomach of all infected birds.[119] The treatment protocol involves a 30-day course of oral amphotericin B administered at an elevated dose. Care should be taken to avoid aspiration of the concentrated amphotericin suspension by the patient. The antifungal suspension is extremely irritating to the respiratory membranes and if aspirated fatal aspiration tracheitis may occur. The author uses a feeding tube to avoid aspiration of the amphotericin suspension by the patient. Research investigating the medication of drinking water with sodium benzoate show some promise in treating larger groups of birds.[120]

Parasitic Diseases

TRICHOMONIASIS. Trichomoniasis is primarily a disease of the upper GI tract of birds. Lesions are usually found in the oral cavity, esophagus, and crop. Rarely, the parasite may be identified in the respiratory tract. This disease seems to be quite common in psittacines in other countries but is rarely

diagnosed in these avian species within the United States. However trichomoniasis is most commonly found in wild birds, especially Columbiformes (pigeons and doves) and raptors (especially those that consume pigeons), in the United States. The parasite may be transmitted at garden bird feeders.[121] The gross lesions caused by this parasite are often difficult to distinguish from those caused by *Candida* spp. While the superficial lesions can often be scraped off the mucosa with little or no bleeding, there are more invasive strains that can damage the mucosa. The parasites can easily be observed in saline wet mounts of the lesions or of crop washes of affected birds. Trichomonads often dry out and are difficult to identify in stained cytologic preparations. Culture methods are more sensitive in detecting the parasites.[122] Hematologic findings vary with the degree of invasion. Treatment with metronidazole, carnidazole, or ronidazole is often effective. Infestations with milder strains of the trichamonas organism are common in pigeons, and are thought to provide a natural vaccination against more virulent strains.[123]

COCCIDIOSIS. Coccidia (*Isospora* spp. and *Eimeria* spp.) are commonly found in many types of birds, with most organisms being host specific.[124] These parasites usually have a direct life cycle. Clinical signs are most severe in very young birds and include weight loss, diarrhea, fecal-pasted vents, and occasionally death. Diagnosis is based on finding oocysts in feces using flotation techniques. Treatment with sulfonamides, amprolium, ponazuril, or toltrazuril may be effective.

CRYPTOSPORIDIUM. *Cryptosporidium* spp. are seldom diagnosed in birds. This organism is generally considered a parasite that affects birds with underlying diseases that suppress the immune system.[125,126] *Cryptosporidium* spp. may result in enteritis, leading to diarrhea, and proventricular infections, resulting in vomiting.[127,128] Organisms may be found in feces using acid-fast stains or by PCR methods. Histopathology findings from affected birds often reveal enteritis or proliferative proventriculitis.[127,128] Treatment of cryptosporidiosis is frequently unsuccessful.[129] Paromomycin, alone or in combination with azithromycin over several weeks did not provide any clinical improvement for respiratory cryptosporidiosis in falcons and thus is considered to have no beneficial effect in this disease syndrome.[130] Halofuginone treatment may inhibit *Cryptosporidium* spp. infections of the bursa of Fabricius and cloaca.[131] Enrofloxacin and paromomycin may have weak prophylactic effects.[132] Control of the disease involves sanitation, nutrition, and controlling underlying disease.

GIARDIASIS. *Giardia psittaci*, a flagellate, is relatively common in budgerigars. The flagellate parasite is often found on routine screening of fecal samples in this species. Most birds are clinically healthy. Young birds may have more severe infections that result in diarrhea, dehydration, and poor growth.[133] Diagnosis is best obtained through wet-mount preparations of the feces, where either the characteristic teardrop-shaped trophozoites or the oval-shaped oocysts may be found. The addition of dilute Lugol's iodine solution may highlight the oocysts. Although the organism is distinct from the typical *Giardia* spp. found in humans, the avian parasite should be considered zoonotic. Treatment with metronidazole is generally effective.

HEXAMITIASIS (SPIRONUCLEOSIS). Although there are frequent references to *Giardia* spp. in cockatiels, *Hexamita (Spironucleus)* appears to be much more common in this species.

There are few published reports regarding this species in psittacines, but it is common in game birds.[124] The organisms are structurally very distinct from *Giardia* spp.[134] The *Hexamita* trophozoites are smaller, move more erratically and toward the narrower end. The protozoal organisms are frequently found in routine wet-mount preparations of the feces of cockatiels. Most birds are subclinical when infected with *Hexamita*. When clinical signs are present, polyuria and/or diarrhea is usually noted. Feather-damaging behavior may occur in some affected cockatiels. Treatment is much more challenging than for *Giardia*. Metronidazole, ronidazole, or carnidazole can be used, but treatment failure is common.

ENCEPHALITOZOONOSIS. *Encephalitozoon hellum* is a microsporidial parasite that occasionally infects the intestine of birds. Encephalitozoonosis is usually diagnosed in small psittacine species (e.g., lovebirds, budgerigars).[135,136] Immunosuppression is thought to be a factor, especially when larger birds are infected.[137] There appears to be a strong association with psittacine beak and feather disease (PBFD) and encephalitozoonosis in birds. When disease is present, it may involve the intestine, liver, and kidneys, with the liver being more affected.[138,139] Diagnosis is generally made at necropsy. This disease is potentially zoonotic and has become a considerable problem in immunocompromised humans, although it is unclear whether human isolates are identical to avian isolates.[136]

COCHLOSOMIASIS. *Cochlosoma* spp. are flagellated protozoans that are sometimes responsible for nestling mortality in finches.[140] The parasite can be carried by adult birds without exhibiting clinical signs. Society finches may be very resistant to the disease and, consequently when they are used as foster parents they will expose other finch species to cochlosomiasis. Finch species, transmission of the disease to the offspring may occur.[124] *Cochlosoma* spp. may be found on wet mounts of feces, and treatment with metronidazole or ronidazole may be effective if there is immediate administration of the prescribed therapeutic agent(s).[141]

NEMATODES. Various nematodes can affect the upper GI tract (*Capillaria* spp., *Spiruroidea* spp.), ventriculus (*Acuaria* spp.), or intestines (*Ascaridia* spp., *Capillaria obsignata*) of birds.[124] These parasites are uncommon in individual pet birds but are often found in wild-caught birds or in those from large aviaries where sanitation is not ideal. Fecal flotation or wet-mount examinations may be used to maximize the chance of finding all important parasites. Often, several samples are required before a parasite is identified. In some cases, eggs are not shed. Clinical signs depend on the location and severity of the infestation. Treatment with ivermectin or pyrantel is often effective. While strict sanitation or periodic deworming is recommended if exposure cannot be controlled.

TAPEWORMS. In wild-caught African grey parrots (*Psittacus* spp.) and cockatoos (*Cacatua* spp.) tapeworms are a relatively common disease diagnosis. The tapeworms may not be easily observed on fecal examination. Weight loss, enteritis, or eosinophilia are clinical signs that are often associated with avian tapeworm infestations. Rarely, the owner may see a proglottid pass in the droppings or the worm "hanging" from the cloaca. Often, wild-caught African grey parrots and cockatoo species that have recently been released from quarantine facilities are routinely treated for tapeworms. Praziquantel is the treatment of choice.

Miscellaneous Diseases

INGLUVIOLITHS. Ingluviolithiasis is an uncommon condition in pet birds. Stones located within the crop are usually smooth, composed of uric acid, and, when cut, exhibit concentric layers. Coprophagy, or more specifically, the consumption of urates, is suspected to be important factor in the development of ingluvial stones. The stones can be surgically removed by performing an ingluviotomy. Reoccurrence can be minimized by housing birds in cages where they have no access to droppings.

GASTRIC NEOPLASIA. Gastric neoplasia has been reported in budgerigars (*Melopsittacus undulatus*); cockatiels; gray-cheeked parakeets (*Brotogeris pyrrhopterus*); a blue and gold macaw (*Ara ararauna*); two Amazon parrots (*Amazona* spp.); and several nonpsittacine birds.[142,143,144] Most birds diagnosed with gastric neoplasia in the case reports listed above were middle aged (3 to 20 years). A majority of the cases were diagnosed post mortem after acute death due to hemorrhage caused by ulceration of the mass. The masses in all of the reported psittacine cases were located in the isthmus between the proventriculus and ventriculus; this is where the gland types gradually shift from the proventricular to the ventricular type. The majority of the reported gastric neoplasia cases were classified as proventricular adenocarcinomas. Although uncommon, gastric neoplasia should be considered a differential diagnosis in any mature bird exhibiting signs of proventricular and/or ventricular dysfunction (e.g., vomiting, weight loss, passage of whole seeds). Radiographically, the diseased proventriculus may be mildly enlarged or misshapen. The results of a barium study in a bird reveals a filling defect that could be caused by a number of disease conditions. However the age of the bird and the location of the mass at the isthmus are highly suggestive of gastric neoplasia (Figure 5-13). An endoscopic or surgical biopsy of the mass

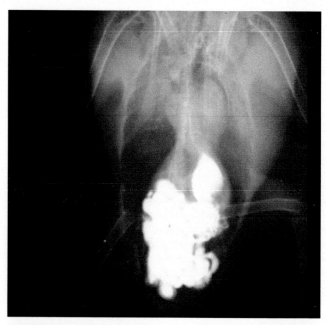

FIGURE 5-13 Contrast study of a parrot. The filling defect at the isthmus was later revealed to be a ventricular carcinoma.

with subsequent histopathological examination of the collected samples is required to confirm the diagnosis. Endoscopic biopsy carries the risk of perforation of the stomach wall. Shallow biopsies can also be nondiagnostic, showing only surface inflammation.

Successful resection of gastric tumors has not been reported; however, since metastases are uncommon, surgical resection could be curative. Because gastric ulceration and subsequent hemorrhage are the primary causes of mortality, sucralfate, a topical GI therapeutic agent that adheres to and provides mucosal protection, may be useful in the management of gastric tumors.

LIVER NEOPLASIA. Neoplasia is an uncommon cause of liver disease. In Amazon parrots, biliary adenocarcinoma has been strongly associated with cloacal papillomas.[93] The liver should be evaluated in birds that have papillomatous disease. In birds with avian leukosis, liver neoplasia (lymphoma) is often diagnosed.[145] Spontaneous lymphoma of the liver is also occasionally seen. Diagnosis of hepatic neoplasia in birds is based on radiography, endoscopy, biopsy, or, most commonly, necropsy. Successful treatment of liver cancer in an avian patient has not been reported.

HYPOVITAMINOSIS A. This is the most common clinically evident nutritional deficiency in pet avian practice. The signs of hypovitaminosis A are often found in the oral cavity: swollen salivary glands, keratin cysts, blunted and thickened choanal papillae, redness in the throat, and increased susceptibility to infection (Figure 5-14). Integumentary signs (hyperkeratosis) may be present as well. A definitive diagnosis of hypovitaminosis A is based on dietary history, typical lesions, and response to therapy. Cytology of affected areas may reveal heavily cornified squamous epithelial cells, with an amber cast. Secondary infections are common due to a breakdown in the surface epithelium's ability to adequately protect the patient. Treatment involves vitamin A supplementation followed by correction of the dietary deficiency.

CROP TRAUMA, BURNS, AND FISTULAE. Improper hand feeding practices or tube feeding can result in serious damage to the crop. If a tube is forced too vigorously or if the wall of the crop is devitalized, the tube may penetrate the crop wall. Food may then leak or be deposited in the subcutaneous tissue surrounding the crop. An alternative form of this condition occurs if food is deposited around the pharynx. Severe cellulitis can also occur as a result of food being deposited; if deposition occurs in the subcutaneous space secondary to trauma, immediate surgery should be performed to flush the area of food debris. Another common reason for thermal crop injury involves the feeding of microwaved baby formula to a neonate that may have hot areas within due to inadequate stirring after removal from the oven. This occasionally occurs in adult birds if they are allowed to drink hot liquids. Initially, edema is present, but this is soon followed by necrosis. As the tissues of the crop slough, they coalesce with the skin. The lesion will then fistulate through the fused surface epithelium and crop mucosa and food will leak out (Figure 5-15). A period of 3 to 5 days is required for the fistula to mature following the initial insult. Endotoxic shock can occur in these cases in addition to the animals being dehydrated and malnourished (e.g., food and water falls out of the crop). Intensive supportive care may be necessary prior to correcting the deficit. A tube can be passed into the defect and down the

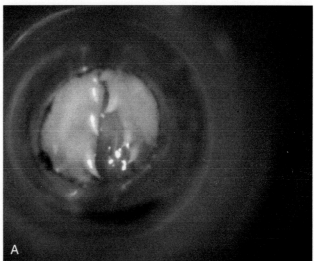

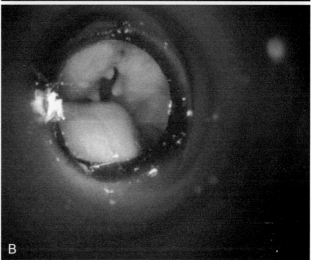

FIGURE 5-14 *A,* View of the choana using a video otoscope. Note the sharp choanal papillae. *B,* View of the choana using a video otoscope. This bird is exhibiting blunted choanal papillae.

esophagus for nutritional support. Eventually, the defect may require surgical repair. In burn cases, the surgery should be delayed several days until the wound begins to contract. Early repair can sometimes be ineffective because the extent of necrosis cannot always be determined. The skin and crop must be dissected from each other. All devitalized tissue must be resected. Up to 50% of the crop wall can be resected in most avian cases without significant impact to the patient. Any subcutaneous debris should be lavaged out. Primary closure of the crop and skin is accomplished using a simple interrupted suture patterns. It is important that the crop and skin are closed in two separate layers. If endotoxic shock is not severe, the prognosis is favorable.

CLOACAL PROLAPSE. Several types of tissues can prolapse through the cloacal orifice. Birds with cloacal papillomas will often have the proliferative tissue protruding from the orifice. In small birds such as budgies, cockatiels, and finches, the oviduct may prolapse from the cloacal opening. Intestinal

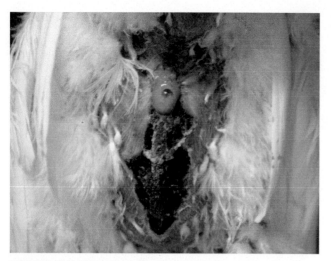

FIGURE 5-15 This Goffin's cockatoo developed a crop burn that fistulated through the skin. When the food was taken away in preparation for surgery, the bird consumed his feces, which is flowing from the fistula. The skin lesions over the sternum were a chronic problem prior to the fistula.

intussusceptions, especially in neonates, will occasionally prolapse through the cloacal opening. True cloacal prolapses occur most frequently in cockatoos, with African greys less frequently affected. The condition is most common in male birds. The cause of these true cloacal prolapses is not known, although abnormal sexual attachment to the owners is often present and has been suggested that there is hormonal influence regarding the underlying cause of this disease condition. Proposed etiologies such as straining due to intestinal disease rarely occur. The prolapse involves tearing of some of the pericloacal connective tissue. The protruding structure is smooth surfaced and red. Initial inspection to determine the nature of the prolapsed tissue is required. A cotton-tipped applicator or other blunt probe can be inserted alongside the prolapsed tissue. If the blunt probe reaches a blind end immediately, the prolapse is most likely cloacal tissue. The prolapse may be replaced and transverse sutures placed across the vent. If there is a prolapsed intestinal intussusception, open surgical treatment is indicated. (Prolapse of the oviduct is a separate problem and is not discussed in this chapter.) Supportive care is provided as needed. Unless the behavioral aspects of this condition are corrected, there is a high rate of recurrence. In these birds, cloacapexy can be performed. For the cloacapexy procedure a ventral abdominal incision is made after which the cloaca is elevated with a blunt probe and sutures are placed to attach the coprodeum to the ribs and body wall. The body wall must be penetrated to ensure adequate adherence to the internal structures so that the pexy does not break down.

HEPATIC LIPIDOSIS. Birds that are maintained on high-fat and/or unbalanced diets will often form deposits of excessive fat. Occasionally, the excessive fat will accumulate in and between the liver cells. This condition is known as hepatic lipidosis. Budgerigars and Amazon parrots appear to be highly susceptible to hepatic lipidosis (and obesity in general). Unlike a similar clinical condition in cats, hepatic lipidosis in birds is not usually associated with anorexia. Instead, the clinical signs of hepatic lipidosis in birds are those associated with chronic, low-grade liver disease. Polyuria, hypoproteinemia, elevated AST, enlarged liver, lipemia, normal CBC, overgrown beak (especially in budgies), and coagulopathies are all clinical characteristics commonly identified in birds diagnosed with hepatic lipidosis.

A tentative diagnosis can often be made from the history, clinical signs, hematology, and evidence of liver disease (e.g., biochemistries, elevated AST and bile acids, radiographs). Definitive diagnosis requires a liver biopsy. The recommended treatment for the affected avian patient is a strict, low-fat, balanced diet. This diet is beneficial for any psittacine and is often prescribed based on a presumptive diagnosis. The bird's normal diet is gradually changed to the prescribed nutritional offerings over a period of 3 to 4 weeks. If the owner has difficulty converting the bird, boarding at the veterinary hospital during the dietary conversion can be helpful. If the diet is already appropriate, restricting food quantity or adding L-carnitine supplementation may be required. Other supportive measures, including antioxidants such as silymarin, may be useful adjuncts to therapy. Prognosis is good for stabilizing the avian patient that has been diagnosed with hepatic lipidosis if the client complies with the dietary recommendations, although in chronic cases hepatic firbrosis may develop, which can be progressive, despite therapy.

HEMOCHROMATOSIS. Hemochromatosis (iron storage disease) is a metabolic disorder involving the deposition of iron-containing pigments into various solid viscera. Originally thought to be associated with excessive iron in the diet, the disease is now attributed to a bird's inability to process generally acceptable levels of dietary iron. The disease commonly affects certain species of birds, including mynahs (*Acridotheres* spp.), toucans (Ramphastidae), birds of paradise (Paradisaeidae), tanagers (Thraupidae), and some other softbill-type birds. Many of the birds affected by this disease are wild caught, making genetics an unlikely contributing factor to the problem. Rarely, a psittacine bird may be diagnosed with hemochromatosis. The liver is the primary organ affected by the disease. In mynahs, the disease takes a more chronic course, with heart and liver failure combining to cause ascites and pulmonary edema. Respiratory distress and abdominal swelling are common clinical findings in generalized hemochromatosis cases. In toucans, the disease presents acutely, and death may occur without prior clinical signs. A tentative diagnosis is often based on the signalment, history, and clinical signs. Additional data may include radiographs (if ascites is not present or after removal of ascitic fluid), ultrasound (when fluid is present), or blood biochemistries. Hematologic values are generally unremarkable. In toucans, severe organ damage often occurs before any biochemistry alterations appear. The value of serum iron, iron binding capacity, serum ferritin, or other blood tests evaluating iron metabolism is questionable at this point. A definitive diagnosis requires a liver (or other organ) biopsy. Hepatic iron levels are also diagnostic. In some birds, clinical improvement and an increase of life expectancy have been accomplished by the combination of dietary iron restriction and phlebotomy. The weekly removal of blood at 1% of the body weight (1 mL/100 g) until clinical signs resolve and then monthly to maintain lower levels has been recommended to manage cases. The hematocrit of the patient should be monitored closely when performing phlebotomy treatments. Deferoxamine may also be used as an iron binding agent to slow iron absorption. Prognosis for long-term survival of avian patients diagnosed with hemachromatosis is guarded. In species predisposed to hemochromatosis, low iron diets are highly recommended with iron content of the food product <150 ppm. Citric acid can enhance iron absorption, therefore citrus fruits should be limited. A nutrition almanac should be consulted to select potential low iron food items to include in a restricted diet.

AFLATOXICOSIS. Aflatoxins, a family of closely related, biologically active mycotoxins, are a common cause of toxic changes to the liver in birds. The toxins occur naturally in animal feeds, including corn, cottonseed, and peanuts.[146] Aflatoxin levels increase when drought or insect damage facilitate invasion of *Aspergillus flavus* and *Aspergillus parasiticus*, which abound in the environment. Acute aflatoxicosis causes a distinct overt clinical disease marked by hepatitis, icterus, hemorrhage, and death. In pet birds, chronic aflatoxin poisoning is more common producing subtle signs that may not be obvious (e.g., cachexia or anorexia, weight loss, biliverdinuria). The immune system is also sensitive to aflatoxins and problems directly related to immunological dysfunction include suppression of the cell-mediated immune response, reduced phagocytosis, and depressed complement and interferon production. In patients that are immunocompromised, clinical signs associated with the disease are attributed to the infectious process rather than the aflatoxin that predisposed the animal to infection.[146] Histopathology often reveals acute centrilobular necrosis or, in chronic cases, mild inflammation and fibrosis. Treatment is focused on removing the source of the aflatoxin, providing supportive care and liver protectants (e.g., milk thistle, lactulose), and controlling opportunistic infections.

LEAD POISONING. Lead poisoning (or plumbism) represents one of the most common toxicoses in pet birds. Many sources of lead have been implicated in avian lead poisoning. In older homes, the deeper layers of paint may contain lead. House paint manufactured after 1980 should be lead free. Weights from curtains, fishing tackle, and even some bird toys contain lead. Costume jewelry, solder, lead shot, pellets from pellet guns, stained glass, and chandeliers are also possible sources of lead. Many of the birds that develop lead toxicity are not confined when their owners are away, and the owners are usually unaware where the animal was exposed to the toxin. Presenting clinical disease signs in affected birds can include seizures, profound depression, polyuria, biliverdinuria, hemoglobinuria (e.g., in Amazon parrots), blindness, or other neurologic conditions. The clinical signs often are acute in their initial presentation. The CBC of a bird with lead toxicosis may show leukocytosis, anemia, hemolysis, or unusual red blood cells. The basophilic stippling often described in mammalian erythrocytes with plumbism does not usually occur in birds. Radiographic images of the avian patient with elevated blood lead levels may show hepatomegaly, nephromegaly, ileus, or metal-dense foreign material in the ventriculus, proventriculus, or intestines. The absence of radiographically evident material does not rule out lead poisoning. Blood lead levels will be elevated, but birds may show clinical signs at much lower levels than mammals. Some laboratories will not detect the levels of lead that can cause signs in birds (>20 µg/dL). Treatment of lead poisoning involves chelation of the metal until all of the lead is removed from the GI tract. Calcium ethylenediaminetetraacetic acid (caEDTA; 35 mg/kg IM [intramuscularly], twice daily, for 3 to 5 d, 3 to 5 d off, and then repeated until cleared) is the drug most commonly used to treat birds for heavy metal poisoning. D-penicillamine can be used alone or in conjunction with CaEDTA. Barium sulfate, hemicellulose, peanut butter, and Pepto Bismol have all been used to speed the elimination of lead objects from the ventriculus. Large lead pellets can be surgically removed via endoscopy, proventriculotomy, or ventriculotomy. In larger waterfowl, an endoscopic technique for removing lead shot from the ventriculus has been described. As with other diseases, supportive and therapy based on clinical presentation is crucial to the successful treatment of lead poisoning. Diazepam or midazolam can be used, as needed, to control seizures.

ACUTE PANCREATIC NECROSIS. Acute pancreatic necrosis is an uncommon condition in pet birds, but obese quaker (monk) parrots *(Myiopsitta monachus)* appear to be particularly susceptible to this condition. In one study, 16.5% of quaker parrot submissions to a pathology service were found to have acute panacreatic necrosis.[147] The cause of acute pancreatic necrosis in unknown, but improved nutrition has been found to reduce the incidence of the disease. Affected birds are usually overweight and will acutely present with severe depression, anorexia, and occasionally polyuria, diarrhea, or vomiting. The white blood cell count and amylase are usually elevated in these cases; glucose may be very high as well. Affected birds may die within a few days of onset of clinical signs associated with acute pancreatic necrosis.

PANCREATITIS. Pancreatitis has been diagnosed in association with zinc toxicosis, herpesvirus infection, adenovirus infection, egg-related coelomitis, and a number of other etiologies. In some cases, the cause of pancreatitis has been considered idiopathic. Clinical signs of pancreatitis in the avian patient are often nonspecific and include anorexia, lethargy, abdominal pain, weight loss, polyuria, polydipsia, and abdominal distension may all be variably seen.[89] Suspicion may be raised based on elevated amylase levels and an inflammatory white blood cell response. Diagnosis requires biopsy. Treatment for birds diagnosed with pancreatitis is supportive.

PANCREATIC EXOCRINE INSUFFICIENCY. This appears to be a rare condition in birds. Clinical signs may include polyphagia, weight loss, and pale bulky droppings (amylorrhea). The feces can be mixed with iodine to determine if there is undigested starch present. Amylase levels may be normal in these cases.[89] Treatment using pancreatic enzymes to predigest food may improve signs while some cases appear to be transient and have a spontaneous resolution.

Mammals

Exotic companion mammals are commonly affected by GI disorders; however, each group has its own common disease conditions. For this reason, the exotic companion mammal

GI diseases are subdivided in this section. Table 5-5 lists clinical signs, diagnostic tests of choice, and differential diagnoses for the various anatomic parts of the exotic small mammal digestive tract.

Sugar Gliders

Sugar gliders have specialized lower incisors that are used for gouging the bark and sap of trees. Since these specialized lower incisors are prominent, they are susceptible to trauma. The lower incisors are not continuously growing teeth as with rodents and therefore should never be trimmed. If the sugar glider's lower incisors are trimmed, a painful infection can possibly occur.[16] These iatrogenic problems are unfortunately common. Extraction of the incisors is complicated, requiring gingivotomy and fine elevation of the tooth root. Placement of synthetic bone matrix is recommended when the incisors have to be removed.

Enteritis in sugar gliders may be due to a variety of causes, including bacterial infections, parasitic infestations, organ dysfunction, malnutrition, or stress. Treatment involves specific therapy for the underlying cause and fluid and nutritional support.[16]

Rectal or cloacal prolapse may occur secondary to tenesmus and is more common in gliders in poor overall health. Care should be taken to identify the prolapsed tissue. Treatment involves reduction of the prolapse and placement of transverse sutures to reduce the width of the cloacal vent, similar to the procedure described for birds and reptiles.[16]

Hedgehogs

Hedgehogs present a challenge to the veterinarian because they roll into an inaccessible ball when frightened. This defensive response makes detection and evaluation of problems more difficult. Hedgehogs should be watched prior to handling to determine behavioral responses, since the actual exam may require anesthesia. They also have a high incidence of neoplasia that should be considered on every differential diagnosis list.

TABLE 5-5

Clinical Signs, Diagnostics, and Differential Disease Diagnoses by Anatomic Site in Mammals

Site	Clinical Signs	Diagnostics	Differentials
Oral Cavity	Anorexia, Dysphagia, Visible lesions, exudates, Hypersalivation, Yawning, Head shaking, Halitosis	Visual examination, Oral swabs, Endoscopy, Biopsy, Radiography, CT	Dental disease, Cheek pouch impaction, Neoplasia
Esophagus	Regurgitation, Weight loss	Radiography, Contrast radiography	Megaesophagus
Stomach	Vomiting (if capable), Anorexia, Abdominal pain, Respiratory distress, Melena	Radiography, Contrast radiography, Ultrasound, Gastroscopy, Exploratory laparotomy	Gastritis, Gastric impaction, Gastric dilatation ± volvulus, Neoplasia, GI stasis
Small Intestine	Diarrhea, Anorexia, Vomiting, Abdominal pain	Radiography, Contrast radiography, Ultrasound, Feces, Exploratory surgery, Biopsy	Enteritis, Intussusception, GI stasis, Neoplasia, Parasites
Large Intestine/cecum	Anorexia, Diarrhea, Reduced feces, Constipation, Abdominal pain	Radiography, Contrast radiography, Ultrasound, Feces, Exploratory surgery	GI stasis, Dysbiosis, Colitis, Mucoid enteropathy, Cecoliths
Rectum/anus	Tenesmus, Protruding tissue	Visual exam, Biopsy	Rectal papillomas, Prolapse
Liver	Vague signs, Icterus, Hepatomegaly	ALT, bile acids, Radiography, Ultrasound, Biopsy	Hepatic lipidosis, Hepatitis, Liver lobe torsion, Hepatic cysts
Pancreas	Hypoglycemia, Vomiting	Blood glucose, Insulin level, Biopsy	Insulinoma, Pancreatitis, Neoplasia

ALT, Alanine aminotransferase; *CT,* computed tomography; *GI,* gastrointestinal.

Hedgehogs tend to have significant problems with periodontal disease. Whether due to their captive diets or a genetic predisposition, many pet hedgehogs present with severe tartar, gingival proliferation, and tooth loss. Preventive health care must include regular dental care.[18] Dental care products should be used to reduce the occurrence of disease affecting the teeth of hedgehogs. The author has used chlorhexidine oral rinses as a preventive product for hedgehog dental disease, with some success. As hedgehogs are usually anesthetized when examined, the teeth should always be examined, scaled, and treated as needed. Extractions are frequently required and often require little elevation of the tooth roots to accomplish. Antibiotic, anti-inflammatory, and analgesic treatments are warranted in hedgehogs diagnosed with dental disease.

Oral neoplasia, especially squamous cell carcinoma, is very common in hedgehogs.[18] The underlying etiology for oral neoplasia in hedgehogs is unknown, but the author suspects that it may be related to the chronic proliferative gingivitis that occurs with dental disease. Diagnosis often occurs late in the disease because owners are unable to regularly examine the oral cavity. The tumors are locally invasive, therefore if complete excision can be achieved, a cure is possible. However, this often requires aggressive surgery (e.g., hemimandibulectomy).

Diarrhea, occasionally encountered in hedgehogs, may be a result of a variety of species of bacteria, including *Salmonella* spp. Alimentary candidiasis, cryptosporidiosis, and various parasites have also been identified, but they are not common disease problems in pet hedgehogs.[18] Sporulated bacterial rods resembling *Clostridium* organisms are often identified in Gram stains of hedgehog feces, even in animals not exhibiting clinical signs of disease.

Obstructions with foreign bodies are uncommon but may occasionally be diagnosed in hedgehogs. Those affected with GI obstruction will present with acute abdominal pain, anorexia, and lethargy; patients may also be in shock. Vomiting is variable in these cases.[18] A thorough diagnostic workup is necessary to confirm a diagnosis of an obstruction. The patient should be stabilized and surgery performed to remove the obstruction.

Hepatic lipidosis may occur in obese hedgehogs that become anorexic.[18] Tentative diagnosis is usually based on the history, clinical signs, and diagnostic workup of the patient. Treatment for heptatic lipidosis includes dietary management (e.g., provide adequate calories short term and weight management long term), hepatoprotectants (e.g., lactulose, milk thistle), and supportive care.

Hepatic neoplasia has also been identified in hedgehogs and may be part of a blood cell neoplasm such as lymphoma, metastatic tumor, or primary liver neoplasm. The author has observed eosinophilic leukemia in one hedgehog that infiltrated all of the viscera including the liver.

Ferrets

Dental disease is relatively common in ferrets. Fractures of the canine teeth are present in a high proportion of adult ferrets. In most ferret cases, in which the canine teeth are fractured, the animal does not exhibit any clinical signs of disease, but if pulp is exposed, tooth root abscesses can occur. A root canal can be performed to prevent the formation of abscesses in an affected tooth (teeth) or the tooth (teeth) can be extracted. Periodontal disease is also common. Treatment should follow standard dental care techniques used in cats.

Oral neoplasia is uncommon in ferrets, with squamous cell carcinoma being the most common tumor type being diagnosed. Squamous cell carcinomas in ferrets are locally aggressive, and wide surgical excision, sometimes including maxillectomy or mandibulectomy, is needed to achieve resolution.[148]

Megaesophagus is an uncommon disease of ferrets. To date, there is no known etiology for this disease in ferrets. Clinical signs in affected animals may include passive regurgitation, weight loss, and secondary respiratory signs (from aspiration). Diagnosis is made on contrast radiography, displaying the widely expanded esophagus in the thorax with the prognosis for these cases being poor. Management is the same as for canine patients however treatment response in ferrets is poor.[148]

Acute or chronic gastritis is one of the most commonly encountered clinical conditions in ferrets. Clinical signs observed in ferrets diagnosed with gastritis may include signs of nausea (e.g., salivation, pawing at the mouth), pain (e.g., bruxism), and abdominal splinting. Some of these signs are nonspecific and are also associated with other disease. Vomiting is uncommon, but ferrets with gastritis may gag. Melena may occur if gastric ulceration is involved. The patient's appetite is usually diminished or absent in affected ferrets, and animals can lose weight at a drastic rate. Common causes of gastritis include *Helicobacter mustelae* infection, ulcerogenic drugs (e.g., nonsteroidal anti-inflammatories), and uremia from renal disease. Gastric foreign bodies can mimic gastritis.

Enteritis is very common in ferrets with affected animals generally exhibiting diarrhea as the primary clinical sign. Anorexia may or may not be present while weight loss and dehydration being the primary disease consequences. A variety of etiologies for enteritis in ferrets have been identified and include viruses, bacteria, parasites, idiopathic inflammation, and neoplasia.[148] Intestinal obstruction is clinically distinct from enteritis and generally presents as an acute abdomen.

Hepatic diseases occasionally occur in ferrets. Clinical signs associated with hepatic disease in ferrets is often nonspecific, including anorexia, weight loss, and general malaise. The alanine aminotransferase level (ALT) is usually elevated in affected ferrets, while icterus is rare.[148] In severe hepatic disease cases, reduced protein levels (e.g., albumin) or glucose may be found. Causes of liver disease in ferrets include neoplasia, lipidosis, and lymphocytic inflammation.

VIRAL DISEASES

EPIZOOTIC CATARRHAL ENTERITIS. Epizootic catarrhal enteritis (ECE), which is attributed to ferret enteric coronavirus (FECV), is a common contagious disease of ferrets. Adult ferrets are most often affected, and the disease usually occurs after a new younger ferret is introduced into the household. In most cases, the younger ferret has a subclinical infection. Initially, a green mucoid diarrhea will develop; hence the origin of "green slime disease." Feces will sometimes have a grainy appearance due to undigested material as a result of an inefficient digestive process. Although morbidity is high, the mortality rate for this disease is low. Hematology may be normal while elevation of hepatic enzymes such as ALT is common. A definitive diagnosis can be achieved histologically or by detecting the virus in feces using PCR testing methods. Treatment is primarily supportive, including antibiotics (these should target *Helicobacter mustelae*), fluid therapy, nutritional support, and separation from other ferrets. After recovery, there may be persistent diarrhea for weeks to months. Corticosteroids may be useful during the recovery phase in which diarrhea or digestive dysfunction (e.g., bird seed stool) is present. More recently, a systemic coronavirus has been identified in ferrets. This disease follows a course similar to feline infectious peritonitis and carries a grave prognosis.[148]

OTHER VIRAL ENTERITIDES. Rotavirus, canine distemper virus, and influenza may also cause enteritis in ferrets. In the case of distemper and influenza, non-GI signs are more prominent presentations of the disease. Rotavirus affects kits and leads to transient green mucoid diarrhea with treatment being supportive.[148]

BACTERIAL DISEASES

HELICOBACTER *GASTRITIS.* *Helicobacter mustelae* is the most common cause of gastritis in ferrets. Nearly all U.S. ferrets are exposed as kits to this bacterium and become persistently infected.[149] Untreated, the infection is lifelong, and gastritis appears to progress with age, although many ferrets with histologically severe gastritis have minimal clinical signs. Often, the onset of clinical disease will correspond to a concurrent illness or surgery. Clinical signs are attributed to gastritis as previously described, with ulceration being common. Definitive diagnosis of helicobacter gastritis depends on histopathology of gastric mucosal biopsy or PCR diagnostics from gastric mucosa or feces. Treatment with "triple therapy" (e.g., amoxicillin 12.5 mg/kg, PO, twice daily [BID]; metronidazole, 20 mg/kg, PO, BID; and bismuth subsalicylate, 0.25 to 0.5 mL, PO, 3 to 4 times daily [TID-QID]), as in humans, is recommended. Sucralfate (50 to 100 mg/kg, PO, TID-QID) can also be used to help minimize the discomfort associated with the gastric ulcers; however sucralfate should be administered as a separate treatment 2 to 4 hours after the other drugs to limit the likelihood that it will decrease absorption of the triple therapeutics. Clarithromycin (12.5 mg/kg, PO, BID-TID), combined with ranitidine bismuth (24 mg/kg, PO, BID), omeprazole (4 mg/kg, PO, once daily [SID]), or metronidazole and omeprazole, is also effective.

PROLIFERATIVE BOWEL DISEASE. Proliferative bowel disease in ferrets is the same disease that swine and hamsters develop due to what was originally identified as a *Campylobacter*-like bacteria, later renamed *Desulfovibrio*. Currently, the organism is called *Lawsonia intracellularis*.[150] Chronic diarrhea is the primary clinical sign associated with this disease. Partial rectal prolapse is inconsistently observed in animals diagnosed with proliferative bowel disease. Weight loss can be dramatic as a result of chronic malabsorption. Young ferrets are most commonly affected but animals of all ages are susceptible. *Lawsonia intracellularis* is difficult to culture, making a definitive diagnosis a challenge although presumptive diagnosis can be made based on the signalment and clinical signs of the patient. Fecal cytology may reveal the typical spiral to curved bacteria, but this does not constitute a definitive diagnosis, especially since *Helicobacter*, another common GI pathogen, is similarly shaped. Chloramphenicol (50 mg/kg BID) is the treatment of choice for *Lawsonia intracellularis*.

Fluid and nutritional support should be provided as well. Since this disease can be difficult to distinguish from *Helicobacter* gastritis, it may be advisable to treat both conditions in ferrets with severe GI disease. Proliferative bowel disease appears to be more of a problem for laboratory ferrets than pet ferrets.

PARASITIC DISEASES

COCCIDIOSIS. Intestinal parasites are rarely diagnosed in ferrets. While nematodes are extremely rare, coccidiosis may be a clinical disease problem, especially in large, densely populated, dynamic ferret populations. In ferret populations diagnosed with coccidiosis morbidity may be high, with significant mortality, with the disease affecting animals of all ages. The most notable clinical signs observed in ferrets diagnosed with coccidiosis include diarrhea, often with frank or digested blood. Dehydration, weakness, lethargy, and weight loss are clinical signs most often associated with severe chronic cases. Fecal examination often reveals sporadic and inconsistent shedding of oocysts. Supportive care and treatment with sulfadimethoxine (25 to 50 mg/kg, PO, SID, for 7 to 10 d) is palliative but may fail to eliminate infection.[151] Coccidiocides, such as ponazuril (10 to 20 mg/kg, PO, SID, for 3 to 5 d), may be more effective.

MISCELLANEOUS DISEASES

GASTRIC/INTESTINAL OBSTRUCTION. Trichobezoars or foreign bodies that cause partial or complete obstruction of the stomach or small intestine are very common in pet ferrets. The size of the ferret's intestinal lumen of ferrets will not allow the passage of apparently small foreign objects. The author has witnessed ferrets die from the ingestion of items as small as a cherry pit. Ferrets are mischievous creatures and will often ingest items that can be harmful. These curious animals have a particular taste for rubber and foam rubber products.[152] In addition, ferret trichobezoars have a tendency be very firm and can lead to chronic gastric, or occasionally acute intestinal, obstruction. Typically, younger ferrets ingest foreign bodies, while middle- to older-age ferrets are diagnosed more often with hairballs. The presenting complaint for gastric obstruction may be chronic weight loss and lack of appetite, with or without vomiting. Although ferrets are physically capable of vomiting, it is an uncommon clinical presentation with foreign body ingestion or hair ball formation. Intestinal obstructions present as an acute severe processes involving anorexia, dehydration, abdominal pain, and severe depression. Diagnosis is based on palpation or radiography. Contrast studies may be performed but should not be considered conclusive. Many of the items ingested by ferrets can absorb barium, making it difficult to visualize the foreign material on contrast films. Confirmation of the disease is made through an exploratory laparotomy. When doubt exists, it is better to err on the side of caution and perform the exploratory surgical procedure. The consequences of a negative abdominal exploratory surgery are much better than the consequences of leaving an obstruction unresolved. The treatment for GI obstruction is a gastrotomy or enterotomy, depending on the site affected. In the case of intestinal obstruction, the surgery should be performed as soon as possible (within hours). The abdominal surgical procedure is similar to that used for dogs or cats, although it is somewhat easier to perform. Intravenous (IV) fluids, antibiotics, and other supportive care are administered as necessary.

EOSINOPHILIC GASTROENTERITIS. Although uncommon in ferrets, this disease appears to be more common in these animals than cats and dogs. Unlike most of the other GI disorders of ferrets, eosinophilic gastroenteritis is most common in mature to older ferrets. The underlying etiology for eosinophilic gastroenteritis is unknown, but is suspected to be a hypersensitivity reaction. The author had one ferret develop this disease approximately 1 week after exhibiting signs of both rabies and distemper vaccination reactions. Clinical signs associated with eosinophilic gastroenteritis include diarrhea, anorexia, vomiting, and weight loss. Peripheral eosinophilia is often observed in the differential white blood cell count. Treatment for eosinophilic gastroenteritis in ferrets consists of using prednisolone at 2 mg/kg, PO, SID, for 1 week and then every other day until resolved, at which time the dose is tapered. Ivermectin was also successful in resolving the disease in one ferret case.[153] Supportive care should be administered as needed.

INFLAMMATORY BOWEL DISEASE. Inflammatory bowel disease is an idopathic lymphoplasmacytic inflammation of the bowel. The source of inflammation may be diet, hypersensitivity reactions, or another abnormal immune response.[148] Inflammatory bowel disease in ferrets may be overlooked because it clinically resembles coronaviral enteritis (e.g., ECE) and other causes of diarrhea. It is also possible that these other disease conditions listed above could initiate the inflammatory response. Another major differential diagnosis for this disease is intestinal lymphoma. Inflammatory bowel disease should be considered if diarrhea persists beyond 6 to 8 weeks. Hematologic test results may reveal a may lymphocytosis, and serum chemistries indicating an increase ALT and globulin concentrations. Ultrasound may reveal thickened bowel wall and enlarged lymph nodes. However, definitive diagnosis requires intestinal biopsies. Treatment is aimed at controlling inflammation and although corticosteroids may be used for antiinflammatory purposes, they may not be effective for long-term management of this disease problem. Azathioprine (0.9 mg/kg, PO, q24 to 72 h) is a useful antiinflammatory therapeutic alternative.[154]

GASTROINTESTINAL LYMPHOMA. Infiltrative lymphoma is a relatively common finding in ferrets. The disease can be very difficult to distinguish from inflammatory bowel disease as it has many of the same disease conditions in the affected animal. While the pathophysiologic responses and imaging results are similar, they are more severe with GI lymphoma. Diagnosis requires biopsy of the affected region(s) of the GI tract (e.g., stomach, intestine), lymph nodes, and occasionally other tissues. When a ferret is diagnosed with gastrointestinal lymphoma the prognosis is poor. However treatment with chemotherapy can be attempted but is usually unsuccessful with this form of lymphoma.[148]

GASTROINTESTINAL ADENOCARCINOMA. Adenocarcinoma is the most common primary GI tumor diagnosed in ferrets. This neoplasm is often locally aggressive and tends to induce a scirrhous response, which may lead to obstruction. Complete excision may be curative if metastasis has not occurred prior to the surgical procedure.[155]

HEPATIC NEOPLASIA. The liver may be the site of either primary or metastatic neoplasia. Metastatic tumors involving the liver can arise from a variety of primary neoplasms. Lymphoma may infiltrate the hepatic tissue

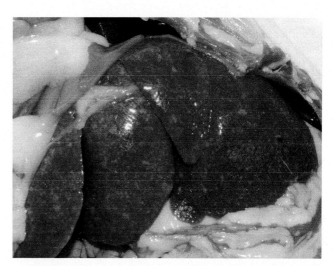

FIGURE 5-16 Liver of a ferret that died from lymphoma.

(Figure 5-16). The most common primary tumor diagnosed in the ferret liver is cystadenoma, with cholangiocarcinoma, hepatocellular carcinoma, and hepatoma less common.[155] Clinical signs associated with ferret hepatic neoplasia range from no clinical signs to nonspecific (e.g., anorexia, weight loss). Serum biochemistry values may suggest hepatocellular damage, and imaging may reveal the mass or masses in the liver. Histopathology is required for a definitive diagnosis the recommended treatment options are a wide surgical excision or lobectomy.

EXOCRINE PANCREATIC NEOPLASIA. Neoplasia of the exocrine pancreas is an uncommon occurrence in ferrets. When present, this tumor type is aggressive, generally resulting in invasion into the surrounding pancreas, seeding the abdomen, and metastasizing to additional organs.[155] Clinical signs may include anorexia, weight loss, or rarely vomiting. In severe cases, abdominal effusion may be present, occasionally exhibiting mast cells.[156] Prognosis is grave and complete surgical excision is unlikely, however this may represent the best treatment option.

Rabbits

Dental Disorders

A wide variety of dental disorders occur in rabbits. Rabbits are hypsodontic; all of the teeth are open rooted and grow continuously throughout the life of the animal. The dental formula for the rabbit is 2-0-3-3/1-0-2-3. Selective breeding for a more rounded head has resulted in these rabbits being predisposed to congenital prognathism. Prognathism can also be acquired when a tooth or its supporting bone is injured. The lower incisors then grow rostral to the upper incisors. When the rabbit's incisors do not occlude properly, the teeth will overgrow. The lower incisors will grow upward like tusks, while the upper incisors curve backward and into the palate. The maloccluded teeth must be trimmed on a regular basis for the rest of the rabbit's life. A preferred treatment method is to extract all of the incisors. Rabbits do very well without the incisors as long as the food is offered in a small size. Some rabbits may develop problems of the nasolacrimal duct as a result of elongated reserve crowns of the upper incisors.[157]

Rabbits also develop problems with the cheek teeth. If the occlusion is not perfect or the diet is inadequately fibrous, the teeth will develop points or spurs, usually on the buccal side of the upper and the lingual side of the lower cheek teeth. Weakened bones, resulting from inadequate vitamin D or calcium, have been a proposed contributor to dental problems in rabbits. Additionally, periodontal disease, abscessation, and other disease associated with these teeth may occur. Clinical signs of rabbit dental disease may include anorexia, dysphagia, and swelling of the face, jaw, or infraorbital area. The small opening of a rabbit's mouth makes examination and therapy of the cheek teeth difficult limiting visualization and access to the oral cavity. A vaginal or nasal speculum with a light source may be used to open the mouth. Anesthesia is required for an in-depth oral examination of the rabbit patient. Skull radiographs are invaluable for evaluation of the reserve crowns of the teeth. Computed tomography (CT) can detect problems that would otherwise go undiagnosed. Small rongeur forceps may be used to trim away spurs on the teeth, or small files can be used to "float the teeth."[158] Preferably, dental burrs on a hobby drill or dental drill can be used to reduce and shape the clinical crown.[22] Abscessed teeth require extraction (Figure 5-17). This is a difficult process in rabbits and either an intraoral or extraoral approach may be used, depending on the case presentation. If multiple cheek teeth require removal, it is preferable to stage the required surgeries, removing only 1 to 4 teeth at a single procedure. Whenever cheek teeth are removed, the opposing tooth should be frequently assessed for overgrowth. All of the dental work performed on rabbits requires general anesthesia and appropriate analgesia. Antibiotic therapy is routinely used for many of the rabbit dental procedures.

Gastrointestinal Stasis Syndrome

Gastrointestinal stasis accounts for a high proportion of rabbit presentations to veterinary clinics. Although it can be a consequence of an inappropriate diet, gastrointestinal stasis syndrome also can be secondary to any number of physiologic conditions including illness, pain, or stress.[159] The term rabbit GI syndrome (RGIS) has been proposed to include a variety of GI conditions in rabbits.[160] Rabbits have extremely sensitive digestive tracts and are hindgut fermenters, as such, have a long and voluminous digestive tract. Dietary fiber, particularly indigestible fiber, is the main factor stimulating motility of the large intestine. Inadequate intake of indigestible fiber, whether due to an inappropriate diet or anorexia secondary to other disease, is the main cause of GI stasis.[159] Pain, drugs, anorexia, and/or just about any other adverse event can also affect GI function. Gastrointestinal stasis is a very common complication during the treatment of other disease conditions in rabbits. When gastrointestinal statsis occurs, a vicious cycle ensues, with further anorexia, dilation of the tract, and pain. Potentially pathogenic bacteria such as *Clostridium* and coliforms, normally present in very low numbers in the cecum, can readily proliferate when slow motility leads to abnormal cecal fermentation and alterations in the pH resulting in a condition called dysbiosis.[159] Dysbiosis can lead to clinical signs ranging from diarrhea to enterotoxemia and death. Carbohydrates provide a substrate for the proliferation of these pathogens. Glucose is required for the production of iota toxin by *Clostridium*.

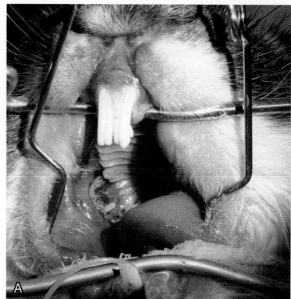

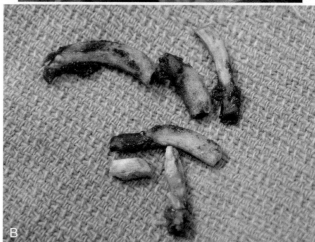

FIGURE 5-17 *A,* Rabbit positioned for dental work. The entire upper right cheek tooth arcade has been extracted. *B,* Severely diseased teeth removed from the rabbit in *A.*

Gastrointestinal stasis should be considered in rabbits that exhibit discomfort, anorexia, and a reduction in stools. Clinical signs of GI stasis typically include a gradual loss in appetite and subsequent reduction in fecal output. There may also be reduced activity, abdominal pain (evidenced by behavior changes, posture changes, and tooth grinding), and weight loss.[159]

Rabbits with GI stasis may have only subtle clinical disease signs recognized during the physical examination. Most rabbits with GI stasis are alert but quiet, with only mild depression. The stomach generally contains ingesta, which is frequently doughy to firm on palpation. The intestines and cecum may contain a large amount of gas, and the colon will have reduced feces. Gut sounds (borborygmi) are generally reduced.[159]

Radiography may be helpful in the diagnosis of GI stasis. A large, ingesta-filled stomach in an anorexic rabbit is suggestive of GI stasis. Severe gas or fluid distension of the stomach is more suggestive of an obstructive process (Figure 5-18). Moderate to severe distension of the intestines and cecum may also be identified.[159] Concurrent and underlying conditions should also be explored.

Treatment of GI stasis involves rehydration of the patient and stomach contents, analgesic therapy, nutritional support, GI prokinetics, and treatment of underlying disorders.[159] Fluid therapy may be administered through the subcutaneous (SC) or IV routes, depending on the severity of the condition and the patient's hydration status. Some of the fluids may be given orally along with assisted feedings as this method of treatment aids in rehydrating the stomach contents as well. Nutritional support is critical in the management of GI stasis.

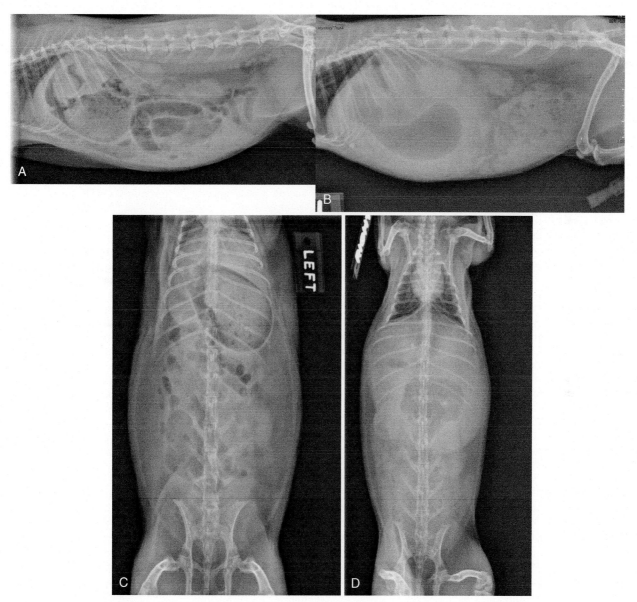

FIGURE 5-18 *A,* Lateral radiograph from a rabbit with moderate GI stasis. Note the moderate distension of the stomach and numerous loops of the intestines. The dried contents of the stomach appear to be pulling away from the wall, leaving a gas "halo." *B,* Lateral projection of a rabbit that presented with acute abdominal pain and vascular compromise. The large, fluid-filled stomach suggested a gastric outflow obstruction. The small mineral particle in the area of the liver was an incidental finding. *C,* Ventro-dorsal radiograph from a rabbit with moderate GI stasis. Note the moderate distension of the stomach and numerous loops of the intestines. The dried contents of the stomach appear to be pulling away from the wall, leaving a gas "halo." *D,* Ventro-dorsal projection of a rabbit that presented with acute abdominal pain and vascular compromise. The large, fluid-filled stomach suggested a gastric outflow obstruction.

Water, hay, and fresh greens should be made available to encourage self-feeding. Generally, syringe feeding will be required, as most of the affected rabbits will be anorexic. Commercial products are available (Critical Care for Herbivores, Oxbow Animal Health, Murdock, NE) for syringe feeding, but the commercial products are unavailable pulverized commercial rabbit diet or canned pumpkin may be used. In rabbits that refuse to swallow the products, a nasogastric tube can be placed and a finer ground product used (Emeraid Herbivore, Lafeber Company, Cornell, IL). Providing nutritional supplementation early in the disease process is essential because it provides fiber to stimulate intestinal motility and nutrients to prevent the onset of hepatic lipidosis, which occurs rapidly in rabbits in a negative-calorie balance.[159]

Gastrointestinal stasis is associated with mild to severe visceral pain. Until the pain is alleviated, most affected rabbits will not begin to eat. Opioid pain relievers are preferred, especially if pain is severe. Buprenorphine (0.03 to 0.05 mg/kg, IM or SC, BID-TID) is commonly used for rabbits that may be in mild to severe visceral pain. NSAIDs should be used with caution because rabbits with GI stasis are at increased risk for reduced renal perfusion and gastric ulceration.

Prokinetic drugs such as cisapride (0.5 mg/kg, PO, BID-TID) and metoclopramide (0.5 mg/kg, PO, BID-TID) may help stimulate the motility of the GI tract. Metoclopramide works primarily at the stomach, while cisapride works on the entire GI tract. There is debate about how useful these drugs are in the management of rabbit patients diagnosed with GI stasis.[159]

Antibiotics may be a useful treatment option if there is evidence of dysbiosis. Metronidazole (20 mg/kg, PO, BID) is effective against most *Clostridium* spp., while enrofloxacin (5 to 10 mg/kg, PO, SID-BID) or trimethoprim sulfamethoxazole (15 to 30 mg/kg, PO, BID) are often effective against coliform bacteria, all of which constitute the primary concerns gastrointestinal infection in these cases. Popular remedies such as lubricants, enzymes, and simethicone appear to have little benefit in the treatment of GI stasis in rabbits.[159] Treatment should be continued for at least 3 to 5 days, with a positive response evidenced by a return of appetite and fecal production. Initially, the feces may appear somewhat abnormal, being misshapen, irregular sized, and mucoid.[159]

Gastric impactions can be a significant component of GI stasis. Rabbits ingest a large amount of hair in the process of grooming, which can accumulate in the stomach. It appears that gastric impactions are primarily due to a motility disorder, with the accumulation of hair or other material occurring as a result of improper gastrointestinal function. Normally, the hair moves through the digestive tract to be removed along with the feces. However, when GI motility is impaired, a large amount of hair can accumulate in the stomach. Since rabbits cannot vomit, affected animals will exhibit anorexia, weight loss, reduction in stool volume and size, and, occasionally, abdominal pain. Dessication of the stomach contents often contributes to the problem. If fluid is then absorbed, the mat of hair and ingesta becomes further compacted and fills the stomach, further reducing the patient's appetite and perpetuating the cycle. Although this condition is frequently referred to as a hairball, wool block, or trichobezoar, gastric impaction does not appear to be initiated by the presence of hair in the stomach.[159]

A diagnosis of gastric impaction in rabbits is based on the history and physical exam findings of dehydration, weight loss, palpable gastric contents, and abdominal pain (sometimes). Radiographs will reveal a stomach full of ingesta even when the animal has not eaten. Often, the gastric contents will pull away from the wall of the stomach, leaving a crescent-shaped gas pocket. Treatment for gastrointestinal impaction should be initiated immediately following the diagnosis. The rare cases that require surgical removal of the impacted material from the GI tract usually carry a poor prognosis.[159] Surgery is required only when a complete obstruction has been identified (see below). The patient's hydration status is a primary concern and fluid therapy should be provided in a manner (e.g., IV, IO, SC) to address required needs. Caution should be used when considering the use of GI motility-enhancing drugs (e.g. metoclopramide, cisapride). The use of metoclopramide and cisapride should be reserved for cases of incomplete obstructions. Syringe or nasogastric feedings with a commercial critical care diet will stimulate gastric motility, help rehydrate the gastric contents, and provide semi-elemental nutrition until the rabbit is eating again. The frequency and amount of feces should increase in 3 to 5 days along with an increased appetite. Prevention of gastric impactions involves feeding a high-fiber diet, brushing the fur, and keeping the rabbit well hydrated.

Acute Gastrointestinal Dilation or Obstruction

True obstructions of the GI tract are relatively rare in rabbits but usually occur due to a compact mat of hair in the small intestine. Unlike GI stasis, rabbits with intestinal obstruction present with an acute abdomen and are painful, shocky, and minimally responsive.[159] Occasionally, the stomach will distend to the point of rupture, resulting in sudden vocalization and death.[159]

Physical examination reveals severe depression, recumbency, and a severely distended stomach. Early in the disease process, these rabbits may be tachypneic and tachycardic but later become hypothermic, bradycardic, and hypotensive.[159] The obstruction frequently consists of a compact mat of hair (trichobezoar) but occasionally will include carpet fibers, plastic, wax, or locust beans. Rabbit intestinal impaction usually occurs in the proximal duodenum but occasionally is diagnosed at the ileocecocolic junction (Figure 5-19).[159]

Radiographs will often reveal the severely distended stomach filled with fluid, gas, or both. Free gas within the abdomen suggests rupture of the stomach and carries a grave prognosis.[159]

Intestinal obstruction condition is a surgical emergency, and the patient should be immediately stabilized and prepared for surgery. Analgesia should be a top priority. A stomach tube should be passed to decompress the stomach as soon as possible which may require sedation or anesthesia to alleviate the distress of the patient. Intravenous or intraosseous (IO) fluid and colloid support should be initiated. In extremely rare cases, when surgery has been declined by the owner, the foreign material may pass through the intestinal tract without surgery.[159]

Surgical treatment of this condition involves exploration of the abdomen to identify and remove the obstruction. When possible, the obstruction should be manipulated into the stomach and removed via gastrotomy. Even with immediate and appropriate surgical care, the prognosis for this condition

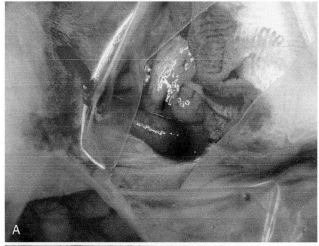

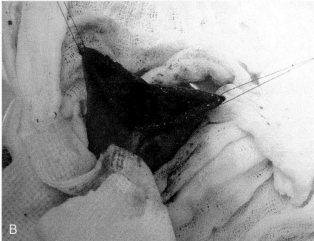

FIGURE 5-19 *A,* The duodenum of the rabbit from Figures 5-18*B,D* at surgery. There was a firm knot of fur obstructing the duodenum. *B,* The stomach of the rabbit from Figures 5-18*B,D* at surgery. There were multiple ulcers and foci of necrosis.

is guarded, as many patients will die in the 48 hours postoperative period from peritonitis, endotoxemia, GI stasis, or acute renal failure.[159]

Diarrhea
Diarrhea is a common disease condition in pet rabbits, and there are a multitude of predisposing factors that contribute to the development of this particular illness. Enteritis is one of the clinical conditions associated with diarrhea in rabbits. Pathogenic or opportunistic bacteria such as *Salmonella* spp. and *E. coli* may be isolated from affected animals, and the effects of these pathogens tend to be more severe in young rabbits. Other cases may involve overgrowth of bacteria normally present in low numbers within the GI tract. This is generally a result of alterations in the GI environment (e.g., dietary changes). Most of these infections will result in a true diarrhea, where there are no solid droppings. When liquid feces are noted, the stool, should be examined for the presence of parasites (e.g., coccidia) and cultured using standard

microbiological techniques. Initial treatment for rabbit's with diarrhea includes fluid therapy, supportive care, trimethoprim-sulfa (15 to 30 mg/kg, PO, BID), and metronidazole (20 mg/kg, PO, BID). Once the pathogenic bacteria have been identified antibiotic therapy based on antimicrobial sensitivities is initiated. Mild enteritis may result from dysbiosis and lead to soft or watery stools which may resolve with a dietary and environmental correction.[159]

In more severe cases, enterotoxemia may occur. Enterotoxemia is caused by an iota toxin produced by *Clostridium spiroforme*. Rabbits with enterotoxemia will have severe, watery diarrhea that soils their perineum and legs and may contain blood. Rabbits with enterotoxemia can rapidly weaken and die, often within 48 hours.[159] Although it is often unrewarding, aggressive treatment that includes IV fluid therapy, antibiotic administration (e.g., metronidazole (20 mg/kg, PO, BID)), toxin-binding drugs (e.g., cholestyramine), and analgesia may be attempted.

Tyzzer's disease, which can also cause enteritis in rabbits also, is caused by *Clostridium piliforme*. This disease causes miliary foci of necrosis in the intestine, liver, and other organs. There is no treatment for Tyzzer's disease at the present time and the diagnosis is usually made on postmortem examination.[161] Tyzzer's disease is discussed in more detail in the rodent section that follows.

Parasitic diseases such as coccidiosis are common causes of diarrhea in young rabbits. Diagnosis of coccidiosis in rabbits is made based on fecal flotation. Coccidiosis can be treated with trimethoprim sulfadimethoxazole (15 to 30 mg/kg, PO, BID for 5 to 7 d) or ponazuril (20 mg/kg, PO, SID for 3 to 5 d); however, ponazuril is preferred as it is coccidiocidal.

Antibiotic-Associated Enteritis or Enterotoxemia
One problem that warrants special attention is antibiotic-associated enteritis. In the author's practice, it is still common to have rabbits and hindgut fermenting rodents present with severe enterotoxemia after being treated with antibiotics by a practitioner unfamiliar with these animals. Diarrhea, shock, and death may occur in rabbit cases of antibiotic-associated enteritis. The microbial flora contained within the intestinal tract of rabbits is a complex ecosystem. When certain antibiotics are used, a specific portion of the GI bacterial population is killed. The result is that other harmful bacterial organisms proliferate. *Clostridium difficile*, in particular, is thought to be responsible for the majority of toxin production in these cases. While it is possible for antibiotic-associated enteritis to happen with any antibiotic, some antimicrobial products are much worse than others. Penicillins, cephalosporins, and macrolide antibiotics should never be used orally in rabbits.[159] While these drugs have been used parenterally without adverse effects, other alternatives should be considered first and foremost. Safer antibiotics include trimethoprim-sulfa, enrofloxacin, and chloramphenicol (not in meat rabbits). Aminoglycosides are safe for the GI microbial flora but still have nephrotoxic side effects, as in other animals. When signs of antibiotic-associated enteritis are encountered, antibiotic therapy should be discontinued and fluid therapy, intestinal absorbants (e.g., cholestyramine, bismuth subsalicylate), and any other necessary supportive care initiated. A high-fiber diet is the most protective factor one can use when rabbits must be treated with antibiotics, as it provides the substrate for the

normal anaerobic microbial flora of the GI tract. *Lactobacillus* products are of questionable efficacy since stomach acid kills most organisms during passage, and *Lactobacillus* spp. are not normal microbial flora for rabbits. Milk-based products, such as yogurt, should be avoided.

Cecotroph Staining

Rabbits produce two types of feces. The first type, the cecotroph, are mucous, gelatinous feces, rich in nutrients. Cecotrophs come from the cecum and are eaten by the rabbit directly from the anus. Normally, the owner never observes cecotrophs. When they are not consumed, cecotrophs will stick in the fur in the perineal area and the cage bedding. The mucoid gelatinous feces are often mistaken for diarrhea by people unfamiliar with cecotrophs.[159] The other type of feces is hard feces, the dry pellet that are found in the bottom of rabbit enclosures. Common causes of the rabbit's failure to consume cecotrophs include obesity, musculoskeletal problems, dental disease, pain, or physical barriers such as Elizabethan collars.[159] Occasionally, the cecotrophs may be abnormal because of changes in GI motility, microbial flora, or pH. In cases of abnormal cecotroph formation, the affected rabbit may not consume the feces.[159] The key distinguishing characteristic of this condition from true diarrhea is that affected rabbits will produce normal hard feces throughout most of the day. There may be a large mat around the anus, resulting in dermatitis. Correction of any contributing factor is the key component to treat this condition. If no physical barrier to cecotroph consumption is identified, dietary changes may be required. Insufficient fiber or excessive carbohydrates are common causes of abnormal cecotroph formation.[159] Pet rabbits provided only pelleted diets, or worse, seed mixtures, often develop this problem. If fed grass hay, most rabbits will have a positive response and start to develop normal cecotrophs within 2 weeks. The pelleted diet can be gradually reintroduced, but with some rabbits, cecotroph staining will reoccur.

Cecoliths

Cecoliths, or abnormal hard masses of cecal contents, do occasionally occur in rabbits. Cecoliths appear to be the result of altered GI motility or an inappropriate diet. Specifically, short fiber length and inappropriate fiber sources, such as psyllium, may be involved.[159] Rabbits that form cecoliths frequently have a history of chronic GI problems. Many are underweight and have reduced muscle mass. There is speculation that *Encephalitozoon cuniculi* may be involved with cecolith formation, as many affected rabbits are serologically positive for this parasite.[159] Diagnosis of this condition is based on palpation of the hard masses in the abdomen, radiography, and history. Treatment involves rehydration and softening of the cecal and colonic contents, feeding high-moisture and high-fiber foods, and promotility drugs.[159] If the cecolith is causing an obstruction, the prognosis is poor. In cecolith obstruction cases, aggressive therapy includes pain relief, IV fluid therapy, careful enema, and surgery is recommended.[159]

Mucoid Enteropathy

Mucoid enteropathy or mucoid enteritis is a common problem in young rabbits and is believed to result from dybiosis of the cecum. Features of this disease include diarrhea, cecal impactions, anorexia, lethargy, and weight loss. The cecum produces excessive amounts of mucus. Feeding a diet high in fiber and low in carbohydrates appears to have a protective effect.[159]

Rectal Papillomas

Rectal papillomas occasionally occur in rabbits. Clinical signs are minimal but include blood-tinged feces, proliferative red tissue protruding from the anus, and mild pain. Rectal papillomas generally are benign. Treatment of the lesions is similar to the treatment of avian cloacal papillomas, although this method is often curative in rabbits.[159]

Rabbit Hemorrhagic Disease

Viral hemorrhagic disease is a severe, fatal disease of rabbits older then 2 months of age. Clinical signs include depression, lethargy, anorexia, and diarrhea. Viral hemorrhagic disease may progress to neurologic signs, bloody nasal discharge, and death.[159] Diagnosis is generally made post mortem using histopathology, electron microscopy, molecular diagnostics, and immunologic testing methodologies. The disease is reportable in the United States.

Coccidiosis

Rabbits can develop both hepatic and intestinal coccidiosis. Clinical disease associated with coccidial infections is generally limited to young rabbits. The presence of the parasite can be determined by finding the oocysts in the feces, but their presence does not always indicate disease. Treatment with ponazuril (20 mg/kg, PO, SID, for 3 to 5 d) appears to be effective.

Neoplasia

Various neoplastic processes have been reported in rabbit GI systems. No specific tumors are particularly common, although neoplasms have been reported in the stomach, intestine, sacculus rotundus, and liver of rabbit patients.[159] Diagnosis may be made based on imaging and biopsy. Unfortunately, there are few clinical data available on the treatment of these disorders.

Liver Lobe Torsion

Reports of live lobe torsions appear to be increasing in pet rabbits. Affected rabbits may present for anorexia, a painful abdomen, and possibly icterus. ALT and gamma-glutamyl-transferase (GGT) values are often elevated, while the hematocrit is often decreased. Radiographs may be of limited value in these cases, however ultrasound is often used to characterize the location of the liver lobe torsion. Surgical removal of the affected liver lobe may resolve this condition if detected in time.[159]

Rodents

Dental and Oral Disease

In the Hystricognathi, dental disease is a common problem. Dental disease accounts for 90% of chinchilla presentations to the author's practice. The incisors of Hystricognathi rarely are presented with the same congenital problems noted in rabbits; instead, incisor fractures or disease of the cheek teeth may influence incisor abnormalities. However it is much more common to encounter diseased cheek teeth in these animals than with incisors. The complex disease process is simply referred to as acquired dental disease (ADD).[22] Dental disease forms when the rate of wear is less than the rate of growth which can lead to more stress on the occlusal surface, slowing the growth of the clinical crown.[25] Underlying causes of ADD may include congenital defects, lack of dietary fiber, and either excessive or inadequate vitamin C.[162] In chinchillas, vitamin C does not appear to be a factor. However, as in rabbits, vitamin D and calcium may be important predisposing factors to dental disease. Prevention of dental disease involves encouraging normal wear of the teeth by feeding fresh leafy vegetables, particularly from monocotyledenous plants.[25]

Numerous clinical aspects of ADD can present. Both the clinical and the reserve crown can overgrow, leading to pressure on the bone surrounding the apices or sharp points that traumatize oral surfaces. Typical intraoral changes include sharp edges, referred to as spurs, hooks, spikes, or points. These sharp enamel edges will typically form on the buccal surface of the maxillary cheek teeth or on the lingual surface of the mandibular cheek teeth. In guinea pigs, the lower cheek teeth angle medially and converge rostrally, therefore when the lower premolars elongate, they can quickly form a bridge that traps the tongue. Naturally an entrapped tongue makes grooming, eating, and even swallowing water very difficult for these animals. Some animals will form irregular growth patterns with altered occlusal surfaces. These are often called wave mouth or step mouth, depending on the configuration.[22] Increased interproximal spaces may form, allowing food and contamination to invade the periodontal ligaments and subsequently form apical abscesses. The reserve crown length may start to distort the supporting bone. Clinical signs of dental disease may include weight loss, dysphagia, alterations in droppings, palpable changes in the mandible or maxilla, pain on palpation, elongated incisors, restriction of jaw movement, ocular discharge, and salivation.[25] Diagnosis of dental disease in Hystricognathi is dependent on using various diagnostic modalities. Oral examination in the conscious patient is very limited. More than half of the potential problems will be missed if this is the only examination method used. Oral examination with anesthesia will allow a much better examination of the patient's teeth (Figure 5-20). The use of an endoscope can facilitate detection of subtler problems. However, radiography and, with increasing frequency, CT are required to fully assess dental disease in these rodents.

Dental disease in guinea pigs and chinchillas carries a poor long-term prognosis. When dental problems can no longer be managed to maintain a good quality of life, euthanasia should be recommended to the owners.[25] Treatment for dental disease includes restoration of the occlusal surfaces by using a burr and drill to reduce and contour the crowns and generally needs to be repeated at 6- to 8-week intervals.[25] In some cases, extraction of teeth may be indicated and may be performed through either an intraoral or extraoral approach.[22] Antibiotic therapy may be indicated if there is evidence of periodontal involvement while analgesics are indicated in all cases of dental disease. Supportive care, including fluids and nutritional support, should be administered as necessary.

Dental disease of Sciurognathi is usually a result of trauma to the incisors. Gnawing on the cage bars, with subsequent loosening of the reserve crowns or fracture of the tooth, is a

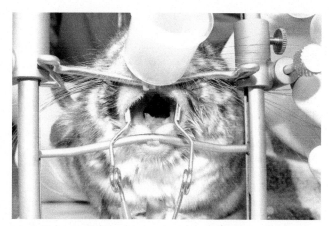

FIGURE 5-20 Chinchilla prepared for dental treatment. The lower right premolar is severely elongated with a rostrally oriented point. The angle of the occlusal plane of the lower left arcade is reversed as well.

common etiology.[163] In prairie dogs, the continuous overstimulation of the tooth bud may result in a pseudo-odontoma. These large knots at the apex of the maxillary incisors often result in compression of the nasal passages and subsequent dyspnea in affected prairie dogs.[22] The crown length for small rodents is often mistakenly thought to be abnormal because the lower incisors are much longer than those located in the maxilla, with an upper-to-lower ratio of 1:3. Normal teeth should not be trimmed.[164] Clipping incisors with nail trimmers or wire cutters can shatter teeth; therefore, the use a dental burr with a dental or hobby drill is recommended. Extraction of incisors can be very difficult in smaller rodents because of the long reserve crown and fragility of the tooth and jaw[163]; however, it is possible in larger species and is considered the treatment of choice for pseudo-odontoma in prairie dogs. Periodontal disease and dental caries can occur in the cheek teeth of Sciurognathi but are probably underdiagnosed because of the difficulty in thoroughly examining the teeth.[22] Gerbils may develop periodontal disease when fed rat and mouse diets for more than 6 months, therefore should only be fed diets labeled for gerbils.[165]

Several different species of rodents maintained in captivity, including hamsters, chipmunks, and pouched rats, have cheek pouches, which can become impacted. Cheek pouch impaction may occur more readily with formulated diets that soften and become doughy when moistened. Cheek pouch impactions often present as persistent swellings on the side of the face.[164] This should not be mistaken for the normal filling of the pouch with food, which is transient. Impacted cheek pouches can be carefully emptied using a cotton-tipped applicator and lavaged with a dilute chlorhexidine solution. If needed, antimicrobial (trimethoprim-sulfadimethoxazole 48 mg/kg, PO, BID) and anti-inflammatory therapy using NSAIDs (meloxicam, 1 to 2 mg/kg, PO, SID) should be prescribed.

Salivary gland swelling can occur in rats with sialodacryoadenitis virus, a coronavirus.[165] Although the clinical signs are largely associated with the eyes and respiratory system, the swollen salivary glands can also cause oral pain. Enlargement of the salivary glands is usually self-limiting, but treatment with NSAIDs (meloxicam, 1 to 2 mg/kg, PO, SID) may be warranted to improve comfort.

Esophageal Conditions

Megaesophagus is a rare disorder of chinchillas. While these animals generally cannot vomit, chinchillas with megaesophagus will regurgitate which predisposes these animals to aspiration pneumonia.[166] The prognosis is grave in these cases.

Gastric Conditions

Gastric dilatation, with or without volvulus, occasionally occurs in guinea pigs. This is usually in association with a generalized GI stasis as described below. Guinea pigs with gastric dilatation will present with severe abdominal distension, pain, shock, and respiratory distress. Radiographs will show a severely gas-dilated stomach, which will be rotated out of position in the case of a volvulus. The diagnosis of gastric dilatation carries a grave prognosis. Immediate care should include pain relief and possibly sedation, decompression using either a stomach tube or a needle, and treatment for shock. See the therapy section below for details on shock therapy. Gastric dilatation may also occur in gerbils and may result from being fed stale or inappropriate diets. Affected gerbils will exhibit abdominal tympany, bruxism, dyspnea, and cardiovascular shock.[167] Gerbils diagnosed with gastric dilatation should be managed using the methods described for guinea pigs.

Hamsters will occasionally develop benign tumors in the stomach or intestine. In the stomach, neoplasms are usually gastric squamous papillomas, and in the intestine, they are typically adenomas.[164] Gerbils have been diagnosed with intestinal adenocarcinomas.[167]

Intestinal Diseases

GASTROINTESTINAL STASIS. Gastrointestinal stasis can occur secondary to many other disorders. It occurs most frequently in the Hystricognathi—in particular, guinea pigs and chinchillas. Ileus is also common in gerbils following anesthesia, malocclusion, or anorexia.[167] Gastrointestinal stasis in rodents is very similar to the syndrome described in rabbits. See the rabbit section for more information.

ANTIBIOTIC-ASSOCIATED ENTERITIS OR ENTEROTOXEMIA. Antibiotic-associated enteritis occurs in rodents as in rabbits. Guinea pigs, chinchillas, and hamsters are particularly susceptible to antibiotic-induced enterotoxemia. The normal predominant bacteria in rodents' intestines are Gram-positive organisms such as *Lactobacillus* spp. and anaerobes such as *Bacteroides* spp. If the normal bacterial flora are significantly reduced by antibiotics, *Clostridium difficile* may proliferate. *Clostridium difficile* produce severe enterotoxins, resulting in diarrhea and death.[164] Chloramphenicol, enrofloxacin, and trimethoprim-sulfa combinations appear to be the safest oral antibiotics to use in rodents.[162]

TYZZER'S DISEASE. Tyzzer's disease, which is caused by *Clostridium piliforme*, is a severe GI and hepatic disease in rodents (and other animals). Gerbils may be particularly susceptible.[165,167] This species of bacteria is an obligate intracellular pathogen, with spores that are extremely stable within the environment.[167] The source of infection is often spore-contaminated food or bedding.[163] Infections are typically spread among animals via the fecal-oral route.[167] Stress caused by overcrowding, poor sanitation, thermal stress, or overbreeding may contribute to the formation of disease.[159] Clinical signs of Tyzzer's disease in rodents may include diarrhea, general malaise, and death. In gerbils, a head tilt may be seen in chronic cases.[167] Young animals typically develop an acute form of the disease, while older animals usually prevent with a more chronic form.[159] Although the *Clostridium piliforme* infection originates in the intestine, dissemination to the liver and other systemic locations may occur with this disease. Diagnosis is usually made post mortem on histopathology, as the organism does not grow well on culture media. An ELISA test can be used to help obtain a diagnosis.[167] Treatment is generally unsuccessful however tetracycline or chloramphenicol may be effective at reducing mortality in group settings.[163,164,167] A carrier state may develop following treatment.[167]

DIARRHEA IN GUINEA PIGS. Pseudotuberculosis, an intestinal infection caused by *Yersinia pseudotuberculosis*, is an uncommon infection in pet guinea pigs.[162] The infection may occur as a result of contamination of the feed by wild birds or rodents. Clinical signs associated with pseudotuberculosis include diarrhea and weight loss over the course of several weeks. This disease is zoonotic, if diagnosed, euthanasia of the patient is recommended to minimize any health risks for the human caretakers.[162]

Coccidiosis in guinea pigs is caused by *Eimeria caviae*. It is an uncommon finding in pet guinea pigs. While affected adults rarely exhibit any clinical signs associated with this parasite, younger guinea pigs may be presented for diarrhea and weight loss. Treatment with trimethoprim sulfadiazine (25 mg/kg, PO, BID, for 5 to 7 d) or ponazuril (20 mg/kg, PO, SID, for 3 to 5 d) and strict sanitation may help alleviate the disease.[162] The author has diagnosed cryptosporidiosis in guinea pigs that was determined to be the cause of chronic diarrhea. Unfortunately, there is no effective treatment for cryptosporidiosis in guinea pigs.

DIARRHEA IN RATS AND MICE. Diarrhea is a common finding in rats and mice and may be associated with a number of different etiologies (e.g., infectious, dietary, hypersensitivity). Unless a specific pathogen (e.g., *Salmonella* spp.) is identified, supportive care, dietary management, and (possibly) antibiotics are usually effective.[163] Viral enteritis, resulting from the mouse hepatitis virus, a coronavirus, may occur in neonates but is rare in pet mice.[163] Pinworms are ubiquitous in mice but generally considered nonpathogenic. If desired, pinworms can be treated using ivermectin (0.4 to 0.8 mg/kg, PO, SC) at high doses. *Spironucleus muris* and *Giardia muris* are two protozoal pathogens that can cause severe diarrhea in mice and should be treated with metronidazole (20 mg/kg, PO, SID-BID).[165]

DIARRHEA IN GERBILS. There are a number of underlying conditions that are known to cause diarrhea in gerbils, including Tyzzer's disease, protozoal enteritis, Gram-negative opportunists, and helminth parasites, such as tapeworms and pinworms.[167] Treatment should follow the same practices outlined for other species of rodents.

DIARRHEA IN HAMSTERS. Proliferative ileitis, caused by *Lawsonia intracellularis*, is a severe disease of weanling hamsters. Clinical disease signs include diarrhea, lethargy, anorexia, and poor hair coat.[164] The unformed feces stains the perineal area and, thus, is where the lay term wet tail originated for this disease (although it is often applied to any diarrhea in hamsters). On palpation, thickened bowel may be identified, and affected hamsters may have intussusceptions, rectal prolapses, and other severe complications.[164] Prognosis is poor for recovery, but treatment with chloramphenicol (50 mg/kg, PO, BID) and supportive care may be effective in some cases. Hamsters with intussusception or prolapses may require surgical care.

Protozoa are normal inhabitants of the intestinal tract of hamsters, although *Giardia* spp. and *Spironucleus* spp. may contribute to enteritis.[164]

The dwarf tapeworm *Hymenolepis nana* may affect hamsters. *Hymenolepis nana* has an indirect life cycle, with fleas or beetles as intermediate hosts and is considered a zoonotic parasite. Most hamsters show no clinical signs associated with this infestation because of low parasite burdens. Diagnosis can be made by observing tapeworm eggs in the feces. Praziquantel may be effective in eliminating this parasite.[164]

HEPATIC CYSTS. Hepatic cysts are occasionally found in the livers of hamsters. This disease condition is usually diagnosed in geriatric hamsters, and the cysts form as developmental defects of the biliary ducts.[165] Although the cysts are benign, they can grow to a very large size and compress the surrounding liver tissue. Diagnosis is determined through palpation, ultrasound, and aspiration of the cysts. Some neoplastic diseases can become cystic, therefore caution should be used when interpreting the examination and diagnostic results. Hepatic cysts can be surgically removed if necessary.

DIAGNOSTICS

Invertebrates

Diagnoses are most often obtained through history and examination in invertebrates. Magnification and focused lighting can greatly enhance examination results, and numerous methods are available to provide optical enhancement, from loupes to videomicroscopes. Some species of invertebrates can be transilluminated to visualize internal structures. Cytologic preparations of samples collected from the animal's body surface are useful for the identification of pathogens and host responses. Imaging can be performed as well, but in some species of invertebrates, the contrast between tissues limits the sensitivity.

Fish

Gastrointestinal disease in fish requires a systematic workup, as in other species. The assessment of fish should always include a thorough history, physical examination, and weight. Diagnostic tests such as hematology and serum/plasma biochemistry panels can be helpful for internal evaluation. Imaging techniques and endoscopy are also possible, particularly for larger fish species. Specific GI workup procedures may also include sampling of feces, gastric lavage, cloacal lavage, swim bladder aspiration, or peritoneal lavage. Collected diagnostic samples can be used for cytology, parasite testing, microbiology, or specific infectious disease testing.[1]

Radiographic images can be taken of larger fish, such as koi, without anesthesia, utilizing a sealed plastic bag with a small amount of their pond water. Foam supports may be used to aid in positioning.[39] Tricaine methanesulfate (100 to 150 mg/L) should be used as an anesthetic agent in cases where patient movement is a concern. Radiography is helpful in detecting swim bladder disorders, spinal or other bone deformities, masses, or ingested foreign objects.[39] The administration of barium can help outline the GI system. However, care must be taken to avoid barium contacting the oral mucous membranes and gills, as this can impair oxygen exchange.[39] Computed tomographic scanning of koi may also be a valuable tool in obtaining a diagnosis.[39]

Ultrasound is useful for imaging larger fish as well. The water that surrounds the fish patient precludes the need for coupling gel. Biopsies can be obtained under ultrasound guidance, although anesthesia may be essential for this technique to minimize pain.[39] The swim bladder is readily identified as a hyperechoic structure if normal and hypoechoic if fluid filled (abnormal).[39]

Endoscopy can be used to assess the GI tract of fish that are large enough for passage of the scope. An endoscope can be used to examine the mouth, esophagus, proximal intestines, and body cavity (through a small incision).[39] Biopsies or other diagnostic samples can be collected under direct visual control with this technique.

Amphibians

A diagnostic workup of an amphibian case should follow a similar process as described for fish. Due to the extremely small size of some animals, magnification may be critical for examining the patient. Transillumination is a useful technique to visualize certain internal structures, albeit in an extremely vague manner. Hematology and biochemistry evaluation may provide useful information, but correlation of the results with the disease process is not always consistent. Imaging techniques as described for fish are possible as well. Although soft tissues have little contrast in amphibian species, the lungs, bones, and mineral-dense foreign material can be readily identified. Endoscopy may be applicable in amphibians of adequate size. Cytology of the mouth, esophagus, stomach, cloaca, or feces may help identify disease conditions associated with the areas/material from which the samples were collected. The same samples can be used for microbiological culture, parasite evaluation, or molecular diagnostics. Pathologic examination of tissues remains the most reliable diagnostic method currently available for amphibians. However, histologic examination of amphibian livers is complicated by extramedullary hematopoiesis and melanin-laden melanomacrophage aggregates.[168]

Reptiles

Reptile cases can be approached in a similar fashion to higher vertebrates; however, patient size can range from very small to very large, therefore differences may result from variation in body mass. An initial patient workup should include a thorough history and physical examination. In smaller species, and for certain anatomic structures, magnification may still be helpful. Small species may be transilluminated, as was noted with amphibians. In large lizards, digital palpation of the cloaca may be helpful. Hematology and biochemistry testing are more consistent for reptile patients than in amphibians but still lack the sensitivity and specificity found with birds and mammals. Generally, the guidelines used for birds in selecting parameters and interpreting hematologic results are useful in reptiles. However, as one would expect, there are

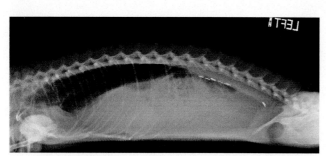

FIGURE 5-21 Lateral radiograph of an iguana with hepatomegaly. The large liver compresses the ventral margin of the lungs. The metallic objects are hemoclips from a previous ovariohysterectomy. The caudo-ventral coelom is occupied by extensive fat bodies.

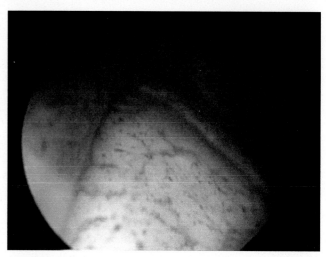

FIGURE 5-22 Endoscopic view of a box turtle liver. Note the pale color and pigment spots. The liver was histologically normal.

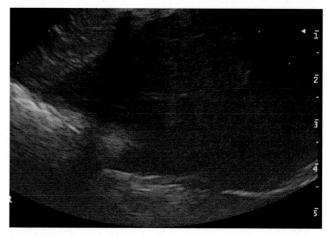

FIGURE 5-23 An ultrasound of the liver of the same iguana in Figure 5-21. After confirming that the liver had a homogeneous texture, a needle biopsy was taken. Histopathology showed lipidosis and mild fibrosis.

significant variation in the physiologic conformation of the different reptile species.

All of the imaging methods previously described for fish and amphibians are beneficial in reptiles. The soft tissues of the reptile body cavity lack contrast, as fat is stored in distinct fat bodies rather than filling the space between organs (Figure 5-21). However, the lungs, bones, and gas patterns or foreign objects within the GI tract can be evaluated. Ultrasound can be used to better distinguish soft tissue structures. The probe can be placed directly on the skin with coupling gel, or the patient can be imaged in a tub of water with the probe on the surface of the plastic. Computed tomographic scans provide superior images, particularly with the use of contrast agents and are especially helpful when examining chelonians, where the shell makes radiographic interpretation difficult and limits the window for ultrasound evaluation.

Most reptile patients are of sufficient size for endoscopic evaluation. The endoscope, depending on the available instrumentation, can access the upper GI tract, cloaca, colon, and coelomic cavity. In addition to direct visualization of the tissues or viscera, endoscopy allows for visually directed biopsy collection. See the avian section below for further information on endoscopy.

Fecal evaluation is very useful as well. Since some reptile species defecate infrequently, the clinician should take advantage of available samples for parasitology, cytology, microbiology, or molecular diagnostics, depending on the presenting problems and/or tentative diagnosis.

Collection of samples for cytologic evaluation, parasite detection, microbiology, or molecular diagnostics may provide the most efficient path to a diagnosis in many circumstances. Histopathology is still the most dependable means of obtaining a diagnosis in reptiles. Samples can be collected from the same sites discussed for cytologic sampling, but a small piece of the tissue must be collected. The oral cavity is readily accessible and swabs are easily obtained from this area. Unfortunately sample will be significantly contaminated, consequently the results should be interpreted with caution. For microbiologic samples, it may be advisable to remove surface debris or even make a small incision in the mucosa and obtain samples below the surface. To increase the chance of a more reliable result, a small piece of tissue can be submitted in sterile saline for the culture. Samples from the esophagus and stomach can be obtained using swabs, lavages, or endoscopic biopsy, utilizing an oral approach. Lower intestinal samples can likewise be obtained by swabs, lavages, or an endoscopic approach through the cloaca.

One can evaluate the liver and pancreas through aspiration or biopsy. Generally, these samples are obtained through endoscopic- or ultrasound-guided collection procedures (Figures 5-22 and 5-23). In some smaller lizards (e.g., leopard gecko) the liver can be observed through the skin and, if necessary, percutaneously aspirated.

Birds

In birds, as in other species, evaluation of the GI tract should follow a systematic evaluation. Since many diseases can be localized to the affected area, a targeted approach to the various sites is applied for avian species.

Oral Diseases

In many cases, the diagnosis is determined based on cytologic or microbiologic examination of swabs or scrapings collected from lesions. The sample should first be examined as a wet preparation in saline and then dried and stained for examination. The normal cytology of the oral cavity will show squamous epithelial cells with low to moderate numbers of Gram-positive bacteria present. Frequently, the etiologic agent responsible for the disease condition will be identified. A microbiological culture and antibiotic sensitivity profile can follow if bacteria appear to be associated with the disease process. Occasionally, histopathology of a biopsy sample may be required to make a diagnosis. Molecular diagnostics are available for the diagnosis of some avian infectious diseases. A general health workup is usually indicated since many diseases involving the oral cavity are opportunistic.

Crop and Esophagus

Cytology and microbiology from crop washes are very useful in diagnosing ingluvial disease. Wet-mount and stained slides should be examined. If visualization of the crop is desired, an endoscope can be passed to visualize the lumen. The crop can also be inflated with air and transilluminated to detect lesions or foreign bodies. Plain or contrast radiography can also be used to visualize the crop.

Gastric Diseases

Diagnosis of gastric diseases is challenging in birds. Plain and contrast radiography are often used to determine the presence and character of gastric problem disease (Figure 5-24). However, a specific diagnosis often depends on aggressive diagnostic techniques such as surgical or endoscopic biopsy, cytology of samples obtained by a wash, or microbiology. Occasionally a causative agent can be identified by examination of the feces for parasites, acid-fast organisms, yeasts, or specific pathogens (e.g., *Macrorhabdus*, Gram-negative bacteria).

Intestinal Diseases

Diagnostic tests that are helpful in determining the cause of intestinal disease include plain or contrast radiography, fecal flotation, fecal wet mount, fecal cytology (including several special stains), fecal culture, plain and contrast radiography, and occasionally, exploratory coelioscopy or coeliotomy.

Cloacal Diseases

The diagnosis of cloacal diseases is often determined by direct visualization of the lesion. The application of 5% acetic acid (vinegar) aids in the visualization of small areas of papillomatous tissue. Cytology, cultures, biopsy, and other techniques may be used to obtain a more specific diagnosis. Cloacaliths may be visualized on radiographs. Cloacal endoscopy using saline infusion can be very useful for detecting and identifying cloacal disease conditions.

Liver Diseases

There are two basic steps in diagnosing liver disease. First, it must be established that liver disease is present and, second, the specific disease affecting the liver must be determined. Liver disease may be is considered based on the history and physical examination. Color changes in the urates, a swollen

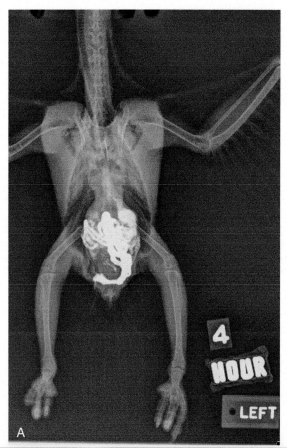

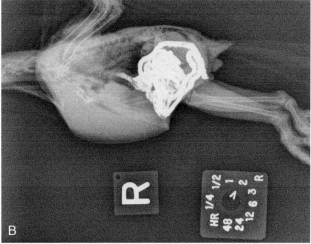

FIGURE 5-24 *A,* GI contrast series of a parrot. The barium is filling most of the digestive tract after 4 hours. *B,* GI contrast series of a parrot. The barium is filling most of the digestive tract after 2 hours.

abdomen, or seizures may suggest the liver is diseased. However, since each of these signs may be related to other causes, other diagnostic tests are necessary to confirm liver involvement. In these cases, radiographs, hematology, biochemistry profiles, or urine analysis may be performed.

If the abdomen is swollen, fluid samples may be collected for analysis. Coelomic fluid formed due to liver disease is generally low in protein, cells, and specific gravity when compared to an inflammatory process such as egg peritonitis. The urine of birds with liver disease is often hyposthenuric, with a specific gravity <1.007. No other significant findings are usually identified in the urine analysis of birds with liver disease.

Imaging of the liver can provide a great deal of information. Radiographs may indicate that the liver is enlarged or smaller than normal. The liver is readily identified in the ventro-dorsal radiographic view. The avian liver is narrow at the heart's apex, forming an hourglass shadow with the heart, and widens toward the caudal border of the organ. The normal liver does not extend outside a line drawn from the scapula to the greater trochanter of the femur.[13] On the lateral view, the liver should not extend caudal to the end of the sternum. Radiographic signs of hepatomegaly include widening of the liver shadow with loss of the hourglass shape, caudal and dorsal displacement of the ventriculus, and alteration of the shape of the liver (Figure 5-25). The liver lobes surround many other viscera, and enlargement of these organs can elevate the liver lobes, thus widening the liver shadow and giving the appearance of hepatomegaly. The position of the ventriculus should aid in distinguishing false enlargement from true hepatomegaly. Radiographs may not be useful in distinguishing liver size in birds with ascites. Positioning birds with ascites for radiographs carries some risk of the fluid

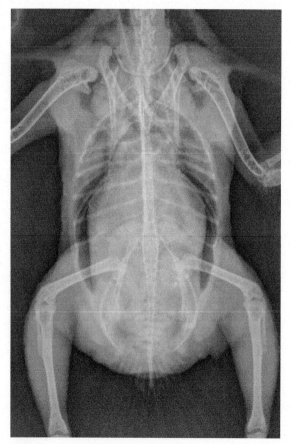

FIGURE 5-25 Ventro-dorsal radiograph of an Amazon parrot with severe liver disease. The abdomen was very distended and the liver was enlarged and very firm.

rupturing into the air sacs and lungs. Ultrasound may be useful in birds with ascites in determining the size and texture of the liver. Ultrasound gives a better assessment of liver uniformity. Although the air sac system presents challenges for ultrasound examination in avian patients, the liver is one organ that can generally be imaged. The enlarged liver or ascites present in some hepatic cases further enhances the imaging window.[13] CT, magnetic resonance imaging, nuclear scintigraphy, positron emission tomography (PET), or other advanced imaging methodologies are used infrequently but can provide superior images of the liver and viscera in select cases (Figure 5-26).[13]

The biochemistry profile in a bird with liver disease may show elevated AST, lactose hydrogenase (LDH), or bile acids; decreased glucose, total protein, and albumin; or may be normal. AST is the preferred liver enzyme for detection of hepatocellular damage. AST is a sensitive indicator of cellular damage, but it is present in muscle tissue as well, therefore elevations in this enzyme may be due to either muscle or liver cell damage.[13] For this reason, AST is usually evaluated in conjunction with CK levels to help determine if muscle or liver is the main source of the enzyme. One should remember that AST has a longer half-life than CK. As the liver and/or muscle damage is repaired, the enzyme levels will return to normal. GGT and glutamyl dehydrogenase (GLDH) are specific indicators of liver disease.[13] Increases in GGT occur with biliary damage or obstruction, and marked elevations occur with bile duct carcinoma.[13] GLDH is a mitochondrial enzyme and elevations occur with severe hepatic damage and necrosis, such as occurs with Pacheco's disease.[13] LDH is neither sensitive nor specific for liver disease and can be elevated with liver, renal, muscle, or other disorders.[13] Alkaline phosphatase has little value in the diagnosis of hepatic disease.[13] Bile acids are sensitive and specific for the liver and give information regarding functional capacity of the liver. It is not necessary to test fasting and postprandial samples in birds. Bile acid analysis is preferred after a 2- to 3-hour fast, but random samples can be used if necessary. Although measurement of bile acids provides the best evaluation of hepatic function, it does not have 100% correlation with hepatic disease.[13] Total proteins and albumin may be reduced in avian patients diagnosed with liver failure.

Once it is determined that a hepatosis is present, a specific diagnosis must be made. Often, a tentative diagnosis may be determined based on history (e.g., obese bird on poor diet = fatty liver) or initial workup (e.g., high white blood cell count = hepatitis). Many organisms can cause hepatitis in birds, including *Chlamydia psittaci*, Gram-negative bacteria, viruses, mycobacteria, and some parasites. Definitive diagnosis of these pathogens requires special tests. Avian chlamydiosis diagnostic tests should be performed on liver patients to rule out this disease. Screening for blood levels of toxins such as lead and aflatoxins is recommended if these diseases are suspected. Concurrent Gram-negative enteritis can be suggestive of Gram-negative hepatitis. If hepatitis secondary to septicemia is suspected, a blood sample should be submitted for culture.

Hepatic biopsy is the only way to definitively diagnose hepatic diseases. The biopsy method used should be selected based on the specific risks and needs of the patient but include endoscopic, surgical, or fine-needle aspiration techniques.

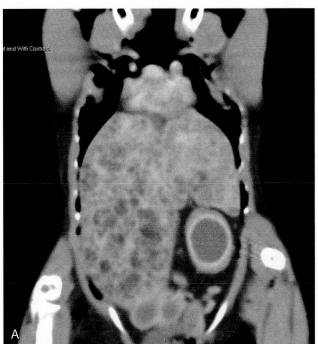

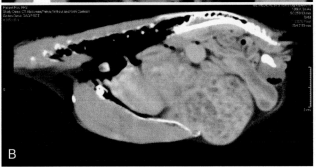

FIGURE 5-26 *A,* CT scan of the parrot from Figure 5-25 with severe hepatic disease. The severe hepatomegaly is much more evident than in the radiographs where the soft tissues were silhouetted and could not be readily distinguished from a mass. The IV iodinated contrast material highlights the fibrous tissue that has developed. *B,* CT scan of the parrot in Figure 5-25 with severe hepatic disease. The severe hepatomegaly is much more evident than in the radiographs where the soft tissues were silhouetted and could not be readily distinguished from a mass. The IV iodinated contrast material highlights the fibrous tissue that has developed.

Samples obtained can be used for cytology, histopathology, or microbiologic examinations.[13] In stable avian patients a liver biopsy is recommended. Microbiologic swabs should be obtained from the liver at the time of biopsy if hepatitis is suspected. Biopsies can be collected during endoscopic examination or through a ventral laparotomy. Impressions are made from the sample, which are then processed for histopathological evaulation. Despite the fact that clotting ability may be compromised, complications related to hemorrhage at the biopsy site are uncommon. If the liver can be visualized or palpated through the skin, a fine-needle aspirate is possible (Figure 5-27). While not as sensitive as histopathology, the fine needle aspirate method is rapid and inexpensive. Liver

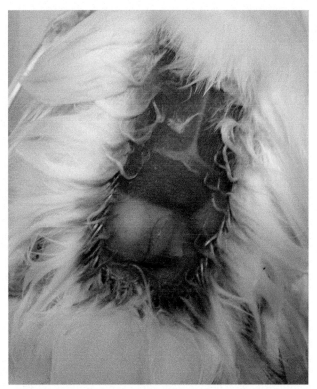

FIGURE 5-27 View of the "abdomen" of a finch. The feathers have been wet to expose the skin. The coelomic viscera are visible through the body wall. The right liver lobe, duodenum, pancreas, and ventriculus can be readily seen. The liver is enlarged, judging by the fact that it extends well beyond the caudal border of the sternum.

aspiration carries the risk of lacerating the organ if restraint is inadequate. The risk of traumatizing the liver while performing a fine needle aspirate can be minimized by anesthetizing the patient. In cases where the bird is a poor surgical or anesthetic risk, the treatment protocol must be based on the tentative diagnosis.

Pancreatic Diseases

Pancreatic disease may be suspected based on signalment or clinical signs. Pale, bulky feces can be mixed with iodine to determine if starch is present. Starch will turn purple/black when mixed with iodine (Figure 5-28). Pancreatic disease may result in hematologic changes, such as elevations in amylase or glucose. Specifically, elevated amylase has a high association with pancreatic disease.[89] Definitive diagnosis of pancreatic disease, much like liver disease, depends on biopsy and histopathology. The duodenal portion of the pancreas is readily accessible and lies dorsal to the ventral body wall, slightly to the right of midline. It can be accessed endoscopically or through a small ventral midline incision. The avian pancreas appears to be tolerant of biopsy, consequently post-biopsy pancreatitis is uncommon.

Endoscopy

While with most mammalian species GI endoscopy requires long flexible endoscopes, in most companion birds the rigid

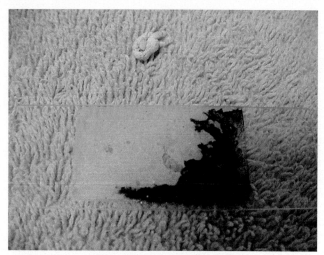

FIGURE 5-28 Amylorrhea from a budgerigar. This bird was passing these pale, white droppings. When mixed with iodine, a purple/black color formed, suggesting the passage of undigested starches.

endoscope can reach all of the accessible sites with superior optics. The intestinal lumen is generally not accessible except for the terminal section leading into the cloaca. As previously mentioned, wet field examination using warmed saline is usually preferred for examination of the GI tract. In most avian cases, GI endoscopy is used for diagnostic purposes, such as specimen collection and direct visualization internal body structures, but it can also be useful for foreign body retrieval.

Ingluvioscopy, or endoscopic examination of the crop, is a relatively simple and noninvasive procedure. While the crop is easily palpated, and to some extent can be visualized externally by wetting and separating the overlying feathers, endoscopy can allow detailed examination of the mucosal surface. Additionally, foreign bodies may rest in the crop if they have been recently ingested or are too large to enter the thoracic esophagus. For the procedure, the patient should be properly anesthetized and placed in dorsal recumbency, preferably with the head elevated and directed toward the endoscopist. The patient should be intubated and the choana packed with gauze or cotton to prevent aspiration of refluxed fluids. The endoscope should be gently inserted into the mouth and slid down the esophagus to the crop. Generally, a sheath should be used to protect the telescope: an examination sheath if only visualization is required and an operating sheath if a more complex procedure is necessary. Air or saline can be infused into the port of the sheath to distend the walls of the esophagus and facilitate examination.

Proventriculoscopy, or gastroscopy, is the endoscopic examination of the proventriculus, isthmus, and ventriculus. This procedure may be a noninvasive procedure via an oral entry in small- to medium-sized psittacids but requires an entry through an ingluviotomy incision in larger birds. The patient is prepared as described for an ingluvioscopy. When an oral approach is used, the scope is passed from the mouth into the crop, as described. At this level of the GI tract, the entry into the thoracic esophagus is required. The scope is gently manipulated into the thoracic esophagus and advanced

into the proventriculus. The procedure for birds requiring ingluvioscopy has the bird in the same position, but the area overlying the crop is prepared for a surgical incision. A small incision is made in the skin and the crop wall, and the telescope and sheath are inserted. From this point, the procedure is the same as described for the oral approach. Saline insufflation aids in examination of the GI tract. The proventriculus is often filled with ingesta, which can make the examination more difficult. Lavaging the ingesta within the proventriculus can improve visualization. Proventricular lavage can be performed using a large-bore catheter or the endoscope sheath as described below. The interior of the proventriculus and ventriculus should be inspected and any diagnostic samples collected or foreign bodies removed. The instruments are removed, and if necessary, the ingluviotomy and skin incisions are closed in a routine manner.

Cloacoscopy, or examination of the cloaca, provides access to the lower digestive tract, urinary tract, and reproductive tract. Generally, this is a diagnostic procedure, although it can also be used for some innovative approaches to treat specific disease conditions. Saline infusion can greatly improve the ability of the endoscopist to examine the cloaca.[169] Cloacal papillomas, common viral-induced lesions in Amazon parrots and macaws, will float into the visual field, resembling sea anemones. These floating lesions can be biopsied using standard biopsy forceps passed through the channel in the operating sheath. These lesions are much easier to identify with the extensive magnification offered by the endoscope.

Mammals

The methodology used to diagnose digestive disorders in mammals varies between the animal groups that comprise companion exotic mammals. The typical approach to diagnosing GI disease described in the section is based on the anatomic/physiologic differences between the small mammal groups.

Sugar Gliders, Hedgehogs, and Small Rodents

Smaller exotic mammalian species can be a diagnostic challenge. Fortunately, the history may be used to guide the required diagnostic plan for that particular patient. In some cases, especially in hedgehogs, the diagnostic plan should be devised prior to the examination, because if the patient has to be anesthetized for the examination, the diagnostic tests and sample collection can be performed at this time. Hedgehogs, and to a lesser extent sugar gliders, cannot be adequately examined when fully conscious. Small rodents vary in their tolerance of handling and manipulation. If oral or dental disease is suspected, all of these smaller species require sedation or anesthesia for adequate examination. In most cases, inhalant anesthetics are used for this purpose, but injectable sedatives may be appropriate in some cases. Blood or other clinical samples should be collected, and any imaging required performed before the patient recovers from anesthesia or sedation. Although the blood values can provide useful information regarding systemic health, they usually do not provide a specific diagnosis. Imaging may include skull or whole-body radiographs, ultrasound, or, occasionally, CT images.

For hedgehog patient, the clinician should always be prepared to perform a dental prophylactic procedure which includes probing of the periodontal pockets to assess for root abscesses or other disease. Tooth extractions are often necessary in hedgehogs and, in most cases, can be performed in a timely manner. For sugar gliders and rodents, dental care may require more planning and diagnostics. The mouth in sugar gliders and rodents is small. The use of an otoscope or endoscope can facilitate complete oral examination in patients with small mouths. The teeth should be probed for periodontal pocketing and skull radiographic images may be a useful diagnostic aid.

Diagnosis of gastric or intestinal disease is usually made based on palpation, imaging, and fecal analysis. Contrast radiography has been successfully used to evaluate the GI system in many species of companion exotic mammals.[170]

Ferrets

Diagnosis of GI conditions in ferrets should follow a logical systematic approach. For any ferret case that is presented with GI disease, the diagnostic approach should begin with a thorough evaluation of general health. A history, physical examination, and hematology and serum biochemistries are warranted for a thorough health assessment of the patient. Any abnormal findings from this initial evaluation should be pursued. Imaging techniques are generally provide relevant information regarding the ferret patient's condition.

In cases of diarrhea, evaluation of the feces may be useful but will often yield less than optimum results relative to other small mammal species. Fecal wet-mount preparations, flotations, or other parasitologic investigations rarely elicits information that will help diagnose abnormal GI conditions affecting ferrets. PCR techniques for specific pathogens such as *Helicobacter mustelae* or ferret enteric coronavirus may be of more use to the veterinarian.[148] Gastric washes or samples collected via gastroscopy may also be used to identify *H. mustelae* or other pathogens.

Plain and contrast radiography, as well as ultrasound, is helpful when localizing a GI problem in ferrets. Radiographs may show size alterations of viscera, gas patterns suggestive of an obstruction, mineralization, or other abnormal physical changes. Contrast studies may help determine if an obstructive process is present but is not always definitive, as some of the foreign objects will absorb the contrast material and look very similar to ingesta. With a skilled operator, ferrets are sonographically "transparent," providing very good images of most of the abdominal viscera. In addition, ultrasound can be used to guide fine-needle aspiration techniques to collect cytologic or microbiologic samples.

In contrast to many exotic species, exploratory laparotomy in ferrets is an extremely useful and highly recommended diagnostic technique. Ferrets are excellent surgical patients. They tolerate anesthesia and surgery well, their body shape allows excellent visualization within the abdomen, and many medical problems are often found within the abdominal cavity. Due to of the frequency of obstructive conditions, and the difficulty in absolutely ruling this disease problem out, exploratory surgeries are frequently performed in ferrets. The consequences of a negative exploratory are far preferable to the consequences of failing to promptly correct an obstruction. Additionally, it is rare to have a completely negative exploratory laparotomy. If an obstruction is not identified, a diagnosis can usually still be made if appropriate biopsies are collected. Depending on the clinical signs and condition of the patient, samples of liver, lymph node, stomach, or intestine may be obtained for histopathological evaluation. It is also common to find concurrent disease processes during exploratory surgery (e.g., adrenal disease, islet cell tumors).

Endoscopy is rarely used in ferrets because of the frequency of open surgery. However, there are applications where endoscopy may be helpful in patient evaluation. Laparoscopic techniques can be used to examine the viscera, and laparoscopy-assisted intestinal biopsies and other techniques are possible with this diagnostic option. Moreover liver biopsies can be readily collected through an endoscopic approach. Gastroscopy may provide a means for removal of smaller foreign bodies or to confirm gastritis by collecting mucosal biopsies.

Rabbits, Guinea Pigs, and Chinchillas

The health of rabbits, guinea pigs, and chinchillas are evaluated in a similar manner as ferrets. Most of these animals are amenable to handling for examination and minor procedures, but sedation is frequently indicated if there is significant pain, distress, or a fractious temperament. Gastrointestinal disease in these species can be roughly divided into "head" disorders and "abdominal" disorders.

The majority of head disorders are diagnosed based on examination and imaging. Occasionally, cytology, histopathology, or other techniques may be used. Examination should include thorough palpation of the head and neck, including the ventral jaw margins (for boney masses or abscesses), lymph nodes, periocular area, and cheeks. The eyes and nose should be examined for excessive tearing or discharge. The incisors can be evaluated by pulling the lips back, but cheek teeth require specialized equivalent to fully evaluate these structures. Although an otoscope can be used to evaluate the mouth it provides a restricted view. A canine vaginal speculum is preferable for oral examination and allows retraction of the buccal mucosa to provide a better view of the mouth. Anesthesia significantly facilitates the oral and dental examination and in chinchillas is essential. Skull radiography or CT will allow evaluation of the reserve crowns and gives an overview of the occlusal surface of the teeth (Figure 5-29). Although patients dental occlusion can be subjectively evaluated, it is helpful to draw reference lines to objectively assess the reserve crown length and occlusal planes.[171] Computed tomographic imaging is very useful when evaluating the head of small mammals, particularly rodents with dental disease.[170]

Diagnosis of abdominal problems begins with the initial pysical examination. Palpation of the abdomen may reveal a firm, doughy, gassy, or fluid-filled stomach or intestines. Pain or splinting may be readily recognized. Auscultation of the abdomen may reveal either hypermotility or hypomotility of the intestinal tract. Radiography is the most important diagnostic test for evaluation of the GI tract of the rabbit and Hystricognath rodents.[172]

Several decisions must be made in the initial evaluation of the rabbit presented with GI disease:
1. Can the rabbit tolerate restraint and manipulation? Occasionally, the patient is very distressed and manual restraint may present added risks. For these cases, sedation using midazolam (0.5 to 1.0 mg/kg, SC) combined with an opioid (buprenorphine, 0.01 to 0.05 mg/kg SC) may help alleviate both pain and distress.

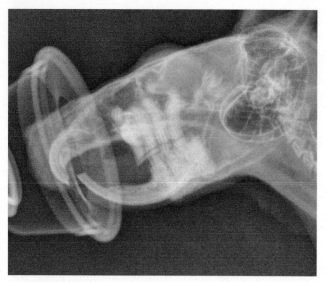

FIGURE 5-29 Lateral projection of the skull of a chinchilla with moderate dental disease. Numerous abnormalities can be seen, including elongation of the reserve crown of the upper incisors, squared-off occlusal plane of the lower incisors, elongation of the reserve crowns of the upper cheek teeth, elongation of the lower cheek teeth with remodeling of the ventral jaw margin, development of points on the rostral edges of the upper premolars, and a caudal shift of the mandibular arcade relative to the maxillary arcade.

2. What type of fluid support is required and how should it be administered? One should determine whether IV access is required and whether colloids are needed to support adequate perfusion.
3. When should a diagnostic workup proceed? This is closely related to the first decision.
4. Can the patient be medically managed or will surgery be required? This decision is based on both clinical and radiographic information.[172]

TREATMENT

Therapy of specific GI disorders has been discussed above with the description of the diseases. Table 5-6 lists an overview of drugs mentioned in the text along with some dosages. Readers are referred to an exotic animal formulary for drug dosages not listed in this chapter.[173] Some general therapeutic approaches and GI surgical procedures are outlined in this section. Table 5-7 lists the more common GI surgical procedures.

Invertebrates

Invertebrates present a tremendous treatment challenge. Although some antibiotic agents can be used, parasitic treatments are often toxic to these species, since common species of invertebrates maintained in captivity are closely related to their own parasites and have common physiology. Few, if any, pharmacologic studies have evaluated the safety and/or efficacy of therapeutic agents used in invertebrate species.

Fish

Drugs can be administered PO, IM, intracoelomically, or topically as baths or dips. The intracoelomic route is useful in treating critically ill patients that require rapid drug distribution. Only nonirritating drugs should be administered by this route.[174] The IM route can be used in nonsedated fish and may be easier to perform for clients.[174] If fish are still eating when presented, the oral route is usually preferred with the prescribed drugs being incorporated into the food. Topical treatments are available in several forms. Tank treatments affects the entire environment. While treating the entire tank is the easiest method to administer therpeutic agents to fish, it is the least preferred because of the negative effects on the biological filter.[174] A good alternative to tank treatments are long-term baths or dips. To perform long-term baths or dips, a separate treatment tank should be set up with a known volume of water from the aquarium. The desired drug is then added to this water, and affected fish are placed in the medicated water for a prescribed length of time. Direct topical treatment of localized lesions are also useful.[174]

Surgery of the coelomic cavity is possible in larger fish. In koi, this is performed through a ventral midline incision. The fish is positioned on foam blocks, and soluble anesthetics (e.g., tricaine methanesulfonate) are administered over the gills with either a syringe or a recirculation system from the tub below the patient.[39] Common GI surgeries include foreign body retrieval, tumor removal and/or biopsy, and swim bladder procedures.

Amphibians

Medical therapies in amphibians are similar to fish. The skin is highly permeable, therefore topical therapy may result in significant absorption of the drug. Fluid therapy can be accomplished through patient soaks. In addition, oral, IM injections, intracoelomic injections, and, in larger species, IV injections are possible. The skin of amphibian species is thin and fragile, consequently care should be taken when giving injections.

Cloacal and rectal prolapse are surgical emergencies. Trauma, parasites, impaction, neoplasia, and foreign bodies should be treated if present. A prolapse must be reduced, which may be facilitated by hypertonic sugar solution. A purse-string suture can be placed around the cloacal opening to retain the reduced prolapse until the tissue heals.[49]

A gastrotomy procedure is sometimes required to remove foreign objects that cannot be treated by gavage or endoscopy. The gastrotomy technique is similar to that described in other species. Fasting for 7 days is recommended if the patient condition allows, and only small meals should be provided for 4 to 6 weeks following the surgical procedure.[49]

Reptiles

Medical therapies in reptiles are similar to those in higher vertebrates. The same routes of administration can be utilized, although with varying ease and effectiveness. Pharmacologic data are available on a number of drugs in a variety of reptile species, but their physiologic diversity makes extrapolating treatments from one species to another a speculative process. The renal portal system in reptiles may allow drugs injected into the rear half of the body to pass through the kidneys before reaching the systemic circulation. The renal portal system leads to the dual theoretical risk of increased renal damage by nephrotoxic drugs and premature elimination of renally excreted drugs. Although there is no direct evidence that these

TABLE 5-6

Dosages of Drugs Listed in the Text

Drug	Species	Dosage[173]
ANTIVIRALS		
Acyclovir	Reptiles	80 mg/kg PO q8 h
	Birds	20-40 mg/kg PO q12 h; 1000 mg/L drinking water
ANTIBIOTICS		
Amoxicillin	Fish	12.5-80 mg/kg PO q12-24 h
	Reptile	10-22 mg/kg PO q12-24 h
	Bird	150-175 mg/kg q4-8 h
	Mammal	15-30 mg/kg PO q12 h; do not use in rabbits, some rodents
Amox/clavulenic acid	Bird	125 mg/kg PO q12 h
	Mammal	12.5-25 mg/kg PO q12 h; do not use in rabbits, some rodents
Azithromycin	Fish	30 mg/kg q24 h
	Reptiles	10 mg/kg q2-7 d
	Birds	10-80 mg/kg PO q24-48 h
	Mammals	15-30 mg/kg PO q24 h; caution in rabbits/rodents
Chloramphenicol	Fish	25-50 mg/kg PO, IM q24 h
	Amphibians	50 mg/kg IM, SC, ICe q12-24 h; 20 mg/L bath changed q24 h
	Reptiles	20-50 mg/kg IM, SC, PO q12-72 h
	Birds	25-50 mg/kg PO q6-12 h
	Mammal	25-50 mg/kg IM, SC, PO q8-12 h
Clarithromycin	Reptiles	15 mg/kg PO q48-72 h
	Birds	60-85 mg/kg PO q24 h
	Mammals	12.5-50 mg/kg PO q12-24 h; caution in rabbits, rodents
Clindamycin	Reptiles	5 mg/kg PO q12 h
	Birds	25-50 mg/kg PO q12 h
	Mammals	5.5-12.5 mg/kg PO q12 h; avoid oral dosing in rabbits, rodents
Clofazamine	Birds	1-12 mg/kg PO q24 h; combined with other drugs
Cycloserine	Birds	5 mg/kg PO q12-24 h; combined with other drugs
Doxycycline	Amphibians	5-50 mg/kg q24 h
	Reptiles	5-50 mg/kg PO q24 h
	Birds	25-50 mg/kg PO q12-24 h
	Mammals	2.5-10 mg/kg PO q12 h
Enrofloxacin	Invertebrates	2.5-20 mg/kg PO, IV, IM q12-24 h
	Fish	2-5-10 mg/kg PO, IM, ICe q24-96 h; 2.5-5 mg/L 5 h bath q24 h
	Amphibians	5-10 mg/kg PO, IM, SC q24 h; 500 mg/L 6-8 h bath q24 h
	Reptiles	5-10 mg/kg PO, IM, SC, ICe q24-72 h
	Birds	5-30 mg/kg PO, IM q12-24 h
	Mammals	2.5-20 mg/kg PO, IM, SC q12-24 h
Ethambutol	Birds	10-30 mg/kg PO q12-24 h; combined with other drugs
Oxalinic acid	Fish	5-50 mg/kg PO, ICe q24 h
Rifabutin	Birds	15-45 mg/kg PO q24 h; combined with other drugs
Sulfadimidine	Fish	75 mg/kg ICe q48 h[182]
	Amphibians	1 g/L bath to effect; change daily
Sulfadimethoxine	Reptiles	90 mg/kg PO, IM once; then 45 mg/kg q24 h
	Birds	25-55 mg/kg PO q24 h
	Mammals	2-50 mg/kg PO q24 h
Trimeth/sulfa	Fish	30 mg/kg PO q24 h
	Amphibians	15 mg/kg PO q24 h
	Reptiles	30 mg/kg PO q24 h
	Birds	20-100 mg/kg PO q8-12 h
	Mammals	5-30 mg/kg PO q12-24 h
ANTIFUNGAL		
Amphotericin B	Amphibians	1 mg/kg ICe q24 h
	Reptiles	0.5-1 mg/kg IV, ICe, in lung q24-72 h
	Birds	1.5 mg/kg IV, IO q8 h
		100 mg/kg PO q12 h; not absorbed; for *Macrorhabdus*
	Mammals	0.1-1 mg/kg IV q8 h
Fluconazole	Amphibians	60 mg/kg PO q24 h
	Reptiles	5 mg/kg PO q24 h
	Birds	5-10 mg/kg PO q12-24 h
	Mammals	5-80 mg/kg PO q24 h

Continued

TABLE 5-6

Dosages of Drugs Listed in the Text—cont'd

Drug	Species	Dosage[173]
Itraconazole	Fish	1-5 mg/kg PO q1-7 d
	Amphibians	10 mg/kg PO q24h; 0.01% in 0.6% saline as 5 min bath q24 h
	Reptiles	5-23.5 mg/kg q24-48 h
	Birds	2.5-10 mg/kg PO q12-24 h; African greys sensitive
	Mammals	2.5-20 mg/kg PO q12-24 h
Ketoconazole	Amphibians	10-20 mg/kg PO q24 h
	Reptiles	15-30 mg/kg PO q24 h
	Birds	10-30 mg/kg PO q12 h
	Mammals	10-40 mg/kg PO q8-24 h
Nystatin	Reptiles	100,000 U/kg PO q24 h; not absorbed from GI tract
	Birds	300,000-600,000 U/kg q8-12 h; not absorbed from GI tract
	Mammals	2,000-90,000 U/kg q8-24 h; not absorbed from GI tract
Sodium benzoate	Birds	1 tsp/L of drinking water for 30 d; caution in heat

ANTIPARASITIC

Drug	Species	Dosage
Amprolium	Birds	250 mg/L drinking water for 7 d
	Mammals	19 mg/kg PO q24 h; 120 mg/L drinking water for 21 d
Carnidazole	Birds	20-50 mg/kg PO once; repeat in 10-14 d
Diclazuril	Birds	10 mg/kg PO q12 h days 0,1,2,4,6,8,10
	Mammals	4 mg/kg SC
Fenbendazole	Fish	6 mg/kg PO q24 h × 1-2 d; repeat in 14 d
	Amphibians	30-50 mg/kg PO q24 h × 1-3 d; repeat in 14 d
	Reptiles	50 mg/kg PO q24 h × 3-5 d; ± repeat in 14 d
	Birds	20-50 mg/kg PO q24 h; USE WITH CAUTION IN BIRDS
	Mammals	10-50 mg/kg PO q24 h × 3-5 d; ± repeat in 14 d
Halofuginone	Birds	1.5 mg/kg
Ivermectin	Amphibians	0.2-0.4 mg/kg PO, SC; repeat in 14 d; use caution
	Reptiles	0.2 mg/kg; not chelonians, crocodilians, skinks, indigo snakes
	Birds	0.2-2 mg/kg; repeat in 10-14 d
	Mammals	0.2-0.5 mg/kg; repeat in 14 d
Levamisole	Fish	10 mg/kg PO q7 d
	Amphibians	10 mg/kg IM, ICe; repeat in 2 wk
	Reptiles	5-10 mg/kg SC, ICe; repeat in 2 wk
	Birds	20-40 mg/kg PO once
	Mammals	10 mg/kg PO; repeat in 14 d
Metronidazole	Fish	50 mg/kg PO q24 h; 6.6-25 mg/L in tank water q24-48 h
	Amphibians	10-20 mg/kg PO q24-48 h
	Reptiles	20-50 mg/kg PO q1-14 d
	Birds	25-50 mg/kg PO q12-24 h
	Mammals	10-70 mg/kg PO q8-14 h
Nitazoxanide	Reptiles	30 mg/kg q24 h (author's anecdotal dosage)
	Mammals	15 mg/kg q12 h (author's anecdotal dosage)
Paromomycin	Amphibians	50-75 mg/kg q24 h
	Reptiles	35-100 mg/kg q24 h
	Birds	100 mg/kg q12 h
	Mammals	165 mg/kg q12 h for 5 d
Praziquantel	Fish	5 mg/kg PO, ICe q24 h × 3 or once and repeat in 14-21 d
	Amphibians	8-24 mg/kg PO, SC, ICe, topical; repeat in 14 d
	Reptiles	5-10 mg/kg PO, SC, IM; repeat in 14 d
	Birds	5-10 mg/kg PO, IM; repeat in 14 d
	Mammals	5-30 mg/kg PO, IM, SC; repeat in 14 d
Pyrantel pamoate	Fish	10 mg/kg in feed
	Amphibians	5 mg/kg PO q14 d
	Reptiles	25 mg/kg q24 h × 3; repeat in 14 d
	Birds	5-20 mg/kg PO; repeat in 14 d
	Mammals	5-50 mg/kg PO; repeat in 14 d
Ronidazole	Amphibians	10 mg/kg q24 h × 10d
	Birds	6-10 mg/kg q24 h × 6-10 d
Spiramycin	Reptiles	160 mg/kg PO q24 h × 10; then 2×/wk for 3 mo
	Birds	250 mg/kg PO q24 h
Toltrazuril	Reptiles	5-15 mg/kg PO q24-48 h
	Birds	7-25 mg/kg PO q24 h; 12.5-25 mg/L of drinking water
	Mammals	2.5-10 mg/kg PO; 25-50 mg/L drinking water

TABLE 5-6

Dosages of Drugs Listed in the Text—cont'd

Drug	Species	Dosage[173]
ANTI-INFLAMMATORY		
Celecoxib	Birds	10 mg/kg q24 h
Tepoxalin	Birds	40 mg/kg q24 h[97]
Prednisolone	Amphibians	5-10 mg/kg IM
	Reptiles	2-5 mg/kg PO, IM
	Birds	2 mg/kg PO q12 h; use with caution
	Mammals	0.25-2.5 mg/kg PO
Azathioprine	Mammals	0.9 mg/kg PO q24-72 h
ANALGESIC		
Buprenorphine	Amphibians	38 mg/kg SC
	Reptiles	0.4-1 mg/kg SC, IM; questionable efficacy
	Mammals	0.01-0.05 mg/kg SC q8-12 h
Fentanyl	Mammals	0.3-.6 mg/kg/h CRI with low-dose ketamine
Ketamine	Mammals	1-2 mg/kg/h CRI with low-dose ketamine
ANESTHETIC		
Tricaine	Fish	15-200 mg/L immersion; low end for sedation
	Amphibians	1 g/L (gill-less species)
SEDATIVE/ANTICONVULSANT		
Diazepam	Reptiles	0.5-2 mg/kg IV, IM
	Birds	0.5-4 mg/kg IV, IM, PO, intranasal
	Mammals	0.5-2 mg/kg IV, IM, PO
Midazolam	Reptiles	0.5-2 mg/kg IM
	Birds	0.1-2 mg/kg IM
	Mammals	0.25-2 mg/kg IM
PROKINETIC		
Cisapride	Reptiles	0.5-2 mg/kg PO q24 h
	Birds	0.25-1.5 mg/kg PO q8 h
	Mammals	0.5 mg /kg PO q12 h
Metoclopramide	Reptiles	0.06-10 mg/kg PO q24 h
	Birds	0.3-2 mg/kg IM, PO q8-12 h
	Mammals	0.2-1 mg/kg IM, SC, PO, q8-12 h
MISCELLANEOUS		
Bismuth subsalicylate	Birds	1-2 mL/kg q12 h
	Mammals	0.5-1.0 mL/kg q6-8 h
CaEDTA	Birds	20-70 mg/kg IM q12 h
Cholestyramine	Mammals	2g/rabbit PO q24 h
Chlorhexidine	Reptiles	Oral rinse solution: 1-2 drops in mouth daily
	Birds	2.6-7.9 mL/L drinking water
Deferoxamine	Birds	20 mg/kg PO q4 h
D-Penicillamine	Birds	50-55 mg/kg PO q24 h
Lactulose	Birds	0.2-1 mL/kg q8-12 h
Mineral oil	Birds	5 mL/kg via gavage
Omeprazole	Mammals	4 mg/kg q24 h
Pancreatic enzymes	Birds	1/8 tsp/kg with moist food or gavaged[178]
Psyllium	Birds	0.5 tsp/60 mL feeding formula
Ranitidine	Mammals	3.5 mg/kg q12 h
Silymarin	Birds	50-150 mg/kg q12 h
Ursodiol	Birds	10-15 mg/kg q24 h[178]
Vitamin A	Reptiles	1000-5000 U/kg IM, PO q7 d × 4
	Birds	2000-33000 U/kg IM, PO q7 d
Zinc ascorbate	Reptiles	1-2 drops in mouth daily

CaEDTA, Calcium ethylenediaminetetraacetic acid; *GI,* gastrointestinal; *ICe,* intracoelomic; *IM,* intramuscular; *IO,* intraosseus; *IV,* intravenous; *PO,* by mouth; *SC,* subcutaneous.

TABLE 5-7

Common Gastrointestinal Surgical Procedures

Procedure	Indications	Species Most Likely to Require Procedure
Oral curettage	Oral lesions	Reptiles Birds
Periodontal treatment	Periodontal disease	Hedgehogs Ferrets Sciurognathi
Coronal reduction	Acquired dental disease	Hystricognathi Rabbits
Dental extraction	Severe periodontal disease Apical abscess Severe acquired dental disease Severe incisor malocclusion Caries	Hedgehogs, Ferrets Rabbits Hystricognathi Sciurognathi
Ingluviotomy	Crop biopsy Access for proventriculoscopy Foreign body removal Fistula repair	Birds
Proventriculotomy	Difficult foreign bodies	Birds
Ventriculotomy	Difficult foreign bodies	Birds
Gastrotomy	Foreign bodies Trichobezoars Gastric biopsy	Ferrets Rabbits Amphibians Reptiles
Enterotomy	Foreign body Intestinal biopsy	Ferrets Rabbits Birds
Enteric plication	Repeated intussusception prolapse	Hamsters
Resection/anasomosis	Necrotic bowel segments	Ferret Hamster Rabbit Birds Reptiles Amphibians
Hepatic biopsy	Liver disease	Birds Reptiles All mammals
Liver lobectomy	Hepatic neoplasia Liver lobe torsion Hepatic cysts	Ferrets Rabbits Hamsters
Reduce prolapse	Cloacal, rectal prolapse	Amphibians Reptiles Birds Hamsters Ferrets
Cloaca/colopexy	Repeated prolapses	Birds Reptiles

potential problems occur in practice, it is generally recommended to inject drugs in the cranial half of the body. Reptiles should be maintained within their POTZ during treatment to optimize metabolism of drugs and immune function.

Surgical treatments used for reptile patients are similar to those used for birds and small mammals. The skin of many reptiles is very tough, and when possible it is recommended that incisions be made between rather than through the scales. Closure of surgical wounds should evert the skin because the scales tend to invert and may impede healing. Common surgical procedures of the digestive system include curettage of oral lesions, gastrotomy, enterotomy, liver biopsy, and cloacal prolapse reduction. In cases of repeated cloacal prolapse, cloacapexy or colopexy may be required.

Birds

Medical therapy in birds is facilitated by the numerous pharmacologic studies and the general homology of avian physiology when compared to that in mammals and reptiles. All routes of administration are applicable in birds. Intraosseous therapy is usually preferred to IV because the cannulas remain in place longer than IV catheters. The limitation of IO drug/fluid administration is that some birds, with concurrent reproductive activity or disease, may have excessively dense bones with no functional marrow cavity. The reluctance of many birds to be restrained and their rapid use of escape and avoidance techniques can complicate longer-term treatments.

Therapeutic Endoscopy

Rigid endoscopy is frequently applied for therapeutic uses in birds. If a foreign body is diagnosed in the crop, it may be grasped with forceps and the entire object slowly removed. Rarely will the foreign body fit through the sheath. Foreign bodies that lodge in the crop are often large and may or may not be readily grasped with the small forceps that can be passed through an operating sheath. Additionally, care must be observed not to traumatize the esophagus when these objects are removed. Occasionally the object can be manipulated up the esophagus and grasped with hemostatic forceps when it enters the mouth.

Foreign bodies within the proventriculus and ventriculus are often small and are in multiple pieces. The ingested objects frequently affect the motility of the GI tract and gastric emptying. Consequently, the stomach is filled with a large amount of detritus and food, along with the foreign bodies. Identification and removal of these foreign objects, one at a time, can be extremely time consuming. Even when a proventriculotomy or ventriculotomy is performed, it can be very difficult to remove the entire contents of the stomach. A procedure called endoscope-assisted gastric lavage (EAGL) is often helpful in these cases.[175] The procedure initially is identical to the procedure described above. However once the endoscope is placed within the proventriculus, the table is tilted so that the head is lower than the body. At this point, higher volumes of warmed saline are infused into the port of the sheath. The fluid is allowed to escape around the instrument, hopefully carrying the debris from the proventriculus and ventriculus. The fluid is caught on a clean white towel so that foreign objects can be readily identified. In some cases, the fluid does not easily escape around the sheath. Consequently with these cases, the telescope must be intermittently removed from the sheath to provide an escape channel for the fluid and foreign material. The infusion and drainage is continued until the fluid escaping from the stomach is clear and no further debris is noted. If an ingluviotomy incision has been made, the area should be lavaged prior to closure.

If available, diode lasers can be used in the wet field to ablate the lesions. Occasionally, concretions of urate salts will become lodged within the cloaca. These urate concretions or uroliths can be observed during the cloacoscopy procedure, and in some cases, crumbled and removed using grasping forceps.

Treatment of Liver Disease

Treatment of the underlying cause of hepatic disease should be initiated if identified. Therapy can also target secondary complications of hepatic dysfunction and support of the remaining hepatic cells.[13] Fluid therapy, nutritional support (e.g., tube feeding), medications that reduce levels of metabolic toxins, and treating secondary problems are essential to a successful treatment response for hepatic disease. Although commonly used for this purpose, lactulose may have little value in the treatment of avian liver disease. The theoretical use of lactulose is based on reducing blood ammonia levels

ammonia that can accumulate in hepatic patients which is considered the primary factor behind the development of hepatic encephalopathy (hepatic encephalopathy has not been confirmed as an avian disease condition).[13] However, there appears to be little risk involved with the use of lactulose in avian patients that have liver disease. The use of milk thistle (active compound: silymarin) as an antioxidant is common, although there is very little scientific research to support its use. *S*-Adenosylmethionine (SAMe) is commonly used in mammals for adjunct therapy for liver disease. The use of SAMe use in birds has not yet been evaluated, and the mammalian products require that the tablets remain intact, which makes compounding this therapeutic agent for small patients (birds) impractical.[13] Ursodiol may be useful to promote choleresis when cholestasis occurs.[13]

Mammals

Inpatient versus Outpatient

In many cases, therapy is usually conducted on an outpatient basis. Outpatient treatment is less stressful for the patient, less expensive for the owner, and equally or more successful for most conditions than hospitalizing the animal. Oral treatments are easily administered by many pet owners, although medical therapy in pet hedgehogs is complicated by their defensive responses. When hedgehogs roll up into a ball presenting only erect spines, administration of medication is nearly impossible. Treatment can be facilitated by using palatable preparations and gentle handling techniques.

Fluid therapy for the outpatient can be accomplished with a combination of SC fluids administered in the hospital or by experienced and/or educated owners at home. When nutritional support is required, most small mammals respond well to syringe feeding. A variety of commercially available critical care diets that are designed to pass through a syringe or tube are available. Unconscious or very depressed patients should not be syringe fed by owners.

In more severe cases, when the required care cannot be administered by the pet owner, hospitalization of the patient is required. Small mammals should be hospitalized away from carnivore sounds and smells. Generally hospitalized small exotic mammals should have a hiding area and access to food and water.

Sedation/Anesthesia/Analgesia

Anesthesia should be avoided in the critically ill patient; however, risk of sedation and/or anesthesia must be weighed against the risk of foregoing diagnostics and treatments or attempting procedures in the conscious animal. Many minor procedures, such as IV or IO catheterization, can be accomplished with the use of sedation alone or with the addition of local analgesia.[160] Many small mammals with GI disease present with mild to severe pain. Opioid drugs are more effective for visceral pain, and NSAIDs have increased toxicity in patients that are dehydrated. Although some opioid agents may have a negative effect on gut motility, pain is more problematic. For most cases, buprenorphine (0.01 to 0.05 mg/kg, SC, BID-TID) is used to treat patients with mild to moderate pain. Fentanyl (F)/ketamine (K) combinations (F: 0.3 to 0.6 mg/kg/h; K: 1 to 2 mg/kg/h) may be added to crystalloid fluids to provide ongoing pain relief for severely painful rabbits.[172] When perfusion deficits are corrected, and if

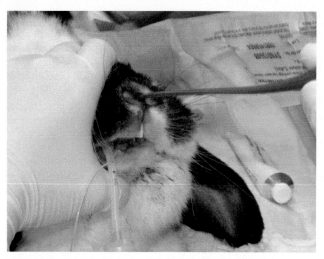

FIGURE 5-30 Placement of a nasogastric tube in the rabbit from Figure 5-18. Generally, this does not require anesthesia. In this case, the extensive dental work was expected to result in anorexia, so the tube was placed before recovery.

inflammatory pain is present, NSAID (meloxicam, 0.2 to 1.0 mg/kg, PO, SID-BID) therapy may be beneficial.

Fluid Therapy

Fluid therapy proceeds in three phases: correction of dehydration deficits, rehydration of the patient, and maintenance.[172] For decompensatory shock, the recommended initial therapy includes hypertonic (7.2%) saline and hetastarch at 3 mL/kg, each administered IV or IO as a slow bolus over 10 minutes, repeated several times until the blood pressure returns to normal.[172] Moreover the patient should be gradually warmed.[176] These guidelines are relatively straightforward and extremely useful for use in small mammals. Although measurement of systolic Doppler blood pressure has been reported in these species and appears to be similar to that in other small mammals. Practitioners may find Doppler blood pressure monitoring more challenging in smaller individuals than in larger animals, particularly hedgehogs and sugar gliders.[176]

Nutritional Support

Early enteral feeding is critical in the management of critically ill or recovering small mammals. Nutritional support decreases pain, helps with motility of the GI tract, and decreases bacterial translocation.[177] Hepatic lipidosis develops quickly in rabbits and rodents but can be often averted with enteral feeding. Syringe feeding is used for most cases. Due to the arrangement of the soft palate and glottis in rabbits and rodents, it is difficult for these patients to aspirate. Critically ill patients will often refuse to swallow food from a syringe therefore a nasogastric tube may be used. These tubes can be less stressful in the critical patient than force-feeding with a syringe. In addition, the placement of the nasogastric tube within the stomach allows for release of gas from within this anatomic structure. Nasogastric tubes can be placed in rabbits and larger rodents (Figure 5-30); however, the size of the tube for guinea pigs and chinchillas is very small, making it difficult to get high-fiber formulas through the tube.

Surgical Treatments

Gastrotomy, enterotomy, and resection/anastomosis are all occasionally required to treat an exotic small animal patient. These procedures appear to be used more often in ferrets, which often recover well following the surgery. Conversely, rabbits and rodents are less tolerant of surgical manipulation of the bowels, and the conditions requiring bowel manipulation are usually more advanced when diagnosed. Techniques used for traditional companion animals are appropriate when surgically treating exotic small mammals.

When treating rectal prolapse, it is important to determine which part of the bowel is exposed.[164] Rectal assessment can be achieved by very gently inserting a slim, urethral swab alongside the prolapsed tissue. If a rectal prolapse is diagnosed, the swab will not enter more than a few millimeters. If the swab enters further into the body cavity, an intestinal prolapse is most likely the diagnosis. Intestinal prolapses require a laparotomy for appropriate reduction and treatment. Rectal prolapses should be assessed for tissue viability. If the prolapsed tissue is viable, it should be replaced and a purse-string suture used so that it remains in place. If the tissue is necrotic, an amputation with a subsequent anastomosis should be performed. The amputation and anastomosis require microsurgical technique in animals the size of a hamster.

REFERENCES

1. Weber ES. Gastroenterology for the piscine patient. *Vet Clin North Am.* 2005;8:247-276.
2. Stoskopf MK. Anatomy. In: Stoskopf MK, ed. *Fish Medicine.* Philadelphia: W.B. Saunders; 1993:2-30.
3. Clayton LA. Amphibian gastroenterology. *Vet Clin North Am Exot Anim.* 2005;8:227-245.
4. Helmer PJ, Whiteside DP. Amphibian anatomy and physiology. In: O'Malley B, ed. *Clinical Anatomy and Physiology of Exotic Species.* Edinburgh: Elsevier; 2005:3-14.
5. Wright KM. Anatomy for the clinician. In: Wright KM, Whitaker BR, eds. *Amphibian Medicine and Captive Husbandry.* Malabar, FL: Krieger Publishing Company; 2001:15-34.
6. O'Malley B. General anatomy and physiology of reptiles. In: O'Malley B, ed. *Clinical Anatomy and Physiology of Exotic Species.* Edinburgh: Elsevier; 2005:17-39.
7. O'Malley B. Tortoises and turtles. In: O'Malley B, ed. *Clinical Anatomy and Physiology of Exotic Species.* Edinburgh: Elsevier; 2005: 41-56.
8. O'Malley B. Snakes. In: O'Malley B, ed. *Clinical Anatomy and Physiology of Exotic Species.* Edinburgh: Elsevier; 2005:77-93.
9. O'Malley B. Lizards. In: O'Malley B, ed. *Clinical Anatomy and Physiology of Exotic Species.* Edinburgh: Elsevier; 2005:57-75.
10. Mitchell MA, Diaz-Figueroa O. Clinical reptile gastroenterology. *Vet Clin North Am Exot Anim.* 2005;8:277-298.
11. King AS, McLelland J. *Birds: Their Structure and Function.* London: Bailliére Tindall; 1984.
12. O'Malley B. Avian anatomy and physiology. In: O'Malley B, ed. *Clinical Anatomy and Physiology of Exotic Species.* Edinburgh: Elsevier; 2005:97-161.
13. Grunkemeyer VL. Advanced diagnostic approaches and current management of avian hepatic disorders. *Vet Clin North Am Exot Anim.* 2010;13(3):413-427.
14. Vella D, Donnelly TM. Basic anatomy, physiology, and husbandry. In: Quesenberry KE, Carpenter JW, eds. *Ferrets, Rabbits, and Rodents: Clinical Medicine and Surgery.* 3rd ed. St. Louis: Elsevier; 2012:157-173.

15. Merck Veterinary Manual Online. Table 16: Selected physiologic data for sugar gliders. Available at: http://www.merckvetmanual.com/mvm/htm/bc/texl16.htm Accessed June 28, 2012.

16. Ness RD, Johnson-Delaney CA. Sugar gliders. In: Quesenberry KE, Carpenter JW, eds. *Ferrets, Rabbits, and Rodents: Clinical Medicine and Surgery*. 3rd ed. St. Louis: Elsevier; 2012:393-410.

17. Heatley JJ. Hedgehogs. In: Mitchell MA, Tully TN, eds. *Manual of Exotic Pet Practice*. St. Louis: Saunders Elsevier; 2009:433-455.

18. Ivey E, Carpenter JW. African hedgehogs. In: Quesenberry KE, Carpenter JW, eds. *Ferrets, Rabbits, and Rodents: Clinical Medicine and Surgery*. 3rd ed. St. Louis: Elsevier; 2012:411-427.

19. Powers LV, Brown SA. Basic anatomy, physiology, and husbandry. In: Quesenberry KE, Carpenter JW, eds. *Ferrets, Rabbits, and Rodents: Clinical Medicine and Surgery*. 3rd ed. St. Louis: Elsevier; 2012:1-12.

20. Lewington JH. Ferrets. In: O'Malley B, ed. *Clinical Anatomy and Physiology of Exotic Species*. Edinburgh: Elsevier; 2005:237-261.

21. O'Malley B. Rabbits. In: O'Malley B, ed. *Clinical Anatomy and Physiology of Exotic Species*. Edinburgh: Elsevier; 2005:173-195.

22. Capello V, Gracis M, Lennox AM. *Rabbit and Rodent Dentistry Handbook*. Lake Worth: Zoological Education Network; 2005.

23. Campbell-Ward ML. Gastrointestinal physiology and nutrition. In: Quesenberry KE, Carpenter JW, eds. *Ferrets, Rabbits, and Rodents: Clinical Medicine and Surgery*. 3rd ed. St. Louis: Elsevier; 2012:183-192.

24. Myers P. Rodentia. *Animal Diversity Web*. University of Michigan Museum of Zoology. 2000; http://animaldiversity.ummz.umich.edu/site/accounts/information/Rodentia.html. Accessed June 28, 2012.

25. Hoefer HL, Crossley DA. Chinchillas. In: Meredith A, Redrobe S, eds. *BSAVA Manual of Exotic Pets*. 4th ed. Gloucester: BSAVA; 2005:63-75.

26. Quesenberry KE, Donnelly TM, Mans C. Biology, husbandry, and clinical techniques of guinea pigs and chinchillas. In: Quesenberry KE, Carpenter JW, eds. *Ferrets, Rabbits, and Rodents: Clinical Medicine and Surgery*. 3rd ed. St. Louis: Elsevier; 2012:279-294.

27. Lennox AM, Bauck L. Basic anatomy, physiology, husbandry, and clinical techniques. In: Quesenberry KE, Carpenter JW, eds. *Ferrets, Rabbits, and Rodents: Clinical Medicine and Surgery*. 3rd ed. St. Louis: Elsevier; 2012:339-353.

28. O'Malley B. Guinea pigs. In: O'Malley B, ed. *Clinical Anatomy and Physiology of Exotic Species*. Edinburgh: Elsevier; 2005:197-208.

29. Pizzi R. Spiders. In: Lewbart G, ed. *Invertebrate Medicine*. Ames: Blackwell; 2006:143-168.

30. McAllister PE. Goldfish, koi, and carp viruses. In: Stoskopf MK, ed. *Fish Medicine*. Philadelphia: W.B. Saunders; 1993:478-486.

31. Noga EJ. *Fish Disease: Diagnosis and Treatment*. St. Louis: Mosby; 1996.

32. McAllister PE, Stoskopf MK. Marina tropical fish viruses. In: Stoskopf MK, ed. *Fish Medicine*. Philadelphia: W.B. Saunders; 1993:642-646.

33. Shotts EB, Nemetz TG. Selected bacterial diseases of salmonids. In: Stoskopf MK, ed. *Fish Medicine*. Philadelphia: W.B. Saunders; 1993:364-372.

34. Stoskopf MK. Bacterial diseases of marine tropical fishes. In: Stoskopf MK, ed. *Fish Medicine*. Philadelphia: W.B. Saunders; 1993:635-639.

35. Chacko AJ. Fungal and algal diseases of salmonids. In: Stoskopf MK, ed. *Fish Medicine*. Philadelphia: W.B. Saunders; 1993:373-379.

36. Stoskopf MK. Parasitic diseases of goldfish, koi, and carp. In: Stoskopf MK, ed. *Fish Medicine*. Philadelphia: W.B. Saunders; 1993:486-490.

37. Cheung P. Parasitic diseases of marine tropical fishes. In: Stoskopf MK, ed. *Fish Medicine*. Philadelphia: W.B. Saunders; 1993:646-658.

38. Stoskopf MK, Gratzek JB, eds. Parasites associated with freshwater tropical fishes. In: *Fish Medicine*. Philadelphia: W.B. Saunders; 1993:573-590.

39. Saint-Erne N. Diagnositc techniques and treatments for internal disorders of koi *(Cyprinus carpio)*. *Vet Clin North Am Exotic Anim*. 2010;13(3):333-347.

40. Post GW. Nutrition and nutritional diseases of salmonids. In: Stoskopf MK, ed. *Fish Medicine*. Philadelphia: W.B. Saunders; 1993:343-358.

41. May EB. Goldfish, koi, and carp neoplasia. In: Stoskopf MK, ed. *Fish Medicine*. Philadelphia: W.B. Saunders; 1993:490-491.

42. Belleau MH. Neoplasias of catfishes. In: Stoskopf MK, ed. *Fish Medicine*. Philadelphia: W.B. Saunders; 1993:531.

43. May EB. Neoplasias of freshwater tropical fishes. In: Stoskopf MK, ed. *Fish Medicine*. Philadelphia: W.B. Saunders; 1993:591-593.

44. Robert J, Gregory CV. Ranaviruses: an emerging threat to ectothermic vertebrates. Report of the First International Symposium on Ranaviruses. Minneapolis, MN. *Dev Comp Immunol*. 2012;36(2):259-261.

45. Taylor SK, Green DE, Wright KM, et al. Bacterial diseases. In: Wright KM, Whitaker BR, eds. *Amphibian Medicine and Captive Husbandry*. Malabar, FL: Krieger Publishing Company; 2001:159-179.

46. Taylor SK. Mycoses. In: Wright KM, Whitaker BR, eds. *Amphibian Medicine and Captive Husbandry*. Malabar, FL: Krieger Publishing Company; 2001:181-191.

47. Poynton SL, Whitaker BR. Protozoa and metazoa infecting amphibians. In: Wright KM, Whitaker BR, eds. *Amphibian Medicine and Captive Husbandry*. Malabar, FL: Krieger Publishing Company; 2001:193-221.

48. Wright KM. Idiopathic syndromes. In: Wright KM, Whitaker BR, eds. *Amphibian Medicine and Captive Husbandry*. Malabar, FL: Krieger Publishing Company; 2001:239-244.

49. Wright KM. Surgical techniques. In: Wright KM, Whitaker BR, eds. *Amphibian Medicine and Captive Husbandry*. Malabar, FL: Krieger Publishing Company; 2001:273-283.

50. Green DE, Harshbarger JC. Spontaneous neoplasia in amphibia. In: Wright KM, Whitaker BR, eds. *Amphibian Medicine and Captive Husbandry*. Malabar, FL: Krieger Publishing Company; 2001:335-400.

51. Reavill DR, Schmidt R. A survey of reptile GI disease from teeth to cloaca. *Proc Annu Conf Assoc Reptile Amphibian Vet*. 2011:138-141.

52. Stenglen MD, Sanders C, Kistler AL, et al. Identification, characterization, and in vivo culture of highly divergent arenaviruses from boa contrictors and annulated tree boas: candidate etiological agents for snake inclusion body disease. *MBio*. 2012;3(4):e00180-12. doi:10.1128/mBio.00180-12.

53. Garner MM, Raymond JT. Methods for diagnosing inclusion body disease in snakes. *Proc Annu Conf Assoc Reptile Amphibian Vet*. 2004:21-25.

54. Origgi FC, Jacobson ER. Diseases of the respiratory tract of chelonians. *Vet Clin North Am Exot Anim*. 2000;3(2):537-549.

55. Johnson AJ, Pessier AP, Wellehan JF, et al. Identification of a novel herpesvirus from a California desert tortoise *(Gopherus agassizii)*. *Vet Microbiol*. 2005;111(1-2):107-116.

56. Hunt CJ. Herpesvirus outbreak in a group of Mediterranean tortoises *(Testudo spp)*. *Vet Clin North Am Exot Anim*. 2006;9(3):569-574.

57. Hervás J, Sánchez-Cordón PJ, de Chacón LF, et al. Hepatitis associated with herpes viral infection in the tortoise *(Testudo horsfieldii)*. *J Vet Med B Infect Dis Vet Public Health*. 2002;49(2):111-114.

58. Origgi FC, Klein PA, Mathes K, et al. Enzyme-linked immunosorbent assay for detecting herpesvirus exposure in Mediterranean tortoises, spur-thighed tortoise *(Testudo graeca)* and Hermann's tortoise *(Testudo hermanni)*. *J Clin Microbiol*. 2001;39(9):3156-3163.

59. Murakami M, Matsuba C, Une Y, et al. Development of species-specific PCR techniques for the detection of tortoise herpesvirus. *J Vet Diagn Invest*. 2001;13(6):513-516.

60. Ritchie B. Virology. In: Mader DR, ed. *Reptile Medicine and Surgery*. 2nd ed. St. Louis, MO: Elsevier; 2006:391-417.

61. Kim DY, Mitchell MA, Bauer RW, et al. An outbreak of adenoviral infection in inland bearded dragons (*Pogona vitticeps*) coinfected with dependovirus and coccidial protozoa (*Isospora* sp.). *J Vet Diagn Invest*. 2002;14(4):332-334.

62. Jacobson ER, Kopit W, Kennedy FA, et al. Coinfection of a bearded dragon, *Pogona vitticeps*, with adenovirus- and dependovirus-like viruses. *Vet Pathol*. 1996;33(3):343-346.

63. Moormann S, Seehusen F, Reckling D, et al. Systemic adenovirus infection in bearded dragons (*Pogona vitticeps*): histological, ultrastructural and molecular findings. *J Comp Pathol*. 2009;141(1): 78-83.

64. Allender MC, Abd-Eldaim M, Schumacher J, et al. PCR prevalence of ranavirus in free-ranging Eastern box turtles (*Terrapene carolina carolina*) at rehabilitation centers in three southeastern US states. *J Wildl Dis*. 2011;47(3):759-764.

65. De Voe R, Geissler K, Elmore S, et al. Ranavirus-associated morbidity and mortality in a group of captive eastern box turtles (*Terrapene carolina carolina*). *J Zoo Wildl Med*. 2004;35(4):534-543.

66. Johnson AJ, Pessier AP, Wellehan JF, et al. Ranavirus infection of free-ranging and captive box turtles and tortoises in the United States. *J Wildl Dis*. 2008;44(4):851-863.

67. Draper CS, Walker RD, Lawler HE. Patterns of oral bacterial infection in captive snakes. *J Am Vet Med Assoc*. 1981;179(11): 1223-1226.

68. Schmidt V, Dyachenko V, Aupperle H, et al. Case report of systemic coccidiosis in a radiated tortoise (*Geochelone radiata*). *Parasitol Res*. 2008;102(3):431-436.

69. Garner MM, Gardiner CH, Wellehan JF, et al. Intranuclear coccidiosis in tortoises: nine cases. *Vet Pathol*. 2006;43(3):311-320.

70. Graczyk TK, Cranfield MR. Experimental transmission of *Cryptosporidium* oocyst isolates from mammals, birds and reptiles to captive snakes. *Vet Res*. 1998;29(2):187-195.

71. O'Donoghue PJ. *Cryptosporidium* and cryptosporidiosis in man and animals. *Int J Parasitol*. 1995;25(2):139-195.

72. Brower AI, Cranfield MR. *Cryptosporidium* sp.-associated enteritis without gastritis in rough green snakes (*Opheodrys aestivus*) and a common garter snake (*Thamnophis sirtalis*). *J Zoo Wildl Med*. 2001; 32(1):101-105.

73. Cimon KY, Oberst RD, Upton SJ, et al. Biliary cryptosporidiosis in two corn snakes (*Elaphe guttata*). *J Vet Diagn Invest*. 1996;8(3): 398-399.

74. Terrell SP, Uhl EW, Funk RS. Proliferative enteritis in leopard geckos (*Eublepharis macularius*) associated with *Cryptosporidium* sp. infection. *J Zoo Wildl Med*. 2003;34(1):69-75.

75. Dillehay DL, Boosinger TR, MacKenzie S. Gastric cryptosporidiosis in a chameleon. *J Am Vet Med Assoc*. 1986;189(9):1139-1140.

76. Deming C, Greiner E, Uhl EW. Prevalence of cryptosporidium infection and characteristics of oocyst shedding in a breeding colony of leopard geckos (*Eublepharis macularius*). *J Zoo Wildl Med*. 2008;39(4):600-607.

77. Kik MJ, van Asten AJ, Lenstra JA, et al. Cloacal prolapse and cystitis in green iguana (*Iguana iguana*) caused by a novel *Cryptosporidium* species. *Vet Parasitol*. 2011;175(1-2):165-167.

78. Uhl EW, Jacobson E, Bartick TE, et al. Aural-pharyngeal polyps associated with *Cryptosporidium* infection in three iguanas (*Iguana iguana*). *Vet Pathol*. 2001;38(2):239-242.

79. Griffin C, Reavill DR, Stacy BA, et al. Cryptosporidiosis caused by two distinct species in Russian tortoises and a pancake tortoise. *Vet Parasitol*. 2010;170(1-2):14-19.

80. Graczyk TK, Cranfield MR. Assessment of the conventional detection of fecal *Cryptosporidium serpentis* oocysts in subclinically infected captive snakes. *Vet Res*. 1996;27(2):185-192.

81. Pedraza-Díaz S, Ortega-Mora LM, Carrión BA, et al. Molecular characterisation of *Cryptosporidium* isolates from pet reptiles. *Vet Parasitol*. 2009;160(3-4):204-210.

82. Fayer R, Graczyk TK, Cranfield MR. Multiple heterogenous isolates of *Cryptosporidium serpentis* from captive snakes are not transmissible to neonatal BALB/c mice (*Mus musculus*). *J Parasitol*. 1995;81(3):482-484.

83. Graczyk TK, Fayer R, Cranfield MR. *Cryptosporidium parvum* is not transmissible to fish, amphibians, or reptiles. *J Parasitol*. 1996;82(5): 748-751.

84. Cranfield MR, Graczyk TK. Cryptosporidiosis. In: Mader DR, ed. *Reptile Medicine and Surgery*. 2nd ed. St. Louis, MO: Elsevier; 2006:756-762.

85. Graczyk TK, Cranfield MR, Bostwick EF. Hyperimmune bovine colostrum treatment of moribund leopard geckos (*Eublepharis macularius*) infected with *Cryptosporidium* sp. *Vet Res*. 1999;30(4):377-382.

86. Graczyk TK, Cranfield MR, Bostwick EF. Successful hyperimmune bovine colostrum treatment of Savanna monitors (*Varanus exanthematicus*) infected with *Cryptosporidium* sp. *J Parasitol*. 2000;86(3): 631-632.

87. Ritter JM, Garner MM, Chilton JA, et al. Gastric neuroendocrine carcinomas in bearded dragons (*Pogona vitticeps*). *Vet Pathol*. 2009;46(6):1109-1116.

88. Lyons JA, Newman SJ, Greenacre CB. A gastric neuroendocrine carcinoma expressing somatostatin in a bearded dragon (*Pogona vitticeps*). *J Vet Diagn Invest*. 2010;22(2):316-320.

89. Speer BL. A clinical look and the avian pancreas in health and disease. *Proc Annu Conf Assoc Avian Vet*. 1998:57-64.

90. Olsen GH. Oral biology and beak disorders of birds. *Vet Clin N Am Exot Anim*. 2003;6:505-521.

91. Graham DL. Internal papillomatous disease. *Proc Annu Conf Assoc Avian Vet*. 1991:141-145.

92. VanDerHeyden N. Psittacine papillomas. *Proc Annu Conf Assoc Avian Vet*. 1988:23-25.

93. Hillyer EV, Moroff S, Hoefer H. Bile duct carcinoma in two out of ten Amazon parrots with cloacal papillomas. *J Assoc Avian Vet*. 1991; 5(2):91-95.

94. Garner MM, Phalen D. Cloacal carcinoma in psittacines: is it herpes all over again? *Proc Annu Conf Assoc Avian Vet*. 2006:21-24.

95. Styles DK, Tomaszewski EK, Jaeger LA, et al. Psittacid herpesviruses associated with mucosal papillomas in neotropical parrots. *Virology*. 2004;32:24-35.

96. Antinoff N, Hottinger HA. Treatment of a cloacal papilloma by mucosal stripping in an Amazon parrot. *Proc Annu Conf Assoc Avian Vet*. 2000:97-100.

97. Gancz AY, Clubb S, Shivaprasad HL. Advanced diagnostic approaches and current management of proventricular dilatation disease. *Vet Clin North Am Exotic An*. 2010;13(3):471-494.

98. Hoppes S, Gray PL, Payne S, et al. The isolation, pathogenesis, diagnosis, transmission, and control of avian bornavirus and proventricular dilatation disease. *Vet Clin North Am Exotic An*. 2010; 13(3):495-508.

99. Dahlhausen R, Aldred S, Colazzi E. Resolution of clinical proventricular dilatation disease by cycloogenase 2 inhibition. *Proc Annu Conf Assoc Avian Vet*. 2002:9-12.

100. Lierz M. Systemic infectious disease. In: Harcourt-Brown N, Chitty J, eds. *BSAVA Manual of Psittacine Birds*. Gloucester: BSAVA; 2005:155-169.

101. Parrott T. New clinical trials using acyclovir. *Proc Annu Conf Assoc Avian Vet*. 1990:237-238.

102. Shivaprasad HL, Palmieri C. Pathology of mycobacteriosis in birds. *Vet Clin North Am Exot Anim*. 2012;15(1):41-55.

103. Dahlhausen R, Soler-Tovar D, Saggese MD. Diagnosis of mycobacterial infections in the exotic pet patient with emphasis on birds. *Vet Clan North Am Exit Anim*. 2012;15(1):71-83.

104. Bur J, Sages MD. Taking a rational approach in the treatment of avian mycobacteriosis. *Vet Clin North Am Exot Anim*. 2012;15(1):57-70.

105. Harcourt-Brown NH. Psittacine birds. In: Tully TM, Dorrestein GM, Jones AK, eds. *Avian Medicine*. 2nd ed. Edinburgh: Elsevier; 2009:138-168.

106. Lane R. Gram stains: theory and practice. *Proc Annu Conf Assoc Avian Vet.* 1991:316-320.
107. Hall RK, Bemis D. A spiral bacterium found in psittacines. *Proc Annu Conf Assoc Avian Vet.* 1995:345-348.
108. Wade L, Bartick T. Pathology of spiral bacteria (*Helicobacter* species) in cockatiels (*Nymphicus hollandicus*). *Proc Annu Conf Assoc Avian Vet.* 2004:345-348.
109. Welle KR. Psittacine spiroform pharyngitis. *Proc Annu Conf Assoc Avian Vet.* 1998:165-169.
110. Dorrestein GM. Passerine birds. In: Tully TM, Dorrestein GM, Jones AK, eds. *Avian Medicine.* 2nd ed. Edinburgh: Elsevier; 2009:169-208.
111. Smith KA, Campbell CT, Murphy J, et al. Compendium of measures to control *Chlamydophila psittaci* infection among humans (psittacosis) and pet birds (avian chlamydiosis). 2010 National Association of State Public Health Veterinarians (NASPHV). *J Exot Pet Med.* 2011;20(1):32-45.
112. Harkinezhad T, Geens T, Vanrompay D. *Chlamydophila psittaci* infections in birds: a review with emphasis on zoonotic consequences. *Vet Microbiol.* 2009;135:68-77.
113. Gerlach H. Chlamydia. In: Ritchie B, Harrison G, Harrison L, eds. *Avian Medicine: Principles and Application.* Lake Worth, FL: Wingers; 1994:984-996.
114. Dahlhausen RA, Radabaugh CS. Detection of *Chlamydia psittaci* infection in pet birds using a molecular based diagnostic assay. *Proc Annu Conf Assoc Avian Vet.* 1997:191-198.
115. Curtis-Velasco M. Candidiasis and cryptococcosis in birds. *Sem Avian Exot Pet Med.* 2000;9(2):75-81.
116. Tomaszewski EK, Loan KS, Snowden KF, et al. Phylogenetic analysis identifies the "megabacterium" of birds as a novel anamorphic ascomycetous yeast, *Macrorhabdus ornithogaster* gen. nov., sp. nov. *Int J Syst Evol Microbiol.* 2003;53:1201-1205.
117. Flammer K, Orosz SE. Avian mycoses: managing these difficult diseases. *Proc Annu Conf Assoc Avian Vet.* 2008:153-163.
118. Lublin A, Mechani S, Malkinson M, et al. A five year survey of megabacteriosis in birds of Israel and a biological control trial. *Proc Annu Conf Assoc Avian Vet.* 1998:241-245.
119. Moore RP, Snowden KF, Phalen DN. Diagnosis, treatment, and prevention of megabacteriosis in the budgerigar (*Melopsittacus undulatus*). *Proc Annu Conf Assoc Avian Vet.* 2001:161-163.
120. Hoppes S. Treatment of *Macrorhabdus ornithogaster* with sodium benzoate in budgerigars (*Melopsittacus undulatus*). *Proc Annu Conf Assoc Avian Vet.* 2011:67.
121. Anderson NL, Grahn RA, Van Hoosear K, et al. Studies of trichomonad protozoa in free ranging songbirds: prevalence of *Trichomonas gallinae* in house finches (*Carpodacus mexicanus*) and corvids and a novel trichomonad in mockingbirds (*Mimus polyglottos*). *Vet Parasit.* 2009;161(3):178-186.
122. Bunbury N, Bell DJ, Jones C, et al. Comparison of the inpouch TF culture system and wet-mount microscopy for *Trichomonas gallinae* in the pink pigeon *Columba mayeri. J Clin Micro.* 2005;43(2):1005-1006.
123. Stabler RM. Protection in pigeons against virulent *Trichomonas gallinae* acquired by infection with milder strains. *J Parasitol.* 1948;34(2):150-151.
124. Donely R. *Avian Medicine and Surgery in Practice: Companion and Aviary Birds.* London: Manson Publishing; 2011.
125. Latimer KS, Steffens WL, Rakich PM, et al. Cryptosporidiosis in four cockatoos with psittacine beak and feather disease. *J Am Vet Med Assoc.* 1992;200(5):707-710.
126. Donely R. Bacterial and parasitic disease of parrots. *Vet Clin North Am Exot Anim.* 2009;12(3):423-431.
127. Goodwin MA, Krabill VA. Diarrhea associated with small-intestinal cryptosporidiosis in a budgerigar and a cockatiel. *Avian Dis.* 1989;33(4):829-833.
128. Makino I, Abe N, Reavill DR. Cryptosporidium avian genotype III as a possible causative agent of chronic vomiting in peach-faced lovebirds (*Agapornis roseicollis*). *Avian Dis.* 2010;54(3):1102-1107.
129. Shahiduzzaman M, Daugschies A. Therapy and prevention of cryptosporidiosis in animals. *Vet Parasitol.* 2012;118(3-4):203-214.
130. van Zeeland YR, Schoemaker NJ, Kik MJ, et al. Upper respiratory tract infection caused by *Cryptosporidium baileyi* in three mixed-bred falcons (*Falco rusticolus* × *Falco cherrug*). *Avian Dis.* 2008;52:357-363.
131. Lindsay DS, Blagburn BL, Sunderman CA, et al. Chemoprophylaxis of cryptosporidiosis in chickens using halofuginone, salinomycin, lasalocid or monensin. *Am J Vet Res.* 1987;48:354-355.
132. Sréter T, Széll Z, Varga I. Anticryptosporidial prophylactic efficacy of enrofloxacin and paromomycin in chickens. *J Parasitol.* 2002;88:209-211.
133. Filippich LJ, McDonnell PA, Munoz E, et al. *Giardia* infection in budgerigars. *Aust Vet J.* 1998;76(4):246-249.
134. Wood AM, Smith HV. Spironucleosis (hexamitiasis, hexamitosis) in the ring-necked pheasant (*Phasianus colchicus*): detection of cysts and description of *Spironucleus meleagridis* in stained smears. *Avian Dis.* 2005;49(1):138-143.
135. Black SS, Steinohrt LA, Bertucci DC, et al. *Encephalitozoon hellem* in budgerigars (*Melopsittacus undulatus*). *Vet Pathol.* 1997;34(3):189-198.
136. Snowden KF, Logan K, Phalen DN. Isolation and characterization of an avian isolate of *Encephalitozoon hellem. Parasitology.* 2000;121(1):9-14.
137. Pulparampil N, Graham D, Phalen D, et al. *Encephalitozoon hellem* in two eclectus parrots (*Eclectus roratus*): identification from archival tissues. *J Eukaryot Microbiol.* 1998;45(6):651-655.
138. Kemp RL, Kluge JP. *Encephalitozoon* sp. in the blue-masked lovebird, *Agapornis personata* (Reichenow): first confirmed report of microsporidan infection in birds. *J Protozool.* 1975;22(4):489-491.
139. Novilla MN. Microsporidian infection in the pied peach-faced lovebird (*Agapornis roseicollis*). *Avian Dis.* 1978;22(1):198-204.
140. Poelma FG, Zwart P, Dorrestein GM, et al. Cochlosomosis, a problem in raising waxbills kept in aviaries [author's translation]. *Tijdschr Diergeneeskd.* 1978;103(11):589-593.
141. Filippich LJ, O'Donoghue PJ. Cochlosoma infections in finches. *Aust Vet J.* 1997;75(8):561-563.
142. Leach MW, Paul-Murphy J, Lowenstine LJ. Three cases of gastric neoplasia in psittacines. *Avian Dis.* 1989;33(1):204-210.
143. Rae MA, Merryman M, Lintner M. Gastric neoplasia in caged birds. *Proc Annu Conf Assoc Avian Vet.* 1992:180-189.
144. Yonemaru K, Sakai H, Asaoka Y, et al. Proventricular adenocarcinoma in a Humboldt penguin (*Spheniscus humboldti*) and a great horned owl (*Bubo virginianus*); identification of origin by mucin histochemistry. *Avian Pathol.* 2004;33(1):77-81.
145. Bauck L. Lymphosarcoma/avian leukosis in pet birds—case reports. *Proc Annu Conf Assoc Avian Vet.* 1986:241-245.
146. Pier AC. Major biological consequences of aflatoxicosis in animal production. *J Anim Sci.* 1992;70(12):3964-3967.
147. Graham DL. Acute pancreatic necrosis in quaker parrots (*Myiopsitta monachus*). *Proc Annu Conf Assoc Avian Vet.* 1994:87-88.
148. Hoefer HL, Fox JG, Bell JA. Gastrointestinal disease. In: Quesenberry KE, Carpenter JW, eds. *Ferrets, Rabbits, and Rodents: Clinical Medicine and Surgery.* 3rd ed. St. Louis, MO: Elsevier; 2012:27-45.
149. Fox JG. Bacterial and mycoplasmal diseases: *Helicobacter mustelae.* In: Fox JG, ed. *Biology and Disease of the Ferret.* 2nd ed. Baltimore, MD: Williams and Wilkins; 1998:327-333.
150. Fox JG. Bacterial and mycoplasmal disease: proliferative bowel disease—*Desulfovibrio* spp. (*Lawsonia intracellularis*). In: Fox JG, ed. *Biology and Disease of the Ferret.* 2nd ed. Baltimore, MD: Williams and Wilkins; 1998:335-339.
151. Sledge DG, Bolin SR, Lim A, et al. Outbreaks of severe enteric disease associated with *Eimeria furonis* infection in ferrets (*Mustela putorius furo*) of 3 densely populated groups. *J Am Vet Med Assoc.* 2011;239(12):1584-1588.

152. Lightfoot T, Rubinstein J, Aiken S, et al. Soft tissue surgery. In: Quesenberry KE, Carpenter JW, eds. *Ferrets, Rabbits, and Rodents: Clinical Medicine and Surgery*. 3rd ed. St. Louis, MO: Elsevier; 2012:27-45.

153. Palley LS, Fox JG. Eosinophilic gastroenteritis in the ferret. In: Kirk RW, Bonagura JD, eds. *Kirk's Current Veterinary Therapy XI, Small Animal Practice*. Philadelphia: Saunders; 1992:1182-1184.

154. Burgess M, Garner M. Clinical aspects of inflammatory bowel disease in ferrets. *Exot DVM*. 2002;4(2):29-34.

155. Antinoff N, Williams BH. Neoplasia. In: Quesenberry KE, Carpenter JW, eds. *Ferrets, Rabbits, and Rodents: Clinical Medicine and Surgery*. 3rd ed. St. Louis, MO: Elsevier; 2012:103-121.

156. Whittington JK, Emerson JA, Satkus TM, et al. Exocrine pancreatic carcinoma and carcinomatosis with abdominal effusion containing mast cells in a ferret (*Mustela putorius furo*). *Vet Clin North Am Exot Anim*. 2006;9:643-650.

157. Harcourt-Brown F. *Rabbit Medicine*. Edinburgh: Butterworth Heinemann; 2002.

158. Lightfoot TL. Molar trimming in rabbits, chinchillas, and guinea pigs. *Proc Natl Am Vet Conf*. 1999:843-844.

159. Oglesbee BL, Jenkins JR. Gastrointestinal diseases. In: Quesenberry KE, Carpenter JW, eds. *Ferrets, Rabbits, and Rodents: Clinical Medicine and Surgery*. 3rd ed. St. Louis, MO: Elsevier; 2012: 193-204.

160. Lichtenberger M, Lennox A. Updates and advanced therapies for gastrointestinal stasis in rabbits. *Vet Clin North Am Exot Anim*. 2010;13(3):525-541.

161. Jenkins JR. Gastrointestinal diseases. In: Hillyer EV, Quesenberry KE, eds. *Ferrets, Rabbits, and Rodents: Clinical Medicine and Surgery*. Philadelphia: W.B. Saunders; 1997:176-188.

162. Flecknell P. Guinea pigs. In: Meredith A, Redrobe S, eds. *BSAVA Manual of Exotic Pets*. 4th ed. Gloucester: BSAVA; 2005: 52-64.

163. Orr HE. Rats and mice. In: Meredith A, Redrobe S, eds. *BSAVA Manual of Exotic Pets*. 4th ed. Gloucester: BSAVA; 2005:13-25.

164. Goodman G. Hamsters. In: Meredith A, Redrobe S, eds. *BSAVA Manual of Exotic Pets*. 4th ed. Gloucester: BSAVA; 2005:26-33.

165. Brown C, Donnelly TM. Disease problems of small rodents. In: Quesenberry KE, Carpenter JW, eds. *Ferrets, Rabbits, and Rodents:*

166. Mans C, Donnelly TM. Disease problems of chinchillas. In: Quesenberry KE, Carpenter JW, eds. *Ferrets, Rabbits, and Rodents: Clinical Medicine and Surgery*. 3rd ed. St. Louis, MO: Elsevier; 2012:311-325.

167. Keeble E. Gerbils. In: Meredith A, Redrobe S, eds. *BSAVA Manual of Exotic Pets*. 4th ed. Gloucester: BSAVA; 2005:34-46.

168. Green DE. Pathology of amphibia. In: Wright KM, Whitaker BR, eds. *Amphibian Medicine and Captive Husbandry*. Malabar, FL: Krieger Publishing Company; 2001:401-486.

169. Taylor M. Examining the avian cloaca using saline infusion cloacoscopy. *Exotic DVM*. 2001;3(3):77-79.

170. Evans EE, Souza MJ. Advanced diagnostic approaches and current management of internal disorders of select species (rodents, sugar gliders, hedgehogs). *Vet Clin North Am Exotic Anim*. 2010;13(3): 453-469.

171. Boehmer E, Crossley D. Objective interpretation of dental disease in rabbits, guinea pigs and chinchillas: use of anatomical reference lines. *Tierärztliche Praxis Kleintiere*. 2009;37:250-260.

172. Lichtenberger M, Lennox A. Emergency and critical care of small mammals. In: Quesenberry KE, Carpenter JW, eds. *Ferrets, Rabbits, and Rodents: Clinical Medicine and Surgery*. 3rd ed. St. Louis, MO: Elsevier; 2012:532-544.

173. Carpenter JW. *Exotic Animal Formulary*. 4th ed. St. Louis, MO: Elsevier; 2013.

174. Stoskopf MK. Freshwater tropical fish pharmacology. In: Stoskopf MK, ed. *Fish Medicine*. Philadelphia, PA: W.B. Saunders; 1993:593-601.

175. Loudis B. Endoscope-assisted gastric lavage. *Proc Annu Conf Assoc Avian Vet*. 2004:83-88.

176. Lennox AM. Emergency and critical care procedures in sugar gliders (*Petaurus breviceps*), African hedgehogs (*Atelerix albiventris*), and prairie dogs (*Cynomys* spp.). *Vet Clin North Am Exot Anim Pract*. 2007;10(2):533-555.

177. Paul-Murphy J. Critical care of the rabbit. *Vet Clin N Am Exot Anim*. 2007;10(2):437-461.

178. Plumb DC. *Plumb's Veterinary Drug Handbook*. 7th ed. Hoboken, NJ: Wiley-Blackwell; 2011.

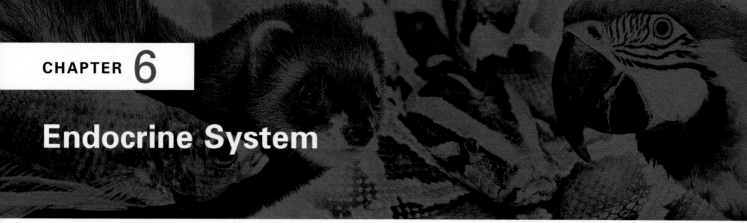

CHAPTER 6

Endocrine System

João Brandão, LMV, MS • Markus Rick, DrMedVet, PhD • Jörg Mayer, DrMedVet, MS, DABVP (Exotic Companion Mammal), DACZM, DECZM (Small Mammal)

INTRODUCTION

Endocrinology is the science that examines hormonal influences on body function.[1] Endocrine glands are specialized tissues/cells that synthesize, store, and release their hormonal secretions directly into blood. Since most endocrine glands lack a duct system (the pancreas, liver, and kidneys are exceptions), they are commonly referred to as ductless glands of internal secretion.[2] The endocrine system can be described by two words of Greek origin: endocrine and hormone. Endocrine means "to separate within," while hormone means "to arouse or excite."[3] The word hormone was first used by Ernest Starling, who described it as a chemical messenger "speeding from cell to cell along the blood stream, coordinating activities and growth of different body parts."[4] Since the introduction of this term, many hormones have been identified and characterized, and others remain to be discovered. Nonetheless, the concept of hormone and hormonal influence on metabolism has a basis in modern medicine.[5]

The endocrine system is a major homeostatic control system.[6] In general, the endocrine system influence on body function is longer lasting than that of both the central and autonomic nervous systems. The primary function of the endocrine system is to maintain normal metabolic function through internal and external environmental variation, a balance achieved through secretion of different hormones, some antagonistic, others synergistic.[6] Each hormone will bind to specific receptors located on or in respective target cells, thus creating hormone-receptor complexes. This binding will cause a measurable change in target cell activity, either through stimulation or inhibition.[1] Endocrinology studies the chemical regulation of virtually all biological phenomena at the molecular, cellular, organismal, and population level, so-called chemical bioregulation.[1] Bioregulation results from interactions of the endocrine system, the central and autonomic nervous systems, the immune system, and most cells of the body (Figure 6-1).[1]

Medical historians have highlighted endocrinology as dating back to the 14th century.[7,8] Some authors describe warriors ingesting parts of their enemies to gain and possess their strength.[9] Although this can be recognized as cannibalism or related to a spiritual belief, some suggest that it could

be considered organotherapy.[9] The credence of increased strength or other physiologic benefits from ingesting body parts could be related to effects from certain tissue hormones. Organotherapists have stated "that a given condition could be successfully treated by the use of an extract."[10] Actually, the concept of organotherapy was a first step in creating endocrinology as it is known and understood today and was first introduced by Charles-Edouard Brown-Séquard, a physiologist and professor at the College de France.[10,11] In 1889, Brown-Séquard first described the theory that chemical messengers could be secreted into blood to exert systemic effects.[11] He demonstrated this concept by administering guinea pig and dog testicular extract to himself, which he believed enhanced his physical strength, intellectual capacity, and sexual potency.[12,13] Although his experimental conclusions were later refuted, the chemical messenger concept still stands to this day.[14] Endocrinology has evolved and advanced since 1889, with early milestones highlighted in Table 6-1.

Both academically and clinically, veterinary endocrinology is a well-established discipline. Although endocrine disorders appear to be involved in ~10% to 20% of canine disease processes, this rate is ~5% (or less) in cats.[3] Endocrinopathies in large animals (e.g., cattle, horses) are often diagnosed as reproductive disorders.[3] There is relatively little information regarding endocrinology in exotic pet medicine, but it is a growing field, as basic medical knowledge of different species continues to evolve. The shear multitude of species and their unique characteristics, as well as a general lack of pathophysiologic understanding, may allow exotic pet endocrinopathies to go undetected or misdiagnosed. Although there is a significant amount of information available regarding exotic species in the basic science literature, it is difficult to extract and apply what is known and/or applies to clinical medicine.

Some exotic species are associated with important endocrine discoveries. For example, in 1849, Arnold Berthold showed that rooster castration led to regression of the wattle and comb.[15] When the testicles were reintroduced to the coelomic cavity, the comb and wattle did not return to their previous appearance; therefore, an "unknown substance" was likely being secreted into blood by the testicles for normal development of the wattle and comb.[15] This experiment led directly to the discovery of testosterone.

Chemical Bioregulation

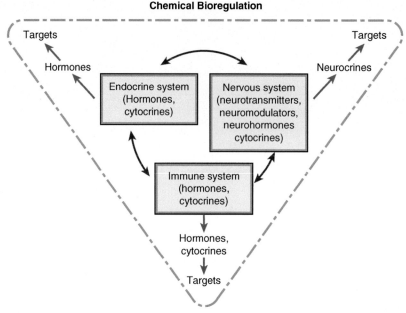

FIGURE 6-1 Chemical regulation. The endocrine system, nervous system, and immune system each secrete its own bioregulators: hormones and neurocrines. However, all of these systems influence each other, and from a homeostatic viewpoint, we can assume that they function as one great bioregulatory system. (Redrawn from Norris DO, Carr JA, eds. *Vertebrate Endocrinology.* 5th ed. Amsterdam: Academic Press, Elsevier; 2013.)

TABLE 6-1
Some Early Endocrine Milestones

1889	Brown-Séquard self-administers testis extracts
1891	Murray treats myxoeedema with thyroid extract
1894	Oliver and Schäefer describe epinephrine
1903	Bayliss and Starling discover secretin
1904	Bouin and Ancel deduce role of the Leydig cell in male phenotypic differentiation
1909	MacCallum and Voetlin discover link between parathyroid glands and calcium metabolism
1913	Farmi and von den Velden treat diabetes insipidus with posterior pituitary extracts
1921	Evans and Long describe growth hormone
1922	Discovery of insulin by Banting and Best

After Medvei VC: A history of endocrinology, 1982. IN Wilson JD: The evolution of endocrinology. *Clinical Endocrinology* 62:389-396, 2005.

This chapter provides current endocrinological knowledge in particular groups of exotic species, with the organization based on organ and/or disease processes. Since the interactions and relationships are between and among different endocrine organs, certain disease processes may affect multiple organ systems. Therefore, the disease process is described in the major organ section influenced by the so-called hypothalamic-pituitary axes. Reference intervals for certain hormones are also presented to aid in the diagnostic evaluation of patients suspected of having an endocrine disorder.

THE HYPOTHALAMUS AND PITUITARY

The hypothalamus is located at the base of the brain, near the third ventricle, extending from a plane immediately anterior to the optic chiasm to one immediately posterior to the mammillary bodies.[16] Although the avian hypothalamus is relatively small (~3% of total brain volume), in humans it represents ~0.3%.[17,18] A comparative morphometric analysis of the hypothalamus among mammals revealed that the volume of this part of the brain is highly correlated with brain size, irrespective of the ecological strategy or evolutionary history of the species considered.[17] Hypothalamic neurosecretory nuclei and the preoptic area produce neurohormones that can be stored in the neurohypophysis.[19] Neurons of these nuclei also connect to either the median eminence or the pars nervosa.[19] These neurohormones are included either as releasing hormones or release-inhibiting hormones, depending on the effects these substances have on the anterior pituitary (adenohypophysis).[19]

In all vertebrates studied, the pituitary is formed by the union of a lobe of the brain floor and a lobe or vesicle of the somatic ectoderm that migrates inward from the oral epithelium or from the upper lip ectoderm (in cyclostomes).[20] The neurohypophysis (posterior pituitary) develops from a downgrowth from the floor of the diencephalon, while the adenohypophysis (anterior pituitary) originates from Rathke's pouch.[21] The somatic ectoderm exhibits further development in an intermediate lobe (which is absent in birds), pars distalis, and pars tuberalis.[20] In teleosts and cyclostomes, another region between the pars intermedia and pars distalis is also present, called the übergangsteil.[20] In elasmobranchs, a ventral lobe extending ventrally from the base of the pars distalis has been described.[20] Once formed, the pituitary is located in the

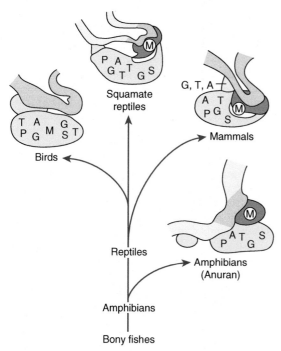

FIGURE 6-2 Comparative anatomy of the tetrapod pituitary. Approximate distributions of cell types secreting tropic hormones as indicated by letters. *A,* Corticotropin; *G,* gonadotropins; *M,* melanotropin; *P,* prolactin; *S,* growth hormone or somatotropin; *T,* thyrotropin. (Redrawn from Schreibman MP in "Vertebrate Endocrinology: Fundamentals and Biomedical Implications. Vol. 1 Morphological Considerations." (P.K.T. Pang and M. Schreibman, Eds.), Academic Press, Orlando, FL. 1986. IN From Norris DO, Carr JA. Vertebrate endocrinology. Fifth edition / ed. Amsterdam: Academic Press, Elsevier, 2013.)

sella turcica, just beneath the hypothalamus, remaining connected to the hypothalamus by a stalk known as the infundibulum.[22] In most species, the anterior lobe comprises ~80% of the gland's weight (Figure 6-2).[3]

Several hypothalamic-pituitary axes have been described including the hypothalamic-pituitary-thyroid (HPT) axis, the hypothalamic-pituitary-adrenal (HPA) axis, and the hypothalamic-pituitary-gonadal (HPG) axis.[19]

Reptiles

The pituitary of most reptiles is well developed and, composed of a pars distalis, pars tuberalis, and a pars intermedia.[1] The pituitary of the Greek tortoise (*Testudo graeca*) and European green lizard (*Lacerta viridis*) appears to be of an intermediate type between amphibians and birds.[23] The pituitary of chelonians resemble the avian pituitary, while the saurian and ophidian pituitary resemble that of the amphibian.[24] A large epithelial lobe is also present in the reptile pituitary and contains the pars glandularis, which is situated below the pars nervosa and the pars intermedia.[23] The pars intermedia is markedly reduced or absent in many lizards and burrowing snakes; however, it is well developed in certain chelonians, crocodilians, snakes, and anoline lizards.[1] The pars glandularis is unique to reptiles and consists of columns of cubical or columnar cells that form distinct acini with central cavities filled with a colloid material.[23] The pars distalis

appears to have two distinct regions.[1] The pars tuberalis is well developed in Rhynchocephalia, chelonian species, and Crocodilia, but reduced or sometimes absent in some species of lizards and absent in adult snakes.[1]

Birds

The avian hypothalamus is relatively small but occupies a large portion of the ventral diencephalon.[18] Anteriorly, the most prominent cell clusters are the preoptic, supraoptic, and paraventricular nuclei, while posteriorly the infundibular nucleus and medial posterior hypothalamic nucleus can be found.[18] As mentioned above, birds lack a pars intermedia; therefore, the adenohypophysis is formed by the pars distalis and a well-developed pars tuberalis, while the neurohypophysis is formed by the pars nervosa, infundibulum, and median eminence.[1,25,26] The human pars intermedia is present in the fetus; however, it is absent or significantly reduced during adulthood.[27] The lack of a pars intermedia has been reported in chickens (*Gallus gallus domesticus*), ducks, and 18 other species of birds.[28] Since birds lack a pars intermedia, melanocyte-stimulating hormones (MSHs) are found in the pars anterior.[20] Initial reports indicated that a cluster of cells corresponding to the pars intermedia was present in the caudal region of the chicken pituitary pars anterior; however, it was later determined that the cephalic third of the chicken's pituitary anterior lobe contained 10 to 20 times more active MSH.[29] The pars distalis is well developed in avian species as in reptiles and is divided into cephalic and caudal lobes.[1] It has been suggested that corticomelanotrophs of the pars distalis are co-responsible for the production of α-MSH and adrenocorticotropic hormone (ACTH) in the duck and chicken.[30–32] The tissue concentration of α-MSH was considered to be very low (10 ng/gland), but there is no information on circulating values in birds.[32,33] A published report indicates that α-MSH is produced locally, not by the pituitary, and acts as an autocrine and/or paracrine hormone in birds.[34] Moreover, there are two distinct areas within the pars anterior of the chicken and duck pituitaries, which are defined as cephalic and caudal lobes.[28] Among 18 different species of 7 different orders of birds, all had distinct regions of the pars anterior, and the two regions appeared to communicate with the hypophysial stalk and pars tuberalis.[28] However, some species-specific characteristics have been reported, mainly at the cytological level.[23]

Mammals

The anatomy and histology of the small mammal hypothalamus and pituitary are similar to those of other mammals.

Functions

Both the hypothalamus and pituitary are responsible for stimulation of several body endocrine activities. Sir Walter Langdon-Brown in 1931 stated that "the pituitary is the director of the endocrine orchestra."[35] However, his statement received some skepticism, since others compare the pituitary to the first fiddle and the hypothalamus to the conductor.[36] Although these analogies appear to simplify the function of these endocrine organs, they are reasonably good descriptions for the roles of the hypothalamus and pituitary in endocrinology. Even in current medical references, the pituitary is often called the "master gland" because of its control over several other endocrine glands. The hypothalamus is responsible for the production of several hormones that, in turn, stimulate pituitary activity (or inactivity). Release or release-inhibiting hormones produced by the hypothalamus are thyrotropin-releasing hormone (TRH), corticotropin-releasing hormone (CRH), dopamine (DA, a prolactin [PRL]-inhibiting hormone), growth hormone (GH)-releasing hormone (GHRH), GH-release-inhibiting hormone (GHIH, also called somatostatin [SS]), gonadotropin-releasing hormone (GnRH), melanocyte-releasing hormone (MRH), and melanocyte release-inhibiting hormone (MRIH). As the names imply, these hormones are responsible for stimulating or inhibiting the secretion of other hormones by positive or negative feedback mechanisms. Following stimulation by specific hypothalamic-releasing hormones, the pituitary synthesizes and secretes (into blood) several different hormones: somatotropin (also known as growth hormone or GH), thyrotropin (thyroid-stimulating hormone [TSH]), corticotropin (ACTH), lactotropin (PRL), the gonadotropins (luteinizing hormone [LH] and follicle-stimulating hormone [FSH]), and in certain species, melanotropin (MSH). The posterior pituitary secretes, but does not synthesize, antidiuretic hormones (ADHs, or vasopressin) and oxytocin. The intermediate lobe (where present) also synthesizes and secretes MSH and ACTH. Although removal of the pituitary is not fatal, it has important actions (as previously stated) in regulating hormonal secretions of other glands (with the notable exception of the pancreas and parathyroid glands).[3]

Due to the close anatomic and physiologic communication between the hypothalamus and pituitary, their functions are intrinsically connected. Activities of both glands can be related to various axes (e.g., HPT axis). The hypothalamus produces TRH, which in turn stimulates the pituitary to synthesize and secrete TSH. Under the influence of TSH, the thyroid produces triiodothyronine (T_3) and thyroxine (T_4). This cascade of events, in turn, is controlled by negative feedback from the different hormones produced. If there is a sufficient amount of T_3 or T_4, production of TSH and TRH is decreased (or inhibited). Most hypothalamic hormones have a stimulating activity, with the exception of GHIH, MRIH, and DA. These hormones have a suppressing effect on the pituitary to decrease the release of GH, α-MSH, and PRL, respectively.

To show the cross activity of hormone effects, pituitary extracts from nonmammalian species have been administered to mammals, leading to similar effects as in their nonmammalian counterparts.[37] These studies also allowed, by paper chromatography, the identification of two types of substances that resembled mammalian oxytocin, both slow and rapid substances that were later identified as arginine[8]-oxytocin or vasotocin.[37]

Disease Processes

Hypothalamic and pituitary dysfunctions have been well described in human medicine but to a lesser extent in veterinary medicine. Due to the physiologic relationship between the pituitary and hypothalamus, most disease processes have some effect on both glands.

Diabetes Insipidus

The word diabetes originates from Greek and was first used by Demetrius of Apameia to mean "to pass or run through" like a siphon.[38,39] In both diabetes mellitus (DM) and diabetes insipidus (DI), one of the most striking clinical signs is polyuria/polydipsia (PU/PD). In the past, due to the lack of

other diagnostic tests, tasting the urine was one method of distinguishing between these two differing conditions.[39] Mellitus means "sweet flavor," while insipidus means "tasteless." Frank described DI in 1974 as "a long-continued abnormally increased secretion of non-saccharine urine, which is not caused by a disease condition of the kidneys."[40] Frank continued to provide contributions to the knowledge of DI and was the first to report the case of a patient who developed polyuria after a gunshot wound to the head, in which the bullet was lodged in the posterior pituitary.[41] This was considered the first clinical evidence of the role of the pituitary in DI.[42]

Under normal conditions, the posterior pituitary produces ADH, also called arginine-vasopressin, and as the name indicates, it promotes antidiuretic effects through promoting renal retention of water. ADH is a nonapeptide (9 amino acids) that inhibits diuresis. This escalates urinary osmolarity by increasing permeability of the renal collecting ducts to water, which is subsequently reabsorbed into the hypertonic renal medullary interstitium.[3] In nonmammalian species, a hormone similar to ADH, vasotocin, is produced. Vasotocin is an oligopeptide homologous to oxytocin and vasopressin, and it is found in all nonmammalian vertebrates (e.g., birds, fishes, amphibians, reptiles) and possibly in mammals during fetal stages of development.[37,43,44]

Clinical signs typically associated with DI in mammals are profound PU/PD.[45] The failure to produce (by hypothalamic nuclei) or secrete (by the posterior pituitary) or the lack of renal effects of ADH can all result in DI. Subdivisions of DI are generally referred to as primary (neurogenic or central DI), nephrogenic DI, dipsogenic DI, or gestational DI. Central DI results from the destruction of ADH production sites in the hypothalamus (i.e., the supraoptic and paraventricular nuclei), loss of major axons that carry ADH to storage sites in the pituitary, or disruption of the ability to release stored ADH.[3] DI is characterized by production of hyposmolar (hyposthenuric) urine, regardless of a strong osmotic stimulus for ADH secretion, a rise in urine osmolarity following administration of exogenous ADH, and the absence of renal disease.[45] In dogs and cats, two types of central DI have been recognized: complete and partial.[46] In the case of complete central DI, there is a total lack of ADH, while in partial central DI, some of the hormone is present.[47] In humans, DI can be idiopathic (50%), genetic (5%), secondary to a tumor, or secondary to inflammatory reactions.[48] Although prevalence in small animals is not published, several causes have been reported: idiopathic, congenital, subsequent to trauma, and neoplasia related.[49–60] There is no reported age, breed, or gender predisposition in dogs and cats: however, young adults (6 mo of age) are most commonly affected.[61]

In nephrogenic DI, the kidneys are unable to concentrate urine despite normal or elevated concentrations of ADH.[62] Nephrogenic DI can be caused by multiple etiologies that result in the inability of the kidneys to respond to ADH.[3] In cases diagnosed with nephrogenic DI, ADH serum levels may be normal or elevated, although a partial or nearly complete lack of renal response occurs.[3]

A temporary state of DI in humans has been described secondary to alcohol ingestion.[63] Alcohol can indeed cause several endocrine abnormalities such as alcohol-induced pseudo-Cushing's syndrome and a syndrome of HPA unresponsiveness, both of which result from long-term alcohol overindulgence. Impairment of testosterone secretion may occur following relatively short-term drinking of alcoholic beverages as well.[64] Alcohol promotes urine production by inhibiting pituitary release of ADH, which leads to dehydration and subsequently the so-called state of hangover (or veisalgia).[65]

REPTILES. To the authors' knowledge, no cases of DI have been reported in reptiles. Nonetheless, this condition may hypothetically occur.

BIRDS. Birds, as mentioned previously, as other nonmammalian species, do not produce vasopressin; instead, they produce arginine vasotocin. Arginine vasotocin is an oligopeptide, homologous to the mammalian oxytocin and vasopressin, produced by neurosecretory cells of the posterior pituitary gland. Arginine vasotocin has vascular and renal tubular antidiuretic effects that are mediated via V_1 (smooth muscle) and V_2 (renal epithelial) receptors.[45,66] There are reports suggesting that vasotocin induces increased aquaporin 2 mRNA and protein biosynthesis in quails.[67]

Although DI is rare in avian species, central DI has been previously reported in an African grey parrot (*Psittacus erithacus*),[45] and nephrogenic DI has been reported in domestic fowl.[68] Genetically selected lines of Japanese quail (*Coturnix japonica*) and chickens with DI have been developed.[69,70] Reports of intracranial neoplasias/lesions and PU/PD have been published, but specific DI diagnostic tests were not performed.[45,71] One of the authors (J.B.) is also aware of two highly suspected clinical cases of DI: a green cheek conure (*Pyrrhura molinae*) with suspected idiopathic nephrogenic DI and an umbrella cockatoo (*Cacatua alba*) with suspected central DI secondary to trauma.

Reported diagnostic tests for DI in birds have been adapted from small animal medicine. As the main clinical sign for DI is PU/PD, it is important to rule out other conditions that can cause such a presentation. In dogs and cats, normal water intake varies between 20 and 70 mL/kg/day, with urine production between 20 and 45 mL/kg/day.[72] In birds, daily requirements vary with species, size, and environmental temperature.[73] In general, ad libitum water consumption is inversely related to body weight.[73] Species that originate from areas where water is not abundant often have lower water intake demands.[73] For example, a budgerigar (*Melopsittacus undulatus*) with an average weight of 30 g requires 5% of its body weight in water per day; however, a house sparrow (*Passer domesticus*) requires ~30%.[73] Since evaporative losses and ad libitum water consumption are inversely proportional to body weight, larger birds are expected to lose weight more slowly than small species when denied water and maintained on a dry diet.[73] Some authors suggest that fluid maintenance for most bird species can be calculated at 100 mL/kg/day.[74] The general, range of renal output in birds is between 100 and 200 mL/kg/day; however, in dehydrated birds, renal output can decrease to 25 mL/kg/day.[75] Nonetheless, species-specific characteristics influence renal output. Moreover, the avian cloaca makes it difficult to solely quantitate the amount of urine produced. After 30 hours of dehydration, in house sparrows' body weights decreased by 12%, plasma osmolarity increased, the glomerular filtration rate (GFR) declined from 7.7 to 3.5 mL/hour, and the urine flow rate declined from 0.2 to 0.03 mL/hour.[76] The rate of water loss in the excreta of hydrated sparrows was 0.2 mL/hour, while in dehydrated

birds it was 0.04 mL/hour.[76] In great horned owls (*Bubo virginianus*) fed mice without water supplementation, the water intake from the mouse content was 43.7 g/kg/day, which led to a water loss in the excreta of 19.7 g/kg/day.[77] When fed poults, water intake was 53.3 g/kg/day, with a water loss of 27.4 g/kg/day.[77] For both types of diets, water lost in the excreta accounted for ~50% of water ingested with food.[77] In healthy pigeons (*Columba livia*) deprived of water for 24 and 48 hours, the weight loss over time was ~6% and 10%, respectively.[78]

One of the most common diagnostic tests performed for differentiating among causes of PU/PD (e.g., DI, psychogenic polydipsia, hyperadrenocorticism) is the water deprivation test.[79] The basis of the water deprivation test is to determine whether vasopressin (or vasotocin in nonmammalian vertebrates) is released in response to dehydration and whether the renal tissue responds to this stimulus.[18,79] Patients with DI become dehydrated but maintain a hyposthenuric urine (decreased osmolality and specific gravity).[80] In the case of psychogenic polydipsia, the urine should concentrate over time.[80] During the water deprivation diagnostic test, water is withheld for a certain amount of time. During that period, the weight is checked at regular intervals, as are urine osmolality and/or specific gravity. In normal pigeons, it is said that a 1-day water deprivation is sufficient to determine normal response. At 24 hours, urine osmolalities >450 mOsmol/kg are considered normal.[79] In Hispaniolan Amazon parrots (*Amazona ventralis*), the urine osmolality measured by vapor pressure osmometry was highly correlated with the specific gravity.[81] An equation was calculated to allow specific gravity results from a medical refractometer to be converted to specific gravity values of Hispaniolan Amazon parrots: USG_{HAp} = 0.201 + 0.798(USG_{ref}), with USG_{HAp} urine specific gravity of Hispaniolan Amazon parrots and USG_{ref} urine specific gravity measured on a reference scale.[81] Use of the reference-canine scale to approximate the osmolality of parrot urine led to an overestimation, with the error increasing as the concentration of urine increased.[81] The feline scale provides a closer approximation to urine osmolality of this species of psittacines but still results in osmolality overestimation.[81] It is important to consider that due to the avian anatomical characteristics, urine will be contaminated with fecal material, therefore artificially affecting values of urine osmolality and specific gravity. Several methods for urine collection have been described; however, some of these methods are invasive and may not be beneficial to the patient.[82] Recommendations indicate that plasma ADH concentrations should be measured at the beginning of study and at 72 hours of water deprivation; ADH concentration >2.2 pg/mL at 24 hours is indicative of a normal ADH release in the pigeon.[18] It is also important to ensure the safety of the patient. An animal suffering from central DI has an uncontrollable need to ingest water, and limiting access to water can be severely detrimental. The water deprivation test in a case of central DI was only reported once. In this case, the bird was weighed and placed in a stainless steel cage with a nonporous perch; food and water were withheld during the test.[45] Plasma electrolytes and osmolality were determined at 0 and 170 minutes; hematocrit was measured at 0, 170, and 480 minutes; and plasma total solid concentration (by refractometry) was measured at 480 minutes.[45] The subjective "clean" urine was occasionally collected within 1 minute after voiding to measure urine supernatant specific gravity and osmolality.[45] Body weight was monitored frequently to determine hydration status.[45] At 170 minutes, 2.14 µg/kg intramuscular (IM) desmopressin (DDAVP, a synthetic ADH) was administered, leading to a noticeable decrease in urination frequency and a urine osmolality increase of >300%.[45] The test was discontinued at 610 minutes when the birds' weight loss reached 6.4%.[45]

As mentioned above, the water deprivation test is useful to distinguish between central DI and psychogenic polydipsia. In the cases of central DI, the animal should be able to conserve water because ADH is commonly produced under normal circumstances; therefore, in the case of water deprivation, the urine osmolality and specific gravity should increase over time. In the case of an African grey parrot with a water intake of 200 mL/day and diagnosed with psychogenic polydipsia, a water deprivation test of 48 hours was performed.[83] Urine osmolality was 115, 710, and 758 mOsmol/kg, while specific gravity was 1.004, 1.023, and 1.026 at times 0, 24, and 48 hours, respectively.[83] Over the 48-hour test, weight loss was ~10% of the bird's initial body weight.[83] All reported changes supported a diagnosis of psychogenic polydipsia and ruled out DI. Although DI appears to be an uncommon disease, it has been reported in birds and likely underdiagnosed.

MAMMALS. Spontaneous DI in exotic small mammal species (rats and rabbits) commonly kept as pets can occur.[84-86] Diagnostic tests similar to those described for birds are also adequate for mammals and may help to distinguish between central DI, nephrogenic DI, and other causes of DI. The use of the water deprivation test for diagnosing psychogenic polydipsia was reported in a laboratory New Zealand white rabbit (*Oryctolagus cuniculus*).[87] However, it is important to consider some characteristics specific to certain small exotic mammal species. In gerbils (*Meriones unguiculatus*), if food is restricted, they naturally become polydipsic (in the absence of DI).[88]

Neoplasia

REPTILES. Pituitary tumors appear to be rare in reptiles. A pituitary cystoadenoma associated with hyperkeratosis, generalized dysecdysis, and intestinal lipidosis was reported in an Everglades ratsnake (*Elaphe obsoleta rossalleni*).[89] When postmortem levels of ACTH were compared with those obtained from antemortem samples and a control clutch mate, no relevant differences were detected. Two cases of pituitary adenomas were reported in a black-headed python (*Aspidites melanocephalus*) and a Dumeril's ground boa (*Acrantophis dumerili*).[90,91] A limited number of publications reporting the presence of pituitary neoplasias in reptiles may be attributed to the fact that brain and pituitary are not commonly evaluated histologically in these species.[89]

BIRDS. Pituitary neoplasias reported in birds are adenocarcinomas, carcinomas, and chromophobe pituitary tumors.[92] The most commonly reported avian neuroendocrine tumors are pituitary adenomas originating from the endocrinologically inactive chromophobe cells of the anterior lobe.[93] Pituitary adenomas and, to a lesser extent, pituitary carcinomas are common in budgerigars.[94-97] A total of 156 cases of primary pituitary adenoma or carcinoma were reported in one study.[96] Pituitary adenomas have been reported in cockatiels (*Nymphicus hollandicus*) and one yellow-napped Amazon parrot

(*Amazona auropalliata*).[93,98,99] Chromophobe adenomas appear to be endocrinologically inactive; therefore, most of the significant functional disturbances occur by virtue of compression atrophy of the pars nervosa and pars distalis or extension into the overlying brain.[2] Clinical signs associated with pituitary neoplasias include exophthalmia (secondary to the extension of neoplastic cells along the optic nerve), polyuria, cere color changes, feather abnormalities, circling, vocalization, and blindness.[92] Somatotroph pituitary tumors have also been reported in budgerigars.[100]

MAMMALS. Although pituitary neoplasms have been reported in multiple species of small exotic mammals (e.g., rabbits, ferrets), the species in which these are most prevalent is rats.[101-103] Several predisposing factors, including age and sex, have been reported. As older female rats are most commonly diagnosed with pituitary neoplasms, it has been suggested that estrogen may play a role in their development.[104] In Sprague-Dawley and Fischer strains, prevalence rates for pituitary tumors have been reported to be 85% and 83% in animals older than 24 months.[105,106] Multiple studies evaluating the prevalence of spontaneous pituitary tumors in control group rats have been published. Among 1857 neoplasms detected in a 1370 control Wistar rat population, 74% were endocrine and reproductive in origin, with pituitary adenoma being the most common (27.7% males, 55% females).[107] In another study, among 930 rats in which 1599 neoplasms were detected, pituitary adenoma was the most commonly detected in 34% of males and 50% of females.[108] Studies have indicated that pituitary adenomas are more common in older rats. In one study comparing the occurrence of tumors in Sprague-Dawley male rats, the most common tumor at 50 weeks was lymphoma, while pituitary adenoma was the most common at 50 to 80 weeks of age and at 2 years.[109] No difference was detected among females. A genetic influence is possible, as one study reported that the highest incidence of neoplasms in young Sprague-Dawley female rats was pituitary tumor, while in Han Wistar rats it was malignant lymphoma.[110] Although significantly lower in prevalence, cases of aggressive infiltrative pituitary tumors have also been reported in rats. The prevalence in one study was 0.42% (11/2609).[111] In rats, PRL-producing pituitary adenomas are the most common, followed by gonadotroph cell adenomas and immunonegative adenomas.[112] Mixed PRL- and GH-producing adenomas have also been described.[112] This prevalence is useful in terms of potential treatment options. The treatment objective in humans is to (1) suppress excessive hormone secretion and its clinical consequences, (2) control tumor mass, (3) preserve or improve residual pituitary function, and (4) prevent disease recurrence or progression.[113] PRL secretion is regulated by DA, also called PRL-inhibitory hormone, by a short-loop feedback mechanism.[3,114] DA reaches the pituitary via hypophysial portal blood that is controlled by PRL itself as well as estrogens and other neuropeptides and neurotransmitters.[115] DA binds to type-2 DA receptors, suppressing the high intrinsic secretory activity of pituitary lactotrophs.[115] Additionally, DA suppresses PRL gene expression and lactotroph proliferation.[115] The most common compounds used in human clinical practice to treat prolactinomas are all DA agonists, including bromocriptine, cabergoline, pergolide, and quinagolide.[113] Cabergoline is usually the DA agonist of choice.[116]

Reports of pituitary adenomas in pet rats and treatment of clinical cases are rare. A 2-year-old intact male albino pet rat presented with a 3-week history of hypodipsia, suspected blindness, and behavioral changes.[112] A pituitary adenoma was diagnosed on magnetic resonance imaging (MRI), and the rat was subsequently treated with carbergoline (0.6 mg/kg, PO, q 72 h).[112] A recheck MRI at 2 months post initiation of treatment revealed a significant decrease in pituitary size.[112] Clinical signs recurred at 8.5 months, and a pituitary adenoma was diagnosed on necropsy.[112]

THE HYPOTHALAMIC-PITUITARY-THYROID AXIS

The thyroid gland is present in all vertebrates and is unique among endocrine glands in that it has extracellular storage of its secretory products (the thyroid hormones). The thyroid gland is among the most highly vascularized of endocrine glands and phylogenetically appears to be one of the oldest. The thyroid hormones are critical players in differentiation, growth, and metabolism.[117,118] Thyroid hormones are necessary for the normal metabolic activity of most body tissues, with a major emphasis on oxygen consumption and thus the basal metabolic rate (BMR).[117] Hormones from the thyroid gland are thought to perform in a manner similar to exercise by increasing the animal's metabolic state, oxygen consumption, and cellular activity, which in turn causes increased heat production and vasodilation.[119] In order to maintain adequate tissue perfusion and nutrient delivery, there is an increase in blood volume, cardiac output, and ventilation, without major effects on blood pressure.[119]

The basic functional unit of the thyroid gland is the follicle, which contains colloid. This colloid is the store for thyroglobulin, a large glycoprotein dimer containing iodotyrosines (that serve as precursors for thyroid hormone biosynthesis).[66] The two main hormones produced by the thyroid are thyroxine (3,5,3′,5′-tetraiodothyronine, or T_4) and lesser amounts of the more active triiodothyronine (3,5,3′-triiodothyronine, or T_3).[120] The thyroid gland also secretes calcitonin, which is involved in calcium and phosphorus homeostasis and skeletal remodeling, along with parathyroid hormone (PTH) and vitamin D.[121] The T_4 may be considered a storage and transport form of thyroid hormones, while T_3 is the more metabolically active form.[122] The T_4 accounts for ~80% of thyroid hormones in the thyroid gland and plasma, and it is converted to T_3 in skeletal muscle, liver, brain, and other target tissues by removal of an outer layer ring 5′ iodine (deiodination).[122] Less than 20% of T_3 is produced in the thyroid.[66] In birds, TRH stimulates GH-releasing action that causes an increase of T_3 due to GH inhibition of T_3 degradation by type-3 deiodinase.[123]

Iodide is essential for normal function of the thyroid, with a minimum human daily iodine intake requirement of 50 μg and a recommended daily intake of 150 μg.[122] Iodide is actively transported from the extracellular fluid into the thyroid follicular cell via a sodium-iodide symporter, a transmembrane channel that is energy dependent, saturable, and requires oxidative metabolism that responds to TSH stimulation.[122,124] After transport, the iodide is oxidized by thyroid peroxidase into a reactive intermediate that is then incorporated into the tyrosine residues of protein (mainly thyroglobulin) by a process called organification.[66] The T_3 and T_4 are synthesized by coupling of two iodotyrosine residues and stored in the colloid until thyroid follicular cells take up thyroglobulin.[124] Thyroid hormones are released into blood when signaled by TSH stimulation.[124]

Thyroid activity is regulated by a negative feedback loop involving the hypothalamus, pituitary, and thyroid gland.[119] TRH is secreted by the hypothalamus after exposure to stress, illness, cold, metabolic demand, or decreased circulating thyroid hormones, mainly T_3.[119,121] TRH stimulates the pituitary to release TSH, which causes the release of T_3 and T_4.[119] Other conditions that can affect this axis include drugs, illness, thyroid disease, pituitary disorders, and age.[121] Thyroid hormones have a negative effect, which is the primary TSH regulatory mechanism, although tonic stimulation of TRH has a permissive role in TSH secretion.[125] It is also suggested that thyroid hormones have a direct negative effect on TRH release from the hypothalamus.[125]

The majority of T_3 and T_4, called total T_3 (TT_3) and total T_4 (TT_4), are bound to the plasma protein (i.e., the thyroxine-binding globulins transthyretin and thyroid-binding albumin).[121] Thyroxine-binding globulins bind ~70% of plasma T_4 and ~75% to 80% of T_3.[121] Only a small fraction of each is freely present in plasma; free thyroxine (fT_4) accounts for 0.02% to 0.03% of TT_4, while free triiodothyronine (fT_3) accounts for ~0.3% of TT_3.[121]

Thyroid hormones have significant effects in multiple organs (e.g., bone, heart).[117] Thyroid hormones are critical for normal bone growth and development, as T_3 stimulates both osteoblast and osteoclast activities.[117,126] Reports indicate that T_3 plays an important role in linear growth and bone maintenance and is essential for normal development of endochondral and intramembranous bone.[127] Thyroidal disease processes are thus known to cause changes in bone growth and development (Table 6-2).[128]

The thyroid gland exhibits both direct and indirect effects on the heart and cardiovascular system (i.e., influences on myocardial contractility and hemodynamics).[129] The first reported relationship between the heart and thyroid was recognized in 1785 by Caleb Hillier Parry, who noted thyroid enlargement and cardiac changes in eight women.[130] The effects caused by thyroid hormones on the heart result from interaction with specific nuclear receptors in cardiac myocytes.[130] Overall, changes in thyroid function influence cardiac action because T_3 exerts a direct effect on cardiac myocytes by binding to nuclear T_3 receptors; T_3 may also influence the sympathetic system by increasing sensitivity, and T_3 leads to hemodynamic alterations in the periphery that result in increased cardiac filling and modification of cardiac contractility.[130] It has been suggested that clinical signs related to the cardiovascular system are major manifestations of thyroid dysfunction in humans; therefore, thyroid function should be assessed in patients with cardiovascular disease.[129] Even minimal but persistent changes in circulating thyroid hormones can cause cardiac changes,[131] and subclinical hyperthyroidism has been correlated with development of atrial fibrillation.[132,133]

Clinical Assessment

Several diagnostic tests associated with thyroid function have been developed over the years, and most are currently being

TABLE 6-2

Clinical Thyroid Diseases and Their Skeletal Consequences in Small Animals

Disease	Thyroid Status			Skeletal Consequences	
	T_4	T_3	TSH	Juvenile	Adult
Hypothyroidism	Low	Low	High	Delayed bone age, growth arrest, short stature	Reduced bone turnover, increased fracture risk
Hyperthyroidism	High	High	Low	Advanced bone age, accelerated growth, premature fusion of growth plates, short stature, craniosynostosis	High bone turnover osteoporosis, increased fracture risk
Resistance to thyroid hormone	High	High	Inappropriately normal or high	Variable	Variable
Activating TSHR mutation	High	High	Low	Short metacarpals and metatarsals, advanced bone age, craniosynostosis	Short metacarpals and metatarsals
Inactivating TSHR mutation	Low	Low	High	Not reported	Not reported
T_4 suppression therapy	Normal	Normal	Low	Not reported	Reduced BMD in postmenopausal women
TSH-β deficiency	Low	Low	Absent	Normal following T4 replacement after birth	Not reported
Subclinical hyperthyroidism	Normal	Normal	Low	Not reported	Increased bone turnover, reduced BMD, increased fracture risk

BMD, Bone mineral density; *RTH,* resistance to thyroid hormone; *TSH,* thyroid-stimulating hormone; *TSRH,* TSH receptor.
From Gogakos AI, Duncan Bassett J, Williams GR. Thyroid and bone. *Arch Biochem Biophys.* 2010;503:129-136.
Validation of this information in exotic animals is needed but is expected to be similar to that of other species.

used in veterinary medicine. The most common initial assessment of thyroid function is based on the measurement of serum thyroid hormones. As previously stated, two different "active" thyroid hormones (in two different states) are available: TT_4, fT_4, TT_3, and fT_3. The first available test to assess thyroid function was TT_4.[134] This test has been available since the 1950s but has been shown to have poor sensitivity and specificity for thyroid disease.[134] In dogs, TT_4 is only useful if the value is normal or elevated.[125] In human medicine, TT_4 is not commonly used because the measurement of TT_4 and TT_3 is unreliable since other nonthyroidal diseases can influence these values. This condition is commonly called euthyroid sick syndrome or nonthyroidal illness syndrome.[135] Euthyroid sick syndrome refers to changes in serum TSH, serum thyroid hormones, and tissue thyroid hormone levels that occur in patients with various nonthyroidal conditions; however, it is not a primary thyroid disease.[136] Euthyroid sick syndrome may occur due to reduced TRH secretion, impaired TSH secretion, decreased thyroid-binding capacity, reduced tissue/cellular thyroid hormone uptake, altered 5'-deiodinase (that converts T_4 to T_3), and altered thyroid hormone receptor expression/signaling (e.g., reduced in skeletal muscle).[137-143] Euthyroid sick syndrome occurs in cases of starvation, sepsis, surgery, myocardial infarction, bypass, bone marrow transplantation, and probably any severe disease.[144] In cases of mild illness, only TT_3 decreases; however, in severe cases, both TT_3 and TT_4 decrease.[144] Among animals, circadian cycles are also included as influencing TT_4 values.[125] It should be noted that in formation of reverse T_3 (rT_3) by the liver or in target cells, where T_4 is deiodinated on the 5 position of the inner ring rather than the 5' position of the outer ring, an "inactive" form of the thyroid hormone is produced rather than an active form. Thus, the basal metabolic rate (BMR) is reduced. The relative hypothyroid state produced is a physiological means of conserving energy during times of food deprivation (starvation) and hibernation.

Discussion regarding the terminology of euthyroid sick syndrome and nonthyroidal illness syndrome has persisted. When the term euthyroid sick syndrome was proposed in the 1980s, the consensus was that patients were euthyroid, and detected thyroid abnormalities had no impact on the adverse physiologic and clinical effects.[145] Reports suggest that a considerable degree of secondary hypothyroid status may be present in some patients; therefore, the terminology of nonthyroidal illness syndrome was suggested.[145] Under this new definition, abnormalities in thyroid function can be defined as low T_3 syndrome, low T_3-low T_4 syndrome, high T_4 syndrome, and other abnormalities.[135] It is possible that the occurrence of nonthyroidal illness syndrome may be a beneficial response (e.g., to reduce metabolic rate) or a maladaptive response (with potential benefit from thyroid hormone replacement therapy).[146] Nonetheless, compelling evidence supporting the use of thyroid hormone replacement therapy in most cases of nonthyroidal illness syndrome is currently lacking.[146] Reductions of TT_4 in humans, dogs, and cats correlate with higher mortality.[125] However, because of the unreliability of the total thyroid hormone measurement, this method has been largely abandoned in human medicine. Conversely, total thyroid hormone measurement is still commonly used in veterinary medicine, particularly in exotic animal medicine.

Measurement of the free hormones is a more up-to-date methodology. Furthermore, when measured by reliable methods, decreases in fT_4 and fT_3 are usually modest when compared to decreases in TT_3 and TT_4 (in the case of euthyroid sick syndrome or nonthyroidal illness syndrome).[138] Similar information has been suggested for dogs.[147] Isolated measurement of serum fT_3 or TT_3 concentrations in dogs is a less meaningful estimate of thyroid function than is measurement of the serum fT_4 or TT_4 concentration.[125] Nonetheless, free thyroid values are also influenced by other nonthyroidal factors.[148] In dogs with severe disease, TT_4 and fT_4 concentrations were commonly lower than reference intervals (59% and 32%, respectively).[149]

Serum TSH measurement in humans is the single most reliable test to diagnose all common forms of hypothyroidism and hyperthyroidism.[150] Initially, TSH measurement was used for assessment of hypothyroid cases (in which the TSH should be elevated). However, with current methodologies, it is possible to detect low values, which are indicative of hyperthyroidism. Approximately 25% of hypothyroidism cases in dogs show normal TSH values.[125] Other studies have shown low correlation between diagnosed hypothyroid dogs and serum TSH values.[149,151] Nonetheless, the use of TSH is a useful diagnostic test in cases of suspected canine hypothyroidism, but dynamic testing may still be necessary to confirm this disease condition.[151] Since euthyroid dogs rarely have elevated TSH (with the exception of the ones recovering from nonthyroidal illness syndrome), elevated TSH is highly indicative of hypothyroidism.[125] In most cases, interpretation of human thyroid function tests with free hormone assays and TSH is straightforward.[152] Other methods used for serum quantification of TSH in both humans and dogs are thyroid autoimmunity. Different antibodies have been described: thyroglobulin autoantibodies (TgAA), antitriiodothyronine (T_3AA), and antithyroxine (T_4AA). Thyroid autoimmunity is useful for the diagnosis of thyroiditis because positive TgAA results are usually associated with underlying thyroiditis.[125] Dogs with T_3AA or T_4AA also have positive TgAA.[125] The use of thyroid autoimmunity is necessary because T_4AA alone may cause a false increase in the TT_4 concentration.[66] This false increase in TT_4 may result in the hypothyroid dog's being within normal reference intervals or even appear hyperthyroid.[66] This false increase occurs when nondialysis (direct) radioimmunoassays (RIAs) are used for serum fT_4; however, this will not happen if fT_4 is measured using a dialysis procedure, because autoantibodies cannot pass through the dialysis membrane and interfere with the assay.[66] To our knowledge, this diagnostic test is not available for other animal species.

Another thyroid function diagnostic test, used primarily for patients considered hypothyroid, is dynamic testing. The concept of dynamic testing is to administer a certain hormone and determine the physiologic response. This is possible due to the HPT axis. In a euthyroid patient, when a certain amount of functional TRH is administered, the pituitary and consequently the thyroid should release TSH and thyroid hormones, respectively. If a functional TSH is administered, thyroid hormone production should also occur. In the case of

euthyroidism, when TSH or TRH is given to the patient, serum levels of T_3 and T_4 should increase. If there is no elevation of serum levels of T_3 and T_4, one can assume that there is glandular dysfunction. Multiple TRH and TSH formulations are commercially available, and it is possible that dynamic effects on different animal species may vary with this testing methodology. Further assessment about the use of different TSH and TRH formulations in exotic species is required.

Among exotic species, limited studies assessing dynamic thyroidal testing have been published. In reptiles, TRH induced an in vivo increase in the plasma T_4 of a Carolina anole (*Anolis carolinensis*).[153] In painted turtles (*Chrysemys picta*), an in vivo TRH stimulation test did not result in increased circulating T_4.[154] In birds, TSH stimulation tests have been shown to be effective in pigeons, multiple psittacine species, and chickens.[155-160] Several of the commercially available TSH stimulation tests (e.g., bovine, canine, human) have been used in chickens. Although canine TSH has been recommended for use in birds, bovine TSH induced a greater postintravenous (post-IV) administration response.[160] TRH and TSH stimulation testing has been reported in multiple mammalian species (e.g., rats, mice, ferrets, guinea pigs).[161-163]

Although further studies are necessary to assess the use of TSH and TRH stimulation studies in exotic species, current information is promising for clinical use. It is suggested that the primary structure of the TRH tripeptide (pGlu-His-Pro-NH$_2$) has been conserved across the vertebrate phylum.[164] Differences between human TSH (hTSH) and that of other species have been reported, but it should be recognized that TSH is a glycoprotein of 211 amino acids (and not a simple tripeptide).[165,166] Although no scientific validation has been reported, if the chemical structure of the TRH is similar across species, this test is more likely to be reliable.

Diagnostic imaging (e.g., nuclear medicine) has long been used for the diagnosis of thyroid dysfunction, specifically cases of hyperthyroidism. Taking advantage of the physiologic iodine/iodide cycle, an isotope with high affinity to the thyroid gland is administered, and uptake by the thyroid gland is either quantified or compared with another organ. A comparative ratio of the isotope uptake is commonly determined using the salivary gland (which removes iodide quickly from blood, perhaps because of its evolutionary proximity to the thyroid gland). Normal ratios have been formulated for small animals and, when elevated, may be indicative of a hyperfunctioning thyroid gland, supporting a possible hyperthyroid diagnosis. Furthermore, scintigraphy is also useful to determine the presence of ectopic thyroid tissue. Reference intervals of thyroid scintigraphy for exotic species have not been well established. Based on literature references, it appears that only cockatiels and rabbits have been investigated to determine possible application of scintigraphy in assessing thyroid health.[167-169]

Other imaging modalities used for thyroid diagnostic testing include ultrasonography (US), computed tomography (CT), and MRI, mainly for the diagnosis of neoplasia. Although these tests have been used to assess the thyroid gland, they may not provide useful information regarding glandular function. In dogs, CT has enjoyed the highest specificity (100%) and MRI the highest sensitivity (93%) for diagnosing thyroid carcinoma; US had considerably lower

TABLE 6-3						
Thyroid Diagnostic Testing Comparisons in the Dog						
Test	**Low TT$_4$**	**Low TT$_3$**	**Low fT$_4$d**	**High TSH**	**Low TT$_4$/High TSH**	**Low fT$_4$d/High TSH**
Sensitivity	89%/100%	10%	98%/80%	76%/87%	67%/87%	74%/80%
Specificity	82%/75%	92%	93%/94%	93%/82%	98%/92%	98%/97%
Accuracy	85%	55%	95%	84%	82%	86%

fT$_4$d, Free thyroxine by equilibrium dialysis; *TSH,* thyroid-stimulating hormone; *T$_4$,* thyroxine; *TT$_3$,* total T$_3$; *TT$_4$,* total T$_4$.
From Ferguson DC. Testing for hypothyroidism in dogs. *Vet Clin North Am Small Anim Pract.* 2007;37:647-669, v.
This information is most likely not correlatable to exotic species but highlights the differences in the specificity and sensitivity of multiple tests in the dog.

results.[170] Investigators suggest that US is adequate as a screening tool for dogs with suspected thyroid carcinoma, but CT or MRI is needed for preoperative diagnosis and staging.[170] No information is available regarding exotic species using these imaging modalities for diagnosing thyroid disease.

The most common imaging techniques used in veterinary medicine for thyroid assessment are US and scintigraphy.[171] However, as in human medicine, CT and MRI also have potential indications in veterinary medicine.[171] In exotic species, due to the lack of research in this field, it is important to investigate and determine normal appearance and findings of thyroid imaging; nonetheless, the benefits of each modality should be similar to those for humans and small animals. Nuclear medicine, although not readily available, is an important diagnostic route for the assessment of thyroid hyperfunction. Although assessment of thyroid function using scintigraphy has only been reported in one guinea pig, one rabbit, and in a study of normal and radiothyroidized cockatiels, a limited number of studies for the assessment of other metabolic functions (e.g., hepatic, renal) have been reported in pigeons and green iguanas (*Iguana iguana*).[167,172-177] Technological developments in nuclear medicine, including the use of pinhole collimators, have been hypothesized as being useful in making this diagnostic test more practicable for exotic animal species.[178]

Other diagnostic testing methods used to assess the thyroid gland include cytology and histopathology. However, these diagnostic tools are used most often for assessing a previously diagnosed dysthyroid state. For example, in the cases of hyperthyroidism, a neoplastic condition may be the underlying cause; thus, determination of histological characteristics is beneficial (Table 6-3).

Reptiles

As in other vertebrates, the reptilian thyroid gland plays an important role in ecdysis, growth, reproduction, BMR regulation, oxygen consumption, endocrine function, hematopoiesis, and tail regeneration.[179] The location and anatomy of the thyroid gland varies among reptilian species.[180] In snakes and chelonians, the thyroid gland is a single unpaired structure located ventral to the trachea, cranial to the heart base, and caudal to the thymus.[180,181] The lizard and crocodilian thyroid gland may be single, bilobed, or paired, and is located in the ventral cervical region.[180]

Functionally, the reptile thyroid gland appears to be similar to that of mammals, with some functions differing in significance and effect. As with birds, it has been suggested that thyroid hormones may influence seasonal testicular regression, which is supported by the identification of thyroid hormone receptors in the testicles of the Italian wall lizard (*Podarcis sicula*).[180,182] Moreover, thyroidectomies in agamids, lacertids, and geckonids resulted in testicular regression.[183,184] Therefore, it has been speculated that testicular activity is controlled by thyroid hormones, androgens, and estrogen.[182,185] Others have hypothesized that thyroid hormones exert their effects at the hypothalamic level, thereby affecting pituitary gonadotropin release.[3] The effects of thyroid activity on the ecdysis of reptiles have long been studied. In the Mohave shovel-nosed snake (*Chionactis occipitalis occipitalis*), a thyroidectomy increased the shedding frequency, whereas administration of injectable thyroxine (8 μg, q48 h, route not specified) prevented shedding.[186] Similar results were reported in thyroidectomized and hypophysectomized common garter snakes (*Thamnophis sirtalis*).[187] Shedding frequency in lizards is increased by elevation of thyroid hormones.[188] It is, however, unclear why certain reptile species react differently to changes in blood thyroid hormone levels.

A limited number of thyroid disease conditions are known to exist in exotic species. At this time, it is believed that thyroid dysfunction may be caused by improper light cycles, hibernation, or thermal gradients.[180] Goiter has been reported in tortoises, particularly, Galapagos (*Chelonoidis nigra*) and Aldabra (*Aldabrachelys gigantea*) tortoises.[180,189-191] In one such case involving a Galapagos tortoise diagnosed with hypothyroidism, the goitered tortoise had TT$_3$ of 0.07 nmol/L and TT$_4$ of 3.73 nmol/L, which were considered low when compared to three suspected euthyroid Galapagos tortoises (control TT$_3$ 0.51 to 1.53 nmol/L; control TT$_4$ 13.9 to 19.82 nmol/L).[189] Although the cause of hypothyroidism was not clearly determined, it was suspected to be secondary to an iodine imbalance.[189] A hypothyroid (type I) goiter is less common in mammals than hyperthyroid toxic (type II), hyperthyroid physiologic (type III), and normothyroid (type IV). The tortoise was managed with levothyroxine (0.02 mg/kg, orally [PO], q48 h).[189] Another case report described an adult sulcata tortoise (*Centrochelys sulcata*) diagnosed with hypothyroidism based on clinical disease and responses to levothyroxine treatment.[192] Mean reference intervals for this species were reported to be TT$_4$ 4 nmol/L, fT$_4$ 4 pmol/L, TT$_3$ 0.15 nmol/L, and fT$_3$ 2.9 pmol/L, which were much lower than the previously mentioned reference intervals for Galapagos tortoises.[193] Reference intervals for other reptilian species have been reported using a commercially available method that is no longer available.[194]

Hyperthyroidism has been reported in a green iguana. Clinical signs included weight loss, polyphagia, hyperactivity, increased aggression, loss of dorsal spines, tachycardia, and a palpable ventral cervical mass.[195] Diagnosis was based on an elevated TT_4 level (30 nmol/L) compared to the reported reference range of 3.81 ± 0.84 nmol/L.[195] The underlying cause of the green iguana's hyperthyroid condition was a functional thyroid follicular adenoma, which was surgically removed.[195] The TT_4 was within the normal range at 173 days following the surgical procedure.[195] One case of hyperthyroidism has been reported in a geriatric corn snake (*Pantherophis guttatus*) that was shedding every 2 weeks.[196] The animal was treated with methimazole (1 mg/kg, PO, q24 h), which resulted in a return to normal ecdysis.[196] Although there was a clinical response to treatment, a definitive diagnosis of hyperthyroidism was not made. One case of hyperthyroidism in an African helmeted turtle (*Pelomedusa subrufa*) with a history of reduced appetite and continuous skin shedding over a 1-year period has been reported.[197] Diagnosis was based on measurement of serum thyroxine concentration, and the animal was treated using transdermal methimazole.[197]

Thyroid neoplasias and other histological abnormalities have been diagnosed in reptile species. Thyroid adenomatous hyperplasia and follicular adenomas have been described in lizard, snake, and chelonian species.[179,195,196,198-204] Thyroid carcinomas have been reported in a Chinese crocodile lizard (*Shinisaurus crocodilurus*), a red-eared slider (*Trachemys scripta elegans*), an Indian black turtle (*Melanochelys [Geoemyda] trijuga*), a rough knob-tail gecko (*Nephrurus amyae*), and a smooth knob-tail gecko (*Nephrurus levis*).[179,205-207] Neoplasms affecting the thyroid gland appear to be uncommon and/or underdiagnosed in reptile species based on large-scale retrospective studies of zoological collections.[208,209]

Birds

Avian thyroid structure and function are similar to those of mammals, and thyroid hormones have been reported to affect reproduction, growth, metabolism, temperature regulation, molting, and other various avian behaviors.[19] The anatomical location of the avian thyroid is different from that in mammals. The thyroid gland is located within or cranial to the thoracic inlet.[210] The avian thyroid gland lies along the ventral aspect of the common carotid artery at the level of the jugular vein and origin of the vertebral artery.[211] The left thyroid is attached to the ventral aspect of the left internal carotid artery, and the right lobe is attached to the internal jugular vein.[211] Although it has been suggested that the avian female thyroid gland is usually larger than that in males, that observation was not reported in budgerigars.[212] However, variable interspecific and individual vascularization of the thyroid gland has been reported in budgerigars and Falconiformes.[210,212]

Avian thyroid diseases have long been reported. Goiter (or thyroid hyperplasia) is an enlargement of the thyroid gland due to abnormal proliferation of epithelial cells lining the follicles as a result of TSH stimulation.[18] It has been speculated that the most common cause of goiter in avian species is iodine deficiency.[18] Historically, budgerigars and pigeons (in particular, White Carneaux) appear to be overrepresented in this category, although prevalence studies are not available.[18,213] In a retrospective study by a specialty pathology service, 30/12,457 avian specimens were morphologically diagnosed with thyroid hyperplasia.[213] Macaws (20/30), in particular blue-and-gold macaws (*Ara ararauna*, 15/30), were overrepresented.[213] It is important to mention again that goiter does not imply a hyper- or hypofunction of the thyroid gland; therefore, a patient may have normal thyroid function.[214] To the authors' knowledge, thyroid function has not been assessed in reported cases of avian goiter. Nonetheless, some clinical signs that have been described (obesity, abnormal vocalization, lethargy, myxedema, and feather abnormalities) may correlate with thyroid dysfunction.[18] Other typical clinical signs such as regurgitation, dyspnea, and circulatory problems appear to be related to a mass effect caused by thyroid hyperplasia on surrounding tissues (including the esophagus, trachea, and vasculature).[18]

Avian thyroid functions have some particularities that make them slightly different from their mammalian counterparts (i.e., TRH is not thyrotropic in adult chickens and therefore does not promote TSH release).[211] In the avian species studied, TSH release is apparently controlled by circulating T_3.[211] Both TSH and GH promote thyroidal T_4/T_3 release.[211] No specific thyroxine-binding globulins are present in birds, as in humans and dogs; therefore, thyroid hormone is bound in blood by either prealbumin or albumin. Since the binding of T_4 to albumin is weak, higher fT_4 levels have been reported for birds (compared to mammals).[211] Historically, the avian HPT axis control appeared to be similar to that of mammals; however, more recently it has been shown that CRH is a more important TSH stimulator in nonmammalian vertebrates.[123] CRH stimulates TSH secretion and therefore T_4 secretion, and corticosterone exhibits a negative feedback on T_4.[215] The most important role of TRH is to stimulate the GH-releasing hormone, which leads to circulating T_3 increase due to inhibition of the T_3 degradation by type-3 deiodinases.[123]

As endocrinology continues to evolve, more information and clarification of thyroid function in exotic animal species will become available. Nonetheless, it should be emphasized that the HPT axis of exotic animal species shares many parallels with mammals with respect to the thyroid structure as well as to the synthesis and metabolism of thyroid hormones.[19]

Avian hypothyroidism has been reported and is a clinical concern for common disease presentations (e.g., feather picking).[18,216,217] A confirmed clinical diagnosis of avian hypothyroidism in a scarlet macaw (*Ara macao*) was achieved using a TSH stimulation test.[218] The patient presented with delayed molt, generalized feather abnormalities, and obesity, and there was a lack of response to the TSH stimulation test.[218] Treatment with levothyroxine (0.2 µg/kg, PO, q12 h) resulted in resolution of clinical signs.[218] Hereditary hypothyroidism has been reported in chickens.[219] Experimentally induced hypothyroidism using radioiodine-131 in cockatiels has also been reported.[159] Interestingly, the cockatiels exhibited mild or no hypercholesterolemia, obesity, or poor feathering at 48 days following thyroid ablation.[159]

Avian hypothyroidism is a "questionable" diagnosis. As stated by Fudge and Speer, "a plasma T_4 submission can appear to be quite "rewarding" to the clinician suspecting avian hypothyroidism, because virtually all assays are often low or at undetectable levels."[220] Due to low physiological values and low sensitivity of available methodologies, TT_4

and TT₃ results tend to be low or below reported normal values. Only one validated thyroid assay method has been developed: a free hormone method used to determine total thyroid hormone concentrations.[194] However, this method is no longer commercially available.

Free thyroid hormone reference intervals have been rarely reported. Although the sample size was small, ranges for fT₄ and fT₃ measured by equilibrium dialysis (ED) have been reported in Hispaniolan Amazon parrots.[221] In quail, it has been suggested that free hormones measured by ED have similar results to humans.[222] This information is promising and may provide additional clinical use in the assessment of thyroid function in birds. Nevertheless, reference intervals for thyroid values are generally lacking for birds; thus, the clinical value of free hormone quantification in avian species is suspect at this point in time.

Hyperthyroidism (like hypothyroidism) is rarely reported for birds. To the authors' knowledge, only one scientific report of hyperthyroidism affecting an avian species has been published. A productive thyroid follicular carcinoma was diagnosed on an adult free-ranging male barred owl (*Strix varia*).[223] Although an ill-defined soft tissue opacity over the plane of the syrinx and great vessels was noted on radiographic examination antemortem, the neoplasm was only detected through postmortem examination.[223] Antemortem total and free thyroid hormones were compared with suspected normal barred owls; the thyroid values were higher than in controls (TT₄ by RIA [nmol/L] 14.14 vs. <2.57, <2.57, 7.71, <2.57; fT₄ by ED [pmol/L] >13 vs. <0.39, <0.39, 2.73, <0.39).[223] These findings, in combination with reactive immunohistochemistry, were supportive of a hyperthyroid state due to a productive thyroid follicular carcinoma.

Mammals

Among small mammals, one species commonly develops thyroid abnormalities (e.g., hyperthyroidism): the guinea pig (*Cavia porcellus*). Although guinea pig thyroid disease has been discussed for many years in the German literature, only recently have such reports been published in English language journals.[224,225] In addition to the recent publication of a clinical case, thyroid neoplasias have also been reported as some of the most common neoplasias (3.6%) detected in guinea pigs by one laboratory service.[226] Age and gender predisposition have not been determined, but it appears that there may be a female bias and a higher predisposition for animals older than 3 years.[224] Several publications have reported normal thyroid reference intervals for guinea pigs, with specific intervals per sex, age, and environment.[227-231] It is important to note that several methodologies were used to obtain the reported reference intervals, which may substantially influence interpretation of the data. Conversely, hypothyroidism is rarely diagnosed in small mammal species. There is only one limited report of hypothyroidism in a guinea pig, and the case description is nonspecific.[224]

Although rabbits are one of the most commonly kept exotic small mammal pets and have long been used in medical research, naturally occurring and induced thyroid dysfunction is rarely reported.[232-237] To the authors' knowledge, the only report of naturally occurring rabbit thyroid dysfunction was published over 85 years ago.[236] Rabbits developed goiter when fed a cabbage (*Brassica oleracea*)-based diet for 2 to 3 months.[236]

Further studies investigating the correlation of goiter in rabbits, ingestion of cabbage, and its treatment with iodine supplementation were performed.[238-240] Although these studies may be of little clinical significance today, one study reported the occurrence of exophthalmos in rabbits that develop cyanide-induced goiter.[241,242] A common cause of rabbit bilateral exophthalmos is a mediastinal mass (e.g., thymoma, thymic lymphoma) that compromises the vascular drainage from the head, leading to a cranial vena caval syndrome.[243] The cause of exophthalmos in rabbits with goiter is unknown, but we can surmise that a cervical mass could compromise the venous return, leading to this clinical finding. Nonetheless, in humans with Graves' disease, exophthalmos also occurs secondary to an orbital tissue inflammation: so-called thyroid-associated ophthalmopathy.[244]

Although rabbit thyroid disorders have not been reported, the authors are aware of several highly suspected cases of thyroid dysfunction. In one case, an 8-year-old spayed female French lop rabbit was presented for a grade III heart murmur.[176] An echocardiogram revealed biatrial enlargement with mitral and tricuspid regurgitation.[176] Hyperexia and weight loss were also reported by the owner.[176] Hyperthyroidism was suspected based on the patient's history, physical examination, and diagnostic test results.[176] Total and free thyroid hormones were quantified using RIA and ED, respectively, performed 1 month apart, prior to treatment.[176] Results were indicative of hyperthyroidism (fT₄ 18 and 28 pmol/L; fT₃ 7.1 and 6.6 pmol/L; TT₄ 48 and 46 nmol/L; TT₃ 0 and 0.3 nmol/L) based on limited reference intervals from non-clinical research.[176,232,234,235,245] Thyroid scintigraphy revealed homogeneous symmetrical uptake with a thyroid to salivary gland ratio of 3:1 (reference interval at 20 min post isotope administration, 1:1).[168,169,176] Hyperthyroidism was diagnosed and oral methimazole (1.25 mg total dose, PO, twice a day) initiated.[176] Serum thyroid hormone values were decreased from initial values at 1 and 6 months (fT₄ 31 and 37 nmol/L; TT₄ 13 and 6 pmol/L).[176] Cardiac function was unchanged at 6 months.[176] The animal died 12 months after diagnosis.[176] Bicavitary effusion, mild myocardial fibrosis, and chronic passive congestion postmortem were indicative of chronic cardiac insufficiency.[176] No evidence of hyperplasia or neoplasia within the thyroid gland was detected. Pituitary cysts were detected, but their clinical significance remains unclear.[176]

Although naturally occurring thyroid disease in rabbits is considered underreported, research studies have shown that thyroid function is adversely affected (i.e., similar to other mammals) in the presence of physiologic stress. Thyroid dysfunction (e.g., euthyroid sick syndrome or nonthyroidal illness) was induced in rabbits that suffered skin wounds through experimental thermal means.[234,246,247] Hypothyroid status was also induced in other groups of rabbits using pharmaceuticals or surgical removal of the thyroid gland.[232,233]

Among other small mammals, only a limited number of case reports have been published related to thyroid disease. One case of concurrent DM and hyperthyroidism has been reported in a chinchilla (*Chinchilla lanigera*).[248] Although correlation between the two conditions is considered unlikely, hyperthyroidism in cats can impair glucose tolerance, potentially leading to peripheral insulin resistance.[248,249]

Ferret hypothyroidism has been diagnosed in 7 cases based on low basal TT₄ values and a limited response (<1.4-fold increase) in TT_4 after a TSH stimulation test.[250] Recently, the use of recombinant hTSH for stimulation testing has been validated in the ferret.[163] Hypothyroid ferrets had similar clinical signs to other endocrinopathies: obesity, lethargy, inactivity, and excessive sleeping behavior.[250] In 2/7 cases, hind limb weakness was also reported; however, this is widely considered a nonspecific clinical sign in extremely ill ferrets.[250] There are at least two reports of thyroid neoplasias identified in ferrets: a C-cell carcinoma (medullary thyroid carcinoma) associated with multiple endocrine neoplasms and a thyroid follicular adenocarcinoma.[251,252] Although productivity was not assessed, in one case, hyperthyroxinemia was considered unlikely because immunohistochemistry indicated a decrease in thyroglobulin production.[251]

Most information available regarding thyroid disease in other rodents (e.g., rats, mice, hamsters) is extrapolated from animal laboratory literature. Thyroid neoplasia, euthyroid sick syndrome or nonthyroidal illness, hypothyroidism, and hyperthyroidism have been reported in rats.[253,254] As with guinea pigs, it is believed that thyroid disease in rodent species is underdiagnosed due to the lack of published information and availability of reliable validated diagnostic tests. As diagnostic tests are developed for exotic small mammals, clinicians will have more available options at their disposal to better assess thyroid function/dysfunction.

Calcium Homeostasis

Calcium is the fifth most abundant element in the body and an essential supplement in that it can only be acquired through dietary sources.[3,255,256] Calcium provides structural strength and support for bones and plays vital roles in many intra- and extracellular reactions.[255] Serum calcium, magnesium, and phosphate levels are closely regulated by the combined effects of several hormones (e.g., PTH, vitamin D, calcitonin, cortisol) on the gastrointestinal tract, bone, and kidneys.[3] Calcium is essential for the proper function of muscles and nerves and activates a series of reactions including fatty acid oxidation, mitochondrial carriers for adenosine triphosphate (ATP) (with magnesium), and glucose-stimulated insulin release.[257] Magnesium, also essential for proper function of muscles and nerves,[257] is a cofactor in over 300 enzymatic reactions, particularly those involving the metabolism of food components, and it is required by all enzymatic reactions involving the energy storage molecule ATP.[257] Phosphorus is a structural component of nucleotide coenzymes: ATP and creatine phosphate.[257]

Within the body, calcium exists intracellularly in all tissues and extracellularly as brushite and hydroxyapatite (in bone).[255] Skeletal bone corresponds to >99% of total body calcium, while nonbone calcium is <1%.[256] Although nonbone calcium exists in small amounts (overall), it is in constant and rapid exchange between extra- and intracellular pools and responsible for a wide number of vital functions that include extra- and intracellular signaling, nerve impulse transmission, and muscle contraction.[256] Despite major fluctuations in dietary calcium including bone dissipation and adsorption, renal excretion, and the additional calcium demand during pregnancy and/or lactation, nonbone calcium is generally maintained within a narrow range.[3] This efficient control is a consequence of the activity of several endocrine glands and their corresponding hormones.

Magnesium is the second most abundant cation in intracellular spaces of vertebrates, and ~50% to 60% of the total can be found in the bone, 40% to 50% in soft tissues, and <1% in extracellular spaces.[258] As with phosphorus and potassium, serum magnesium levels do not accurately reflect actual body stores because of the relatively small amounts found in plasma. Approximately 30% of plasma magnesium is protein bound; therefore, reduced albumin levels may falsely decrease the serum reading even if actual levels are within normal limits.[258] Magnesium is a cofactor promoting several enzymatic reactions within cells, and during carbohydrate metabolism it helps the body produce and use ATP (i.e., the magnesium of ATP helps it to interface with various ATPases).[259] Signs of hypomagnesemia are similar to those observed with hypokalemia (e.g., respiratory muscle paralysis, complete heart block, coma).[260,261] Hypomagnesemia can also cause a secondary hypocalcemia, which remains resistant to calcium supplementation until magnesium levels are corrected. A patient with hypocalcemia due to hypomagnesemia may exhibit a high, normal, or low PTH level. Magnesium deficiency in humans induces reversible failure of PTH secretion and increases peripheral PTH degradation and resistance to PTH.[262–267]

Richard Owen first recognized the parathyroid gland in 1850 while performing a necropsy on an Indian rhinoceros (*Rhinoceros unicornis*).[268–270] The first description of this gland in humans was made by Ivar Sandström in 1880.[270,271] The parathyroid gland is often referred to as the "last anatomical discovery."[271] The number of isolated parathyroid glands varies with species. While most mammalian species have 2, 3, or 4 glands, some may have more: the African palm civet (*Nandinia binotata*) and fossa (*Cryptoprocta ferox*) have 6; the green monkey (*Chlorocebus sabaeus*), 8; and the collared fruit bat (*Cynonycteris collaris*), 10.[272] However, it is often difficult to identify the parathyroid glands from the thyroid.[272] In the majority of avian species in which the parathyroid gland has been described, there is one lobe on each side of the trachea, lying in contact with the thyroid or near the posterior pole.[273] Some species possess two separate parathyroid glands or exhibit a singular bilobed structure.[273] Although there are also variations among reptiles, the parathyroid glands are usually separate from the thyroid: the anterior pair associated with the carotid artery and the posterior pair with the aortic arch.[180] Parathyroid glands are absent in fish.[3]

In other land vertebrates (e.g., humans), the parathyroid glands are primarily responsible for calcium homeostasis, controlling strict regulation between the plasma calcium concentration and appropriate skeletal mineralization/demineralization.[268] Parathyroid chief cells synthesize and release PTH, which is an 84-amino-acid peptide, in response to hypocalcemia.[268] PTH mobilizes calcium by increasing calcium reabsorption from bone and by increasing calcium reabsorption in proximal tubules of the kidneys (mainly), the ascending thick limb of the loop of Henle, and the distal tubules, and it stimulates hydroxylation of vitamin D_3 (25-hydroxycholecalciferol from the liver) to form 1,25-dihydroxycholecalciferol (also called calcitriol; the active form of vitamin D) by stimulating activity of renal 1α-hydroxylase.[268] In small intermittent doses, PTH has anabolic functions and it is used to treat osteoporosis in humans.[274] While the PTH is classically considered to be a bone catabolic agent, when delivered intermittently at low doses PTH potently stimulates cortical and trabecular bone growth in humans.[274]

Several forms of vitamin D exist: vitamin D_1, vitamin D_2 or ergocalciferol (present in plants), reduced vitamin D_2, vitamin D_3 or cholecalciferol, calcidiol or 25-hydroxycholecalciferol, and calcitriol or 1,25-dihydroxycholecalciferol.[3] In humans, vitamin D is ingested from a few natural food sources (e.g., fortified foods, supplements).[275] The two naturally occurring vitamin D forms are cholecalciferol (vitamin D_3) from animal sources and ergocalciferol (vitamin D_2) from plants.[276] Vitamin D can also be synthesized in exposed skin from sunlight (ultraviolet B [UVB] radiation) exposure, which converts 7-dehydrocholesterol (7-DHC), a cholesterol-like precursor, into vitamin D.[276] The vitamin D prohormone is first metabolized to 25-hydroxychocalciferol in the liver (an endocrinologically unregulated step) and then further activated to 1,25-dihydroxycholecalciferol by 1α-hydroxylase in the kidneys or inactivated to 24,25-dihydroxycholecalciferol by renal 24-hydroxylase.[276]

UVB light (270- to 315-nm range) is necessary for the conversion of 7-DHC by the skin to the previtamin D_3, which then undergoes thermal isomerization to vitamin D_3 over the course of ~3 days.[277] The UVB intensity that reaches the skin of animals depends on latitude and altitude, hair coat, and, in the case of captive animals, light that may be provided in their enclosure.[277] The ability to form vitamin D_3 from skin varies with species (e.g., in dogs and cats, exposure to UVB light does not significantly increase the dermal vitamin D_3 concentration, but in rats it may lead to a 40-fold increase in vitamin D_3).[277] This species variability may be related to the presence of a 7-DHC-D7-reductase, an enzyme capable of degrading 7-DHC.[277] In most herbivores, the skin is capable of producing vitamin D_3 in response to UVB skin irradiation.[277]

Vitamin D function and metabolism have been well studied in mammals and birds but are relatively underinvestigated in reptiles.[278] However, reports indicate that lizards and snakes possess 25-hydroxycholecalciferol-1α-hydroxylase activity and vitamin D-dependent calcium-binding proteins in kidney tissue.[279,280] Hypercalcemia was induced in a yellow monitor (*Varanus flavescens*) and a checkered keelback (*Xenochrophis [Natrix] piscator*) by vitamin D_3 intraperitoneal administration.[281-283] Similar to mammals, 1,25-dihydroxycholecalciferol has also been shown to be the major metabolite of vitamin D and may represent the vitamin D storage form in the eastern bearded dragon (*Pogona barbata*).[278]

Although a detailed review is beyond the scope of this chapter, there has been a long discussion regarding the term vitamin D. Since its first discovery, considerable knowledge about this fat-soluble vitamin and its metabolism has evolved, which has led to more questions regarding its identity.[284] Some authors suggest that vitamin D is truly a vitamin, because "insufficient amounts in the diet may cause deficiency diseases."[285] In turn, 25-hydroxychocalciferol is appropriately described as a prehormone (a glandular secretory product), itself having little or no inherent biologic potency, but it is converted peripherally to an active hormone.[285] Other authors defend that vitamin D is indeed a hormone.[286-288]

Major physiological effects of 1,25-dihydroxycholecalciferol are increasing calcium, magnesium, and phosphate intestinal absorption; increasing renal calcium and phosphate reabsorption; and increasing bone resorption.[3] In general terms, 1,25-dihydroxycholecalciferol assists PTH in performing its functions, and since it is a steroid (and PTH is a protein), PTH deficiency can be treated through oral administration of vitamin D.[3]

A third major hormone involved in calcium homeostasis is calcitonin. This hormone is produced in nonmammalians by ultimobranchial bodies.[3] The ultimobranchial bodies of mammals are included in the thyroid and are called parafollicular cells.[3] The PTH and active form of vitamin D, however, are considered to be far more important to calcium homeostasis than calcitonin. In general, glucocorticoids are thought to exert negative influences on calcium homeostasis by (1) reducing intestinal calcium absorption, (2) enhancing bone resorption, and (3) reducing PTH-stimulated renal calcium reabsorption (Figures 6-3 and 6-4).

Reptiles

Calcium is an essential element for every living animal, but calcium imbalances may be more problematic and common in reptiles. Metabolic bone disease (MBD) is a broad term that includes a large number of conditions including fibrous osteodystrophy, hypertrophic osteodystrophy, hypertrophic osteopathy, nutritional secondary hyperparathyroidism, osteomalacia, osteopetrosis, osteoporosis, Paget's disease, panosteitis, renal secondary hyperparathyroidism, and rickets.[289] The disease conditions listed above are the result of abnormal physiologic levels and/or function of minerals such as calcium, phosphorus, and magnesium or vitamin D and PTH. This vitamin D "system" appears to be similar between reptiles and mammals.[278]

The pathogenicity of MBD in reptiles starts with nutritional and environmental factors that create deficits in the plasma calcium concentration. A decrease in plasma calcium concentration stimulates the parathyroid glands to release PTH, which in turn results in the release of cytokines from osteoblasts, thereby activating osteoclasts that resorb bone, thus correcting the plasma concentration.[290] Over time, this reduces bone density, leading to secondary disease conditions.[290]

Nutritional secondary hyperparathyroidism is the most common MBD diagnosed in captive reptile species.[289] This condition commonly occurs due to poor husbandry conditions, often the result of owners unaware of proper animal care.[291] Most mammals are able to obtain vitamin D from their diet; however, many lizards and chelonians are unable to obtain this essential physiologic component solely from dietary sources.[292] The ability of reptiles to absorb dietary vitamin D appears to vary among species, especially with heliothermic reptiles (animals that display basking behaviors in sunlight).[292] Reptiles are ectotherms and therefore unable to generate their own internal body temperature. Nonetheless, many are capable of maintaining relatively high and constant body temperatures through behavioral adjustments.[293] The basking behavior, for example, allows reptiles to receive sun exposure to increase their body temperature. There are many forms of animal basking behaviors that are obvious adaptations to the individual species' natural environment.[294] However, it has been shown that for the Murray River turtle (*Emydura signata*), basking did not apparently increase body temperature.[295] Since basking behavior may be life threatening (i.e., increased exposure to predation), some researchers

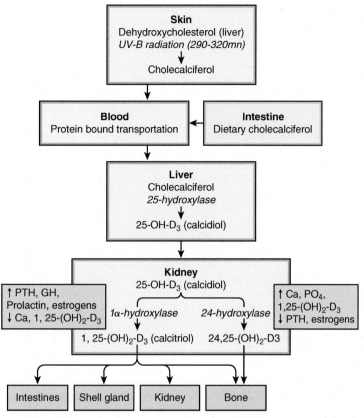

FIGURE 6-3 Vitamin D metabolism in birds. $\downarrow$, Down-regulation; $\uparrow$, up-regulation; *Ca,* calcium; *GH,* growth hormone; *PO₄,* phosphate; *PTH,* parathyroid hormone. (From de Matos R. Calcium metabolism in birds. *Vet Clin North Am Exot Anim Pract.* 2008;11: 59-82.)

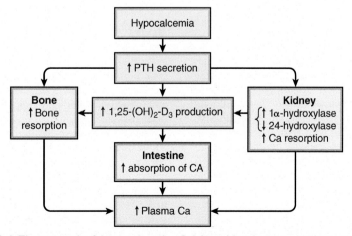

FIGURE 6-4 The control of hypocalcemia. Calcium blood concentrations are restored mainly by the actions of PTH and 1,25(OH)₂D₃ in the bone, kidneys, and intestinal tract. $\uparrow$, Up-regulation; *Ca,* calcium; *PTH,* parathyroid hormone. (From de Matos R. Calcium metabolism in birds. *Vet Clin North Am Exot Anim Pract.* 2008;11:59-82.)

defend that there should be other benefits to this behavior.[296] One is light exposure and, thus, endogenous vitamin D production.[297] In their native environment, reptiles have ample opportunity to bask in the sun and generate vitamin D; however, in captivity, they may not have adequate exposure to UVB light.[277] Inadequate exposure to UVB light may be a consequence of owner ignorance, inappropriate enclosure preparation, defective equipment, and/or lack of proper dietary supplementation. Interestingly, it has been shown in panther chameleons *(Furcifer pardalis)* that UVB exposure time correlates inversely to dietary vitamin D_3 supplementation.[296,297] In both indoor and outdoor conditions, chameleons would increase the length of UVB exposure when fed a lower vitamin D_3-enriched diet.[296,297] To the authors' knowledge, no subsequent publication has reported a similar finding in another reptile species.

It has been anecdotally suggested that some crepuscular species (e.g., leopard geckos [*Eublepharis macularius*]) or carnivorous species (e.g., snakes) do not require UVB exposure. Although information on this subject appears limited, and species-specific variations appear to exist, some suggest that depending on species, UVB exposure may be beneficial.[292] In corn snakes *(Pantherophis guttatus)*, the plasma 25-hydroxycholecalciferol concentration significantly increased in animals exposed to supplemental UVB lighting for a period of 4 weeks, whereas control snakes that were not exposed to UVB failed to show similar results.[298] Conversely, in female ball pythons *(Python regius)*, no association was demonstrated between exposure to UVB radiation and the plasma 25-hydroxycholecalciferol or ionized calcium concentrations.[299] The need for appropriate plasma concentrations of vitamin D_3 is so important that the skin of some nocturnal species of lizards, such as the Mediterranean house gecko *(Hemidactylus turcicus)*, has developed the ability to synthesize the hormone in minimal light conditions, whereas other species can modify their basking to compensate for variations in dietary amounts of vitamin D_3.[300] Inland bearded dragons *(Pogona vitticeps)*, a species commonly diagnosed with MBD, have been shown to maintain similar values of ionized and total plasma calcium as well as vitamin D when deprived of UVB exposure for at least 83 days.[301] Although there is variation in the results of UVB studies regarding UVB exposure among reptile species, it is strongly recommended that appropriate sources of UVB light be provided for reptiles maintained in captivity.

Clinical presentation of reptilian MBD is variable, and clinical signs are often nonspecific. Common signs include, but are not limited to, anorexia, lethargy, inability to fully lift the body from the ground, shell deformity or soft shell (in chelonians), dystocia, and constipation.[302,303] Pathological fractures of limbs and ribs and demineralization of the mandible and maxilla leading to facial deformities are common in lizards.[303] If acute hypocalcemia is present, neurological signs (e.g., tremors, seizures, tetany) can occur.[302] Although clinical signs and history may be supportive of MBD, due to unspecific characteristics of the clinical signs, several diagnostic tests are recommended. Imaging, in particular, radiography, is useful for the assessment of a reptile patient in which MBD is a top differential disease diagnosis. Radiographic imaging not only allows for the detection of potential pathological fractures, it also provides a means to evaluate skeletal density. In lizards with MDB, bone loss, limb and mandibular

deformities, and swelling of surrounding soft tissues are common clinical disease signs.[304] Nonetheless, radiographic examination may not provide a definitive diagnosis for MBD in reptiles. Radiographic evidence is usually present in MBD cases where calcium bone depletion has occurred, but if the disease process is not chronic, radiographic images of the patient's skeletal structure may appear normal.

Quantification of plasma calcium is considered essential when trying to diagnose MBD. Due to the different forms of calcium in the body, assessment of total calcium and ionized calcium is beneficial, with interpretations from each being complementary. Multiple species-dependent reference intervals can be found in the current literature. Seasonal variations have also been reported.[305] Presently, several commercial laboratories offer tests that quantitate circulating vitamin D, and several published studies have provided normal reference intervals of these hormones in reptiles.[306–308] Although PTH serum levels can be quantitated and these tests are commercially available, reference intervals have not been well established for reptile species.

Treatment of MBD includes both stabilizing the patient and correcting underlying husbandry and dietary factors.[292] Secondary disease conditions including dehydration and pain should be controlled in an appropriate manner. Renal disease is often a secondary and often life-threatening condition associated with MBD. Therefore, renal function must be assessed, monitored, and treated (if necessary) when MBD is considered a differential or definitive diagnosis. If hypocalcemia is detected, calcium supplementation should be provided. The most efficient route of calcium administration in reptiles has not been determined. It is suggested that parenteral calcium administration can lead to soft tissue mineralization and permanent damage to arteries, renal tubules, and other soft tissues.[303,309] IM administration of calcium and appropriate seizure modification therapy are recommended when a patient presents with hypocalcemic seizures, muscle tremors, or flaccid paresis. However, this should be switched to oral calcium as soon as the patient is stable.[310] Depending on severity of the condition, calcium supplementation may be required for extended time periods. Vitamin D administration is controversial due to the risk of intoxication and metastatic calcification.[303]

Birds

Although calcium deficits are not diagnosed as often in birds as reptiles, hypocalcemia is considered a common disease presentation. As in mammals, avian calcium metabolism is controlled by PTH, calcitonin, and vitamin D; however, estrogen and prostaglandins play important roles in avian calcium homeostasis.[311]

Avian PTH has an 88-amino-acid sequence, as opposed to 84 in mammals, but both have a similar biologically active region.[255] It appears that the average avian PTH blood concentration is lower than in mammals and can be determined using mammalian assays.[255] Birds appear to be more sensitive to PTH than mammals, responding to IV injections of PTH with an immediate (minutes) rise in blood calcium; however, it is unclear why birds respond faster than mammals.[255,311] Birds normally reabsorb more than 98% of filtered calcium in the kidneys.[312] IV calcium or exogenous PTH causes increased renal calcium excretion; however, in some birds, removal of the parathyroid gland increases renal calcium excretion (as would be expected).[312] Avian calcitonin is produced by the ultimobranchial glands, which are anatomically distinct from the parathyroid glands.[313] Moreover, blood levels of calcitonin are typically much higher in birds than in mammals.[313] Contradictory published information regarding the function of calcitonin in avian species has led to controversy. In starlings *(Sturnus vulgaris)*, salmon calcitonin did not induce significant changes in serum calcium or renal calcium excretion.[312,314] Other authors have shown that chickens show a lack of response to calcitonin administration.[315-317] However, in pigeons treated with salmon calcitonin, the plasma calcium levels exhibit a progressive decline from day 1 to day 5, and by day 15, levels become more or less similar to control values.[318] The ultimobranchial gland of pigeons exhibits no morphological changes up to day 5, but nuclear volume of ultimobranchial cells exhibits a decrease on day 10, which continues to progress to day 15.[318] The influence of calcitonin in avian calcium homeostasis continues to be questionable. Interestingly, in pigeons injected with ovine PRL, hypercalcemia was induced.[319] The slight calcium decrease, which was observed on day 15 in that study, was linked to hyperactivity of ultimobranchial cells, which secreted increased amounts of calcitonin to counteract the prolonged hypercalcemic challenge.[319]

Another difference between calcium homeostasis in birds and mammals relates to vitamin D metabolism. Other than 1,25-hydroxycholecalciferol, birds can also utilize 24,25-dihydroxycholecalciferol, which is inactive in mammals.[255] The 24,25-dihydroxycholecalciferol metabolite, although considered a stage of vitamin D inactivation, inhibits mammalian PTH secretion, but it is essential for normal growth plate chondrocyte development in birds and appears to be important in egg-laying fowl.[255]

As estrogen increases at the time of sexual maturity in support of egg laying and egg production, the osteoblasts change from forming lamellar cortical bone to producing spicules of nonstructural medullary bone (in the endosteal surface) that can fill the entire bone cavity.[255] Medullary bone formation occurs through this estrogenic effect apparently without much of a vitamin D influence; however, complete mineralization can only occur if vitamin D levels are adequate.[255]

Among the different species of pet birds, African grey parrots are commonly affected, as hypocalcemia syndrome in these animals has long been described.[18,320] Although the exact etiology of this syndrome remains unknown, several theories have been suggested. It is said that skeletal demineralization does not occur when low serum calcium levels are maintained.[18] African grey parrots have significantly lower total calcium, albumin, and total protein levels than Amazon parrots.[321] The parathyroid gland may be damaged due to a virus leading to an inability to mobilize skeletal calcium.[322] Renal calcium loss may be responsible for the hypocalcemia; however, no clear evidence of the pathophysiology associated with this disorder has been produced.[323] A dietary insufficiency of calcium and vitamin D, in combination with an excess fat intake, which may prevent intestinal calcium absorption, has been hypothesized.[320] Nonetheless, the etiology of this condition remains largely unknown.

A recent report described a case of hypocalcemia in an African grey parrot that was nonresponsive to calcium supplementation as well as vitamins A, D, and E supplementation, regardless of route.[320] Magnesium levels were quantitated and were determined to be low.[320] Once magnesium supplementation was provided, calcium and magnesium levels resolved and no further seizures were detected.[320] This case was similar to previously described hypomagnesemia in avian species (chickens) that led to hypocalcemia and insufficient 1,25-dihydroxycholecalciferol production.[324,325] Magnesium deficiency induces reversible failure of human PTH secretion, and it increases peripheral PTH degradation and resistance to PTH.[262-267] Magnesium is apparently needed for proper parathyroid gland function. Although hypomagnesemia was only reported once in a psittacine species, magnesium may be an important factor in the hypocalcemic syndrome of African grey parrots. Reference intervals for African grey parrots and Hispaniolan Amazon parrots have been reported.[326]

Birds, as egg layers, have seasonal/temporary demands for more calcium. The average amount of calcium in the chicken eggshell ranges from 1.5 to 2.0 g.[327] Calcium is withdrawn from blood at the rate of ~100 mg/hour during shell calcification.[327] In order to provide enough calcium for egg formation, there is a marked increase in plasma protein, which leads to a significant increase in total available calcium; ~40% of plasma calcium is normally protein bound.[3,18,328] Avian ionized plasma calcium has shown a sigmoidal pattern over the ovulation cycle.[329] It reaches a peak within 3 to 6 hours of oviposition and then falls to low levels until the next oviposition.[329]

Mammals

Among small mammals, information regarding the influence of UVB in the production of endogenous vitamin D is limited; however, some recent research projects have investigated this topic. In guinea pigs, exposure to long-term UVB radiation caused a significant increase in serum 25-hydroxycholecalciferol.[330] Findings from this study demonstrated that guinea pigs provided with artificial supplementation of UVB light produced and maintained significantly higher serum 25-hydroxy vitamin D_3 (OHD_3) levels (~3 times the control group) compared to those without UVB supplementation.[330] It is important to mention that an increased corneal thickness in both eyes was found in the UVB-supplemented group in comparison to the control group; however, no apparent negative clinical or pathologic side effects could be found.[330] Chinchillas also have the ability to produce endogenous 25-hydroxycholecalciferol through photobiochemical synthesis following exposure to artificial UVB light.[330,331] Eight-week-old chinchillas exposed to 12-hour UVB supplementation for 16 days had significantly higher 25-hydroxycholecalciferol (189 ± 102.7 nmol/L) when compared with those not provided with UVB radiation (87.8 ± 34.4 nmol/L).[331] Interestingly, both guinea pigs and chinchillas are native to the Andes Mountains, a high altitude and low latitude with ample access to sunlight and natural UVB radiation in their home range.[330] Other species from the same area, such as llamas *(Lama glama)* and alpacas *(Vicugna pacos)*, have been found to be highly susceptible to vitamin D deficiency.[277] These camelids have a thick hair coat and pigmentation that protect them from the intense solar radiation present in their natural environment; however, when transferred to lower altitudes or higher latitudes where solar radiation is much lower, serum vitamin D concentrations decline to low levels, especially during winter.[277]

In domestic rabbits, calcium metabolism is somewhat independent of vitamin D, because rabbits are known to passively absorb calcium from the intestine and maintain a total serum calcium concentration that is 30% to 50% higher than that reported for other mammals, potentially due to the high calcium demand of life-long dental growth.[332] In an experimental design, exposure to UVB radiation produced by artificial light significantly increased serum 25-hydroxycholecalciferol concentration in juvenile rabbits, approximately double that of the control group (66.4 ± 14.3 nmol/L vs. 31.7 ± 9.9 nmol/L, respectively).[332] Because vitamin D is an essential hormone in vertebrates, these findings suggest that the provision of supplemental UVB radiation to captive rabbits might be important.

In humans, some authors suggest that <50 nmol/L serum 25-hydroxycholecalciferol should be considered deficient.[330] If this were to be true for other mammals, the rabbits and the guinea pigs in the previously mentioned studies would be considered deficient. However, significant differences between humans and small mammals exist. More studies investigating the effect of 25-hydroxycholecalciferol and the consequence of hypovitaminosis D in small mammals are needed, but based on the current literature, UVB supplementation may be recommended for rabbits, guinea pigs, and chinchillas.

ENDOCRINE PANCREAS

The pancreas is a glandular organ having an exocrine influence on digestive physiology as well as an endocrine influence in vertebrate animals. For the purpose of this chapter, only the endocrine pancreas is discussed.

The endocrine pancreas is composed of nests of cells known as the islets of Langerhans.[3] In mammals, several types of cells are present: alpha (α) cells responsible for glucagon production, beta (β) cells that produce insulin and amylin, delta (δ) cells that produce somatostatin, pancreatic polypeptide (PP) cells, and epsilon (ϵ) cells that produce ghrelin.[333-335] Not all of the cells and hormones described above for mammals have been reported in avian and reptilian species.[336-340] The ϵ cells have been recently described in humans, and ghrelin has been reported in the pancreas of reptiles and birds and appears to play a role in feeding behavior.[341,342] Cellular distribution within rat islets is typically represented with α, δ, and PP cells peripherally arranged around a central core of β cells.[343] The classic function of hormones produced by the pancreatic islets is glucose homeostasis.[334] Insulin, a polypeptide hormone of 51-amino-acid residues, promotes the absorption of glucose from blood to muscle and adipocytes. In the liver, insulin promotes glycogen biosynthesis by stimulating glycogen synthetase and inhibiting glycogen phosphorylase. In adipose tissue, glucose can be converted to fatty acids, but its main function is to provide hydrocarbons for the glycerol backbone in triglyceride formation.[344] Concurrently, insulin suppresses fuel mobilization by inhibition of glycogen breakdown by the liver, amino acid release from muscle, and free fatty acid (FFA) release from adipose tissue.[344] In addition to glucose uptake, insulin promotes nucleoside, amino acid, potassium, magnesium, and phosphate uptake into its target cells. Glucagon, also a peptide hormone, has the opposite effect of insulin on glucose homeostasis, leading to an increase in blood glucose when the animal is deprived of food. This effect is mainly provided by the liver, for few glucagon receptors are found on other mammalian tissues. Although produced by the pancreas, glucagon is generally secreted at significantly lower amounts than insulin, and it also functions to slow gastric emptying and promote satiety.[344] Glucagon, unlike insulin, has other synergistic hormones (e.g., GH, epinephrine, cortisol); therefore, there is less of a need for this hormone. In the liver, glucagon binds to a 7-transmembrane G-protein-linked glycoprotein receptor, stimulates cyclic adenosine monophosphate (cAMP) production, and may also activate the phosphatidylinositol signaling pathway.[344] Through a subsequent cascade of intracellular events, glucagon stimulates the glycogen to break down glucose and hepatic gluconeogenic enzymes. Through these processes, glucose is released into the blood.

Glucagon may also stimulate fatty acid release from adipose tissue in certain animal species, but in mammals, this role is modest (compared to epinephrine and cortisol).[344] Glucagon is considered to be a hyperglycemic hormone, and in some animals, it is also considered to be ketogenic.[344] Conversely, insulin is hypoglycemic and antiketotic. Somatostatin, also known as GH-inhibiting hormone, regulates insulin and glucagon release in a paracrine fashion. In other areas of the body, somatostatin can affect neurotransmission and cell proliferation. Via its paracrine action in the pancreas, somatostatin inhibits the release of both insulin and glucagon.[344]

Among common diseases affecting the endocrine pancreas, functional neoplasias tend to be the most common. Insulinomas are often functional β-cell insulin-secreting tumors.[345] This condition has been well documented in ferrets as well as some other exotic animal species. DM is another endocrinopathy that occasionally affects exotic species. DM is perhaps the most investigated endocrine disease of humans and also occurs with a high incidence in dogs and cats.

Neoplasia

Reptiles

One case report involving a reptile species (savannah monitor [*Varanus exanthematicus*]) has described a functional islet-cell neoplasia in which the patient presented with clinical illness and elevated insulin levels.[346] On postmortem, hepatic metastases and multifocal hepatic cholangiocarcinomas were detected.[346]

Mammals

As previously indicated, insulinoma is an endocrinologically active insulin-secreting tumor of the pancreatic β cells.[3,347,348] Hyperinsulinemia causes hypoglycemia by increased uptake of glucose by muscle tissue, fat, and the liver (all insulin target cells) and suppression of hepatic glycogenolysis and gluconeogenesis.[349] Neoplastic hyperfunctioning islet cells continue to produce insulin due to lack of negative feedback.[349] The first report of islet tumors in humans was by Nicholls in 1902, but clinical hyperinsulinism was only reported by Fletcher and Campbell in 1922.[350] Insulinoma has been reported in humans and several animal species including laboratory, exotic, and wild animals.[350-353] Although uncommon in dogs, insulinoma is the most common islet-cell neoplasia of dogs and is often highly metastatic, primarily affecting the regional lymph nodes and liver.[349,353] Insulinomas in cats appear to be rare, based on the number of published reports.[353,354] Among exotic species, insulinomas are one of the two most common neoplasias of middle-aged to older ferrets.[355,356] Insulinomas are considered the most common reported neoplasias of ferrets, with an incidence of ~25% of all neoplasms diagnosed.[356] In a retrospective ferret neoplasm study from Japan, the most common tumor reported was insulinoma (211/945).[357] Insulinomas in ferrets tend to be benign and nonmetastatic, although local metastases have been reported.[355] It is suggested that ferrets may be predisposed to insulinomas because of inappropriate diet, but there is no scientific evidence to support this theory.[355]

Both spontaneous and induced insulinomas have been reported in laboratory rats. Insulinoma induction in rats has been caused by diabetogenic agents (streptozotocin, nicotinamide, and alloxan), radiation, electrofusion, and BK virus.[358-360] Evidence indicates that in rats and hamsters, subcutaneous (SC) implantation of induced insulinoma fragments leads to hypoglycemia and hyperinsulinemia on new hosts.[361-363] Under these settings, metastasis has not been reported, which could be indicative of a low metastatic rate for this tumor.[362,363] In late stages of the disease, rats exhibited clinical signs of hypoglycemia, tachypnea, and partial limb paralysis.[350] After resection of the mass, a significant blood glucose increase and gradual return to normal values were noticed.[362] In one study, despite careful resection, local reoccurrence was detected.[363] The prevalence of spontaneous islet-cell adenoma in aged laboratory rats appears to be low, with pancreatic islet-cell adenomas reported to represent 2% to 6% of all tumors.[107,364,365] In retrospective studies on spontaneous neoplasms in young rats, insulinomas are not reported, which may show that older animals are more susceptible to this disease condition.[109,110,366]

There have been three case reports of insulinomas in guinea pigs.[367] Insulinomas do not appear to be a common clinical problem in guinea pigs, with only one case being diagnosed in vivo. In one rabbit case, in which an insulinoma was diagnosed, a serendipitous diagnosis was obtained during a study assessing the usefulness of blood glucose measurement in pet rabbits.[368]

Hypoglycemia alone is not necessarily diagnostic for insulinoma in small mammals since it can be related to other conditions including sepsis, hepatic disease, glucose-utilizing tumors, hypoadrenocorticism, hypoglycemic medications, storage diseases, and neonatal hypoglycemia.[348,354,369] Hypoglycemia may be counteracted by the release of cathecholamines, glucagon, and corticosteroids, as well as by normal glucose fluctuations.[345,348] A concurrent hypoglycemia with hyperinsulinemia is highly indicative of insulinoma, but there is no clear consensus on the paired glucose:insulin ratio value.[348,349,354] Historically, diagnosis of insulinoma depended on confirming the Whipple's triad, which consisted of demonstrating subnormal blood glucose, recognizing clinical signs of hypoglycemia, and the reversibility of signs after resolution of hypoglycemia.[345] However, it is believed that for ferret patients, hypoglycemia without evidence of other conditions is highly indicative of insulinoma, in part because of ferrets' high prevalence for this disease condition. Nonetheless, further diagnostic testing should be performed in order to confirm the tentative insulinoma diagnosis. Paired measurement of insulin and glucose is recommended to determine potential paradoxical values. High values of insulin in the presence of hypoglycemia are rare. Fructosamine concentrations can be used to assess chronic hypoglycemia, since

fructosamine levels reflect the blood glucose concentrations over the previous 1- to 2-week period.[345] It has been shown that dogs with insulinomas have significantly lower fructosamine concentrations than normal animals.[348,370,371] Such evidence in exotic mammals has not been reported, but reference intervals have been established.[372,373] A definitive diagnosis of insulinoma is only achieved through histopathological evaluation of diseased tissue.[345]

It is said that a prolonged and profound hypoglycemia can adversely affect nerve function, cause the development of peripheral neuropathies, and promote seizures.[374,375] Brain lesions have been reported in several species as a consequence of hypoglycemia caused by both induced and spontaneous insulinomas.[354,376,377] In a cat in which an insulinoma was suspected, neurological deficits (disorientation, inconsistent menace response, and aggressiveness) were attributed to hypoglycemia, although the disease condition was not confirmed.[354] Neuronal death in the superficial layer of the cerebral cortex and hypothalamus dentate gyrus was diagnosed through histopathological evaluation of a dog's brain tissue and was believed to be caused by ischemic-type neuronal death as a result of the hypocalcemia.[376] The correlation between hypoglycemia and neuropathies has been studied in rats under laboratory conditions. Several studies have shown that a blood glucose below 45 mg/dL (2.5 mmol/L) for at least 12 hours results in peripheral nerve axonal degeneration, with subsequent reduction of nerve conduction velocity (although both the brain and peripheral neurons can supposedly adapt to prolonged hypoglycemia).[374] Although brain adaptability is not completely understood, it appears that up-regulation of GLUT-1 (the blood-brain barrier glucose transport protein) may increase glucose extraction from blood.[374] In hibernating animals, the brain can switch to ketone body utilization (rather than glucose utilization) as a major means of energy production during hypoglycemia, thus sparing the breakdown of muscle protein for hepatic glucose production.[328] Peripheral neuropathies appear to be related to the duration and severity of hypoglycemia.[377] In rats, axonal de- and regeneration and de- and remyelination of the sciatic, tibial, and sural nerves have been reported.[377] Three-month-old male Wistar rats with induced insulinoma became hypoglycemic and developed sciatic and peroneal nerve endoneurial ischemia/hypoxia as well as endoneurial necrosis of the sciatic nerve, which caused hind limb paresis in 2/12 animals.[360] Further studies showed that hypoglycemia is related to increased myelinated axonal damage, while hyperinsulinemia is related to increased densities of small myelinated axons and endoneurial microvessels (with microangiopathic changes).[378]

The treatment option for insulinoma in ferrets, and hypothetically in rats, may be either surgical or medical. Surgical removal of an insulinoma may provide a definitive treatment; however, there is a high probability of disease recurrence. It is also possible that undetected insulinomas may not be removed at the time of surgery, and therefore the condition may persist.[379] Prior to surgery, US is advisable in order to determine whether a lesion is detected.[380] Although the sensitivity of this test is unknown in ferrets, in dogs, US was able to detect 5/14 insulinomas in confirmed cases.[380] The use of CT and single-photon emission CT was also evaluated in the canine cases of insulinoma, and these tests identified tumors in 10/14 and 6/14 subject animals, respectively.[380] This canine study concluded that US should be used as an initial evaluation of canine hypoglycemia, but other diagnostic imaging techniques are reliable.[380]

Ferret insulinomas do not commonly metastasize, but spread via local invasion to the liver, spleen, and regional lymph nodes has been reported.[367] Conversely, canine insulinomas often exhibit metastatic behavior.[345,349,381] A useful diagnostic test in the case of insulinoma metastasis is scintigraphy with indium-111, a radioisotope with high affinity for somatostatin.[349] This diagnostic test has not been validated for ferret use; therefore, its effectiveness in this species is unknown.

Surgical removal of an insulinoma may be performed with nodulectomy and/or partial pancreatectomy. One study assessed these 2 different surgical modalities (pancreatic nodulectomy [n = 27] or pancreatic nodulectomy combined with partial pancreatectomy [n = 29]) and their comparison to medical management with prednisolone and/or diazoxide.[382] Mean disease-free intervals for each group were 234, 365, and 22 days, respectively.[382] Mean survival times for each group were 456, 668, and 186 days, respectively.[382] Nonetheless, it is important to consider that pancreatic nodulectomy combined with partial pancreatectomy is obviously a more invasive procedure and for this particular study involved a 25% to 50% removal of the pancreas. Furthermore, recurrence of insulinoma is possible (and likely) if there is incomplete removal of the tumor. In ferrets, as many as 52% (26/50) of the animals remained hypoglycemic after surgery, and the reported disease-free intervals ranged from 0 to 23.5 months.[356] Surgical removal of the lesion or partial removal of the pancreas can also induce DM.

Medical management is traditionally performed using glucocorticoids (prednisolone or prednisone). These pharmaceuticals increase the blood glucose level by increasing hepatic gluconeogenesis, decreasing glucose uptake by peripheral tissues, and inhibiting insulin binding to its receptors.[356] This treatment option does not truly treat the condition; instead, it provides an alternative source of glucose to the body, thus counteracting the hyperinsulinemic state. Diazoxide, an arteriolar dilator used to treat hypertensive emergencies, is another alternative treatment. This drug is a nondiuretic benzothiadiazide that also inhibits pancreatic insulin secretion by decreasing the intracellular release of ionized calcium, which subsequently prevents release of insulin from insulin granules. In addition, by stimulating epinephrine release, diazoxide promotes hepatic gluconeogenesis and glycogenolysis and decreases cellular glucose uptake.[356]

Chemotherapeutic regimes for insulinoma have been described for ferrets. In ferrets, doxorubicin has been prescribed for insulinoma and is used in a similar manner as that to treat lymphoma.[356] Precise catheterization is mandatory for doxorubicin administration due to local site effects of the chemotherapeutic agent, with a recommended IV dose of 30 mg/m² every 3 weeks; the cumulative dose should stay below 240 mg/m².[356]

Recently, newer treatment options for insulinoma in ferrets have surfaced, but their use remains hypothetical, and scientific assessment of efficacy and potential side effects is required. Octreotide, a synthetic long-acting analog of somatostatin, inhibits insulin, glucagon, secretin, gastrin, and motilin secretion; therefore, it may be useful for insulinoma cases unresponsive to palliative treatment. Published reports

indicate that canine insulinoma cells have a high affinity for octreotide, but their use in ferrets is anecdotal.[345,356] Two newer chemotherapeutic agents have been hypothesized: streptozotocin and alloxan. Streptozotocin is a nitrosourea commonly used to treat unresectable metastatic insulinomas in humans because it is specifically cytotoxic to pancreatic β cells.[345] In the first canine trial, high nephrotoxicity was documented, but subsequent studies indicated that streptozotocin could be used safely in dogs when aggressive 0.9% saline diuresis is employed.[345] However, streptozotocin use in ferrets is questionable since concerns about potential renal toxicity remain. Streptozotocin is commonly used in the laboratory setting to induce DM in rats and rabbits.[383] Alloxan, another chemotherapeutic agent, also has a direct toxic effect on pancreatic β cells; however, other toxicities (e.g., renal, hepatic, pulmonary) have been reported, and alloxan requires aggressive fluid therapy during administration to prevent renal tubular necrosis.[384] Alloxan use has not been validated in ferrets. Toceranib phosphate is a chemotherapeutic agent commonly used for treatment of canine mast cell tumors.[385] Toceranib is a small-molecule inhibitor of a variety of tyrosine kinases expressed on the cell surface and is closely related to sunitinib (another small-molecule inhibitor).[386] Sunitinib has been shown to be effective when used to treat insulinomas in humans.[386] Further evaluation of toceranib is recommended to evaluate its effectiveness in treating animals diagnosed with insulinomas.

Diabetes Mellitus

DM results from a lack of or deficiency in insulin or an inability of insulin to properly facilitate the transport of glucose (nucleosides, potassium, magnesium, phosphate, and amino acids) into target cells. In many cases in which DM has been diagnosed, insulin target cells (primarily muscle, adipocytes, and liver tissue) either lack appropriate insulin receptors or the receptors are down-regulated. This endocrine disorder is a well-studied human disease, in part because of its worldwide distribution and increasing prevalence. DM was first described in 1500 BC.[387] Since then, several forms of DM have been described: types 1 and 2 and gestational. Type-1 DM, sometimes called insulin dependent or juvenile, is largely an autoimmune disease causing immunologically mediated destruction of pancreatic β cells. DM is a common chronic disease of childhood, with a prevalence of <5 in every 100,000 individuals in Eastern countries and 39.9/100,000 in European and other Western countries.[388] Approximately 10% of adults who present with DM have type 1 rather than the more common type 2 (adult-onset diabetes), which is not autoimmune.[388] Type-2 DM is a metabolic disorder characterized by hyperglycemia with insulin resistance. It was estimated in 2013 that more than 382 million human beings are affected by type-2 DM.[389] Conversely, gestational diabetes, which tends to be more physiologic, occurs in women without a previous history of DM and is characterized by the development of high blood glucose levels during pregnancy.

There are specific characteristics regarding rodent insulin and insulin receptors, in particular, receptors belonging to the suborder Hystricomorpha. Published reports indicate that insulin receptors of mammals, other than rodents, share a common epitope with the human insulin receptor.[390] Rodent insulin receptors, however, appear to be different in the 485- to 599-amino-acid sequence of the α subunit. Furthermore, the Hystricomorpha insulin molecule exhibits immunological property differences and a higher growth-promoting activity.[391] The insulin and carboxy-terminal regions of glucagon in guinea pigs and degus (*Octodon degus*) are highly divergent from those of other mammals, with insulin being only 1% to 10% as biologically active as insulin from other mammals.[392,393] The range of endocrine axis anomalies in guinea pigs indicates that their lineage may have branched off before divergence among other rodents.[394] To compensate for this characteristic, degus have increased insulin receptors and potentially higher insulin concentrations.[392] Due to these anomalies, it is not recommended that diabetic rodents be treated with porcine insulin.

Reptiles

DM has been suggested by some to occur in reptiles,[196,395] most notably red-eared sliders (*Trachemys scripta elegans*), desert tortoises (*Gopherus agassizii*), Chinese water dragons (*Physignathus cocincinus*), western pond turtles (*Actinemys marmorata*), Exuma Island iguanas (*Cyclura cychlura figginsi*), inland bearded dragons, and the green iguana.[396] It is believed that persistent, marked hyperglycemia (>200 mg/dL [11.1 mmol/L] with or without glucosuria) should be considered indicative of reptilian DM.[396] However, hyperglycemia has not been established as a consistent or specific indicator of pancreatic disease or DM in reptiles, for elevations in blood glucose are often related to other metabolic conditions, systemic diseases, and/or physiologic variables.[396] Although several cases of reptile DM have been reported, there is a lack of peer-reviewed publications to support the occurrence of this disease in this group of animals.

Another emerging condition that may cause marked hyperglycemia in inland bearded dragons is gastric neuroendocrine adenocarcinoma, a highly malignant neoplasia.[397,398] The prevalence of this condition in a retrospective pathological review of bearded dragon presentations was reported to be 1.5%.[397] In bearded dragons, this neoplasia may overproduce somatostatin, which in humans suppresses secretion of insulin, glucagon, PP, and gastrin and reduces gastric acid secretion, gastric motility, intestinal motility, and gallbladder contraction.[399] These combined effects produce a characteristic human diabetic syndrome of hypochlorhydria, pancreatic exocrine insufficiency, and gallstones.[399]

Birds

DM has indeed been reported in birds, but it is considered an uncommon disease. A characteristic of the avian pancreas to note is the pancreatic insulin content being ~1/6 that of the mammalian pancreas in granivorous birds, while the glucagon content is ~2 to 5 times greater.[18] In fact, circulating plasma glucagon concentrations are 10 to 50 times higher in birds than in mammals.[18] Birds also maintain higher plasma glucose levels than other vertebrates of similar body mass. Moreover, plasma glucose appears to be largely insensitive to insulin regulation in granivorous species.[338] Conversely, raptor species may be more insulin dependent.[18] Furthermore, some raptor species have high circulating β-hydroxybutyrate titers, a naturally occurring ketone body produced from fatty acids in the liver. Elevated plasma concentrations of this fatty acid by-product in mammals is correlated with high insulin resistance.[400]

Chickens normally have approximately twice the plasma glucose concentration of mammals, experiencing only minor changes during short-term and/or prolonged starvation.[401] These findings indicate that avian glucose regulation is unorthodox, compared to other vertebrate species, and it is not well understood.[401] An important difference between chicken and sparrow glucose transporters (GLUTs) and mammalian GLUTs is that these birds appear to lack the predominant mammalian GLUT found in plasma membranes of insulin-sensitive cells (i.e., GLUT-4).[402] The absence of this insulin-responsive GLUT may be the main factor causing high avian blood glucose levels and insulin insensitivity.[402] It is believed that glucagon is a more effective glucose regulator in granivorous species than is insulin, and based on limited data, it is thought that DM is not caused by insulin deficiency.[18] However, as in mammals, exposing the avian pancreas to exogenous glucose inhibited glucagon release from caudal and cranial regions by 27%, but unlike insulin, birds appear to be quite sensitive to glucagon and respond with increased plasma glucose, triglyceride, glycerol, and FFA levels.[338]

Ducks and chickens appear to withstand the surgical removal of the pancreas better than mammals, leading to a mild and temporarily induced DM.[403] In addition, chickens appear to be resistant to diabetogenic drugs (e.g., streptozotocin, alloxan), which may indicate that chicken pancreatic β cells are highly protected.[401] Pigeons, fowl, ducks, hawks, and quail are reported to have a higher resistance to insulin than mammals, requiring larger doses than mammals to induce seizure activity.[403] The administration of 40 μg/kg porcine insulin to 8-day-old chicks led to a slight reduction in plasma glucose but increased uptake of glucose by insulin-sensitive tissues.[404] The administration of 80 μg/kg of chicken insulin administered to adult mourning doves (*Zenaida macroura*) had no effect on tissue glucose uptake, despite a slight decrease in plasma levels.[402,405]

DM has been reported in a nanday conure (*Nandayus nenday*), a chestnut-fronted macaw (*Ara severus*), budgerigars, toco toucans (*Ramphastos toco*), an African grey parrot, a red-tailed hawk (*Buteo jamaicensis*), a cockatiel, an emperor penguin (*Aptenodytes forsteri*), and a blue-and-gold macaw (*Ara ararauna*).[406-414]

The most striking clinical signs of psittacine species diagnosed with DM included PU/PD and weight loss with normal food intake.[18] A tentative diagnosis of DM can made by demonstrating hyperglycemia and glucosuria, although a definitive diagnosis can only be determined by demonstrating persistent hyperglycemia.[18] Other authors suggest that blood glucose levels above 800 mg/dL (44.4 mmol/L) are diagnostic, and most birds present with values well above 1000 mg/dL (55 mmol/L).[415] Pancreatic biopsies are recommended but not commonly performed.[415]

There have been no scientific studies assessing the use of different insulin products to treat DM in birds; however, some anecdotal use of bovine and porcine protamine-zinc, glipizide, and human recombinant insulin has been reported.[415] Further avian studies are needed to scientifically validate the up-to-date and commercially available insulin products used to treat avian DM.

Mammals

Although DM has been reported in several exotic mammalian species, this condition appears to be rare and consequently has a low prevalence.[416] Some rodents, in particular, species belonging to the suborder Hystricomorpha, have some unique characteristics regarding physiology associated with DM. In guinea pigs and degus, the insulin and carboxy-terminal regions of glucagon are highly divergent from that of other mammals, with insulin being only 1% to 10% as biologically active as that of other species.[392,393] To compensate for this characteristic, degus have increased insulin receptors and potentially higher insulin concentrations.[392] It is important to mention that diabetic rats and mice are resistant to porcine and human insulin.[417] In Lewis rats, BALB/c mice, and athymic BALB/c mice, both IV porcine and human insulin were unable to restore normoglycemia in immunocompetent diabetic rodents, even at doses that may be lethal to humans.[418] Although this information is not available for guinea pigs, some evidence has been reported that guinea pig insulin is different from other mammalian insulins. It has been shown that physical properties of guinea pig insulin are unique and different from those of bovine and porcine insulin, and it is likely that physical differences produce changes in physiologic activity.[419] Guinea pig antibodies have intense reactions to porcine or bovine insulin.[420] Although not scientifically validated, there are concerns regarding the use of pig insulin to treat DM in small exotic mammals; therefore, the use of this product is not recommended due to potential and severe side effects.

Spontaneous DM in guinea pigs has been reported in a laboratory colony and in a pet guinea pig.[421-423] Transient DM has been tentatively diagnosed in two related inbred strains of guinea pigs exhibiting clinical signs of PU/PD, mild obesity, and decreased breeding performance.[424,413] Preliminary studies revealed an increased blood glucose concentration, and histological analyses showed severe degeneration of pancreatic islet cells without mononuclear cell infiltration.[424] Transient DM without requiring insulin treatment has been proposed as a potential condition.[425]

Degus may be one of the most common exotic small mammal species that develop spontaneous diabetes during obesity.[426] In a retrospective study of degu diseases, DM was reported in 12/300, with a majority of animals (10/12) being 2 years old or older.[427] This condition appears to be related to inappropriate diet (including fruits and pelleted feeds high in starch) and thus obesity.[416] DM in degus is suspected to be similar to the adult-onset noninsulin-dependent (type II) variety in humans and may be associated with islet amyloidosis or a viral component.[416] Cataract formation is a common clinical sign.[416] Another interesting and unique characteristic of DM in degus has been suggested. Amyloid ("amylin") deposition, derived from either pancreatic β cells or islet amyloid polypeptides (IAPPs), is the single most typical islet alteration in type-2 diabetes.[428] Degus are an exception to the rule in that islet amyloid does not occur in species with apparently nonfibrillogenic IAPPs.[428] Direct amino acid sequence analysis of purified degu islet amyloid showed that the fibril protein in this species is derived from insulin, which is similar to human amyloid protein, although in humans, fibril protein may also be of iatrogenic origin since it is associated with repeated insulin injections.[428]

DM, resembling type 2, has been diagnosed in two chinchillas.[429] The chinchillas' blood glucose levels were four times the upper normal limit, and they developed glucosuria and ketonuria.[429] Both animals experienced an initial improvement following insulin treatment but subsequently died. Pathological diagnosis indicated that one animal had pancreatic atrophy and islet cell vacuolation, while the other was diagnosed with a pancreatic adenoma.[429]

Rabbits are used for diabetes research, and cases of spontaneous DM in New Zealand white rabbits have been reported.[430] However, spontaneous DM appears to be rare in rabbits. In a study assessing the usefulness of determining blood glucose levels in pet rabbits, no cases of DM were suspected in the 907 rabbits investigated.[368]

Although the most common endogenous pancreatic disease of ferrets is insulinoma, DM has also been reported, with the most common cause being iatrogenic following surgical removal of an insulinoma.[431] This condition tends to be transient, with insulin and glucose levels normalizing over a period of time. However, normalization of insulin levels may be due to recurrence of the insulinoma. Ferrets with DM may nonetheless require insulin therapy depending on severity of illness and the length of time necessary for resolution. Spontaneous DM unrelated to pancreatectomy and/or spontaneous pancreatitis has been reported.[432-436] There is also one case report of spontaneous DM in a black-footed ferret (Mustela nigripes).[437]

It is common practice to use point-of-care units for the quantification of blood glucose concentrations in exotic small mammal patients. This method is useful and convenient, primarily because of the small amounts of blood required, and results are obtained as soon as the test strip is inserted into the machine. Several studies have assessed the reliability and performance of these units in small exotic animal species.[368,438-440] It is important to recognize that rabbit blood glucose is commonly determined using a portable blood glucose meter (used for humans), while ferrets require a veterinary-specific blood glucose unit set on "canine."[438,439] As for other animals, small exotic mammals diagnosed with DM require insulin treatment. Medical management using insulin in different mammalian species requires further assessment, but the most common insulin products used are neutral protamine Hagerdorn (NPH), ultralente, glargine, and detemir.[416] Some of these medications may no longer be commercially available. Overall, the objective of insulin therapy is to achieve blood glucose levels <300 mg/dL (16.7 mmol/L),[416] and patients are best hospitalized until blood glucose is stabilized to between 125 and 200 mg/dL (6.9 and 11.1 mmol/L).[416]

THE HYPOTHALAMIC-PITUITARY-ADRENAL AXIS

The adrenal glands were first described by Bartolomeus Eustachius (1520-1574), but at that time, no explanation for their function was provided.[441] Early authors suggested an involvement of the nervous system in adrenal function as well as an association with sexual function.[442] However, not until the 19th century were two distinguishable sections of these glands noted: the cortex and medulla.[441] There are significant histological and functional differences between these two distinct areas of the adrenal glands. The cortex comprises three zones: zonae glomerulosa (also called the zona arcuata in dogs and cats), fasciculata, and reticularis.[3,443] The major bioactive mineralocorticoid in humans is aldosterone, which is synthesized in the zona glomerulosa.[3,443] The inner zonae fasciculata and reticularis produce, respectively, cortisol (a glucocorticoid) and the adrenal androgens (dehydroepiandrosterone [DHEA] and androstenedione).[3,443] To a varying degree, the three zones of the adrenal cortex zones are regulated by circulating levels of potassium and angiotensin II (aldosterone) and ACTH released from the anterior pituitary (cortisol).[3,443] The medulla is composed of a "sponge-like" network of chromaffin cells or pheochromocytes and small groups of nerve cells (paraganglia).[3] Paraganglia are considered specialized ganglia of the sympathetic nervous system.[3] The medulla is responsible for the production of epinephrine, norepinephrine, and small amounts of DA.[444-446]

Among small exotic mammal species, ferrets are well known for their development of clinical signs associated with adrenal disease.[447] There are some rather unique anatomical characteristics of the ferret adrenal gland that may be related to its predisposition for disease. As in other mammals, ferrets possess zonae glomerulosa, fasciculata, and reticularis.[448] Ferrets, and a few other carnivores, also have two extra less prominent layers, zonae intermedia and juxtamedullaris, the functions of which are less well understood.[449] In the zona intermedia, located between the zonae glomerulosa and fasciculata, cells are smaller than in either of the adjacent zones.[448] The zona juxtamedullaris is composed of a few cells with similar morphology to the cells of the inner zona fasciculata and are found between the zona reticularis and the medulla.[448] In mice, an extra layer, the X zone, is adjacent to the medulla.[450] In mice and ferrets, the neoplastic adrenocortical cells, which functionally resemble gonadal steroidogenic cells, arise from progenitors in the subcapsular or juxtamedullary region.[451] Although other factors most likely influence the development of adrenal neoplasias in ferrets, these unique anatomical characteristics of ferrets and mice may be significant predisposing factors. In birds, there is no distinct division between the medulla and cortex within the adrenal glands; instead, adrenocortical and chromaffin tissues intermingle, although the chromaffin tissue is primarily located in the center of the gland.[452]

As in other glands, adrenal function is controlled by a cascade of hormonal stimulation (the HPA axis), and under normal conditions negative feedback mechanisms are a part of axis control. The HPA serves both in the resting state to maintain homeostasis and, in the case of metabolic, physical, and/or emotional stress, to enhance endocrine control of the organism.[453] The paraventricular nucleus of the hypothalamus produces and secretes ADH, which is stored in the posterior pituitary, and the hypothalamus synthesizes CRH, which is released into the hypothalamo-hypophyseal portal system. Moreover, both hormones ADH and ACTH are known to stimulate the anterior lobe of the pituitary to secrete ACTH, which next acts on the adrenal cortex to induce production of the glucocorticoid hormones cortisol and corticosterone. Sufficient serum levels of glucocorticoid hormones provide a negative feedback to the hypothalamus and pituitary, causing a decrease in CRH and ACTH.

A number of steroid hormones have been isolated from the adrenal tissue, but those of physiological significance include cortisol (hydrocortisone), corticosterone, deoxycorticosterone, aldosterone, and the adrenal androgens.[3] In birds, rats, and mice, corticosterone is secreted in higher amounts than cortisol,[3] and avian aldosterone is produced in small amounts.[454] The HPA axis of birds appears to be functionally and anatomically different from that of mammals.[454]

Pheochromocytoma

Pheochromocytomas are tumors that arise from adrenal medullary pheochromocytes (chromaffin cells).[455] Eighty-five percent of human pheochromocytomas originate from chromaffin cells, while 18% arise from extra-adrenal tissues.[456] Pheochromocytomas are often interchangeable with paragangliomas, although underlying differences in genetics, clinical presentation, and malignant potential exist.[457] Intra-adrenal tumors are frequently classified as pheochromocytomas, while extra-adrenal chromaffin neoplasms are called paragangliomas (or extra-adrenal pheochromocytomas).[458] The adrenal glands of birds are innervated by preganglionic sympathetic fibers that originate from the thoracic and synsacral splanchnic nerves and, according to some authors, by parasympathetic fibers (i.e., the vagus nerve via the celiac plexus).[459] Parasympathetic innervation of the adrenal gland has not been identified in mammals.

Published reports indicate that pheochromocytomas are the most common adrenal medulla neoplasia in animals.[460] However, pheochromocytomas are diagnosed through necropsy examination in fewer than half of animal patients in whom this tumor type is identified and in 30% to 60% of human patients at autopsy.[3] Variable results among reports support the belief that the prevalence of pheochromocytomas in humans has not precisely been determined.[461] Although prevalence studies are also lacking in veterinary medicine, pheochromocytomas nonetheless appear to be most common in dogs and cattle.[462] Pheochromocytomas appear to be sporadic in other species (i.e., among 3.7 million slaughtered pigs in Great Britain, only one pheochromocytoma was reported).[462] These findings from the UK should be considered suspect since it is mainly young pigs that are slaughtered, and postmortem examination is not complete.[462] However, pheochromocytomas have been reported in several captive and wild species including dog (*Canis lupus familiaris*),[463] cat (*Felis catus*),[464] ferret,[252] pig (*Sus scrofa domesticus*),[462] cow (*Bos primigenius*),[465] horse (*Equus ferus caballus*),[466] sheep (*Ovis aries*),[467] goat (*Capra aegagrus hircus*),[468] mouse (*Mus musculus*),[469] rat (*Rattus norvegicus*),[470] jaguar (*Panthera onca*),[471,472] clouded leopard (*Neofelis nebulosa*),[473] coatimundi (*Nasua nasua*),[474] tiger quoll (*Dasyurus maculatus*),[473] maned wolf (*Chrysocyon brachyurus*),[475] Asian raccoon dog (*Nyctereutes procyonoides*, suspected familial form),[476] hippopotamus (*Hippopotamus amphibius*),[477] white rhinoceros (*Ceratotherium simum*),[478,479] African elephant (*Loxodonta africana*),[460] desert warthog (*Phacochoerus aethiopicus*),[480] European mouflon (*Ovis orientalis musimon*),[481] ring-tailed lemur (*Lemur catta*),[482,483] fat-tailed dwarf lemur (*Cheirogaleus medius*),[484] red-fronted lemur (*Eulemur rufifrons*),[484] cotton-top tamarin (*Saguinus oedipus oedipus*),[485,486] golden lion tamarin (*Leontopithecus rosalia*),[486,487] mantled howler (*Alouatta palliata*),[487] black howler (*Alouatta caraya*),[486] brown spider monkey (*Ateles hybridus*),[487] Geoffroy's spider monkey (*Ateles geoffroyi*),[486] rhesus macaque (*Macaca mulatta*),[488] coypu (*Myocastor coypu*),[489] North American river otter (*Lontra canadensis*)[490], sea otter (*Enhydra lutris*),[491] and Atlantic spotted dolphin (*Stenella frontalis*).[492] Pheochromocytomas appear to be rarely reported in birds, although this tumor type has been diagnosed in the nicobar pigeon (*Caloenas nicobarica*), chicken, and budgerigar.[493-495] Metastatic characteristics were only reported with the budgerigar.[495]

Clinical signs are considered nonspecific in animals with pheochromocytomas but include generalized weakness and episodic collapse, and to a lesser degree, panting, tachypnea, and seizures.[455] Clinical manifestations of pheochromocytomas are associated with the hormones produced by the tumor, hormonal release patterns, and individual variations in catecholamine sensitivity.[461] The common clinical signs associated with pheochromocytomas involve overproduction of norepinephrine and/or epinephrine and subsequent consequences of this hormonal release. In a 50-year retrospective study of clinically unsuspected pheochromocytomas in humans, hypertension was the most common clinical finding (22/54).[496]

Hyperadrenocorticism

Ferret hyperadrenocorticism, commonly called adrenal gland disease, is arguably the most well-studied endocrinopathy of exotic small mammals. Ferret adrenal gland disease is a form of hyperadrenocorticism caused by adrenal tissue hypertrophy and/or neoplasm within the adrenal cortex that overproduces one or more steroid hormones (e.g., glucocorticoids, mineralocorticoids, androgens).[356] It is important to mention that this condition is not considered to be the same as Cushing's syndrome (or disease), which is characterized by elevated cortisol levels that result from an ACTH-secreting pituitary tumor or a cortisol-secreting adrenal tumor.[356] With Cushing's disease, the contralateral adrenal gland is frequently atrophied, which is not a common occurrence in ferrets.[356] In one report, ~85% of ferrets with hyperadrenocorticism had only one enlarged adrenal gland, in the absence of contralateral atrophy, and the remaining 15% had bilateral adrenal involvement.[497] There appears to be a high prevalence of adrenal disease in ferrets, with one retrospective study reporting 107 adrenocortical cell tumors out of a total of 639 neoplasms.[498] There are indications that ferret adrenal gland disease is being diagnosed more often, with a reported rise from 30% in 1993 to 70% in 2003.[499] In Japan, 207/945 neoplasms were diagnosed as adrenal gland tumors.[357] However, in the UK, ferret adrenal disease is seldom diagnosed.[497]

As mentioned above, some unique anatomic and physiologic characteristics of the ferret adrenal gland may influence the occurrence of this disease process. Nonetheless, other factors are also important with the development of this condition in ferrets. It is suggested that removal of gonadal tissue at an early age may have an influence on the development of ferret adrenal disease.[500] In the United States, it is common practice to remove ferret gonadal tissue at 6 weeks of age, as opposed to European countries (e.g., The Netherlands) where this procedure is performed later in life, at ~1 year of age.[500,501] It is suggested that the interval between neutering age and age of diagnosis in the Dutch ferret population (3.5 ± 1.8 y) was similar to that in the American population (3.3 ± 1.4 y); however, because Dutch ferrets are neutered later, there is a later age of diagnosis (5.1 ± 1.9 y).[501] This study shows that a predisposing factor related to the development of hyperadrenocorticism in ferrets may be neutering, independent of the age at which it is performed (Table 6-4).

Furthermore, pituitary gonadotropic hormones (LH and FSH) also appear to have an influence on the pathogenesis of hyperadrenocorticism in ferrets.[497] Ferret adrenal disease develops from the expression of LH receptors (LHRs) on sex-steroid-producing adrenocortical cells.[497] Research investigations have shown that certain inbred mice (e.g., DBA/2J, CE) develop sex-steroid-producing adrenocortical tumors following gonadectomy.[502,503] This adrenal response is thought

---

TABLE 6-4

Comparison of Gonadectomy-Induced Adrenocortical Neoplasia in Domestic Ferrets and Three Mouse Models

	Ferrets	Inbred Strains of Mice (e.g., DBA2/J, CE)	Inhibin-α Promoter-SV40 T-Antigen Transgenic Mice	Inhibin-α Null Mice
Tumor location within adrenal	Variable, often near corticomedullary junction	Subcapsular	Subcapsular and X zone	Subcapsular and X zone
Histology	Nodular hyperplasia, adenomas, and carcinomas; spindle cell component or myxoid differentiation might be present	Nodular adenomas and carcinomas; composed of spindle-shaped α cells and sex-steroid-producing B cells	Carcinomas, spindle-shaped α cells, and sex-steroid-producing B cells	Carcinomas, spindle-shaped α cells, and sex-steroid-producing B cells
Latency	3.5 y	1-6 mo	5-7 mo	5-7 mo
Incidence or penetrance	Reported incidence varies (0.5%-20%)	Penetrance of 40%-100%, depending on the strain	Penetrance approaches 100%	Penetrance approaches 100%
Sex steroids produced	Estrogen, androstenedione, 17-hydroxyprogesterone, DHEAS	Estrogen (DBA/2J, CE, NU/J) or androgens (CE)	Estrogen	Estrogen
Molecular markers	LHR, GATA4, inhibin-α, ERα, vimentin	LHR, GATA4, inhibin-α, P450c17	LHR, GATA4, inhibin-α	LHR, P450c17, aromatase

DHEAS, Dehydroepiandrosterone sulfate; *ERα*, estrogen receptor α; *GATA4*, GATA-binding protein 4; *LHR*, luteinizing hormone receptor.
From Bielinska M, Kiiveri S, Parviainen H, et al. Gonadectomy-induced adrenocortical neoplasia in the domestic ferret *(Mustela putorius furo)* and laboratory mouse. *Vet Pathol.* 2006;43:97-117.

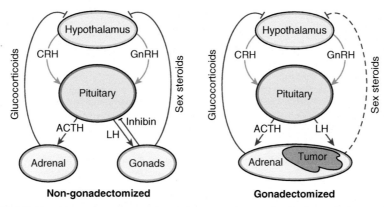

Non-gonadectomized   **Gonadectomized**

FIGURE 6-5 Hormone secretion and regulatory pathways in the hypothalamo-pituitary-adrenal-gonadal axes of nongonadectomized and gonadectomized animals. Positive regulation *(solid line)* and negative regulation *(dashed line).* Following gonadectomy, feedback inhibition of the hypothalamus by sex steroids is reduced, as indicated by the *dashed line.* (From Bielinska M, Kiiveri S, Parviainen H, et al. Gonadectomy-induced adrenocortical neoplasia in the domestic ferret *[Mustela putorius furo]* and laboratory mouse. *Vet Pathol.* 2006;43:97-117.)

to result from an unopposed increase in circulating gonadotropins and/or a decrease in factor(s) of gonadal origin.[502] Although the exact cell origin related to adrenocortical neoplasia in ferrets and mice remains unknown, some reasonable hypotheses have been forwarded. It is possible that the adrenal gland contains gonadal progenitor tissue, and the cell of origin could be a multipotential progenitor cell population capable of differentiation into either adrenocortical or gonadal-like steroidogenic cells, depending on hormonal influences and other environmental factors.[451] It is also possible that neoplastic progenitors are of extra-adrenal origin and invade the adrenal capsule by direct contact or via the bloodstream.[451] These characteristics support differences between ferrets and certain mice strains compared to other small exotic mammals. These are specific characteristics related to the high incidence of adrenocortical neoplasms (Figure 6-5).

Several diagnostic tests are available for evaluating adrenal disease in ferret patients. US is considered the gold standard for evaluating adrenal size relative to normal and clinical disease conditions, and this diagnostic imaging modality has been reasonably well established within veterinary practice. US examination allows evaluation of the size, shape, and structure of the adrenal glands as well as surrounding tissues.[356] In a retrospective study of US examinations of ferrets with adrenal disease, this diagnostic imaging test was considered useful for the diagnosis of adrenal disease.[504] Although vascular invasion was not detected, evidence of such may potentially be detected using a Doppler-enhanced image and thus would be useful when determining a patient treatment plan. Reference intervals of normal adrenal size measured by US have been reported (Table 6-5). In general, when examined using US imaging, the adrenal glands may be classified as abnormal when the gland has a rounded appearance, there is an increase in size of the cranial/caudal pole (thickness >3.9 mm), a heterogeneous structure is observed, an increased

echogenicity occurs, and/or signs of mineralization are detected.[507]

Another useful diagnostic test recommended to assess a ferret patient for adrenal disease is blood level measurement of estradiol, androstenedione, and 17α-hydroxyprogesterone.[356] In neutered ferrets, estradiol, androstenedione, and 17α-hydroxyprogesterone are normally found in minute quantities, but may be elevated in patients with adrenocortical disease.[356] These androgenic hormones may also be elevated by unrelated causes (e.g., season of year); therefore, depending on the case, their diagnostic value may be suspect. As these clinical signs in the female ferret can also occur with an ovarian remnant, which can be difficult to visualize by US, one of the authors (J.M.) suggests the use of the human chorionic gonadotropin (hCG) stimulation test in order to be able to differentiate between hyperadrenocorticism and an ovarian remnant (Figure 6-6).

Treatment options for adrenocortical disease include surgical or medical management. Surgical management has been well described, and it is a long-standing practice. Medical management is commonly performed using GnRH agonist drugs (which cause down-regulation of GnRH receptors [GnRHRs] in the adenohypophysis; see the HPG axis section below for further information). Comparison between surgical adrenalectomy and medical management with deslorelin implants has shown that deslorelin-treated ferrets had longer periods free of clinical signs (16.5 mo, *n* = 35) than surgical cases (13.6 mo, *n* = 54).[508] Recently, a new medical modality, a GnRH vaccine developed for wildlife species, has been used to treat ferret adrenal disease.[509] This medication provided relief from adrenal disease by causing production of antibodies to GnRH, probably suppressing production and/or release of LH.[509] The GnRH vaccine was more effective when administered to animals that had not developed overt clinical signs of adrenal disease.[509] However, many vaccinated animals with adrenal disease signs showed a clinical resolution, allowing

TABLE 6-5

Measurements of Ferret Adrenal Glands Using Ultrasonography

Side	Number	Length	Width	Depth or Thickness	Reference	Characteristics
Left	12 Ferrets	7.4 ± 1.0 mm	3.7 ± 0.4 mm	2.8 ± 0.4 mm	Neuwirth, et al. 1997[505]	Female
Right	12 Ferrets	7.5 ± 1.2 mm	3.7 ± 0.6 mm	2.8 ± 0.4 mm	Neuwirth, et al. 1997[505]	Female
Left	14 Ferrets	8.6 ± 1.2 mm	4.2 ± 0.6 mm	3.0 ± 0.6 mm	Neuwirth, et al. 1997[505]	Male
Right	14 Ferrets	8.9 ± 1.6 mm	3.8 ± 0.6 mm	3.0 ± 0.8 mm	Neuwirth, et al. 1997[505]	Male
Left	20 Ferrets	7.2 ± 1.8 mm	2.8 ± 0.5 mm		O'Brien, et al. 1996[506]	Healthy
Right	20 Ferrets	7.6 ± 1.8 mm	2.6 ± 0.4 mm		O'Brien, et al. 1996[506]	Healthy
Left	21 Glands	6.1 ± 1.0 mm		2.9 ± 0.5 mm	Kuijten, et al. 2007[507]	Healthy
Right	20 Glands	7.8 ± 1.4 mm		2.5 ± 0.6 mm	Kuijten, et al. 2007[507]	Healthy
Left	28 Glands	9.2 ± 3.2 mm		6.3 ± 3.0 mm	Kuijten, et al. 2007[507]	With hyperadrenocorticism
Right	19 Glands	8.5 ± 2.5 mm		5.2 ± 3.3 mm	Kuijten, et al. 2007[507]	With hyperadrenocorticism

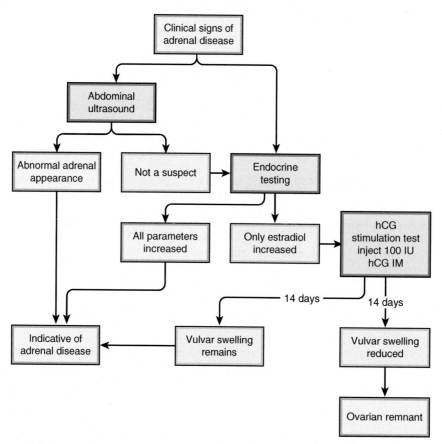

FIGURE 6-6 Practical flow chart of a possible differentiation method between hyperadrenocorticism and ovarian remnant in the female ferret.

ferrets to return to an acceptable quality of life.[497] It should be noted that injection site reactions were observed in some patients.[509] Although scientific validation is lacking, the use of GnRH agonists or GnRH vaccines early in a ferret's life may prevent occurrence of this disease altogether.

Hypertestosteronism secondary to adrenal neoplasia and hyperplasia, with increased sexual and aggressive behavior, has been reported in two older neutered rabbits.[510] It has been said that in normal rabbits, the adrenal glands secrete appreciable amounts of sex steroids.[510]

THE HYPOTHALAMIC-PITUITARY-GONADAL AXIS

The relationship between the endocrine system and the gonads starts during the animal's development and persists throughout life. The interests of endocrinologists in sex differentiation and development have long existed.[511] As mentioned in the introduction to this chapter, the birth of endocrinology occurred in 1891 with Charles Edouard Brown-Séquard, who proposed the concept of "internal secretions" (later known to be testosterone).[511] One of the first demonstrations of the relationship between the gonads and sexual differentiation was shown in a rooster. Berthold showed that rooster caponization would cause decreased comb size, reduced interest in hens, and reduced aggressive behaviors.[512,513] Those effects could be reversed with testicular reimplantation, even if denervated.[512] These internal secretions, provided by the gonads, were named sex hormones and were later divided into male hormones (controlling dependent male characteristics) and female hormones (controlling dependent female characteristics).[511]

Males of most vertebrate species have two testicles, and females have two ovaries, with birds being an exception since females of the majority of avian species have only one developed ovary. Both ovaries and oviducts are present during embryogenesis in birds; however, the left side continues to develop while the right side regresses. Species from a total of 16 avian orders have been reported to preserve bilateral ovaries and oviducts.[514,515] Female Cooper's hawks (*Accipiter cooperii*) have been said to have two ovaries but only a left oviduct.[516] Bilateral ovaries were detected in other species of hawks, but it was explained that in some of these animals, the right side reproductive tract was still undergoing regression.[516,517] Bilateral ovaries are more common in *Accipiter* spp. than in Stringiformes.[518] Kiwis have two functional ovaries, but only the left oviduct receives the follicles from both ovaries.[514,519] It was found that successful ovulation from either ovary, or from both ovaries alternately within the same laying season, is a normal occurrence.[514] If two follicles are growing simultaneously on separate ovaries, one will temporarily arrest growth at a 40- to 50-mm diameter to allow room in the body cavity for the formation of a single large egg.[514,519,520] Vestigial remnants of right oviducts were found in 3/51 kiwis.[514]

In many species of oviparous reptiles, gonadal sex differentiation depends on the incubation temperature of the eggs.[521] Temperature-dependent sex determination (TSD) occurs in crocodilians, the majority of turtles, some lizards, and the two species of *Sphenodon*.[521] In TSD reptiles, the embryo's sex is determined by the incubation temperature during the early and middle incubation period, not by sex chromosomes.[94] Feminization of the gonads by exogenous estrogens at a male-producing temperature, and masculinization of gonads by antiestrogens and aromatase inhibitors at a female-producing temperature, have demonstrated the involvement of estrogens in ovarian differentiation.[521]

In rats, there is a strong correlation between uterine disease and mammary gland tumor development in intact females, mainly after 1 year of age. In general terms, ovariohysterectomy or ovariectomy (depending on the age of the individual) is considered the treatment of choice for the prevention of uterine disease and mammary tumors.[522] It may also be part of the treatment plan for an animal suffering from these diseases.[522] In dogs, it is said that virtually all complications associated with performing ovariohysterectomy are due to the removal of the uterus.[523] Therefore, with the exception of animals suffering from uterine disease, ovariectomy should

be the treatment of choice, according to some authors.[522] The frequency of mammary tumors in ovariectomized rats is significantly lower than in sexually intact rats (2/47 vs. 24/49, respectively), as well as the frequency of pituitary adenomas (2/46 vs. 27/41, respectively).[524] In rats that are ovariectomized by 90 days of life, the incidence of mammary tumors and pituitary chromophobe tumors was 4%, while intact rats had an incidence of 47% (mammary tumors) and 66% (pituitary tumors).[522] Removal of ovaries before middle-age onset (~5 to 7 mo) inhibited development of spontaneous mammary tumors by 95%.[525] Only one mammary tumor was observed in 19 ovariectomized animals, while 47 tumors developed in 42 nonovariectomized animals.[525] Tumor incidence was reduced from 73.8% to 5.3%.[525] In a retrospective study assessing the effect of ovariohysterectomy and castration between 90 and 180 days in pet rats, the incidence of suspected or histopathology-confirmed mammary tumors in intact male and female rats combined was 24.8%, compared to 6.2% in the spayed and castrated rats combined.[526] Therefore, in this study, castration or ovariohysterectomy between 90 and 180 days had protective effects against the development of mammary tumors.[526] Surgical descriptions of ovariectomy and ovariohysterectomy have been previously published.[522,527] A study assessing the effects of ovariectomy in the serum levels of progesterone showed that in the ovariectomized rat, the progesterone remains in the systemic circulation for 25 days.[528,529] In order to decrease the progesterone levels, ovariectomy would have to be performed along with adrenalectomy.[528] In the ovariectomized rat, the ACTH controls the progesterone level; however, the ACTH does not have a direct effect on the ovarian progesterone.[528] Although the function of adrenal progesterone is not completely understood, some studies have suggested that adrenals and the placenta can maintain a pregnancy.[530] It is said that it is possible to support pregnancy from the blastocyst stage to full fetal development with steroid analogs that do not cross react in RIA of hormones being produced from the adrenal and placenta or the placenta alone.[530] Ovo-implantation in the guinea pig on the 6th to 7th day postcoitum was not affected by ovariectomy on days 3 to 7 postcoitum.[531] If the ovaries are removed on the 2nd day after mating, however, implantation did not occur unless at least one injection of progesterone was given.[531] In the ovariectomized guinea pigs, the embryos develop normally for several days but may regress after day 14 unless progesterone is supplied, permitting further growth.[531] No evidence was found of delayed implantation.[531] So, although very unlikely, it is important to consider that some small mammals may still remain physiologically capable of reproducing for a certain amount of time after ovariectomy.

Nevertheless, reproduction is regulated primarily by the HPG axis, which coordinates specific gonadal events by regulating circulating gonadotropins.[1] The hypothalamus produces GnRH, which stimulates the anterior pituitary to secrete FSH and LH.[3] It is possible that FSH and LH production is also influenced by a gonadotropin inhibitory hormone (GnIH), but such has not been well established.[1] GnRH is released in a pulsatile fashion, which is essential for normal release of LH and FSH.[3] For a few decades, it was thought that GnRH was a unique structure, with a primary role in regulating gonadotropin release; however, other homologous

TABLE 6-6

Summary of Generalized Hormone Actions in Mammalian Reproduction (Eutheria)

Hormone	Action in	
	Females	**Males**
GnRH	Stimulation of FSH and LH secretion	Stimulation of FSH and LH secretion
FSH	Initiation of follicle growth; conversion of androgen to estrogen; synthesis of inhibin and P450aro	Initiation of spermatogenesis; secretion of androgen-binding protein, STP, and inhibin by Sertoli cells; conversion of androgen to estrogen by Sertoli cells
LH	Androgen synthesis; ovulation; formation of corpus luteum from granulosa; secretion of progesterone initiated in corpus luteum	Androgen secretion by interstitial cells (Leydig)
Prolactin	Synthesis of milk	Stimulation of certain sex accessory structures (with androgen)
Oxytocin	Contraction of uterine smooth muscle; menstrual sloughing; birth; orgasm; milk ejection from mammary	Ejaculation of sperm; orgasm
Androgens	Precursors for estrogen synthesis; stimulation of sexual behavior	Completion of FSH-initiated spermatogenesis; stimulation of prostate gland and other sex accessory structures; stimulation of secondary sexual characters, such as beard growth in man
Estrogens	Stimulates proliferation of endometrium; induces LH surge; sensitizes uterus to oxytocin; role in negative feedback on pituitary release; may be primate luteolytic factor (estrone); may induce PRL surge; maintains pregnancy	Conversions from androgens; induces male hypothalamus; stimulates sexual behavior
Progesterone	Maintains secretory phase of uterus; inhibits release of gonadotropins from adenohypophysis; maintains pregnancy	
Prostaglandins	Causes corpus luteum to degenerate at end of luteal phase (not in primate); may be involved in birth initiation (induction of labor)	Ejaculation
Relaxin	Softens pelvic ligaments and cervix; possible role in lactation	
Chorionic gonadotropin	Stimulates corpus luteum to produce progesterone	
Chorionic somatomammotropin	Stimulates mammary gland to synthesize milk during late pregnancy; GH-like (somatotropin) actions on metabolism	
Inhibin (Sertoli cell factor, folliculostatin)	Inhibits FSH secretion from pituitary	Inhibits FSH secretion from pituitary

FSH, Follicle-stimulating hormone; *GH,* growth hormone; *GnRH,* gonadotropin-releasing hormone; *LH,* luteinizing hormone; *P450$_{aro}$,* P450-aromatase; *PRL,* prolactin.
From Norris DO, Carr JA, eds. *Vertebrate Endocrinology.* 5th ed. Amsterdam: Academic Press, Elsevier; 2013.

ligands of the GnRHR exist.[532] More than 20 natural variants of mammalian GnRH have been identified in different species, which may compete for binding and/or have their own receptors.[532] These GnRH forms have apparently common and divergent functions.[532] If GnRH is released in large amounts, the GnRHRs are down-regulated, leading to a cessation of LH production.[3] Depending on the animal gender, FSH and LH will have different effects. General effects of different hormones involved in mammalian reproduction are summarized in Table 6-6.

Medical Management of the HPG Axis

Due to the cascade of events controlled by the HPG axis and the presence of negative feedback control, medical

management of disease or abnormal activity of this endocrine pathway becomes possible, with the most common drugs used being those that cause extensive negative feedback and thus stop final production of gonadal steroid precursors in the adrenal glands or those in the gonads themselves.

It is a physiologic response to decrease production of hormones, if such hormones are present in the body. Therefore, if a chemically GnRH-like drug is provided exogenously, the hypothalamus will stop or endogenously decrease producing GnRH. Drugs that have this effect are called GnRH agonists, because they have an affinity for GnRHRs. GnRH agonists are derived from native GnRH by substitution of a D-amino acid for the native L-amino acid at position 6 in the decapeptide.[533] In normal physiologic conditions, the anterior pituitary requires pulsatile stimulation by GnRH to synthesize and appropriately release the gonadotropins LH and FSH.[534] Agonists of GnRH are delivered in a continuous mode to turn off reproductive function by inhibiting gonadotropin production in a normal pulsatile fashion, thus lowering sex steroid production, resulting in medical castration.[534,535] It is important to mention that administration of a GnRH agonist causes an initial agonistic action, or the "flare" response, followed by down-regulation of GnRHRs. The flare response occurs because of the release of preexisting gonadotropins already stored in the pituitary.[533] Such agonists are characterized by poor pharmacokinetic properties, often requiring repeated administration or special formulations.[536] Hormonal or chemical castration using GnRHR agonists became a well-established strategy for the treatment of hormone-dependent cancers.[536] The two most commonly used GnRHR agonists in exotic animal medicine are deslorelin and leuprolide. Leuprolide acetate is a synthetic peptide available in multiple commercial formulations. Daily injections of leuprolide acetate were first introduced for the palliative treatment of advanced human prostate cancer in 1985, with the depot formulation later being developed to reduce the need for regular injections.[537] Leuprolide is used to treat a wide range of sex-hormone-related disorders in humans, including advanced prostatic cancer, endometriosis, and precocious puberty.[538] Leuprolide acetate acts primarily on the anterior pituitary, leading to a transient early rise in gonadotropin release; however, with continued use or continuous release, as discussed above, leuprolide causes pituitary desensitization and/or down-regulation, leading to suppressed circulating levels of gonadotropins and sex hormones.[539] For its use in humans, this compound has been formulated as a depot formulation (1, 3, and 4 mo) to provide long-term treatment for reproductive diseases.[540] The hydrophilic leuprorelin is held in biodegradable highly lipophilic synthetic polymer microspheres, allowing for release over a defined length of time depending on the polymer used.[540] This drug has also been used and studied in exotic animals. The use of leuprolide has been assessed in ferrets for the treatment of adrenal disease, the treatment of ovarian cysts in guinea pigs, and the control of excessive/abnormal egg laying and ovarian neoplasia.[541-545] The use of leuprolide in ferrets has alleviated clinical signs associated with adrenal gland disease.[546] Although no scientific study has been published, it appears that leuprolide may be useful for the treatment of ovarian cysts in guinea pigs.[542] Effects of leuprolide on plasma androstenedione, plasma 17β-estradiol, and fecal 17β-estradiol were assessed in Hispaniolan Amazon parrots, which led to the decrease of plasma sex hormones for <21 days.[547] In female cockatiels, treatment with leuprolide resulted in delayed egg laying for 12 to 19 days.[541] In pigeons, no effect on egg laying or sex hormone levels was detected at tested doses.[548] In chickens, leuprolide induced molt and decreased progesterone, which was indicative of ovarian regression.[549] Leuprolide has been experimentally used in male iguanas to decrease testosterone levels, but at tested doses, no effect was detected.[550] However, there has been anecdotal evidence of leuprolide treatment reducing aggression in male iguanas.[540] One report of presumptive anaphylactic shock was reported in two elf owls (*Micrathene whitneyi*) after the administration of leuprolide acetate.[541]

Deslorelin, a synthetic GnRH analog that differs from natural GnRH in its amino acid sequence by having D-tryptophan in position 6 rather than glycine and proethylamide rather than glycineamide at position 9, is believed to be 10 times more potent than the naturally occurring compound.[552] Although deslorelin is more often used in animals than humans, some attention has been given to this compound for human medicine.[553,554] Deslorelin implants are commercially available in different countries as a 4.7- or 9.4-mg slow-release long-acting SC implant, and a number of research investigations have been completed using this drug on exotic animal species.[552] This medication is available as an SC implant that provides treatment over a period of time, capable of postponing estrus in bitches and suppressing reproductive function in dogs.[555] Deslorelin has been well studied for the treatment of adrenal disease in ferrets and appears to be a promising treatment to temporarily resolve clinical signs and decrease plasma steroid hormone concentrations; nonetheless, it may not decrease tumor growth in some cases.[556] It is reported that a 4.7-mg deslorelin implant placed subcutaneously caused cessation of clinical signs in clinically affected ferrets for 13.7 ± 3.5 months (range 8.5 to 20.5 mo, $n = 15$) and 17.6 ± 5 mo (range 8 to 30 mo, $n = 30$).[556,557] Comparison between surgical adrenalectomy and medical management with deslorelin showed that deslorelin-treated ferrets remained free of clinical signs for longer periods (16.5 mo, $n = 35$) than that in surgical cases (13.6 mo, $n = 54$).[508] Deslorelin implants have been compared with medroxyprogesterone (MPA), proligestone, and hCG.[558] Deslorelin caused treatment-induced ovarian quiescence of 698 ± 122 days in 5 female ferrets, while MPA caused 94 ± 18 days, proligestone 99 ± 40 days, and hCG 53 ± 9 days.[558] Deslorelin implants are considered a viable alternative to the physical neutering of ferrets.[559]

Common conditions in guinea pigs related to the HPG axis are ovarian cysts. Ovarian serous cystadenoma or cystic rete ovarii is often diagnosed. Reports of ovarian cysts in guinea pigs between 3 months and 5 years of age indicate that 66% to 75% of sows are affected.[560] Ovarian cysts are also common in aged rats, cattle, and women.[561] Ovarian cysts are classified by either their location of origin (periovarian or intraovarian) or according to cause (physiologic, infectious, or neoplastic).[545] The rete ovarii is a network of tubules and cords that arises from the mesonephros, which is homologous with the rete testis of male mammals.[545] Tubules begin in the periovarian tissue, enter the ovary at the hilus, and spread to varying degrees throughout the ovary, which is divided into 3 sections: extraovarian rete, intraovarian rete, and connecting rete.[545] In general, five types of cysts can be found in the ovaries of various laboratory animal species: (1) follicular, (2) luteal, (3) inclusion, (4) parovarian, and (5) those of the rete ovarii.[561] In guinea pigs, classification criteria for atretic follicles have been suggested: (1) the granulosa layer became loose, and some apoptotic bodies began to appear; (2) granulosa cells were massively eliminated; (3) theca interna cells differentiated; and (4) the residual follicular cells degenerated.[562]

In guinea pigs, as in most mammals, follicles start to develop simultaneously, but most become atretic.[563] During the luteal phase of the estrous cycle, two waves of follicular growth are initiated, and although most become atretic, a few gain dominance and, toward the end of the luteal phase, ovulate.[563] The mature follicle continues to develop and produces steroids (estradiol, testosterone, and progesterone).[545] The cyst may eventually become nonsteroidogenic, allowing the normal ovulatory cycle to resume.[545]

Between days 13 and 15 of the guinea pig estrous cycle, low serum progesterone levels and rising utero-ovarian blood flow and serum estrogen levels occur, resulting from a dramatic increase in the number of viable follicles.[564] As viable follicles increase, the number of atretic follicles in each size population decreases.[564] It is suggested that as luteal activity declines during the last half of the estrous cycle, follicular recruitment and growth are stimulated.[564] Concomitant elevations in ovarian blood flow have a supportive role in follicular development, while the subsequent elevation in serum estrogen serves as an index of follicular maturation.[564]

The use of deslorelin (4.7 mg, SC) in guinea pigs did not cause a significant change in cyst size ($n = 7$).[565] It is said that localization and physiologic activity of GnRH and its receptors may be unique in guinea pigs.[566] However, in another study, guinea pigs that received SC deslorelin implants developed altered estrous signs: the average time to opening of the vaginal membrane was delayed; after opening, vaginas were found to be variably opened and closed; a significant reduction in progesterone and cessation of progesterone cyclical variation was observed; and plasma estrogen remained high during the whole experimental period.[567] This study showed that cessation of the estrous cycle by the deslorelin implant might be useful in preventing pregnancy in guinea pigs.[567] Limited studies of the use of deslorelin in other exotic mammalian species are available, and in rabbits only one case is known. A male rabbit received a 4.7-mg deslorelin implant subcutaneously for reproductive control.[568] For 7 months, testosterone levels decreased significantly, after which the hormone levels became elevated.[568] Female rats with 4.7-mg deslorelin SC implants ($n = 3$) reproduced for a period of only 1 year, while the control group ($n = 1$) had 100% reproductive success for a longer period of time.[569] It is thought that long-term deslorelin implants in rats may interfere with normal female cyclicity, thus affecting the preantral follicle population.[566]

Deslorelin has also been investigated in pigeons, chickens, and quail. In Japanese quail ($n = 20$), 4.7 mg deslorelin (SC) caused a reversible decrease in egg laying for ~70 days.[570] In chickens, a 4.7-mg implant (SC) caused egg-laying inhibition for 180 days (range 125 to 237, $n = 10$), while a 9.4-mg implant (SC) caused egg-laying inhibition of at least 357 days ($n = 10$; incomplete study at the time of submission).[571] A 4.7-mg implant (IM) in pigeons ($n = 10$ males and 10 females) was shown to be effective in controlling egg laying for 49 days and decreased serum LH levels for at least 84 days in females and at least 56 days in males.[572] Although deslorelin implants are commonly placed subcutaneously, in the above-mentioned pigeon study, the implant was placed intramuscularly and a relatively short effect was reported (compared to other studies). The absorption of the pharmaceutical, its route of administration, and pharmacokinetics will certainly influence the activity of this compound.

Clinical use of deslorelin implants for the control of reproductive behavior or reproductive neoplasia has been reported by several authors.[542,552,573] However, it is important to remember that GnRH appears to vary among animal species, which may have an influence on the different responses reported with GnRH agonists. At least eight forms of GnRHRs have been characterized among vertebrates, and several classes of vertebrates have two or more forms of GnRH.[574] In birds, several GnRH chemical forms have also been identified, including a chicken GnRH-I and chicken GnRH-II.[575] It has been shown that ostriches have a possible third form of GnRH found in hypothalamic and extrahypothalamic brain tissues.[576] It has been suggested that the chicken GnRH-II peptide is phylogenetically old. Despite the presence of chicken GnRH-II across many species and phyla, including mammals, its function is still unclear.[575] As an example, a chicken GnRH-II-like molecule has been identified in stump-tailed macaque (*Macaca arctoides*) and rhesus macaque (*Macaca mulatta*); however, its function is unknown.[577] In white-crowned sparrows (*Zonotrichia leucophrys*), it is suggested that both GnRH molecules have a behavior role; however, it seems that the influence of each type is independent of the other.[578] A GnIH has been isolated from the quail.[579,580] A published report states that GnIH interacts with GnRH to time release of gonadotropins and thus time-reproductive activity in birds and mammals.[581] It is unclear whether natural differences among species and responses to synthetic GnRH agonists may be related to the presence or absence of different GnRH molecules.

There is only one clinical case report of the use of a deslorelin implant (4.7 mg, SC) in reptiles: an inland bearded dragon for aggression control. A significant decrease in blood testosterone levels was determined at 2 months postimplant, and the owner reported decreased aggressive behavior over that period of time.[582]

ACKNOWLEDGMENT

The authors thank Dr. Larry R. Engelking for his thoughtful comments on the manuscript.

REFERENCES

1. Norris DO. *Vertebrate Endocrinology*. 4th ed. San Diego: Academic Press; 2007.
2. Capen CC. Tumors of the endocrine glands. In: *Tumors in Domestic Animals*. Ames, IA: Iowa State Press; 2008:607-696.
3. Engelking L, Rebar AH. *Metabolic and Endocrine Physiology*. Jackson, WY: CRC Press; 2012.
4. Starling EH. The Croonian Lectures on the chemical correlation of the functions of the body. *Lancet*. 1905;166:339-341.
5. Parkhill T. One hundred years of hormones. *Science in Parliament*. 2005;6(6):62.
6. Marty MS, Carney EW, Rowlands JC. Endocrine disruption: historical perspectives and its impact on the future of toxicology testing. *Toxicol Sci*. 2011;120(suppl 1):S93-S108.
7. Fisher DA. A short history of pediatric endocrinology in North America. *Pediatr Res*. 2004;55:716-726.
8. Medvei VC. *A History of Endocrinology*. Hingham, MA: Springer; 1982.
9. Medvei VC. Prehistoric times. In: *A History of Endocrinology*. Hingham, MA: Springer; 1982:11-13.
10. Borell M. Organotherapy, British physiology, and discovery of the internal secretions. *J Hist Biol*. 1976;9(2):235-268.
11. Wilson JD. The evolution of endocrinology. *Clin Endocrinol (Oxf)*. 2005;62:389-396.

12. Brown-Séquard CE. The effects produced in men by the injection of extracts of the testes of guinea pigs and dogs. *Compte Rendu Societe Biol.* 1899;1:415-419.
13. Brown-Séquard CE. The effects produced on man by subcutaneous injections of a liquid obtained from the testicules of animals. *Lancet.* 1899;2:105-107.
14. Cussons AJ, Bhagat CI, Fletcher SJ, et al. Brown-Sequard revisited: a lesson from history on the placebo effect of androgen treatment. *Med J Aust.* 2002;177:678-679.
15. Freeman ER, Bloom DA, McGuire EJ. A brief history of testosterone. *J Urol.* 2001;165:371-373.
16. Daniel PM. Anatomy of the hypothalamus and pituitary gland. *J Clin Pathol Suppl (Assoc Clin Pathol).* 1976;7:1-7.
17. Hofman MA, Swaab DF. The human hypothalamus: comparative morphometry and photoperiodic influences. *Prog Brain Res.* 1992;93:133-147, discussion 148-139.
18. Lumeij JT. Endocrinology. In: Ritchie BW, Harrison GJ, Harrison LR, eds. *Avian Medicine: Principles and Application.* Lake Worth, FL: Wingers Publishing; 1994:582-606.
19. Norris DO, Carr JA, eds. *Vertebrate Endocrinology.* 5th ed. Amsterdam: Academic Press, Elsevier; 2013.
20. Gorbman A. Comparative anatomy and physiology of the anterior pituitary. *Q Rev Biol.* 1941;16:294-310.
21. Ball JN, Baker BI. The pituitary gland: anatomy and histophysiology. In: Hoar WS, Randall DJ, eds. *Fish Physiology.* Vol 2. New York: Academic Press; 1969;1-3.
22. Goodman HM. Pituitary gland. In: Goodman HM, ed. *Basic Medical Endocrinology.* China: Academic Press; 2010:29.
23. Herring P. Further observations upon the comparative anatomy and physiology of the pituitary body. *Exp Physiol.* 1913;6:73-108.
24. Gentes L. Recherches sur L'Hypophyse et le Sac Vasculaire des Vertebres: Féret et Fils, 1907.
25. Ritchie M. Neuroanatomy and physiology of the avian hypothalamic/pituitary axis: clinical aspects. *Vet Clin North Am Exot Anim Pract.* 2014;17:13-22.
26. Scanes CG. Introduction to endocrinology: pituitary gland. In: Whittow GC, ed. *Sturkie's Avian Physiology.* 5th ed. San Diego: Academic Press; 2000:437-460.
27. Silman R, Chard T, Lowry P, et al. Human foetal pituitary peptides and parturition. *Nature.* 1976;260(5553):716-718.
28. Rahn H, Painter BT. A comparative histology of the bird pituitary. *Anat Rec.* 1941;79:297-311.
29. Kleinholz LH, Rahn H. The distribution of intermedin in the pars anterior of the chicken pituitary. *Proc Natl Acad Sci.* 1939;25:145-147.
30. Iturriza FC, Estivariz FE, Levitin HP. Coexistence of α-melanocyte-stimulating hormone and adrenocorticotrophin in all cells containing either of the two hormones in the duck pituitary. *Gen Comp Endocrinol.* 1980;42:110-115.
31. Castro MG, Estivariz FE, Iturriza FC. The regulation of the corticomelanotropic cell activity in aves. III—effect of various peptides on the release of MSH from dispersed, perfused duck pituitary cells. Cosecretion of ACTH with MSH. *Comp Biochem Physiol C.* 1988;91:389-393.
32. Hayashi H, Imai K, Imai K. Characterization of chicken ACTH and α-MSH: The primary sequence of chicken ACTH is more similar to *Xenopus* ACTH than to other avian ACTH. *Gen Comp Endocrinol.* 1991;82:434-443.
33. Panin M, Giurisato M, Peruffo A, et al. Immunofluorescence evidence of melanotrophs in the pituitary of four odontocete species. An immunohistochemical study and a critical review of the literature. *Ann Anat.* 2013;195:512-521.
34. Takeuchi S, Takahashi S, Okimoto R, et al. Avian melanocortin system: α-MSH may act as an autocrine/paracrine hormone. *Ann NY Acad Sci.* 2003;994:366-372.
35. Welbourn RB. *The History of Endocrine Surgery.* New York, NY: Praeger Publishing; 1990.
36. Hubble D. The endocrine orchestra. *Br Med J.* 1961;1:523-528.
37. Heller H, Pickering BT. Neurohypophysial hormones of non-mammalian vertebrates. *J Physiol.* 1961;155:98-114.
38. Henschen F. On the term diabetes in the works of Aretaeus and Galen. *Med Hist.* 1969;13:190-192.
39. Eknoyan G. A history of diabetes insipidus: paving the road to internal water balance. *Am J Kidney Dis.* 2010;56:1175-1183.
40. Rowntree LG. The differential diagnosis of polyuria, with special reference to diabetes insipidus. *Med Clin North Am.* 1921;5:439-453.
41. Frank E. Uber beziehungen der hypophyse zum diabetes insipidus. *Berl Klin Wochenschr.* 1912;9:1-15.
42. Sever MS, Namal A, Eknoyan G. Erich Frank (1884-1957): unsung pioneer in nephrology. *Am J Kidney Dis.* 2011;58:654-665.
43. Rice GE. Plasma arginine vasotocin concentrations in the lizard *Varanus gouldii* (gray) following water loading, salt loading, and dehydration. *Gen Comp Endocrinol.* 1982;47:1-6.
44. Ervin MG, Amico JA, Leake RD, et al. Arginine vasotocin and a novel oxytocin-vasotocin-like material in plasma of human newborns. *Biol Neonate.* 1988;53:17-22.
45. Starkey SR, Wood C, de Matos R, et al. Central diabetes insipidus in an African grey parrot. *J Am Vet Med Assoc.* 2010;237:415-419.
46. Rijnberk A. Diabetes insipidus. In: Ettinger SJ, Feldman EC, eds. *Textbook of Veterinary Internal Medicine: Diseases of the Dog and the Cat.* St. Louis, MO: Elsevier/Saunders; 2010:1502-1507.
47. Aroch I, Mazaki-Tovi M, Shemesh O, et al. Central diabetes insipidus in five cats: clinical presentation, diagnosis and oral desmopressin therapy. *J Feline Med Surg.* 2005;7:333-339.
48. Al-Tubaikh JA. Diabetes insipidus. In: *Internal Medicine: An Illustrated Radiological Guide.* Berlin: Springer; 2010:370-372.
49. Burnie A, Dunn J. A case of central diabetes insipidus in the cat: diagnosis and treatment. *J Small Anim Pract.* 1982;23:237-241.
50. Court MH, Watson ADJ. Idiopathic neurogenic diabetes insipidus in a cat. *Aust Vet J.* 1983;60:245-247.
51. Green R, Farrow C. Diabetes insipidus in a cat. *J Am Vet Med Assoc.* 1974;164:524.
52. Pittari JM. Central diabetes insipidus in a cat. *Feline Pract.* 1996;24:18.
53. Winterbotham J, Mason KV. Congenital diabetes insipidus in a kitten. *J Small Anim Pract.* 1983;24:569-573.
54. Smith J, Elwood C. Traumatic partial hypopituitarism in a cat. *J Small Anim Pract.* 2004;45:405-409.
55. Rogers W, Valdez H, Anderson B, et al. Partial deficiency of antidiuretic hormone in a cat. *J Am Vet Med Assoc.* 1977;170:545-547.
56. Campbell F, Bredhauer B. Trauma-induced central diabetes insipidus in a cat. *Aust Vet J.* 2005;83:732-735.
57. Foley C, Bracker K, Drellich S. Hypothalamic-pituitary axis deficiency following traumatic brain injury in a dog. *J Vet Emerg Crit Care.* 2009;19:269-274.
58. Oliveira KM, Fukushima FB, Oliveira CM, et al. Head trauma as a possible cause of central diabetes insipidus in a cat. *J Feline Med Surg.* 2013;15:155-159.
59. Simpson CJ, Mansfield CS, Milne ME, et al. Central diabetes insipidus in a cat with central nervous system B cell lymphoma. *J Feline Med Surg.* 2011;13:787-792.
60. Lee KI, Park HM. Central diabetic insipidus associated with suspected pituitary gland tumor in a dog. *Korean J Vet Res.* 2011;51:319-323.
61. Greco DS. Pituitary deficiencies. *Topics Compan Anim Med.* 2012;27:2-7.
62. Bichet DG. Nephrogenic diabetes insipidus. *Am J Med.* 1998;105:431-442.
63. Roberts KE. Mechanism of dehydration following alcohol ingestion. *Arch Intern Med.* 1963;112:154-157.
64. Wright J. 6 Endocrine effects of alcohol. *Clin Endocrinol Metab.* 1978;7:351-367.

65. Swift R, Davidson D. Alcohol hangover. *Alcohol Health Res World.* 1998;22:54-60.

66. Feldman EC, Nelson RW. *Canine and Feline Endocrinology and Reproduction.* 3rd ed. St. Louis, MO: Elsevier Health Sciences; 2004.

67. Nishimura H. Urine concentration and avian aquaporin water channels. *Pflugers Arch.* 2008;456:755-768.

68. Braun EJ, Stallone JN. The occurrence of nephrogenic diabetes insipidus in domestic fowl. *Am J Physiol.* 1989;256:F639-F645.

69. Minvielle F, Grossmann R, Gourichon D. Development and performances of a Japanese quail line homozygous for the diabetes insipidus *(di)* mutation. *Poult Sci.* 2007;86:249-254.

70. Dunson WA, Buss EG, Sawyer WH, et al. Hereditary polydipsia and polyuria in chickens. *Am J Physiol.* 1972;222:1167-1176.

71. Kuenzel WJ, Helms CW. Hyperphagia, polydipsia, and other effects of hypothalamic lesions in the white-throated sparrow, *Zonotrichia albicollis. Condor.* 1970;72:66-75.

72. Barsanti JA. Diagnostic approach to polyuria and polydipsia. In: Bonagura JD, ed. *Current Veterinary Therapy XIII.* Philadelphia: W.B. Saunders; 2000:831.

73. Bartholomew GA, Cade TJ. The water economy of land birds. *The Auk.* 1963;80:504-539.

74. Orosz SE. Clinical avian nutrition. *Vet Clin North Am Exot Anim Pract.* 2014;17:397-413.

75. Lumeij JT. Nephrology. In: Ritchie BW, Harrison GJ, Harrison LR, eds. *Avian Medicine: Principles and Application.* Lake Worth, FL: Wingers Publishing; 1994:538-555.

76. Goldstein DL, Braun EJ. Contributions of the kidneys and intestines to water conservation, and plasma levels of antidiuretic hormone, during dehydration in house sparrows *(Passer domesticus). J Comp Physiol B.* 1988;158:353-361.

77. Duke GE, Ciganek JG, Evanson OA. Food consumption and energy, water, and nitrogen budgets in captive great-horned owls *(Bubo virginianus). Comp Biochem Physiol A Comp Physiol.* 1973;44: 283-292.

78. Martin HD, Kollias GV. Evaluation of water deprivation and fluid therapy in pigeons. *J Zoo Wildl Med.* 1989;20:173-177.

79. Alberts H, Halsema WB, de Bruijne JJ, et al. A water deprivation test for the differentiation of polyuric disorders in birds. *Avian Pathol.* 1988;17:385-389.

80. Guzman D. Renal disease. In: Mayer J, Donnelly TM, eds. *Clinical Veterinary Advisor, Birds and Exotic Pets. 1: Clinical Veterinary Advisor.* Philadelphia: Elsevier Health Sciences; 2013:228-229.

81. Brock AP, Grunkemeyer VL, Fry MM, et al. Comparison of osmolality and refractometric readings of Hispaniolan Amazon parrot *(Amazona ventralis)* urine. *J Avian Med Surg.* 2013;27: 264-268.

82. Kurien BT, Everds NE, Scofield RH. Experimental animal urine collection: a review. *Lab Anim.* 2004;38:333-361.

83. Lumeij J, Westerhof I. The use of the water deprivation test for the diagnosis of apparent psychogenic polydipsia in a socially deprived African grey parrot *(Psittacus erithacus erithacus). Avian Pathol.* 1988;17:875-878.

84. Cheng K, Friesen H, Martin J. Neurophysin in rats with hereditary hypothalamic diabetes insipidus (Brattleboro strain). *Endocrinology.* 1972;90:1055-1063.

85. Kalimo H, Rinne U. Ultrastructural studies on the hypothalamic neurosecretory neurons of the rat. II. The hypothalamo-neurohypophysial system in rats with hereditary hypothalamic diabetes insipidus. *Z Zellforsch Mikrosk Anat.* 1972;134(2):205-225.

86. Boorman GA, Bree MM. Diabetes insipidus syndrome in a rabbit. *J Am Vet Med Assoc.* 1969;155:1218-1220.

87. Potter MP, Borkowski GL. Apparent psychogenic polydipsia and secondary polyuria in laboratory-housed New Zealand White rabbits. *J Am Assoc Lab Anim Sci.* 1998;37:87-89.

88. Kutscher CL, Stillman RD, Weiss IP. Food-deprivation polydipsia in gerbils *(Meriones unguiculatus). Physiol Behav.* 1968;3:667-671.

89. Dadone LI, Klaphake E, Garner MM, et al. Pituitary cystadenoma, enterolipidosis, and cutaneous mycosis in an Everglades ratsnake *(Elaphe obsoleta rossalleni). J Zoo Wildl Med.* 2010;41:538-541.

90. Linn MJ, McNamara T, Seinberg JJ, et al. Pituitary adenoma in a black-headed python *(Aspidites melanocephalus). Proc Am Assoc Zoo Vet Annu Meet.* 1996;1996:449.

91. Gyimesi SS, Garner MM. Pituitary adenoma in a Dumeril's ground boa, *Acrantophis dumerili. J Herpetol Med Surg.* 2007;17:16-18.

92. Reavill DR. Tumors of pet birds. *Vet Clin North Am Exot Anim Pract.* 2004;7:537-560.

93. Romagnano A, Mashima TY, Barnes HJ, et al. Pituitary adenoma in an Amazon parrot. *J Avian Med Surg.* 1995;9(4):263-270.

94. O'Malley B. *Clinical Anatomy and Physiology of Exotic Species.* London: W.B. Saunders; 2005.

95. Schlumberger HG. Neoplasia in the parakeet. I. Spontaneous chromophobe pituitary tumors. *Cancer Res.* 1954;14:237-245.

96. Schlumberger HG. Tumors characteristic for certain animal species: a review. *Cancer Res.* 1957;17:823-832.

97. Dezfoulian O, Abbasi M, Azarabad H, et al. Cerebral neuroblastoma and pituitary adenocarcinoma in two budgerigars *(Melopsittacus undulatus). Avian Dis.* 2011;55:704-708.

98. Wheler C. Pituitary tumors in cockatiels. *J Assoc Avian Vet.* 1992;6:92.

99. Curtis-Velasco M. Pituitary adenoma in a cockatiel *(Nymphicus hollandicus). J Assoc Avian Vet.* 1992;6:21-22.

100. Langohr IM, Garner MM, Kiupel M. Somatotroph pituitary tumors in budgerigars *(Melopsittacus undulatus). Vet Pathol.* 2012;49:503-507.

101. Lipman NS, Zhao ZB, Andrutis KA, et al. Prolactin-secreting pituitary adenomas with mammary dysplasia in New Zealand White rabbits. *Lab Anim Sci.* 1994;44:114-120.

102. Sikoski P, Trybus J, Cline JM, et al. Cystic mammary adenocarcinoma associated with a prolactin-secreting pituitary adenoma in a New Zealand White rabbit *(Oryctolagus cuniculus). Comp Med.* 2008;58:297-300.

103. Schoemaker NJ, van der Hage MH, Flik G, et al. Morphology of the pituitary gland in ferrets *(Mustela putorius furo)* with hyperadrenocorticism. *J Comp Pathol.* 2004;130:255-265.

104. Richardson VCG. *Diseases of Small Domestic Rodents.* 2nd ed. Oxford, UK; Malden, MA: Blackwell Publishing; 2003.

105. McComb DJ, Kovacs K, Beri J, et al. Pituitary adenomas in old Sprague-Dawley rats: a histologic, ultrastructural, and immunocytochemical study. *J Natl Cancer Inst.* 1984;73:1143-1166.

106. Burek JD. *Pathology of Geriatric Rats: A Morphological and Experimental Study of the Age-Associated Lesions in Aging BN/Bi, WAG/Rij, and (WAG × BN)F b1 s Rats.* West Palm Beach, FL: CRC Press; 1978.

107. Walsh K, Poteracki J. Spontaneous neoplasms in control Wistar rats. *Toxicol Sci.* 1994;22:65-72.

108. Poteracki J, Walsh KM. Spontaneous neoplasms in control Wistar rats: a comparison of reviews. *Toxicol Sci.* 1998;45:1-8.

109. Son WC, Gopinath C. Early occurrence of spontaneous tumors in CD-1 mice and Sprague-Dawley rats. *Toxicol Pathol.* 2004;32: 371-374.

110. Son WC, Bell D, Taylor I, et al. Profile of early occurring spontaneous tumors in Han Wistar rats. *Toxicol Pathol.* 2010;38: 292-296.

111. Magnusson G, Majeed SK, Gopinath C. Infiltrating pituitary neoplasms in the rat. *Lab Anim.* 1979;13:111-113.

112. Mayer J, Sato A, Kiupel M, et al. Extralabel use of cabergoline in the treatment of a pituitary adenoma in a rat. *J Am Vet Med Assoc.* 2011;239:656-660.

113. Gillam MP, Molitch ME, Lombardi G, et al. Advances in the treatment of prolactinomas. *Endocr Rev.* 2006;27:485-534.

114. Fitzgerald P, Dinan TG. Prolactin and dopamine: what is the connection? A review article. *J Psychopharmacol.* 2008;22:12-19.

115. Ben-Jonathan N, Hnasko R. Dopamine as a prolactin (PRL) inhibitor. *Endocrin Rev.* 2001;22:724-763.

116. Webster J. Clinical management of prolactinomas. *Best Pract Res Clin Endocrinol Metab*. 1999;13:395-408.

117. Yen PM. Physiological and molecular basis of thyroid hormone action. *Physiol Rev*. 2001;81:1097-1142.

118. Zhang J, Lazar MA. The mechanism of action of thyroid hormones. *Annu Rev Physiol*. 2000;62:439-466.

119. Noble KA. Thyroid storm. *J Perianesth Nurs*. 2006;21:119-122, quiz 123-115.

120. Westgren U, Melander A, Wåhlin E, et al. Divergent effects of 6-propylthiouracil on 3,5,3′-triiodothyronine (T₃) and 3,3′,5′-triiodothyronine (RT₃) serum levels in man. *Acta Endocrinologica*. 1977;85:345-350.

121. Little JW. Thyroid disorders. Part I: hyperthyroidism. *Oral Surg Oral Med Oral Pathol Oral Radiol Endod*. 2006;101:276-284.

122. Mazzaferri EL, Amdur RJ. Thyroid and parathyroid physiology. In: Amdur RJ, Mazzaferri EL, eds. *Essentials of Thyroid Cancer Management*. Berlin: Springer; 2005:7-17.

123. McNabb FMA. Thyroids. In: Scanes CG, ed. *Sturkie's Avian Physiology*. San Diego: Academic Press; 2015:535-547.

124. Spitzweg C, Morris JC. The sodium iodide symporter: its pathophysiological and therapeutic implications. *Clin Endocrinol (Oxf)*. 2002;57:559-574.

125. Ferguson DC. Testing for hypothyroidism in dogs. *Vet Clin North Am Small Anim Pract*. 2007;37:647-669, v.

126. Allain TJ, McGregor AM. Thyroid hormones and bone. *J Endocrinol*. 1993;139:9-18.

127. Duncan Bassett J, Williams GR. The molecular actions of thyroid hormone in bone. *Trends Endocrinol Metab*. 2003;14:356-364.

128. Gogakos AI, Duncan Bassett J, Williams GR. Thyroid and bone. *Arch Biochem Biophys*. 2010;503:129-136.

129. Klein I, Ojamaa K. Thyroid hormone and the cardiovascular system. *N Engl J Med*. 2001;344:501-509.

130. Kahaly GJ, Dillmann WH. Thyroid hormone action in the heart. *Endocr Rev*. 2005;26:704-728.

131. Biondi B, Palmieri EA, Lombardi G, et al. Effects of subclinical thyroid dysfunction on the heart. *Ann Intern Med*. 2002;137:904-914.

132. Carrero JJ, Qureshi AR, Axelsson J, et al. Clinical and biochemical implications of low thyroid hormone levels (total and free forms) in euthyroid patients with chronic kidney disease. *J Intern Med*. 2007;262:690-701.

133. Cappola AR, Fried LP, Arnold AM, et al. Thyroid status, cardiovascular risk, and mortality in older adults. *JAMA*. 2006;295:1033-1041.

134. Haarburger D. Thyroid disease: thyroid function tests and interpretation. *Contin Med Ed*. 2012;30(7):241-243.

135. Chopra IJ. Euthyroid sick syndrome: is it a misnomer? *J Clin Endocrinol Metab*. 1997;82:329-334.

136. McDermott MT. *Endocrine Secrets*. 6th ed. Philadelphia: Elsevier Health Sciences; 2013.

137. Economidou F, Douka E, Tzanela M, et al. Thyroid function during critical illness. *Hormones (Athens)*. 2011;10:117-124.

138. Warner MH, Beckett GJ. Mechanisms behind the non-thyroidal illness syndrome: an update. *J Endocrinol*. 2010;205:1-13.

139. Fliers E, Guldenaar SE, Wiersinga WM, et al. Decreased hypothalamic thyrotropin-releasing hormone gene expression in patients with nonthyroidal illness. *J Clin Endocrinol Metab*. 1997;82:4032-4036.

140. Jirasakuldech B, Schussler GC, Yap MG, et al. A characteristic serpin cleavage product of thyroxine-binding globulin appears in sepsis sera. *J Clin Endocrinol Metab*. 2000;85:3996-3999.

141. Boelen A, Kwakkel J, Wieland CW, et al. Impaired bacterial clearance in type 3 deiodinase-deficient mice infected with *Streptococcus pneumoniae*. *Endocrinology*. 2009;150:1984-1990.

142. St Germain DL, Galton VA, Hernandez A. Minireview: defining the roles of the iodothyronine deiodinases: current concepts and challenges. *Endocrinology*. 2009;150:1097-1107.

143. Lado-Abeal J, Romero A, Castro-Piedras I, et al. Thyroid hormone receptors are down-regulated in skeletal muscle of patients with non-thyroidal illness syndrome secondary to non-septic shock. *Eur J Endocrinol*. 2010;163:765-773.

144. De Groot LJ. Dangerous dogmas in medicine: the nonthyroidal illness syndrome. *J Clin Endocrinol Metab*. 1999;84:151-164.

145. Chopra IJ. Nonthyroidal illness syndrome or euthyroid sick syndrome? *Endocr Pract*. 1996;2:45-52.

146. Koulouri O, Moran C, Halsall D, et al. Pitfalls in the measurement and interpretation of thyroid function tests. *Best Pract Res Clin Endocrinol Metab*. 2013;27:745-762.

147. Scott-Moncrieff JC. Hypothyroidism. In: Ettinger SJ, Feldman EC, eds. *Textbook of Veterinary Internal Medicine: Diseases of the Dog and the Cat*. 7th ed. St. Louis, MO: Elsevier/Saunders; 2010:1751-1761.

148. Midgley JE, Moon CR, Wilkins TA. Validity of analog free thyroxin immunoassays. Part II. *Clin Chem*. 1987;33:2145-2152.

149. Torres SM, Feeney DA, Lekcharoensuk C, et al. Comparison of colloid, thyroid follicular epithelium, and thyroid hormone concentrations in healthy and severely sick dogs. *J Am Vet Med Assoc*. 2003;222:1079-1085.

150. Ladenson PW, Singer PA, Ain KB, et al. American Thyroid Association guidelines for detection of thyroid dysfunction. *Arch Intern Med*. 2000;160:1573-1575.

151. Ramsey I, Evans H, Herrtage M. Thyroid-stimulating hormone and total thyroxine concentrations in euthyroid, sick euthyroid and hypothyroid dogs. *J Small Anim Pract*. 1997;38:540-545.

152. Dayan CM. Interpretation of thyroid function tests. *Lancet*. 2001;357:619-624.

153. Licht P, Denver RJ. Effects of TRH on hormone release from pituitaries of the lizard, *Anolis carolinensis*. *Gen Comp Endocrinol*. 1988;70:355-362.

154. Sawin CT, Bacharach P, Lance V. Thyrotropin-releasing hormone and thyrotropin in the control of thyroid function in the turtle, *Chrysemys picta*. *Gen Comp Endocrinol*. 1981;45:7-11.

155. Lothrop CD Jr, Loomis MR, Olsen JH. Thyrotropin stimulation test for evaluation of thyroid function in psittacine birds. *J Am Vet Med Assoc*. 1985;186:47-48.

156. Lumeij JT, Westerhof I. Clinical evaluation of thyroid function in racing pigeons (*Columba livia domestica*). *Avian Pathol*. 1988;17:63-70.

157. Williamson R, Davison T. The effect of a single injection of thyrotrophin on serum concentrations of thyroxine, triiodothyronine, and reverse triiodothyronine in the immature chicken (*Gallus domesticus*). *Gen Comp Endocrinol*. 1985;58:109-113.

158. Zenoble R, Kemppainen R, Young D, et al. Endocrine responses of healthy parrots to ACTH and thyroid stimulating hormone. *J Am Vet Med Assoc*. 1985;187:1116-1118.

159. Harms CA, Hoskinson JJ, Bruyette DS, et al. Development of an experimental model of hypothyroidism in cockatiels (*Nymphicus hollandicus*). *Am J Vet Res*. 1994;55:399-404.

160. Greenacre CB, Jaques JT. TSH Testing in birds using canine, bovine, or human TSH. *Proc Assoc Avian Vet*. 2011;2011:49.

161. Heard DJ, Collins B, Chen DL, et al. Thyroid and adrenal function tests in adult male ferrets. *Am J Vet Res*. 1990;51:32-35.

162. Colzani RM, Alex S, Fang SL, et al. The effect of recombinant human thyrotropin (rhTSH) on thyroid function in mice and rats. *Thyroid*. 1998;8:797-801.

163. Mayer J, Wagner R, Mitchell MA, et al. Use of recombinant human thyroid-stimulating hormone for evaluation of thyroid function in guinea pigs (*Cavia porcellus*). *J Am Vet Med Assoc*. 2013;242:346-349.

164. Galas L, Raoult E, Tonon M-C, et al. TRH acts as a multifunctional hypophysiotropic factor in vertebrates. *Gen Comp Endocrinol*. 2009;164:40-50.

165. Szkudlinski MW, Fremont V, Ronin C, et al. Thyroid-stimulating hormone and thyroid-stimulating hormone receptor structure-function relationships. *Physiol Rev*. 2002;82:473-502.

166. Bentley PJ. *Comparative Vertebrate Endocrinology.* 3rd ed. Cambridge, UK; New York: Cambridge University Press; 1998.
167. Harms CA, Hoskinson JJ, Bruyette DS, et al. Technetium-99m and iodine-131 thyroid scintigraphy in normal and radiothyroidectomized cockatiels *(Nymphicus hollandicus). Vet Radiol Ultrasound.* 1994;35:473-478.
168. Brandao J, Ellison M, Beaufrere H, et al. Thyroid scintigraphy determined by technetium-99m pertechnetate in euthyroid New Zealand White rabbits *(Oryctolagus cuniculus). Proc Int Conf Avian Herpetol Exot Mammal Med.* 2015;313.
169. Brandao J, Ellison M, Beaufrere H, et al. *Quantitative 99m-technetium pertechnetate thyroid scintigraphy in euthyroid New Zealand White rabbits* (Oryctolagus cuniculus). Proceedings of the American College of Veterinary Radiology Annual Conference. St. Louis: American College of Veterinary Radiology; 2014.
170. Taeymans O, Penninck DG, Peters RM. Comparison between clinical, ultrasound, CT, MRI, and pathology findings in dogs presented for suspected thyroid carcinoma. *Vet Radiol Ultrasound.* 2013;54:61-70.
171. Taeymans O, Peremans K, Saunders JH. Thyroid imaging in the dog: current status and future directions. *J Vet Intern Med.* 2007;21:673-684.
172. Mayer J, Hunt K, Eshar D, et al. Thyroid scintigraphy in a guinea pig with suspected hyperthyroidism. *Exotic DVM.* 2009;11:25-29.
173. Schumacher J, Toal RL. Advanced radiography and ultrasonography in reptiles. *Sem Avian Exotic Pet Med.* 2001;10:162-168.
174. Grizzle J, Hadley TL, Rotstein DS, et al. Effects of dietary milk thistle on blood parameters, liver pathology, and hepatobiliary scintigraphy in White Carneaux pigeons *(Columba livia)* challenged with B₁ aflatoxin. *J Avian Med Surg.* 2009;23:114-124.
175. Hadley TL, Daniel GB, Rotstein DS, et al. Evaluation of hepatobiliary scintigraphy as an indicator of hepatic function in domestic pigeons *(Columba livia)* before and after exposure to ethylene glycol. *Vet Radiol Ultrasound.* 2007;48:155-162.
176. Brandao J, Rick M, Blair R, et al. Idiopathic hyperthyroidism in a pet rabbit *(Oryctolagus cuniculus). Proc Int Conf Avian Herpetol Exot Mammal Med.* 2015;372.
177. Greer LL, Daniel GB, Shearn-Bochsler VI, et al. Evaluation of the use of technetium Tc 99m diethylenetriamine pentaacetic acid and technetium Tc 99m dimercaptosuccinic acid for scintigraphic imaging of the kidneys in green iguanas *(Iguana iguana). Am J Vet Res.* 2005;66:87-92.
178. Young K, Daniel GB, Bahr A. Application of the pin-hole collimator in small animal nuclear scintigraphy: a review. *Vet Radiol Ultrasound.* 1997;38:83-93.
179. Hadfield CA, Clayton LA, Clancy MM, et al. Proliferative thyroid lesions in three diplodactylid geckos: *Nephrurus amyae, Nephrurus levis,* and *Oedura marmorata. J Zoo Wildl Med.* 2012;43:131-140.
180. Rivera S, Lock B. The reptilian thyroid and parathyroid glands. *Vet Clin North Am Exot Anim Pract.* 2008;11:163-175, viii.
181. Lynn WG. Structure and functions of the thyroid gland in reptiles. *Am Midl Nat.* 1960;62(2):309-326.
182. Cardone A, Angelini F, Esposito T, et al. The expression of androgen receptor messenger RNA is regulated by tri-iodothyronine in lizard testis. *J Steroid Biochem Mol Biol.* 2000;72:133-141.
183. Plowman MM, Lynn WG. The role of the thyroid in testicular function in the gecko, *Coleonyx variegatus. Gen Comp Endocrinol.* 1973;20:342-346.
184. Haldar-Misra C, Thapliyal JP. Thyroid in reproduction of reptiles. *Gen Comp Endocrinol.* 1981;43:537-542.
185. Flood DE, Fernandino JI, Langlois VS. Thyroid hormones in male reproductive development: Evidence for direct crosstalk between the androgen and thyroid hormone axes. *Gen Comp Endocrinol.* 2013;192:2-14.
186. Chiu KW, Lynn WG. The role of the thyroid in skin-shedding in the shovel-nosed snake, *Chionactis occipitalis. Gen Comp Endocrinol.* 1970;14:467-474.
187. Chiu K, Lynn WG. Observations on thyroidal control of sloughing in the garter snake, *Thamnophis sirtalis. Copeia.* 1972;1:158-163.
188. Maas AK 3rd. Vesicular, ulcerative, and necrotic dermatitis of reptiles. *Vet Clin North Am Exot Anim Pract.* 2013;16:737-755.
189. Norton TM, Jacobson ER, Caligiuri R, et al. Medical management of a Galapagos tortoise *(Geochelone elephantopus)* with hypothyroidism. *J Zoo Wildl Med.* 1989;20(2):212-216.
190. Jacobson ER. Causes of mortality and diseases in tortoises: a review. *J Zoo Wildl Med.* 1994;25:2-17.
191. Frye F, Dutra F. Hypothyroidism in turtles and tortoises. *Vet Med Small Anim Clin.* 1974;69:990.
192. Franco KH, Hoover JP. Levothyroxine as a treatment for presumed hypothyroidism in an adult male African spurred tortoise *(Centrochelys* [formerly *Geochelone] sulcata). J Herp Med Surg.* 2009;19:42-44.
193. Franco K, Famini D, Hoover J, et al. Serum thyroid hormone values for African spurred tortoises *(Centrochelys* [formerly *Geochelone] sulcata). J Herpetol Med Surg.* 2009;19:47-49.
194. Greenacre CB, Young DW, Behrend EN, et al. Validation of a novel high-sensitivity radioimmunoassay procedure for measurement of total thyroxine concentration in psittacine birds and snakes. *Am J Vet Res.* 2001;62:1750-1754.
195. Hernandez-Divers SJ, Knott CD, MacDonald J. Diagnosis and surgical treatment of thyroid adenoma-induced hyperthyroidism in a green iguana *(Iguana iguana). J Zoo Wildl Med.* 2001;32:465-475.
196. Frye FL. *Biomedical and Surgical Aspects of Captive Reptile Husbandry.* 2nd ed. Malabar, FL: Krieger Publishing; 1991.
197. Kubiak M. Hyperthyroidism diagnosis and treatment in an African helmeted turtle. *Proc Int Conf Avian Herpetol Exot Mammal Med.* 2015;421.
198. Garner MM, Hernandez-Divers SM, Raymond JT. Reptile neoplasia: a retrospective study of case submissions to a specialty diagnostic service. *Vet Clin North Am.* 2004;7:653-671.
199. Griffin C. Possible thyroid hyperplasia in a green iguana *(Iguana iguana). Abstr Assoc Rept Amphib Vet.* 2006;2006:1-38.
200. Gyimesi ZS, Garner MM, Burns RB. Goiter and thyroid disease in captive Kirtland's snakes *(Clonophis kirtlandii). J Herp Med Surg.* 2008;18:75-80.
201. Kolle P, Hoffman R. Thyroid adenoma in a stinkpot *(Sternotherus odoratus). Abstr Eur Assoc Zoo Wildl Vet.* 2002;2002:71-72.
202. Raiti P. Chronic renal disease, pseudogout and thyroid adenoma in a male Chaco tortoise *(Geochelone chilensis). Abstr Proc Assoc Rept Amphib Vet.* 2008;2008:62-64.
203. Ramsay EC, Munson L, Lowenstine L, et al. A retrospective study of neoplasia in a collection of captive snakes. *J Zoo Wildl Med.* 1996;27(1):28-34.
204. Hernandez-Divers SM, Garner MM. Neoplasia of reptiles with an emphasis on lizards. *Vet Clin North Am Exot Anim Pract.* 2003;6:251-273.
205. Cowan DF. Diseases of captive reptiles. *J Am Vet Med Assoc.* 1968;153:848-859.
206. Gal J, Csiko G, Pasztor I, et al. First description of papillary carcinoma in the thyroid gland of a red-eared slider *(Trachemys scripta elegans). Acta Vet Hungar.* 2010;58:69-73.
207. Whiteside D, Garner M. Thyroid adenocarcinoma in a crocodile lizard, *Shinisaurus crocodilurus. J Herp Med Surg.* 2001;11:13-16.
208. Sykes JMt, Trupkiewicz JG. Reptile neoplasia at the Philadelphia Zoological Garden, 1901-2002. *J Zoo Wildl Med.* 2006;37:11-19.
209. Catao-Dias J, Nichols D. Neoplasia in snakes at the National Zoological Park, Washington, DC (1978-1997). *J Comp Pathol.* 1999;120:89-95.
210. Radek T, Piasecki T. Topography and arterial supply of the thyroid and the parathyroid glands in selected species of Falconiformes. *Anat Histol Embryol.* 2007;36:241-249.
211. Merryman JI, Buckles EL. The avian thyroid gland. Part one: a review of the anatomy and physiology. *J Avian Med Surg.* 1998;12(4):234-237.

212. Radek T, Piasecki T. The topographical anatomy and arterial supply of the thyroid and parathyroid glands in the budgerigar *(Melopsittacus undulatus). Folia Morphol.* 2004;63:163-171.

213. Schmidt RE, Reavill DR. Thyroid hyperplasia in birds. *J Avian Med Surg.* 2002;16:111-114.

214. Chen AY, Bernet VJ, Carty SE, et al. American Thyroid Association statement on optimal surgical management of goiter. *Thyroid.* 2014;24:181-189.

215. Decuypere E, Van As P, Van der Geyten S, et al. Thyroid hormone availability and activity in avian species: a review. *Domest Anim Endocrinol.* 2005;29:63-77.

216. Koski MA. Dermatologic diseases in psittacine birds: an investigational approach. *Sem Avian Exotic Pet Med.* 2002;11:105-124.

217. Burgmann PM. Common psittacine dermatologic diseases. *Sem Avian Exotic Pet Med.* 1995;4:169-183.

218. Oglesbee BL. Hypothyroidism in a scarlet macaw. *J Am Vet Med Assoc.* 1992;201:1599-1601.

219. Cole RK. Hereditary hypothyroidism in the domestic fowl. *Genetics.* 1966;53:1021-1033.

220. Fudge AM, Speer B. Selected controversial topics in avian diagnostic testing. *Sem Avian Exotic Pet Med.* 2001;10:96-101.

221. Brandao J, Rick M, Beaufrere H, et al. Free and total thyroid hormones reference interval in the Hispaniolan Amazon parrot. *Proc Assoc Avian Vet.* 2014;2014:29.

222. McNabb FM, Hughes TE. The role of serum binding proteins in determining free thyroid hormone concentrations during development in quail. *Endocrinology.* 1983;113:957-963.

223. Brandao J, Manickam B, Blas-Machado U, et al. Productive thyroid follicular carcinoma in a wild barred owl *(Strix varia). J Vet Diagn Invest.* 2012;24:1145-1150.

224. Mayer J, Wagner R, Taeymans O. Advanced diagnostic approaches and current management of thyroid pathologies in guinea pigs. *Vet Clin North Am Exot Anim Pract.* 2010;13:509-523.

225. Brandão J, Vergneau-Grosset C, Mayer J. Hyperthyroidism and hyperparathyroidism in guinea pigs *(Cavia porcellus). Vet Clin North Am.* 2013;16:407-420.

226. Gibbons PM, Garner MM, Kiupel M. Morphological and immunohistochemical characterization of spontaneous thyroid gland neoplasms in guinea pigs *(Cavia porcellus). Vet Pathol.* 2012;50:334-342.

227. Fredholm DV, Cagle LA, Johnston MS. Evaluation of precision and establishment of reference ranges for plasma thyroxine using a point-of-care analyzer in healthy guinea pigs *(Cavia porcellus). J Exot Pet Med.* 2012;21:87-93.

228. Muller K, Muller E, Klein R, et al. Serum thyroxine concentrations in clinically healthy pet guinea pigs *(Cavia porcellus). Vet Clin Pathol.* 2009;38:507-510.

229. Castro MI, Alex S, Young RA, et al. Total and free serum thyroid hormone concentrations in fetal and adult pregnant and nonpregnant guinea pigs. *Endocrinology.* 1986;118:533-537.

230. Anderson RR, Nixon DA, Akasha MA. Total and free thyroxine and triiodothyronine in blood serum of mammals. *Comp Biochem Physiol A Comp Physiol.* 1988;89:401-404.

231. Quimby FW. *The Clinical Chemistry of Laboratory Animals.* 2nd ed. Philadelphia: Taylor & Francis; 1999.

232. Kilicarslan H, Bagcivan I, Yildirim MK, et al. Effect of hypothyroidism on the NO/cGMP pathway of corpus cavernosum in rabbits. *J Sex Med.* 2006;3:830-837.

233. Kowalczyk E, Urbanowicz J, Kopff M, et al. Elements of oxidation/reduction balance in experimental hypothyroidism. *Endokrynol Pol.* 2011;62:220-223.

234. Mebis L, Debaveye Y, Ellger B, et al. Changes in the central component of the hypothalamus-pituitary-thyroid axis in a rabbit model of prolonged critical illness. *Crit Care.* 2009;13(5):R147.

235. Mustafa S, Al-Bader MD, Elgazzar AH, et al. Effect of hyperthermia on the function of thyroid gland. *Eur J Appl Physiol.* 2008;103:285-288.

236. Chesney AM, Clawson TA, Webster B. Endemic goitre in rabbits. I. incidence and characteristics. *Bull Johns Hopkins Hosp.* 1928;43:261-277.

237. Kasavina B, Ukhina T, Mironov V. Effect of experimental hyperthyroidism on lysosomal membrane function and structural organization of the rabbit cornea. *Bull Exp Biol Med.* 1983;95:734-737.

238. Carpenter KJ. David Marine and the problem of goiter. *J Nutr.* 2005;135:675-680.

239. Marine D, Baumann E, Spence AW, et al. Further studies on etiology of goiter with particular reference to the action of cyanides. *Exp Biol Med.* 1932;29:772-775.

240. Marine D, Baumann EJ, Cipra A. Studies on simple goiter produced by cabbage and other vegetables. *Exp Biol Med.* 1929;26:822-824.

241. Marine D, Spence A, Cipra A. Production of goiter and exophthalmos in rabbits by administration of cyanide. *Exp Biol Med.* 1932;29:822-823.

242. Marine D, Rosen S, Cipra A. Further studies on the exophthalmos in rabbits produced by methyl cyanide. *Exp Biol Med.* 1933;30:649-651.

243. Van der Woerdt A. Ophthalmologic disease in small pet mammals. In: Quesenberry K, Carpenter JW, eds. *Ferrets, Rabbits, and Rodents: Clinical Medicine and Surgery.* 3rd ed. St. Louis, MO: Elsevier/Saunders; 2012:523-531.

244. Hatton MP, Rubin PA. The pathophysiology of thyroid-associated ophthalmopathy. *Ophthalmol Clin North Am.* 2002;15:113-119.

245. DePaolo LV, Masoro EJ. Endocrine hormones in laboratory animals. In: Loeb WF, Quimby FW, eds. *The Clinical Chemistry of Laboratory Animals.* 1st ed. New York: Pergamon Press; 1989:279-308.

246. Mebis L, Eerdekens A, Güiza F, et al. Contribution of nutritional deficit to the pathogenesis of the nonthyroidal illness syndrome in critical illness: a rabbit model study. *Endocrinology.* 2012;153:973-984.

247. Weekers F, Van Herck E, Coopmans W, et al. A novel in vivo rabbit model of hypercatabolic critical illness reveals a biphasic neuroendocrine stress response. *Endocrinology.* 2002;143:764-774.

248. Fritsche R, Simova-Curd S, Clauss M, et al. Hyperthyroidism in connection with suspected diabetes mellitus in a chinchilla *(Chinchilla laniger). Vet Rec.* 2008;163:454-456.

249. Hoenig M, Ferguson D. Impairment of glucose tolerance in hyperthyroid cats. *J Endocrinol.* 1989;121:249-251.

250. Wagner R. Hypothyroidism in ferrets. *Proc Assoc Exotic Mammal Vet Conf.* 2012;2012:29-31.

251. Wills TB, Bohn AA, Finch NP, et al. Thyroid follicular adenocarcinoma in a ferret. *Vet Clin Pathol.* 2005;34:405-408.

252. Fox JG, Dangler CA, Snyder SB, et al. C-cell carcinoma (medullary thyroid carcinoma) associated with multiple endocrine neoplasms in a ferret *(Mustela putorius). Vet Pathol.* 2000;37:278-282.

253. Thorson L. Thyroid diseases in rodent species. *Vet Clin North Am Exot Anim Pract.* 2014;17:51-67.

254. Bray GA, York DA. Thyroid function of genetically obese rats. *Endocrinology.* 1971;88:1095-1099.

255. de Matos R. Calcium metabolism in birds. *Vet Clin North Am Exot Anim Pract.* 2008;11:59-82, vi.

256. Peacock M. Calcium metabolism in health and disease. *Clin J Am Soc Nephrol.* 2010;5(suppl 1):S23-S30.

257. Huskisson E, Maggini S, Ruf M. The role of vitamins and minerals in energy metabolism and well-being. *J Int Med Res.* 2007;35:277-289.

258. Nishizawa Y, Morii H, Durlach J. *New Perspectives in Magnesium Research.* London: Springer; 2007.

259. Saris NE, Mervaala E, Karppanen H, et al. Magnesium. An update on physiological, clinical and analytical aspects. *Clin Chim Acta.* 2000;294:1-26.

260. Kingston ME, Al-Siba'i MB, Skooge WC. Clinical manifestations of hypomagnesemia. *Crit Care Med.* 1986;14:950-954.

261. Agus ZS. Hypomagnesemia. *J Am Soc Nephrol.* 1999;10:1616-1622.
262. Anast CS, Mohs JM, Kaplan SL, et al. Evidence for parathyroid failure in magnesium deficiency. *Science.* 1972;177:606-608.
263. Anast CS, Winnacker JL, Forte LR, et al. Impaired release of parathyroid hormone in magnesium deficiency. *J Clin Endocrinol Metab.* 1976;42:707-717.
264. Suh SM, Tashjian AH Jr, Matsuo N, et al. Pathogenesis of hypocalcemia in primary hypomagnesemia: normal end-organ responsiveness to parathyroid hormone, impaired parathyroid gland function. *J Clin Invest.* 1973;52:153.
265. Mori S, Harada S-i, Okazaki R, et al. Hypomagnesemia with increased metabolism of parathyroid hormone and reduced responsiveness to calcitropic hormones. *Intern Med.* 1992;31(6):820-824.
266. Raisz LG. Effect of phosphate, calcium and magnesium on bone resorption and hormonal responses in tissue culture. *Endocrinology.* 1969;85:446-452.
267. Rude RK, Oldham SB, Singer FR. Functional hypoparathyroidism and parathyroid hormone end-organ resistance in human magnesium deficiency. *Clin Endocrinol (Oxf).* 1976;5:209-224.
268. Akerstrom G, Hellman P, Hessman O, et al. Parathyroid glands in calcium regulation and human disease. *Ann NY Acad Sci.* 2005;1040:53-58.
269. Cave A. The glands of Owen. *St Bartholomew Hosp J.* 1953;57:131-133.
270. Giddings CE, Rimmer J, Weir N. History of parathyroid gland surgery: an historical case series. *J Laryngol Otol.* 2009;123:1075-1081.
271. Johansson H. Parathyroid history and the Uppsala anatomist Ivar Sandstrom. *Med Secoli.* 2008;21:387-401.
272. Forsyth D. The comparative anatomy, gross and minute, of the thyroid and parathyroid glands in mammals and birds: part I. *J Anat Physiol.* 1908;42:141.
273. Forsyth D. The comparative anatomy, gross and minute, of the thyroid and parathyroid glands in mammals and birds: part II. *J Anat Physiol.* 1908;42:302-319.
274. Morley P, Whitfield JF, Willick GE. Parathyroid hormone: an anabolic treatment for osteoporosis. *Curr Pharm Des.* 2001;7:671-687.
275. Giovannucci E. The epidemiology of vitamin D and cancer incidence and mortality: a review (United States). *Cancer Causes Control.* 2005;16:83-95.
276. Cui Y, Rohan TE. Vitamin D, calcium, and breast cancer risk: a review. *Cancer Epidemiol Biomarkers Prev.* 2006;15:1427-1437.
277. Dittmer KE, Thompson KG. Vitamin D metabolism and rickets in domestic animals: a review. *Vet Pathol.* 2011;48:389-407.
278. Laing C, Fraser D. The vitamin D system in iguanian lizards. *Comp Biochem Physiol B Biochem Mol Biol.* 1999;123:373-379.
279. Henry H, Norman AW. Presence of renal 25-hydroxyvitamin-D-1-hydroxylase in species of all vertebrate classes. *Comp Biochem Physiol B.* 1975;50:431-434.
280. Rhoten WB, Bruns ME, Christakos S. Presence and localization of two vitamin D-dependent calcium binding proteins in kidneys of higher vertebrates. *Endocrinology.* 1985;117:674-683.
281. Swarup K, Pandey A, Srivastav AK. Calcaemic responses in the yellow monitor, *Varanus flavescens* to vitamin D$_3$ administration. *Acta Physiol Hung.* 1986;70:375-377.
282. Srivastav AK, Rani L. Phosphocalcic response to vitamin D$_3$ treatment in freshwater snake, *Natrix piscator. Zool Sci.* 1988;5:893-895.
283. Srivastav AK, Srivastav SK, Singh S, et al. Effect of various vitamin D metabolites on serum calcium and inorganic phosphate in the freshwater snake *Natrix piscator. Gen Comp Endocrinol.* 1995;100:49-52.
284. DeLuca HF. History of the discovery of vitamin D and its active metabolites. *Bonekey Rep.* 2014;3:479.
285. Vieth R. Why "vitamin D" is not a hormone, and not a synonym for 1, 25-dihydroxy-vitamin D, its analogs or deltanoids. *J Steroid Biochem Mol Biol.* 2004;89:571-573.
286. DeLuca HF. The transformation of a vitamin into a hormone: the vitamin D story. *Harvey Lect.* 1979;75:333-379.
287. Kodicek E. The story of vitamin D from vitamin to hormone. *Lancet.* 1974;303:325-329.
288. Bikle DD. Vitamin D: newly discovered actions require reconsideration of physiologic requirements. *Trends Endocrinol Metab.* 2010;21:375-384.
289. Mader DR. Metabolic bone disease. In: Mader DR, ed. *Reptile Medicine and Surgery.* 2nd ed. St. Louis, MO: Elsevier/Saunders; 2006:841-851.
290. McWilliams D. Nutrition research on calcium homeostasis. I. Lizards (with recommendations). *Int Zoo Yearb.* 2005;39:69-77.
291. Hoby S, Wenker C, Robert N, et al. Nutritional metabolic bone disease in juvenile veiled chameleons (*Chamaeleo calyptratus*) and its prevention. *J Nutr.* 2010;140:1923-1931.
292. Hedley J. Metabolic bone disease in reptiles: Part 1. *Compan Anim.* 2012;17:52-54.
293. Huey RB, Slatkin M. Cost and benefits of lizard thermoregulation. *Q Rev Biol.* 1976;51:363-384.
294. Brattstrom BH. Body temperatures of reptiles. *Am Mid Nat.* 1965;73:376-422.
295. Manning B, Grigg GC. Basking is not of thermoregulatory significance in the "basking" freshwater turtle *Emydura signata. Copeia.* 1997;3:579.
296. Karsten KB, Ferguson GW, Chen TC, et al. Panther chameleons, *Furcifer pardalis,* behaviorally regulate optimal exposure to UV depending on dietary vitamin D$_3$ status. *Physiol Biochem Zool.* 2009;82:218-225.
297. Ferguson GW, Gehrmann WH, Karsten KB, et al. Do panther chameleons bask to regulate endogenous vitamin D$_3$ production? *Physiol Biochem Zool.* 2003;76:52-59.
298. Acierno MJ, Mitchell MA, Zachariah TT, et al. Effects of ultraviolet radiation on plasma 25-hydroxyvitamin D$_3$ concentrations in corn snakes (*Elaphe guttata*). *Am J Vet Res.* 2008;69:294-297.
299. Hedley J, Eatwell K. The effects of UV light on calcium metabolism in ball pythons (*Python regius*). *Vet Rec.* 2013;173(14):345.
300. Acierno MJ, Mitchell MA, Roundtree MK, et al. Effects of ultraviolet radiation on 25-hydroxyvitamin D$_3$ synthesis in red-eared slider turtles (*Trachemys scripta elegans*). *Am J Vet Res.* 2006;67:2046-2049.
301. Ooninx D, van de Wal M, Bosch G, et al. Blood vitamin D$_3$ metabolite concentrations of adult female bearded dragons (*Pogona vitticeps*) remain stable after ceasing UVB exposure. *Comp Biochem Physiol B Biochem Mol Biol.* 2013;165:196-200.
302. Hedley J. Metabolic bone disease in reptiles: part 2. *Compan Anim.* 2012;17:38-41.
303. Mans C, Braun J. Update on common nutritional disorders of captive reptiles. *Vet Clin North Am Exot Anim Pract.* 2014;17:369-395.
304. Banzato T, Hellebuyck T, Van Caelenberg A, et al. A review of diagnostic imaging of snakes and lizards. *Vet Rec.* 2013;173:43-49.
305. Eatwell K. Variations in the concentration of ionised calcium in the plasma of captive tortoises (*Testudo* species). *Vet Rec.* 2009;165:82-84.
306. Eatwell K. Plasma concentrations of 25-hydroxycholecalciferol in 22 captive tortoises (*Testudo* species). *Vet Rec.* 2008;162:342-345.
307. Selleri P, Di Girolamo N. Plasma 25-hydroxyvitamin D$_3$ concentrations in Hermann's tortoises (*Testudo hermanni*) exposed to natural sunlight and two artificial ultraviolet radiation sources. *Am J Vet Res.* 2012;73:1781-1786.
308. Stringer EM, Harms CA, Beasley JF, et al. Comparison of ionized calcium, parathyroid hormone, and 25-hydroxyvitamin D in rehabilitating and healthy wild green sea turtles (*Chelonia mydas*). *J Herpetol Med Surg.* 2010;20:122-127.

309. Gibbons PM. Advances in reptile clinical therapeutics. *J Exot Pet Med.* 2014;23:21-38.

310. Martinez-Jimenez D, Hernandez-Divers SJ. Emergency care of reptiles. *Vet Clin North Am Exot Anim Pract.* 2007;10:557-585.

311. Stanford M. Calcium metabolism. In: Harrison GJ, Lightfoot TL, eds. *Clinical Avian Medicine.* Palm Beach, FL: Spix Publishing; 2006:141-152.

312. Goldstein DL, Skadhauge E. Renal and extrarenal regulation of body fluid composition. In: Whittow GC, ed. *Sturkie's Avian Physiology.* 5th ed. San Diego: Academic Press; 2000:265-298.

313. Johnston MS, Ivey ES. Parathyroid and ultimobranchial glands: calcium metabolism in birds. *Sem Avian Exotic Pet Med.* 2002;11: 84-93.

314. Clark NB, Wideman RF Jr. Calcitonin stimulation of urine flow and sodium excretion in the starling. *Am J Physiol.* 1980;238:R406-R412.

315. Candlish JK, Taylor TG. The response-time to the parathyroid hormone in the laying fowl. *J Endocrinol.* 1970;48:143-144.

316. Kraintz L, Intscher K. Effect of calcitonin on the domestic fowl. *Can J Physiol Pharmacol.* 1969;47:313-315.

317. Urist MR. Avian parathyroid physiology: including a special comment on calcitonin. *Am Zool.* 1967;7:883-895.

318. Yadav S, Srivastav AK. Influence of calcitonin administration on ultimobranchial and parathyroid glands of pigeon, *Columba livia. Microsc Res Tech.* 2009;72:380-384.

319. Srivastav AK, Yadav S. Prolactin effects on ultimobranchial and parathyroid glands in pigeon. *North-West J Zool.* 2008;4:300-310.

320. Kirchgessner MS, Tully TN Jr, Nevarez J, et al. Magnesium therapy in a hypocalcemic African grey parrot (*Psittacus erithacus*). *J Avian Med Surg.* 2012;26:17-21.

321. Lumeij JT. Relation of plasma calcium to total protein and albumin in African grey (*Psittacus erithacus*) and Amazon (*Amazona* spp.) parrots. *Avian Pathol.* 1990;19:661-667.

322. Rosskopf WJ, Woerpel RW, Lane RA. The hypocalcemia syndrome in African greys: an updated clinical viewpoint. *Proc Annu Conf Assoc Avian Vet.* 1985;1985:129-131.

323. McDonald LJ. Hypocalcemic seizures in an African grey parrot. *Can Vet J.* 1988;29:928-930.

324. Weaver VM, Welsh J. 1, 25-dihydroxycholecalciferol supplementation prevents hypocalcemia in magnesium-deficient chicks. *J Nutr.* 1993;123:764-771.

325. Weaver VM, Welsh JJ. Vitamin D metabolism in magnesium deficient chicks. *Nutr Res.* 1989;9:1363-1369.

326. de Carvalho FM, Gaunt SD, Kearney MT, et al. Reference intervals of plasma calcium, phosphorus, and magnesium for African grey parrots (*Psittacus erithacus*) and Hispaniolan parrots (*Amazona ventralis*). *J Zoo Wildl Med.* 2009;40:675-679.

327. Hertelendy F, Taylor T. Changes in blood calcium associated with egg shell calcification in the domestic fowl 1. chances in the total calcium. *Poult Sci.* 1961;40:108-114.

328. Engelking LR. *Textbook of Veterinary Physiological Chemistry.* 3rd ed. Waltham, MA: Academic Press/Elsevier; 2015.

329. Luck MR, Scanes CG. Plasma levels of ionized calcium in the laying hen (*Gallus domesticus*). *Comp Biochem Physiol A Physiol.* 1979;63:177-181.

330. Watson MK, Stern AW, Labelle AL, et al. Evaluating the clinical and physiological effects of long term ultraviolet B radiation on guinea pigs (*Cavia porcellus*). *PLoS ONE.* 2014;9:e114413.

331. Rivas AE, Mitchell MA, Flower J, et al. Effects of ultraviolet radiation on serum 25-hydroxyvitamin D concentrations in captive chinchillas (*Chinchilla laniger*). *J Exot Pet Med.* 2014;75:380-384.

332. Emerson JA, Whittington JK, Allender MC, et al. Effects of ultraviolet radiation produced from artificial lights on serum 25-hydroxyvitamin D concentration in captive domestic rabbits (*Oryctolagus cuniculi*). *Am J Vet Res.* 2014;75:380-384.

333. Elayat AA, el-Naggar MM, Tahir M. An immunocytochemical and morphometric study of the rat pancreatic islets. *J Anat.* 1995;186:629.

334. Andralojc KM, Mercalli A, Nowak KW, et al. Ghrelin-producing epsilon cells in the developing and adult human pancreas. *Diabetologia.* 2009;52:486-493.

335. Wierup N, Svensson H, Mulder H, et al. The ghrelin cell: a novel developmentally regulated islet cell in the human pancreas. *Regul Pept.* 2002;107:63-69.

336. Kobayashi S, Fujita T. Fine structure of mammalian and avian pancreatic islets with special reference to D cells and nervous elements. *Z Zellforsch Mikrosk Anat.* 1969;100:340-363.

337. Kimmel JR, Hayden LJ, Pollock HG. Isolation and characterization of a new pancreatic polypeptide hormone. *J Biol Chem.* 1975; 250:9369-9376.

338. Braun EJ, Sweazea KL. Glucose regulation in birds. *Comp Biochem Physiol B Biochem Mol Biol.* 2008;151:1-9.

339. Guha B, Ghosh A. A cytomorphological study of the endocrine pancreas of some Indian birds. *Gen Comp Endocrinol.* 1978;34: 38-44.

340. Penhos JC, Ramey E. Studies on the endocrine pancreas of amphibians and reptiles. *Am Zool.* 1973;13:667-698.

341. Kaiya H, Darras VM, Kangawa K. Ghrelin in birds: its structure, distribution, function. *J Poult Sci.* 2007;44:1-18.

342. Kaiya H, Sakata I, Kojima M, et al. Structural determination and histochemical localization of ghrelin in the red-eared slider turtle, *Trachemys scripta elegans. Gen Comp Endocrinol.* 2004;138:50-57.

343. Brelje TC, Scharp DW, Sorenson RL. Three-dimensional imaging of intact isolated islets of Langerhans with confocal microscopy. *Diabetes.* 1989;38:808-814.

344. Nussey SS, Whitehead SA. *Endocrinology: An Integrated Approach.* Oxford: CRC Press; 2013.

345. Goutal CM, Brugmann BL, Ryan KA. Insulinoma in dogs: a review. *J Am Anim Hosp Assoc.* 2012;48:151-163.

346. Naples LM, Langan JN, Mylniczenko ND, et al. Islet cell tumor in a savannah monitor (*Varanus exanthematicus*). *J Herpetol Med Surg.* 2009;19:97-105.

347. Polton GA, White RN, Brearley MJ, et al. Improved survival in a retrospective cohort of 28 dogs with insulinoma. *J Small Anim Pract.* 2007;48:151-156.

348. Mellanby RJ, Herrtage ME. Insulinoma in a normoglycaemic dog with low serum fructosamine. *J Small Anim Pract.* 2002;43:506-508.

349. Lester NV, Newell SM, Hill RC, et al. Scintigraphic diagnosis of insulinoma in a dog. *Vet Radiol Ultrasound.* 1999;40:174-178.

350. Grant CS. Gastrointestinal endocrine tumours. Insulinoma. *Baillieres Clin Gastroenterol.* 1996;10:645-671.

351. Malta M, Luppi M, Oliveira R, et al. Malignant insulinoma in a crab-eating fox (*Cerdocyon thous*). *Braz J Vet Pathol.* 2008; 1:25-27.

352. Elvestad K, Henriques UV, Kroustrup JP. Insulin-producing islet cell tumor in an ectopic pancreas of a red fox (*Vulpes vulpes*). *J Wildl Dis.* 1984;20:70-72.

353. Hess RS. Insulin-secreting islet cell neoplasia. In: Ettinger SJ, Feldman EC, eds. *Textbook of Veterinary Internal Medicine: Diseases of the Dog and the Cat.* 7th ed. St. Louis, MO: Elsevier/Saunders; 2010:1779-1782.

354. Kraje AC. Hypoglycemia and irreversible neurologic complications in a cat with insulinoma. *J Am Vet Med Assoc.* 2003;223:812-814, 810.

355. Vinke CM, Schoemaker NJ. The welfare of ferrets (*Mustela putorius furo* T): a review on the housing and management of pet ferrets. *Appl Anim Behav Sci.* 2012;139(3-4):155-168.

356. Chen S. Advanced diagnostic approaches and current medical management of insulinomas and adrenocortical disease in ferrets (*Mustela putorius furo*). *Vet Clin North Am Exot Anim Pract.* 2010;13:439-452.

357. Miwa Y, Kurosawa A, Ogawa H, et al. Neoplasitic diseases in ferrets in Japan: a questionnaire study for 2000 to 2005. *J Vet Med Sci.* 2009;71:397-402.

358. Inoue C, Shiga K, Takasawa S, et al. Evolutionary conservation of the insulinoma gene *rig* and its possible function. *Proc Natl Acad Sci.* 1987;84:6659-6662.

359. Skelin M, Rupnik M, Cencic A. Pancreatic β cell lines and their applications in diabetes mellitus research. *ALTEX.* 2010;27:105-113.

360. Sugimoto K, Shoji M, Yasujima M, et al. Peripheral nerve endoneurial microangiopathy and necrosis in rats with insulinoma. *Acta Neuropathol.* 2004;108:503-514.

361. Novikoff AB, Yam A, Novikoff PM. Cytochemical study of secretory process in transplantable insulinoma of Syrian golden hamster. *Proc Natl Acad Sci.* 1975;72:4501-4505.

362. Chick WL, Warren S, Chute RN, et al. A transplantable insulinoma in the rat. *Proc Natl Acad Sci.* 1977;74:628-632.

363. Flatt PR, Tan KS, Bailey CJ, et al. Effects of transplantation and resection of a radiation-induced rat insulinoma on glucose homeostasis and the endocrine pancreas. *Br J Cancer.* 1986;54:685-692.

364. Bomhard E, Karbe E, Loeser E. Spontaneous tumors of 2000 Wistar TNO/W.70 rats in two-year carcinogenicity studies. *J Environ Pathol Toxicol Oncol.* 1986;7:35-52.

365. Bomhard E. Frequency of spontaneous tumors in Wistar rats in 30-months studies. *Exp Toxicol Pathol.* 1992;44:381-392.

366. Ikezaki S, Takagi M, Tamura K. Natural occurrence of neoplastic lesions in young Sprague-Dawley rats. *J Toxicol Pathol.* 2011;24:37-40.

367. Hess LR, Ravich ML, Reavill DR. Diagnosis and treatment of an insulinoma in a guinea pig *(Cavia porcellus).* *J Am Vet Med Assoc.* 2013;242:522-526.

368. Harcourt-Brown F, Harcourt-Brown S. Clinical value of blood glucose measurement in pet rabbits. *Vet Rec.* 2012;170:674.

369. Syme HM, Scott-Moncrieff JC. Chronic hypoglycaemia in a hunting dog due to secondary hypoadrenocorticism. *J Small Anim Pract.* 1998;39:348-351.

370. Loste A, Marca MC, Perez M, et al. Clinical value of fructosamine measurements in non-healthy dogs. *Vet Res Commun.* 2001;25:109-115.

371. Thoresen SI, Aleksandersen M, Lonaas L, et al. Pancreatic insulin-secreting carcinoma in a dog: fructosamine for determining persistent hypoglycaemia. *J Small Anim Pract.* 1995;36:282-286.

372. Hein J, Spreyer F, Sauter-Louis C, et al. Reference ranges for laboratory parameters in ferrets. *Vet Rec.* 2012;171:218-223.

373. Jenkins JR. Ferret metabolic testing. In: Fudge AM, ed. *Laboratory Medicine: Avian and Exotic Pets.* Philadelphia: W.B. Saunders; 2000:305-309.

374. Strachan MW, Deary IJ, Ewing FM, et al. Acute hypoglycemia impairs the functioning of the central but not peripheral nervous system. *Physiol Behav.* 2001;72:83-92.

375. Sugimoto K, Yagihashi S. Peripheral nerve pathology in rats with streptozotocin-induced insulinoma. *Acta Neuropathol.* 1996;91:616-623.

376. Shimada A, Morita T, Ikeda N, et al. Hypoglycaemic brain lesions in a dog with insulinoma. *J Comp Pathol.* 2000;122:67-71.

377. Mohseni S. Hypoglycemic neuropathy. *Acta Neuropathol.* 2001;102:413-421.

378. Sugimoto K, Baba M, Suda T, et al. Peripheral neuropathy and microangiopathy in rats with insulinoma: association with chronic hyperinsulinemia. *Diabetes Metab Res Rev.* 2003;19:392-400.

379. Caplan ER, Peterson ME, Mullen HS, et al. Diagnosis and treatment of insulin-secreting pancreatic islet cell tumors in ferrets: 57 cases (1986-1994). *J Am Vet Med Assoc.* 1996;209:1741-1745.

380. Robben JH, Pollak YW, Kirpensteijn J, et al. Comparison of ultrasonography, computed tomography, and single-photon emission computed tomography for the detection and localization of canine insulinoma. *J Vet Intern Med.* 2005;19:15-22.

381. Trifonidou MA, Kirpensteijn J, Robben JH. A retrospective evaluation of 51 dogs with insulinoma. *Vet Q.* 1998;20(suppl 1):S114-S115.

382. Weiss CA, Williams BH, Scott MV. Insulinoma in the ferret: clinical findings and treatment comparison of 66 cases. *J Am Anim Hosp Assoc.* 1998;34:471-475.

383. Akbarzadeh A, Norouzian D, Mehrabi MR, et al. Induction of diabetes by streptozotocin in rats. *Indian J Clin Biochem.* 2007;22:60-64.

384. Chen S. Pancreatic endocrinopathies in ferrets. *Vet Clin North Am Exot Anim Pract.* 2008;11:107-123, vii.

385. London CA, Malpas PB, Wood-Follis SL, et al. Multi-center, placebo-controlled, double-blind, randomized study of oral toceranib phosphate (SU11654), a receptor tyrosine kinase inhibitor, for the treatment of dogs with recurrent (either local or distant) mast cell tumor following surgical excision. *Clin Cancer Res.* 2009;15:3856-3865.

386. London C, Mathie T, Stingle N, et al. Preliminary evidence for biologic activity of toceranib phosphate (Palladia®) in solid tumours. *Vet Comp Oncol.* 2012;10:194-205.

387. Poretsky L. *Principles of Diabetes Mellitus.* New York: Springer; 2010.

388. Herold KC, Vignali DA, Cooke A, et al. Type 1 diabetes: translating mechanistic observations into effective clinical outcomes. *Nat Rev Immunol.* 2013;13:243-256.

389. Shi Y, Hu FB. The global implications of diabetes and cancer. *Lancet.* 2014;383:1947-1948.

390. Tong ZQ, Jack E, Moule M, et al. Rodent insulin receptors are immunologically different from other mammalian insulin receptors. *Gen Comp Endocrinol.* 1994;94:374-381.

391. Vera F, Zenuto RR, Antenucci CD. Decreased glucose tolerance but normal blood glucose levels in the field in the caviomorph rodent *Ctenomys talarum*: the role of stress and physical activity. *Comp Biochem Physiol A Mol Integr Physiol.* 2008;151:232-238.

392. Edwards MS. Nutrition and behavior of degus *(Octodon degus).* *Vet Clin North Am.* 2009;12:237-253.

393. Opazo JC, Soto-Gamboa M, Bozinovic F. Blood glucose concentration in caviomorph rodents. *Comp Biochem Physiol A Mol Integr Physiol.* 2004;137:57-64.

394. Taymans SE, DeVries AC, DeVries MB, et al. The hypothalamic-pituitary-adrenal axis of prairie voles *(Microtus ochrogaster)*: evidence for target tissue glucocorticoid resistance. *Gen Comp Endocrinol.* 1997;106:48-61.

395. Barten SL. Lizards. In: Mader DR, ed. *Reptile Medicine and Surgery.* 2nd ed. St. Louis, MO: Elsevier/Saunders; 2006:59-77.

396. Stahl SJ. Hyperglycemia in reptiles. In: Mader DR, ed. *Reptile Medicine and Surgery.* 2nd ed. St. Louis, MO: Elsevier/Saunders; 2006:822-830.

397. Ritter JM, Garner MM, Chilton JA, et al. Gastric neuroendocrine carcinomas in bearded dragons *(Pogona vitticeps).* *Vet Pathol.* 2009;46:1109-1116.

398. Mans C. Clinical update on diagnosis and management of disorders of the digestive system of reptiles. *J Exot Pet Med.* 2013;22:141-162.

399. Lyons JA, Newman SJ, Greenacre CB, et al. A gastric neuroendocrine carcinoma expressing somatostatin in a bearded dragon *(Pogona vitticeps).* *J Vet Diagn Invest.* 2010;22:316-320.

400. Sweazea KL, McMurtry JP, Elsey RM, et al. Comparison of metabolic substrates in alligators and several birds of prey. *Zoology.* 2014;117:253-260.

401. Akiba Y, Chida Y, Takahashi T, et al. Persistent hypoglycemia induced by continuous insulin infusion in broiler chickens. *Br Poult Sci.* 1999;40:701-705.

402. Sweazea KL, Braun EJ. Glucose transporter expression in English sparrows *(Passer domesticus).* *Comp Biochem Physiol B Biochem Mol Biol.* 2006;144:263-270.

403. Chen K, Anderson RC, Maze N. Susceptibility of birds to insulin as compared with mammals. *J Pharmacol Exp Ther.* 1945;84:74-77.

404. Tokushima Y, Takahashi K, Sato K, et al. Glucose uptake in vivo in skeletal muscles of insulin-injected chicks. *Comp Biochem Physiol B Biochem Mol Biol.* 2005;141:43-48.

405. Sweazea KL, McMurtry JP, Braun EJ. Inhibition of lipolysis does not affect insulin sensitivity to glucose uptake in the mourning dove. *Comp Biochem Physiol B Biochem Mol Biol.* 2006;144:387-394.
406. Desmarchelier M, Langlois I. Diabetes mellitus in a nanday conure *(Nandayus nenday). J Avian Med Surg.* 2008;22:246-254.
407. Pilny AA, Luong R. Diabetes mellitus in a chestnut-fronted macaw *(Ara severa). J Avian Med Surg.* 2005;19:297-302.
408. Appleby R. Diabetes mellitus in a budgerigar *(Melopsittacus undulatus). Vet Rec.* 1984;115:652-653.
409. Altman R, Kirmayer A. Diabetes mellitus in the avian species. *J Am Anim Hosp Assoc.* 1976;12:531-537.
410. Ryan C, Walder E, Howard E. Diabetes-mellitus and islet cell-carcinoma in a parakeet. *J Am Anim Hosp Assoc.* 1982;18:139-142.
411. Douglass E. Diabetes mellitus in a toco toucan. *Mod Vet Pract.* 1981;62:293-295.
412. Candeletta SC, Homer BL, Garner MM, et al. Diabetes mellitus associated with chronic lymphocytic pancreatitis in an African grey parrot *(Psittacus erithacus erithacus). J Assoc Avian Vet.* 1993;7:39-43.
413. Wallner-Pendleton EA, Rogers D, Epple A. Diabetes mellitus in a red-tailed hawk *(Buteo jamaicensis). Avian Pathol.* 1993;22:631-635.
414. Pollock CG, Pledger T. Diabetes mellitus in avian species. *Proc Annu Conf Assoc Avian Vet.* 2001;2001:151-154.
415. Pilny AA. The avian pancreas in health and disease. *Vet Clin North Am Exot Anim Pract.* 2008;11:25-34, v-vi.
416. Campbell-Ward ML, Rand J, et al. Diabetes mellitus in other species. In: Rand J, Behrend E, Gunn-Moore D, eds. *Clinical Endocrinology of Companion Animals.* 1st ed. Ames, IA: John Wiley & Sons; 2013:191-200.
417. Pepper AR, Gall C, Mazzuca DM, et al. Diabetic rats and mice are resistant to porcine and human insulin: flawed experimental models for testing islet xenografts. *Xenotransplantation.* 2009;16:502-510.
418. Schneider MK, Seebach JD. Xenotransplantation literature update: November 2009-January 2010. *Xenotransplantation.* 2010;17:166-170.
419. Zimmerman AE, Moule ML, Yip CC. Guinea pig insulin II. Biological activity. *J Biol Chem.* 1974;249:4026-4029.
420. Roth J, Gorden P, Pastan I. "Big insulin": a new component of plasma insulin detected by immunoassay. *Proc Natl Acad Sci.* 1968;61(1):138.
421. Vannevel J. Diabetes mellitus in a 3-year-old, intact, female guinea pig. *Can Vet J.* 1998;39:503.
422. Belis JA, Curley RM, Lang CM. Bladder dysfunction in the spontaneously diabetic male Abyssinian-Hartley guinea pig. *Pharmacology.* 1996;53:66-70.
423. Ewringmann A, Göbel T. Diabetes mellitus bei kaninchen, meerschweinchen und chinchilla. *Kleintierpraxis.* 1998;43:337-348.
424. Glage S, Kamino K, Jörns A, et al. Hereditary hyperglycaemia and pancreatic degeneration in guinea pigs. *J Exp Anim Sci.* 2007;43:309-317.
425. Hawkins MG, Bishop CR. Disease problems of guinea pigs. In: Quesenberry KE, Carpenter JW, eds. *Ferrets, Rabbits, and Rodents: Clinical Medicine and Surgery.* 3rd ed. St. Louis, MO: Elsevier/Saunders; 2012:295-310.
426. Spear G, Caple M, Sutherland L. The pancreas in the degu. *Exp Mol Pathol.* 1984;40:295-310.
427. Jekl V, Hauptman K, Knotek Z. Diseases in pet degus: a retrospective study in 300 animals. *J Small Anim Pract.* 2011;52:107-112.
428. Westermark P. Amyloid in the islets of Langerhans: thoughts and some historical aspects. *Ups J Med Sci.* 2011;116:81-89.
429. Mans C, Donnelly TM. Disease problems of chinchillas. In: Quesenberry K, Carpenter JW, eds. *Ferrets, Rabbits, and Rodents: Clinical Medicine and Surgery.* 3rd ed. St. Louis, MO: Elsevier/Saunders; 2012:311-325.
430. Roth S, Conaway H. Animal model of human disease. Spontaneous diabetes mellitus in the New Zealand White rabbit. *Am J Pathol.* 1982;109:359.
431. Rosenthal KL, Wire NR. Endocrine diseases. In: Quesenberry K, Carpenter JW, eds. *Ferrets, Rabbits, and Rodents: Clinical Medicine and Surgery.* 3rd ed. St. Louis, MO: Elsevier/Saunders; 2012:86-102.
432. Benoit-Biancamano MO, Morin M, Langlois I. Histopathologic lesions of diabetes mellitus in a domestic ferret. *Can Vet J.* 2005;46:895-897.
433. Phair KA, Carpenter JW, Schermerhorn T, et al. Diabetic ketoacidosis with concurrent pancreatitis, pancreatic β islet cell tumor, and adrenal disease in an obese ferret *(Mustela putorius furo). J Am Assoc Lab Anim Sci.* 2011;50(4):531.
434. Boari A, Papa V, Di Silverio F, et al. Type 1 diabetes mellitus and hyperadrenocorticism in a ferret. *Vet Res Commun.* 2010;34:107-110.
435. Hess L. Insulin glargine treatment of a ferret with diabetes mellitus. *J Am Vet Med Assoc.* 2012;241:1490-1494.
436. Mitchell SCG, Michael M, Reavill DR. Spontaneous pancreatitis in the ferret *(Mustela putorius furo). Proc Assoc Exotic Mammals Vet.* 2012;2012:39.
437. Carpenter JW, Novilla MN. Diabetes mellitus in a black-footed ferret. *J Am Vet Med Assoc.* 1977;171:890-893.
438. Petritz OA, Antinoff N, Chen S, et al. Evaluation of portable blood glucose meters for measurement of blood glucose concentration in ferrets *(Mustela putorius furo). J Am Vet Med Assoc.* 2013;242:350-354.
439. Selleri P, Di Girolamo N, Novari G. Performance of two portable meters and a benchtop analyzer for blood glucose concentration measurement in rabbits. *J Am Vet Med Assoc.* 2014;245:87-98.
440. Selleri P, Di Girolamo N. Point-of-care blood gases, electrolytes, chemistries, hemoglobin, and hematocrit measurement in venous samples from pet rabbits. *J Am Anim Hosp Assoc.* 2014;50:305-314.
441. Lippi D, et al. Historical background or de quibusdam renum glandulis: the history of adrenals. In: Valeri A, Bergamini C, Bellantone R, et al., eds. *Surgery of the Adrenal Gland.* Milan: Springer-Verlag Italia; 2012:1-14.
442. Leoutsakos B, Leoutsakos A. The adrenal glands: a brief historical perspective. *Hormones (Athens).* 2008;7:334-336.
443. Galac S, Reusch C, Kooistra H, et al. Adrenals. In: Rijnberk A, Kooistra HS, eds. *Clinical Endocrinology of Dogs and Cats: An Illustrated Text.* Hannover: Schlütersche; 2010;93-154.
444. Fung MM, Viveros OH, O'Connor DT. Diseases of the adrenal medulla. *Acta Physiol (Oxf).* 2008;192:325-335.
445. Hartman FA, Brownell KA. The hormone of the adrenal cortex. *Exp Biol Med.* 1930;27:938-939.
446. Viveros OH, Diliberto EJ, Hazum E, et al. Opiate-like materials in the adrenal medulla: evidence for storage and secretion with catecholamines. *Mol Pharmacol.* 1979;16:1101-1108.
447. Miller CL, Marini RP, Fox JG. Diseases of the endocrine system. In: Fox JG, Marini RP, eds. *Biology and Diseases of the Ferret.* 3rd ed. Ames, IA: Wiley-Blackwell; 2014:377-400.
448. Holmes RL. The adrenal glands of the ferret, *Mustela putorius. J Anat.* 1961;95:325-336.
449. Bielinska M, Parviainen H, Kiiveri S, et al. Review paper: origin and molecular pathology of adrenocortical neoplasms. *Vet Pathol.* 2009;46:194-210.
450. Deacon CF, Mosley W, Jones IC. The X zone of the mouse adrenal cortex of the Swiss albino strain. *Gen Comp Endocrinol.* 1986;61:87-99.
451. Bielinska M, Kiiveri S, Parviainen H, et al. Gonadectomy-induced adrenocortical neoplasia in the domestic ferret *(Mustela putorius furo)* and laboratory mouse. *Vet Pathol.* 2006;43:97-117.
452. Carsia RV, Harvey S. Adrenals. In: Whittow GC, ed. *Sturkie's Avian Physiology.* San Diego: Academic Press; 2000:489-538.
453. Honour JW. Hypothalamic-pituitary-adrenal axis. *Respir Med.* 1994;88(suppl 1):9-15.
454. de Matos R. Adrenal steroid metabolism in birds: anatomy, physiology, and clinical considerations. *Vet Clin North Am Exot Anim Pract.* 2008;11:35-57, vi.

455. Herrera M, Nelson RW. Pheochromocytoma. In: Ettinger SJ, Feldman EC, eds. *Textbook of Veterinary Internal Medicine: Diseases of the Dog and the Cat.* 7th ed. St. Louis, MO: Elsevier/Saunders; 2010:1865-1871.
456. Manger WM, Eisenhofer G. Pheochromocytoma: diagnosis and management update. *Curr Hypertens Rep.* 2004;6:477-484.
457. Waguespack SG, Rich T, Grubbs E, et al. A current review of the etiology, diagnosis, and treatment of pediatric pheochromocytoma and paraganglioma. *J Clin Endocrinol Metab.* 2010;95:2023-2037.
458. Disick GI, Palese MA. Extra-adrenal pheochromocytoma: diagnosis and management. *Curr Urol Rep.* 2007;8:83-88.
459. Ritchie M, Pilny AA. The anatomy and physiology of the avian endocrine system. *Vet Clin North Am Exot Anim Pract.* 2008;11:1-14, v.
460. Bonar CJ, Lewandowski AH, Arafah B, et al. Pheochromocytoma in an aged female African elephant (*Loxodonta africana*). *J Zoo Wildl Med.* 2005;36:719-723.
461. Bravo EL, Tagle R. Pheochromocytoma: state-of-the-art and future prospects. *Endocr Rev.* 2003;24:539-553.
462. Martinez J, Galindo-Cardiel I, Diez-Padrisa M, et al. Malignant pheochromocytoma in a pig. *J Vet Diagn Invest.* 2012;24:207-210.
463. Gilson SD, Withrow SJ, Wheeler SL, et al. Pheochromocytoma in 50 dogs. *J Vet Intern Med.* 1994;8:228-232.
464. Chun R, Jakovljevic S, Morrison WB, et al. Apocrine gland adenocarcinoma and pheochromocytoma in a cat. *J Am Anim Hosp Assoc.* 1997;33:33-36.
465. West JL. Bovine pheochromocytoma: case report and review of literature. *Am J Vet Res.* 1975;36:1371-1373.
466. Yovich JV, Horney FD, Hardee GE. Pheochromocytoma in the horse and measurement of norepinephrine levels in horses. *Can Vet J.* 1984;25:21-25.
467. Aydogan A, Ozmen O. A pheochromocytoma case in a 6-year-old sheep. *Revue Med Vet.* 2012;163:536-538.
468. Lohr CV. One hundred two tumors in 100 goats (1987-2011). *Vet Pathol.* 2013;50:668-675.
469. Tischler AS, Sheldon W, Gray R. Immunohistochemical and morphological characterization of spontaneously occurring pheochromocytomas in the aging mouse. *Vet Pathol.* 1996;33:512-520.
470. Collins BR. Endocrine diseases of rodents. *Vet Clin North Am Exot Anim Pract.* 2008;11:153-162, vii-viii.
471. Port CD, Maschgan ER, Pond J, et al. Multiple neoplasia in a jaguar (*Panthera onca*). *J Comp Pathol.* 1981;91:115-122.
472. Hope K, Deem SL. Retrospective study of morbidity and mortality of captive jaguars (*Panthera onca*) in North America: 1982-2002. *Zoo Biol.* 2006;25:501-512.
473. Chu P-Y, Zhuo Y-X, Wang F-I, et al. Spontaneous neoplasms in zoo mammals, birds and reptiles in Taiwan—a 10-year survey. *Anim Biol.* 2012;62:95-110.
474. Reppas GP, Bodley KB, Watson GF, et al. Phaeochromocytoma in two coatimundi (*Nasua nasua*). *Vet Rec.* 2001;148:806-809.
475. Munson L, Montali RJ. High prevalence of ovarian tumors in maned wolves (*Chrysocyon brachyurus*) at the National Zoological Park. *J Zoo Wildl Med.* 1991;22:125-129.
476. Sills RC, Dunstan RW, Watson GL, et al. Pheochromocytomas in two raccoon dogs. *Vet Pathol.* 1988;25:178-179.
477. Duncan M, Grahn BH, Wilcock BP, et al. Pheochromocytoma associated with hypertensive lesions in a river hippopotamus (*Hippopotamus amphibius*). *J Zoo Wildl Med.* 1994;25:575-579.
478. Bertelsen MF, Steele SL, Grondahl C, et al. Pheochromocytoma in a white rhinoceros (*Ceratotherium simum*). *J Zoo Wildl Med.* 2011;42:521-523.
479. Stringer EM, De Voe RS, Linder K, et al. Vesiculobullous skin reaction temporally related to firocoxib treatment in a white rhinoceros (*Ceratotherium simum*). *J Zoo Wildl Med.* 2012;43:186-189.
480. Cole G, Suedmeyer WK, Johnson G. Pheochromocytoma in an African warthog (*Phacochoerus aethiopicus*). *J Zoo Wildl Med.* 2008;39:663-666.
481. Griner LA. Thyroid medullary carcinoma and pheochromocytoma in an aged European mouflon (*Ovis ammon musimon*). *J Zoo Anim Med.* 1981;12:117-120.
482. Reichard TA, Ensley PK, Henrick MJ. Pheochromocytoma in a ring-tailed lemur (*Lemur catta*). *Proc Am Assoc Zoo Vet.* 1981;1981:44-45.
483. Spelman LH, Osborn KG, Anderson MP. Pathogenesis of hemosiderosis in lemurs: role of dietary iron, tannin, and ascorbic acid. *Zoo Biol.* 1989;8:239-251.
484. Remick AK, Van Wettere AJ, Williams CV. Neoplasia in prosimians: case series from a captive prosimian population and literature review. *Vet Pathol.* 2009;46:746-772.
485. Brack M. Adrenal gland tumours in two cotton-top tamarins (*Saguinus oedipus oedipus*). *Lab Anim.* 2000;34:106-110.
486. Juan-Salles C, Ramos-Vara JA, Garner MM. Pheochromocytoma in six New World primates. *Vet Pathol.* 2009;46:662-666.
487. Dias JL, Montali RJ, Strandberg JD, et al. Endocrine neoplasia in New World primates. *J Med Primatol.* 1996;25:34-41.
488. Vogel P, Fritz D. Cardiomyopathy associated with angiomatous pheochromocytoma in a rhesus macaque (*Macaca mulatta*). *Vet Pathol.* 2003;40:468-473.
489. Wadsworth PF, Jones DM, Pugsley SL. A survey of mammalian and avian neoplasms at the Zoological Society of London. *J Zoo Anim Med.* 1985;16:73-80.
490. Schlanser JR, Patterson JS, Kiupel M, et al. Disseminated pheochromocytoma in a North American river otter (*Lontra canadensis*). *J Zoo Wildl Med.* 2012;43:407-411.
491. Stetzer E, Williams TD, Nightingale JW. Cholangiocellular adenocarcinoma, leiomyoma, and pheochromocytoma in a sea otter. *J Am Vet Med Assoc.* 1981;179:1283-1284.
492. Estep JS, Baumgartner RE, Townsend F, et al. Malignant seminoma with metastasis, Sertoli cell tumor, and pheochromocytoma in a spotted dolphin (*Stenella frontalis*) and malignant seminoma with metastasis in a bottlenose dolphin (*Tursiops truncatus*). *Vet Pathol.* 2005;42:357-359.
493. Sonnenfield JM, Carpenter JW, Garner MM, et al. Pheochromocytoma in a Nicobar pigeon (*Caloenas nicobarica*). *J Avian Med Surg.* 2002;16:306-308.
494. Campbell JG. *Tumours of the Fowl.* London: William Heinemann Medical Books Ltd.; 1969.
495. Hahn KA, Jones MP, Petersen MG, et al. Metastatic pheochromocytoma in a parakeet. *Avian Dis.* 1997;41:751-754.
496. Sutton MG, Sheps SG, Lie JT. Prevalence of clinically unsuspected pheochromocytoma. Review of a 50-year autopsy series. *Mayo Clin Proc.* 1981;56:354-360.
497. Schoemaker NJ, Teerds KJ, Mol JA, et al. The role of luteinizing hormone in the pathogenesis of hyperadrenocorticism in neutered ferrets. *Mol Cell Endocrinol.* 2002;197:117-125.
498. Li X, Fox JG, Padrid PA. Neoplastic diseases in ferrets: 574 cases (1968-1997). *J Am Vet Med Assoc.* 1998;212:1402-1406.
499. Simone-Freilicher E. Adrenal gland disease in ferrets. *Vet Clin North Am Exot Anim Pract.* 2008;11:125-137, vii.
500. Vinke CM, van Deijk R, Houx BB, et al. The effects of surgical and chemical castration on intermale aggression, sexual behaviour and play behaviour in the male ferret (*Mustela putorius furo*). *Appl Anim Behav Sci.* 2008;115:104-121.
501. Shoemaker NJ, Schuurmans M, Moorman H, et al. Correlation between age at neutering and age at onset of hyperadrenocorticism in ferrets. *J Am Vet Med Assoc.* 2000;216:195-197.
502. Bielinska M, Genova E, Boime I, et al. Nude mice as a model for gonadotropin-induced adrenocortical neoplasia. *Endocr Res.* 2004;30:913-917.
503. Beuschlein F, Galac S, Wilson DB. Animal models of adrenocortical tumorigenesis. *Mol Cell Endocrinol.* 2012;351:78-86.
504. Besso JG, Tidwell AS, Gliatto JM. Retrospective review of the ultrasonographic features of adrenal lesions in 21 ferrets. *Vet Radiol Ultrasound.* 2000;41:345-352.

505. Neuwirth L, Collins B, Calderwood-Mays M, et al. Adrenal ultrasonography correlated with histopathology in ferrets. *Vet Radiol Ultrasound*. 1997;38:69-74.

506. O'Brien RT, Paul-Murphy J, Dubielzig RR. Ultrasonography of adrenal glands in normal ferrets. *Vet Radiol Ultrasound*. 1996;37:445-448.

507. Kuijten AM, Schoemaker NJ, Voorhout G. Ultrasonographic visualization of the adrenal glands of healthy ferrets and ferrets with hyperadrenocorticism. *J Am Anim Hosp Assoc*. 2007;43:78-84.

508. Lennox AM, Wagner R. Comparison of 4.7-mg deslorelin implants and surgery for the treatment of adrenocortical disease in ferrets. *J Exot Pet Med*. 2012;21:332-335.

509. Miller LA, Fagerstone KA, Wagner RA, et al. Use of a GnRH vaccine, GonaCon™, for prevention and treatment of adrenocortical disease (ACD) in domestic ferrets. *Vaccine*. 2013;31:4619-4623.

510. Lennox AM, Chitty J. Adrenal neoplasia and hyperplasia as a cause of hypertestosteronism in two rabbits. *J Exot Pet Med*. 2006;15:56-58.

511. Oudshoorn N. Endocrinologists and the conceptualization of sex, 1920-1940. *J Hist Biol*. 1990;23:163-186.

512. Dotson JL, Brown RT. The history of the development of anabolic-androgenic steroids. *Pediatr Clin North Am*. 2007;54:761-769.

513. Schlinger BA, Soma KK, Saldanha C. Advances in avian behavioral endocrinology. *The Auk*. 2001;118:283-289.

514. Kinsky FC. The consistent presence of paired ovaries in the kiwi (*Apteryx*) with some discussion of this condition in other birds. *J Für Ornithol*. 1971;112(3):334-357.

515. Coles BH. *Essentials of Avian Medicine and Surgery*. 3rd ed. Oxford, UK; Ames, IA: Blackwell Publishing; 2007.

516. Fitzpatrick F. Unilateral and bilateral ovaries in raptorial birds. *Wilson Bull*. 1934;46:19-22.

517. Boehm EF. Bilateral ovaries in Australian hawks. *Emu*. 1942;42:251.

518. Blanco J, Bird DM, Samour JH. Reproductive. In: Bildstein KL, Bird DM, eds. *Raptor Research and Management Techniques*. Surrey, British Colombia; Blaine, WI: Hancock House; 2007:286-292.

519. Calder WA. The kiwi and egg design: evolution as a package deal. *Bioscience*. 1979;29:461-467.

520. Jensen T, Durrant B. Assessment of reproductive status and ovulation in female brown kiwi (*Apteryx mantelli*) using fecal steroids and ovarian follicle size. *Zoo Biol*. 2006;25:25-34.

521. Pieau C, Dorizzi M. Oestrogens and temperature-dependent sex determination in reptiles: all is in the gonads. *J Endocrinol*. 2004;181:367-377.

522. Bennett RA. Soft tissue surgery. In: Quesenberry KE, Carpenter JW, eds. *Ferrets, Rabbits, and Rodents: Clinical Medicine and Surgery*. St. Louis, MO: Elsevier/Saunders; 2012:373-391.

523. Van Goethem B, Schaefers-Okkens A, Kirpensteijn J. Making a rational choice between ovariectomy and ovariohysterectomy in the dog: a discussion of the benefits of either technique. *Vet Surg*. 2006;35:136-143.

524. Hotchkiss C. Effect of surgical removal of subcutaneous tumors on survival of rats. *J Am Vet Med Assoc*. 1995;206:1575-1579.

525. Planas-Silva MD, Rutherford TM, Stone MC. Prevention of age-related spontaneous mammary tumors in outbred rats by late ovariectomy. *Cancer Detect Prev*. 2008;32:65-71.

526. Greenacre C, Mccleery B, Jones MP, et al. Effect of spaying or neutering between 90 and 180 days of age on occurrence of spontaneous mammary fibroadenoma in pet rats (*Rattus norvegicus*). *Proc Int Conf Avian Herpetol Exot Mammal Med*. 2015;2015:444.

527. Steele MS, Bennett RA. Clinical technique: dorsal ovariectomy in rodents. *J Exot Pet Med*. 2011;20:222-226.

528. Resko JA. Endocrine control of adrenal progesterone secretion in the ovariectomized rat. *Science*. 1969;164:70-71.

529. Feder HH, Resko JA, Goy RW. Progesterone levels in the arterial plasma of pre-ovulatory and ovariectomized rats. *J Endocrinol*. 1968;41:563-569.

530. Macdonald GJ. Maintenance of pregnancy in ovariectomized rats with steroid analogs and the reproductive ability of the progeny. *Biol Reprod*. 1982;27:261-267.

531. Deanesly R. Implantation and early pregnancy in ovariectomized guinea-pigs. *J Reprod Fertil*. 1960;1:242-248.

532. Schneider F, Tomek W, Grundker C. Gonadotropin-releasing hormone (GnRH) and its natural analogues: a review. *Theriogenology*. 2006;66:691-709.

533. Magon N. Gonadotropin releasing hormone agonists: Expanding vistas. *Indian J Endocrinol Metab*. 2011;15:261-267.

534. Harrison GS, Wierman ME, Nett TM, et al. Gonadotropin-releasing hormone and its receptor in normal and malignant cells. *Endocr Relat Cancer*. 2004;11:725-748.

535. Huirne JA, Lambalk CB. Gonadotropin-releasing-hormone-receptor antagonists. *Lancet*. 2001;358:1793-1803.

536. Katsila T, Balafas E, Liapakis G, et al. Evaluation of a stable gonadotropin-releasing hormone analog in mice for the treatment of endocrine disorders and prostate cancer. *J Pharmacol Exp Ther*. 2011;336:613-623.

537. Sharifi R, Bruskewitz RC, Gittleman MC, et al. Leuprolide acetate 22.5 mg 12-week depot formulation in the treatment of patients with advanced prostate cancer. *Clin Ther*. 1996;18:647-657.

538. Plosker GL, Brogden RN. Leuprorelin. A review of its pharmacology and therapeutic use in prostatic cancer, endometriosis and other sex hormone-related disorders. *Drugs*. 1994;48:930-967.

539. Chrisp P, Sorkin EM. Leuprorelin. A review of its pharmacology and therapeutic use in prostatic disorders. *Drugs Aging*. 1991;1:487-509.

540. Mitchell MA. Leuprolide acetate. *Sem Avian Exotic Pet Med*. 2005;14(2):153-155.

541. Millam J, Finney H. Leuprolide acetate can reversibly prevent egg laying in cockatiels (*Nymphicus hollandicus*). *Zoo Biol*. 1994;13:149-155.

542. Keller KA, Beaufrere H, Brandao J, et al. Long-term management of ovarian neoplasia in two cockatiels (*Nymphicus hollandicus*). *J Avian Med Surg*. 2013;27:44-52.

543. Millam JR, Finney HL. Leuprolide acetate can reversibly prevent egg laying in cockatiels (*Nymphicus hollandicus*). *Zoo Biol*. 1994;13:149-155.

544. Mans C, Sladky KK. Clinical management of an ectopic egg in a Timneh African grey parrot (*Psittacus erithacus timneh*). *J Am Vet Med Assoc*. 2013;242:963-968.

545. Bean AD. Ovarian cysts in the guinea pig (*Cavia porcellus*). *Vet Clin North Am Exot Anim Pract*. 2013;16:757-776.

546. Wagner RA, Bailey EM, Schneider JF, et al. Leuprolide acetate treatment of adrenocortical disease in ferrets. *J Am Vet Med Assoc*. 2001;218:1272-1274.

547. Klaphake E, Fecteau K, Dewit M, et al. Effects of leuprolide acetate on selected blood and fecal sex hormones in Hispaniolan Amazon parrots (*Amazona ventralis*). *J Avian Med Surg*. 2009;23:253-262.

548. Mans C, Pilny A. Use of GnRH-agonists for medical management of reproductive disorders in birds. *Vet Clin North Am*. 2014;17:23-33.

549. Dickerman RW, Wise TH, Bahr JM. Effect of ovarian regression and molt on plasma concentrations of thymosin β_4 in domestic hens (*Gallus domesticus*). *Domest Anim Endocrinol*. 1992;9(4):297-304.

550. Kirchgessner M, Mitchell M, Domenzain L, et al. Evaluating the effect of leuprolide acetate on testosterone levels in captive male green iguanas (*Iguana iguana*). *J Herpetol Med Surg*. 2009;19:128-131.

551. Stringer EM, De Voe RS, Loomis MR. Suspected anaphylaxis to leuprolide acetate depot in two elf owls (*Micrathene whitneyi*). *J Zoo Wildl Med*. 2011;42:166-168.

552. Johnson JG III. Therapeutic review: deslorelin acetate subcutaneous implant. *J Exot Pet Med*. 2013;22:82-84.

553. Conn PM, Crowley WF Jr. Gonadotropin-releasing hormone and its analogs. *Annu Rev Med*. 1994;45:391-405.

554. Trigg T, Doyle A, Walsh J, et al. A review of advances in the use of the GnRH agonist deslorelin in control of reproduction. *Theriogenology*. 2006;66:1507-1512.

555. Trigg T, Wright P, Armour A, et al. Use of a GnRH analogue implant to produce reversible long-term suppression of reproductive function in male and female domestic dogs. *J Reprod Fertil Suppl*. 2001;57:255-261.

556. Wagner RA, Piche CA, Jochle W, et al. Clinical and endocrine responses to treatment with deslorelin acetate implants in ferrets with adrenocortical disease. *Am J Vet Res*. 2005;66:910-914.

557. Wagner RA, Finkler MR, Fecteau KA, et al. The treatment of adrenal cortical disease in ferrets with 4.7-mg deslorelin acetate implants. *J Exot Pet Med*. 2009;18:146-152.

558. Prohaczik A, Kulcsar M, Trigg T, et al. Comparison of four treatments to suppress ovarian activity in ferrets *(Mustela putorius furo)*. *Vet Rec*. 2010;166:74-78.

559. Schoemaker N, Van Deijk R, Muijlaert B, et al. Use of a gonadotropin releasing hormone agonist implant as an alternative for surgical castration in male ferrets *(Mustela putorius furo)*. *Theriogenology*. 2008;70:161-167.

560. Pilny A. Ovarian cystic disease in guinea pigs. *Vet Clin North Am Exot Anim Pract*. 2014;17:69-75.

561. Keller LS, Griffith JW, Lang CM. Reproductive failure associated with cystic rete ovarii in guinea pigs. *Vet Pathol*. 1987;24:335-339.

562. Wang W, Liu H-l, Tian W, et al. Morphologic observation and classification criteria of atretic follicles in guinea pigs. *J Zhejiang Univ Sci B*. 2010;11:307-314.

563. Shi F, Watanabe G, Trewin AL, et al. Localization of ovarian inhibin/activin subunits in follicular dominance during the estrous cycle of guinea pigs. *Zoolog Sci*. 2000;17:1311-1320.

564. Garris DR, Foreman D. Follicular growth and atresia during the last half of the luteal phase of the guinea pig estrous cycle: relation to serum progesterone and estradiol levels and utero-ovarian blood flow. *Endocrinology*. 1984;115:73-77.

565. Schuetzenhofer G, Goericke-Pesch S, Wehrend A. Effects of deslorelin implants on ovarian cysts in guinea pigs. *Schweiz Arch Tierheilkd*. 2011;153:416-417.

566. Risi E. Control of reproduction in ferrets, rabbits and rodents. *Reprod Domest Anim*. 2014;49:81-86.

567. Kohutova S, Jekl V, Knotek Z, et al. The effect of deslorelin acetate on the oestrous cycle of female guinea pigs. *Vet Med (Praha)*. 2015;60:155-160.

568. Arlt S, Spankowski S, Kaufmann T, et al. Fertility control in a male rabbit using a deslorelin implant. A case report. *World Rabbit Sci*. 2010;18:179-182.

569. Grosset C, Peters S, Peron F, et al. Contraceptive effect and potential side-effects of deslorelin acetate implants in rats *(Rattus norvegicus)*: Preliminary observations. *Can J Vet Res*. 2012;76:209.

570. Petritz OA, Sanchez-Migallon Guzman D, Paul-Murphy J, et al. Evaluation of the efficacy and safety of single administration of 4.7-mg deslorelin acetate implants on egg production and plasma sex hormones in Japanese quail *(Coturnix coturnix japonica)*. *Am J Vet Res*. 2013;74:316-323.

571. Noonan B, Johnson P, de Matos R. Evaluation of egg-laying suppression effects of the GnRH agonist deslorelin in domestic chickens. *Proc Annu Conf Assoc Avian Vet*. 2012;2012:321.

572. Cowan ML, Martin GB, Monks DJ, et al. Inhibition of the reproductive system by deslorelin in male and female pigeons *(Columba livia)*. *J Avian Med Surg*. 2014;28:102-108.

573. de Matos R. Investigation of the chemopreventive effects of deslorelin in domestic chickens with high prevalence of ovarian cancer. *Proc Int Conf Avian Herpetol Exot Mammal Med*. 2013;2013:90.

574. Kuenzel WJ. Central nervous system regulation of gonadal development in the avian male. *Poult Sci*. 2000;79:1679-1688.

575. Ottinger MA, Murray RB. Endocrinology of the avian reproductive system. *J Avian Med Surg*. 1995;9:242-250.

576. Powell RC, Jach H, Millar RP, et al. Identification of Gln8-GnRH and His5, Trp7, Tyr8-GnRH in the hypothalamus and extrahypothalamic brain of the ostrich *(Struthio camelus)*. *Peptides*. 1986;8:185-190.

577. Lescheid DW, Terasawa E, Abler LA, et al. A second form of gonadotropin-releasing hormone (GnRH) with characteristics of chicken GnRH-II is present in the primate brain. *Endocrinology*. 1997;138(12):5618-5629.

578. Maney DL, Richardson RD, Wingfield JC. Central administration of chicken gonadotropin-releasing hormone-II enhances courtship behavior in a female sparrow. *Horm Behav*. 1997;32:11-18.

579. Tsutsui K, Saigoh E, Ukena K, et al. A novel avian hypothalamic peptide inhibiting gonadotropin release. *Biochem Biophys Res Commun*. 2000;275:661-667.

580. Ukena K, Ubuka T, Tsutsui K. Distribution of a novel avian gonadotropin-inhibitory hormone in the quail brain. *Cell Tissue Res*. 2003;312:73-79.

581. Bentley GE, Kriegsfeld LJ, Osugi T, et al. Interactions of gonadotropin-releasing hormone (GnRH) and gonadotropin-inhibitory hormone (GnIH) in birds and mammals. *J Exp Zool A Comp Exp Biol*. 2006;305:807-814.

582. Rowland M. Use of a deslorelin implant to control aggression in a male bearded dragon *(Pogona vitticeps)*. *Vet Rec*. 2011;169:127.

APPENDIX

Reptiles

Hypothalamus-Pituitary-Adrenal and Hypothalamus-Pituitary-Gonadal Axis-Related Hormones

Species	Corticosterone (nmol/L)	Progesterone (nmol/L)	17β-Estradiol (pmol/L)	Testosterone (nmol/L)	Methodology	Information	Reference
Gopher tortoise (*Gopherus polyphemus*)		Egg layers 9.7 ± 2.5 (4.0-18.8)§ (n = 13) Not egg layers 6.4 ± 1.1 (0-13.3)§			RIA	Wild females, May to November, blood collected within 5 min after being discovered in the trap	1
Yellow-blotched map turtle (*Graptemys flavimaculata*)	Female 1.1 ± 0.23 (0-6.6)§ (n = 49) Male 1.5 ± 0.26 (0-8.6)§ (n = 60)				RIA	Wild, basal value from sample collected immediately after capture	2
Marine iguana (*Amblyrhynchus cristatus*)				Nonbreeding 0.05 ± 0.025† (n = 17) Breeding 0.33 ± 0.082† (n = 17)	RIA	Wild, male, undisturbed populations, breeding season (July), nonbreeding season (December)	3
Marine iguana (*Amblyrhynchus cristatus*)				Nonbreeding 0.08 ± 0.055† (n = 15) Breeding 1.50 ± 0.460† (n = 15)	RIA	Wild, male, undisturbed populations, breeding season (July), nonbreeding season (December)	3
Green sea turtle (*Chelonia mydas*)				Fall ~0.10‖ Spring 0.94-1.35‡	RIA	Captive breeding colony	4
Eastern bearded dragon (*Pogona barbata*)	Vitellogenic 3.6 ± 0.78† (n = 6) Gravid 9.6 ± 2.98† (n = 8) Not gravid/vitellogenic 5.7 ± 2.05† (n = 11)	Vitellogenic 39.1 ± 14.2† (n = 6) Gravid 32.4 ± 15.9† (n = 8) Not gravid/vitellogenic 33.8 ± 14.5† (n = 11)			RIA	Females, reproductive status identified on palpation (vitellogenic, gravid, not gravid, or vitellogenic)	5
Eastern bearded dragon (*Pogona barbata*)	5.2 ± 1.82† (n = 19)	0.9 ± 0.01 (0.7-1.8)§ (n = 20)		0.35 ± 0.076 (0.07-1.07)§ (n = 13)	RIA	Male, without previous manipulation	5
Duvaucel's gecko (*Hoplodactylus duvaucelii*)	Summer 16.7 ± 4.28† (n = 9) Winter 19.6 ± 2.86† (n = 10) Spring 3.7 ± 0.89† (n = 5)				RIA	Captive females, several seasons of the year	6

Continued

Hypothalamus-Pituitary-Adrenal and Hypothalamus-Pituitary-Gonadal Axis-Related Hormones—cont'd

Species	Corticosterone (nmol/L)	Progesterone (nmol/L)	17β-Estradiol (pmol/L)	Testosterone (nmol/L)	Methodology	Information	Reference
Duvaucel's gecko (Hoplodactylus duvaucelii)	Summer 4.1 ± 1.13† (n = 8) Winter 13.9 ± 3.69† (n = 8) Spring 7.5 ± 1.24† (n = 14)				RIA	Wild females, several seasons of the year	6
Blotched blue-tongued lizard (Tiliqua nigrolutea)		2nd Semester of gestation 40.4 ± 4.0† Late summer, prior to parturition 14.0 ± 2.8†	Spring 1010.0 ± 135.3† November (ovulation) 2624.4 ± 391.5†	Mating season 0.22 ± 0.022† Quiescent 0.16 ± 0.011†	RIA	Wild-caught females, different reproductive stages, reproductively active (n = 8), quiescent (n = 8)	7
Shingleback lizard (Tiliqua rugosa)		1st Pregnancy trimester 1.8‖ 2nd Pregnancy trimester 7.2‖ 3rd Pregnancy trimester 0.9‖ Nonpregnant 0.2‖			RIA	6 gravid females, wild caught	8
Green sea turtle (Chelonia mydas)	Females capable of breeding 3.0 ± 0.84† Post last clutch 1.3 ± 0.61†			Females capable of breeding 0.03 ± 0.002† Post last clutch 0.01 ± 0.006†	RIA	Adult wild females, n = 23	9
Green sea turtle (Chelonia mydas)	<2 Min of capture 2.0‖ (n = 5) 3-4 H of confinement 7.8‖ (n = 5)				RIA	Clinically healthy juvenile animals	10,11
Loggerhead sea turtle (Caretta caretta)	<15 Min from capture 1.6‖ 3 H of confinement ~17.3‖				RIA	Animals captured by tangle net	10,12
Loggerhead sea turtle (Caretta caretta)	~0.6-5.8‡ (n = 54)	~0.6-1‡ (n = 54)		~0.004-0.024‡ (n = 54)	RIA	Females, <3 min from capture	10,13
American alligator (Alligator mississippiensis)	<5 Min from capture ~2.9‖ (n = 6) 4 H of confinement ~17.3‖ (n = 6)			0.0003-1.77‡ (n = 6)	RIA	Males	10,14
American alligator (Alligator mississippiensis)	<15 Min from capture 2.5‖ (n = 21)				N/A	Males	10,15
American alligator (Alligator mississippiensis)	<15 Min from capture 1.0‖ (n = 44)				N/A	Females	10,15

Species				Assay	Notes	References
American alligator (*Alligator mississippiensis*)	<10 Min from capture 2.3‖ (n = 5) 4 H of confinement 36.4‖ (n = 5)	<10 Min from capture ~2128.6‖ (n = 5) 22 H of confinement ~1394.6‖ (n = 5)		RIA	Females	10,16
American alligator (*Alligator mississippiensis*)	~1.5-21.7‡ (n = 61)	~1137.7-~2238.7‡ (n = 61)	~0.17-~1.22‡ (n = 61)	RIA	Females, <15 min from capture	10,17
American alligator (*Alligator mississippiensis*)	<2 Min from capture 2.3-3.1‡ (n = 35) 2 H of confinement ~72.3-104.4‡ (n = 35)	<2 Min from capture 33.8-107.3‡ (n = 35) 2 H of confinement ~29.4-66.1‡ (n = 35)	0.25-0.80‡ (n = 35) ~0.31-0.69‡ (n = 35)	RIA	Juveniles, no variation between early- and late-evening capture	10,18
Tuatara (*Sphenodon punctatus*)	<10 Min from capture 0.32-5.9‡ 3 H of confinement 32.5‖			N/A	Males, values varied with season but not time of the day	10
Tuatara (*Sphenodon punctatus*)	<10 Min from capture 1.5-12.9‡ 3 H of confinement 31.8‖			N/A	Females, values varied with season but not with time of the day	10
Tuatara (*Sphenodon punctatus*)	3.7-13.4‡			N/A	Juveniles, seasonal variation in juvenile females but not juvenile males, <20 min from capture	10,19
Ornate crevice-dragon (*Ctenophorus ornatus*)	~1.5-433.5‡			N/A	Values varied with season, <3 min from capture	10
Six-lined racerunner (*Aspidoscelis sexlineata*)	<57.8‖			N/A	Male, values varied with season, <5 min from capture	10
Six-lined racerunner (*Aspidoscelis sexlineata*)	~11.6-49.1‡			N/A	Female, values did not vary with season or reproductive condition, <5 min from capture	10
Desert grassland whiptail lizard (*Aspidoscelis uniparens*)	~5.8-18.8‡			N/A	Female, value declined during vitellogenesis, <5 min from capture	10
Common gecko (*Woodworthia maculatus*)	~1.5-18.8‡			N/A	Female, value varied with season, <14 min from capture	10

Continued

Hypothalamus-Pituitary-Adrenal and Hypothalamus-Pituitary-Gonadal Axis-Related Hormones—cont'd

Species	Corticosterone (nmol/L)	Progesterone (nmol/L)	17β-Estradiol (pmol/L)	Testosterone (nmol/L)	Methodology	Information	Reference
Italian wall lizard (*Podarcis siculus*)	<1 Min from capture ~43.4-260.1‡ 6 H of confinement ~161.8-491.3‡				N/A	Male, value varied with season or reproductive cycle	10
Western fence lizard (*Sceloporus occidentalis*)	<1 Min from capture 33.2‖ 1 H of confinement ~23.1‖				N/A	Male, unparasitized animals	10
Western fence lizard (*Sceloporus occidentalis*)	<1 Min from capture ~8.7-34.7‡ 1 H of confinement ~28.9-130.1‡				N/A	No consistent variation with season or site	10
Ornate tree lizard (*Urosaurus ornatus*)	<1 Min from capture ~5.8‖ 4 H of confinement ~63.6‖				N/A	Males, significant elevation during the first 10 min of confinement	10
Ornate tree lizard (*Urosaurus ornatus*)	5.8-48.3‡				N/A	Males, significant variation with season, reproductive condition, and site, <5 min from capture	10
Ornate tree lizard (*Urosaurus ornatus*)	11.9-65.9‡				N/A	Females, significant variation with season, reproductive condition, and site, <5 min from capture	10
Ornate tree lizard (*Urosaurus ornatus*)	~21.7-54.9‡				N/A	Juveniles, <5 min from capture	10
Red-sided garter snake (*Thamnophis sirtalis parietalis*)	<1 Min from capture ~231.2‖ 6 H of confinement ~144.5‖				N/A	Females, significant decline after 1 h of confinement	10

RIA, Radioimmunoassay.

*Values are provided as mean/median values and reference interval.

†Values are provided as mean/median and standard error/standard deviation of the mean.

‡Values are provided as range.

§Values are provided as mean/median, standard error/standard deviation of the mean, and reference interval.

‖Mean/median.

Glucose Metabolism Hormones and Other Related Molecules

	Insulin (pmol/L)	Glucagon (ng/L)	Glucose (mg/dL; mmol/L)	Methodology	Source of Animals	Fasted/Time of Fast	Reference
Asp viper (*Vipera aspis*)	75.3 ± 8.6† (n = 3)		39.3 ± 0.5† mg/dL (n = 3); 2.18 ± 0.03† (n = 3)	Insulin RIA Glucose ion-selective electrodes	Adult male	Fed one mouse within the last 24 h	20
Indian flapshell turtle (*Lissemys punctata*)	58.8‖			Insulin RIA Glucose spectrophotometry	Adult females	Ad libitum food	21
Italian wall lizard (*Podarcis sicula*)	10.1‖			RIA	Adult male	N/A	22
American alligator (*Alligator mississippiensis*)	145.6 ± 27.7† (n = 8)	33.3 ± 1.72† (n = 8)	89.7 ± 3.4† mg/dL (n = 8); 4.98 ± 0.19† mmol/L (n = 8)	Insulin and glucagon RIA Glucose spectrophotometry	Captive juveniles	16 d	23
Indian flapshell turtle (*Lissemys punctata*)	Summer ~33.7‖ (n = 12) Winter ~70.3‖ (n = 12)		Summer ~90‖ mg/dL (n = 12); ~5‖ mmol/L (n = 12) Winter ~45‖ mg/dL (n = 12); ~2.5‖ mmol/L (n = 12)	Insulin RIA Glucose spectrophotometry	Wild adults	Ad libitum food	24

RIA, Radioimmunoassay.

*Values are provided as mean/median values and reference interval.

†Values are provided as mean/median and standard error/standard deviation of the mean.

‡Values are provided as range.

§Values are provided as mean/median, standard error/standard deviation of the mean, and reference interval.

‖Mean/median.

Calcium Metabolism Hormones and Other Related Molecules

Species	PTH (pmol/L)	25-Hydroxycholecalciferol (nmol/L)	1,25-Dihydroxycholecalciferol (nmol/L)	Total Calcium (mg/dL; mmol/L)	Ionized Calcium (mmol/L)	Magnesium (mg/dL; mmol/L)	Methodology	Information	Reference
Green sea turtle (Chelonia mydas)	2.95 (1.31-3.96)* (n = 10)	27.5 (17.2-64.6)* (n = 10)			0.63 (0.55-0.72)* (n = 10)		RIA	Wild juvenile animals in rehabilitation	25
Green sea turtle (Chelonia mydas)	0.75 (0.04-2.28)* (n = 10)	36 (16.1-72.1)* (n = 10)			1.05 (0.87-1.23)* (n = 10)		RIA	Suspected healthy wild animals accidentally captured	25
Green iguana (Iguana iguana)					Males 1.32‖ (n = 29) Gravid females 1.21‖ (n = 21) Nongravid females 1.30‖ (n = 17)		iCa i-stat	Captive, 2 to 4 y old, 29 males, 17 nongravid females, and 21 gravid females	26
Testudo sp.				12.52 (8.2-13.28)* mg/dL (n = 25) 3.13 (2.05-3.32)* mmol/L (n = 25)	1.32 (1.26-1.38)* (n = 25)		iCa ion-selective electrode measurement	Originally wild caught but in captivity for several years, males (n = 11) and females (n = 14); Hermann's tortoises, Testudo hermanni boettgeri; spur-thighed tortoises, Testudo graeca ibera; marginated tortoises, Testudo marginata; Horsfield tortoises, Testudo horsfieldi	27

Species			Method	Population	Ref
Ball python (Python regius)	No UVB exposure 197 ± 35† (n = 8) 70 d UVB exposure 203.5 ± 13.8† (n = 6)	No UVB exposure 1.84 ± 0.05† (n = 8) 70 d UVB exposure 1.78 ± 0.07† (n = 6)	N/A	Captive, >4 y old; exposed to UVB (n = 6 females); not exposed to UVB (n = 3 females and 5 males)	28
Loggerhead sea turtle (Caretta caretta)	7 ± 1.2† mg/dL (n = 7) 1.75 ± 0.3† mmol/L (n = 7)	4.68 ± 1.08† mg/dL (n = 7) 1.95 ± 0.45† mmol/L (n = 7)	Clinical analyzer	Captive juvenile females	29
Inland bearded dragon (Pogona vitticeps)	With UVB supplementation 17.72 ± 4† mg/dL (n = 8); 4.43 ± 1† mmol/L 83 d without UVB 13.88 ± 0.36† mg/dL (n = 10); 3.47 ± 0.09† mmol/L	With UVB supplementation 1.3 ± 0.1† (n = 4) 83 d without UVB 1.48 ± 0.1† (n = 10)	TCAutomation clinical analyzer, iCa clinical analyzer	Captive adult female	30
Inland bearded dragon (Pogona vitticeps)	UVB exposure 178.4 ± 9† No UVB exposure 9.9 ± 1.3†	UVB exposure 1.205 ± 0.100† No UVB exposure 0.229 ± 0.025†	RIA	Captive raised, 6 mo old, n = 40 males and 44 females	31
Green sea turtle (Chelonia mydas)	7.56 (3.24-10.92)* mg/dL (n = 28) 1.89 (0.81-2.73)* mmol/L (n = 28)	9.74 (3.77-23.28)* mg/dL (n = 28) 4.06 (1.57-9.7)* mmol/L (n = 28)	Commercial kits	Wild caught	32

Continued

Calcium Metabolism Hormones and Other Related Molecules—cont'd

Species	PTH (pmol/L)	25-Hydroxycholecalciferol (nmol/L)	1,25-Dihydroxycholecalciferol (nmol/L)	Total Calcium (mg/dL; mmol/L)	Ionized Calcium (mmol/L)	Magnesium (mg/dL; mmol/L)	Methodology	Information	Reference
Veiled chameleon (Chamaeleo calyptratus)		UVB exposure 142[||] With Ca and vitamin A 160[||] With Ca, vitamin A, cholecalciferol, and UVB >250[||] With Ca, vitamin A, and cholecalciferol 102[||]		UVB exposure 8.8[||] mg/dL 2.2[||] mmol/L No UVB exposure 8[||] mg/dL 2[||] mmol/L With Ca, vitamin A, and UVB 11.2[||] mg/dL 2.8[||] mmol/L With Ca and vitamin A 12.4[||] mg/dL 3.1[||] mmol/L With Ca, vitamin A, cholecalciferol, and UVB 12.4[||] mg/dL 3.1[||] mmol/L With Ca, vitamin A, and cholecalciferol) 18.4[||] mg/dL 4.6[||] mmol/L			TCAutomation clinical analyzer, 25(OH)D$_3$ HPLC	6 mo old, captive reared (n = 29 males, 27 females)	33
Corn snake (Pantherophis guttatus)		No UVB supplementation 57.33 ± 45.59 (0-132)[§] (n = 12) With 28 d UVB supplementation 196.0 ± 16.73 (121–232)[§] (n = 12)					RIA	Captive, not fed during the study	34
Red-eared slider (Trachemys scripta elegans)		No UVB supplementation 10.7 ± 3.4 (5-14)[§] (n = 6) 30 d UVB supplementation 71.7 ± 46.9 (34-155)[§] (n = 6)						Yearlings, captive	35
Ricord's iguana (Cyclura ricordii)		554 ± 275 (250-1118)[§] (n = 22)	504 ± 174 (185-785)[§] (n = 12)					Wild caught	36
Rhinoceros iguana (Cyclura cornuta)		332 ± 47 (260-369)[§] (n = 7)	195 ± 62 (112-307)[§] (n = 7)					Wild caught	36

Species				Analyte/Method	Animals	Reference
Rhinoceros iguana (Cyclura cornuta)	317 ± 81 (220-519)[§] (n = 13); 317 ± 99 (78-432)[§] (n = 12)				Captive	36
Indoor iguanian lizard	44 ± 25[†] (n = 12)	11.2 ± 2[†] mg/dL (n = 13); 2.8 ± 0.5[†] nmol/L		25(OH)D Competitive protein-binding assay	Pogona barbata (1), Physignathus lesueurii lesueurii (2), Chlamydosaurus kingii (4), Iguana iguana (2), Brachulophus fasciatus (4)	37
Outdoor iguanian lizard	105 ± 70[†] (n = 26)	10.28 ± 2[†] mg/dL (n = 25); 2.57 ± 0.5[†] nmol/L		25(OH)D Competitive protein-binding assay	Pogona barbata (7), Physignathus lesueurii lesueurii (12), Chlamydosaurus kingii (1), Iguana iguana (2), Cyclura cornuta cornura (4)	37
Fijian iguana (Brachylophus sp.)	78 ± 47[†] (n = 21)	11.84 ± 2[†] mg/dL (n = 14); 2.96 ± 0.5[†] nmol/L		25(OH)D Competitive protein-binding assay	Brachyluphus fasciatus (10), Brachylophus vitiensis (11)	37
Komodo dragon (Varanus komodoensis)	164 (4-324)* (n = 54)	14.16 (12-17.6)* mg/dL (n = 52); 3.54 (3-4.4)* mmol/L	3.22 (2.02-4.46)* mg/dL (n = 48); 1.34 (0.84-1.86)* mmol/L (n = 48)	TCAutomation spectrophotometric assay method 25(OH)D$_3$ RIA	Captive and wild animals	38

HPLC, High-performance liquid chromatography; iCa, ionized calcium; PTH, parathyroid hormone; RIA, radioimmunoassay; UVB, ultraviolet B.

*Values are provided as mean/median values and reference interval.

[†]Values are provided as mean/median and standard error/standard deviation of the mean.

[‡]Values are provided as range.

[§]Values are provided as mean/median, standard error/standard deviation of the mean, and reference interval.

[‖]Mean/median.

Hypothalamus-Pituitary-Thyroid Axis-Related Hormones

Species	TT$_4$ (nmol/L)	TT$_3$ (nmol/L)	fT$_4$ (pmol/L)	fT$_3$ (pmol/L)	Methodology	Target Population	Reference
Desert tortoise (*Gopherus agassizii*)	Females 0.55 ± 0.1† to 3.69 ± 0.3† (n = 28) Males 0.46 ± 0.11† to 3.15 ± 0.36† (n = 22)				RIA	Captive population, housed outdoors	39
Green iguana (*Iguana iguana*)	2.98-4.65‡ (n = 7)				Fluorescence polarization immunoassay	Clinically healthy, 2 to 8 y old	40
American alligators (*Alligator mississippiensis*)	0.53-25.4‡	0.05-0.89‡			RIA	Juvenile, wild population	41
Russian tortoise (*Testudo horsfieldii*)	8.88 ± 1.29‡ (n = 4)	0.89 ± 0.09† (n = 4)			RIA	Adult males, at 34°C, active, digging, and looking for shelter	42
Corn snake (*Pantherophis guttatus*)	2.75 (0.45-6.06)* (n = 10)				RIA for fT$_4$	Methodology no longer commercially available	43
Ball python (*Python regius*)	2.58 (0.93-4.79)* (n = 11)				RIA for fT$_4$	Methodology no longer commercially available	43
Milk snake (*Lampropeltis triangulum*)	1.88 (0.27-2.94)* (n = 11)				RIA for fT$_4$	Methodology no longer commercially available	43
Boa constrictor (*Boa constrictor*)	2.5 (≤0.24-3.98)* (n = 10)				RIA for fT$_4$	Methodology no longer commercially available	43
Galapagos tortoises (*Chelonoidis nigra*)	13.90-19.82‡ (n = 3)	0.51-1.53‡ (n = 2)			RIA	Clinically healthy	44
African spurred tortoise (*Geochelone sulcata*)	4‖ (n = 12)	0.15‖ (n = 12)	4‖ (n = 12)	2.9‖ (n = 12)	N/A	Clinically healthy	45
Green sea turtle (*Chelonia mydas*)	10.43 ± 0.9† to 13.51 ± 0.7† (n = 8)				RIA	Measured throughout the day at 3 different time points, laboratory-acclimated immature animals	46
Kemp's Ridley turtle (*Lepidochelys kempii*)	4.76 ± 0.5† to 5.9 ± 0.9† (n = 8)				RIA	Measured throughout the day at 3 different time points, laboratory-acclimated immature animals	46
Italian wall lizard (*Podarcis sicula*)	1.44 ± 0.06†	1.99 ± 0.09†			RIA	Adult males	22

RIA, Radioimmunoassay.
*Values are provided as mean/median values and reference interval.
†Values are provided as mean/median and standard error/standard deviation of the mean.
‡Values are provided as range.
§Values are provided as mean/median, standard error/standard deviation of the mean, and reference interval.
‖Mean/median.

Birds

Hypothalamus-Pituitary-Adrenal and Hypothalamus-Pituitary-Gonadal Axis-Related Hormones

Species	Corticosterone (nmol/L)	Progesterone (nmol/L)	17β-Estradiol- (pmol/L)	Testosterone (nmol/L)	Methodology	Information	Reference
Pekin duck (*Anas platyrhynchos domesticus*)	69.4 ± 23.1[†] (*n* = 5)				RIA	15-mo-old healthy male white Pekin ducks	47
Chicken (*Gallus gallus domesticus*)	23.1 ± 2.9[†] (*n* = 5)				RIA	13-mo-old healthy male Ross roster	47
Willow tit (*Poecile montanus*)	Adult males 52.0 ± 8.7[†] (*n* = 20) Adult females 37.6 ± 5.8[†] (*n* = 13) Juvenile males 66.5 ± 8.7[†] (*n* = 24) Juvenile females 75.1 ± 8.7[†] (*n* = 25)			Adult males 0.59 ± 0.06[†] (*n* = 20) Adult females 0.57 ± 0.04[†] (*n* = 13) Juvenile males 0.69 ± 0.07[†] (*n* = 24) Juvenile females 0.95 ± 0.14[†] (*n* = 25)	RIA	Free-living winter willow tits: adult males (*n* = 20), adult females (*n* = 13), juvenile males (*n* = 24), and juvenile females (*n* = 25)	48
American kestrel (*Falco sparverius*)	T_0 9.5 ± 1.3[†] (*n* = 10) T_{10} 36.3 ± 6.5[†] (*n* = 10)				RIA	Captive raised adult 1 y old, baseline at T_0 and after 10 min (T_{10}) of handling	49
Adélie penguin (*Pygoscelis adeliae*)	16.8 ± 1.2 (2.3-75.4)[§] (*n* = 113)				RIA	Wild caught	50
Red-lored Amazon parrots (*Amazona autumnalis*)	30.6 ± 9.5[†] (*n* = 12)				Direct assay	Captive birds	51
Blue-fronted Amazon (*Amazona aestiva*)	60.4 ± 26.9[†] (*n* = 12)				Direct assay	Captive birds	51
African grey parrot (*Psittacus erithacus*)	64.5 ± 24.0[†] (*n* = 12)				Direct assay	Captive birds	51
Hispaniolan Amazon parrots (*Amazona ventralis*)	Awake 97.4 ± 8.2[†] (*n* = 40) Anesthetized 57.2 ± 5.7[†] (*n* = 40)				RIA	Research colony	52
Scarlet macaw (*Ara macao*)	6-26[†] (*n* = 5)					Suspected healthy animals	53
Harlequin duck (*Histrionicus histrionicus*)	69.7-118.5[‡] (*n* = 3)				RIA	Wild-caught captive females	54
Hispaniolan Amazon parrots (*Amazona ventralis*)			277.7 ± 14.7[†] (*n* = 11)		RIA	Nonbreeding (4 males, 7 females) adults, research colony	55

Continued

Hypothalamus-Pituitary-Adrenal and Hypothalamus-Pituitary-Gonadal Axis-Related Hormones—cont'd

Species	Corticosterone (nmol/L)	Progesterone (nmol/L)	17β-Estradiol- (pmol/L)	Testosterone (nmol/L)	Methodology	Information	Reference
Chicken (Gallus gallus domesticus)			451.4 (132.1-1042.3)*		RIA	Ovulatory cycle, Rhode Island Red × South Carolina White Leghorn	56
Turkey (Meleagris gallopavo)		3.5 ± 1.1† (n = 4)	81.6 ± 10.4† (n = 4)		RIA	Laying female turkeys, 4 to 5 h after oviposition	57
Japanese quail (Coturnix japonica)		At ovulation 3.6 ± 1.1† (n = 5) / 12 H prior to ovulation 2.2 ± 0.3† (n = 5) / 22 H prior to ovulation 2.5 ± 0.5† (n = 5)	At ovulation 260.6 ± 58.7† (n = 5) / 12 H prior to ovulation 400.0 ± 77.1† (n = 5) / 22 H prior to ovulation 664.3 ± 44.0† (n = 5)	At ovulation 0.51 ± 0.24† (n = 5) / 12 H prior to ovulation 0.92 ± 0.21† (n = 5) / 22 H prior to ovulation 1.54 ± 0.34† (n = 5)	RIA	Laying females	58
King penguin (Aptenodytes patagonicus)		5.6 ± 0.3† (n = 6)	807.4 ± 40.4† (n = 6)	High 0.14 ± 0.01† (n = 6) / Low 0.01 ± 0.001† (n = 6)	RIA with chromotography	Wild caught	59
White-throated sparrow (Zonotrichia albicollis)	Free living 19.3 ± 2.9† (n = 26) / Captive 47.5 ± 8.4† (n = 24)				RIA	Wild caught	60
White-crowned sparrow (Zonotrichia leucophrys)	Free living 3.4 ± 0.9† (n = 26) / Captive 14.2 ± 2.9† (n = 24)				RIA	Wild caught	60
Gentoo penguin (Pygoscelis papua)		Male 7.6 ± 0.9† (n = 5) / Female 2.7 ± 0.6† (n = 5)	Male 600 ± 40† (n = 5) / Female 1230 ± 70† (n = 5)	Male 0.6 ± 0.23† (n = 5) / Female 0.21 ± 0.02† (n = 5)	RIA	During nest building	61
Chicken (Gallus gallus domesticus)	Laying 84.7 ± 16.5† (n = 5) / Maximal molt 539.9 ± 66.8† (n = 5)	Laying 3.5 ± 0.2† (n = 25) / Maximal molt 1.9 ± 0.1† (n = 25)	Laying 608.5 ± 32.7† (n = 25) / Maximal molt 242.6 ± 33.8† (n = 25)		RIA	White leghorn hens, winter	62
Chicken (Gallus gallus domesticus)			1057.0 ± 157.8† (n = 10)		Enzyme immunoassay	Cornish hens, 34 wk old	63
Chicken (Gallus gallus domesticus)			1379.9 ± 359.7† (n = 10)		Enzyme immunoassay	Leghorn hens, 34 wk old	63

RIA, Radioimmunoassay.
*Values are provided as mean/median values and reference interval.
†Values are provided as mean/median and standard error/standard deviation of the mean.
‡Values are provided as range.
§Values are provided as mean/median, standard error/standard deviation of the mean, and reference interval.
||Mean/median.

Glucose Metabolism Hormones and Other Related Molecules

	Insulin (pmol/L)	Fructosamine (µmol/L)	Glucagon (ng/L)	Glucose (mg/dL; mmol/L)	Methodology	Information	Fasted/Time of Fast	Reference
Amazona sp.		122 (60-154)* (n = 24)		259 (212.6-297.3)* mg/dL (n = 24); 14.4 (11.8-16.5)* mmol/L (n = 24)				64
Blue-fronted Amazon (*Amazona aestiva*)		129 (114-154)* (n = 6)		277.5 (257.7-297.3)* mg/dL (n = 9); 15.4 (14.3-16.5)* mmol/L (n = 9)				64
Orange-winged Amazon (*Amazona amazonica*)		106 (60-135)* (n = 9)		255.9 (212.6-284.7)* mg/dL (n = 9); 14.2 (11.8-15.8)* mmol/L (n = 9)				64
Yellow-headed Amazon (*Amazona oratrix*)		112 (86-150)* (n = 5)		259.5 (237.8-275.7)* mg/dL (n = 5); 14.4 (13.2-15.3)* mmol/L (n = 5)				64
Yellow-crowned Amazon (*Amazona ochrocephala*)		125 (104-128)* (n = 4)		257.7 (239.6-259.5)* mg/dL (n = 4); 14.3 (13.3-14.4)* mmol/L (n = 4)				64
Cockatiel (*Nymphicus hollandicus*)		108 (80-172)* (n = 11)		336.9 (291.9-425.2)* mg/dL (n = 11); 18.7 (16.2-23.6)* mmol/L (n = 11)				64
Chicken (*Gallus gallus domesticus*)	182.4 ± 25.8† (n = 6)		238 ± 27† (n = 12)	331 ± 19† mg/dL (n = 12); 18.4 ± 1.06† mmol/L (n = 12)			No	65
Chicken (*Gallus gallus domesticus*)							No	66
Bald eagle (*Haliaeetus leucocephalus*)	187.7 ± 43.9† (n = 4)		74.8 ± 24.4† (n = 4)	324.3 ± 16.8† mg/dL (n = 4); 18.0 ± 0.93† mmol/L (n = 4)	Glucose spectrophotometry, glucagon and insulin RIA	From a wildlife center	Yes/24 h	23
Great horned owl (*Bubo virginianus*)	30.2 ± 14.5† (n = 6)		64.8 ± 4.00† (n = 6)	360.4 ± 11.9† mg/dL (n = 6); 20.0 ± 0.66† mmol/L (n = 6)	Glucose spectrophotometry, glucagon, and insulin RIA	From a wildlife center	Yes/24 h	23
Red-tailed hawk (*Buteo jamaicensis*)	205.7 ± 43.6† (n = 5)		44.2 ± 8.5† (n = 5)	355 ± 17.8† mg/dL (n = 5); 19.7 ± 0.99† mmol/L (n = 5)	Glucose spectrophotometry, glucagon, and insulin RIA	From a wildlife center	Yes/24 h	23
Garden warbler (*Sylvia borin*)	27.3 ± 5.7† (n = 6)		2500 ± 500† (n = 6)	~288 mg/dL‖ (n = 6); ~16‖ mmol/L (n = 6)	Glucose photometry, insulin, and glucagon RIA	Captive, indoor conditions		67
King penguin (*Aptenodytes patagonicus*)	Fed 111 ± 11† (n = 9) Fasted for 24 h 43 ± 5† (n = 9)		Fed 542.9 ± 87† (n = 9) Fasted for 4 d 327.1 ± 52.2† (n = 9) Fasted for 14 d 341 ± 38.3† (n = 9)			Wild-caught chicks	Yes	68

RIA, Radioimmunoassay.
*Values are provided as mean/median values and reference interval.
†Values are provided as mean/median and standard error/standard deviation of the mean.
‡Values are provided as range.
§Values are provided as mean/median, standard error/standard deviation of the mean, and reference interval.
‖Mean/median.

Calcium Metabolism Hormones and Other Related Molecules

Species	Calcitonin (ng/L)	PTH (pmol/L)	25-Hydroxycholecalciferol (nmol/L)	Total Calcium (mg/dL; mmol/L)	Ionized Calcium (mmol/L)	Magnesium (mg/dL; mmol/L)	Methodology	Information	Reference
Humboldt penguins (*Spheniscus humboldti*)		0.8 (0-1.1)* (*n* = 14)	3.7 (1-10)* (*n* = 14)		1.21 (1.20-1.38)* (*n* = 33)		iCa i-Stat / PTH immunoradiometric assay / 25-Hydroxycholecalciferol RIA	Juvenile, captive	69
Thick-billed parrot (*Rhynchopsitta pachyrhyncha*)		19.8 (0-65.68)* (*n* = 51)	19.04 (5.2-51)* (*n* = 45)	7.52 (5.48-8.36)* mg/dL (*n* = 51); 1.88 (1.37-2.09)* mmol/L (*n* = 51)	1.12 (0.82-1.3)* (*n* = 46)		iCa Nova 8 electrolyte analyzer / PTH and 25-Hydroxycholecalciferol RIA	Captive, 15 different institutions	70
Chicken (*Gallus gallus domesticus*)	32 ± 7.7† (*n* = 10)	10.7 ± 1.7† (*n* = 10)	287.04 ± 79.8† (*n* = 10)				RIA	Cornish hens	63
Chicken (*Gallus gallus domesticus*)	22 ± 5.5† (*n* = 10)	25.5 ± 1.4† (*n* = 10)	244.61 ± 29.9† (*n* = 10)				RIA	Leghorn hens	63
Gyr × Peregrine hybrid falcons (*Falco sp.*)		<0.01-0.26‡ (*n* = 10)	13.2-26.3‡ (*n* = 10)	7.64-8.84‡ mg/dL (*n* = 10); 1.91-2.21‡ mmol/L (*n* = 10)	0.78-0.96‡ (*n* = 10)			Males, captive bred, fed whole prey	71
Gyr × Peregrine hybrid falcons (*Falco sp.*)		<0.01-1.10‡ (*n* = 10)	8.1-38.4‡ (*n* = 10)	7.8-9.28‡ mg/dL (*n* = 10); 1.95-2.32‡ mmol/L (*n* = 10)	0.86-1‡ (*n* = 10)			Males, captive bred, fed whole prey with 10% red meat	71

Species		Method	Setting	Ref
Hyacinth macaw (*Anodorhynchus hyacinthinus*)	8.8 ± 1.6 (7.6-11.6)* mg/dL (n = 7); 2.2 ± 0.4 (1.9-2.9)* mmol/L (n = 7)	3.36 ± 1.4 (2.52-5.6)* mg/dL (n = 7); 1.2 ± 0.5 (0.9-2)* mmol/L (n = 7)	Atomic emission spectrometry	Captive zoo animals	72
Blue-and-yellow macaw (*Ara ararauna*)	9.2 ± 1.6 (6.8-12.8)* mg/dL (n = 17); 2.3 ± 0.4 (1.7-3.2)* mmol/L (n = 17)	2.8 ± 0.56 (0.7-1.4)* mg/dL (n = 17); 1 ± 0.2 (0.7-1.4)* mmol/L (n = 17)	Atomic emission spectrometry	Captive zoo animals	72
Green-winged macaw (*Ara chloropterus*)	9.2 ± 1.2 (8-11.6)* mg/dL (n = 8); 2.3 ± 0.3 (2-2.9)* mmol/L (n = 8)	3.64 ± 1.4 (2.52-6.16)* mg/dL (n = 8); 1.3 ± 0.5 (0.9-2.2)* mmol/L (n = 8)	Atomic emission spectrometry	Captive zoo animals	72
Hispaniolan Amazon parrots (*Amazona ventralis*)	8.80-10.40‡ mg/dL (n = 26); 2.20-2.60‡ mmol/L (n = 26)	1.80-3.10‡ mg/dL (n = 26); 0.74-1.27‡ mmol/L (n = 26)	Olympus Model AU640e	Research colony	73
African grey parrot (*Psittacus erithacus*)	8.20-20.20‡ mg/dL (n = 24); 2.05-5.05‡ mmol/L (n = 24)	2.10-3.40‡ mg/dL (n = 24); 0.82-1.4‡ mmol/L (n = 24)	Olympus Model AU640e	Breeding colony	73

iCa, Ionized calcium; *PTH*, parathyroid hormone; *RIA*, radioimmunoassay.

*Values are provided as mean/median values and reference interval.

†Values are provided as mean/median and standard error/standard deviation of the mean.

‡Values are provided as range.

§Values are provided as mean/median, standard error/standard deviation of the mean, and reference interval.

‖Mean/median.

Hypothalamus-Pituitary-Thyroid Axis-Related Hormones

Species	TT$_4$ (nmol/L)	TT$_3$ (nmol/L)	fT$_4$ (pmol/L)	fT$_3$ (pmol/L)	Methodology	Target Population	Reference
Pekin duck (Anas platyrhynchos domesticus)	15.44 ± 2.57† (n = 5)				RIA	15-Mo-old healthy male white Pekin ducks	47
Chicken (Gallus gallus domesticus)	16.73 ± 2.57† (n = 5)				RIA	15-mo-old healthy male white Pekin ducks	47
Chicken (Gallus gallus domesticus)	Laying females 16.8 ± 0.82† (n = 47) Maximal molt 26.35 ± 1.07† (n = 47)	Laying females 0.42 ± 0.02† (n = 47) Maximal molt 0.84 ± 0.05† (n = 47)			RIA	White leghorn hens, winter	62
Iberian imperial eagle (Aquila adalberti)	26.8 ± 18.5 (5.1-64.4)§ (n = 12)				Quimioluminescence	Captive adult	74
Pigeon (Columba livia)	6-35‡ (n = 24)				RIA	Healthy adult	75
White-tailed eagle (Haliaeetus albicilla)	1.54-4.63‡ (n = 5)				RIA	1 healthy, 4 pinching off syndrome	76
Herring gull (Larus argentatus)	30.89 (14.16-70.79)* (n = 155)				Solid-phase competitive binding enzyme assay	Adult, wild, multiple breeding colonies	77
Ring-necked dove (Streptopelia capicola)	21.62 ± 0.78† (n = 8)	6.9 ± 0.46† (n = 8)	9.01 ± 1.16† (n = 8)	4.61 ± 0.77† (n = 8)	TT$_4$ and TT$_3$ RIA, fT$_4$ and fT$_3$ ED	Adult animals, breeding colony	78
Japanese quail (Coturnix japonica)	28.96 ± 4.89† (n = 8)	14.75 ± 0.16† (n = 8)	1.54 ± 0.26† (n = 8)	12.9 ± 0.46† (n = 8)	TT$_4$ and TTT$_3$ RIA, fT$_4$ and fT$_3$ ED	Breeding colony	78
Barred owl (Strix varia)	<2.57-7.72‡ (n = 4)		<0.39-2.70‡ (n = 4)		fT$_4$ ED, TT$_4$ RIA	Potential unhealthy status	79

Species				Methodology	Description	Ref
American kestrel *(Falco sparverius)*	Male 7.59 ± 0.471† (n = 13), Female 8.14 ± 0.51† (n = 18)	Male 1.55 ± 0.15† (n = 13), Female 1.93 ± 0.14† (n = 18)		RIA	Captive, nestling, control group	80
American kestrel *(Falco sparverius)*	Male 7.12 ± 0.34† (n = 5), Female 5.58 ± 0.45† (n = 12)	Male 1.34 ± 0.11† (n = 8), Female 1.49 ± 0.14† (n = 13)		RIA	Captive, adults, control group	80
King penguin *(Aptenodytes patagonicus)*	Fed 8.40 ± 1.11† (n = 9), Fasted for 14 d 0.98 ± 0.31† (n = 9)	Fed 1.17 ± 0.29† (n = 9), Fasted for 14 d 2.00 ± 0.29† (n = 9)			Wild-caught juveniles	68
Congo African grey parrot *(Psittacus erithacus)*	3.18 (2.02-5.06)* (n = 12)			RIA for fT$_4$, methodology no longer commercially available	Healthy nonmolting adult	43
Moluccan cockatoo *(Cacatua moluccensis)*	4.66 (2.04-6.29)* (n = 11)			RIA for fT$_4$, methodology no longer commercially available	Healthy nonmolting adult	43
Blue and gold macaw *(Ara ararauna)*	3.36 (2.02-4.85)* (n = 11)			RIA for fT$_4$, methodology no longer commercially available	Healthy nonmolting adult	43
Umbrella cockatoo *(Cacatua alba)*	4.61 (2.86-5.96)* (n = 5)			RIA for fT$_4$, methodology no longer commercially available	Healthy nonmolting adult	43
Yellow-headed Amazon parrot *(Amazona oratrix)*	5.05 (2.49-7.68)* (n = 10)			RIA for fT$_4$, methodology no longer commercially available	Healthy nonmolting adult	43
Blue-fronted Amazon parrot *(Amazona aestiva)*	10.7 (3.17-24.5)* (n = 9)			RIA for fT$_4$, methodology no longer commercially available	Healthy nonmolting adult	43
Hispaniolan Amazon parrot *(Amazona ventralis)*	1.7-8.2‡ (n = 18)	0.6-7‡ (n = 20)	6.64-15.14‡ (n = 20)	fT$_4$ and fT$_3$ ED, TT$_4$ and TT$_3$ RIA	Research colony	81
Ostrich *(Struthio camelus)*	19.66 ± 1.91† (n = 8)	2.29 ± 0.17† (n = 8)		RIA	Healthy, 3 mo old, male	82

ED, Equilibrium dialysis; *fT$_3$,* free triiodothyronine; *fT$_4$,* free thyroxine; *RIA,* radioimmunoassay; *TT$_3$,* total T$_3$; *TT$_4$,* total T$_4$.
*Values are provided as mean/median values and reference interval.
†Values are provided as mean/median and standard error/standard deviation of the mean.
‡Values are provided as range.
§Values are provided as mean/median, standard error/standard deviation of the mean, and reference interval.
||Mean/median.

Mammals

Hypothalamus-Pituitary-Adrenal and Hypothalamus-Pituitary-Gonadal Axis-Related Hormones

Species	Cortisol (nmol/L)	Corticosterone (nmol/L)	Aldosterone (pmol/L)	Progesterone (nmol/L)	17β-Estradiol (pmol/L)	Testosterone (nmol/L)	Methodology	Information	Reference
Guinea pig (*Cavia porcellus*)	138.0-827.7‡						Unknown	Male	83
				3.2∥			Unknown	Female, basal	83
				28.6∥			Unknown	Female, estrus	83
				22.3-25.4‡			Unknown	Female, diestrus, d 8-12	83
					110.1∥		Unknown	Female, diestrus	83
					256.9∥		Unknown	Female, estrus	83
Rabbit (*Oryctolagus cuniculus*)	88.3 ± 16.6†		299.6 ± 52.7†				Unknown	Unknown	83
			1387∥				Unknown	Male, early morning	83
				<3.2∥			Unknown	Male, late afternoon	83
				25.4∥			Unknown	Female, basal	83
							Unknown	Female, 6 h after coitus	83
				47.7-63.6°			Unknown	Female, 10 d after coitus	83
					11.01∥		Unknown	Female, basal, preovulatory	83
						0.10-0.17‡	Unknown	Male, peak at 4 to 5 h cycle	83
	54.6 ± 22.1† (*n* = 20)					0.07 ± 0.023†	Unknown	Grimaud rabbit, housed at 20°C	84
	56.8 ± 24.8† (*n* = 20)					0.06 ± 0.022†	Unknown	Grimaud rabbit, 71 d old	84
	47.7 ± 13.8† (*n* = 20)					0.04 ± 0.017†	Unknown	Grimaud rabbit, 85 d old	84
	71.7-104.8‡	44.51∥				0.01-0.02‡	Unknown	Unknown	85
					11.01∥ Growth phase 0.5 Ca% diet 2011.9 ± 93.2† (*n* = 12) 1 Ca% diet 2001.3 ± 112.7† (*n* = 12)		Unknown	New Zealand Whites, growth phase on different Ca% diet	86
					Plateau phase 0.5 Ca% diet 1502.5 ± 53.2† (*n* = 12) 1 Ca% diet 1493.0 ± 49.2† (*n* = 12)		Unknown	New Zealand Whites, plateau phase on different Ca% diet	86

Species	Value 1	Value 2	Value 3	Method	Group	Ref
Ferret (*Mustela putorius furo*)						
		220.2-256.9‡		Unknown	Female, estrus	83
		36.7-220.2‡		Unknown	Female, pregnant	83
	6.7 ± 5.9 (2.1-15.9)§ (n = 5)	817.80 ± 433.9 (170-1 377.00)§ (n = 5)		Unknown	Females with ovarian or uterine tumors	87
	1.3 ± 1.3 (0.6-1.0)§ (n = 6)	83.50 ± 32.53 (<73-136.00)§ (n = 6)		Unknown	Healthy, intact female	87
	1.0 ± 0.4 (0.6-1.0)§ (n = 6)	73.17 ± 0.41 (<73-74.00)§ (n = 6)		Unknown	Healthy, spayed female	87
	3.5 ± 8.2 (0.6-23.9)§ (n = 8)	274.75 ± 192.4 (133-716.00)§ (n = 8)		Unknown	Females with clinical symptoms of hyperestrogenism	87
	48.7 ± 20.1 (2.2-63.6)§ (n = 6)	144.00 ± 48.33 (<73-215.00)§ (n = 6)		Unknown	Females with clinical symptoms of hyperestrogenism treated with hCG	87
	0.004‖			Magnetic-antibody immunoassay	Adult male, fall	88
	0.61‖			Magnetic-antibody immunoassay	Adult male, spring	88
Rat (*Rattus norvegicus*)						
			374.4-574.1‡	Unknown	Male Sprague-Dawley, late light period	83
			25.0-149.8‡	Unknown	Male Sprague-Dawley, late dark period	83
			1747.2‖	Unknown	Female Sprague-Dawley, late light period	83
			424.3‖	Unknown	Female Sprague-Dawley, late dark period	83
			332.9-970.9‡	Unknown	Male Sprague-Dawley, late light period	83
			110.9-305.1‡	Unknown	Male Sprague-Dawley, middle light period	83
			277.4-416.1‡	Unknown	Male Sprague-Dawley, 9-10 AM	83

Continued

Hypothalamus-Pituitary-Adrenal and Hypothalamus-Pituitary-Gonadal Axis-Related Hormones—cont'd

Species	Cortisol (nmol/L)	Corticosterone (nmol/L)	Aldosterone (pmol/L)	Progesterone (nmol/L)	17β-Estradiol (pmol/L)	Testosterone (nmol/L)	Methodology	Information	Reference
	693.5-970.9‡						Unknown	Female Sprague-Dawley, 9-10 AM	83
			233.1 ± 36.1†				Unknown	F344 male	83
			826.7 ± 138.7†				Unknown	Long-Evans, female, early morning	83
			726.8 ± 102.6†				Unknown	Wistar, male, late morning	83
				3.2-15.9‡			Unknown	Female, early proestrus	83
				127.2-159‡			Unknown	Female, late proestrus, estrus	83
				63.6-95.4‡			Unknown	Female, first diestrus d	83
					<36.7||		Unknown	Female, basal	83
					73.4-110.1‡		Unknown	Female, 2nd diestrus d	83
					146.8-183.5‡	0.10||	Unknown	Female, proestrus	83
						<0.04||	Unknown	Male, 1330-1600 h	83
						17.35-20.82‡	Unknown	Male, 2130 h	83
							Unknown	Female, proestrus	83
						3.47||	Unknown	Female, estrus	83
Degu (Octodon degus)	413.9||	37.44||					Unknown		85
Chinchilla (Chinchilla lanigera)				21.8 ± 9.6† (n = 5)			RIA	Pregnant female, d 0-9	89
				5.4 ± 0.7† (n = 4)			RIA	Pregnant female, d 10-19	89
				24.4 ± 6.7† (n = 8)			RIA	Pregnant female, d 20-29	89
				6.2 ± 1.9† (n = 7)			RIA	Pregnant female, d 30-39	89
				0.5 ± 0.4† (n = 6)			RIA	Pregnant female, d 50-59	89
				5.4 ± 0.9† (n = 8)			RIA	Pregnant female, d 60-69	89
				16.2 ± 3.6† (n = 5)			RIA	Pregnant female, d 70-79	89
				4.7 ± 3.3† (n = 6)			RIA	Pregnant female, d 90-99	89

hCG, Human chorionic gonadotropin; RIA, radioimmunoassay.

*Values are provided as mean/median values and reference interval.

†Values are provided as mean/median and standard error/standard deviation of the mean.

‡Values are provided as range.

§Values are provided as mean/median, standard error/standard deviation of the mean, and reference interval.

||Mean/median.

Glucose Metabolism Hormones and Other Related Molecules

	Insulin (pmol/L)	Fructosamine (µmol/L)	Glucagon (ng/L)	Glucose (mg/dL, mmol/L)	Glycated Hemoglobin (%)	Methodology	Information	Fasted/Time of Fast	Reference
Ferret (*Mustela putorius furo*)									
	67.5-137.6‡ (n = 14)			91.4-110.3‡ mg/dL (n = 14); 5.1-6.1‡ mmol/L (n = 14)		RIA	Pet	Unknown	90
		163 (121.1-201.6)* (n = 105)		108.1 (54-153.2)* mg/dL (n = 105); 6 (3-8.5)* mmol/L (n = 105)		Nonenzymatic color assay	Pet	Unknown	91
	45.9-126.3‡ (n = 15)					RIA	Unknown	Yes/4 hr	92
	33.0-310.7‡ (n = 30)					Immunoreactive insulin RIA	Unknown	Yes/overnight	92
	35.9-251.1‡					N/A	Unknown	Unknown	92
	71.8-287‡					N/A	Unknown	Unknown	83
	34.4-321.4‡					N/A	Unknown	Unknown	93,94
Rabbit (*Oryctolagus cuniculus*)									
	~193.7‖ (n = 5)		~145‖ (n = 5)	~117‖ mg/dL (n = 5); ~6.5‖ mmol/L (n = 5)		Unknown	Laboratory (New Zealand White)	Yes/16 h	95
	57.4 ± 14.4† (n = 12)			131 ± 2† mg/dL (n = 12); 7.3 ± 0.1† mmol/L (n = 12)		Unknown	Laboratory (albino rex rabbits)	No	96
	19.2 ± 4.2† (n = 12)	287 ± 25† (n = 12)		104.3 ± 4.7† mg/dL (n = 12); 5.8 ± 0.3† mmol/L (n = 12)		Fructosamine kinetic method, insulin chemiluminescence	Laboratory (New Zealand White)	Yes/12 h	97
	144.2 ± 1.4† (n = 12)	288 ± 8.6† (n = 12)		99 ± 8† mg/dL (n = 12); 5.5 ± 0.5† mmol/L (n = 12)	2.41 ± 0.6†% (n = 12)	Insulin chemiluminescence, fructosamine, calorimetric	Laboratory	Yes/24 h	98
	145.7 ± 4.3† (n = 13)	272 ± 7.8b† (n = 13)		90.1 ± 5† mg/dL (n = 13); 5 ± 0.3† mmol/L (n = 13)	2.76 ± 0.5†% (n = 13)	Insulin chemiluminescence, fructosamine, calorimetric, glycated hemoglobin, HPLC	Laboratory	Yes/24 h	98

Continued

Glucose Metabolism Hormones and Other Related Molecules—cont'd

	Insulin (pmol/L)	Fructosamine (µmol/L)	Glucagon (ng/L)	Glucose (mg/dL; mmol/L)	Glycated Hemoglobin (%)	Methodology	Information	Fasted/Time of Fast	Reference
Guinea pig (*Cavia porcellus*)		134-271‡		89-287‡ mg/dL; 4.9-15.9‡ mmol/L		Unknown	Unknown		99
Rat (*Rattus norvegicus*)									
	373.1 ± 43.1† (n = 32)		160 ± 7† (n = 18)	150 ± 5† mg/dL (n = 32); 8.3 ± 0.3† mmol/L (n = 32)		Unknown	Female laboratory rats	No	100
	28.7 ± 14.4† (n = 7)		187 ± 10† (n = 10)	112 ± 5† mg/dL (n = 17); 6.2 ± 0.3† mmol/L (n = 17)		Unknown	Female laboratory rats	Yes/48 h	100
	296.3 ± 29.4† (n = 11)			114.3 ± 3.2† mg/dL (n = 11); 6.3 ± 02† mmol/L (n = 11)		Unknown	Laboratory Wistar male	Unknown	101
	172.2 ± 14.4† (n = 17)			77.4 ± 4† mg/dL (n = 17); 4.3 ± 0.2† mmol/L (n = 17)		Unknown	Laboratory Wistar male	Yes/16 h	101

HPLC, High-performance liquid chromatography; *RIA*, radioimmunoassay.

*Values are provided as mean/median values and reference interval.

†Values are provided as mean/median and standard error/standard deviation of the mean.

‡Values are provided as range.

§Values are provided as mean/median, standard error/standard deviation of the mean, and reference interval.

‖Mean/median.

Calcium Metabolism Hormones and Other Related Molecules

Species	Calcitonin (ng/L)	PTH (pmol/L)	25-Hydroxycholecalciferol (nmol/L)	1,25-Dihydroxycholecalciferol (pmol/L)	Total Calcium (mg/dL; mmol/L)	Ionized Calcium (mmol/L)	Magnesium (mg/dL; mmol/L)	Methodology	Information	Reference
Rat (*Rattus norvegicus*)	100‖							Unknown	Sprague-Dawley, 1 mo, male	83
	<90‖							Unknown	F344, 6 Wk	83
	300-3800‡									83
									F344, 6.5 Mo, female	
	200-1000‡							Unknown	F344, 9 Mo	83
	200-16,500‡							Unknown	F344, 15 Mo, female	83
	>14,000‡							Unknown	F344, 27 Mo	83
	200-500‡							Unknown	Wistar, 6-8 mo, male	83
	450-1100‡							Unknown	Wistar, 6-8 mo, female	83
	400-900‡							Unknown	Wistar, 12-14 mo, male	83
	700-1800‡							Unknown	Wistar, 12-14 mo, female	83
	100‖							Unknown	Sprague-Dawley, 1 mo	83
	500-1500‡							Unknown	Holtzman, adult male	83
	440 ± 160†	14.7-18.9‡						Unknown	Long-Evans, adult male	83
		<5.25-42‡						Unknown	Sprague-Dawley, male	83
								Unknown	Sprague-Dawley, female	83
		21-63‡						Unknown	Wistar, male	83
		5.25-15.75‡						Unknown	Wistar, female	83
		31.5-73.5‡						Unknown	F344, male	83
		7.35-18.9‡						Unknown	Sherman, male	83
		15.5 ± 0.5†						Unknown	Black hooded/Ztn	83
				180 ± 9.6†				Unknown	Sprague-Dawley, male	83
				288 ± 57.6†				Unknown	Wistar, male	83
				230.4 ± 40.8†				Unknown	Wistar, female	83

Continued

Calcium Metabolism Hormones and Other Related Molecules—cont'd

Species	Calcitonin (ng/L)	PTH (pmol/L)	25-Hydroxychole-calciferol (nmol/L)	1,25-Dihydroxychole-calciferol (pmol/L)	Total Calcium (mg/dL; mmol/L)	Ionized Calcium (mmol/L)	Magnesium (mg/dL; mmol/L)	Methodology	Information	Reference
Rabbit (*Oryctolagus cuniculus*)				88.8 ± 12†				Unknown	Unknown	83
			No UVB supplementation at day 0 29.7 ± 14.9† (n = 4) No UVB supplementation d 14 31.7 ± 9.9† (n = 4)					Unknown	6 Wk old, dwarf mixed breed	102
			D 0 prior to UVB exposure 38.8 ± 21.4† (n = 5) D 14, after UVB exposure 66.4 ± 14.3† (n = 5)	125.8 ± 9.8† (n = 19)				Unknown	6 Wk old, dwarf mixed breed	102
		2.83 ± 0.34† (n = 9)				1.71 ± 0.02† (n = 9)		Immunoradiometric	White New Zealands of both sexes, aged 9-15 mo	103
								Immunoradiometric	White New Zealands of both sexes, aged 9-15 mo	104
		3.31 ± 0.64† (n = 10)				1.69 ± 0.02† (n = 10)		Immunoradiometric	White New Zealands of both sexes, aged 9-15 mo	104
						1.67-1.85‡ (n = 44)		i-stat	Unknown	105
							2.11 ± 0.28† mg/dL (n = 110); 0.92 ± 0.12† mmol/L (n = 110)	Clinical analyzer	Male, New Zealand White, 4-7 mo	106

Calcium Metabolism Hormones and Other Related Molecules—cont'd

Species	Calcitonin (ng/L)	PTH (pmol/L)	25-Hydroxychole-calciferol (nmol/L)	1,25-Dihydroxychole-calciferol (pmol/L)	Total Calcium (mg/dL; mmol/L)	Ionized Calcium (mmol/L)	Magnesium (mg/dL; mmol/L)	Methodology	Information	Reference
					Adults 14.4 ± 0.4† mg/dL (n = 42); 3.6 ± 0.1† mmol/L (n = 42) Juveniles 15.2 ± 0.4† mg/dL (n = 28); 3.8 ± 0.1† mmol/L (n = 28)		Adults 4.68 ± 0.24† mg/dL (n = 42); 1.95 ± 0.1† mmol/L (n = 42) Juveniles 4.68 ± 0.29† mg/dL (n = 28); 1.95 ± 0.12† mmol/L (n = 28)	Clinical analyzer	Animals from rabbitries, New Zealand White (n = 59), mixed breed (n = 11), males (n = 40), and females (n = 30)	107
		0.5 Ca% diet 7.81 ± 0.77† (n = 12) 1 Ca% diet 6.03 ± 0.95† (n = 12)		0.5 Ca% diet 197.5 ± 12.2† pmol/L (n = 12) 1 Ca% diet 129.6 ± 11.5† pmol/L (n = 12)	0.5 Ca% diet 13.2 ± 0.40† mg/dL (n = 12); 3.3 ± 0.1† mmol/L (n = 12) 1 Ca% diet 14.5 ± 0.08† mg/dL (n = 12); 3.63 ± 0.02† mmol/L (n = 12)	0.5 Ca% diet 1.75 ± 0.02† (n = 12) 1 Ca% diet 1.76 ± 0.01† (n = 12)		Total calcium atomic absorption PTH Immunoradiometry assay Vitamin D RIA	New Zealand Whites, fed two different diets during growth phase	86
		0.5 Ca% diet 6.21 ± 0.73† (n = 12) 1 Ca% diet 3.79 ± 0.43† (n = 12)		0.5 Ca% diet 197.5 ± 12.2† (n = 12) 1 Ca% diet 129.6 ± 11.5† (n = 12)	0.5 Ca% diet 14.2 ± 0.2† mg/dL (n = 12); 3.55 ± 0.05† mmol/L (n = 12) 1 Ca% diet 14.52 ± 0.08† mg/dL (n = 12); 3.63 ± 0.02† mmol/L (n = 12)	0.5 Ca% diet 1.74 ± 0.04† (n = 12) 1 Ca% diet 1.75 ± 0.03† (n = 12)		Total calcium atomic absorption PTH Immunoradiometry assay Vitamin D RIA	New Zealand Whites, fed two different diets during plateau phase	86
					Nonpregnant female 15.57 ± 0.36† mg/dL (n = 15); 3.89 ± 0.09† mmol/L (n = 15)		Nonpregnant female 2.03 ± 0.01† mg/dL (n = 15); 0.88 ± 0.01† mmol/L (n = 15)	Spectrophotometric	Angora	108

Continued

Species	Calcitonin (ng/L)	PTH (pmol/L)	25-Hydroxycholecalciferol (nmol/L)	1,25-Dihydroxycholecalciferol (pmol/L)	Total Calcium (mg/dL; mmol/L)	Ionized Calcium (mmol/L)	Magnesium (mg/dL; mmol/L)	Methodology	Information	Reference
					Pregnant female 13.06 ± 0.24† mg/dL (n = 15); 3.27 ± 0.06† mmol/L (n = 15) Male 14.66 ± 0.36† mg/dL (n = 15); 3.67 ± 0.09† mmol/L (n = 15)		Pregnant female 2.07 ± 0.21† mg/dL (n = 15); 0.9 ± 0.09† mmol/L (n = 15) Male 2.16 ± 0.06† mg/dL (n = 15); 0.94 ± 0.03† mmol/L (n = 15)			
					Nonpregnant 16.35 ± 0.32† mg/dL (n = 30); 4.09 ± 0.08† mmol/L (n = 30) Pregnant 13.9 ± 0.14† mg/dL (n = 30); 3.48 ± 0.04† mmol/L (n = 30)		Nonpregnant 2.22 ± 0.02† mg/dL (n = 30); 0.97 ± 0.01† mmol/L (n = 30) Pregnant 2.32 ± 0.02† mg/dL (n = 30); 1.01 ± 0.01† mmol/L (n = 30)	Spectrophotometric	Domestic	109
					11.40 ± 0.29† mg/dL (n = 15); 2.85 ± 0.07† mmol/L (n = 15)		3.28 ± 0.23† mg/dL (n = 15); 1.43 ± 0.1† mmol/L (n = 15)	Clinical analyzer	Unknown breeds of 3, 4, and over 5 mo of age	110
Chinchilla (Chinchilla lanigera)			Pre-UVB exposure 110.7 ± 39.5 (63-158)§ (n = 5) Post-16 d UVB exposure 189 ± 102.7 (91-319)§ (n = 5)		9.0 ± 1.47 (6.1-10.8)§ mg/dL (n = 10); 2.25 ± 0.37 (1.53-2.7)§ mmol/L (n = 10)			RIA	8 wk of age	111

Calcium Metabolism Hormones and Other Related Molecules—cont'd

Species	Calcitonin (ng/L)	PTH (pmol/L)	25-Hydroxycholecalciferol (nmol/L)	1,25-Dihydroxycholecalciferol (pmol/L)	Total Calcium (mg/dL; mmol/L)	Ionized Calcium (mmol/L)	Magnesium (mg/dL; mmol/L)	Methodology	Information	Reference
			No UVB exposure at d 0 92.2 ± 52 (31-166)§ (n = 5) No UVB exposure at d 16 87.8 ± 34.4 (53-126)§ (n = 5)		9.0 ± 1.47 (6.1-10.8)§ mg/dL (n = 10); 2.25 ± 0.37 (1.5-2.7)§ mmol/L (n = 10)			RIA	8 wk of age	111
					9.5 ± 0.9 (7.4-11.5)§ mg/dL (n = 16); 2.38 ± 0.23 (1.85-2.88)§ mmol/L (n = 16)		3.8 ± 0.2 (3.3-4.2)§ mg/dL (n = 16); 1.56 ± 0.08 (1.36-1.73)§ mmol/L (n = 16)	Colorimetric	Commercial purpose (fur), 16 adult males	112
					9.28 ± 1.52† mg/dL (n = 20); 2.32 ± 0.38† mmol/L (n = 20)		2.9 ± 0.41† mg/dL (n = 20); 1.21 ± 0.17† mmol/L(n=20)	Spectrometry	Commercial purpose, 2-4 y female	113
Guinea pig (Cavia porcellus)			36.33 ± 24.42 (10-114)§ (n = 6)			1.52 ± 0.07 (1.35-1.65)§ (n = 6)		RIA	14 to 16 wk, female intact Hartley, no UVB supplementation	114
			101.49 ± 21.81 (67-165)§ (n = 6)			1.58 ± 0.09 (1.29-1.74)§ (n = 6)		RIA	14 to 16 wk, female intact Hartley, UVB supplemented for 6 mo	114
					2.58-3.16‡ mmol/L (n = 58); 10.32-12.64‡ mg/dL (n = 58)		1.73-3.84‡ mg/dL (n = 58); 0.72-1.60‡ (n = 58) mmol/L	Clinical analyzer	Healthy pets, 24 males, 34 females, ranging from 8 wk to 5 y	115

PTH, Parathyroid hormone; *RIA,* radioimmunoassay.

*Values are provided as mean/median values and reference interval.

†Values are provided as mean/median and standard error/standard deviation of the mean.

‡Values are provided as range.

§Values are provided as mean/median, standard error/standard deviation of the mean, and reference interval.

||Mean/median.

Hypothalamus-Pituitary-Thyroid Axis-Related Hormones

Species	TT₄ (nmol/L)	TT₃ (nmol/L)	fT₄ (pmol/L)	fT₃ (pmol/L)	TSH (mIU/L)	Methodology	Target Population	Reference
Guinea pig (Cavia porcellus)	51.99 (29.09-74.90)* (n = 63)					Quimioluminescence	Laboratory (Duncan-Hartley strain)	116
	53.67 (38.74-68.60)* (n = 60)					Quimioluminescence	Pet	116
	Female 25.74 (14.16-64.35)* (n = 16) Male 28.31 (14.16-57.92)* (n = 16) Castrated male 34.75 (19.31-66.92)* (n = 8) Overall 27.03 (14.16-66.92)* (n = 40)		15.06 ± 1.16†			Unknown	Laboratory	117
						Chemiluminescence	Pet	118
	32.18-41.18‡ (n = 19)	0.6-0.68‡ (n = 19)	16.21-26.13‡ (n = 19)	3.40-3.99‡ (n = 19)		RIA	Laboratory	119
	58.43 ± 5.57† (n = 10)	0.49 ± 0.02† (n = 10)	8.62 ± 7.34† (n = 10)	3.44 ± 1.66† (n = 10)		RIA	Unknown	120
	9.05 (7.39-16.99)* (n = 10)					RIA	Pet, 10 intact 1 y olds (6 females, 4 males)	121
	Males 37.32 ± 7.72† Females 41.18 ± 9.01†	Males 0.6 ± 0.26† Females 0.68 ± 0.15†	Male 16.22 ± 5.28† Female 17.12 ± 3.22†	Male 3.95 ± 0.54† Female 3.99 ± 0.9†		Unknown	Unknown	83
Rabbit (Oryctolagus cuniculus)	21.88-30.89‡	1.99-2.2‡				Unknown	Unknown	83
			26.1 ± 3† (n = 5)	7.3 ± 0.2† (n = 10)		RIA	Laboratory New Zealand White, 10 wk old	122
	~35 ± 15† (n = 10)	~1.3 ± 0.5† (n = 10)			~4.3 ± 1.2† (n = 10)	RIA	Male laboratory New Zealand White, extrapolated from graph	123
Rat (Rattus norvegicus)	38.61-90.09‡	0.38-1.54‡				Unknown	Sprague-Dawley, male	83
	38.61-90.09‡	1.23-1.54‡				Unknown	Sprague-Dawley, female	83
	32.18-90.09‡	0.46-1.54‡				Unknown	Wistar, male	83
	65.64 ± 5.15†	1.01 ± 0.05†				Unknown	Long-Evans, male	83
	63.06 ± 1.29†	1.28 ± 0.05†				Unknown	Long-Evans, female	83
	41.18 ± 1.29†	0.84 ± 0.05†				Unknown	Black hooded/Ztn, male	83
			28.47 ± 0.71†	3.20 ± 0.13†		Unknown	Sprague-Dawley, adult	83
	31.53 ± 2.45†	0.76 ± 0.04†				TT₄ Larsen's method, TT₃ RIA	Male Wistar rat	124

Hypothalamus-Pituitary-Thyroid Axis-Related Hormones—cont'd

Species	TT4 (nmol/L)	TT3 (nmol/L)	fT4 (pmol/L)	fT3 (pmol/L)	TSH (mIU/L)	Methodology	Target Population	Reference
Ferret (*Mustela putorius furo*)								
	18.0 ± 3.6† (n = 14)					Solid-phase competitive RIA	Laboratory, 9 females, 5 males	125
	25.5 ± 6.1† (n = 11)					Solid-phase competitive RIA	Pets, 5 females, 6 males	125
	19.3-38.61‡					Unknown	Unknown	83
	Male 41.7 ± 21.24† (n = 31) Female 24.07 ± 10.17† (n = 13)	Male 0.89 ± 0.14† (n = 31) Female 0.81 ± 0.2† (n = 13)				RIA	Commercial vendor, specific pathogen free for *Salmonella*, *Campylobacter*, and parasites, 31 males (27 intact, 4 castrated), 13 females	126
	23.44-37.19‡ (n = 14)	0.98-1.36‡ (n = 14)				RIA	Intact female pets, 9 to 35 mo, hospitalized for ovariectomy, either 3 to 10 d after the beginning of heat (n = 5) or 9 to 21 d after, with hCG-inducted ovulation (n = 6) or out of breeding season (in winter when females were in anoestrus; n = 3)	90
	27 (15.9-42.0)* (n = 94)					Chemiluminescence	Clinically healthy pets	91
	22.53 ± 4.63† (n = 8)	1.04 ± 0.17† (n = 8)				RIA	Adult male, laboratory	127
	24.45 ± 6.44† (n = 5)	1.08 ± 0.14† (n = 5)				RIA	Adult male, laboratory	127
	32.56 ± 11.97† (n = 8)	1.25 ± 0.27† (n = 8)				RIA	Adult male, laboratory	127
	37.97 ± 10.17† (n = 5)	1.43 ± 0.35† (n = 5)				RIA	Adult male, laboratory	127
	45 ± 19†	1.08 ± 0.15†				Magnetic-antibody immunoassay	Adult female laboratory, extrapolated from graphic	88

hCG, Human chorionic gonadotropin; *RIA*, radioimmunoassay; *TT₃*, total triiodothyronine; *TT₃*, total triiodothyronine; *TT₄*, total thyroxine.
*Values are provided as mean/median values and reference interval.
†Values are provided as mean/median and standard error/standard deviation of the mean.
‡Values are provided as range.
§Values are provided as mean/median, standard error/standard deviation of the mean, and reference interval.
‖Mean/median.

REFERENCES FOR APPENDIX

1. Ott JA, Mendonca MT, Guyer C, et al. Seasonal changes in sex and adrenal steroid hormones of gopher tortoises (*Gopherus polyphemus*). *Gen Comp Endocrinol.* 2000;117:299-312.
2. Selman W, Jawor JM, Qualls CP. Seasonal variation of corticosterone levels in *Graptemys flavimaculata*, an imperiled freshwater turtle. *Copeia.* 2012;2012:698-705.
3. French SS, DeNardo DF, Greives TJ, et al. Human disturbance alters endocrine and immune responses in the Galapagos marine iguana (*Amblyrhynchus cristatus*). *Horm Behav.* 2010;58:792-799.
4. Licht P, Wood JF, Wood FE. Annual and diurnal cycles in plasma testosterone and thyroxine in the male green sea turtle *Chelonia mydas*. *Gen Comp Endocrinol.* 1985;57:335-344.
5. Cree A, Amey AP, Whittier JM. Lack of consistent hormonal responses to capture during the breeding season of the bearded dragon, *Pogona barbata*. *Comp Biochem Physiol A Mol Integr Physiol.* 2000;126:275-285.
6. Barry M, Cockrem JF, Brunton DH. Seasonal variation in plasma corticosterone concentrations in wild and captive adult Duvaucel's geckos (*Hoplodactylus duvaucelii*) in New Zealand. *Aust J Zool.* 2010;58:234-242.
7. Edwards A, Jones SM. Changes in plasma progesterone, estrogen, and testosterone concentrations throughout the reproductive cycle in female viviparous blue-tongued skinks, *Tiliqua nigrolutea* (Scincidae), in Tasmania. *Gen Comp Endocrinol.* 2001;122:260-269.
8. Bourne AR, Stewart BJ, Watson TG. Changes in blood progesterone concentration during pregnancy in the lizard *Tiliqua* (*Trachydosaurus*) *rugosa*. *Comp Biochem Physiol A Comp Physiol.* 1986;84:581-583.
9. Hamann M, Jessop T, Limpus C, et al. Interactions among endocrinology, seasonal reproductive cycles and the nesting biology of the female green sea turtle. *Mar Biol.* 2002;140:823-830.
10. Tyrrell C, Cree A. Relationships between corticosterone concentration and season, time of day and confinement in a wild reptile (tuatara, *Sphenodon punctatus*). *Gen Comp Endocrinol.* 1998;110:97-108.
11. Aguirre AA, Balazs GH, Spraker TR, et al. Adrenal and hematological responses to stress in juvenile green turtles (*Chelonia mydas*) with and without fibropapillomas. *Physiol Zool.* 1995:831-854.
12. Gregory LF, Gross TS, Bolten AB, et al. Plasma corticosterone concentrations associated with acute captivity stress in wild loggerhead sea turtles (*Caretta caretta*). *Gen Comp Endocrinol.* 1996;104:312-320.
13. Whittier JM, Corrie F, Limpus C. Plasma steroid profiles in nesting loggerhead turtles (*Caretta caretta*) in Queensland, Australia: Relationship to nesting episode and season. *Gen Comp Endocrinol.* 1997;106:39-47.
14. Lance VA, Elsey RM. Stress-induced suppression of testosterone secretion in male alligators. *J Exp Zoolog.* 1986;239:241-246.
15. Elsey RM, Joanen T, McNease L, et al. Stress and plasma corticosterone levels in the American alligator—relationships with stocking density and nesting success. *Comp Biochem Physiol A Physiol.* 1990;95:55-63.
16. Elsey RM, Lance VA, Joanen T, et al. Acute stress suppresses plasma estradiol levels in female alligators (*Alligator mississippiensis*). *Comp Biochem Physiol A Physiol.* 1991;100:649-651.
17. Guillette LJ Jr, Woodward AR, Crain DA, et al. The reproductive cycle of the female American alligator (*Alligator mississippiensis*). *Gen Comp Endocrinol.* 1997;108:87-101.
18. Guillette LJ Jr, Crain DA, Rooney AA, et al. Effect of acute stress on plasma concentrations of sex and stress hormones in juvenile alligators living in control and contaminated lakes. *J Herpetol.* 1997;31(3):347-353.
19. Tyrrell C, Cree A. Plasma corticosterone concentrations in wild and captive juvenile tuatara (*Sphenodon punctatus*). *NZ J Zool.* 1994;21:407-416.
20. Masini MA, Maria Uva B. Glucose, insulin and renin activity after sodium loading and depletion in *Vipera aspis*. *Comp Biochem Physiol C Pharmacol Toxicol Endocrinol.* 1996;113:375-380.
21. Sarkar H, Sarkar S, Maiti B. Diabetogenic effects of streptozotocin on endocrine pancreatic islets, adrenal and carbohydrate profiles in turtles, *Lissemys punctata punctata* (Bonnoterre) (Reptilia: Chelonia). *Ital J Zool.* 2013;80:12-34.
22. Sciarrillo R, Laforgia V, Cavagnuolo A, et al. Effects of administration of glucagon on the plasma and hepatic contents of the thyroid hormones in the lizard *Podarcis sicula*. *Ital J Zool.* 1999;66:323-327.
23. Sweazea KL, McMurtry JP, Elsey RM, et al. Comparison of metabolic substrates in alligators and several birds of prey. *Zoology.* 2014;117:253-260.
24. Sarkar HP, Maiti BR. Summer and winter changes in the pancreatic endocrine cells, hormones and carbohydrate metabolism of the softshelled turtle *Lissemys punctata punctata* Bonnoterre (Reptilia, Chelonia). *Ital J Zool.* 2011;78:304-319.
25. Stringer EM, Harms CA, Beasley JF, et al. Comparison of ionized calcium, parathyroid hormone, and 25-hydroxyvitamin D in rehabilitating and healthy wild green sea turtles (*Chelonia mydas*). *J Herpetol Med Surg.* 2010;20:122-127.
26. Nevarez JG, Mitchell MA, Le Blanc C, et al. Determination of plasma biochemistries, ionised calcium, vitamin D_3 and hematocrit values in captive green iguanas (*Iguana iguana*) from El Salvador. *Proc Assoc Reptile Amphib Vet: 9th Annu Conf.* 2012;2012:2002.
27. Eatwell K. Calcium and phosphorus values and their derivatives in captive tortoises (*Testudo* species). *J Small Anim Pract.* 2010;51:472-475.
28. Hedley J, Eatwell K. The effects of UV light on calcium metabolism in ball pythons (*Python regius*). *Vet Rec.* 2013;173:345.
29. Eisenhawer E, Courtney CH, Raskin RE, et al. Relationship between separation time of plasma from heparinized whole blood on plasma biochemical analytes of loggerhead sea turtles (*Caretta caretta*). *J Zoo Wildl Med.* 2008;39:208-215.
30. Oonincx D, van de Wal M, Bosch G, et al. Blood vitamin D_3 metabolite concentrations of adult female bearded dragons (*Pogona vitticeps*) remain stable after ceasing UVB exposure. *Comp Biochem Physiol B Biochem Mol Biol.* 2013;165:196-200.
31. Oonincx D, Stevens Y, van den Borne J, et al. Effects of vitamin D_3 supplementation and UVB exposure on the growth and plasma concentration of vitamin D_3 metabolites in juvenile bearded dragons (*Pogona vitticeps*). *Comp Biochem Physiol B Biochem Mol Biol.* 2010;156:122-128.
32. Hamann M, Schäuble CS, Simons T, et al. Demographic and health parameters of green sea turtles *Chelonia mydas* foraging in the Gulf of Carpentaria, Australia. *Endangered Species Res.* 2006;2:81-88.
33. Hoby S, Wenker C, Robert N, et al. Nutritional metabolic bone disease in juvenile veiled chameleons (*Chamaeleo calyptratus*) and its prevention. *J Nutr.* 2010;140:1923-1931.
34. Acierno MJ, Mitchell MA, Zachariah TT, et al. Effects of ultraviolet radiation on plasma 25-hydroxyvitamin D_3 concentrations in corn snakes (*Elaphe guttata*). *Am J Vet Res.* 2008;69:294-297.
35. Acierno MJ, Mitchell MA, Roundtree MK, et al. Effects of ultraviolet radiation on 25-hydroxyvitamin D_3 synthesis in red-eared slider turtles (*Trachemys scripta elegans*). *Am J Vet Res.* 2006;67:2046-2049.
36. Ramer JC, Maria R, Reichard T, et al. Vitamin D status of wild Ricord's iguanas (*Cyclura ricordii*) and captive and wild rhinoceros iguanas (*Cyclura cornuta cornuta*) in the Dominican Republic. *J Zoo Wildl Med.* 2005;36:188-191.
37. Laing CJ, Trube A, Shea GM, et al. The requirement for natural sunlight to prevent vitamin D deficiency in iguanian lizards. *J Zoo Wildl Med.* 2001;32:342-348.
38. Gillespie D, Frye FL, Stockham SL, et al. Blood values in wild and captive Komodo dragons (*Varanus komodoensis*). *Zoo Biol.* 2000;19:495-509.

39. Kohel KA, MacKenzie DS, Rostal DC, et al. Seasonality in plasma thyroxine in the desert tortoise, *Gopherus agassizii*. *Gen Comp Endocrinol*. 2001;121:214-222.

40. Hernandez-Divers SJ, Knott CD, MacDonald J. Diagnosis and surgical treatment of thyroid adenoma-induced hyperthyroidism in a green iguana (*Iguana iguana*). *J Zoo Wildl Med*. 2001;32:465-475.

41. Boggs AS, Hamlin HJ, Lowers RH, et al. Seasonal variation in plasma thyroid hormone concentrations in coastal versus inland populations of juvenile American alligators (*Alligator mississippiensis*): influence of plasma iodide concentrations. *Gen Comp Endocrinol*. 2011;174:362-369.

42. Balletto E, Cherchi MA, Melodia F, et al. Temperature-dependent thyroid hormone biosynthesis in *Testudo horsfieldi* Gray. *Gen Comp Endocrinol*. 1979;39:548-561.

43. Greenacre CB, Young DW, Behrend EN, et al. Validation of a novel high-sensitivity radioimmunoassay procedure for measurement of total thyroxine concentration in psittacine birds and snakes. *Am J Vet Res*. 2001;62:1750-1754.

44. Norton TM, Jacobson ER, Caligiuri R, et al. Medical management of a Galapagos tortoise (*Geochelone elephantopus*) with hypothyroidism. *J Zoo Wildl Med*. 1989;20:212-216.

45. Franco K, Famini D, Hoover J, et al. Serum thyroid hormone values for African spurred tortoises (*Centrochelys* [formerly *Geochelone*] *sulcata*). *J Herpetol Med Surg*. 2009;19:47-49.

46. Moon D-Y, Owens DW, MacKenzie DS. The effects of fasting and increased feeding on plasma thyroid hormones, glucose, and total protein in sea turtles. *Zoolog Sci*. 1999;16:579-586.

47. Spano JS, Pedersoli WM, Kemppainen RJ, et al. Baseline hematologic, endocrine, and clinical chemistry values in ducks and roosters. *Avian Dis*. 1987;31:800-803.

48. Silverin B, Viebke PA, Westin J. Plasma levels of luteinizing hormone and steroid hormones in free-living winter groups of willow tits (*Parus montanus*). *Horm Behav*. 1984;18:367-379.

49. Love OP, Bird DM, Shutt LJ. Corticosterone levels during postnatal development in captive American kestrels (*Falco sparverius*). *Gen Comp Endocrinol*. 2003;130:135-141.

50. Vleck CM, Vertalino N, Vleck D, et al. Stress, corticosterone, and heterophil to lymphocyte ratios in free-living Adelie penguins. *Condor*. 2000;102:392-400.

51. Zenoble R, Kemppainen R, Young D, et al. Endocrine responses of healthy parrots to ACTH and thyroid stimulating hormone. *J Am Vet Med Assoc*. 1985;187:1116-1118.

52. Heatley JJ, Oliver JW, Hosgood G, et al. Serum corticosterone concentrations in response to restraint, anesthesia, and skin testing in Hispaniolan Amazon parrots (*Amazona ventralis*). *J Avian Med Surg*. 2000;14:172-176.

53. Cornelissen H, Verhofstad A. Adrenal neoplasia in a scarlet macaw (*Ara macao*) with clinical signs of hyperadrenocorticism. *J Avian Med Surg*. 1999;13:92-97.

54. Nilsson PB, Hollmen TE, Atkinson S, et al. Effects of ACTH, capture, and short term confinement on glucocorticoid concentrations in harlequin ducks (*Histrionicus histrionicus*). *Comp Biochem Physiol A Mol Integr Physiol*. 2008;149:275-283.

55. Klaphake E, Fecteau K, Dewit M, et al. Effects of leuprolide acetate on selected blood and fecal sex hormones in Hispaniolan Amazon parrots (*Amazona ventralis*). *J Avian Med Surg*. 2009;23:253-262.

56. Peterson A, Common R. Estrone and estradiol concentrations in peripheral plasma of laying hens as determined by radioimmunoassay. *Can J Zool*. 1972;50:395-404.

57. Camper PM, Burke WH. Serum estradiol and progesterone levels of the laying turkey hen following acute treatment with mammalian luteinizing hormone or follicle-stimulating hormone. *Gen Comp Endocrinol*. 1977;31:224-232.

58. Doi O, Takai T, Nakamura T, et al. Changes in the pituitary and plasma LH, plasma and follicular progesterone and estradiol, and plasma testosterone and estrone concentrations during the ovula-

59. Mauget R, Jouventin P, Lacroix A, et al. Plasma LH and steroid hormones in king penguin (*Aptenodytes patagonicus*) during the onset of the breeding cycle. *Gen Comp Endocrinol*. 1994;93:36-43.

60. Marra PP, Lampe KT, Tedford BL. Plasma corticosterone levels in two species of *Zonotrichia* sparrows under captive and free-living conditions. *Wilson Bull*. 1995;107(2):296-305.

61. Williams TD. Reproductive endocrinology of macaroni (*Eudyptes chrysolophus*) and gentoo (*Pygoscelis papua*) penguins: I. Seasonal changes in plasma levels of gonadal steroids and LH in breeding adults. *Gen Comp Endocrinol*. 1992;85:230-240.

62. Hoshino S, Suzuki M, Kakegawa T, et al. Changes in plasma thyroid hormones, luteinizing hormone (LH), estradiol, progesterone and corticosterone of laying hens during a forced molt. *Comp Biochem Physiol A Physiol*. 1988;90:355-359.

63. Preda C, Budica C, Dojana N. Effect of various levels of dietary calcium on blood calcium concentration and hormonal status in White Cornish and White Leghorn hens. *Bull Univ Agric Sci Vet Med Cluj-Napoca Vet Med*. 2014;71:182-186.

64. Kothe R, Mischke R. Fructosamine concentration in blood plasma of psittacides—relevance for diagnostics of diabetes? *Prakt Tierarzt*. 2009;90(2):102-109.

65. Freeman B, Langslow D. Responses of plasma glucose, free fatty acids and glucagon to cobalt and nickel chlorides by *Gallus domesticus*. *Comp Biochem Physiol A Physiol*. 1973;46:427-436.

66. Langslow DR, Freeman BM, Buchanan KD. Responses of plasma glucose, free fatty acids, glucagon and insulin to synthalin A by *Gallus domesticus*. *Comp Biochem Physiol A Comp Physiol*. 1973;46:437-445.

67. Totzke U, Hubinger A, Korthaus G, et al. Fasting increases the plasma glucagon response in the migratory garden warbler (*Sylvia borin*). *Gen Comp Endocrinol*. 1999;115:116-121.

68. Le Ninan F, Cherel Y, Robin JP, et al. Early changes in plasma hormones and metabolites during fasting in king penguin chicks. *J Comp Physiol B*. 1988;158:395-401.

69. Adkesson MJ, Langan JN. Metabolic bone disease in juvenile Humboldt penguins (*Spheniscus humboldti*): investigation of ionized calcium, parathyroid hormone, and vitamin D_3 as diagnostic parameters. *J Zoo Wildl Med*. 2007;38:85-92.

70. Howard LL, Kass PH, Lamberski N, et al. Serum concentrations of ionized calcium, vitamin D_3, and parathyroid hormone in captive thick-billed parrots (*Rhynchopsitta pachyrhyncha*). *J Zoo Wildl Med*. 2004;35:147-153.

71. Kubiak M, Forbes N. Effects of diet on total calcium, vitamin D and parathyroid hormone in falcons. *Vet Rec*. 2012;2012:54.

72. Polo FJ, Peinado VI, Viscor G, et al. Hematologic and plasma chemistry values in captive psittacine birds. *Avian Dis*. 1998;42:523-535.

73. de Carvalho FM, Gaunt SD, Kearney MT, et al. Reference intervals of plasma calcium, phosphorus, and magnesium for African grey parrots (*Psittacus erithacus*) and Hispaniolan parrots (*Amazona ventralis*). *J Zoo Wildl Med*. 2009;40:675-679.

74. Garcia-Montijano M, Garcia A, Lemus JA, et al. Blood chemistry, protein electrophoresis, and hematologic values of captive Spanish imperial eagles (*Aquila adalberti*). *J Zoo Wildl Med*. 2002;33:112-117.

75. Lumeij JT, Westerhof I. Clinical evaluation of thyroid function in racing pigeons (*Columba livia domestica*). *Avian Pathol*. 1988;17:63-70.

76. Müller K, Schettler E, Gerlach H, et al. Investigations on the aetiology of pinching off syndrome in four white-tailed sea eagles (*Haliaeetus albicilla*) from Germany. *Avian Pathol*. 2007;36:235-243.

77. Fox GA, Jeffrey DA, Williams KS, et al. Health of herring gulls (*Larus argentatus*) in relation to breeding location in the early 1990s. I. Biochemical measures. *J Toxicol Environ Health A*. 2007;70:1443-1470.

78. McNabb FM, Lyons LJ, Hughes TE. Free thyroid hormones in altricial (ring doves) versus precocial (Japanese quail) development. *Endocrinology.* 1984;115:2133-2136.

79. Brandao J, Manickam B, Blas-Machado U, et al. Productive thyroid follicular carcinoma in a wild barred owl *(Strix varia). J Vet Diagn Invest.* 2012;24:1145-1150.

80. Smits JE, Fernie KJ, Bortolotti GR, et al. Thyroid hormone suppression and cell-mediated immunomodulation in American kestrels *(Falco sparverius)* exposed to PCBs. *Arch Environ Contam Toxicol.* 2002;43:338-344.

81. Brandao J, Rick M, Beaufrere H, et al. Free and total thyroid hormones reference interval in the Hispaniolan Amazon parrot. *Proc Assoc Avian Vet.* 2014;2014:29.

82. Nazifi S, Mosleh N, Nili H, et al. Diurnal variations in serum biochemical parameters and their correlations with thyroid hormones in ostrich chicks *(Struthio camelus). Comp Clin Pathol.* 2012;21:1669-1675.

83. Quimby FW. *The Clinical Chemistry of Laboratory Animals.* 2nd ed. Philadelphia: Taylor & Francis; 1999.

84. Chiericato GM, Boiti C, Canali C, et al. Effects of heat stress and age on growth performance and endocrine status of male rabbit. *World Rabbit Sci.* 1995;3:125-131.

85. Suckow MA, Stevens KA, Wilson RP. *The Laboratory Rabbit, Guinea Pig, Hamster, and Other Rodents.* 1st ed. London; Waltham, MA: Academic Press/Elsevier; 2012.

86. Norris S, Pettifor J, Gray D, et al. Calcium metabolism and bone mass in female rabbits during skeletal maturation: effects of dietary calcium intake. *Bone.* 2001;29:62-69.

87. Hauptman K, Jekl V, Dorrestein G, et al. Comparison of estradiol and progesterone serum levels in ferrets suffering from hyperoestrogenism and ovarian neoplasia. *Vet Med (Praha).* 2009;54:532-536.

88. Kastner R, Kastner D, Apfelbach R. Developmental patterns of thyroid hormones and testosterone in ferrets. *Horm Metab Res.* 1987;19:194-196.

89. Gromadzka-Ostrowska J, Zalewska B, Szylarska-Gozdz E. Peripheral plasma progesterone concentration and haematological indices during normal pregnancy of chinchillas *(Chinchilla laniger,* M.). *Comp Biochem Physiol A Comp Physiol.* 1985;82:661-665.

90. Prohaczik A, Kulcsar M, Huszenicza G. Metabolic and endocrine characteristics of pregnancy toxemia in the ferret. *Vet Med (Praha).* 2009;54:75-80.

91. Hein J, Spreyer F, Sauter-Louis C, et al. Reference ranges for laboratory parameters in ferrets. *Vet Rec.* 2012;171:218-223.

92. Rosenthal KL, Wire NR. Endocrine diseases In: Quesenberry K,Carpenter JW, eds. *Ferrets, Rabbits, and Rodents: Clinical Medicine and Surgery.* 3rd ed. St. Louis, MO: Elsevier/Saunders; 2012; 86-102.

93. Mann F, Stockham S, Freeman M, et al. Reference intervals for insulin concentrations and insulin: glucose ratios in the serum of ferrets. *Scientifur.* 1995;19:289.

94. Lloyd CG, Lewis WG. Two cases of pancreatic neoplasia in British ferrets *(Mustela putorius furo). J Small Anim Pract.* 2004;45: 558-562.

95. Knudtzon J. Plasma levels of glucagon, insulin, glucose and free fatty acids in rabbits during laboratory handling procedures. *Z Versuchstierkund.* 1984;26:123.

96. Heding LG, Anderson H. Increased serum immunoreactive insulin in rabbits fed a protein- and mineral-rich diet. *Diabetologia.* 1973;9:282-286.

97. Helfenstein T, Fonseca FA, Ihara SS, et al. Impaired glucose tolerance plus hyperlipidaemia induced by diet promotes retina microaneurysms in New Zealand rabbits. *Int J Exp Pathol.* 2011;92:40-49.

98. Ersan B, Ok M. Importance of fasting serum glucose, haemoglobin A1c and fructosamine in the diagnosis of diabetes. *Eurasian J Vet Sci.* 2011;27:13-18.

99. Quesenberry K, Donnelly T, Mans C. Biology, husbandry, and clinical techniques of guinea pigs and chinchillas. In: Quesenberry K,Carpenter JW, eds. *Ferrets, Rabbits, and Rodents: Clinical Medicine and Surgery.* St. Louis, MO: Elsevier/Saunders; 2012;279-294.

100. Saudek CD, Finkowski M, Knopp RH. Plasma glucagon and insulin in rat pregnancy. Roles in glucose homeostasis. *J Clin Invest.* 1975;55:180.

101. Junod A, Lambert AE, Stauffacher W, et al. Diabetogenic action of streptozotocin: relationship of dose to metabolic response. *J Clin Invest.* 1969;48:2129-2139.

102. Emerson JA, Whittington JK, Allender MC, et al. Effects of ultraviolet radiation produced from artificial lights on serum 25-hydroxyvitamin D concentration in captive domestic rabbits *(Oryctolagus cuniculi). Am J Vet Res.* 2014;75:380-384.

103. Bas S, Bas A, Lopez I, et al. Nutritional secondary hyperparathyroidism in rabbits. *Domest Anim Endocrinol.* 2005;28:380-390.

104. Bas S, Aguilera-Tejero E, Estepa JC, et al. The influence of acute and chronic hypercalcemia on the parathyroid hormone response to hypocalcemia in rabbits. *Eur J Endocrinol.* 2002;146:411-418.

105. Ardiaca M, Bonvehi C, Montesinos A. Point-of-care blood gas and electrolyte analysis in rabbits. *Vet Clin North Am Exot Anim Pract.* 2013;16:175-195.

106. Hewitt CD, Innes DJ, Savory J, et al. Normal biochemical and hematological values in New Zealand White rabbits. *Clin Chem.* 1989;35:1777-1779.

107. Burnett N, Mathura K, Metivier K, et al. An investigation into haematological and serum chemistry parameters of rabbits in Trinidad. *World Rabbit Sci.* 2006;14(3):175–87.

108. Cetin N, Bekyürek T, Cetin E. Effects of sex, pregnancy and season on some haematological and biochemical blood values in Angora rabbits. *Scand J Lab Anim Sci.* 2009;36:155–62.

109. Al-Eissa M. Effect of gestation and season on the haematological and biochemical parameters in domestic rabbit *(Oryctolagus cuniculus). Br Biotechnol J.* 2011;1:10-17.

110. Elamin KM. Age and sex effects on blood biochemical profile of local rabbits in Sudan. *Wayamba J Anim Sci.* 2013;5:548–553.

111. Rivas AE, Mitchell MA, Flower J, et al. Effects of ultraviolet radiation on serum 25-hydroxyvitamin D concentrations in captive chinchillas *(Chinchilla laniger). J Exot Pet Med.* 2014;75:380-384.

112. Oliveira Silva TD, Kreutz LC, Barcellos LJG, et al. Reference values for chinchilla *(Chinchilla laniger)* blood cells and serum biochemical parameters. *Ciência Rural.* 2005;35:602-606.

113. Muszczyński Z, Sulik M, Ogoński T, et al. Plasma concentration of calcium, magnesium and phosphorus in chinchilla with and without tooth overgrowth. *Folia Biol.* 2009;58:107-111.

114. Watson MK, Stern AW, Labelle AL, et al. Evaluating the clinical and physiological effects of long term ultraviolet B radiation on guinea pigs *(Cavia porcellus). PLoS ONE.* 2014;9:e114413.

115. Hein J, Hartmann K. Reference ranges for laboratory parameters in guinea pigs. *Tierarztl Prax Ausg K Kleintiere Heimtiere.* 2003; 31:383-389.

116. Fredholm DV, Cagle LA, Johnston MS. Evaluation of precision and establishment of reference ranges for plasma thyroxine using a point-of-care analyzer in healthy guinea pigs *(Cavia porcellus). J Exot Pet Med.* 2012;21:87-93.

117. Binah O, Rubinstein I, Gilat E. Effects of thyroid hormone on the action potential and membrane currents of guinea pig ventricular myocytes. *Pflugers Arch.* 1987;409:214-216.

118. Muller K, Muller E, Klein R, et al. Serum thyroxine concentrations in clinically healthy pet guinea pigs *(Cavia porcellus). Vet Clin Pathol.* 2009;38:507-510.

119. Castro MI, Alex S, Young RA, et al. Total and free serum thyroid hormone concentrations in fetal and adult pregnant and nonpregnant guinea pigs. *Endocrinology.* 1986;118:533-537.

120. Anderson RR, Nixon DA, Akasha MA. Total and free thyroxine and triiodothyronine in blood serum of mammals. *Comp Biochem Physiol A Comp Physiol.* 1988;89:401-404.

121. Mayer J, Wagner R, Mitchell MA, et al. Use of recombinant human thyroid-stimulating hormone for evaluation of thyroid function in guinea pigs *(Cavia porcellus)*. *J Am Vet Med Assoc*. 2013;242:346-349.

122. Mustafa S, Al-Bader MD, Elgazzar AH, et al. Effect of hyperthermia on the function of thyroid gland. *Eur J Appl Physiol*. 2008;103:285-288.

123. Mebis L, Debaveye Y, Ellger B, et al. Changes in the central component of the hypothalamus-pituitary-thyroid axis in a rabbit model of prolonged critical illness. *Critical Care*. 2009;13:R147.

124. Takeuchi A, Suzuki M, Tsuchiya S. Effect of thyroidectomy on the secretory profiles of growth hormone, thyrotropin and corticosterone in the rat. *Endocrinol Jpn*. 1978;25:381-390.

125. Mayer J, Wagner R, Mitchell MA, et al. Use of recombinant human thyroid-stimulating hormone for thyrotropin stimulation testing in euthyroid ferrets. *J Am Vet Med Assoc*. 2013;243:1432-1435.

126. Garibaldi BA, Pecquet Goad ME, Fox JG, et al. Serum thyroxine and triiodothyronine radioimmunoassay values in the normal ferret. *Lab Anim Sci*. 1988;38:455-458.

127. Heard DJ, Collins B, Chen DL, et al. Thyroid and adrenal function tests in adult male ferrets. *Am J Vet Res*. 1990;51:32-35.

CHAPTER 7

Musculoskeletal System

Michael S. McFadden, MS, DVM, DACVS

INTRODUCTION

Exotic animal species are commonly presented for disorders of the musculoskeletal system. Despite the wide variety of species that may be called "exotic" animals, there are many musculoskeletal diseases that share common etiologies with domestic species. Veterinarians that treat and care for exotic animals should be knowledgeable of the many common musculoskeletal diseases reported in domestic species (e.g., canine, feline) to use as a reference and a guide. In many cases, the same diagnostic approach and treatments used for domestic species can be applied to an exotic animal patient; however, there will be certain cases where the pathophysiology and treatment are more specific to the exotic patient. Once a strong knowledge base in the diagnosis and treatment of musculoskeletal diseases in domestic species is established, the diseases and diagnostics that are unique to exotic animal musculoskeletal diseases can be added to form a complete understanding of musculoskeletal disease.

ANATOMY AND PHYSIOLOGY

A basic understanding of anatomy and physiology of exotic animals is crucial to understanding musculoskeletal diseases. There are many anatomic differences between exotic species specifically related to the musculoskeletal system, which can affect diagnosis and treatment of different diseases. This includes differences in body organization (e.g., limb number, limb function), skeletal type (e.g., endoskeleton vs. exoskeleton), and histologic differences in bone structure that may affect bone healing (e.g., bones in reptiles vs. birds vs. mammals). Any veterinarian working with exotic animals must develop a basic understanding of the anatomy and physiology of the species that he or she works with. Due to the large number and diversity of species characterized as "exotic animals," only a brief review of the anatomy relevant to the musculoskeletal system is presented here.

Invertebrates

Invertebrates are the largest group of animals on Earth, with over 1 million species described.[1] Arachnids (e.g., spiders and scorpions), myriapods (e.g., centipedes and millipedes), and insects are commonly kept as pets or as display animals and more commonly presented for veterinary care. As the name of the group implies, all of these animals lack a vertebral column and spinal cord but also have an exoskeleton, making them unique compared to other species of exotic animals (vertebrates) when discussing the musculoskeletal system.

The arachnid body plan is divided into a prosoma and an opisthoma.[1,2] The prosoma (cephalothorax) is comprised of a fused head and thorax, while the opisthoma represents the abdominal segment and contains the majority of the internal organs. The prosoma is covered ventrally by a sternal plate and dorsally by the carapace. The appendages originate from the prosoma and include the chelicerae, pedipalps, and legs. The chelicerae are the first appendages and have a distal movable fang. The pedipalps resemble legs but lack a metatarsal segment and are not used in locomotion. Instead, they are predominantly used as a sensory organ and to manipulate prey. There are four pairs of legs that attach between the carapace and sternum of the prosoma. Each leg contains seven segments (coxa, trochanter, femur, patella, tibia, metatarsus, and tarsus), and the distal segment contains a tarsal claw. Spider muscles are striated but contain few mitochondria.[2] This allows brief periods of rapid movement, although the muscles will rapidly fatigue. Approximately two-thirds of the prosoma are occupied by muscles. These attach to a central carapacial apodeme and are responsible for the movement of the limbs and assist with the function of the sucking stomach. Each limb contains approximately 30 individual muscles. Both flexor and extensor muscle groups are present; however, major joints rely on muscles for flexion and (increasing) hemolymph pressure within the limbs for extension.[2]

Myriapods have a body plan that is elongated with several body segments.[1] Each segment, with the exception of the head and anal segments, has one (centipedes) or two (millipedes) pairs of legs. Millipedes are cylindrical in shape with a hard calcified exoskeleton, while centipedes are dorso-ventrally flattened.

Insect body plans are divided into the head, thorax, and abdomen. Three pairs of legs originate from the thorax. Each leg has six segments (coxae, trochanter, femur, tibia, tarsus, and pretarsus) and ends with a pair of tarsal claws.[1] The wings also originate from the thorax and can vary in number, with most insects having one or two pairs; however, some species do not have wings or their wings are modified into accessory structures to cover the functional wings (e.g., elytra in coleopterans) or serve as stabilizers during flight (e.g., halteres in dipterans).

Vertebrates

Animals commonly kept as exotic pets include ornamental fish, amphibians, reptiles, birds, and small mammals (e.g., ferrets, rabbits, rodents, and marsupials). While these animals are all classified as vertebrates, there is significant variation in the anatomy and physiology of the musculoskeletal system between these groups.

Fish

Fish are the largest class of vertebrates, with more than 25,000 different species worldwide and more than 1000 different species being commonly kept in captivity.[3] Fish have a variety of body plans. The more commonly kept species are fusiform, but fish can also be laterally compressed (e.g., angelfish), dorso-ventrally compressed (e.g., rays), or have an eel form (e.g., moray eel).[4] The image of a fusiform fish is what most people think of when they imagine the "typical fish"; however, there can even be significant variations to this body plan. Fusiform fish have three basic body regions: the head, trunk, and tail. The head extends to the caudal margin of the opercula (gill coverings), the trunk continues to the caudal portion of the peritoneal cavity, and the muscular tail starts at the anal opening and extends caudally.[4] Most common fish have two sets of paired fins (pectoral and pelvic) and three unpaired fins (dorsal, anal, and caudal) that aid in balance, steering, and locomotion. These fins can be modified in different taxa to adapt to certain niches or act as part of their defense system. The skeletal system of fish can be variable but in most fish is composed of true bone, with the same basic components of mammalian skeletons.[4] As in mammals, fish have three basic types of muscle fibers: involuntary smooth muscle, cardiac muscle, and skeletal muscle. Skeletal muscle can be further divided into dark and light muscles. Light muscle is found in higher proportions in most fish and is responsible for quick rapid movements. Dark muscle, thought to be involved in maintaining sustained swimming, has a higher lipid content and more mitochondria present per cell. Dark muscle is found in different proportions based on the lifestyle of the fish but is usually in highest abundance underlying fins used for propulsion.[5] Clinically, the differences in muscle types can play a role in drug metabolism if intramuscular injections are used.[4,5]

Cartilage plays an important role in the musculoskeletal system of fish. Elasmobranchs (e.g., sharks and rays) have a skeleton composed almost entirely of cartilage, while other species have skeletal systems that begin as hyaline cartilage and ossify as the animal matures.[5]

Amphibians

The class Amphibia includes the orders Anura (frogs and toads), Caudata (salamanders and newts), and Gymnophonia (caecilians). Although there are thousands (>7000 species) of different species of amphibians, only a small number are kept as pets or display animals.[6] Clinicians should remember that both larval and adult forms exist and there can be significant differences between the two in regard to diseases and treatments. Since larval forms are less commonly presented for veterinary care, the anatomy of larval forms is not covered here.

The caecilian body structure resembles that of an annelid worm due to the absence of limbs and presence of cutaneous folds.[7] There is little variation to this body plan; however,

some aquatic species have a dorsal fin. Caecilians lack pectoral and pelvic girdles and do not have a sacrum.

Newts and salamanders generally have four limbs, with a variable number of toes; however, some species lack hind limbs.[7] Most salamanders have tails with cleavage planes to allow autotomy as a method to escape predation. The vertebral column is poorly differentiated into cervical, trunk, sacral, caudal sacral, and caudal regions.

Frogs and toads have similar basic body plans. They have four limbs, although the length of the hind limbs can vary depending on locomotory adaptations, with longer hind limbs allowing greater jumping ability.[6,7] The forelimbs possess a fused radius and ulna (radioulna) and the hind limbs have a fused tibia and fibula (tibiofibula). The forelimbs have four phalanges on each foot, while the hind limbs have five phalanges. The vertebral column is separated into three fused segments (presacral, sacral, and postsacral). A true sacrum is lacking and the highly modified pelvic girdle is fused to the caudal aspect of the postsacral vertebrae.

Reptiles

Reptiles are another diverse group of animals that may be kept as pets. There is a high degree of variability in the anatomy and physiology between the different orders, with some groups being more similar to birds (e.g., crocodilians) than other groups of reptiles. Reptiles commonly presented to veterinarians include crocodilians, snakes, lizards, and chelonians (turtles and tortoises).

There are a variety of snakes that are available in the reptile trade; however, snakes have a body plan that is similar across species (>3400 species).[8] The skull of a snake is adapted to ingest large prey items, so it lacks a mandibular symphysis. The vertebral column consists of several hundred vertebrae, with very little variation along the length of the animal. Large groups of epaxial muscles are present along the length of the animal, with multiple attachments to aid in locomotion. Snakes do not have a sternum; instead, their ribs connect to their ventral scales to allow locomotion. Some groups have vestigial pelvic and hind limb remnants, including external spurs, that are used in courtship and mating.[9]

Although the body structure in most snakes is very similar, there are adaptations in locomotion and locomotory types.[9] Lateral undulation involves contractions of one side of the body and bending of the spinal column. This is the fastest form of locomotion in snakes. Rectilinear locomotion involves symmetrical muscle contraction in waves to move forward in a caterpillar-like fashion. Concertina locomotion involves pulling up the body into bends and then straightening out the body forward from the bends. This is done in an alternating fashion to move forward or up trees, as in arboreal species. Sidewinding locomotion is similar to lateral undulation but only two points of the snake's body are in contact with the substrate, and the snake travels in a diagonal direction in relation to the tracts left in the substrate. It is important to recognize that the method of locomotion can vary depending on species, and each species can display more than one type of locomotion depending on the substrate they are on.

Lizards are comprised of over 4000 species, and 30 to 50 species can be commonly found in the pet trade.[10] The musculoskeletal system is similar across most lizard species. They have well-developed extremities (except legless lizards) and tails that are well adapted for different locomotion strategies (e.g., running, climbing, and swimming). Most lizards have a rib attached to every vertebral body, except the sacral vertebrae.[11]

One aspect of the skeletal system that is common in many lizard species is tail autotomy. Species that have tail autotomy develop fracture planes through the vertebral bodies and neural arches of each caudal vertebra. These planes are composed of cartilage or other connective tissue and form after the caudal vertebrae have ossified. However, not all species of lizards have tail autotomy and some species, such as the green iguana (*Iguana iguana*), lose their fracture planes as they mature because these areas are replaced by bone.[11] There is some regenerative capacity for individuals that lose their tails, although the tails are usually shorter, blunter, and discolored.

Chelonians (turtles and tortoises) are one of the most recognizable groups of animals due to their shells. There are over 285 species of chelonians in the world and they are the only tetrapod that has both their pelvic and pectoral girdles within their rib cage and encased in bone.[12,13] The shell consists of an upper carapace and lower plastron connected by boney bridges. Many species, particularly aquatic species, have variations to their shell where large portions of the boney carapace and plastron are replaced with thick leathery skin.[13] Chelonians have both thoracic and lumbar ribs incorporated into their shell and no sternum is present. The trunk vertebrae are fused together but the cervical vertebrae move independently and allow the chelonian to retract its head into its shell. Modified pectoral and pelvic girdles are present and fused to the carapace. The pectoral girdle consists of the epiplastron (clavicle), entoplastron (interclavicle), scapula, acromion process, and coracoid bone. The pelvic girdle consists of paired ilium, ischium, and pubic bones. The humerus and femur are reduced in length and the limbs extend more laterally than mammalian limbs.

Birds

Birds are a very diverse group of animals and many different species may be encountered by veterinarians. The complexity of specific anatomic variations is not covered here but, instead, basic principles of psittacines and passerines are introduced to form a general knowledge base that may then be extrapolated to other species.[14]

There are some fundamental adaptations of the avian musculoskeletal system that have evolved to enable flight. These modifications have produced a strong lightweight skeleton with two main types of bones: pneumatic bones and medullary bones. Pneumatic bones are linked with the air sacs and are located in the skull, vertebrae, pelvis, sternum, ribs, and humerus.[15,16] Medullary bones are long bones with large medullary cavities and thin cortices. Interconnecting spicules extend across the medullary canal for strength and support while minimizing weight. Avian bones also have a higher calcium content to increase the strength of the thin cortices.[14] Medullary bone can undergo changes in response to estrogen and serve as a calcium store during egg-laying. Radiographically, these regions of the long bones will appear homogenously hypercalcified.[17] The appearance of the medullary bone during the egg-laying period can be mistaken for a pathologic process.

There are two main muscle types in birds: white muscle, which is similar to mammalian muscle tissue, and red muscle.[15,16] White muscles are focally innervated by one nerve fiber. Red muscle fibers are innervated by multiple nerve fibers, have larger numbers of mitochondria, have an extensive capillary bed, and contain large amounts of myoglobin. Most muscle groups contain mixes of these two muscle types. Muscles with a higher proportion of red muscle fibers are better suited for sustained effort, while white muscle fibers are more powerful but have less endurance.[16] Proportions of each type of muscle fiber may vary between species or even change within a species at different times of the year.[15]

The avian thoracic limb is also highly adapted for flight. The thoracic girdle is composed of specialized scapulae, coracoid bones, and clavicles. These are important for proper wing function, and fractures of these bones alter a bird's posture and ability to hold its wings in the proper orientation required to achieve lift during flight. Large superficial pectoral muscles are responsible for strong down strokes of the wings that generate thrust during flight. These muscles can comprise up to 20% of the body weight and can be useful in the assessment of overall body condition.[16] The skeletal anatomy of the thoracic limb includes a short stout humerus, paired radius and ulna, carpal bones, and carpometacarpus. The carpal bones are significantly reduced compared to mammalian skeletons. The carpus consists of the radial and ulnar carpal bones and the remainder of the carpal bones have fused to form the carpometacarpus. There are three digits present: the alular, the major digit, and the minor digit. The major digit has a proximal and distal phalanx, while the other digits are made up of a single phalanx.[15,16]

The pelvic limb is composed of the femur, tibiotarsus and fibula, distal tarsal bones, and metatarsal bones, which are fused to form the tarsometatarsus. There are four digits with a variable number of phalanges. Digit I has two phalanges and originates from the medial aspect of the distal tarsometatarsus. Digits II, III, and IV have three, four, and five phalanges, respectively, and originate from the trochlea at the end of the tarsometatarsus.[15,16] Functionally, the pelvic limbs are used for perching, movement while on the ground, climbing, and capturing and manipulating food items in certain species. Any injuries to a limb can cause weight shifting to the contralateral limb. It is important that any injuries be addressed quickly to prevent complications associated with abnormal weight distribution.

Mammals

Small mammals commonly kept as pets include ferrets (*Mustela putorius furo*), rabbits (*Oryctolagus cuniculus*), small rodents (mice [*Mus musculus*], rats [*Rattus norvegicus*], chinchillas [*Chinchilla lanigera*], guinea pigs [*Cavia porcellus*]), sugar gliders (*Petaurus breviceps*), and hedgehogs (*Atelerix albiventris*).

Ferrets have a slender elongated body with a lightweight, strong, flexible skeleton. The skeleton is very similar to dogs and cats with the exception of the spine. Ferrets have 15 thoracic vertebrae and a variable number of lumbar vertebrae that ranges from five to seven.[18]

Rabbits have a lightweight skeleton surrounded by very well-developed powerful muscles that make them prone to fractures. The skeleton of rabbits represents only 7% to 8% of their body weight (compared with 12% to 13% in cats), while their muscle mass accounts for 50% of their body weight. The hind limb musculature alone can account for up to 13% of the body mass, giving rabbits the strong powerful hind limbs needed to accelerate quickly and maintain high speeds to avoid predators. If patients are not adequately restrained and supported, their powerful hind limbs can kick with sufficient force to cause fractures of the lumbar spine and damage to the spinal cord. The number of thoracic and lumbar vertebrae in rabbits can vary, and the spinal cord extends into the sacral spinal canal.[19,20]

Variations in the musculoskeletal system of hedgehogs include fusion of the distal radius and ulna and the complex system of muscles involved in positioning of the spines. The frontodorsalis muscle, panniculus carnosus muscle, caudodorsalis muscle, and orbicularis muscle function to allow the hedgehog to roll into a ball and have the entire body protected by spines except for a 1-cm-diameter ventral opening.[21]

Small rodents have been extensively used in biomedical research, and texts detailing their anatomy have been published and are recommended to clinicians interested in specific anatomic variations in these species.[22,23]

DIAGNOSTICS

Diagnostic imaging of invertebrates is usually unrewarding. There is very little difference in the density of the soft tissues of these animals and standard radiographs provide little information. Magnetic resonance imaging (MRI) studies have been performed using 7.7 Tesla magnets in arachnids.[2] Although these provided excellent images, long acquisition times of these magnets and the relative rarity of these types of magnets do not make MRI a clinically useful diagnostic tool in invertebrates. Contrast studies have also been described in myriapods, but this was primarily to assess the gastrointestinal (GI) tract.[24]

Radiographs can be performed in fish but are usually done to examine internal organs (e.g., GI tract, swim bladder). The value of radiographs for assessing the musculoskeletal system of fish is limited, with few exceptions (e.g., spinal fractures). Diagnostic procedures in fish related to the musculoskeletal system are mainly limited to muscle biopsies of lesions caused by bacteria, parasites, or neoplasia. Complete blood counts (CBCs) and biochemistry profiles may have value for further characterizing inflammation in the muscle (e.g., leukocytosis, increased creatine kinase [CK]).

Radiographic examination for orthopedic disease in most other vertebrates is straightforward and, in many cases, follows guidelines for obtaining radiographs of the axial and appendicular skeleton in domestic species.[25]

Radiographic imaging is considered routine when evaluating reptile and amphibian patients with musculoskeletal abnormalities. Radiographs can be used to assess bone density in metabolic bone disease (MBD) as well as evaluate the skeletal system for any fractures or luxations. Standard radiographic equipment can be used, although in many amphibians and small reptiles, dental radiography is preferred. Dental film is a nonscreen film that has a high speed and comes in a variety of sizes. These are often useful for whole-body images in smaller species or detailed focal areas of interest in larger species.[26] These films can be used with standard radiographic units or special dental radiography units.

When radiographing reptiles and amphibians, certain aspects of their anatomy require special considerations. In snakes, it is preferred that multiple exposures are taken of the different segments (lengths) of the snake instead of a single image of the snake coiled up. Sedation or immobilization with proper restraint will provide proper lateral and dorso-ventral projections.

Radiographs are an important diagnostic tool in birds. In most cases, diagnostic imaging of birds is performed under general anesthesia or sedation, and restraint boards can be used to help provide consistent positioning and diagnostic images. Dental radiography units and films are useful for many of the small passerines.[14,27]

Computed tomography (CT) and MRI studies have been performed in reptiles and amphibians; however, availability, cost, and the need for sedation or anesthesia are limiting factors for pursuing these imaging modalities. Newer CT scans allow very rapid acquisition of images, often making anesthesia or sedation unnecessary. The main benefit of CT over conventional radiography is the increased sensitivity and ability to create three-dimensional (3D) reconstructions (Figure 7-1). An added benefit in chelonians is the ability to perform cross-sectional examination of various structures without superimposition of the dense bones of the carapace and plastron. A case series demonstrating lesions that were missed on plain radiographs but detected on CT scans has been published.[21] A radiated tortoise was diagnosed with a shoulder luxation following a CT scan and two snapping turtles were diagnosed with fractures that were not seen on plain film radiographs.

Computed tomography and MRI images can also be helpful for diagnosing musculoskeletal abnormalities of

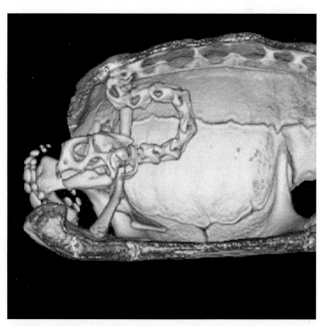

FIGURE 7-1 A three-dimensional (3D) CT reconstruction in an African spurred tortoise *(Centrochelys sulcata)*. 3D reconstructions can be performed in order to thoroughly assess the musculoskeletal system.

the avian musculoskeletal system. These advanced imaging modalities offer a higher sensitivity than plain film radiography and lesions that are not visible on plain films can be easily seen. The main drawbacks of these modalities are cost and general lack of availability to most general practitioners.

Nuclear scintigraphy can be used in reptiles, birds, and mammals to detect variations in blood flow to the musculoskeletal system. This diagnostic test will allow a very sensitive indication of changes in blood flow, but the presence of "hot spots" has a low specificity and often must be followed up with additional imaging of the area in question.[28]

Joint aspirates and cytological evaluation of joint fluid has been used in exotic pet species with joint disease and should be used to evaluate any swollen or painful joint. Sterile preparation of the skin over the joint of interest is critical to prevent iatrogenic introduction of skin microflora. Assessment of joint fluid includes color, volume, viscosity, protein concentration, total cell count, and differential cell count.[29,30] This can help differentiate degenerative joint disease, immune-mediated polyarthritis, and septic arthritis. Normal joint fluid should be clear, viscous, and poorly cellular (limited to small amounts of mononuclear cells). There should be a dense eosinophilic background, and cells will often be seen in a linear arrangement referred to as windrowing. Inflammatory joint fluid is often turgid, has decreased viscosity, and contains increased amounts of neutrophils or heterophils and mononuclear cells. In many cases of septic arthritis, infectious agents are not seen on cytological examination of the joint fluid, although culture is recommended for any abnormal joint samples. Many exotics have very small volumes of joint fluid available for diagnostics, even in an effusive joint. If there is only a small volume of fluid available, a small amount of sterile saline can be aspirated into the syringe after slides are prepared. The saline and any remaining joint fluid in the needle and hub can be submitted for culture and antimicrobial sensitivity testing.

In many myopathies, clinical suspicion of infectious agents usually warrants aspirates and cultures of affected tissues, and muscle biopsies are not needed. However, in some myopathies, muscle biopsies can aid in the diagnosis, especially in animals that are presented for wasting or weakness. Careful planning is needed due to the relative lack of a large muscle mass in many smaller species of exotic animals.

Bone biopsies from exotic animals can be collected in a similar fashion to mammals using bone biopsy instruments of the appropriate size for the patient. In smaller species, hypodermic needles can be used. The bone can be submitted for histopathology or for culture and antimicrobial sensitivity testing in cases of osteomyelitis.

CBC Hematological and biochemistry testing can be used to provide some insight into how the musculoskeletal system is responding to certain diseases processes. Inflammatory leukograms, characterized by a heterophilia (neutrophilia) and monocytosis, are not uncommon in exotic animal patients with myositis, osteomyelitis, and septic joints. Aspartate aminotransferase (AST) and CK are enzymes that are commonly used in exotic animal patients to evaluate disease processes affecting the muscles. Alkaline phosphatase (ALP) is a enzyme found in many different tissues but is commonly elevated in young, fast-growing exotic animal patients because of bone growth in animals with fractures or osteomyelitis. Uric acid

is an end product of protein catabolism. Elevations in uric acid are commonly seen in birds and reptiles with gout. Articular forms of gout commonly present of these species as swellings of the joints and distal limbs.

NUTRITIONAL DISORDERS OF THE MUSCULOSKELETAL SYSTEM

Husbandry

Proper husbandry is a critical component of keeping exotic animals. Unfortunately, many of the exotic pets presented for veterinary care have problems directly related to inappropriate husbandry. Temperature, humidity, diet, and proper lighting are all very important, and each species has specific requirements that must be met. Improper husbandry practices can be a significant cause of musculoskeletal problems in many commonly kept exotic species.

Metabolic Bone Disease

Metabolic bone disease (MBD) is a broad term used to describe a group of medical disorders affecting the development, integrity, and function of bones. This term encompasses many medical conditions that have closely related etiologies, including osteoporosis, osteomalacia, rickets, fibrous osteodystrophy, and nutritional (and renal) secondary hyperparathyroidism. The pathophysiology is similar and MBD has been seen in amphibians, reptiles, birds, and mammals. In all species, MBD involves derangements of blood calcium levels. Calcium homeostasis is carefully controlled through feedback mechanisms involving concentrations of ionized calcium, phosphorus, parathyroid hormone (PTH), vitamin D_3 (calcitriol), and calcitonin. Abnormalities in any of these factors can lead to clinical abnormalities. Proper diet and husbandry practices are essential to maintaining proper calcium homeostasis, and each species can have unique requirements for calcium and vitamin D_3.

Calcium is found in the body in three forms. Calcium in bone is stored as hydroxyapatite, and this accounts for 99% of the total calcium stores in the body. A majority of the remaining 1% is found in the intracellular compartment; less than 0.1% of the body's calcium is found in the extracellular fluid.[31]

Calcium in the extracellular fluid exists in three forms. Ionized calcium, which is the physiologically active form, is responsible for important functions such as bone homeostasis, muscle contraction, nerve conduction, and blood coagulation. This accounts for 20% to 60% of the calcium in the extracellular fluid. Approximately 40% of the extracellular calcium is protein bound. Protein bound calcium is physiologically inactive and mainly believed to be a buffer system for ionized calcium. The remaining calcium is bound to ions (lactate, citrate, bicarbonate), and the role of this form of calcium is unknown.[31]

Dietary calcium intake is an important part of maintaining proper extracellular calcium concentrations. Without adequate calcium in the diet, there will be decreased calcium absorption regardless of other factors that help regulate calcium levels. Diets should be modified so that there is sufficient calcium present for that species, while minimizing other factors that can alter dietary calcium absorption such as phosphorus, oxalates, and phytates. High phosphorus concentrations can lead to a disturbance in the calcium-phosphorus ratio. Under normal conditions, this ratio should be positive (2 : 1 or greater). Excessive phosphate binds calcium, thus lowering the ionized calcium in the blood and triggering PTH release. Phytates (found in soy) and oxalates (found in spinach, rhubarb, cabbage, and beet greens) can bind to calcium in the intestine and decrease calcium absorption.[32,33]

Depletion of ionized calcium concentrations in the blood stimulates the parathyroid glands to release PTH, which acts on osteoclasts to resorb bone and increase calcium levels in the blood. Over time, the chronic depletion of calcium from bones causes weakening of the skeletal system and pathologic fractures. Parathyroid hormone also acts on the kidneys to enhance calcium reabsorption and increase phosphorus excretion and also affects calcium absorption in the intestine by up-regulating enzymes responsible for producing activated vitamin D_3 in the kidneys.

Vitamin D_3 (calcitriol) is an important component of calcium homeostasis, and it is important to understand the complex metabolism of vitamin D in order to prevent MBD. Under natural conditions, 7-dehydrocholesterol is converted to cholecalciferol in the skin when exposed to ultraviolet (UV) B radiation. Cholecalciferol is converted to calcidiol (25-hydroxycholecalciferol) in the liver and then further converted into the active form of calcitriol (1,25-dihydroxycholecalciferol) in the kidneys.[34-37] This is a temperature-dependent process, so it is important that ectotherms (e.g., reptiles and amphibians) are provided an appropriate environmental temperature. Calcitriol is responsible for increasing calcium absorption in the GI tract, increasing calcium reabsorption in the kidneys, increasing phosphorus excretion in the kidneys, and increasing release of calcium from bone. In the absence of appropriate UV light exposure, these animals are unable to synthesize appropriate levels of vitamin D_3 and have decreased calcium absorption. Fortunately, in most species, vitamin D can be supplemented in the diet and will be readily absorbed. There are two variations of vitamin D that can be supplemented: vitamin D_2, ergocalciferol, is produced by plants and vitamin D_3, calcitriol, is produced by animals. There are variations in the bioavailability and activity of the different forms of vitamin D in different species, which is important to consider if supplementation is needed.

Reptiles and Amphibians
In reptiles and amphibians, the main causes of MBD are nutritional and renal disorders and have been termed nutritional MBD (NMBD) and renal MBD (RMBD).[35]

NMBD or nutritional secondary hyperparathyroidism (NSHP) is the more common cause of MBD in reptiles and amphibians. This is often due to dietary and husbandry mismanagement. Deficiencies of dietary calcium and vitamin D_3 and excessive dietary phosphorus are commonly seen.[10,32,38]

Carnivorous reptiles and amphibians can develop a deficiency in ingested calcium when fed diets consisting of skeletal muscle without bone or unsupplemented insects. Herbivorous reptiles and amphibians can develop calcium deficiencies if not exposed to UV-B light and/or fed a diet deficient in calcium or containing excessive amounts of phosphorus.[32]

Although much less common, renal disease can also be a contributing factor in RMBD. The kidneys play an important role in phosphate excretion. Renal disease leads to a decreased glomerular filtration and hyperphosphatemia develops. Elevated levels of phosphorus lead to decreased ionized calcium levels, stimulation of PTH secretion, and release of calcium from bone. In addition, the kidneys are the final site in the activation of vitamin D_3 into calcitriol. With chronic renal disease, the formation of calcitriol is reduced and calcium homeostasis is altered. Finally, a large amount of calcium filtered through the glomeruli from the plasma is reabsorbed in the renal tubules and therefore renal disease will lead to an increased loss of calcium in the urine.[39] Because of the importance of the kidneys in calcium homeostasis, renal function should be assessed in any patients with MDB, particularly if they are not responding to therapy. In reptiles and amphibians, an inverse calcium-phosphorus ratio in the blood is indicative for renal disease, in particular in the absence of excessive dietary phosphorus intake.

Signs of MBD in reptiles and amphibians are directly related to the functions of calcium in the body. In states of hypocalcemia, calcium is removed from the bones to increase blood calcium concentrations. If the calcium deficiency is not resolved, long-term removal of calcium from the bones leads to osteopenia and weakens the integrity of the bone. Signs attributed to this include mandibular deformity, abnormal posture, splayed legs, scoliosis, fibrous osteodystrophy of the long bones and mandible (rubber jaw), and pathologic fractures.[10,35,38,40] Calcium is also important in neuromuscular function; therefore, reptiles and amphibians with MBD can show signs such as tremors, disorientation, and ataxia. Hypocalcemia can also lead to depolarization of nerves, and in severe hypocalcemia cases, seizures can occur. Finally, calcium's effect on smooth muscle can lead to signs such as bloating and cloacal or rectal prolapse.[35]

A diagnosis of NSHP can be made through various methods. A thorough history, including diet and husbandry, should always be taken. Understanding specific requirements for each species becomes important to recognize deficiencies such as a history of an improper diet (e.g., low calcium and high phosphorus) or a lack of UV light exposure or vitamin D supplementation.[10] Once a clinical suspicion of NSHP has been made, additional diagnostic tests can be performed to help confirm the diagnosis and determine the severity of the disease. Radiographs can be evaluated for abnormally shaped bones, thin cortices, overall loss of bone density, angular limb deformities, luxations, or fractures[10,34,35,41] (Figure 7-2). It is important to note that radiographs only detect 30% or greater change in bone density.[34] Other imaging modalities such as dual-energy X-ray absorptiometry (DXA) scans and CT scans have shown some promise but are not readily available to most practitioners. Blood biochemistry can be evaluated for total calcium and phosphorus, ionized calcium, and calcium-phosphorus ratios. Total calcium and phosphorus concentrations are typically within reference ranges for affected animals.[10,40] However, as the disease progresses, continued depletion of calcium stores can lead to hypocalcemia, hyperphosphatemia, and an abnormal calcium-phosphorus ratio. Ionized calcium concentrations might be best for identifying acute changes in calcium homeostasis. Unfortunately, few

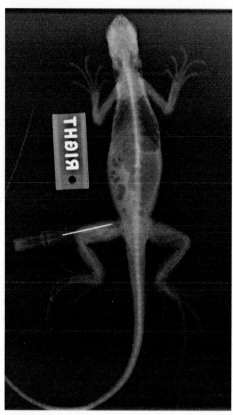

FIGURE 7-2 Severe metabolic bone disease in a green iguana *(Iguana iguana)*. There is a decrease in overall bone density and multiple pathologic fractures. An intraosseus catheter was inserted in the right femur and may have caused additional pathologic fractures.

ionized calcium concentration references are available for amphibians and reptiles.

Treatment of NSHP involves supplementation of calcium and vitamin D_3 (in carnivorous species) or exposure to UVB (in herbivorous species) as well as correction of the underlying husbandry problems.[10,35,40] Calcium can be supplemented orally (PO) or injected parenterally. Parenteral routes are preferred for acute hypocalcemic tetany but should not be used for long-term supplementation, because they can lead to muscle necrosis and metastatic tissue calcification. Instead the oral route is recommended for supplementation, once vitamin D deficiency has been corrected if present, in order to ensure intestinal calcium absorption. Calcium glubionate can be administered orally to reptiles or as a daily bath for amphibians that are difficult to medicate.[40] There are concerns regarding calcium injections causing pain, muscle necrosis, and kidney damage, so long-term calcium injections are not recommended.[34,35]

Salmon calcitonin (SCT) has been used to treat osteoporosis in postmenopausal women and has also been used with success in green iguanas with NSHP. Calcitonin has been found to have a negative effect on the parathyroid glands by decreasing the release of PTH, decreasing osteoclast activity, and increasing osteoblast activity. SCT has also been found to decrease bone pain by augmenting bone mass and reducing

the treatment time required for animals to recover from NSHP. Calcitonin and SCT decrease serum calcium concentrations through their effect on PTH and by increasing renal excretion of calcium. Therefore, hypocalcemia is a side effect of SCT use, and it should only be used when normal calcium concentrations can be maintained through supplementation and dietary modification.[34,35] While SCT has shown promise for the treatment of NSHP in reptiles, the role of calcitonin in amphibians is not completely understood and it may not be effective in treating amphibians with NSHP.[40,41]

Husbandry modification is as important in treating NSHP as initial calcium and vitamin D_3 supplementation. Without modification of the diet and husbandry, treatment will be unrewarding. Care must be taken to select the appropriate diets for carnivorous, herbivorous, and omnivorous species.

Nutrient composition of various prey species has been previously published.[32] Insects commonly available as food for reptiles and amphibians are relatively high in phosphorus and low in calcium.[10,32,34,35,40] Unlike whole-vertebrate prey, insect exoskeletons do not contain the high concentrations of calcium that are present in vertebrate endoskeletons. Insects can be supplemented with calcium by gut loading or dusting prior to feeding. Gut loading involves feeding prey items a high calcium diet for 48 hours prior to being offered as food. Many different calcium and vitamin supplement powders are commercially available and can be dusted on the prey item immediately prior to being offered to an amphibian or reptile.[32]

Dietary modification for herbivorous reptiles involves selecting the appropriate food items to offer. The calcium-phosphorus ratio is known for many fruits, vegetables, and leafy greens commonly fed to reptiles and should be 1.5:1 to 2:1.[12] Selecting the appropriate food items and supplementation with calcium powders will ensure adequate dietary calcium intake in herbivorous reptiles. When feeding omnivorous reptiles, a combination of the outlined herbivore and carnivore strategies can be used to ensure adequate calcium and vitamin D_3 intake and an optimum calcium-phosphorus ratio.

The link between calcium homeostasis and UV radiation is well established in reptiles, but there is some debate whether all reptiles need UV light exposure. Some snakes (e.g., ball python, *Python regius*) are not believed to rely on UV light exposure, and there are a number of reptilian species that are nocturnal in the wild.[36] Corn snakes *(Pantherophis guttatus)* exposed to UVB radiation had significantly higher vitamin D_3 plasma concentrations than control snakes. Fortunately, MDB is uncommon in snakes, and the changes in vitamin D_3 after UVB exposure may not be clinically relevant. Nocturnal species may rely more heavily on dietary vitamin D_3 and they may have a more sensitive mechanism for photobiosynthesis of vitamin D_3 to compensate for limited light exposure.[42] Although the relationship between UVB exposure and calcium homeostasis has been studied in reptiles, this relationship has not been well studied in amphibians but may play an important role in some species.[40]

Exposure to full-spectrum lighting, including UVB radiation, is highly recommended for reptiles and is particularly important in herbivorous reptiles, suffering from NSHP, which do not ingest any dietary vitam D_3 and instead rely on UVB dependent endogenous synthesis of vitamin D_3. There

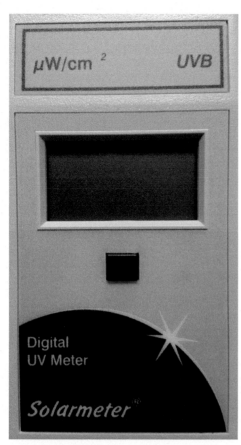

FIGURE 7-3 An ultraviolet (UV) B meter can be used during routine health examinations to evaluate the amount of UVB radiation being produced by a light bulb.

is no debate that exposure to natural sunlight is the best source of UVB radiation, but in some instances, it may not be possible or practical. Many UVB radiation-producing bulbs are available, but lights with specific UVB radiation output in the range of 280 to 320 nm are most desired.[43] The placement of the lights should be within 6 to 18 inches from the animal, and caretakers must be aware that any plastic or glass in between the light and the animal can filter out the desired UVB wavelengths. The output of UVB radiation in this range from any light source decays over time, so bulbs should be replaced every 6 to 12 months. There are many different brands of UVB-producing lights available, and not all the bulbs meet their claims. Veterinarians may consider purchasing an UVB radiation meter (Figure 7-3) to measure the amount of UVB radiation produced by their client's light bulbs.

In addition to providing full-spectrum lighting to photosynthesize vitamin D, vitamin D should be supplemented in the diet of carnivorous and omnivorous reptiles.

Birds

Many health problems in birds can also be linked to improper nutrition.[44] MBD is also an important nutritional deficiency in birds. The pathophysiology of NSHP in birds is similar to that described for amphibians and reptiles and can be due to inadequate calcium intake, inappropriate calcium-phosphorus ratios, inadequate exposure to UVB radiation, or a deficiency of vitamin D_3. There are some important differences in calcium metabolism in birds, and these are primarily associated with egg-laying in females.

As was described for amphibians and reptiles, PTH is responsible for calcium release from bones in response to hypocalcemia in birds. Birds appear to be especially sensitive to PTH compared to mammals. The reason why birds are more sensitive to the effects of PTH is not known, but it is believed to be an adaptive response associated with egg-laying since the hypercalcemic effects of PTH are greater in egg-laying hens compared with roosters.[33,37]

In birds, vitamin D is important in maintaining normal blood calcium levels through its effects on the intestines, kidneys, oviducts, and bone. The metabolism and regulation of vitamin D_3 in birds are similar to other species; however, there are some differences. In birds, two forms of vitamin D are metabolically active. In the kidney, 25-hydroxycholecalciferol is converted to 1,25-dihydroxycholecalciferol and 24,25-dihydroxycholecalciferol. In mammals, 24,25-dihydroxycholecalciferol has little activity, while in birds it appears to be important for egg-laying.[37] As was noted previously, vitamin D is produced in plants (vitamin D_2) and animals (vitamin D_3), and while mammals are able to utilize both forms, vitamin D_2 has 10% the efficacy of vitamin D_3 in birds.[33,37] Therefore, any vitamin supplementation provided to birds should be in the form of vitamin D_3.

A unique aspect of avian calcium metabolism allows birds to produce large calcium-rich eggshells.[33] Each egg can represent 10% to 20% of the total body calcium stores, and smaller species lay proportionally larger eggs with more shell. Estrogen plays an important role in calcium metabolism in egg-laying hens and can affect calcium storage, mobilization, and transportation. During egg-laying, the main sources of calcium are bone and dietary calcium.[16,33] Rising estrogen levels during sexual maturity alter the function of osteoblasts, leading to the formation of spicules within the medullary cavities. These spicules can eventually replace the entire medullary canal and act as a calcium store. This can be initiated without vitamin D_3, but complete mineralization of medullary bone requires adequate vitamin D_3 concentrations.[17,33,45] Medullary bone is most prominent in the long bones of the pelvic limb, although it can also be seen in the thoracic limbs.[33] During egg production, PTH and vitamin D_3 are responsible for mobilization of calcium from the medullary bone. As estrogen levels decline, osteoblast activity is reversed, medullary bone disappears, and the structure of normal cortical bone returns.

Dietary requirements of calcium, phosphorus, and vitamin D for birds have been extensively studied in poultry, but care must be used when extrapolating these studies to other avian species (e.g., passerines and psittacines).[33] The effects of calcium deficiencies are well known and excessive calcium can lead to renal disease; therefore, selecting an appropriate diet is very important. The calcium-phosphorus ratio in a bird's diet should be 1.5-2.0:1. Seed diets are low in calcium, and some seed-only diets can have a calcium-phosphorus ratio as low as 1:10.[15,45,46] High-fat content in some seeds can interfere with calcium absorption and exacerbate the problem.[47] Total dietary calcium requirements can vary depending on species, age, reproductive status, and vitamin D concentrations. General recommendations range between 0.3% and 0.7%; levels above 0.7% can lead to toxicity in some species.[33,48] Seeds commonly fed to birds provide 0.1% to 0.3% calcium, while many commercially available diets provide calcium in excess of 0.7%. Grains and seeds that are frequently fed to psittacine are low in calcium, have very little vitamin D_3, contain excessive phosphorus, and contain excess fat.[37] Calcium can easily be supplemented in caged birds in the form of a cuttlebone or mineral block.[14] An all-meat (muscle) carnivorous bird diet can have a calcium-phosphorus ratio as high as 1:20.[47] To reduce the likelihood of NSHP in these birds, it is important to include bones and viscera in these diets to provide a more appropriate calcium-phosphorus ratio. As was noted with amphibians and reptiles, invertebrate prey have a poor calcium-phosphorus ratio, so it is important to gut load or dust the prey before offering them to a bird.[48] Because of these different potential dietary complications, it is important for a veterinarian to understand the needs of each species they work with and to formulate the appropriate combination of food items to prevent calcium deficiency.

Vitamin D can be consumed in the diet or synthesized with appropriate exposure to UVB radiation. Birds with adequate UVB exposure do not have specific dietary vitamin D requirements, and as little as 30 minutes of exposure to direct sunlight is sufficient for endogenous vitamin D production.[33] Due to differences in natural habitats, there are species differences in UVB light requirements, with South American species being less dependent on UVB exposure to maintain adequate vitamin D production, compared to other species such as African grey parrots.[33,37] For birds that are housed indoors with little or no exposure to natural sunlight, Vitamin D must be supplemented in the diet and is therefore contained in commercially available pelleted bird diets. Like dietary calcium, dietary vitamin D requirements can vary depending on species, age, breeding status, and dietary calcium-phosphorus levels. Dietary requirements for vitamin D will be higher in cases of low dietary calcium intake or if the calcium-phosphorus ratio is outside the optimal range.[33]

Diagnosis of NSHP in birds is based on history, clinical signs, physical examination, blood work, and radiographs. Clinical signs can include reproductive abnormalities such as egg binding, abnormal eggs (e.g., soft or misshapen), or poor reproductive performance. Osteomalacia, limb deformities, and pathologic fractures are commonly observed. Neurologic signs such as weakness, ataxia, paralysis, or seizures may also be seen.[33,37] Some animals may also present for beak abnormalities or angular limb deformities, particularly of the proximal tibiotarsus.[46] Plasma calcium levels must be evaluated carefully along with history and physical exam findings, since animals with significant NSHP can be normocalcemic. Radiographs of affected birds can show decreased mineral density, angular limb deformities, and pathologic fractures.[33,49]

Measuring vitamin D and PTH concentrations can also be helpful in confirming NSHP. Vitamin D is easily measured and assays used in humans can be used for birds because of the homology between avian and mammalian vitamin D metabolites. 25-Hydroxycholecalciferol is the preferred metabolite to measure, due to its longer half-life.[33,37,49,50] Unlike vitamin D, there are structural differences in PTH that make measuring it more difficult across species. In humans, different PTH assays are available, and there is some

variation regarding the portion of the PTH molecule that is detected by each assay. PTH assays that concentrate on measuring the entire PTH molecule, or the mid or terminal segments, are not recommended. A PTH assay that measures the 1–34N section of PTH shows the most promise for use in birds due to the homology of PTH in this region with mammals. 1–34N assays have been used in grey parrots with consistent results.[51] Results of vitamin D and PTH assays should always be interpreted within the context of ionized calcium, diet, UVB exposure, and reproductive activity.[37,49,51]

Chronic stimulation of PTH secretion can lead to parathyroid hyperplasia. One retrospective study evaluating parathyroid lesions in birds found that 80% of the cases of parathyroid hyperplasia occurred in psittacines, with the highest incidence occurring in African grey parrots.[51]

Management of NSHP in birds is similar to that described for reptiles, including supplementing calcium and vitamin D_3 while simultaneously correcting the underlying husbandry and dietary deficiencies. Pathologic fractures and some limb deformities can be addressed. Acute cases of hypocalcemia can be treated with calcium gluconate administered intramuscularly and supportive care. The prognosis will depend on the severity of boney abnormalities and response to treatment.

Mammals

Mammals are less commonly diagnosed with NSHP compared to reptiles and birds, although clinical disease associated with abnormal calcium homeostasis can be seen. NSHP has been reported in nonhuman primates, exotic cats, skunks, guinea pigs, opossums, rabbits, and sugar gliders.[48]

Rabbits have some unique aspects regarding calcium metabolism. Total blood calcium is 30% to 50% higher in rabbits than other mammals. Normal total calcium levels are between 13 and 15 mg/dL and ionized calcium is 1.71 +/− 0.11 mmol/L.[52] In most mammals, PTH release is triggered when ionized calcium levels fall below 1.2 mmol/L, but in rabbits this value is 1.7 mmol/L.

Another difference in calcium metabolism in rabbits occurs in the intestinal tract. In other mammals, calcium absorption in the GI tract involves a vitamin D_3-regulated active transport system. In the rabbit, there is passive diffusion of calcium along a concentration gradient between the blood and intestinal lumen that accounts for the majority of the calcium absorption in this species. This causes an increase in calcium absorption in proportion to the amount in the diet and is independent of vitamin D_3 concentrations.[52-54]

Regulation of calcium in rabbits is similar to other species and is dependent on PTH and vitamin D_3. Due to the higher circulating concentrations of calcium and the ability to absorb greater amounts of calcium in the GI tract, rabbits must be able to excrete large amounts of calcium. In rabbits, the kidneys play a significant role in excreting calcium in the urine. During periods of high calcium intake, the kidney is capable of increasing the fractional excretion of calcium into the urine.[55] Urine from rabbits is normally cloudy in appearance and contains calcium crystals.

Despite the efficiency in which rabbits are able to absorb calcium from their GI tract, rabbits can suffer from calcium deficiencies and develop NSHP. Rabbits suffering from NSHP can present with enlarged joints, crooked legs, enlargement of the costochondral junctions, and pathologic fractures of the appendicular skeleton.[56] More commonly, rabbits fed calcium-deficient diets have altered mineral deposition in the mandibles. This leads to loss of alveolar bone and loosening of the teeth.[52,54] Dental disease is among the most common medical problems in rabbits. There is some debate regarding the etiology of acquired dental disease (ADD). Differentials include lack of dietary fiber and dental wear. Rabbits with ADD often have decreased blood serum calcium levels and elevated PTH levels, compared to rabbits without dental disease, suggesting that ADD may, in part, be due to NSHP. Many rabbits with dental disease also have skulls with poor bone quality; these changes can be assessed on skull radiographs.[57,58] In severe cases of NSHP in rabbits, other bones are affected, particularly the spine.[54] Other clinical signs that can be seen in rabbits that are fed low-calcium diets include weakness, depression, ataxia, anorexia, convulsions, and seizures.

Because of the unusual calcium metabolism of rabbits, special attention should be given to the dietary concentrations of calcium and vitamin D and the calcium-phosphorus ratio. Calcium levels in the diet should range between 0.6% and 1%. This can be best provided using a mixture of Timothy grass hay, commercial Timothy pellets, and fresh vegetables.[52,54]

Fibrous osteodystrophy has been documented in two guinea pigs, although many more undocumented cases are likely.[59,60] As with other species, this disease process involves excessive parathyroid activity, leading to osteoclastic resorption of bone. In the few reports of this disease in exotic small mammals, the process appears to be linked to an inappropriate Ca-P ratio or a calcium-deficient diet. Diets with low Ca-P ratios have been linked to changes in growth rates, joint stiffness, and calcification of soft tissues. Clinical signs include anorexia, lethargy, cachexia, difficulty walking, and lameness due to pathologic fractures. Fibrous osteodystrophy can have a similar clinical presentation as vitamin C deficiency, so it is important for the clinician to rule out scurvy in these cases. Diagnosis is based on dietary history, clinical signs, blood calcium, 25-hydroxyvitamin D, and parathyroid levels.[59] Radiographs can be used to show osteopenia and pathologic fractures, which can occur in both the axial and appendicular skeletons. Treatment involves the provision of oral calcium, cage rest (to avoid pathologic fractures), and correcting the underlying husbandry deficiencies.

Sugar gliders are another exotic mammal species that is commonly presented for MBD. Improper husbandry and nutrition (e.g., low calcium and vitamin D_3, high phosphorus) are the most common factors leading to illness in this species.[61,62] Affected sugar gliders are often fed an improper diet comprised of phosphorus-rich meat, mealworms, and fruit. Because sugar gliders are nocturnal, it is expected that they are more dependent on dietary vitamin D_3 than the vitamin D_3 acquired from exposure to UVB radiation.[63] Sugar gliders with MBD commonly present with acute collapse, central nervous system (CNS) abnormalities, or seizures. Some individuals may exhibit hind limb weakness, and osteoporosis can be seen radiographically.[61-63] Diets fed to sugar gliders should contain a minimum of 1% calcium, 0.5% phosphorus, and 1500 IU/kg vitamin D_3.[63] Any insects added to the diet should be gut loaded or coated with a calcium supplement, as previously described.

If the problem is identified early in the disease process, patients may respond to cage rest, parenteral calcium, vitamin D_3 supplementation, and correcting dietary deficiencies.

OTHER NUTRITIONAL DISORDERS OF THE MUSCULOSKELETAL SYSTEM

Fish

Vitamin deficiencies in fish can lead to musculoskeletal abnormalities. Vitamin D deficiencies in fish lead to changes in muscle tissue. Lesions can be seen in white muscle and can lead to tetany. Vitamin E deficiency has been shown to cause muscular dystrophy in carp.[64]

Reptiles and Amphibians

Although NSHP is the most common cause of musculoskeletal disease in reptiles and amphibians, other vitamin and mineral deficiencies can lead to musculoskeletal abnormalities. In vertebrates, vitamin A plays an important role in vision, growth, cellular differentiation, immune response, and reproduction. Vitamin A deficiencies can lead to squamous metaplasia and impaired immune function.[65]

Excessive vitamin A has also been linked to musculoskeletal disease in amphibians. Hypervitaminosis A can lead to clinical signs similar to those seen with NSHP, including bone pain, skeletal malformations, and spontaneous fractures.[40,66-68] Excessive vitamin A in the diet may compete with other fat-soluble vitamins at the sites of absorption. This can lead to relative deficiencies in vitamin D, which is the likely etiology of the skeletal abnormalities noted with excessive vitamin A intake.[67] Amphibians also utilize lipoproteins in the transport of active vitamin D metabolites. This mechanism can be affected by imbalances of fatty acids and fats and can affect utilization of vitamin D_3 in individuals that have adequate dietary intake and absorption of vitamin D_3.[41] High levels of vitamin A are found in rodents that are commonly offered as prey items.[66] In the wild, many species are not likely to survive on a diet composed exclusively of rodents; thus, hypervitaminosis A is not observed in free-ranging individuals. However, hypervitaminosis A can become a clinical problem when these species are fed an exclusive rodent diet.[40]

Spindly leg syndrome, or skeletal and muscular underdevelopment, is a complex disease process that is not completely understood. This syndrome is predominantly seen in anurans, although it has also been reported in a crocodile newt (*Tylototriton shanjing*). It may also be overlooked in caecilians due to the absence of forelimbs. In anurans, apparently healthy larval forms fail to complete metamorphosis. In affected animals, the hind limbs may be normal or have varus or valgus deformities, while the forelimbs are extremely thin and delicate or fail to erupt.[40,68,69] Affected animals usually die within a few days. Many suspected etiologies have been proposed for spindly leg syndrome, including nutritional deficiencies; however, the exact etiology is unknown. Vitamin B has been shown to play a role in the development of spindly leg, and supplementation of vitamin B complex reduces the incidence of the disease.[40,69] Unfortunately, supplementation of vitamin B complex in affected individuals will not alter the outcome once signs are present. Other factors that have been proposed to play a role in the disease process include genetics (e.g., inbreeding, interspecific hybridization), environment (e.g., overcrowding, toxins), and trauma.

Birds

Vitamin E deficiency in birds has been associated with muscle weakness.[45,47] Clinical signs include muscle weakness, localized wing paralysis, poor digestion, and embryonic and hatchling mortalities. Clinically affected birds have been found to respond to vitamin E supplementation.[47] Gross lesions associated with vitamin E and selenium deficiencies include white streaks and patches in striated muscles. Histologically, there is muscle degeneration without inflammation. Individual muscle fibers are enlarged, hypercontracted, and have loss of striations.[70]

Mammals

Hypovitaminosis E has been shown to cause muscular dystrophy in rabbits due to degeneration and necrosis of skeletal muscle fibers. Rabbits with vitamin E deficiency have increased plasma concentrations of CK and cholesterol. Long-term storage of feed can decrease vitamin E content. Offering fresh food or supplementing the diet with vitamin E–rich leafy green vegetables or wheat germ can prevent this problem.[56]

Scurvy (hypovitaminosis C) is an important nutritional musculoskeletal disease in guinea pigs.[59,71] Guinea pigs, like humans and primates, are unable to synthesize vitamin C due to an enzyme deficiency (L-gulonolactone oxidase) and require supplementation in their diet. Vitamin C deficiency leads to defective type-IV collagen, elastin, and laminin. This can lead to a variety of clinical signs including lethargy, joint swelling, lameness, delayed wound healing, hemorrhage, anorexia, loosening of teeth and malocclusion, lethargy, and a poor hair coat. Diagnosis is often based on history and clinical signs. Radiographs often demonstrate changes to the costochondral junctions and widening of the epiphyses of the long bones. Serum vitamin C levels can also be measured to confirm the diagnosis.[59] Treatment involves supportive care, the provision of analgesics, and vitamin C supplementation (50 to 100 mg/kg PO). Dietary requirements of vitamin C in guinea pigs range from 15 to 45 mg/guinea pig/day.[72] Many commercial diets available for guinea pigs contain appropriate levels of vitamin C; however, vitamin C is not typically stable in diets 90 days postmilling. One exception is Oxbow guinea pig pellets (Oxbow Animal Health, Murdock, NE), which have microencapsulated vitamin C that remains stable for 1 year from milling. Fresh vegetables (e.g., bell pepper, kale) and fruits (e.g., oranges) that are high in vitamin C can be added to the diet to supplement vitamin C concentrations. Vitamin C tablets can also be crushed and sprinkled over the food to ensure adequate dosing.

MYOPATHIES

Fish

Myopathies in fish can be the result of bacterial or parasitic infections. Mycobacteriosis can lead to nodules in muscle that can cause deformities. Diagnosis is based on clinical signs, presence of acid-fast bacteria in tissue sections, and culturing of the organisms.[73] Fish can serve as an intermediate host for many cestodes, and wild-caught ornamental fish may have larvae encysted in muscle tissue. These can be seen as incidental findings on postmortem examinations. Adult or larval nematodes can also be found encysted in muscle. Treatment involves using nematocides such as fenbendazole in food.[74]

Amphibians and Reptiles

Myopathies associated with different infectious organisms including fungi, bacteria, viruses, protozoa, and trematodes have been seen in amphibians. Many of these reports involve wild amphibian populations; however, there are some instances of captive wild-caught individuals exhibiting infectious myopathies.

The captive habitats of many amphibians are an ideal environment for fungal growth, although there are surprisingly few reports of fungal diseases in amphibians.[68,75-78] *Ichthyophonus* spp. are pleomorphic fungi, although there is some debate regarding their exact taxonomic classification. Infection with *Ichthyophonus* spp. has been seen in many amphibian species from different areas. Affected animals are often lethargic and present with swellings of the proximal hind limbs. The skeletal muscles of infested amphibians are grossly abnormal with areas of gray and black. Histologic review of affected muscle will reveal fungal elements within muscle tissues. Chronic infections are often accompanied by intense foci of granulomatous inflammation, although in some species, the inflammatory response is minimal.[76] Lesions are typically localized to the skeletal muscle, with no lesions present in any other tissues.

Another case report of fungal myositis was documented in a captive female tiger salamander (*Ambystoma tigrinum*). A granulomatous lesion was found in the lumbar musculature. Fungal elements were seen on histopathology, but fungal cultures were not performed and a positive identification was not established. Based on the morphologic description, the causative agent was believed to be *Cladosporium* spp. No reports exist of successful treatment of fungal myositis in amphibians, and all published reports are composed of gross and histopathologic lesions seen at necropsy.

Fungal myositis has also been reported in reptiles.[79] A nonpigmented fungus with hyphae dissecting between myocytes and leading to myonecrosis was seen in a group of brown anoles (*Anolis sagrei*). Although cultures were performed, a definitive identification was not made, but the etiologic agent was suspected to be the *Chrysosporium* anamorph of *Nannizziopsis vriesii* (CANV). This organism has been recently reclassified into several different genera depending on the species affected, including *Nannizziopsis* spp. (lizards) and *Ophidiomyces ophiodiicola* (snakes). These fungi typically invade through the skin but can then develop deep infections in muscle. Severe infections have been reported in bearded dragons (*Pogona vitticeps*) and green iguanas. Itraconazole (5 mg/kg, PO, SID) and voriconazole (10 mg/kg, PO, SID) have been used to treat affected reptiles, although voriconazole is considered to be the safer and more effective treatment.

Viral diseases are commonly found in amphibians, and many of them result in systemic disease. The herpesvirus associated with Lucke's tumors is one of the most studied. This virus is seen in wild populations of anurans and is associated with the development of renal adenocarcinoma in affected animals. Iridoviruses (e.g., ranavirus) have also been well studied in amphibians. These viruses tend to be associated with significant die-offs in wild populations. There is only a single report of a viral myositis in frogs.[80] Two captive spring peepers *(Pseudacris crucifer)* had degeneration and necrosis of skeletal muscle. Some of the necrotic myofibers had eosinophilic intranuclear inclusion bodies that were believed to be a parvovirus.

Mycobacterial infections in poikilotherms are important because they can cause debilitating disease in the host animal and are also potentially zoonotic. All amphibians are susceptible to developing mycobacteriosis; however, the incidence of disease appears highest in aquatic species. African clawed frogs *(Xenopus laevis)* in both the pet trade and laboratory may be affected. The most common clinical signs for these frogs are swellings and ulcers in the digits, often leading to granulomas in the muscle and bones. Generalized muscle atrophy secondary to cachexia is also common. It is important to recognize that terrestrial species of amphibians are also susceptible to infection. A captive African bullfrog *(Pyxicephalus adspersus)* that presented for swelling of the hind limb with ulcerations of the skin was diagnosed with mycobacteriosis.[81] Necropsy showed granulomas in the liver, lungs, adipose tissue, and skeletal muscles. Many different species of mycobacterium (e.g., *Mycobacterium fortuitum*, *M. marinum*, *M. chelonae*) have been isolated from amphibians.[82] Mycobacteria are difficult to culture and diagnosis is typically based on acid-fast staining and polymerase chain reaction (PCR) testing. There is no effective treatment for mycobacteriosis in amphibians.

Mycobacterial infections have also been reported in snakes, lizards, and chelonians. Mycobacteriosis is typically a systemic disease, but some reports describe localized lesions (e.g., lesions of the limbs and joints).[83] A bearded dragon presented for swellings of the limbs and joints; however, once diagnostic imaging (e.g., radiographs, endoscopy) was performed, additional lesions were seen in the lungs and other organs. Staining of joint aspirates showed acid-fast, rod-shaped bacteria typical of *Mycobacterium* sp.[84] Mycobacterial infections were also seen in the joints of a group of Egyptian spiny-tailed lizards *(Uromastyx aegyptia)* and the bones and joints of a Kemp's ridley sea turtle *(Lepidochelys kempii)*.[85,86]

Myositis associated with microsporidia infection has been reported in captive European toads *(Bufo bufo)*.[68] Microsporidia are very small spore-forming fungi that were once considered to be protozoa. These organisms are obligate intracellular parasites. Microsporidia do not commonly infect amphibians; however, spores can be found in many tissues, including muscle. Most diagnoses are made postmortem. A group of long-term captive common toads were found to have microsporidia spores in striated muscles.[68,87] These animals showed progressive wasting, and necropsies demonstrated lesions in all of the skeletal muscles. Ligaments, tendons, and cardiac and smooth muscles were unaffected. Pale streaks were seen on gross examination of the muscles and spores of *Pleistophora myotropica* were seen on histopathologic examination of affected muscle fibers.

Protozoal myopathies have also been documented in reptiles. Cyst-like masses associated with *Pleistophora* sp. microsporidians have been reported in snakes, turtles, and lizards.[88] Bearded dragons that are poor-doers have been found to be infected with microsporidians. Affected animals are often severely dehydrated and have significant muscle atrophy.

Differential diagnoses for this type of presentation in bearded dragons should also include atadenovirus and *Isospora amphiboluri*. *Entamoeba invadens* is a protozoan that is considered to be a common inhabitant of the intestinal tract of many different species of reptiles, especiallychelonians; however, this parasite can also cause severe disease, including ulcerative enteritis and hepatitis. Cysts are passed in the feces and transmission is via the fecal-oral route. Amoebic enterocolitis is a systemic disease following excystation and has been reported in lizards, snakes, and chelonians.[88-90] Systemic infection is common and cysts can be seen in the liver, kidneys, and lungs. Acute myonecrosis was evident on necropsy of wild-caught leopard tortoises *(Stigmochelys pardalis)* and a common water monitor *(Varanus salvator)*, although this is not a common finding in other *E. invadens* infections.[89,90]

Encysted trematodes can also cause myositis in amphibians, and over 20 genera of trematodes are believed to affect amphibians.[68] In these cases, the amphibians serve as an intermediate host for another predator. Gross lesions consist of small 0.5- to 2-mm spherical cysts or granulomas that are white or black in color. Histologically, a thin layer of inflammatory cells will be found surrounding the encysted trematodes. These lesions are often reported as incidental findings at necropsy, but ova may be detected on a fecal smear or tracheal wash if the amphibian is the definitive host of the parasite. Treatment can be attempted using praziquantel (5 to 8 mg/kg, SC or IM, once and then repeated 14 d later), although in some cases, the death of the trematodes can cause a fatal anaphylaxis in the host.[87]

Not all myopathies are caused by infectious agents or parasites. A nutritional myopathy was reported in a population of satanic leaf-tailed geckos *(Uroplatus phantasticus)*.[91] Multifocal skeletal myofibrillar degeneration and necrosis were suspected to be associated with vitamin E and selenium deficiencies. Although vitamin E and selenium assays were not performed, the remaining colony responded to treatment with vitamin E supplementation. Nutritional myopathies have also been suspected in green iguanas, although, again, they were not definitively confirmed using appropriate assays.[38,92] A nutritional myopathy was also suspected in a veiled chameleon *(Chamaeleo calyptratus)* that had a 1-year history of a progressive inability to use its tongue. Postmortem examination showed changes in several muscles of mastication, the tongue, heart, and orbit. These changes were similar to lesions seen in production animals that are associated with deficiencies in vitamin E and selenium (white muscle disease).[93] In another veiled chameleon case, a fibrosing myopathy was identified.[94] A chronic, active, noninflammatory myopathy affecting the temporal muscles was found in this single captive chameleon. There were less dramatic changes in the pterygoid and masseter muscles. The animal developed lockjaw and was eventually found dead despite attempts at supportive care. The exact etiology was not determined.

Birds

Bacterial and fungal infections are common in birds, and myositis can occur through extension of the disease from the air sacs, hematogenous spread of the organism, or penetrating injuries.[46,70] Viral myositis is uncommon in birds, although some acute polyomaviral infections can lead to muscle pallor and hemorrhage.

Mycobacteria are ubiquitous environmental saprophytes. These pathogens can enter a host through oral, respiratory, or dermal routes and spread hematogenously to other organs. Reports of musculoskeletal involvement vary, from 2% to 93% of cases affecting the bones. Clinical signs include chronic weight loss, muscle wasting, severe atrophy of the pectoral muscles, and acute or chronic lameness (e.g., shifting leg lameness). Granulomatous lesions can be present in the bones or joints, and the carpometacarpal and elbow joints are most commonly affected (Figure 7-4). The skin overlying the affected joints is often thickened or ulcerated. Diagnosis is based on the presence of acid-fast microorganisms in granulomatous lesions, mycobacterial cultures, and PCR.[95,96] Proper husbandry and long-term antibiotics are essential to treatment, if treatment is pursued. It is important that clients be made aware that this pathogen is zoonotic and there is a risk that they may be exposed to it when in direct contact with their pet or cleaning up after it. Not all disinfectants are effective against mycobacteria, and higher concentrations and longer contact times are often required to clear mycobacteria from the environment to prevent reinfection during treatment. There are only a few documented cases of successfully treating mycobacterial infections in birds, and many of the current dosing regimens were extrapolated from human medicine. Mycobacteria can quickly develop resistance to antibiotics, making multidrug protocols necessary. Long-term treatment is required, although there is no current standard for length of treatment in birds.[97]

Parasitic diseases can lead to myopathies in several bird species. Sarcocystosis is a systemic disease that affects multiple organ systems. *Sarcocystis* spp. have an obligate two-host life cycle that involves a definitive host (usually a carnivore) and an intermediate host (herbivorous or insectivorous birds) that has mature cysts in its muscles. In the United States, this occurs most commonly in warmer areas where opossums (*Didelphis virginiana*) are the definitive hosts.[98] Intermediate hosts become infected by ingesting insects that have fed on opossum feces or when the insects contaminate the bird's food

with sporocysts. Bird-to-bird transmission does not occur.[70] Some intermediate hosts have evolved along with the parasite and definitive host and may not show clinical signs; however, naïve species exposed to *Sarcocystis* spp. show clinical signs, and in the case of psittacines, infections have a high mortality rate.[46,70,98,99] Clinical signs can be associated with the respiratory system, CNS, or musculoskeletal system. Severe myositis can lead to swelling and lameness; however, some infected birds may not show any clinical signs and are just found dead.[46,98] Diagnosis can be made using the indirect fluorescent antibody test to detect exposure to *Sarcocystis falcatula*; however, some birds presenting with respiratory signs may have an acute infection and insufficient time to mount an immune response. Other diagnostic tests that may be used to evaluate the bird patient with sarcocystosis include creatine phosphokinase (CK), AST, and muscle biopsies.[46] In a recent case series, 45.4% (5/11) of birds with sarcocystosis were found to have the muscular form. All five birds had profound muscle weakness, extreme elevations in CK and AST, and 80% (4/5) had positive antibodies to *S. falcatula*. Forty percent (2/5) of the birds recovered; however, one relapsed and died secondary to pulmonary aspergillosis.[98]

Leukocytozoon is a protozoal parasite of erythrocytes and leukocytes. In some cases, disruption of cardiac and skeletal muscles can occur. Clinical signs include anorexia and weakness.[46]

Mammals

Disseminated idiopathic myofasciitis is an inflammatory myopathy in young ferrets. The average age at onset is 10 months, although the age range of affected animals can vary from 5 months to 4 years. The onset of clinical signs is acute and rapidly progressive over 12 to 36 hours. The most common signs reported in affected animals include lethargy, pyrexia, depression, inappetence, recumbency, ataxia, paresis, and pain associated with movement or palpation. Affected animals have mature neutrophilic leukocytosis with white blood cell counts ranging from 9000 cells/µL to 80,000 cells/µL or higher. Despite the changes seen in the muscle and fascia, AST and CK levels are not significantly elevated. Grossly, white streaks can be seen in the heart, diaphragm, intercostal muscles, and lumbar and hind limb muscles. Atrophy of the limb muscles is common. Histopathologic examination of affected tissues demonstrates multifocal suppurative to pyogranulomatous inflammation in the fascia between the skeletal muscle fibers. Rarely is there necrosis of the muscle fibers themselves, which may explain the absence of changes in AST or CK activity. Diagnosis is based on clinical suspicion and can be confirmed with biopsies of the hind limb muscles. The cause of this disease is unknown, although some ferrets respond to long-term immunosuppression with prednisolone (1 to 2 mg/kg, PO, q24 h) and cyclophosphamide (10 mg/kg, PO, SC). The overall prognosis is grave for these cases.[100,101]

NEOPLASIA

Obtaining a diagnosis of neoplasia in exotic pets is similar to domestic species.[102] Unfortunately, many exotics pets will not show overt clinical signs related to neoplasia until late in the disease process.[103] Physical examination findings

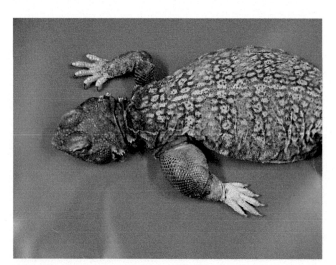

FIGURE 7-4 A Mali uromastyx *(Uromastyx maliensis)* with a granuloma in the left elbow. A mixed fungal/bacterial infection was isolated from the granuloma.

should allow assessment of the location, size, and general invasiveness of the mass. Neoplastic diseases of the musculoskeletal system will often cause swelling and lameness and, in the case of birds, may cause inability or reluctance to fly. When working to confirm a diagnosis, the goal should be to evaluate the tumor type, clinical and biologic behavior, and any systemic effects or metastasis associated with the tumor.

If there is any suspicion of neoplasia, a definitive diagnosis is needed to determine the best form of therapy, and careful planning is needed to obtain diagnostic samples. Fine-needle aspirates (FNAs) are easy to obtain, are associated with low morbidity, and results can be obtained quickly. Often, FNAs can be done without sedation and results are available within 24 hours. Drawbacks of FNAs include difficulty in evaluation of tissue architecture, invasiveness, and mitotic index.[103] Like domestic species, some tumor types in exotic pets exfoliate well and can be diagnosed based on cytology, while others require examination of the tissue architecture to determine a definitive diagnosis. If the results of FNA and cytology are inconclusive, a biopsy and histologic evaluation of the tissue is needed. Biopsies can be obtained using different techniques, including core biopsies, incisional biopsies, and excisional biopsies. Proper planning is needed prior to collecting the samples to ensure they will be adequate for histopathologic examination. Ideally, the tissue is taken at the peripheral margin of the mass to allow the pathologist an opportunity to evaluate the invasiveness of the tumor into adjacent tissues. If surgery is indicated once a diagnosis is made, it is important to remember that the previous biopsy site(s) must also be resected with the same margins as the original mass. Careful planning is needed at the time the biopsies are taken to prevent significantly increasing the margins required during the definitive surgical procedure. It is strongly recommended to submit biopsy samples to pathologists with experience in exotics species.

Once a definitive diagnosis of the tumor is made, staging to assess the patient for metastatic disease is important; this may affect which treatment option, if any, is pursued. In general, blood work (CBC and biochemistry), aspirates of the regional lymph nodes, and radiographic assessment of the thorax for metastasis are recommended, although the staging plan can vary based on tumor diagnosis and species involved. In some cases, imaging of the tumor is indicated, especially for surgical planning. This can include radiographs or advanced imaging such as CT or MRI. Contrast images are especially helpful in these cases and can be used to delineate the neoplastic tissue from normal tissue.

Tumors of the musculoskeletal system often involve muscle, supporting structures (synovium), bone, and cartilage. Muscle and other soft tissue biopsies can be taken using core biopsies, punch biopsies, or taking wedges of the affected tissues. Biopsies of bone and cartilage often require Jamshidi bone marrow biopsy needles or Michele trephines. In smaller species, or areas of weak or thin bone, it is possible to obtain bone and cartilage biopsies with spinal needles, bone marrow needles, or hypodermic needles.[104,105] Bone biopsies obtained with Jamshidi biopsy needles in small mammals have been shown to provide an accurate diagnosis when compared to histopathology samples obtained by surgical resection or amputation.[106]

Therapies for neoplastic diseases in exotic animals include surgical resection, chemotherapy, and radiation therapy. When deciding which therapy is indicated, it is important to understand the biology of the tumor, anatomic considerations of the species affected, and benefits and drawbacks of each treatment modality. Familiarity with species differences will help in the assessment of tumors, as some tumors tend to be benign in behavior in one species but potentially malignant in another species.[103]

The anatomic limitations of exotic animals, especially their small size, are important to consider when developing a treatment plan. For example, vascular access can be very difficult to obtain in some species, and special vascular access systems are needed in order to deliver intravenous chemotherapy.[102] Unfortunately, there are few large-scale reviews of neoplastic diseases in exotic animals, and much of the information that is available on treatment is from individual case reports, data taken from laboratory animals with experimentally induced tumors, or extrapolated from domestic species.[102,107] This makes it very difficult to determine an accurate prognosis for each tumor type in different species with different modalities.

Invertebrates

Neoplasia has been reported in many different invertebrate species. Causes can include environmental factors, genetics, irradiation, and metabolic disturbances. However, neoplastic disease is uncommon in the exotic species of invertebrates usually kept in captivity, even for practitioners that regularly work with invertebrates.[108]

Fish

Rhabdomyosarcoma, rhabdomyoma, chondroma, chondrosarcoma, and osteosarcoma have been reported in fish.[3,109] Neoplasia in fish can be associated with viruses, chemical or biologic agents, hormones, age, sex, and genetic predispositions within groups of animals. The treatment of neoplasia in fish is restricted to surgical resection, as chemotherapy and radiation are not practical.[109] No reports of attempted treatment of neoplasms affecting the musculoskeletal system were found.

Reptiles and Amphibians

Neoplastic disease in amphibians has been well documented.[110] Amphibians have been used in research to study the effects of potential carcinogens due to their sensitivity to toxins. Tumors in amphibians found to affect the musculoskeletal system include fibromas, fibromyxomas, fibrosarcomas, and rhabdomyosarcomas. There is one report of an osteosarcoma in an amphibian; however, there is some debate regarding the exact etiology of this lesion. Treatment options are limited and no reports of successful chemotherapeutic treatment have been reported. Surgical excision of the primary mass would be the treatment of choice if it was determined to be amendable to surgical excision.[111]

Reptiles are becoming increasingly popular as pets, and with improved husbandry practices, they are living longer than their wild counterparts. As a result, reptiles are more commonly diagnosed with neoplasia. Diagnosis is similar to domestic species and any mass should be aspirated or biopsied.[112]

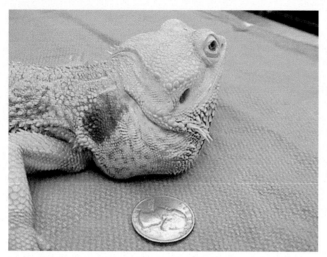

FIGURE 7-5 A ventral cervical fibrosarcoma in a bearded dragon *(Pogona vitticeps).*

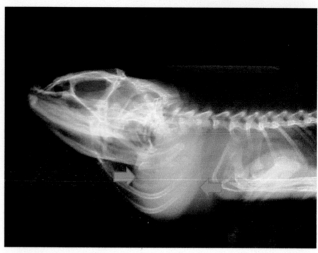

FIGURE 7-6 Radiographic image of the bearded dragon *(Pogona vitticeps)* seen in Figure 7-5 with a fibrosarcoma (arrows).

There are many individual case reports describing neoplasia in reptiles, and several review articles describe neoplasia in large collections over time.[113-119] Overall, there is a low prevalence of tumors found to be affecting the musculoskeletal system of reptiles, including chondrosarcomas, fibrosarcomas, osteosarcomas, osteochondromas, and rhabdomyosarcomas (Figures 7-5 and 7-6). Rhabdomyosarcomas were diagnosed in two snakes and five lizards in one review.[113] In two of these cases, the tumor was within the coelomic cavity and involved the body wall; it was unclear whether this was the result of a primary tumor or metastatic disease. Osteosarcomas have been reported in snakes and lizards. In snakes, they have been found in the vertebral column, and one snake had a solitary mesenteric mass that may have been a primary extraskeletal osteosarcoma. Morphologically, these tumors were similar in appearance to those described in higher vertebrates. Chondrosarcomas have been reported in snakes. They often arise from vertebral articulations, are locally invasive, and in some cases are associated with pathologic spinal fractures and paralysis. A chondrosarcoma was also described in a plate lizard *(Gerrhosaurus major)* with an invasive lesion in the proximal humerus.

To date, there is no specific case report of neoplasia directly associated with the musculoskeletal system of turtles or tortoises. Some of the previously noted retrospective reviews were either limited to snakes and lizards or only lizards, but even the review that included chelonians did not include any specific cases of musculoskeletal neoplasia.[113] Interestingly, in that study, the overall prevalence of neoplasia in chelonians (2.7%) was considerably lower than both lizards (8.5%) and snakes (15%).

Many reports and retrospective studies on neoplasia in reptiles summarize postmortem examination findings. Relatively few antemortem diagnoses are reported in the literature, and there are very limited reports of attempted treatments. Surgery is often the treatment of choice in tumors that are resectable, although detailed information regarding adequate margins required for different neoplasms has not been described. Chemotherapy, radiation therapy, intralesional therapy, and photodynamic therapy in reptiles are limited.[114,120]

Birds

Neoplastic diseases are more commonly encountered in birds due to our increasing knowledge base and the improved quality of avian medicine. Unfortunately, there is still very little information available regarding the prognoses for these cases or "best" treatment options. Tumors that affect the musculoskeletal system can be primary tumors or the result of metastasis from other parts of the body. Tumors of the musculoskeletal system in birds include osteomas, osteosarcomas, chondromas, chondrosarcomas, rhabdomyomas, rhabdomyosarcomas, fibrosarcomas, hemangiosarcomas, and synovial cell sarcomas.[46,121,122]

A recent review found 41 cases of primary bone tumors in birds; 18 of these cases were from poultry or wildlife. Of the cases reported in pet birds, osteomas, osteosarcomas, a chondroma, and a chondrosarcoma were reported. The tumors were located on the head, thoracic limb, pelvic girdle, and pelvic limb.[121] Rhabdomyosarcomas and synovial cell sarcomas have also been reported.[123,124]

Osteomas are benign growths arising from the surface of the bone and are composed of accumulations of cancellous or compact bone. They are seen sporadically in pet birds and are most commonly associated with the skull or vertebrae, although they can also be found on the wing.[70] Osteomas have been reported in a peach-faced lovebird *(Agapornis roseicollis)*, cockatiels, and budgerigars. Osteosarcomas are malignant tumors that primarily occur on the long bones of the legs and wings. Osteosarcomas involving the axial skeleton and head have also been reported. Species with documented cases of osteosarcoma include an Amazon parrot *(Amazona* sp.*)*, gang-gang cockatoo *(Callocephalon fimbriatum)*, sulfur-crested cockatoo *(Cacatua galerita)*, budgerigar, and an umbrella cockatoo *(Cacatua alba)*.[121] Unlike dogs and cats where osteosarcomas metastasize very early in the disease process, the biologic behavior of this cancer in birds may be less aggressive.[121] In one study of 1008 caged birds, six had osteosarcoma, but metastatic disease was uncommon.[121,125] In 10 other cases of osteosarcoma in birds (including poultry), only four mention metastasis and only one case had metastasis to the lungs.[121] In one case where treatment was described, an osteosarcoma on the head of a female blue-fronted Amazon parrot (*Amazona aestiva*) was treated with surgical debulking and doxorubicin. There was no recurrence noted 20 months after the procedure.[122]

Chondromas are uncommon tumors arising from cartilage. Only one case has been documented in a pet bird (an adult female parakeet). The bird presented for a head tilt and a mass compressing a cerebral hemisphere that extended into the brain parenchyma.[122] Chondrosarcomas are comprised of poorly differentiated cartilage, and there is only a single case report of this tumor type in a psittacine (yellow-collared macaw *[Primolius auricollis]*).[121]

Primary tumors of the skeletal muscle are uncommon in birds.[122] In pet birds, rhabdomyosarcomas have only been reported in two budgerigars. One case involved a 7-year-old male budgerigar with orbital swelling and exophthalmia. A retrobulbar mass was found and it was confirmed to be a rhabdomyosarcoma at necropsy.[123]

Synovial cell sarcoma is rarely reported in birds. Affected animals present with proliferative masses that lead to the destruction of the joint(s), with lysis of the adjacent epiphyses.[122] Synovial cell sarcoma has been reported in a sulphur-crested cockatoo that presented with a swollen elbow joint. An amputation was performed, but the bird returned 6 months after surgery with evidence of metastasis. Necropsy showed metastatic disease to multiple organs.[126]

In most cases, the surgical removal of a mass is the treatment of choice for tumors involving the musculoskeletal system of birds. Amputation does increase the likelihood of obtaining wide surgical margins and limiting the potential for metastasis. If the tumor cannot be removed with wide margins, surgery may still be an option to palliate clinical signs or to reduce tumor burden and increase the likelihood that chemotherapy or radiation therapy will be more effective. With the exception of the case using doxorubicin for an osteosarcoma, there are no other reports of chemotherapy being used to treat cancer in the skeletal system of pet birds.[122] To date, there have been no reports of radiation therapy being used to treat musculoskeletal cancer in pet birds, although this could be a viable option for some cases.

Mammals

Neoplasms of the musculoskeletal system in ferrets include chordomas, chondrosarcomas, osteomas, osteosarcomas, and rhabdomyosarcomas.[105,127,128] Chordomas arise from notochord remnants and are usually found at the distal extent of the tail. Chondrosarcomas also occur in the tail. Because these two neoplasms can be difficult to differentiate grossly, special staining is required to definitively diagnose these tumors. The treatment of choice for both of these cancers is tail amputation. To ensure sufficient margins, it is generally recommended to amputate the tail a minimum of 3 to 4 vertebrae proximal to the tumor. Osteomas commonly arise from the flat bones of the skull and ribs. Although these tumors are

benign in behavior, displacement and/or compression of surrounding structures can lead to clinical signs. Surgical resection is the treatment of choice and is curative if resection is complete.[105,128,129] Osteosarcomas are rarely reported in ferrets. Amputation of the affected limb is the treatment of choice and is well tolerated. Unlike osteosarcoma in domestic species where metastasis is common, metastasis of osteosarcoma in ferrets is not documented.[128] Tumors of skeletal muscle are rare, but rhabdomyosarcomas have been reported. Treatment is radical excision, if possible, or amputation if the lesion is located on the limbs.[127,128]

Rabbits

Skeletal and extraskeletal osteosarcomas have been reported in rabbits but are rare. Clinical signs are dependent on the area that is affected. Osteosarcomas of the mandible have been reported and lead to anorexia, weight loss, and nasal discharge. The biologic behavior of osteosarcoma in rabbits is not well defined but metastasis to the lungs, pleura, peritoneum, heart, liver, and musculature of the abdominal and thoracic walls have been reported. Recommended treatment includes aggressive resection and chemotherapy.[56,130]

Other Small Mammals

Even though neoplasia is a common clinical problem in many exotic small mammals (e.g., mice, rats, chinchillas, guinea pigs, hedgehogs, and sugar gliders), neoplasms involving the musculoskeletal system are quite rare. There are only a few documented cases of osteosarcoma in hedgehogs, but there is limited information on these cases regarding diagnosis, biologic behavior, or treatment.[131,132] A single case report documented the treatment of an extraskeletal osteosarcoma in a hedgehog. A mass on the caudodorsal flank was incompletely excised and diagnosed as an extraskeletal osteosarcoma. Two months after surgery, the animal died and a necropsy showed metastatic lesions in the spleen, liver, and lungs.[133]

JOINT DISEASE

Joint disease can be caused by a variety of physical disorders and diseases. Arthritis (e.g., osteoarthritis, septic arthritis, and immune-mediated arthropathies), joint instability, and gout can all lead to pain, joint swelling, and lameness. A complete understanding of the different joint diseases and a systematic workup will help differentiate each type of joint disease and guide treatment.

Arthritis, or inflammation of one or more joints, is a very common cause of musculoskeletal disease in many species. There are many different types of arthritis, depending on the etiology and number of joints involved. With all types of arthritis, there is damage and breakdown of the articular cartilage leading to pain, swelling, and alteration of the normal range of motion. The main forms of arthritis that are seen in veterinary patients include osteoarthritis, septic arthritis, and immune-mediated polyarthritis.

Osteoarthritis occurs through two mechanisms: (1) normal forces acting on an abnormal joint (luxation, articular fracture with a malunion, incongruity) and (2) abnormal forces acting on a normal joint (excessive concussive forces leading to cartilage damage). The normal aging process leads to water and proteoglycan loss from the cartilage, which leads to thinning and erosion of the cartilage. This has been termed primary osteoarthritis and accounts for a large proportion of osteoarthritis cases in people. Secondary osteoarthritis occurs when there is an abnormality in the cartilage such as incongruity, injury, or instability. Normal forces acting through these joints cause cartilage degeneration and erosions.

Septic arthritis refers to an active infection (usually bacterial) within the joint. This type of arthritis occurs with exogenous inoculation or hematogenous spread of infectious agents into the joint, and their presence leads to activation of the inflammatory cascade. Enzymes and by-products released as part of the inflammatory response degrade articular cartilage, leading to cartilage loss, further degeneration of the joint, and loss of joint function.

Immune-mediated polyarthritis can be divided into erosive and nonerosive forms. Erosive forms occur when the cell-mediated response of the inflammatory cascade is activated. T-cell activation results in the release of cytokines that ultimately leads to the release of collagenases and proteases that degrade the articular cartilage. Nonerosive polyarthritis is a type-III hypersensitivity reaction that leads to immune complex deposition in the periarticular tissues. This results in local tissue damage, an increase in neutrophils within the joints, and cartilage damage.

Joint instability occurs when supporting tendons and ligaments no longer function and there are changes in the anatomic relationship between adjacent bones. In minor cases, there may be some palpable instability with mild subluxation, while in more severe cases, complete joint luxation may occur. A majority of these cases is the direct result of a traumatic injury; however, some chronic inflammatory or infectious diseases can also result in the breakdown of tendons, ligaments, and other supporting structures, leading to alterations in limb positioning and gait. There are also several cases of congenital or developmental joint instability and luxation. Treatment of joint instability depends on the etiology. In some cases, the joints can be reduced and stabilized, while in others, irreparable damage has occurred or the joint cannot be reduced and arthrodesis or amputation is required.

Reptiles and Amphibians

There are relatively few cases of documented joint disease in reptiles and amphibians in the veterinary literature. Any reptile or amphibian presented for painful or swollen joints should be evaluated in a systematic manner to determine the etiology of the joint disease. Differential diagnoses for joint disease should be similar to higher vertebrates and include septic arthritis, gout, neoplasia, osteoarthritis, polyarthropathy, or luxation.[6] Radiographs and joint aspirates can be performed to make a definitive diagnosis. In certain cases, other imaging modalities may be helpful.

There are no reports of naturally occurring osteoarthritis reported in amphibians. However, experimental models of induced osteoarthritis in adult newts showed that these animals do develop osteoarthritis in a similar manner to other species in response to instability or introduction of collagenase into the joint.[134] The newts were able to regenerate their articular cartilage and restore normal tissue integrity and function. This has not been evaluated in anurans.

Degenerative bone and articular changes may be seen in older reptiles.[135] Only a small number of cases are documented in the veterinary literature, although this is not an uncommon problem. Osteoarthritis was diagnosed in a sea turtle with a chronic shoulder luxation.[136] The animal was emaciated and anemic, but no other significant lesions were found. The authors concluded that the osteoarthritis was severe enough that it affected the animal's ability to forage for food.

Septic arthritis is common in green iguanas and other lizards.[38] The interphalangeal joints are most often affected. Clinical signs include lameness and painful swollen joints. Radiographs show lysis of the epiphyses and widening of the joint spaces. In some cases, subluxation or luxation of the joint may occur. Joint aspirates can be used to obtain a definitive diagnosis, and culture of the joint fluid can be used to guide antibiotic treatment. Treatment with supportive care, antibiotics, and rest is successful in many cases. In severe cases, an arthrotomy with lavage and debridement of the joint is required. Antibiotic-impregnated polymethylmethacrylate (PMMA) beads can be used for the treatment of septic arthritis.[137] Septic arthritis has been reported in crocodilians and chelonians.[138-141] A postmortem examination in a tortoise euthanized for urinary tract obstruction revealed abscessation of both coxofemoral joints with *Corynebacterium* being cultured from the joints.[141] This was believed to be the primary cause of the urinary tract obstruction. There are also reports of sea turtles with septic arthritis that had lesions extending to surrounding long bones, causing osteomyelitis.[142,143] An outbreak of mycoplasmosis emerged in a colony of captive American alligators (*Alligator mississipiensis*) in Florida. This outbreak caused pneumonia, pericarditis, and multifocal arthritis and was responsible for the death or euthanasia of 60 individuals. The causative agent, *Mycoplasma alligatoris*, was cultured from both ill and dead alligators and was identified in synovial tissues. A similar *Mycoplasma* infection was seen in Nile crocodiles (*Crocodylus niloticus*).[140] These crocodilian cases should remind the clinician that aerobic culture may be insufficient for obtaining a diagnosis and that additional testing (e.g., PCR testing for *Mycoplasma*) may be necessary.

Gout is a condition where uric acid precipitates in various tissues (visceral and articular). Uric acid is the end product of protein metabolism is terrestrial reptiles and it is secreted into the urine by the renal tubules. If the concentration of uric acid in the blood (or other tissues) becomes persistently elevated above 25 mg/dL, insoluble crystals form and are deposited in the body.[10,144] These crystals form white nodules that are visible grossly. Crystallization of uric acid in the joints leads to pain and inflammation and is termed articular gout. If the crystallization occurs in the tissue around the joint, it is termed periarticular gout. In reptiles, gout has been associated with renal tubular disease, dehydration, and inappropriate levels of protein in the diet (e.g., feeding herbivorous reptiles high [animal] protein meals).[10]

Diagnosis of gout is based on history, physical examination, blood work, FNA and cytology, and radiographs. Many affected animals are weak and lethargic, with a poor body condition. Physical examination often reveals subcutaneous nodules near the joints, and these areas can be painful when palpated (Figures 7-7 and 7-8). Radiographs can show lysis of the affected joints and radiopaque nodules may be visualized. Blood work may show elevated uric acid concentrations; however, in some cases, uric acid concentrations may have normalized by the time the animal is presented (i.e., normal uric acid concentrations do not rule out gout). Definitive diagnosis requires microscopic examination of crystals from the joints or nodules (Figure 7-9).

Treatment of gout includes fluid therapy to correct dehydration, analgesics, and the correction of any nutritional imbalances (e.g., herbivorous reptiles are only offered plant-based protein). Unfortunately, once the urate crystals are deposited, they are rarely resorbed and treatment is aimed at prevention of additional crystal formation and progression of the disease. Allorpurinol (20 to 25 mg/kg, PO, q24 h) may be used to treat reptiles with persistently elevated uric acid concentrations. Probenicid has been recommended for gout cases in reptiles too, but it may be detrimental in animals with compromised renal function.

Visceral gout has been reported in amphibians, and one case of articular gout has been reported in an African bullfrog.[69] The animal was presented for a swollen digit that was painful on palpation. Urate crystals were seen on material expressed from the digit. Histopathologic examination of the digit showed chronic inflammation surrounding urate crystals. The animal remained in a captive collection and the cause was never determined.

Proliferative spinal osteopathy affects the joints of the spinal column and has been described in turtles, lizards, and (most commonly) snakes.[145,146] The exact cause remains unclear, but many different etiologies have been proposed, including trauma, nutritional deficiencies, viral infections, neoplasia, and bacterial infections. Many of the lesions can cause spinal cord compression or nerve root compression, and animals may present for neurologic abnormalities. Clinical signs vary, depending on the location and extent of the lesion(s), and can include stiffness, scoliosis, and kyphosis. Spinal lesions can lead to weakness and affect spinal reflexes. In severe cases, this can affect an animal's ability to move, strike, constrict, or swallow prey. Radiographs show segmental vertebral bone proliferation with exostosis predominantly on the ventro-lateral aspects of the vertebrae (Figure 7-10). Biopsy of affected bone for culture and histopathology is recommended as are blood cultures, since there can be a strong correlation between blood and bone culture results[145,146] (Figure 7-11).

There appears to be three distinct histologic groups of animals with spinal osteopathy, despite the similarities in clinical signs and radiographic and gross lesions. One group has strong evidence of bacterial osteoarthritis (septic arthritis). These animals have bacteria present on histopathology and have positive bone and blood cultures. Bacteria commonly isolated in these cases include *Streptococcus* spp., *Salmonella* spp., *Edwardsiella* spp., and *Citrobacter* spp.[146] The second group has noninflammatory osteoarthrosis mixed with multiple small foci of inflammation without histologic evidence

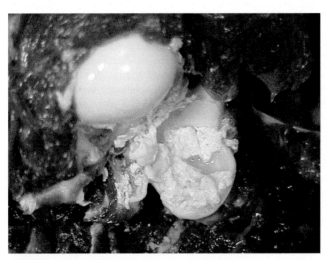

FIGURE 7-7 Severe gout in the coxofemoral joint of an African spurred tortoise *(Centrochelys sulcata)*.

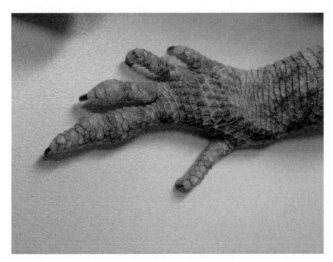

FIGURE 7-8 Articular gout in a bearded dragon *(Pogona vitticeps)*.

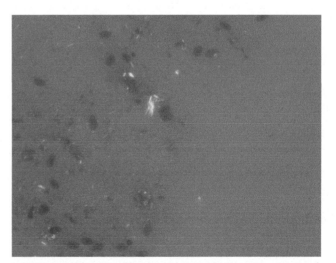

FIGURE 7-9 Aspirate cytology from the soft tissue swelling of the digit from the bearded dragon *(Pogona vitticeps)* in Figure 7-8 (40×, polarizing filter). Numerous birefringent, needle-shaped crystals are present within the background. These are consistent with urate crystals.

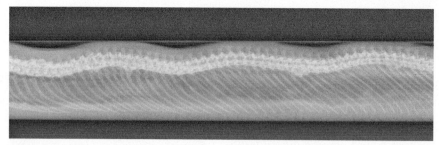

FIGURE 7-10 The radiographic appearance of spinal osteopathy in a red-tail boa *(Boa constrictor).*

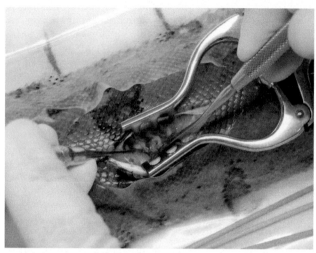

FIGURE 7-11 Surgical approach to the spinal canal in a red-tail boa *(Boa constrictor)* with spinal osteopathy. Samples of irregular bone can be taken for histopathology, culture, and sensitivity.

of bacteria. The inflammation seen is suggestive of previous, chronic, low grade osteoarthritis. Some of these animals may have positive blood cultures. The third group has degenerative osteoarthritis and ankylosis with minimal to no inflammation. No bacteria are seen on histopathology in these cases, and blood and bone cultures are routinely negative. While it is possible that these three different groups may represent unrelated diseases, it is also possible that they may represent bacterial osteoarthritis at different stages, ranging from acute to chronic. Septic arthritis and osteomyelitis can cause the early lesions associated with active infections. These infections can alter the morphology of the bone and joint surfaces, leaving abnormal ankylosed joints once the infection and inflammation resolve.[146]

Treatment of spinal osteopathy involves long-term antibiotic therapy, and early recognition is essential for a favorable long-term prognosis. Antibiotic agents with good bone penetration should be selected and administered. Antibiotic-impregnated beads can also be used in selected cases, and the antibiotic medication impregnated within the PMMA should be based on culture and antibiotic sensitivity results. Analgesia should also be implemented. Overall, the prognosis for these cases is poor, since animals are often presented with advanced clinical disease.[145]

Stifle instability in an amphibian has been documented in a single case in a wild-caught American bullfrog *(Rana catesbeiana).*[147] The injury was presumed to be traumatic, but the exact cause was undetermined. The type of injury was not described, although from the description, it was presumed that there were tears in the cranial cruciate ligament, medial collateral ligament, and meniscus. Intra-articular inspection was not performed. Joint stabilization was performed in a manner similar to a modified retinacular imbrication technique used to treat cranial cruciate-deficient stifles in dogs. Because frogs lack gastrocnemius sesamoid bones and fabellofemoral ligaments, the proximal sutures were anchored in the soft tissue of the distal femur. Tibial bone tunnels were also not used, so the distal sutures were placed in the soft tissues of the proximal tibia. There is a similar report involving a spur-thighed tortoise *(Testudo graeca)* that was presented for acute left hind limb lameness.[148] Stifle instability was diagnosed based on clinical findings and diagnostic imaging. A modification of the over the top method for cranial cruciate reconstruction using a vastus muscle autograft was performed, with lateral imbrication of the joint capsule.

Birds

Degenerative changes in the joints of older birds are not uncommon. Causes may include previous trauma, infection, or a previous history of metabolic conditions such as MBD or gout. Grossly, joints will have areas of cartilage erosion with osteophytes and fibrosis of the joint capsule. The joint itself will be variably thickened depending on the chronicity and severity of the lesion(s).[70]

Septic arthritis in birds may be due to a variety of bacteria.[70] Infections can occur in any synovial joint. Affected birds will have swollen and painful joints with reduced mobility. Inflammatory cells infiltrate the synovium, causing thickening and fibrosis.[70] Aspirates of the joints will contain exudate, fibrin, heterophils, and macrophages.

Articular gout also occurs in birds. Affected birds usually present with vague clinical signs, or they may present with white deposits that are visible under the skin of the distal pelvic limbs and feet. Like reptiles, the treatment is frustrating and many animals do not fully recover. Allopurinol (10 to 30 mg/kg, PO, q24 h) has been suggested for treatment in order to reduce plasma uric acid levels.[45,70] Nonsteroidal analgesics (meloxicam, 0.5 mg/kg, PO, q12-24 h) should be used to control pain, if kidney function is normal.

Joint instability has been documented in birds. Stifle luxations have been treated successfully in an African grey parrot, a trumpeter hornbill, a Moluccan cockatoo, a barn owl, and a monk parakeet using a variety of techniques.[149-151] In addition, metacarpophalangeal luxations have been managed with arthrodeses in raptors.[152]

Mammals

Elbow luxations are common in ferrets and can occur spontaneously or be secondary to trauma. Affected ferrets will have a forelimb lameness, and a swollen painful elbow joint will be palpable during the orthopedic examination.[153] Closed reduction should be attempted under heavy sedation or general anesthesia. In dogs, closed reduction followed by splinting the leg with the elbow in extension is often successful. Dogs have a well-developed anconeal process, and when the elbow is placed in extension, the anconeal process articulates with the supratrochlear foramen, helping to maintain the elbow in proper reduction. Ferrets do not have a well-developed anconeal process, and closed reduction with external coaptation alone often results in reluxation. Additional stabilization with a transarticular pin, cross-pinning, or a transarticular extraskeletal fixator is often required. Once reduction is achieved, the elbow should be placed in 100° to 110° of flexion and an intramedullary (IM) pin inserted at the caudal aspect of the ulna, through the articular surface of the elbow joint, and into the humeral condyle (Figure 7-12). External coaptation is used for additional support. After 2 to 3 weeks, the transarticular pin can be removed, although the external coaptation should be continued for 2 to 3 weeks after pin removal.[154]

Unlike dogs, cranial cruciate ligament tears are not commonly seen in ferrets. Few anecdotal reports exist and surgery is rarely required. Diagnosis is similar to dogs, by documenting cranial translation of the tibia (cranial drawer). Like cats with documented cranial cruciate tears, ferrets can be managed without surgery and often respond to cage rest and anti-inflammatories.

Splay leg or hip dysplasia is a developmental condition observed in young rabbits ranging in age from a few days to a few months. It has also been diagnosed in older rabbits. Affected animals are unable to adduct their hind limbs or ambulate normally. In young developing rabbits, the hind limb anatomy is altered, which leads to changes in the angles of inclination of the proximal femur, subluxation of the coxofemoral joints, valgus deformities, and patellar luxations.[56] Early identification of the problem and treatment using splinting and hobbling can be attempted. Amputation can be performed if the condition is unilateral; however, most cases are bilateral and the response to treatment is poor, so euthanasia is often recommended. The etiology behind this condition is not completely understood, but both genetic and environmental factors likely play a role in the disease process.[20,56] The role of adequate nest box flooring has been shown to affect the incidence of hip dysplasia in rabbits; therefore, young rabbits should be raised on nonslip flooring.[155]

Joint instability can also occur in rabbits. There is a single report of bilateral cranial cruciate tears in a rabbit. A female intact rabbit was presented for right hind limb lameness. Cranial drawer was present and extra-articular stabilization was performed. The rabbit presented again 4 months later with left hind limb lameness and the procedure was repeated on the left hind limb. Long-term follow-up showed the rabbit had normal behavior with no pain on palpation or manipulation of either hind limb.[156] There are also anecdotal reports of successful conservative management of suspected cruciate injuries in rabbits. A traumatic shoulder luxation was also treated nonsurgically by the author (Figures 7-13 and 7-14).

Osteoarthritis is commonly diagnosed in older rabbits. Clinical signs include lameness and reluctance to move. Osteoarthritis has been extensively studied in rabbits in the laboratory setting, as a model for other species. Management of chronic osteoarthritis is similar to domestic species. Weight loss and nonsteroidal anti-inflammatories (meloxicam, 0.5 mg/kg PO q12-24h or 1 mg/kg PO q24h) are the hallmarks of treatment. Hyaluronic acid injections have been used in experimental studies and decreased cartilage degeneration. Glucosamine, chondroitin, green-lipped muscles, and omega-3 fatty acid supplementation have also been used with variable results.[157]

Ulcerative pododermatitis (sore hocks) can be another cause of lameness in rabbits. Lesions occur on the plantar aspects of the rear feet. Causes include obesity, lack of exercise, and improper husbandry (dirty or inappropriate flooring). Because rabbits do not have foot pads, it is important that they are housed on an appropriate substrate (e.g., some form of padded substrate such as a recycled paper bedding is recommended). Treatment is aimed at correcting the underlying cause and relieving pressure form the affected area(s).[20]

Osteoarthritis can occur spontaneously in guinea pigs or may be secondary to other diseases. Obesity and improper exercise are common predisposing factors. Treatment is palliative and includes weight loss, pain management, physical therapy, and providing clean, dry bedding.[59] Glucosamine and

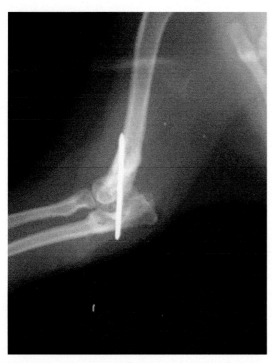

FIGURE 7-12 A lateral postoperative radiograph showing proper placement of a transarticular pin following an elbow luxation in a ferret *(Mustela putorius furo)*. (Photo courtesy of R. Avery Bennett.)

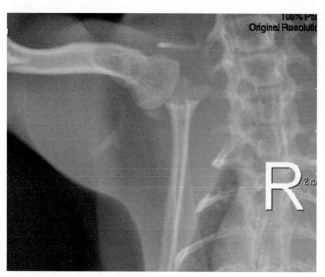

FIGURE 7-13 A radiographic image showing a lateral shoulder luxation in a domestic rabbit *(Oryctolagus cuniculus)* following a traumatic injury.

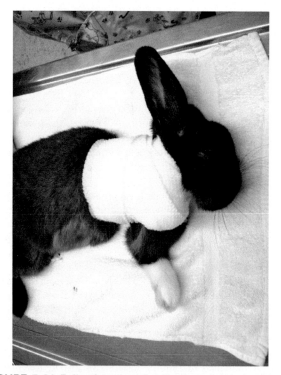

FIGURE 7-14 Following closed reduction of the shoulder, a velpeau sling was placed to hold the shoulder in reduction. After 4 weeks, the sling was removed and the shoulder remained in proper reduction.

chondroitin have been effective in inhibiting progression of osteoarthritis in experimental studies using guinea pigs.[158]

Like rabbits, guinea pigs can also suffer from pododermatitis. In addition to the underlying causes discussed in rabbits, vitamin C deficiencies may also play a role. Treatment should be focused on addressing the underlying cause(s), topically

managing the affected areas, providing analgesics, and supplementing the guinea pig with vitamin C.[71] In moderate to severe cases, surgery is recommended to decrease convalescence time and improve prognosis.[72]

Osteonecrosis of the femoral head occurs in rats, and they have been used extensively as a model for Legg-Calve-Perthes disease in humans. In experimental studies, rats that were forced to stand to reach food or water were predisposed to developing lesions in the femoral head, suggesting that excessive mechanical stress can predispose rats to developing osteonecrosis of the femoral head.[159,160] Strains of rats with hypertension were also found to have a higher incidence of bone necrosis and ossification disorders, compared to normotensive controls. This suggests, as with other species, the disease is multifactorial.[161]

OSTEOMYELITIS

Osteomyelitis is an infection of the bone or medullary canal. *Staphylococcus* spp., *Streptococcus* spp., and gram-negative aerobic bacteria are the most common bacteria isolated from bone infections, although there is some variation of organisms isolated depending on the species. Anaerobic infections are less common but should be suspected in cases of apparent infection with negative aerobic cultures. Examples of anaerobic bacteria that have been associated with bone infections include *Bacteroides* spp., *Fusobacterium* spp., *Actinomyces* spp., *Clostridium* spp., and *Peptococcus* spp. Many infections are associated with a single species of bacteria, although 30% to 60% of cases may have multiple organisms isolated.[162] Fungal osteomyelitis is less common, but cases of osteomyelitis with *Cryptococcus* spp., *Coccidioides* spp., *Aspergillus* spp., *Penicillium* spp., *Blastomyces* spp., *and Histoplasma* spp. have been reported. Osteomyelitis can occur as a result of direct inoculation of the bacteria into the bone through a penetrating wound or open fracture or through hematogenous spread from infections that started in the skin, respiratory system, oral cavity, or GI tract.

Animals with hematogenous osteomyelitis present with swelling of the affected area(s), lameness, and bone pain. A thorough physical examination should be performed to determine the source of the infection. Nonhematogenous osteomyelitis typically occurs after a traumatic injury, so many cases may still have a wound, laceration, or surgical incision that is edematous, erythematous, and painful. With either form of osteomyelitis, systemic signs such as lethargy and inappetance can be seen. Chronic nonhematogenous osteomyelitis can be seen weeks, months, or years after an initial injury. Implants used for internal fixation of fractures can act as a nidus of infection, or a sequestrum may be present. Animals can present with a swelling over the previous injury site and draining tracts are commonly seen. Radiographs and cultures of tissue samples or surgical implants can be used to confirm a diagnosis of osteomyelitis. Fungal osteomyelitis is often diagnosed based on aspirates of the affected area, and many fungal organisms can be easily identified on cytology.

Treatment involves aggressive debridement of any nonviable tissue and removal of any boney sequestra and surgical implants. Antibiotic agents with good bone penetration are selected based on culture and antibiotic sensitivity results. Antibiotic-impregnated PMMA beads can also be used in the treatment of osteomyelitis to achieve high levels of antibiotics within the affected tissue without systemic side effects. Non-hematogenous osteomyelitis typically has a favorable prognosis, while hematogenous osteomyelitis and fungal osteomyelitis have guarded-to-poor prognoses.

Osteomyelitis is common in reptiles and is usually associated with *Salmonella* spp., *Mycobacterium* spp., *Mycoplasma* spp., and various fungal organisms.[163,164] Although osteomyelitis is a common reason reptiles are presented to veterinarians, there are relatively few case reports describing the clinical course of the disease and response to treatment. *Salmonella* spp. in reptiles are usually discussed in the context of zoonosis; however, there are a number of reports of clinical disease in reptiles due to *Salmonella* infections.[163] *Salmonella arizonae* was isolated from osteomyelitis lesions in a group of captive rattlesnakes. The 19 rattlesnakes were monitored over a 5-year period with annual radiographs. Seven individuals had lesions at the beginning of the study and six died or were euthanized by the end of the study due to the progression of the lesions. Three snakes developed lesions during the study period, although no treatment was administered to any of the snakes.[165] A study done to determine the health status of wild spiny-tailed lizards found several individuals with osteomyelitis that were believed to be associated with previous fight injuries. *Escherichia coli*, *Klebsiella* spp., *Proteus* spp., and *Staphylococcus* spp. were isolated from the boney lesions.[166] *Mycobacterium* spp. have been isolated from osteomyelitis lesions in many different species of reptiles.[163] An unidentified atypical *Mycobacterium* was isolated from the tibia of a bearded dragon.[167] Despite amputation of the affected limb, the animal died after new lesions were found in other organs. A new species of *Mycoplasma* has been isolated from feral iguanas in Florida.[168] Spinal abscesses were seen in two feral iguanas during a necropsy. The strain of *Mycoplasma* that was isolated was different from previously described species. Unfortunately, no clinical information was provided regarding the case.

Fungal osteomyelitis was reported in a population of Marlborough green geckos *(Heteropholis manukanus)*.[169] Several digits had skin lesions and histopathology showed branching nonseptate hyphae. There was necrosis of several digits and mycotic osteomyelitis. Fungal osteomyelitis was also reported in a chameleon.[170] An open wound over the mandible resulted in osteomyelitis of both hemimandibles. *Aspergillus* spp. was isolated from the wound and the animal was treated with aggressive debridement followed by itraconazole. It is important to screen osteomyelitis samples (biopsies) from reptiles for fungal pathogens, as they appear more commonly in this group than in other vertebrates.

Shell infections commonly affect chelonians. Superficial lesions can progress to deep infections and osteomyelitis of the underlying bone. Bacterial, fungal, or mixed infections can occur. Aggressive debridement is important in the treatment of these lesions and healing can take months or years. Vacuum-assisted closure (VAC) has been reported in a deep shell abscess as a method for treating the wound while decreasing the time required for the lesion to heal.[171]

Osteomyelitis in birds can occur as a result of local or systemic infection. Aerobic and anaerobic bacteria, fungi (*Aspergillus* spp. and *Candida* spp.), and mycobacteria have all been associated with osteomyelitis in birds.[46,70] Affected animals often present with painful, swollen lesions over the infected bone(s) and may show pelvic limb lameness or be unable or reluctant to fly. In severe cases, pathologic fractures can occur.[70] Radiographs of the affected areas are often diagnostic and show clearly defined areas of boney lysis with a significant periosteal reaction. Abscesses can develop in the bone that are usually caseous and difficult to drain.

Treatment involves surgical debridement to remove any necrotic bone and pus. Antibiotic-impregnated PMMA beads can be placed at the site of the infection to provide high levels of antibiotics at the site of infection. Many different antibiotics can be mixed with the PMMA; however, ideally, antibiotic selection should be based on culture and antibiotic sensitivity results. Systemic antibiotics should also be used to manage these cases, and therapy may be needed for several months in order to completely clear the infection.

There are no specific cases of osteomyelitis in exotic small mammals documented in the literature. However, this is not an uncommon problem and like dogs and cats is usually associated with open fractures or following open reduction and internal fixation of closed fractures. Treatment involves thorough debridement of the affected area, removal of implants, and appropriate antibiotic therapy.

TRAUMA

Invertebrates

Trauma is one of the most common causes of morbidity and mortality in captive spiders.[2] Wounds can lead to rapid loss of hemolymph and exsanguination. The location of the lacerations can determine the extent of the hemorrhage and loss of hemolymph. Large lacerations on the lateral opisthoma can be relatively well tolerated, while a much smaller laceration on the dorsal opisthoma can lead to rapid hemolymph loss. Similarly, the location of a wound on the legs can affect the amount of hemolymph that may be lost. Wounds at the base of the legs or appendages will result in more serious hemolymph loss than more distal wounds. Wounds and lacerations should be closed using cyanoacrylate tissue adhesives, as sutures are ineffective and can result in greater trauma.

If limb injuries are severe and hemostasis is not possible, the limb can be removed by inducing autonomy or by amputation proximal to the injury. Autonomy is a natural defense mechanism and is a voluntary action that occurs between the coxa and trochanter. Contraction of the tissues prevents hemolymph loss. Performing autonomy in anesthetized animals may prevent these normal events, leading to continued hemolymph loss. Amputation is different from autonomy and can be done using scissors and several layers of cyanoacrylate adhesive to seal the wound. Limb regeneration will occur during the next molt (ecdysis) with both limb autonomy and limb amputation.

Many of these principles mentioned for arachnids can be applied to other invertebrates such as scorpions, myriapods, and insects. Traumatic injuries are common and hemolymph loss is a serious concern. Again, cyanoacrylate adhesives can be used to treat these injuries and sutures are not recommended. Limb amputations can be performed for serious injuries that cannot be treated more conservatively.

Vertebrates

Bone Composition, Bone Healing, and Fracture Repair

Understanding bone biology and fracture healing is important when addressing fractures. Bone composition, bone structure, and mechanisms of bone healing are all important in fracture fixation, and differences in these principles do exist between species. These differences can affect fracture configurations and may affect bone healing.

Bones are a mixture of organic and inorganic materials. The inorganic material consists of calcium hydroxyapatite, which gives bone its strength and rigidity.[172] The amount of calcium in a bone can vary between species, and this ultimately affects bone strength, stiffness, and density. Bird bones have a higher calcium content (16%) compared to mammalian bones (10%), which is thought to contribute to the brittle nature of bird bones. The clinical significance of this is that in birds, fractures are more likely to be comminuted, and the more brittle nature of the bones can make internal fixation more challenging.[15] The organic component of bone consists of cells (osteocytes, osteoblasts, and osteoclasts) and the extracellular matrix (glycoproteins, proteoglycans, and collagen).

Bones of virtually all vertebrates from fish to mammals have cortices that are arranged into one or more stratified zones of lamellar or nonlamellar bone. The layering of the cortex is a result of rebuilding and remodeling that occurs during skeletal growth.[173] Cortical (also known as compact or osteonal) and cancellous (also known as trabecular or spongy) bone are the two types of bone that are most commonly described in textbooks and articles addressing bone structure. Cortical bone is often described as longitudinally oriented cylindrical haversian systems with a central canal surrounded by concentric boney lamellae. These are also known as osteons. This forms the dense shafts of the diaphysis of a long bone. Cancellous bone is described as a network of fine irregular plates, rods, and struts called trabeculae that are separated by spaces filled with bone marrow and hematopoietic cells. Cancellous bone typically occupies the metaphysis of long bones and is projected into the medullary canal. This description of bone is oversimplified and is concentrated on the bone structure seen in higher mammals. There is considerable variation in the structural arrangement of bone between species. There is also some variation in the arrangement within species and even within regions of the same bone.[174] When comparing bone structure between different species, three major structural arrangements exist: lamellar, laminar, and haversian system types. Lamellar bone is composed of several lamellae, or thin plate-like structures, concentrically arranged around the medullary canal. Laminar bone is composed of several laminae concentrically arranged around the medullary canal. Each lamina is composed of lamellae separated from adjacent laminae by canals. Haversian system types are composed of osteons running parallel with the axis of the bone. These are surrounded by lamellae or laminae. Each system may occur within bone alone or in combination with other systems within the same bone.[174]

Fish bones are formed in a similar fashion as mammals (direct ossification of dermal bone or perichondral ossification of hyaline cartilage).[5] These are considered cellular bones that contain osteocytes and lacunae within the ossified matrix. In these bones, osteoblasts and osteoclasts appear in a similar fashion to mammals.[5] In addition, some fish have tissues that are considered in between cartilage and bones (acellular bone). Acellular bones are devoid of osteocytes and are derived from perichondral ossification or dermal ossification. Acelluar bone is surrounded by fibrous periosteum and an osteogenic layer of osteoblasts.

The description of the bones in amphibians is limited to bullfrog femurs.[174] The femurs of bullfrogs have poorly developed lamellar bone with three general divisions. External circumferential lamellae surround the bone and contain round-to-oval lacunae with poorly developed canaliculi. A central ring consists of concentric indistinct lamellae with large radiating canals. The internal circumferential lamellae surround the medullary canal and are poorly developed. Other samples of the same species showed some variation, including variation or absence of external and internal concentric lamellae and reduction or absence of radiating canals.

The cortex in bones of snakes and lizards contains bone of periosteal and endosteal origin. Seasons or periodic growth leads to layering or laminar arrangement. Cortical bones of snakes and lizards are composed of a mixture of lamellar and nonlamellar bone with no haversian systems. There are two major differences in cortical bone of snakes and lizards compared to other reptiles: (1) the presence of compact bone that is virtually nonvascular with a marked reduction of vascular channels and (2) a limited amount of cancellous trabeculae.[173] The cortex in chelonian and crocodilian bones is arranged in circumferential broad laminae each containing rows of vascular canals. Each lamination is a result of periods of growth, and in young individuals, the cortex may be composed of a single laminae with the number increasing as the animal ages.[173] Chelonians and crocodilian bones also contain incomplete haversian systems that are limited to localized areas of the cortex.[173,174] The metaphysis of long bones is composed of cancellous bone that is structurally different from cancellous bone seen in mammals. No descriptions of the reptile periosteum were found.

Birds also have cancellous and cortical bone. Cortical bone is arranged in mixed patterns of lamellae and incomplete haversian systems.[172,174,175] External and internal circumferential lamellae are present in most species.[174] The number and arrangement of haversian systems vary considerably between species. Also, the periosteum and endosteum of birds contain very few cells and lack significant biologic activity. Egg-laying female birds have specialized medullary bone within the marrow cavities of nonpneumatic bone. As egg-laying nears, spicules and trabeculae develop from the endosteum and serve as a calcium store that can be quickly mobilized to meet the demands of egg formation.[70]

In mammals, there is considerable variation in arrangement of the bone cortices. Lower mammals such as opossums have bone that is rudimentary in appearance. Incomplete lamellar bands surround the cortex followed by incomplete haversian systems. Internal circumferential lamellae are present but incomplete. In rats, there is a wide distinct band of external circumferential lamellae followed by a second wide band of incomplete haversian systems. The internal circumferential lamellae are poorly defined. In rabbits, the external circumferential lamellae are present in some areas and indistinct in others. A wide central ring exists that is composed of both incomplete and well-developed haversian systems. Well-developed internal circumferential lamellae surround the medullary canal. Higher mammals, such as mink, skunks, felids, and canids, have well-developed external and internal circumferential lamellae with a mixture of complete and incomplete haversian systems. The proportion of complete haversian systems increases in these species. Periosteum covers the outer cortex of all bones and a layer of endosteum covers the inner surface of the medullary canal. In mammals, the periosteum and endosteum contain osteogenic cells responsible for growth, repair, and remodeling.[172,176]

Bone Healing

Bone healing occurs by different mechanisms, depending on contact between fracture fragments and stability. There are also potential inter- and intraspecies differences in bone healing. The classic description of bone healing is through formation of a callus (secondary or indirect bone healing). When the fracture occurs, a hematoma develops at the fracture site. The cells within the hematoma initiate an inflammatory response and release cytokines. Once the inflammatory phase subsides, pluripotent mesenchymal cells arising from the periosteum, endosteum, and surrounding soft tissues are induced and differentiate into fibroblasts, chondroblasts, and osteoblasts. These cells produce fibrous tissue, cartilage, and woven bone, respectively. This results in the formation of a callus that bridges the fracture and continuously reorganizes into progressively stiffer tissue until a boney callus bridges the fracture. The later stages can be evaluated radiographically, and clinical healing is complete when the boney callus bridges the fracture gap.

Primary or direct healing occurs through contact healing and gap healing. Contact healing requires a gap <0.01 mm, absolute stability, and no interfragmentary motion. Lamellar bone is directly deposited in the normal axial direction of the bone. This process is started by the formation of cutting cones at the ends of osteons, with osteoclasts lining the tip of the cutting cones and osteoblasts forming at the base. These cutting cones advance across the fracture line at a rate of 70 to 100 μm per day. This is also known as haversian remodeling and results in new haversian systems crossing the fracture line. Gap healing occurs when the fracture gap is <1 mm and there is no motion at the fracture site. The fracture fills directly with intramembranous bone. The newly formed lamellar bone is oriented perpendicularly to the long axis of the bone and is later reorganized through haversian remodeling. When direct bone healing is evaluated radiographically to assess for healing, there is minimal to no callus present. The fracture lines that are present after the initial stabilization become less distinct over time and eventually disappear.

The considerable variation in bone structure may affect how the fractures heal. Many species lack haversian systems, while in others, they are incomplete. Due to the arrangement of cutting cones with the osteon during direct bone healing, this type of healing may not occur in species that do not have well-developed haversian systems. Direct bone healing has not been studied in birds or reptiles; however, in birds when fractures are stabilized with plates, there appears to be minimal callus produced during the healing period. This suggests that direct healing may be possible in birds.[177-179] Direct bone

healing is commonly seen in mammals after anatomic reduction and rigid fixation of fractured long bones.

The mechanism of indirect bone healing is similar between species, although some differences exist. The main differences noted between species are the rate of repair and the relative contribution of the periosteum, endosteum, and surrounding soft tissues to the healing process.

Reptile and amphibian fractures take the longest to heal and, in some cases, can take as long as 6 to 30 months.[180] In one study, full union of tibial fractures took 50% longer in lizards compared to rats, and full bony union was not seen in frogs during the study period. Interestingly, although some amphibians are capable of complete limb regeneration, fracture healing occurs through indirect bone healing, and if a significant fracture gap is present, a nonunion will occur.[181] Also, fracture healing in lizards maintained at lower environmental temperatures (26° C) took longer to heal compared to lizards kept within their preferred optimal temperature zone (32° C to 37° C).[164,182] Although there is some variation, most mammalian fractures heal in 4 to 12 weeks. Avian fractures heal the fastest (2 to 8 weeks).[180,183]

In reptile and amphibian fractures, a majority of the hematoma and subsequent callus is derived from the periosteum. In avian fractures, the callus is derived from the periosteum and the endosteum. The endosteal callus provides rapid rigid support in well-aligned bones and the periosteal callus provides secondary support.[178,184] Compared to other species, mammalian fractures appear to derive a larger contribution to healing from the soft tissues that surround the fracture.[182] These differences can be important in fracture repair and may affect the implants that are selected in order to minimize any detrimental effects on the endosteum or periosteum.

Principles of Fracture Repair

The principles of fracture repair are similar regardless of species. Reduction of the fracture with correct anatomic alignment, rigid immobilization, and preservation of the soft tissues must be achieved. All fractures have forces acting on them such as bending, rotation, axial load (compression and tension), and shear. The method chosen to immobilize fractures must be able to counteract all forces acting on the fracture site. The methods for fixation can vary, and in some cases, the options available are limited due to the size of the patient, anatomy, skill of the veterinarian in orthopedic surgery, and expense (for the owner as well as to the veterinarian). External coaptation, internal fixation, and external skeletal fixation (ESF) have all been applied in exotics species. External coaptation refers to the use of a sling, splint, bandage, or cast to immobilize the fracture. Internal fixation refers to the use of orthopedic implants such as an IM pin, orthopedic wire, bone plate and screws, and interlocking nails. ESF refers to the use of fixation pins that are inserted percutaneously through the cortices of the bone and are connected externally to a bar or acrylic. Minimally invasive osteosynthesis is also becoming more common in veterinary orthopedics and can be applied in select exotics cases. In all cases of fracture repair, it is important to restrict the animal's activity until the fracture is healed. Any additional movement can cause bandage complications or stress implants leading to implant failure. Other complications that can be encountered with fracture repair include osteomyelitis, malunion, delayed union, nonunion, and diseases in other limbs due to change in weight bearing (e.g., bumblefoot in birds).

External Coaptation

External coaptation is a simple, inexpensive technique that can be used to stabilize certain fractures. In many cases, external coaptation is chosen when surgery is not possible due to patient size or finances. In other cases, external coaptation is applied as a temporary method of immobilization to prevent further injury until surgical stabilization can be performed. To be effective, the splint or cast must immobilize the joint above and below the fracture, and a properly applied splint or cast will counteract bending and rotational forces but will not counteract axial forces applied to the fracture. In domestic species, this typically limits the use of splints and casts to the distal extremities, since the shoulder joint and coxofemoral joint are very difficult to immobilize. In some exotics species, external coaptation can be used for fractures of the humerus and femur more successfully. Ideally, external coaptation is limited to simple, closed minimally displaced fractures.

Although there are some variations, the bandages used for external coaptation have many similar components regardless of the species. Cast padding, conforming cotton roll gauze, and an outer protective layer such as Vet Wrap (3M Corp., St. Paul, MN) or elasticon are used in most cases. Cast padding is the primary layer and is used to protect soft tissues. Any wounds that are present from the initial injury should be treated appropriately with a debriding or nonadherent dressing based on the type of wound. Particular attention should be given to any skin irritation or areas over boney prominences, since these can quickly turn into significant pressure sores. Extra cast padding should be placed over these areas; however, excessive cast padding can lead to instability and movement within the bandage, so a careful balance must be met. When placing cast padding, it should be snug to prevent the bandage from slipping. In most cases, it is impossible to place the cast padding too tight since most brands will tear before they reach sufficient tension to cause vascular compression and constriction of the distal limb. After the cast padding is applied, the conforming roll gauze is used to gently compress the cast padding to help provide immobilization. Unlike the cast padding, the roll gauze can be placed too tight, causing constriction of the distal limb. Splints can be made from a variety of materials depending on the species and area on which the splint is applied. Prefabricated plastic or metal splints are available or a splint can be made from casting material, thermoplastic polymers, syringe cases, or tongue depressors. The splints are applied on top of the roll gauze and are secured with additional roll gauze or tape. A protective layer of elastic bandage is placed over the splint. Most prefabricated splints require the limb to be placed in extension, and long-term immobilization in extension can lead to decreased range of motion in the joints following bandage removal. This can ultimately affect the animal's ability to ambulate normally. Some authors suggest splinting limbs in normal walking angles so that any long-term effects of immobilization on limb function are minimized.[185] In some exotics (e.g., amphibians, reptiles, and birds), the fractured limb can be bandaged against the body or tail instead of using a rigid splint.

Bandages must be monitored carefully after they are applied to ensure that they do not cause any constriction of the distal extremity. They must also be monitored for the duration of treatment to ensure that they do not slip, fall off, or become wet or soiled. If any of these occur, they must be evaluated immediately and the bandage and splint replaced.

Complications associated with external coaptation involve the development of skin irritation, pressure sores, or full-thickness wounds. Any animal that has a bandage, splint, or cast should have the area checked regularly to identify any areas of irritation early before significant wounds are present. In some cases, the soft tissue wounds caused by the bandages can be worse than the original injury, requiring amputation in severe cases. Other complications of external coaptation are atrophy and contracture of the musculature and decreased range of motion in the joints due to long-term immobilization. This is of particular concern for any young growing animal. In these cases, external splints applied during development can lead to angular limb deformities. Finally, since closed reduction is often used when external coaptation is selected, anatomic apposition is not always achieved and malunions can develop. The severity of the malunion and magnitude of any alterations in limb alignment can determine if the malunion causes any functional deficits. To minimize the complications associated with immobilization, external coaptation should be removed as soon as possible and rehabilitation should be started to regain range of motion and muscle mass.

Internal Fixation

Internal fixation involves placement of orthopedic implants to provide rigid immobilization. Orthopedic wire, Kirschner wires (K wires), IM pins, polymer rods, interlocking nails, and plates and screws are common orthopedic implants that can be all applied to exotic animals. Many of these techniques are technically difficult to perform and require advanced training. The techniques are described briefly here for completeness; however, individuals without sufficient training in using these techniques should consider referral when appropriate.

Orthopedic implants are made of 316L stainless steel or titanium alloys. The composition of 316L stainless steel and the method in which the metal is manufactured will determine the mechanical properties of the implant, specifically, stiffness, strength, and ductility. Cold working and annealing can be used to attain the desired properties for each type of implant and allow variations between implant types. For example, orthopedic wire is more ductile than bone plates, which are in turn more ductile than IM pins. Orthopedic implants can also be made of titanium alloys. Titanium implants have a higher strength-to-weight ratio than stainless steel, have improved corrosion resistance, and produce less tissue reaction. Other advantages include increased flexibility compared to steel, which reduces stress protection when applied to bone, and increased resistance to infection. The main disadvantage of titanium implants is the increased cost compared to stainless steel.

IM pins can be used for diaphyseal fractures in long bones, with the exception of the radius. Placing an IM pin in the radius in most species would require penetration of the articular surface of the carpus or elbow. One notable exception to this rule occurs in birds. IM pins can be placed in a retrograde manner in birds, with the pin exiting distally without significant damage to the carpus. Benefits of IM pins include the relatively low cost of the implants, and placing pins does not require a significant investment of specialized equipment. Biomechanical advantages of IM pins include resistance to bending in all directions and placement in the center of the bone is biomechanically advantageous, particularly in comminuted fractures where a fracture gap is present. Disadvantages of IM pins include poor resistance to axial loads and rotational forces; these pins should always be combined with another form of fixation to counteract these forces. Pins can be used in combination with plates, orthopedic wire, or external skeletal fixators. The most common pins used in veterinary medicine are K wires and Steinmann pins. K wires are available in sizes from 0.028 to 0.062 inch and Steinmann pins are available from 1/16 to 1/4 inch, making them versatile for patients of many different sizes. In very small patients, spinal needles can be used as IM pins; they are available in multiple sizes as small as 25 gauge.[186]

IM polymer rods have similar properties to IM pins and are still used in some exotic species.[178] These pins can be made from high-density polymer rods or polypropylene welding rods. These are lightweight (13% lighter than stainless steel), easily sterilized, and inexpensive. These rods can be inserted using a shuttle technique and do not interfere with joint function, since neither end penetrates the proximal or distal cortex. The polymer rods are not as stiff as stainless steel, and micromotion may occur at the fracture site and delay healing. Other disadvantages include the technical difficulty in applying these rods, the length of the pin is limited to the length of the longer fracture fragment, and removal, if required, would necessitate an osteotomy because the rod will be completely imbedded within the diaphysis.

Orthopedic wire has many applications in fracture repair. The most common uses for orthopedic wire in fracture fixation are for cerclage (or hemicerclage) wire and interfragmentary wire. Cerclage wire can be used in long oblique or spiral fractures where the length of the fracture line is at least twice the diameter of the bone and the entire boney column can be reconstructed. Cerclage wire should never be used as a sole method of fixation, but properly placed cerclage wire can provide interfragmentary compression and counteract rotational and axial forces when combined with an IM pin. Rules for the use of cerclage wires include placing a minimum of two wires and spacing them the appropriate distance from each other and from the fracture ends. Cerclage wires are often applied improperly, which can have negative impacts on fracture reduction and bone healing. If the boney column is not reconstructed or if soft tissue is trapped between the wire and the bone, the wires will loosen and decrease fracture stability and disrupt the periosteal blood supply. Hemicerclage wire and interfragmentary wire are utilized in certain short oblique and transverse fractures to prevent rotation, secure bone fragments, and stabilize fissures.

Interlocking nails are pins placed in the medullary canal and locked in place with screws or bolts placed through the proximal and distal fracture fragments. These screws or bolts also pass through special holes within the nail to allow the interlocking nails to counteract all forces acting on the fracture. The pin itself resists bending in a similar fashion as an IM pin, and the screws or bolts passing through cortices into the nail counteract rotation and axial forces. Like IM pins, the use of interlocking nails is contraindicated for the radius, although it can be used for other diaphyseal bone fractures. The largest nail that fits in the medullary canal should be used. Many different sizes are available, ranging from 4.0 to 10 mm, although for most exotic animals the surgeon will be limited to the 4.0-mm nails.

Stabilization of fractures with bone plates and screws is one of the most common methods of internal fixation for diaphyseal fractures. The goal of fixation with bone plates and screws is to achieve early return to function and decreased morbidity that can be seen with other fixation systems. Implant design and application methods are adapting to decrease surgical trauma and maintain optimal bone biology to augment fracture healing.

Plates can be load-sharing or -bearing devices. Neutralization plates neutralize the physiologic forces acting on a section of bone that has been anatomically reconstructed and stabilized. Indications for neutralization include reducible comminuted fractures and long oblique fractures. Compression can be achieved through proper use of a compression plate. Compressing the fragments together will eliminate any gap at the fracture and lead to direct bone healing with minimal to no callus production. Compression is limited to transverse and short oblique fractures, since compressing long oblique fractures will lead to shear and displacement of the fracture ends. Buttress or bridging plates span a nonreducible comminuted fracture. The function of the plate is to maintain length and alignment and prevent axial deformity by resisting bending, shear, and torsional forces acting on the fracture.

There are a wide variety of plates available in veterinary orthopedic surgery. Semitubular plates, veterinary cuttable plates (VCPs), dynamic compression plates (DCPs), limited contact DCPs (LC-DCP), and locking compression plates (LCPs) have all been used in exotic animals. In general, plates are available in sizes from 1.5-mm round hole to 5.5-mm LCPs. The use of plates in exotic animals is often limited by patient size. A general rule in plate fixation is to limit the size of the screw core diameter to 40% of the width of the bone.[187] Using this guideline, 1.5-mm round hole plates, 1.5- to 2.0-mm VCPs, and 2.0 compression plates can be used in many exotic animals with a minimal bone diameter of 3 mm (Figure 7-15). VCPs are versatile plates that have many properties that make them well suited for use in exotic animals. These plates are available in two sizes (1.5/2.0 and 2.0/2.7) based on the screws that can be used with the plates. They are available in one length of 50 holes and can be cut at the time of surgery, depending on the length of the bone that needs to be plated. The holes are spaced close together to allow a sufficient number of cortices to be captured with screws when small fracture fragments are present, and they can be stacked in situations when increased strength is needed. A major disadvantage of plate fixation is the expense associated with their application. Plating systems require a large initial investment for drills, drill bits, guides, taps, and plate benders in addition to an adequate inventory of implants and screws. This results in higher costs to clients, making plating systems less desirable to many veterinarians. Plating systems also require an extensive approach to the bone, which interrupts the soft tissues around the bone. Minimally invasive

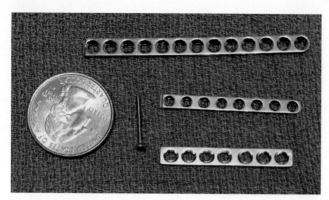

FIGURE 7-15 Bone plates available for small exotic species. A 1.5/2.0-mm VCP, 1.5-mm VCP, and 2.0-mm DCP are shown. A 1.5-mm cortical bone screw is also shown.

plating techniques can minimize the amount of soft tissue disruption and could be applied to certain exotics cases.

External Skeletal Fixation

External Skeletal Fixation requires the placement of two to four transcutaneous pins into each major fracture fragment and connecting those pins to a connecting bar or rod with special clamps. There are a variety of systems available for use in veterinary surgery, with variations on clamp design. The stainless steel fixation pins are inserted through small skin incisions and penetrate both cortices of the proximal and distal major fragments. If the pin only exits the skin on one side of the limb, it is a half pin; however, if it exits the skin on either side of the fracture, it is a full pin. A minimum of two pins and no more than four pins should be placed in each fragment. Any additional pins after the fourth pin will not add any biomechanical advantage and only add to patient morbidity. Threaded pins are recommended over smooth pins to prevent premature loosening, and most current systems utilize positive profile threaded pins. Important principles must be followed when placing fixation pins to maximize results. The pins should be inserted at low revolutions per minutes (rpm; 150 to 300) to minimize any chance for thermal necrosis at the bone implant interface. If the pins are placed at a high speed and there is thermal necrosis, the pins will prematurely loosen as the bone at the implant interface is resorbed. Hand chucks can be used to place the pins; however, this leads to wobble and can also lead to premature loosening. Connecting bars can be made from a variety of materials including carbon fiber, aluminum, titanium, acrylic, PMMA, or epoxy resins. Acrylic, epoxy, and PMMA connecting bars are particularly useful in exotic animals due to their ease of application, low cost, and light weight. Once the fixation pins are in place, various types of tubing (e.g., penrose drains or anesthesia tubing) are filled with acrylic or PMMA while the fracture is held in reduction. Similarly, the epoxy resin can be molded around the fixation pins while the fracture is reduced. The number and configuration of connecting bars can vary depending on the fracture and arrangement of fixation pins. Modifications of the traditional ESF systems such as secured pin intramedullary dorsal epoxy resin (SPIDER) fixators can be applied to exotic species.

A major benefit of ESF systems is their versatility, as they can be used in most long bone fractures, mandibular fractures, and even some spinal fractures. The components are less expensive than plating systems and there is a significant reduction in the equipment required to apply an external fixator. In some cases, an orthopedic drill is helpful, but in many cases, particularly exotic animal cases, fixation pins can be placed using a standard hand chuck. There is also considerable versatility in the systems to allow them to be applied to many different-sized patients. In general, the diameter of the fixation pins should not exceed 25% to 30% of the bone diameter. IMEX Veterinary (Longview, Texas) produces a miniature ESF system with positive profile pins ranging from 0.9 to 2.5 mm that can be used in a variety of small exotic animal patients with bones as narrow as 3.6 mm. These pins can be used with connecting bars and clamps or connected with acrylic or epoxy. In smaller exotic animals, hypodermic needles or spinal needles have been used as fixation pins and connected with epoxy or acrylic.[186,188] The ability to adapt ESF to very small patients, and its affordability, has made ESF a favorite method of fixation among exotic animal veterinarians.

Disadvantages of ESF systems include patient morbidity associated with transcutaneous fixation pins and the need for bandages to protect the fixator. Patient morbidity varies depending on the fracture. ESF placed on the femur has a higher morbidity due to the muscle mass through which the pins must be placed. Bandages for external fixators are important to protect the pins, clamps, and connecting bars and to keep the pin tracts clean. These bandages must be changed and the pin tracts inspected regularly, which can add to costs associated with the treatment.

MANAGEMENT OF TRAUMATIC MUSCULOSKELETAL INJURIES AND FRACTURE MANAGEMENT

Fish

Orthopedic surgical procedures are not commonly performed on fish. There is a single case report describing the repair of a traumatic symphyseal fracture in a moray eel.[189] The authors modified the technique used commonly for similar injuries in mammals. Instead of orthopedic wire, a strand of suture was used and passed through hypodermic needles to stabilize the mandible. In domestic species, intact canine teeth are important to prevent slipping or loosening of the wire. Because eels lack large lower canine teeth, and some teeth were lost due to trauma, a small tunnel was drilled in each hemimandible, and an additional suture was passed through the tunnels and secured.

Reptiles and Amphibians

Traumatic injuries are common in amphibians. These injuries can be associated with inappropriate husbandry, inappropriate handling, or conflict with other animals in the terrarium. Although lacerations and abrasions are more common, skeletal injuries including fractures and traumatic amputations can occur[190] (Figure 7-16). Traumatic amputations can involve the digits, limbs, or tail and can be a result of cage-mate aggression or injury related to the limb being entrapped in

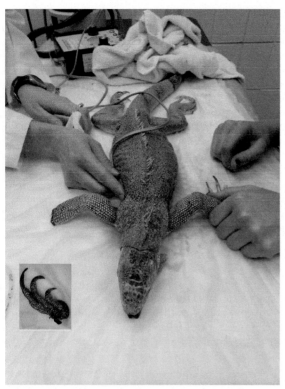

FIGURE 7-16 A green iguana *(Iguana iguana)* with a traumatic amputation of the right distal forelimb due to cagemate aggression.

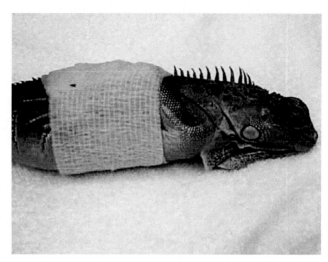

FIGURE 7-17 A forelimb splint in a green iguana *(Iguana iguana).*

the enclosure. In rare cases, this can be due to self-mutilation. Treatment of traumatic amputations is often limited to first aid and administration of antibiotics, if indicated. Direct pressure, hemostatic powders, or ligation of vessels may be needed to stop bleeding, although in most instances, the bleeding has stopped by the time the animal is presented for veterinary care.

A unique aspect of the musculoskeletal system of amphibians, and to a lesser extent reptiles, is the ability to regenerate limbs. The ability of amphibians to regenerate limbs is highest in the larval forms, and the capacity for regeneration decreases as they approach metamorphosis.[68] Adult anurans have limited regenerative abilities; however, the axolotl *(Ambystoma mexicanum)* has been shown to be able to perfectly regenerate complex body parts after experimental amputations into adulthood.[181] Reptiles' regenerative capabilities are limited to tail regeneration in lizards after autonomy.

Many fractures seen in reptiles and amphibians are secondary to MBD, and any individual presenting with a fracture should be closely evaluated for evidence of MBD. Pathologic fractures are often comminuted, although greenstick or folding fractures can also be seen. Successful treatment of these fractures relies heavily on restoring normal calcium metabolism to prevent further bone demineralization. Traumatic fractures can also be seen in reptiles and amphibians and are usually caused by low impact trauma that leads to simple fractures. An exception to this occurs in chelonians that are presented after high impact trauma such as being hit by a car or run over by a lawnmower. These fractures are often open and comminuted with significant soft tissue trauma.

Skeletal injuries may be obvious on initial examination, as in the case of a chelonian after being run over by a car, or they can be very subtle. Postural abnormalities, lameness, swelling, or changes in the alignment of the limbs can be a sign of a fracture or luxation affecting the appendicular skeleton. As with other species, reptiles or amphibians presenting with fractures may have additional injuries; therefore, a complete assessment should be performed. The fracture should only be addressed after any life-threatening abnormalities have been corrected. In most cases, palpation and radiography can be used to confirm the presence of a fracture.

External coaptation is the most common method used for stabilizing fractures in reptiles and amphibians, especially for simple fractures. General principles used for external coaptation in mammals can be applied; however, care must be taken to prevent damage to the fragile skin of amphibians. Also, due to the moist environment that most amphibians require, care must be taken when choosing bandaging materials, since some can swell or shrink when moistened. The bandage should be changed regularly to assess the patient for any skin irritation, and radiographs can be taken to assess the presence of a callus and determine when the bone is healed. Forelimb fractures can be retracted caudally and secured to the lateral body wall in a similar fashion as described for applying a splint (e.g., cast padding, roll gauze, and elastic bandage) (Figure 7-17). If these types of bandages are used, care must be taken not to restrict the animal's breathing. Hind limb fractures can be immobilized by pulling the limb caudally and securing it to the tail (Figure 7-18). Careful application is needed to prevent tail autonomy or incorporation of the vent into the bandage.

The size of most amphibian patients limits our ability to apply orthopedic implants. Amputation is often recommended for the treatment of comminuted or open fractures that would not be amenable to external coaptation.[190,191] Frogs tolerate missing forelimbs and hind limbs, although some functions such as mating and ecdysis may be impaired. Newts and salamanders can regenerate lost limbs, so amputation does not affect their long-term function. There are reports of internal

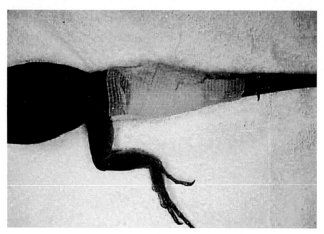

FIGURE 7-18 A rear limb splint in a green iguana *(Iguana iguana).*

fixation used to repair a femur fracture in an American bull-frog and the use of an ESF to repair bilateral tibial fractures in an American bullfrog.[192,193] The femur fracture was repaired using a method not commonly used in other species. Trans-cortical K wires were placed in the fracture fragments and a threaded IM pin was placed alongside the femur. Suture was used to secure the apparatus and then PMMA bone cement was used to cover the apparatus and bond the K wires to the IM pin. This technique resembles an ESF construct that is commonly used in exotic animals when transcortical pins are secured to a PMMA or acrylic connecting bar. In this instance, the connecting bar of PMMA was immediately adjacent to the bone and the soft tissues were closed over the apparatus, with no pins protruding through the skin. This allowed early return to an aquatic environment and also gave some mechanical advantage by minimizing the distance from the fixation construct to the bone. The report using an ESF for the bilateral tibial fractures used small K wires and acrylic connecting bars in a standard fashion.

Traumatic injuries can be seen in wild, farmed, and captive crocodilians. Many of these injuries are the direct result of fights with other individuals.[139] Fractures and amputations can be seen, and in many cases, they will heal without complications. Fracture fixation in crocodilians can be a challenge due to their large size, demeanor, and aquatic environment. Internal fixation with pins, plates, and screws is preferred.

Fractures of the appendicular skeleton in reptiles are often simple fractures that result from low impact forces. In many cases, the fractures are secondary to NSHP and medical management and restoration of calcium homeostasis is an important aspect of fracture treatment. Due to the simple nature of many of these fractures, external coaptation is often successful, especially in cases of NSHP where bone quality is poor. A variety of materials can be used to form splints, depending on the patient size and location of the fracture. Proximal fractures (humerus and femur) in chelonians represent a unique obstacle for external coaptation, since a bandage or splint cannot immobilize the proximal joints. In these cases, the fractured limb can be secured by folding it into a normal position and replacing it into its reduced position within the shell. Open reduction and internal fixation is indicated

for more complicated fractures or those in which external coaptation is not tolerated or possible (e.g., aquatic and semi-aquatic reptiles).[186] Virtually all methods of internal fixation have been applied to reptiles, and the surgical approaches and principles of these techniques are similar to mammals, with some minor differences.[186] When placing ESF constructs in many reptiles, the orientation of the pins should be in a cranial-to-caudal direction that is parallel to the substrate, instead of a medial-to-lateral orientation used in mammals. Bone plating has been performed in larger reptiles. In some species, the long bones are curved, which makes precise plate contouring challenging. For these cases, reconstruction plates that allow contouring in multiple planes may be preferred. An alternative would be to use locking plates since they do not require the plate to be contoured exactly to the surface of the bone.

Shell Fractures

The chelonian shell is a dynamic, metabolically active structure composed of 60 dermal bones covered with keratinized epidermal scutes.[171] Traumatic injuries of the chelonian shell are very common after the patients are hit by cars, run over by lawnmowers, or attacked by dogs or other carnivores.[180] A detailed understanding of anatomy is important because shell fractures can affect other body systems. The ribs, pelvic and pectoral girdles, and spine are incorporated into the shell and fractures can affect all these skeletal components.[180] Chelonians with shell fractures crossing the dorsal midline should be examined carefully for evidence of paresis or paralysis of the hind limbs, as this would carry a guarded-to-grave prognosis. Culture and antibiotic sensitivity testing of the fractured area(s) and antibiotic therapy are crucial for most shell fractures, since they are open fractures and are susceptible to developing osteomyelitis. In addition, many shell fractures communicate with the coelomic cavity and any infection can affect the viscera within the coelomic cavity. Because chelonians do not have a diaphragm, their breathing will not be affected by fractures that penetrate the coelomic cavity. However, any damage or contamination to the lung tissue itself could lead to complications and affect the prognosis. Broad-spectrum antibiotics should be started until the culture and antibiotic sensitivity results are available and aggressive wound therapy should be performed to decrease gross contamination and nonviable tissues. Additional supportive care, including fluid therapy, analgesics, and nutritional support, should also be provided.

There are many different techniques for managing shell fractures. The initial care should be concentrated on triage, stabilization, and wound care. Many traumatic shell injuries are associated with significant wounds (Figure 7-19). Proper wound care with copious lavage and debridement are needed before the shell fracture repair can be planned. Sterile isotonic lavage solutions are preferred; however, chlorhexidine and iodine solutions can be used as long as the proper dilutions are made to prevent cytotoxicity or delays in wound healing. Other wound management techniques used in other species can be applied to chelonians too, including wet-to-dry bandages, sugar bandages, honey bandages, or negative pressure wound therapy, depending on the nature of the wound. Epoxy resin and fiberglass patches were once the standard treatment for shell fractures; however, these methods have been

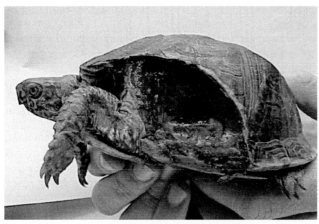

FIGURE 7-19 Traumatic shell injury in a box turtle *(Terrapene carolina).*

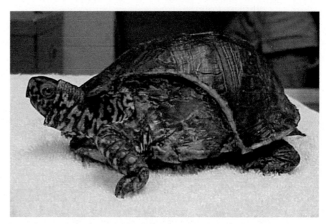

FIGURE 7-21 With time and patience, even extensive shell injuries will heal. The shell of the box turtle *(Terrapene carolina)* in Figure 7-19 completely healed after 6 months of wound management.

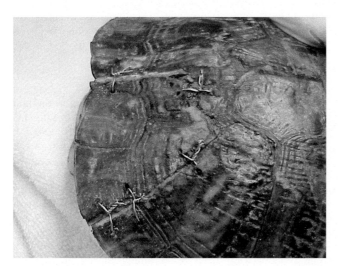

FIGURE 7-20 Orthopedic wire used to reduce a carapacial shell fracture.

associated with abscesses and osteomyelitis that developed underneath the patches, so these techniques are no longer recommended.[194] Many other techniques have been developed using orthopedic screws, orthopedic wire, bone plates, and cable ties. Screws and orthopedic wire are a simple, inexpensive method of reducing a fracture(s) and allowing continued wound care.[195] Bone screws are placed on each side of the fracture and orthopedic wire is wrapped around the screws. As the wire is tightened, it will provide compression across the fracture (Figure 7-20). Similar techniques can be used using epoxy and cable ties.[196] After reduction of the fracture(s), cable tie mounts are epoxied to the opposite sides of the carapace. A cable tie is fed through the ends mounted to the carapace and the end of a second cable tie and then secured. With either technique, the wounds can be treated as the fractures heal and the implants can be easily removed. Once radiographs and follow-up examinations determine when the shell fracture is healed, the surgical hardware can be removed. Shell fractures in chelonians can take 3 to 6 months to heal (Figure 7-21).

Birds

Orthopedic injuries are common in companion birds and result from falls; impact with windows, walls, or ceiling fans; or from crushing injuries such as being stepped on or bites from dogs or cats.[197,198] Like most other species, the orthopedic injuries themselves are not life threatening and patient stabilization is important before considering any orthopedic repair.[178] Once the patient is stabilized, a systemic orthopedic exam can be performed to localize the location of the injury. In many cases, the location is apparent, but other injuries may be more subtle. Symmetry, range of motion, ability to perch, proper positioning of the wings, and overall body posture can be used to assess for abnormalities. Careful palpation for swelling, pain, and crepitus along all long bones can be done to determine where the problems are, and all joints should be assessed for normal range of motion. If the injury is unilateral, the contralateral limb can be used for comparison, especially for subtle injuries or for those with less experience in avian palpation.

Once the orthopedic exam is complete, radiographs can be used to confirm the presence of any fractures and a plan for fracture management can be developed. Options for fracture repair include all the methods previously covered. Species, size, location of the fracture, and fracture configuration are all important determinants when developing a fracture management plan. Although avian bones have been described as being brittle and having thin cortices that are difficult to work with, there are reports of the successful management of avian fractures with nearly all types of fixation methods.[178] Early return to function is important to prevent scarring, contracture, ankylosis, or adhesions that may affect long-term function.[178,198]

External Coaptation

Several specific bandaging techniques are available for managing musculoskeletal injuries in birds. Figure-of-eight bandages, tape splints, ball bandages, and snowshoe splints can all be applied to immobilize fractures (Figure 7-22).[14] A figure-of-eight bandage is one of the most common bandages applied to birds, and it can be used to immobilize the wing

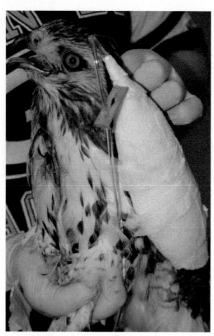

FIGURE 7-22 A figure-eight bandage used to immobilize the left wing of a red-tailed hawk (Buteo jamaicensis).

for fractures of the pectoral girdle and select fractures of the long bones of the thoracic limb. Proper application is important and mistakes are commonly made when applying a figure-of-eight bandage.[14]

Splinting can be used in selected fractures; however, cases in which splints are used should be critically evaluated to ensure splinting is the most appropriate choice. Many fractures are splinted when there are better options, and in some cases, splinting may be detrimental. Tape splints can be used to immobilize fractures of the tibiotarsus or tarsometatarsus on very small birds weighing up to 150 g. Once the fracture is reduced, a piece of tape is applied to one side of the limb, with the joints above and below incorporated into the tape area. The tape is then folded over to immobilize the fracture. Additional support (e.g., paper clip, wooden dowel) can be added to the tape.[14] Ball bandages and snowshoe splints can be applied to immobilize digit fractures. Ball bandages are made by placing 2 × 2 or 4 × 4 gauze pads in a wad and placing them under the foot (with the toes grasping the material). Elastic bandage can then be wrapped around the foot to secure the bandage. Shoe splints can be made using tongue depressors. The toes are extended (flattened) and taped to the tongue depressor.

Internal Fixation

Optimum results for anatomic fracture healing and normal limb function occurs with internal fixation.[178] Although the principles of fracture repair in birds are similar to other species, the calcium content of avian bone is higher than mammals to allow for thinner, stronger cortices. This important adaptation to produce a strong lightweight skeleton necessary for flight also leads to brittle bones that shatter and lead to comminuted fractures. IM pins, cerclage wire, and plates can all be applied to avian long bone fractures. Unlike many mammals where a majority of implants are left in place, the increased weight of stainless steel implants can impair a

bird's ability to fly and implant removal is often recommended.[178] Other materials have been used in place of IM pins to help reduce the weight of the implants, including polypropylene rods and high-density polymer rods. These rods are inert, easily sterilized, do not need to be removed after the fracture is healed, and weigh 13% of the weight of a comparably sized stainless steel IM pin. Because of the sizes available, polymer rods are not intended for fracture fixation in birds that weigh <75 g.[178]

The use of bone plates for fracture repair in birds has historically been discouraged, but many successful cases of bone plating have been described.[178] Bone plate fixation offers early return to function with reduced callus formation, which are important features to consider when repairing fractures in birds. Semitubular plates, VCPs, DCPs, LC-LDPs, and LCPs have all been used to manage fractures in birds. Some special considerations have to be made when repairing fractures in birds to prevent complications. Drill bits used for avian fractures must be sharp and straight, with no wobble. If dull drill bits are used, they often require added pressure during drilling and can lead to iatrogenic fractures. Any wobble or bends in the drill bit can also lead to iatrogenic fractures or decreased pullout strength of the implants.

External Skeletal Fixation

The use of linear and hybrid ESF is a very common method for fracture management in birds. In many fractures, an IM pin can be incorporated into the ESF to increase the strength of the construct. Acrylic or PMMA connecting bars are popular with bird cases due to their light weight, ease of application, and reduced costs, since special fixator clamps are not needed.[197] As previously mentioned, positive profile pins are available in many sizes and can accommodate patients with bones as narrow as 3.6 mm.

Specific Fractures of the Thoracic Limb

The avian pectoral girdle is commonly injured when a bird flies into an object such as a window or wall. Coracoid fractures are often managed with a figure-of-eight bandage combined with a body wrap for approximately 3 weeks and then assessed radiographically for union.[197,199] Regular physical therapy is important in order to prevent contraction of the patagium, which would prohibit normal wing extension following healing of the coracoid fracture. In rare cases, internal fixation using IM pinning or plating (Figures 7-23 and 7-24) can be performed, especially if return to normal flight is essential, although there is the potential for significant morbidity with the surgical approach.[178] Fractures of the clavicle and scapula are less common than coracoid fractures, but they are treated in a similar manner.

Proximal humeral fractures can also be managed using a figure-eight bandage combined with a body wrap. However, fractures managed in this manner may result in rotational deformity due to the pull of the strong pectoral muscles on the proximal fragment, leading to a malunion and decreased flight ability.[178,199] If return to flight is essential, or if there is significant displacement, open reduction and fixation with cross pins or a tension band can be performed.[197] Figure-eight bandages are not appropriate for mid-diaphyseal and distal humeral fractures; instead, these are ideally managed with ESF or internal fixation.[184,197,199] IM pins placed in the humerus should be placed in a retrograde manner, with the tip of the

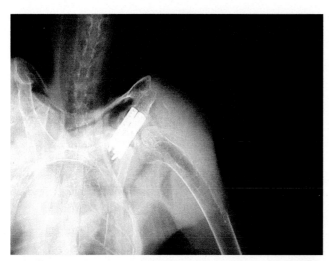

FIGURE 7-23 Ventro-dorsal radiographic image of a repaired coracoid fracture using bone plates.

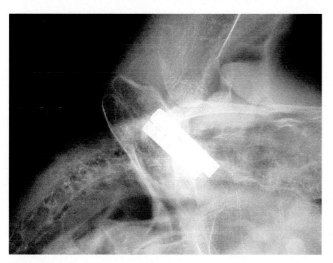

FIGURE 7-24 Lateral radiographic image of a repaired coracoid fracture using bone plates.

pin exiting the deltoid crest. Distal humeral fractures can be treated with cross pins.[178] Care must be taken when placing percutaneous ESF pins in the humerus. Many important neurovascular structures are present on the medial and lateral aspects of the humerus, and safe corridors for pin placement have not been established in birds.

Fractures of the radius and ulna can be managed in a variety of ways depending on the fracture configuration. External coaptation can be used if the radius *or* the ulna is fractured, the other bone is intact, and the fractured bone is minimally displaced.[178,199] The intact bone will help keep the fractured bone in proper alignment and will aid in stability of the fracture during healing. Some proximal radial fractures can be managed conservatively with a figure-of-eight bandage due to the large muscle mass that overlies the bone. This mass of tissue will help with apposition, alignment, and blood supply. External coaptation should be used for 2 to 3 weeks and then rehabilitation initiated. In most cases, wraps can be removed after 3 to 4 weeks.[197,199] If the radius and ulna are both fractured, there is poor alignment, or if they are nonreducible, ESF or internal fixation is indicated. Fixation of both

bones is not required, and fixation of the radius alone is often sufficient; however, stabilizing both bones will lead to decreased healing times.[197] Unlike most other species where IM pin placement in the radius is contraindicated, an IM pin can be placed in a retrograde manner, aimed distally while the carpus is held in flexion. The IM pin will exit just cranial to the carpal joint and therefore not lead to complications from penetrating the joint. IM pins in the ulna should be placed in a normograde fashion from a point distal to the elbow and aimed distally. Care must be taken not to penetrate the distal cortex and cause iatrogenic trauma to the carpus.[178] A unique complication of radius and ulnar fractures in birds that can be clinically important is the development of synostosis between the radius and ulna. Rotation of the radius around the ulna is necessary for proper lift and descent during flight. If a synostosis forms and rotation is restricted, patients may not return to normal flight.[197,199] Plating often results in superior stability that can reduce callus formation and potentially reduce the risk of synostosis. However, the size of the patient may limit a surgeon's ability to place a plate. One study evaluating maxillofacial plating systems for use in radius and ulnar fractures in birds showed that the smaller plates were not designed to counteract the loads on the ulna and there was a high incidence of implant failure.[200]

Fractures of the carpometacarpal bones are usually high impact injuries and present as comminuted, open fractures that are more difficult to treat than other long bone fractures. An additional complicating factor is the lack of soft tissue coverage. External coaptation, ESF with IM pins, and combinations of these treatments have been described.[197,199] IM pins in the metacarpus can be inserted in a normograde fashion, but care must be taken to prevent iatrogenic trauma to the carpus.[178] Careful soft tissue dissection in this area is critical to prevent necrosis of the wing distal to the carpus if the vascular supply is compromised.[178]

Specific Fractures of the Pelvic Limb

Pelvis and synsacrum fractures can lead to neurologic abnormalities, and surgery for these types of injuries is often performed to free entrapped nerves. Prognosis is favorable with simple fractures.[198]

Fractures of the proximal femur, including the femoral head and neck, can be managed with femoral head and neck ostectomies; there is a good prognosis for return to normal function in these cases.[201] Some fractures of the femur can be managed with external coaptation, such as spica splints or modified Ehmer slings, although this will not counteract all forces acting on the fracture, since the hip joint is very difficult to immobilize and may be better suited as an addition to internal fixation techniques such as IM pinning.[178] Many diaphyseal fractures can be repaired using a combination of IM pins and ESF. Normograde or retrograde pinning of the femur can be done, although normograde pinning may decrease the risk of sciatic entrapment.[178] ESF pins should be placed from craniolateral to caudomedial to avoid important neurovascular bundles. Proximal pins should be placed just distal to the dorsal acetabular rim and distal pins through the condyles.[197] Plating can be used in selected patients based on fracture configuration and patient size. Distal fractures can be repaired using cross pins.[178,198]

The tibiotarsus is the most commonly fractured long bone of the avian pelvic limb.[178,197,198] Fractures of the tibiotarsus are most often repaired using an IM pin with the addition of an ESF to prevent rotation. In birds weighing less than 150 g, IM pins and external coaptation can be used.[197] IM pin placement in the tibiotarsus can be done either normograde or retrograde, although normograde placement starting at the craniomedial aspect of the proximal tibia is preferred and well tolerated by patients. Other options include plates, Schroeder-Thomas splints, and interlocking nails (Figure 7-25). Distal tibiotarsal fractures can be challenging due to the small size of the distal fracture fragment. A transarticular SPIDER ESF was successfully used in an American coot (*Fulica americana*) by the author (Figure 7-26).

Tarsometatarsal fractures can be repaired with ESF or splints. IM pinning is difficult in this bone, because there are no good points of entry.[178] Care must be taken to prevent damage to the flexor tendons, and postoperatively the toes should be able to move freely to prevent entrapment of the flexor tendons in the callus.

Phalangeal fractures can be managed with splints or ball bandages; however, this can lead to adhesion formation between the flexor tendons and surrounding tissues resulting in immobility of the affected digits. Cage rest without rigid fixation can be used for simple closed fractures. Compound fractures have a poor prognosis and digit amputation is sometimes required.[198]

Complications noted with pelvic limb fractures in birds are similar to those reported in other species, including malunions, nonunions, delayed unions, and osteomyelitis. Bumblefoot (pododermatitis) is a complication that can be seen after a traumatic injury that is unique to birds. Any injury to a pelvic limb will cause increased weight bearing on the contralateral limb. This results in increased pressure on the plantar aspect of the foot and the formation of pressure sores.[198] Poor diet, obesity, lack of exercise, and hard perching surfaces can also lead to the development of bumblefoot. Bumblefoot typically starts as mild erythematous lesions, but can quickly progress to abscessation and full-thickness skin ulcerations. In severe cases, the tendons and tendon sheaths become infected, osteomyelitis develops, and septic arthritis occurs. Any practitioner repairing fractures or other injuries of the pelvic limb should be aware of the risk of bumblefoot developing and take precautions to prevent formation of lesions, such as controlling calorie intake and providing perches with artificial turf and padding. Treatment of bumblefoot is aimed at alleviating any pressure from the affected area of the foot and treating any wounds or infections. Covering perches with astroturf or similar carpeting will create a surface that constantly shifts pressure to different areas of the foot; ball bandages can also be used to redistribute pressure away from the plantar aspect of the foot.[198] Standard wound care techniques can be used to promote healing; however, in some cases surgery may be needed to close the defect. In large defects, single pedicle advancement flaps created from the webbing can be used.

The prognosis for a fractured bone in a bird is variable and depends on the intended function of the patient following surgical repair. Pet birds and birds intended to remain in captivity have a good prognosis, since return to normal flight is not an absolute necessity. Any wildlife in which return to

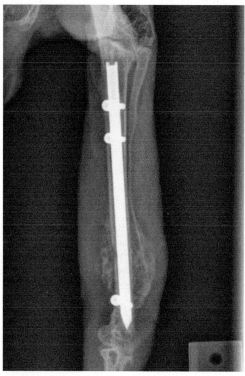

FIGURE 7-25 A postoperative radiograph showing the use of an interlocking nail to repair a tibiotarsal fracture in a red-tailed hawk (*Buteo jamaicensis*).

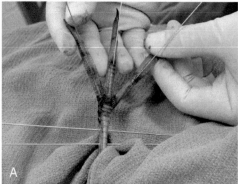
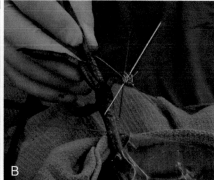
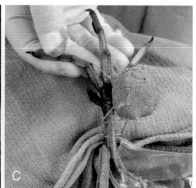

FIGURE 7-26 *A-C.* Intraoperative images showing the application of a secured pin intramedullary dorsal epoxy resin (SPIDER) fixator in an American coot (*Fulica americana*).

the wild is the ultimate goal require few, if any, imperfections in the repair or healing process. In 51 surgically treated humeral fractures in raptors, only 18 healed and only 12 achieved full flight.[202] Similarly, malunions of the pelvic limbs may affect the bird's ability to hunt or obtain food. In 18 surgically treated tibiotarsal fractures, only four birds were released.[202] Articular fractures carry a guarded-to-grave prognosis because most will have long-term effects on joint function, ranging from development of osteoarthritis to ankylosis. Open fractures also have a worse prognosis due to the development of osteomyelitis. Fractures of the distal extremities have a more guarded prognosis due to the tenuous blood supply and scarcity of soft tissue to provide extraosseous blood supply to aid in healing.[178]

Mammals

Fractures are common in exotic small mammals due to their size and delicate skeletons. Falls, getting stepped on, bites from other animals, and getting limbs caught in cages are all common traumatic injuries that can lead to fractures. Fracture management in exotic small mammals is based on the same principles used for dogs and cats. In addition, many exotic small mammals, particularly rabbits, have been extensively used as models of fracture repair and bone healing for humans, and some controlled studies have been performed specifically investigating fracture management in these species.[153,154,203] As with any animal that has sustained a traumatic injury, systemic life-threatening problems should be identified and addressed before moving on to the orthopedic injuries that may be present. Any signs of shock should be treated, neurologic injuries assessed, and appropriate pain management administered. Keep in mind that most exotic small mammals are prey species that respond to stress and pain stimuli in different manners from other species such as dogs and cats. It is very important to minimize stress and to anticipate analgesic needs of the patients, even though they may not be overtly showing signs of pain.[154] Any obvious fractures can be stabilized with a simple splint while a systemic evaluation is performed. Once the patient is stabilized, a systematic orthopedic examination can be completed and radiographs of any areas of instability, pain, crepitus, swelling, or other signs consistent with a fracture can be performed.

The methods of fracture fixation used in other species can be adapted to exotic small mammals. The method selected should be based on the availability of the fixation system, costs, surgeon's experience, species, and patient size. As previously mentioned, there is considerable variation in bone structure between species. Some mammals have well-developed haversian systems, while others, especially rodents, have primitive bone systems. These differences may affect how the bone heals and may play a role in how the fracture is best treated.

External coaptation is an important aspect of fracture management in exotic small mammals, especially in species that are too small for commercially available orthopedic implants. Basic principles of external coaptation can be applied to exotic small mammals. The joint proximal and distal to the fracture must be immobilized, and there are many different types of materials that can be used to provide rigid immobilization. There are also a number of potential complications associated with external coaptation that should be considered, including delayed union, nonunions, and malunions. Splints and bandages can also lead to extensive wounds that may be more devastating than the original fracture. Care must be taken during splint application to supply adequate padding to avoid pressure sores and prevent any constriction of the extremity that can affect venous drainage or perfusion to the distal limb. Regular bandage changes are important to catch any developing wounds so that they can be treated and the bandage can be adapted to prevent further skin irritation. The owners must carefully monitor their pet to ensure that there are no sudden changes in discomfort or pain associated with the bandage, and they must be instructed to keep the bandage clean and dry at all times.

IM pinning can be done in many of the different exotic small mammals presented to veterinarians. K wires are available as small as 0.028 inches (0.071 cm), making IM pinning possible in very small patients. When placing IM pins, 70% of the medullary canal should be filled; therefore, a 0.028-inch K wire can be inserted into a medullary canal as small as 1 to 2 mm. External coaptation, cerclage wire, hemicerclage wire, and simple ESF frames can be added to IM pins to counteract all forces acting on the fracture site.

Bone plates have been used in many small mammals. Due to patient size, 1.5/2.0 veterinary cuttable plates are most commonly used. Other plates such as 2.0/2.7 veterinary cuttable plates and 2.0 DCP or LC-DCP plates can also be used; however, these plates may be too stiff for smaller species.

ESF is versatile and can be adapted to many different species and fracture configurations. Because of its relative low cost compared with plating systems, ESF is one of the most commonly used methods for fracture fixation in exotic small mammal orthopedics (Figure 7-27). It is important to remember the principles for insertion of the fixation pins to achieve the best results and limit patient morbidity. Commercially available ESF systems can be used in many exotic small mammals; however, in cases where the patients are too small for these systems, ESF can be constructed from spinal needles or hypodermic needles and acrylic.

REPAIR OF SPECIFIC FRACTURES

Fractures of the thoracic limb can involve any bone from the scapula to the digits. Scapular fractures are usually managed conservatively unless the articular surface of the glenoid cavity is involved. Anatomic reduction is preferred to minimize the changes to the articular surface that can lead to secondary degenerative joint disease. For these types of fractures, open reduction and stabilization with pins and wire are recommended.

Humeral fractures can occur at the proximal physis, diaphysis, and distal metaphysis. Because the humerus is located adjacent to the thoracic cavity, a careful assessment of the thoracic cavity should be performed, and radiographic evaluation of the thorax is recommended with most humeral fractures. Rib fractures, pulmonary contusions, and pneumothorax damage are commonly associated with trauma to the thoracic limb. Proximal physeal fractures are reduced and stabilized with cross pins to minimize disruption to the growth plate. Diaphyseal fractures are common and can pose a challenge to even experienced orthopedic surgeons. External coaptation is avoided, if possible, because it is difficult to

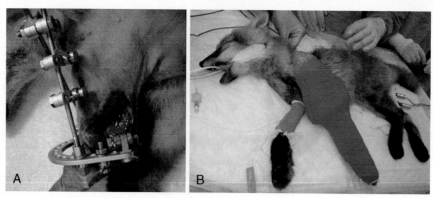

FIGURE 7-27 The application of a hybrid external fixator in a red fox *(Vulpes vulpes)*. A hybrid fixator was chosen due to the proximity of the fracture to the elbow joint. An ESF is also advantageous in traumatic open fractures with large wounds.

adequately immobilize the shoulder joint, and malunions are possible.

A careful review of the anatomy is important prior to any attempts at surgical stabilization. Along the medial diaphysis are many important neurovascular structures, including the brachial artery and vein and the median, ulnar, and musculo-cutaneous nerves. Laterally, the radial nerve courses across the distal diaphysis.[204] Diaphyseal fractures can be repaired with bone plates or ESF. Bone plates can be applied to the medial, lateral, or cranial surface of the bone and can be challenging due to the shape of the humerus. If an ESF is chosen, care must be taken to avoid the previously mentioned neurovascular structures when the fixation pins are placed.

Radial fractures are commonly reported in mammals. Because there is minimal soft tissue coverage over the distal radius, open radial fractures are frequently observed. In general, the radius is the primary weight-bearing bone in mammals, and fractures of the ulna are not specifically addressed unless the articular surface of the elbow is involved or there is a displaced fracture of the olecranon. These can be managed with bone plates or a pin and tension band. Radial fractures can be repaired using external coaptation, bone plates, and ESF. In toy-breed dogs, much like exotic small mammals, there is a higher incidence of nonunions for distal radial and ulnar fractures because of a lack of soft tissue coverage and a poor extraosseous blood supply during healing. External coaptation is not recommended for these types of injuries. IM pinning in the radius cannot be performed without passing through the carpus or elbow; this is therefore also not recommended. Plates are a recommended method of managing these injuries and they can be applied to the cranial or medial surface of the radius. Although applying bone plates on the medial aspect can have a biomechanical advantage, cranial application is easier in exotic small mammals. Type-Ib ESF is most commonly used in radial fractures, although type-Ia or type-II ESF can be used.

Metacarpal fractures are less commonly seen in exotic small mammals than in dogs or cats. Most of these injuries can be managed with splints or soft padded bandages. Internal fixation is usually not possible due to the small size of the bone. Digit amputation may be necessary in cases with chronic pain or arthritis secondary to articular damage or ligamentous injuries.

Fractures of the pelvic limb can involve the pelvis, coxo-femoral joint, femur, or tibia and fibula. Pelvic fractures can appear dramatic and daunting on radiographs because multiple fractures are always present. However, in most cases, only fractures of the weight-bearing arch need to be repaired. This represents acetabular fractures, fractures of the ilium, and fractures or luxations of the sacrum or sacroiliac joint. Fractures of the pubis are rarely repaired unless there is an avulsion of the prepubic tendon and herniation of the urinary bladder. Ischial fractures are rarely addressed. Although surgery may be the preferred treatment, most cases with pelvic fractures can be managed conservatively. Malunions that form can lead to narrowing of the pelvic canal and dystocia or chronic constipation. Ilial body fractures should be repaired with bone plates or interfragmentary wire in exotic small mammals. Acetabular fractures can be repaired with bone plates, pins, and PMMA, or, in situations where the patient is too small for implants or the fracture is comminuted and anatomic reduction is not possible, a femoral head and neck ostectomy (FHO).

Femoral fractures can involve the capital physis, femoral neck, diaphysis, and distal metaphysis and physis. Most cases of capital physeal or femoral neck fractures in exotic small mammals must be managed with an FHO due to patient size; these patients have a good prognosis with this procedure. External coaptation of diaphyseal fractures is to be avoided due to the significant displacement that is often seen in femoral fractures and the inability to immobilize the hip joint. Diaphyseal fractures of the femur can be managed with plates, ESF, IM pins, or a combination of implants. Care must be taken when placing IM pins to avoid the sciatic nerve, as it courses over the trochanteric fossa. Bone plates are applied to the lateral surface of the femur to avoid neurovascular structures on the medial side and also to take advantage of the biomechanical advantage of plating the tension surface of the bone. ESF pins are placed through the lateral aspect of the femur; one disadvantage of ESF in the femur is the high morbidity associated with pin placement through the musculature of the hind limb. Distal metaphyseal and physeal fractures can be treated with cross pins.

Tibial fractures, similar to radial fractures, are commonly open fractures due to the lack of soft tissue covering most of the medial aspect of the tibia. Tibial fractures can be treated with external coaptation, IM pins, bones plates, ESF, or interlocking nails. IM pins and interlocking nails can be inserted in a normograde fashion through a small medial parapatellar incision. The pin is placed cranial to the tibial plateau on the medial side of the tibial epiphysis and directed distally. Bone plates and ESF fixation pins are placed medially to avoid the musculature on the lateral aspect of the tibia. Careful dissection is needed to avoid the medial saphenous artery, vein, and nerve, as they cross the medial tibial diaphysis. Metatarsal and digit fractures are managed in a similar fashion to metacarpal fractures.

Complications associated with fracture repair can occur due to inappropriate choice of implants, improper placement of the implants, poor owner compliance with postoperative instructions, or in some cases bad luck. Delayed unions, nonunions, and malunions can all occur. Depending on the severity of the complication, treatment may not be required, the fracture may need revision, or, in the worst case, amputation may be needed. In general, exotic small mammal patients tolerate amputation well and techniques for amputations are adapted from dogs and cats. Leaving a stump generally leads to repetitive trauma and should be avoided if possible. Forelimb amputations should be done at the shoulder joint or in addition to the removal of the scapula. Hind limb amputation should be done at the level of the proximal femoral diaphysis or by disarticulation of the coxofemoral joint.

MISCELLANEOUS

Amphibians

Congenital anomalies such as limb deformities and supernumerary limbs can affect the musculoskeletal system of amphibians. While many of these reports occur in wild populations, some of these species are kept by hobbyists and there are some reports of similar defects in captive larvae.[68] In anurans, supernumerary limbs have been linked to dermal penetration and encystment of trematodes, although irradiation of sperm or eggs has also been shown to produce supernumerary limbs experimentally.[205] Many different congenital limb deformities were reported in wild populations of northern crested newts *(Triturus cristatus)*. Up to 35% of the otherwise healthy population was affected and had defects of the distal limbs. Defects included supernumerary phalanges, fused carpal bones, and distorted phalanges. Another population of firebelly newts *(Cynops orientalis)* also showed defects, including supernumerary limbs, digits, and tails in some animals and missing limbs or digits in others. Sixty percent of individuals in a population of western slimy salamanders *(Plethodon albagula)* were found to have deformities of the distal limbs, including syndactyly and duplication of the carpi and digits. Nearby populations of the same salamanders were unaffected. The cause of these abnormalities is not known, but elevated water temperatures, water pH, and toxins have been implicated.

Reptile

Congenital abnormalities of the musculoskeletal system have also been documented in crocodilians.[139] Deformities of the head, limbs, and tail have been seen and are believed to be associated with incubation temperature rather than genetics.

REFERENCES

1. Zachariah T, Mitchell M. Invertebrates. In: Mitchell M, Tully T, eds. *Manual of Exotic Pet Practice*. St. Louis: Saunders; 2009.
2. Pizzi R. Spiders. In: Lewbart G, ed. *Invertebrate Medicine*. Oxford: Wiley-Blackwell; 2012:187-221.
3. Miller S, Mitchell M. Ornamental fish. In: Mitchell M, Tully T, eds. *Manual of Exotic Pet Practice*. St. Louis: Saunders; 2009.
4. Stoskopf M. Anatomy. In: Stoskopf M, ed. *Fish Medicine*. Philadelphia: WB Saunders; 1993:2-4.
5. Stoskopf M. Fish Histology. In: Stoskopf M, ed. *Fish Medicine*. Philadelphia: Saunders; 1993:33-35.
6. Mylniczenko, N. Amphibians. In: Mitchell M, Tully T, eds. *Manual of Exotic Pet Practice*. St. Louis: Saunders; 2009.
7. Wright K. Anatomy for the clinician. In: Wright K, Whitaker B, eds. *Amphibian Medicine and Captive Husbandry*. Malabar, FL: Krieger; 2001.
8. Mitchell M. Snakes. In: Mitchell M, Tully T, eds. *Manual of Exotic Pet Practice*. St. Louis: Saunders; 2009.
9. Funk R. Snakes. In: Mader D, ed. *Reptile Medicine and Surgery*. St. Louis: Saunders; 2006:42-58.
10. Nevarez J. Lizards. In: Mitchell M, Tully T, eds. *Manual of Exotic Pet Practice*. St. Louis: Saunders; 2009.
11. Barten SL. Lizards. In: Mader D, ed. *Reptile Medicine and Surgery*. St. Louis: Saunders; 2006:59-77.
12. Kirchgessner M, Mitchell M. Chelonians. In: Mitchell M, Tully T, eds. *Manual of Exotic Pet Practice*. St. Louis: Saunders; 2009.
13. Boyer T, Boyer D. Turtles, tortoises, and terrapins. In: Mader D, ed. *Reptile Medicine and Surgery*. St. Louis: Saunders; 2006:78-99.
14. Tully T. Birds. In: Mitchell M, Tully T, eds. *Manual of Exotic Pet Practice*. St. Louis: Saunders; 2009:250-298.
15. Macwhirter P. Basic anatomy, physiology and nutrition. In: Tully T, Dorrenstein G, Jones A, eds. *Handbook of Avian Medicine*. Edinburgh: Saunders; 2009:25-55.
16. Dyce K, Sack W, Wensing C. Avian anatomy. In: *Textbook of Veterinary Anatomy*. Philadelphia: Saunders; 2002:799-824.
17. Krautwald-Junghanns M, Pees M. Imaging techniques. In: Tully T, Dorrenstein G, Jones A, eds. *Handbook of Avian Medicine*. Edinburgh: Saunders; 2009:85-100.
18. Powers L, Brown S. Basic anatomy, physiology, and husbandry. In: Quesenberry K, Carpenter J, eds. *Ferrets, Rabbits, and Rodents: Clinical Medicine and Surgery*. St. Louis: Elsevier; 2012:1-12.
19. Vella D, Donnelly T. Basic anatomy, physiology, and husbandry. In: Quesenberry K, Carpenter J, eds. *Ferrets, Rabbits, and Rodents: Clinical Medicine and Surgery*. 3rd ed. St. Louis: Elsevier; 2012: 157-173.
20. Vennen K, Mitchell M. Rabbits. In: Mitchell M, Tully T, eds. *Manual of Exotic Pet Practice*. St. Louis: Saunders; 2009:375-405.
21. Abou-Madi N, Scrivani PV, Kollias GV, et al. Diagnosis of skeletal injuries in chelonians using computed tomography. *J Zoo Wildl Med.* 2004;35:226-231.
22. Popesko P, Rajtova V, Horak J. *A Colour Atlas of the Anatomy of Small Laboratory Animals: Rat, Mouse, and Hamster.* Vol 2. Bratislava: Wolfe Publishing; 1992.
23. Popesko P, Rajtova V, Horak J. *A Colour Atlas of the Anatomy of Small Laboratory Animals: Rabbit and Guniea Pig.* Vol 1. Bratislava: Wolfe Publishing; 1992.
24. Chitty J. Myriapods (centipedes and millipedes). In: Lewbart G, ed. *Invertebrate Medicine*. Oxford: Wiley-Blackwell; 2012:255-265.
25. Williams J. Orthopedic radiography in exotic animal practice. *Vet Clin North Am Exot Anim Pract.* 2001;5(1):1-22.
26. Stetter M. Diagnostic imaging of amphibians. In: Whitaker B, Wright K, eds. *Amphibian Medicine and Captive Husbandry*. Malabar, FL: Krieger; 2001:253-272.
27. Doneley B. Clinical techniques. In: Doneley B, ed. *Avian Medicine and Surgery in Practice: Companion and Aviary Birds*. London: Manson; 2011:55-68.

28. Silverman S. Diagnostic imaging. In: Mader D, ed. *Reptile Medicine and Surgery*. St. Louis: Saunders; 2006:471-489.
29. Hernandez-Divers S. Diagnostic techniques. In: Mader D, ed. *Reptile Medicine and Surgery*. St. Louis: Saunders; 2006:490-532.
30. Alleman A, Kupprion E. Cytologic diagnosis of disease in reptiles. *Vet Clin North Am Exot Anim Pract*. 2007;10(1):155-186.
31. Schenck P, Chew DJ, Nagode LA, et al. Disorders of calcium: hypercalcemia and hypocalcemia. In: Dibartola S, ed. *Fluid, Electrolyte, and Acid-Base Disorders in Small Animal Practice*. St. Louis: Saunders; 2006:120-194.
32. Donoghue S. Nutrition. In: Mader D, ed. *Reptile Medicine and Surgery*. St. Louis: Saunders; 2006.
33. McDonald D. Nutritional considerations. In: Harrison G, Lightfoot T, eds. *Clinical Avian Medicine*. Palm Beach, FL: Spix; 2006: 86-107.
34. Klaphake E. A fresh look at metabolic bone disease in reptiles and amphibians. *Vet Clin North Am Exot Anim Pract*. 2010;13(3):375-392.
35. Mader D. Metabolic bone disease. In: Mader D, ed. *Reptile Medicine and Surgery*. St. Louis: Saunders; 2006.
36. Acierno MJ, Mitchell MA, Zachariah TT, et al. Effects of ultraviolet radiation on plasma 25-hydroxyvitamin D3 concentrations in corn snakes (*Elaphe guttata*). *Am J Vet Res*. 2008;69:294-297.
37. de Matos R. Calcium metabolism in birds. *Vet Clin North Am Exot Anim Pract*. 2008;11:59-82.
38. Maxwell L. Infectious and noninfectious diseases. In: Jacobson E, ed. *Biology, Husbandry, and Medicine of the Green Iguana*. Malabar, FL: Krieger; 2003:108-132.
39. Stiffler D. Amphibian calcium metabolism. *J Exp Biol*. 1993;184:47-61.
40. Wright K, Whitaker B. Nutritional disorders. In: Whitaker B, Wright K, eds. *Amphibian Medicine and Captive Husbandry*. Malabar, FL: Krieger; 2001.
41. Wright K, Whitaker B. Metabolic bone disease in amphibians. *Exotic DVM*. 1999;1(6):23-26.
42. Carman EN, Ferguson GW, Geiirmann WH, et al. Photobiosynthetic opportunity and ability for UV-B generated vitamin D synthesis in free-living house geckos (*Hemidactulys turcicus*) and Texas spiny lizards (*Sceloporus olivaceous*). *Copei*. 2000;1:245-250.
43. Brames H, Baines F. Reptile lighting is a process not a bulb. *Exotic DVM*. 2007;9.3:29-36.
44. Doneley B. The physical examination. In: Doneley B, ed. *Avian Medicine and Surgery in Practice: Companion and Aviary Birds*. London: Manson; 2011:40-54.
45. Harcourt-Brown N. Psittacine birds. In: Tully T, Dorrenstein G, Jones A, eds. *Handbook of Avian Medicine*. Edinburgh: Saunders; 2009:138-168.
46. Doneley B. Disorders of the musculoskeletal system. In: Doneley B, ed. *Avian Medicine and Surgery in Practice: Companion and Aviary Birds*. London: Manson Publishing; 2011:148-155.
47. Macwhirter P. Malnutrition. In: Ritchie B, Harrison G, Harrison L, eds. *Avian Medicine: Principles and Application*. Lake Worth, FL: Wingers Publishing; 1994.
48. Hanley C, Wilson G, Hernandez-Divers S. Secondary nutritional hyperparathyroidism associated with vitamin D deficiency in two domestic skunks (*Mephitis mephitis*). *Vet Rec*. 2004;155:233-237.
49. Stanford M. Calcium metabolism. In: Harrison G, Lightfoot T, eds. *Clinical Avian Medicine*. Palm Springs, FL: Spix; 2006:141-151.
50. Rosol T, Chew DJ, Nagode LA, et al. Pathophysiology of calcium metabolism. *Vet Clin Pathol*. 1995;24(2):49-63.
51. Stanford M. Clinical pathology of hypocalcaemia in adult grey parrots (*Psittacus erithacus*). *Vet Rec*. 2007;161:456-457.
52. Eckerman-Ross C. Hormonal regulation and calcium metabolism in the rabbit. *Vet Clin North Am Exot Anim Pract*. 2008;11: 139-152.
53. Redrobe S. Calcium metabolism in rabbits. *Sem Avian Exot Pet Med*. 2002;11(2):94-101.
54. Harcourt-Brown F. Calcium metabolism in rabbits. *Exotic DVM*. 2005;6(2):11-14.
55. Whiting S, Quamme G. Effects of dietary calcium on renal calcium, magnesium, and phosphate excretion by the rabbit. *Miner Electrolyte Metab*. 1984;10:217-221.
56. Fisher P, Carpenter J. Neurologic and musculoskeletal disease. In: Quesenberry K, Carpenter J, eds. *Ferrets, Rabbits, and Rodents: Clinical Medicine and Surgery*. St. Louis: Elsevier; 2012.
57. Harcourt-Brown F. Parathyroid hormone, haematological and biochemical parameters in relation to dental disease and husbandry in rabbits. *J Small Anim Pract*. 2001;42(3):130-136.
58. Harcourt-Brown F. Update on metabolic bone disease in rabbits. *Exotic DVM*. 2002;4(3):43-46.
59. Hawkins M. Disease problems in guinea pigs. In: Quesenberry K, Carpenter J, eds. *Ferrets, Rabbits, and Rodents: Clinical Medicine and Surgery*. St. Louis: Elsevier; 2012:295-338.
60. Schwarz T, Stork CK, Megahy IW, et al. Osteodystrophia fibrosa in two guinea pigs. *J Am Vet Med Assoc*. 2001;219(1):63-66.
61. Johnson-Delaney C. Medical update for sugar gliders. *Exotic DVM*. 2000;2(3):91-93.
62. Lennox A. Emergency and critical care procedures in sugar gliders (*Petaurus breviceps*), African hedgehogs (*Atelerix albiventris*), and prairie dogs (*Cynomys* spp.). *Vet Clin North Am Exot Anim Pract*. 2007;10:533-555.
63. Ness R, Johnson-Delaney C. Sugar gliders. In: Quesenberry K, Carpenter J, eds. *Ferrets, Rabbits, and Rodents: Clinical Medicine and Surgery*. St. Louis: Elsevier; 2012:393-428.
64. Stewart L. Nutrition of koi, carp, and goldfish. In: Stoskopf M, ed. *Fish Medicine*. Philadelphia: Saunders; 1993.
65. Sim RR, Sullivan KE, Valdes EV, et al. A comparison of oral and topical vitamin a supplementation in African foam-nesting frogs (*Chiromantis xerampelina*). *J Zoo Wildl Med*. 2010;41(3):456-460.
66. Douglas T, Pennino M, Dierenfeld E, et al. Vitamins E and A, and proximate composition of whole mice and rats used as feed. *Comp Biochem Physiol*. 1994;107(2):419-424.
67. National Research Council. *Vitamin Tolerance of Animals*. Washington, DC: National Research Council; 1987.
68. Green D. Pathology of Amphibia. In: Wright K, Whitaker B, eds. *Amphibian medicine and captive husbandry*. Malabar: Krieger; 2001.
69. Wright K. Idiopathic syndromes. In: Wright K, Whitaker B, eds. *Amphibian Medicine and Captive Husbandry*. Malabar, FL: Krieger; 2001.
70. Schmidt R, Reavill D, Phalen D. Musculoskeletal system. In: *Pathology of Pet and Aviary Birds*. Ames: Iowa State Press; 2003:149-164.
71. Riggs S. Guinea pigs. In: Mitchell M, Tully T, eds. *Manual of Exotic Pet Practice*. St. Louis: Saunders; 2009:456-473.
72. Jenkins J. Diseases of geriatric guinea pigs and chinchillas. *Vet Clin North Am Exot Anim Pract*. 2010;13:85-93.
73. Stoskopf M. Bacterial disease of freshwater tropical fishes. In: Stoskopf M, ed. *Fish Medicine*. Philadelphia: Saunders; 1993.
74. Gratzek J. Parasites associated with freshwater tropical fishes. In: Stoskopf M, ed. *Fish Medicine*. Philadelphia: Saunders; 1993.
75. Mikaelian I, Ouellet M, Pauli B, et al. *Ichthyophonus*-like infection in wild amphibians from Quebec, Canada. *Dis Aquat Organ*. 2000; 40:195-201.
76. Herman R. *Ichthyophonus*-like infection in newts (*Notophthalmus viridescens rafinesque*). *J Wildl Dis*. 1984;20(1):55-56.
77. Migaki G, Frye F. Mycotic granuloma in a tiger salamander. *J Wildl Dis*. 1975;11:525-528.
78. Taylor S. Mycoses. In: Whitaker B, Wright K, eds. *Amphibian Medicine and Captive Husbandry*. Malabar, FL: Krieger; 2001:181-191.
79. Burcham G, Miller M, Hickok T. Pathology in practice: mycotic dermatitis, cellulitis, and myositis. *J Am Vet Med Assoc*. 2011; 139(10):1305-1307.

80. Raymond J, Reichard T, Shellabrager W, et al. Inclusion body myositis in spring peepers *(Pseudacris crucifer)*. *J Vet Diagn Invest.* 2002;14(6):501-503.

81. Pizzi R, Miller J. Amputation of a *Mycobacterium marinum*-infected hindlimb in an African bullfrog *(Pyxicephalus adspersus)*. *Vet Rec.* 2005;156:747-748.

82. Taylor SK, Green DE, Wright KM, et al. Bacterial diseases. In: Whitaker B, Wright K, eds. *Amphibian Medicine and Captive Husbandry*. Malabar, FL: Krieger; 2001:159-179.

83. Reavill D, Schmidt R. Mycobacterial lesions in fish, amphibians, reptiles, rodents, lagomorphs, and ferrets with reference to animal models. *Vet Clin North Am Exot Anim Pract.* 2012;15: 25-40.

84. Girling S, Fraser M. Systemic mycobacteriosis in an inland bearded dragon *(Pogona vitticeps)*. *Vet Rec.* 2007;160:526-528.

85. Morales P, Dunker F. Fish tuberculosis, *Mycobacterium marinum* in a group of Egyptian spiny-tailed lizards *(Uromastyx aegyptius)*. *J Herpetol Med Surg.* 2001;11:27-30.

86. Greer LL, Strandberg JD, Whitaker BR. *Mycobacterium chelonae* osteoarthritis in a Kemp's ridley sea turtle *(Lepidochelys kempii)*. *J Wildl Dis.* 2003;39(3):736-741.

87. Poynton S, Whitaker B. Protozoa and metazoa infecting amphibians. In: Whitaker B, Wright K, eds. *Amphibian Medicine and Captive Husbandry*. Malabar, FL: Krieger; 2001:193-221.

88. Greiner E, Mader D. Parasitology. In: Mader D, ed. *Reptile Medicine and Surgery*. St. Louis: Saunders; 2006:343-364.

89. Chia MY, Jeng CR, Hsiao SH, et al. *Entamoeba invadens* myositis in a common water monitor lizard *(Varanus salvator)*. *Vet Pathol.* 2009;46(4):673-676.

90. Philbey A. Amoebic enterocolitis and acute myonecrosis in leopard tortoises *(Geochelone pardalis)*. *Vet Rec.* 2006;158(16):567-569.

91. Gabor LJ. Nutritional degenerative myopathy in a population of captive bred *Uroplatus phantasticus* (satanic leaf-tailed geckoes). *J Vet Diagn Invest.* 2005;17:71-73.

92. Farnsworth R, Brannian JR, Fletcher K, et al. A vitamin E-selenium responsive condition in a green iguana. *J Zoo Anim Med.* 1986;17: 42-45.

93. Cole GA, Rao DB, Steinberg H, et al. Suspected vitamin E and selenium deficiency in a veiled chameleon, *Chamaeleo calyptratus*. *J Herpetol Med Surg.* 2008;18(3/4):113-116.

94. Rowland M. Fibrosing myopathy of the temporal muscles causing lockjaw in a veiled chameleon. *Vet Rec.* 2011;169:527.

95. Dahlhausen B, Soler-Tovar D, Saggese M. Diagnosis of micobacterial infections in the exotic pet patient with emphasis on birds. *Vet Clin North Am Exot Anim Pract.* 2012;15:71-83.

96. Pollock C. Implications of mycobacteria in clinical disorders. In: Harrison G, Lightfoot T, eds. *Clinical Avian Medicine*. Palm Beach, FL: Spix; 2006:681-690.

97. Buur J, Saggese M. Taking a rational approach in the treatment of avian mycobacteriosis. *Vet Clin North Am Exot Anim Pract.* 2012;15: 57-70.

98. Villar D, Kramer M, Howard L, et al. Clinical presentation and pathology of sarcocystosis in Psittaciform birds: 11 cases. *Avian Dis.* 2008;52:187-194.

99. Ecco R, Luppi MM, Malta MC, et al. An outbreak of sarcocystosis in psittacines and a pigeon in a zoological collection in Brazil. *Avian Dis.* 2008;52(1):706-710.

100. Antinoff N, Giovanella C. Musculoskeletal and neurologic diseases. In: Quesenberry K, Carpenter J, eds. *Ferrets, Rabbits, and Rodents: Clinical Medicine and Surgery*. St. Louis: Elsevier; 2012: 132-140.

101. Ramsell K, Garner M. Disseminated idiopathic myofasciitis in ferrets. *Vet Clin North Am Exot Anim Pract.* 2010;13:561-575.

102. Graham J, Kent M, Thoen A. Current therapies in exotic animal oncology. *Vet Clin North Am Exot Anim Pract.* 2004;7:757-781.

103. Mehler S, Bennett R. Surgical oncology of exotic animals. *Vet Clin North Am Exot Anim Pract.* 2004;7:783-805.

104. Antinoff N. Special considerations in oncology of exotics. Proceedings of the American College of Veterinary Internal Medicine. 1999. Chicago.

105. Antinoff N, Hahn K. Ferret oncology: diseases, diagnostics, and therapeutics. *Vet Clin North Am Exot Anim Pract.* 2004;7:579-625.

106. Powers BE, LaRue SM, Withrow SJ, et al. Jamshidi needle biopsy for diagnosis of bone lesions in small animals. *J Am Vet Med Assoc.* 1988;193(2):205-210.

107. Kent M. The use of chemotherapy in exotic animals. *Vet Clin North Am Exot Anim Pract.* 2004;7:807-820.

108. Cooper J. Oncology of invertebrates. *Vet Clin North Am Exot Anim Pract.* 2004;7:697-703.

109. Groff J. Neoplasia in fishes. *Vet Clin North Am Exot Anim Pract.* 2004;7:705-756.

110. Green D, Harshbarger J. Spontaneous neoplasia in Amphibia. In: Whitaker B, Wright K, eds. *Amphibian Medicine and Captive Husbandry*. Malabar, FL: Krieger; 2001.

111. Stacy B, Parker J. Amphibian oncology. *Vet Clin North Am Exot Anim Pract.* 2004;7:673-695.

112. Hernandez-Divers S, Garner M. Reptile neoplasia. *Exotic DVM.* 2002;4.3:90-94.

113. Garner M, Hernandez-Divers S, Raymond J. Reptile neoplasia: a retrospective study of case submissions to a specialty diagnostic service. *Vet Clin North Am Exot Anim Pract.* 2004;7:653-671.

114. Hernandez-Divers S, Garner M. Neoplasia of reptiles with an emphasis on lizards. *Vet Clin North Am Exot Anim Pract.* 2003;6: 251-273.

115. Ramsay E, Munson L, Lowenstine L. A retrospective study of neoplasia in a collection of captive snakes. *J Zoo Wildl Med.* 1996;27(1):28-34.

116. Catao J, Nichols D. Neoplasia in snakes at the National Zoologic Park, Washington, DC (1978-1997). *J Comp Pathol.* 1999;120: 89-95.

117. Cowan M, Monks DJ, Raidal SR. Osteosarcoma in a Woma python *(Aspidites ramsayi)*. *Aust Vet J.* 2011;89:520-523.

118. Honour S, Ayroud M, Wheler C. Metastatic chondrosarcoma and subcutaneous granulomas in a grey rat snake *(Elaphe obsoleta obsoleta)*. *Can Vet J.* 1993;34:238-240.

119. Oros J, Monagas P, Andrada Borzolino MA, et al. Metastatic fibrosarcoma in a captive Saharan horned viper *(Cerastes cerastes)* with high hepatic levels of cadmium. *Vet Rec.* 2009;164(22):690-692.

120. Langan J, Adams W, Patton S. Radioation and intralesional chemotherapy for a fibrosarcoma in a boa constrictor *Boa constrictor ortoni*. *J Herpetol Med Surg.* 2001;11(1):4-8.

121. Dittmer KE, French AF, Thompson DJ, et al. Primary bone tumors in birds: a review and description of two new cases. *Avian Dis.* 2012; 56(2):422-426.

122. Reavill D. Tumors of pet birds. *Vet Clin North Am Exot Anim Pract.* 2004;7:537-560.

123. Gulbahar MY, Ozak A, Guvenc T, et al. Retrobulbar rhabdomyosarcoma in a budgerigar *(Melopsittacus undulatus)*. *Avian Pathol.* 2005;34(6):486-488.

124. Raphael B, Nguyen H. Metastasizing rhabdomyosarcoma in a budgerigar. *J Am Vet Med Assoc.* 1980;9:925-926.

125. Arnall L. Further experiences with cagebirds. *Vet Rec.* 1961;73: 1146-1154.

126. Van Der Horst H, Van Der Hage M, Wolvekamp P, et al. Synovial cell sarcoma in a sulfur-crested cockatoo *(Cacatua galerita)*. *Avian Pathol.* 1996;25:179-186.

127. Sakai H, Maruyama M, Hirata A, et al. Rhabdomyosarcoma in a ferret *(Mustela putorius furo)*. *J Vet Med Sci.* 2004;66(1):95-96.

128. Antinoff N, Williams B. Neoplasia. In: Quesenberry K, Carpenter J, eds. *Ferrets, Rabbits, and Rodents: Clinical Medicine and Surgery*. St. Louis: Elsevier; 2012.

129. Jensen W, Myers R, Liu C. Osteoma in a ferret. *J Am Vet Med Assoc.* 1985;187(12):1375-1376.

130. Heatly J, Smith A. Spontaneous neoplasms of lagomorphs. *Vet Clin North Am Exot Anim Pract.* 2004;7:561-577.

131. Greenacre C. Spontaneous tumors of small mammals. *Vet Clin North Am Exot Anim Pract.* 2004;7:627-651.

132. Ivey E, Carpenter J. African hedgehogs. In: Quesenberry K, Carpenter J, eds. *Ferrets, Rabbits, and Rodents: Clinical Medicine and Surgery.* St. Louis: Elsevier; 2012.

133. Phair K, Carpenter JW, Marrow J, et al. Management of extraskeletal osteosarcoma in an African hedgehog (*Atelerix albiventris*). *J Exotic Pet Med* 2011;20(2):151-155.

134. Geyer M, Borchardt T, Schreiyack C, et al. Endogenous regeneration after collagenase-induced knee joint damage in the adult newt *Notophthalmus viridescens. Ann Rheum Dis.* 2011;70(1):214-220.

135. Pare J, Lentini A. Reptile geriatrics. *Vet Clin North Am Exot Anim Pract.* 2010;13:15-25.

136. Raidal S, Shearer P, Prince R. Chronic shoulder osteoarthritis in a loggerhead turtle (*Caretta caretta*). *Aust Vet J.* 2006;84:231-234.

137. Bennett R. Antibiotic PMMA beads for septic arthritis in a green iguana. *Exotic DVM.* 1999;1.3:27-28.

138. Brown DR, Nogueira MF, Schoeb TR, et al. Pathology of experimental mycoplasmosis in American alligators. *J Wildl Dis.* 2001;37(4):671-679.

139. Nevarez J. Crocodilians. In: Mitchell M, Tully T, eds. *Manual of Exotic Pet Practice.* St. Louis: Saunders; 2009:113-135.

140. Jacobson E. Bacterial diseases of reptiles. In: Jacobson E, ed. *Infectious Diseases and Pathology of Reptiles.* Boca Raton, FL: CRC; 2007:461-526.

141. Philbey AW, Lawrie AM, Allison CJ, et al. Lower urinary tract obstruction in a Mediterranean spur-thighed tortoise (*Testudo graeca*) with coxofemoral arthritis. *Vet Rec.* 2006;159(15):492-494.

142. Ogden JA, Rhodan AG, Conlogue GJ, et al. Pathobiology of septic arthritis and contiguous osteomyelitis in a leatherback turtle (*Dermochelys coriacea*). *J Wildl Dis.* 1981;17(2):277-287.

143. Guthrie A, George J, deMaar TW. Bilateral chronic shoulder infections in an adult green sea turtle (*Chelonia mydas*). *J Herpetol Med Surg.* 2010;20(4):105-108.

144. Mader D. Gout. In: Mader D, ed. *Reptile Medicine and Surgery.* St. Louis: Saunders; 2006:793-800.

145. Fitzgerald K, Vera R. Spinal osteopathy. In: Mader D, ed. *Reptile Medicine and Surgery.* St. Louis: Saunders; 2006:906-912.

146. Isaza R, Garner M, Jacobson E. Proliferative osteoarthritis and osteoarthrosis in 15 snakes. *J Zoo Wildl Med.* 2000;31(1):20-27.

147. Van Bonn W. Clinical technique: extra-articular surgical stifle stabilization of an American bullfrog (*Rana catesbeiana*). *J Exotic Pet Med.* 2009;18(1):36-39.

148. Hernandez-Divers S. Diagnosis and surgical repair of stifle luxation in a spur-thighed tortoise (*Testudo graeca*). *J Zoo Wildl Med.* 2002;33(2):125-130.

149. Bowles HL, Zantop DW. A novel surgical technique for luxation repair of the femorotibial joint in a monk parakeet (*Myiopsitta monachus*). *J Avian Med Surg.* 2002;16(1):34-38.

150. Chinnadurai SK, Spodnick G, Degernes L, et al. Use of extracapsular stabilization technique to repair cruciate ligament ruptures in two avian species. *J Avian Med Surg.* 2009;23(4):307-313.

151. Rosenthal K, Hillyer E, Mathiessen D. Stifle luxation repair in a Moluccan cockatoo and a barn owl. *J Assoc Avian Vet.* 1994;8(4):173-178.

152. Van Wettere A, Redig P. Arthrodesis as a treatment for metacarpophalangeal joint luxation in 2 raptors. *J Avian Med Surg.* 2004;18(1):23-29.

153. Ritzman T, Knapp D. Ferret orthopedics. *Vet Clin North Am Exot Anim Pract.* 2002;5(1):129-155.

154. Zehnder A, Kapatkin A. Orthopedics in small mammals. In: Quesenberry K, Carpenter J, eds. *Ferrets Rabbits, and Rodents: Clinical Medicine and Surgery.* St. Louis: Elsevier; 2012:472-484.

155. Owiny JR, Vandewoude S, Painter JT, et al. Hip dysplasia in rabbits: association with nest box flooring. *Comp Med.* 2001;51(1):85-88.

156. Zuijlen M, Vrolijk P, van der Heyden M. Bilateral successive cranial cruciate ligament rupture treated by extracapsular stabilization surgery in a pet rabbit (*Oryctolagus cuniculus*). *J Exotic Pet Med.* 2012;19(3):245-248.

157. Lennox A. Care of the geriatric rabbit. *Vet Clin North Am Exot Anim Pract.* 2010;13:123-133.

158. Taniguchi S, Ryu J, Seki M, et al. Long-term oral administration of glucosamine or chondroitin sulfate reduces destruction of cartilage and up-regulation of MMP-3 mRNA in a model of spontaneous osteoarthritis in Hartley guinea pigs. *J Orthop Res.* 2012;30(5):673-678.

159. Mihara K, Hirano T. Standing is a causative factor in osteonecrosis of the femoral head in growing rats. *J Pediatr Orthop.* 1998;18(5):665-669.

160. Suehiro M, Hirano T, Mihara K, et al. Etiologic factors in femoral head osteonecrosis in growing rats. *J Orthop Sci.* 2000;5(1):52-56.

161. Iwasaki K, Hirano T. Osteonecrosis and ossification disturbance of the femoral head in spontaneously hypertensive rats. *Nihon Seikeigeka Gakkai Zasshi.* 1988;62(11):1003-1010.

162. Bubenik L. Osteomyelitis. In: Bojrab M, ed. *Mechanisms of Disease in Small Animal Surgery.* Jackson, WY: Teton New Media; 2010:558-564.

163. Chinnadurai S, DeVoe R. Selected infectious disease of reptiles. *Vet Clin North Am Exot Anim Pract.* 2009;12:583-596.

164. Raftery A. Reptile orthopedic medicine and surgery. *J Exotic Pet Med.* 2011;20(2):107-116.

165. Ramsay EC, Daniel GB, Tryon BW, et al. Osteomyelitis associated with *Salmonella enterica* ss *arizonae* in a colony of ridgenose rattlesnakes (*Crotalus willardi*). *J Zoo Wildl Med.* 2002;33(4):301-310.

166. Naldo J, Libanan N, Samour J. Health assessment of a spiny-tailed lizard (*Uromastyx* spp.) population in Abu Dhabi, United Arab Emirates. *J Zoo Wildl Med.* 2009;40(3):445-452.

167. Kramer M. Granulomatous osteomyelitis associated with atypical mycobacteriosis in a bearded dragon (*Pogona vitticeps*). *Vet Clin North Am Exot Anim Pract.* 2006;9:563-568.

168. Brown DR, Demcovitz DL, Potter SM, et al. *Mycoplasma iguanae* sp. nov., from a green iguana (*Iguana iguana*) with vertebral disease. *Int J Syst Evol Microbiol.* 2006;56(4):761-764.

169. Gartrell B, Hare K. Mycotic dermatitis with digital gangrene and osteomyelitis, and protozoal intestinal parasitism in Malborough green geckos (*Naultinus manukanus*). *N Z Vet J.* 2005;53(5):363-367.

170. Heatly J, Mitchell M, Willia J, et al. Fungal periodontal osteomyelitis in a chameleon, *Furcifur pardalis. J Herpetol Med Surg.* 2001;11(4):7-12.

171. Adkesson MJ, Travis EK, Weber MA, et al. Vacuum-assisted closure for treatment of a deep shell abscess and osteomyelitis in a tortoise. *J Am Vet Med Assoc.* 2007;231:1249-1254.

172. Dunning D. Basic mammalian bone anatomy and healing. *Vet Clin North Am Exot Anim Pract.* 2002;5(1):115-128.

173. Enlow D. The bone of reptiles. In: Gans C, ed. *Biology of the Reptilia.* London: Academic Press; 1969:45-80.

174. Foote J. The comparative histology of femoral bones. *Trans Am Microsc Soc.* 1911;30(2 [Apr.]):87-140.

175. Fletcher OJ, Abdul-Aziz T, Barnes HJ. Skeletal system. In: Fletcher OJ, Abdul-Aziz T, eds. *Avian Histopathology.* 3rd ed. Am Assoc Avian Pathol; 2008:58-79.

176. Bliss S, Rawlinson J, Todhunter R. Tissues of the musculoskeletal system. In: Tobias K, Johnston S, eds. *Veterinary Surgery: Small Animal.* St. Louis: Elsevier; 2012:553-564.

177. Martin H, Ritchie B. Orthopedic surgical techniques. In: Ritchie B, Harrison G, Harrison L, eds. *Avian Medicine: Principles and Application.* Lake Worth, FL: Wingers; 1994:1137-1169.

178. Bennett R, Kuzman A. Fracture management in birds. *J Zoo Wildl Med.* 1992;23(1):5-38.

179. Kuzman A, Hunter B. A new technique for avian fracture repair using intramedullary polymethylmethacrylate and bone plate fixation. *J Am Anim Hosp Assoc*. 1991;27:239-248.

180. Mitchell M. Diagnosis and management of reptile orthopedic injuries. *Vet Clin North Am Exot Anim Pract*. 2002;5(1):97-114.

181. Hutchison C, Pilote M, Roy S. The axolotl limb: a model for bone development, regeneration, and fracture healing. *Bone*. 2007;40:45-56.

182. Pritchard J, Ruzicka A. Comparison of fracture repair in the frog, lizard, and rat. *J Anat*. 1950;84:236-261.

183. Tully T. Basic avian bone growth and healing. *Vet Clin North Am Exot Anim Pract*. 2002;5(1):23-30.

184. West PG, Rowland PR, Budsberg SC, et al. Histomorphometric and angiographic analysis of bone healing in the humerus of pigeons. *Am J Vet Res*. 1996;57(7):1010-1015.

185. Mader DR, Bennett RA, Funk RS, et al. Surgery. In: Mader D, ed. *Reptile Medicine and Surgery*. St. Louis: Saunders Elsevier; 2006:581-630.

186. Bennett R. Fracture management. In: Mader D, ed. *Reptile Medicine and Surgery*. Philadelphia: Saunders; 1996:281-286.

187. Koch D. Screws and plates. In: Johnson A, Houlton J, Vannini R, eds. *AO Principles of Fracture Management in the Dog and Cat*. Switzerland: AO Publishing; 2005.

188. Wellehan JF, Zens MS, Bright AA, et al. Type I skeletal fixation of radial fractures in microchiropterans. *J Zoo Wildl Med*. 2001;32(4):487-493.

189. Travis E, Mylniczenko N, Greenwell M. Treatment of a traumatic mandibular symphyseal fracture and facial tissue loss in a laced moray eel. *Exotic DVM*. 2004;6.5:31-35.

190. Wright K. Trauma. In: Wright K, Whitaker B, eds. *Amphibian Medicine and Captive Husbandry*. Malabar, FL: Krieger; 2001.

191. Wright K. Surgical techniques. In: Whitaker B, Wright K, eds. *Amphibian Medicine and Captive Husbandry*. Malabar, FL: Krieger; 2001:273-283.

192. Johnson D. External fixation of bilateral tibial fractures in an American bullfrog. *Exotic DVM*. 2003;5(2):27-30.

193. Royal LW, Grafinger MS, Lascelles BD, et al. Internal fixation of a femur fracture in an American bullfrog. *J Am Vet Med Assoc*. 2007;230(8):1201-1204.

194. Barten SL. Shell damage. In: Mader D, ed. *Reptile Medicine and Surgery*. St. Louis: Saunders Elsevier; 2006:893-899.

195. Fleming G. Clinical technique: chelonian shell repair. *J Exotic Pet Med*. 2008;17(4):246-258.

196. Forrester H, Satta J. Easy shell repair. *Exotic DVM*. 2005;6(6):13.

197. Helmer P, Redig P. Surgical resolution of orthopedic disorders. In: *Clinical Avian Medicine*. Palm Beach, FL: Spix Publishing; 2006:761-773.

198. Harcourt-Brown N. Orthopedic conditions that affect the avian pelvic limb. *Vet Clin North Am Exot Anim Pract*. 2002;5(1):49-81.

199. Orosz S. Clinical considerations of the thoracic limb. *Vet Clin North Am Exot Anim Pract*. 2002;5(1):31-48.

200. Christen C, Fischer I, von Rechenberg B, et al. Evaluation of a maxillofacial miniplate compact 1.0 for stabilization of the ulna in experimentally induced ulnar and radial fractures in pigeons (*Columba liva*). *J Avian Med Surg*. 2005;19(3):185-190.

201. Burgdorf-Moisuk A, Whittington JK, Bennett RA, et al. Successful management of simple fractures of the femoral neck with femoral head and neck excision arthroplasty in two free-living avian species. *J Avian Med Surg*. 2011;25(3):210-215.

202. Redig P. A clinical review of orthopedic techniques used in the rehabilitation of raptors. In: Fowler M, ed. *Zoo and Wildlife Medicine*. Philadelphia: Saunders; 1986:388-401.

203. Barron HW, McBride M, Martinez-Jimenez D, et al. Comparison of two methods of long bone fracture repair in rabbits. *J Exotic Pet Med*. 2010;19(2):183-188.

204. Piermattei D, Johnson K. *An Atlas of Surgical Approaches to the Bones and Joints of the Dog and Cat*. 4th ed. Philadelphia: Saunders; 2004.

205. Sessions S, Ruth S. Explanation for naturally occuring supernumerary limbs in amphibians. *J Exp Zool*. 1990;254(1):38-47.

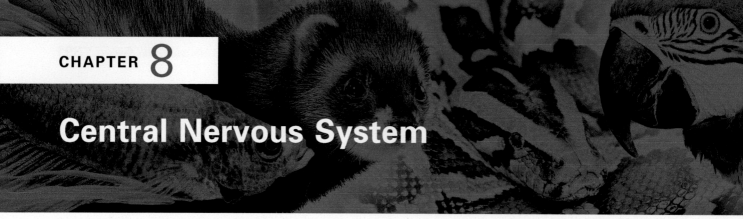

CHAPTER 8

Central Nervous System

Thomas N. Tully, Jr., DVM, MS, DABVP (Avian), DECZM (Avian)

INTRODUCTION

The most difficult case presentations to diagnose, in any animal, are those that involve the nervous system. Neurologic disease is especially frustrating for veterinarians that treat companion exotic species because of the lack of basic knowledge regarding the nervous system and associated clinical signs that result from nerve deficits. As with all exotic species that present with disease, it is imperative that the examiner use a knowledge base of the body system involved to determine what is both normal and abnormal. By interpreting the clinical signs associated with a disease process and correlating these findings to the animal's normal function, one can start developing a differential list of possible causes of the presenting complaint. The evaluation of a patient that is presented with neurologic signs relies heavily on a complete and thorough history, obtained from the owner, and physical examination. The physical examination must include a neurologic workup and evaluation. In many neurologic cases involving companion exotic animals, it is extremely difficult to definitively diagnose an underlying disease problem due to the lack of basic medical information, number of species treated, diminutive size of many patients, and inability to utilize diagnostic tests that may help determine a diagnosis.

The generalized presentation of many neurologic cases and the difficulty in diagnosing and treating disease conditions that led to the patient's condition should be communicated to that animal's owner. The pet owner must be made aware that many neurologic conditions are terminal or result in disease conditions that never completely resolve. Although advances in diagnostic technology have improved the veterinarian's ability to diagnose diseases that affect the nervous system of companion exotic species, these advances do not benefit all animals covered in this chapter. It is beneficial to use diagnostic tests that provide results on the smallest of patients, thereby allowing the veterinarian more latitude in requesting tests that require blood or diagnostic imaging.

The veterinary community has much to learn regarding neurologic diseases and treatment in companion exotic animals. Again, a major problem lies with the various species within this large group of animals that in many cases respond differently to certain medications than do dogs and cats. An example of inconsistent patient response to medication is the inability of African grey parrots to obtain any therapeutic benefits of oral phenobarbital suspension. These problems are compounded due to the lack of scientific studies that validate therapeutic effectiveness and unsubstantiated clinical recommendations through anecdotal patient response. Naturally, there are many variables that affect the treatment of neurologic disease in companion exotic patients; therefore, it can be difficult to determine the primary reason for a positive patient response. There is still much to learn and many scientific studies that need to be performed before significant progress is made in understanding neurologic disease in companion exotic species and appropriate treatment recommendations can be made. This chapter on the central nervous system (CNS) provides current information as it relates to the many exotic animal species that may be treated in the companion animal hospital. Knowledge of the basic anatomy and physiology of the CNS will help one with diagnosing disease problems and provide direction toward appropriate therapeutic measures. Available diagnostic techniques that will lead to a definitive diagnosis are ever expanding. An overview of these tests and what they provide is extremely important to the veterinarian trying to gain information on the patient's condition and cause of the problem. Neurologic diseases and current treatment of those illnesses provide a resource for the clinician to reference when determining a differential disease list for the patient presenting with clinical signs consistent with neurologic disease.

ANATOMY AND PHYSIOLOGY

Invertebrates

Flatworms

Turbellarians or flatworms are believed to be the first group of animals to have developed encephalization and a true brain.[1] The flatworm brain is commonly bilobed; however, if surrounded by a capsule, it may appear globular.[1] Nerve strands connect both the dorsal and lateral trunks and the animal is innervated by a "nerve net" composed of several plexuses.[2,3] The brain controls rostral reflexes, asexual reproduction, and sexual maturation.[1] Flatworms are considered the first group of animals to have a true brain and also the first to have a semblance of a spinal cord.[1] Their brain is consolidated, with clusters of nerve cell bodies at the anterior

392

end, from which 2 ventral nerves course the length of the body where nerve branches extend.[4]

Cephalopods

Cephalopods as a group include nautilus, cuttlefish, squid, and octopus. In general, cephalopods have a well-developed nervous system. The brain anatomy and location between cephalopod species is slightly different, but using the octopus as an example, it is located in a hard cartilaginous cavity between the eyes.[5] The subesophageal part of the brain is thought to control the muscle groups.[6] Although the octopus has well-developed optic and ocular nerves, there is a degree of autonomy of its arms, mantle, and buccal cavity movement from the CNS.[6,7]

Spiders

Although there are many species of spiders, the fundamental anatomic and physiologic description of the CNS described in this section is based on the sedentary spider, *Poecilotheria*. The CNS is located at the cranial aspect of the animal and is comprised of a large unified cephalothoracic nerve mass.[8] This nerve mass is considered the brain or supraesophageal ganglion and a ventral subesophageal bundle.[9] The ventral subesophageal nerve bundle contains a pair of large pedipalps, 4 pairs of leg ganglionic masses, and 11 pairs of small abdominal ganglia.[9] The CNS of the spider is typical of most arthropods, as the cellular cortex encapsulates a highly complex neuropile.[10] The nervous tissue within the CNS of a spider is composed of fibrous matter (50% to 60%), cellular rind (25% to 35%), and glial tissue (5% to 25%).[9]

The center of the nervous tissue contains the neuropile and fiber tracts. There are no nerve cell bodies in the nervous tissue core, which contains processes of motor and interneurons along with branches of sensory neurons.[9] These processes are derived from parallel fiber tracts that have no synaptic terminus.[10] Thus, the neuropile, being the sole location of neuronal contacts, is the primary location for integration processes.[11] Two distinct neuropile are found in spiders and other arthropods and they are diffuse and granular and classified depending on fiber configuration.

The diffuse neuropile comprises the largest amount of neuropile tissue and is involved in the processes of large and small motor neurons and interneurons and axon termination of sensory neurons.[9] Fibers within the diffuse neuropile may combine as nerve tracts and occur in a wide variety of sizes, averaging ~8 μm.[9] The ventral region of the neuropile contains the terminus of the sensory neurons, while the dorsal region contains the dendritic and axonal processes of motor and larger interneurons.[9]

The structured neuropile is found in the ventral aspect of the nervous tissue mass and is sensory in nature. The irregularly shaped, dense masses of fine nerve fibers or ganglia are located most often in the spider's legs and pedipalpal ganglia.[9]

A critical element of the spider neuron is the neurofibril, which is also found in other invertebrates.[10] The neurofibrils are integral components of the basal parts of the stem processes of larger motor neurons and interneurons.[9]

The large motor neurons have a central cell body and an axon that enters into a peripheral nerve. A single stem process characteristically emanates from each cell of the motor neurons and may be lengthy (800 μm), extending from the ventral to dorsal neuropile.[9] These single stem processes divide in the dorsal neuropile into dendrites and axons, with the axons entering peripheral nerves.[9] There are 4 types of motor neurons identified in the spider.[9]

The majority of nervous tissue within the larger diffuse neuropile is composed of type B and D cells of interneuronal processes.[9] Type D neurons are often unipolar and are found in large quantities in the dorsal neuropile. Type B neurons extend processes to the neuropile of adjacent ganglia or central neuropile.

Spiders have interganglionic, ipsilateral, and contralateral neurons that innervate the legs and provide the basis of motor function.[9] Sensory perception is through peripheral axons that enter a ganglion principally from the ventral region of the neuropile, similar to insects.[9]

The magnitude of sensory innervation in spiders is evident in the trichobothria or tactile hairs on their legs. These ultrasensitive trichobothria can detect low velocity air currents and vibration, which is useful in hunting prey.[12] Chemosensitive hairs on the end of the legs also allow the spider to evaluate prey before eating and the surrounding environment for safety. A tarsal organ on each leg serves as a means to evaluate humidity within the animal's environment.[12] While the short body and copula hairs on the tarsi are not innervated, all large articulated hairs have triple innervation. During ecdysis, innervation of the large articulated hair is maintained through a dendritic connection between the old and new hair.[12]

Fish

The anatomic composition of the fish brain includes the hindbrain (cerebellum and medulla), midbrain (optic lobes), and forebrain (olfactory lobes). Most fish have a relatively small brain in relation to their body size. The forebrain consists mainly of the olfactory lobes and, depending on species/group of fish, varies in size. In fish species, in which the sense of smell is important to their survival, such as cyclostomes and elasmobranchs, the olfactory lobes are large, as opposed to teleosts, in which this part of the brain is small. Smell in fish is accomplished when sensory receptor cells, innervated by the olfactory nerve, are stimulated in the olfactory organs.[13] The olfactory organs are called nares and are paired bilateral structures in most fish, composed of olfactory chambers. Olfactory epithelia or lamellae line the olfactory chambers and increase the surface area from which fish can smell. Water is drawn through the anterior nares over the lamellae lining the olfactory chambers and then released back into the surrounding environment through the posterior nares.[13] A cerebrum or pair of cerebral hemispheres may be present along with the pituitary. While the pituitary is critical in hormone production, the cerebral tissue appears to be associated primarily with smell in fish.

The optic lobes originate in the midbrain and, similar to the olfactory lobes, vary in size depending on the importance of sight for a particular species of fish. The midbrain is considered the area of learning and assimilation of information within the fish brain. In mammalian species, the cerebral hemispheres in the forebrain are where knowledge is gained.

The hindbrain in fish is comprised of the cerebellum and medulla. The cerebellum helps maintain equilibrium and coordination as well as regulate muscle control after the initiation of muscle activity. The medulla, as with other

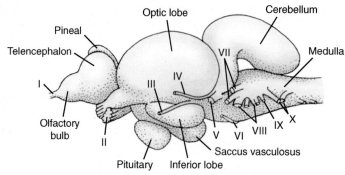

FIGURE 8-1 Fish brain and cranial nerves.

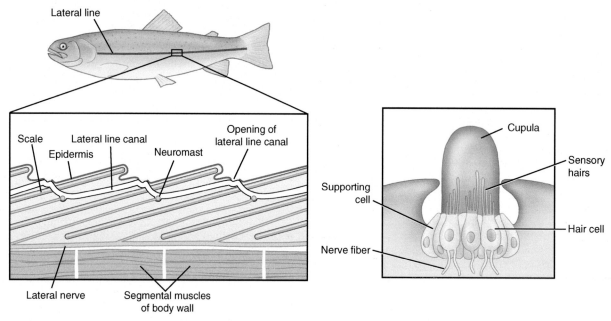

FIGURE 8-2 Fish lateral line system.

TABLE 8-1	
Fish Cranial Nerves	
1. Olfactory	Sensory: connecting nasal organs to olfactory lobes
2. Optic	Sensory: connecting eyes with the optic lobes
3. Oculomotor	Muscles
4. Trochlear	Muscles
5. Trigeminal	Sensory and muscles
6. Abducens	Muscles
7. Facial	Sensory and muscles
8. Auditory	Sensory: connecting the brain with the inner ear, balance
9. Glossopharyngeal	Sensory: connecting the brain with the gills and oral cavity
10. Vagus	Mixed, intestines, gills, heart, lateral line

Data from Bernstein JJ. Anatomy and physiology of the central nervous system. In: Hoar WS, Randall DJ, eds. *Fish Physiology*. Vol 4. San Diego, CA: Academic Press; 1971:5-70.

vertebrates, regulates organ function and serves as a transmission site for nerve signals from the forebrain and midbrain to the rest of the body.

The spinal cord in most fish extends from the hindbrain to the caudal vertebra through the neural canal.[13] This bundle of nervous tissue is protected by the neural canal within the spinal column. Originating at each vertebra is one pair of spinal nerves. Fish have 10 pairs of cranial nerves (CNs) (Figure 8-1 and Table 8-1).

The cephalic lateral line system is an external sensory system in fish that is used to detect subtle water movement and pressure gradients.[14] The neuromast is considered the smallest functional anatomical structure of the lateral line.[14] This sensory structure is composed of a hair cell epithelium and a cupula through which the ciliary bundles of the hair cells "feel" the water in which the animal swims.[14] The neuromast is superficial, found on the head, body, and tail fin, and embedded in lateral-line canals (Figure 8-2).[14] The neuromast embedded in the lateral-line canals communicate to the surrounding water through pores filled with endolymphic fluid. The lateral-line sensory system aids fish in finding food, avoiding predators and obstacles, and for schooling behavior.

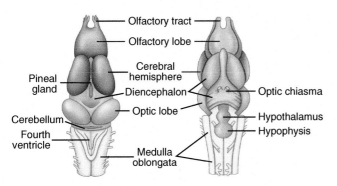

Olfactory tract
Olfactory lobe
Cerebral hemisphere
Pineal gland
Diencephalon
Optic lobe
Cerebellum
Fourth ventricle
Medulla oblongata
Optic chiasma
Hypothalamus
Hypophysis

FIGURE 8-3 Amphibian brain.

TABLE 8-2
Amphibian Cranial Nerves

1. Olfactory	Somatic sensory
2. Opticus	Somatic sensory
3. Oculomotor	Somatic motor
4. Trochlear	Somatic motor
5. Trigeminal	Somatic sensory (ophthalmic nerve and maxillaris nerve) Visceral motor (mandibularis nerve)
6. Abducens	Somatic motor
7. Facial	Visceral sensory (palatinus nerve) Visceral motor (hyomandibularis nerve)
8. Statoacousticus	Somatic sensory and motor
9. Glossopharyngeus	Sensory: connecting the brain with the gills and oral cavity
10. Vagus	Somatic, visceral sensory, visceral motor
11. Accessorius	Motor
12. Hypoglossus	Motor

Data from Oksche A, Ueck M. The nervous system. In: Lofts B, ed. *Physiology of the Amphia*. Vol 3. New York, NY: Academic Press; 1976:312-404.

The lateral line is located along the body wall in the greatest concentration toward the areas of greatest predator danger.

Amphibians

The CNS of most amphibians consists of the brain and spinal cord. The brain is divided into the forebrain, midbrain, and hindbrain (Figure 8-3). For vertebrates, the amphibian brain still maintains a somewhat primitive form. White matter is found on the outer aspect of the ventricles in association with neuronal aggregation.[15] Although there is organizational and functional variability of neurological systems between different amphibian orders and families, the basic anatomy and physiology between all species is reviewed in this chapter. The olfactory lobes (bulbus olfactorius), cerebral hemispheres (telencephalon), and the diencephalon incorporate the amphibian forebrain. The olfactory lobes are located at the anterior aspect of the brain; their primary function is to manage the sense of smell. An amphibian's memory and thought processes are formed in the cerebral hemispheres, which also controls voluntary and spontaneous activity. Also in the forebrain is the diencephalon, centered between the optic lobes and caudal to the cerebral hemispheres. The ventral tissue of the diencephalon contains the focal communication center of the autonomic nervous system. The pair of optic lobes primarily maintains the sense of sight, has control of eye muscles, and comprises the majority of the midbrain. The hindbrain includes the cerebellum, which controls balance and the function of autonomic and voluntary movements. The medulla oblongata (rhombencephalon) is also part of the hindbrain and manages involuntary actions of the animals. The spinal cord extends from the foramen magnum through the vertebral neural canal and terminates in the last vertebral body as the filum terminale.

The midbrain and medulla control the vital physiologic responses to internal and external stimuli. Therefore, in amphibians, the midbrain performs activity that is generated in the forebrain of higher vertebrates.[16] The forebrain in this group of animals does not communicate with centers caudle to the midbrain; consequently, decerebrated frogs can feed, breed, and swim. Electronic stimulation of the forebrain does not result in motor activity.[15] It is speculated that the amphibian forebrain's primary function is to coordinate various sensory data.[15] In some amphibian orders, there is evidence of the development of a basal cortex and some telencephalic regions, including a subsequent proliferation in ascending nonolfactory thalamotelencephalic fibers.[15] The cortical

development leads to the possibility that amphibians may be able to learn; however, they do not have a reptile pallial cortex.[15] In a frog's brain, the 3 main cortices have been described as the telencephalic cortex, mesencephalic tectum, and the cerebellum.[17] The mesencephalic primordial cells develop into the bipartite central corpus and lateral auricular lobes that form the cerebellum.[15]

The mesencephalon is composed of the dorsal tectum (integrates optic impulses with impulses from tactile organs, lateral-line components, and proprioceptive systems) and basal tegmental section (transmits motor impulses to the CNS and controls locomotion).[15,16] The neural pathways to and from the tectum are afferent (optic), ascending (spinal cord, medulla), and efferent (thalamus, basal tegmental section, medulla).[15] The diencephalon of amphibian species is divided into 3 parts: epithalamus (habenular ganglia and their commissure, choroid plexus of the 3rd ventricle, pineal organ, and posthabenular pars intercalaris), thalamus, and hypothalamus.[15]

Through investigative studies, it has been shown that the amphibian CNS has significant regenerative properties.[18] After partial brain resection and transection of the spinal cord in amphibian species, nerve regeneration and hyperplasia were evident.[19,20] In a study involving spinal cord resection, optimal function (normal motor reactions) returned to animals 30 to 50 days following surgery, although complete recovery was not achieved.[20]

At this time, it is generally considered that amphibians have 12 pairs of CNs; however, CN XII (hypoglossal nerve) may be considered a spino-occipital nerve originating from the spinal cord (Table 8-2).[15,21,22] Historically, frogs and other amphibian species were thought to have 10 pairs of CNs. Thus, there are some species variations relating to spinal nerve development (i.e., CN III and IV are absent in species with reduced ocular function) and the total number of spinal nerves present.[15] In amphibians, CN V (trigeminal n.) is formed by two brachial nerves, and CN X (vagus n.) is comprised of more than one brachial nerve.[15]

Reptiles

Similar to other higher vertebrates, the brain and spinal cord comprise the CNS of reptile species. Surrounding the brain, reptile species have subdural and epidural spaces. Depending on species, the brain may have more (e.g., lizards, aquatic turtles) or less (e.g., snakes) space between the neural tissue and wall of the brain case.[23] The cerebral spinal fluid (CSF) is formed by the tela choroidea, which is found in the dorsal midbrain. As with amphibians, the spinal cord of reptiles extends from the foramen magnum through almost the entire length of the vertebral canal. The reptile brain can be divided into 3 sections: the forebrain (olfactory nerve and bulb, cerebrum, pineal complex, pituitary), the midbrain (optic tectum), and hindbrain (cerebellum, pons, choroid plexus, medulla). The forebrain includes both the telencephalon and diencephalon and is a neural center for smell, taste, and sensory-motor interpretation. The telencephalon contains the olfactory tracts and bulbs, cerebral hemispheres, dorsal ventricular ridge, lateral ventricles, CN 0, or nervus terminalis and CN 1 (olfactory n.).[23] The cerebral hemispheres of reptile species lack the cortical folding found in mammals. Although the neocortex is not found in most reptile species, chelonians have an internal ventricular ridge that is considered to be a rudimentary analog.[24] All senses except the olfactory, which is direct, send neural transmissions to the cerebral hemispheres through the thalamus.[23] Located within the diencephalon are the hypothalamus, thalamus, infundibulum, pituitary gland, pineal complex, optic chiasma, CN II (optic n.), and CN III (oculomotor n.).[23] The pineal complex that is composed of an epiphysis and parietal eye will extend from the brain by a thin stem to the dorsal skull to an area demarcated by the pineal scale.[23] In reptiles, the pineal gland is both sensory and secretory. The pineal complex, including the pineal gland, regulates pigmentation and circadian rhythms.[23] The pineal complex is underdeveloped in snake and crocodilian species.[25] The midbrain or mesencephalon contains the areas for visual processing and neuroendocrine processes. Contained within the mesencephalon are the tectum (optic lobes), tegmentum, 3rd ventricle, cerebral aqueduct, and CN IV (trochlear n.).[23] Optic processing, and to a lesser degree auditory processing, occurs in the tectum (optic lobes) within the midbrain. Reptile species are thought to hear at lower auditory frequencies, with neural target areas being located in the medulla oblongata, cerebellum, tectum, and thalamus.[23] The hindbrain includes the metencephalon and myelencephalon, which contains the neural tissue associated with hearing, balance, and physiological homeostasis.[23] The cerebellum, anterior medulla, 4th ventricle, CN V (trigeminal n.), CN VI (abducens n.), CN VII (facial n.), CN VIII (statoacoustic n.), CN IX (glossopharyngeal n.), and CN X (vagus n.) are found in the metencephalon. Cerebellar function in reptiles is similar to that in other vertebrates, integrating sensory and motor stimuli and preserving balance.[23] As with other parts of the brain, the cerebellum varies in size among reptile species. Reptiles that live on the ground generally have a smaller cerebellum relative to reptilian species that climb or live in the water.[23] The crocodilian cerebellum is larger and more complex than other reptile species.[26] The myelencephalon contains the medulla

oblongata, CN XI (spinal accessory n.), and CN XII (hypoglossal n.).

Reptiles are considered to have 12 to 13 CNs, except for snakes, which have 11 to 12 (Table 8-3).[23] In reptile species in which legs are absent, the spinal accessory nerve has a very reduced presence or is not found.[27] The nervus terminalis has been classified as CN 0 and tracts with CN I, the olfactory nerve.[23] There is a paucity of information regarding the function of the nervus terminalis relative to the other CNs identified in reptile species. However, it is generally considered that CN 0 functions in a manner similar to an analogous structures found in other lower vertebrates by actions involving gonadotropin-releasing hormones.[28] The olfactory and vomeronasal (VMN) physiologic synergy is especially important in reptile species. The terminus of CN I is the olfactory cortex of the telencephalon via the olfactory tracts.[23] An accessary olfactory tract allows the VMN organ (in snake and lizard species) to access the cerebrum.[23]

As with other vertebrates, the spinal cord courses through the vertebral column within the spinal canal. Depending on reptile species, there is a variation in the amount of luminal space within the spinal canal that the spinal cord incorporates (i.e., 50% in alligators).[29] The spinal cord in reptiles functions very similarly to other vertebrates and is expanded at the areas that correspond to the cranial and caudal nerve plexuses (e.g., brachial, sacral).[23]

Birds

The avian brain consists of the proencephalon (telencephalon and diencephalon) and the caudal brain (medulla, pons, and mesencephalon) (Figure 8-4).[30] The avian caudal brain had a similar evolutionary development to that of mammals, but the proencephalon is anatomically different,[31] although it performs functions similar to those of mammalian species.[31] The cortical cells, necessary for processing gathered sensory information, are found within the cerebral cortex of birds, as well as reptiles, and not on the surface. The cerebral cortex of the avian brain is considered lissencephalic or smooth, as opposed to the undulating gyri and sulci found in mammals.[31]

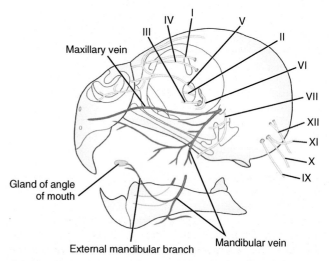

FIGURE 8-4 Avian cranial nerves. (From Tully TN. Neurology and ophthalmology. In Harcourt-Brown N, Chitty J, eds. *BSAVA Manual of Psittacine Birds,* ed. 2, Gloucester, UK: BSAVA 2005:234.)

TABLE 8-3

Cranial Nerves of Reptile Species

Cranial Nerve	Function	Clinical Assessment
CN 0 Nervus terminalis	Innervation nasal epithelial vasculature; chemosensory for GnRH	
CN I Olfactory/VMN nerve branch	Smell, from nasal sacs and VMN organ	Avoidance of noxious odors (e.g., alcohol); move toward food when eyes covered
CN II Optic	Sight, from the retina to thalamus and optic tectum	Menace response
CN III Oculomotor	Movement of eye; iris and ciliary body control	Coordinated eye movement, PLR
CN IV Trochlear	Movement of eye; anterior/dorsal	Coordinated eye movement; observe for strabismus
CN V Trigeminal • Ophthalmic • Maxillary • Mandibular	Sensory skin surrounding • Eye • Mouth • Sensory pits Controls • Jaw adductor muscles • Muscles of skin around teeth (snakes) • Intermandibularis muscle	Ophthalmic/maxillary • Feel stimulus to face, lower lid, nasal region Mandibular • Normal jaw closure
CN VI Abducens	Movement of eye posterior	Coordinated eye movement; observe for strabismus
CN VI Facial	Sensory skin and muscle, ear, upper maxilla, pharynx Control • Superficial neck muscles • Mandibular depressor	Normal • Lid movement • Opening of mouth
CN VIII Statoacoustic	Balance/hearing, sensory • Inner ear	Observe for clinical deficits • Induced spontaneous nystagmus • Torticollis • Abnormal posture • Delayed righting reflex
CN IX Glossopharyngeal	Taste/sensation • Pharynx Controls • Tongue muscles	Swallowing reflex; normal tongue function
CN X Vagus	Sensory/motor • Glottis • Heart • Viscera	Apply pressure to both eyes to induce bradycardia; swallowing reflex; normal glottis function
CN XI Spinal accessory	Controls • Trapezius muscle • Sternomastoid muscle	Condition of dorsal neck and shoulder muscles is difficult to determine in snakes and chelonians
CN XII Hypoglossal	Controls • Hyoid muscles • Tongue	Observe for normal tongue function

CN, Cranial nerve; *GnRH*, gonadotropin-releasing hormone; *PLR*, pupillary light response; *VMN*, vomeronasal.
Wyneken J. Reptilan neurology anatomy and function. *Vet Clin North Am Exot Anim Pract.* 2007;10:837-853.

The spinal cord is the same length as the vertebral column, and the spinal cord segment is at the same point as the vertebral column segment.[30,32] Spinal nerves course laterally through the vertebral foramen in birds. Moreover, birds do not have a cauda equina due to the fact that their spinal cord is as long as the spinal canal.[31] The lack of a cauda equina increases the difficulty of performing a myelogram in this group of animals. The 2 enlargements noted in the spinal cord of most birds correspond to the nerve concentrations formed from the brachial (thoracic limb) and lumbosacral (pelvic limb) plexuses. The glycogen body is found in the lumbosacral cord of birds and is a collection of periependymal

glycogen cells with nests of argentaffin cells.[31,32] There are nerve terminals within the glycogen body that are involved with both sensory and neurosecretory functions.[33]

The spinal cord in birds is similar to that in mammals, except that the dura mater is separate from the periosteal lining.[31] In the space formed by the separation of the dura and periosteal lining, an epidural space in the cervical and thoracic regions is filled with gelatinous tissue.[31] Birds also have an internal vertebral venous plexus that courses the entire length of the vertebral column.[31,32] The long ascending and long descending pathways of avian species have not been studied to the extent of those in mammals, but there is enough

TABLE 8-4

Long Ascending and Long Descending Pathways of Birds

Long Ascending Pathways	
Pathway	**Action**
Dorsal column	Information from body wall Touch, pressure, kinesthesia Proprioception of the joints
Dorso-lateral ascending bundle	Unconscious proprioception of wing
Ventro-lateral ascending bundle	Unconscious proprioception of body
Dorso-lateral fasciculus	Transmit tactile information
Spinoreticular tract	Delivery of pain information
Propriospinal system	Sense of nonlocalized pain

Long Descending Pathways	
Pathway	**Action**
Lateral reticulospinal tract	Visceral motor function
Rubrospinal tract	Enhance flexor tone of muscles
Cerebrospinal tract	Provides upper motor neuron input to motor neurons in ventral horn of cervical region
Vestibulospinal tract	Flight and ability to move freely in three-dimensional space
Reticulospinal tract	Altering somatic and visceral motor tone
Tectospinal tract	Coordination of reflex movements between eyes and upper body, primarily cervical area

Tully TN. Neurology and ophthalmology. In: Harcout-Brown N, Chitty J, eds. *BSAVA Manual of Psittacine Birds.* 2nd ed. Gloucester, UK: BSAVA Publishing; 2005:234-235.

TABLE 8-5

Avian Cranial Nerves and Associated Signs of Dysfunction

Cranial Nerve	Signs of Dysfunction
CN I Olfactory	Impaired smell
CN II Optic	Impaired sight
CN III Oculomotor	Ventro-lateral deviation (motor) Drooped upper eyelid (motor) Dilated pupil (parasympathetic)
CN IV Trochlear	Dorso-lateral deviation
CN V Trigeminal	Facial hypoesthesia; wide palpebral fissure; unable to close jaw
CN VI Abducens	Medial deviation; third eyelid immobility
CN VII Facial	Asymmetry of face; poor taste; decreased secretions of most glands of head
CN VIII Vestibulocochlear	Impaired hearing; nystagmus; head tilt
CN IX Glossopharyngeal	Poor taste and feel; dysphagia; voice loss
CN X Vagus	Regurgitation; voice change; increased heart rate; no crop mobility
CN XI Accessory	Poor neck movement
CN XII Hypoglossal	Tongue deviation

Orosz SE. Principles of avian clinical neuroanatomy. *Sem Avian Exot Pet Med.* 1996;5:127-139.

evidence to correlate the pathways with their mammalian counterparts and to speculate on, if not verify, their actions in birds (Table 8-4).[30-32]

A thorough knowledge and examination of an avian patient's CNs should be performed if there is suspected involvement of the CNS with the presenting disease condition. If a single CN is involved, the lesion is easier to localize than if there is multiple nerve pathology.[30] Patients with CNS lesions often present with clinical signs affecting proprioception, pain localization, and upper motor neuron abnormalities, but the mental status of the bird is not altered.[30] It is imperative that the person performing the neurologic examination on the avian patient be knowledgeable about the location and function of the CNs. The above information and knowledge of the major ascending and descending tracts, found in Table 8-4, will significantly aid in determining whether the neurologic deficit(s) can be localized to a particular area within the CNS.[31] The 12 CNs found in birds and associated signs of dysfunction are found in Table 8-5.

Mammals

As with the other taxa that are discussed within this text and in particular this chapter, the companion animal veterinarian

will see many species of small exotic mammals. Although not inclusive, the group of small exotic mammals commonly maintained as companion animals consists of rats, rabbits, hamsters, guinea pigs, hedgehogs, ferrets, and sugar gliders. This section on basic mammalian anatomy and function of the CNS provides information that is relatively consistent across all species. The brain of small mammals consists of a forebrain (telencephalon and diencephalon), midbrain (mesencephalon), and hindbrain (rhombencephalon) (Figure 8-5).[34] The cerebrum, consisting of the cerebral cortices and basal nuclei, is the most prevalent anatomical structure of the rabbit brain and, for the most part, other small exotic companion mammals.[35] Similar to birds, rabbits and other small mammals (e.g., rats, mice) have a cerebral cortex that is lissencephalic.[36] Ventral to the telencephalon is the diencephalon. The structures of the diencephalon are the metathalamus, thalamus, hypothalamus, pineal gland, and pituitary gland.[34] Caudal to the midbrain is the mesencephalon, which regulates the visual (rostral colliculi) and auditory (caudal colliculi) reflexes.[34] Smell is the only sense that does not have to course through the thalamus to reach the cerebral cortex.[37] The medial geniculate nuclei are primarily auditory conduits, while the lateral geniculate nuclei are visual. The combined medial and lateral geniculate nuclei are the metathalamus.[34] The hindbrain (rhombencephalon) contains the cerebellum, pons, and medulla.[34] To further delineate the hindbrain, the

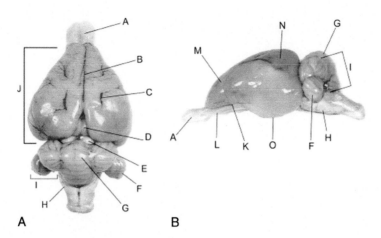

FIGURE 8-5 *A,* Dorsal and *B,* lateral view of the unpreserved brain of a New Zealand white domestic rabbit *(Oryctolagus cuniculus).* A—Olfactory bulb. B—Longitudinal fissure. C—Marginal sulcus. D—Rostral colliculus. F—Cerebellar paraflocculus. G—Cerebellar vermis. H—Medulla. I—Cerebellar hemisphere. J—Cerebral cortex. K—Lateral rhinal sulcus. L—Olfactory peduncle. M—Frontal lobe of cerebrum. N—Occipital lobe of cerebrum. O—Pyriform lobe of cerebrum. (Osofsky A, LaCouteur RA, Vernau KM. Functional neuroanatomy of the domestic rabbit *(Oryctolagus cuniculus). Vet Clin N Am Exot Anim Pract.* 2007;10:723.)

cerebellum and pons are classified as the metencephalon, and the medulla is the myelencephalon.[35] It is important for veterinarians to know the anatomy and physiology associated with disease processes as they relate to rabbits and other small exotic mammalian species. Examples of the importance of knowing the origins of disease pathology and subsequent clinical signs on presentation are encephalitozoonosis and central extension of otitis infections. Both of these diseases affect the brainstem, or more specifically the anatomical structures that form the brainstem, which include the thalamus, hypothalamus, midbrain, pons, and medulla.[35]

The spinal cord of small exotic mammals is similar to that of other mammalian species. The spinal cord is protected by the meninges: dura mater, arachnoid mater, and pia mater. Between the arachnoid and pia mater is the subarachnoid space that contains the cerebrospinal fluid. The composition of the central cord, composed of white matter (myelinated axons of ascending and descending tracts) and gray matter (nerve cell bodies, unmyelinated/slightly myelinated axons), is consistent across the species of small mammals treated in veterinary hospitals.[34,35]

As with other animals, the knowledge of the CNs of small exotic mammals is extremely important when performing a neurologic examination to localize a lesion associated with the disease condition (Table 8-6).

DISEASES

Invertebrates

As a group, there are few neurologic diseases that have been specially identified affecting invertebrates. Overall, in the captive setting, typical causes of neurologic disease signs such as ataxia, paralysis, and disorientation are associated with adverse environmental conditions (e.g., water quality), trauma, inadequate nutrition, or toxin exposure. At this time, the study of invertebrate diseases and associated clinical presentations is in its infancy. It has been common practice to remove the dead and dying animals and replace them without putting much effort towards determining the underlying disease process. Even with a concern, how would one examine an invertebrate that is exhibiting neurological disease signs? In the last 20 to 30 years, there has been an increase in large-scale aquaculture farms raising shrimp and crawfish. When such farms have a disease problem, the diagnostic test of choice is pathology. A necropsy examination is the most rapid and intensive method to determine a disease diagnosis. There has also been a continued interest in aquaria (especially saltwater invertebrates) and an increasing popularity of spiders, insects, scorpions, centipedes, and millipedes being maintained as "companion animals" during this same time period. Many of the invertebrate species are expensive, thereby causing the owner to seek professional assistance in determining the diagnosis of an ill animal so that proper treatment can be initiated. As previously mentioned, there are few specific neurologic disease conditions identified at this time that affect invertebrates, and the neurologic diagnostic techniques used for these animals are rudimentary but continuing to develop. Over time, veterinary medical understanding of neurologic conditions that affect this large group of animals will expand along with the ability to diagnose and treat the diseases that cause these signs.

Spiders

DEHYDRATION. Spiders that are alive but cannot move their legs may be dehydrated due to a reduction in hemolymph pressure.[12] A thorough history is essential in trying to determine if the animal has had access to an adequate water supply.

TOXINS. As with most invertebrates, exposure to toxins, either within the environment (e.g., insecticides) or through prey, is a common cause of neurologic signs and death.

TABLE 8-6	
Small Exotic Mammal Cranial Nerves and Associated Functions	
Cranial Nerve	**Function**
CN I Olfactory	Smell
CN II Optic	Sensory pathway for vision
CN III Oculomotor	Innervation of the eye • Motor fibers, extrinsic striated muscles of the eye • Parasympathetic fibers, intrinsic ocular muscles
CN IV Trochlear	Innervation of the dorsal oblique muscle
CN V Trigeminal	Sensory innervation • Ophthalmic nerve • Maxillary nerve Sensory and motor innervation • Mandibular
CN VI Abducens	Innervation, lateral rectus and retractor bulbi eye muscles
CN VII Facial	Motor function • Mouth and head (facial expression) Minor sensory function • Palate and rostral 2/3 tongue (taste) Parasympathetic innervation • Lacrimal glands • Salivary glands
CN VIII Vestibulocochlear	Sensory Cochlear branch • Hearing Vestibular branch • Orientation of the head relative to gravity The only CN that does not exit the skull
CN IX Glossopharyngeal	Motor function • Pharyngeal muscle control Sensory function • Caudal third of tongue (taste) • Pharyngeal muscosa Parasympathetic innervation • Parotid salivary gland
CN X Vagus	Motor function • Pharyngeal muscles • Laryngeal muscles Sensory function • Caudal pharynx • Larynx • Abdominal viscera Parasympathetic innervation • Thoracic viscera • Abdominal viscera
CN XI Accessory	Motor function • Cleidomastoid muscle • Sternomastoid muscle • Trapezius muscle
CN XII Hypoglossal	Motor function • Tongue • Hyoid muscles

Osofsky A, LeCouteur RA, Vernau KM. Functional neuroanatomy of the domestic rabbit *(Oryctolagus cuniculus). Vet Clin North Am Exot Anim Pract.* 2007;10:713-730.

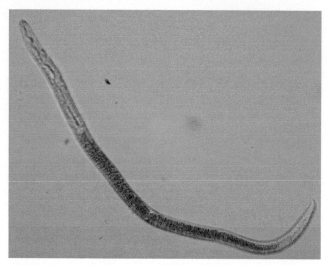

FIGURE 8-6 Photomicrograph of a panagrolaimidae nematode. These are often noted with increased mucoid discharge around the mouthparts of infected spiders. (Courtesy A. Velasco, The University of Adelaide.)

Common neurologic signs associated with toxin exposure in invertebrates are ataxia, paresis, paralysis, disorientation, lack of movement, twitching, and death. Common insecticides (e.g., fipronil) and nicotine (i.e., on the hands of heavy smokers) have been implicated in spider toxicities that caused neurologic signs and death.[12]

PANAGROLAIMIDAE NEMATODES. Panagrolaimidae nematodes can infect many tarantula species, both wild-caught and captive individuals (Figure 8-6). The onset of clinical signs of a nematode infection begins with anorexia and lethargy, progressing to a point of the animal maintaining a "flexed leg" position, with death occurring within weeks to a few months.[12] Some infected tarantulas will appear to stand on the tips of their legs and have a mucoid substance around their mouthparts.[12] The exact life cycle of this parasite is unknown but threatens captive spider populations. Treatment at this time is ineffective; therefore, preventing the introduction of this parasite into a captive population is essential. A quarantine period of at least 30 days is required for all new tarantula acquisitions prior to placing them into an established colony.

MERMITHIDAE NEMATODES. The Mermithidae nematode is rare in tarantulas and primarily found in wild-caught individuals. Infected animals may have behavior changes (i.e., don't move when approached) and become lethargic.[38] Since the nematodes multiply in the opisthosoma prior to killing the host, affected individuals usually display a significantly enlarged opisthosoma.[12] Spiders infected with this nematode display stunted development of their external anatomic structures (e.g., legs).

POMPILIDAE WASPS AND SPHECIDAE MUD DAUBERS. Both the Pompilidae wasps and Sphecidae mud daubers paralyze tarantulas and other spiders with their sting, prior to laying an egg on the immobilized animal. The egg hatches and the larva feeds on the paralyzed spider. Pompilidae wasps attach to tarantulas, while Sphecidae mud daubers most often parasitize Theridiidae and Araneidae spiders.[12] Both types of parasitism most often occur in wild spiders.

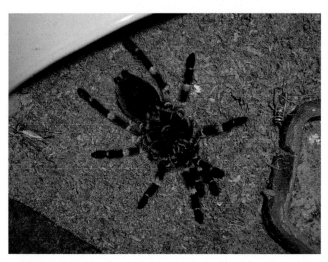

FIGURE 8-7 Tarantula on its back; normal ecdysis. (Courtesy Trevor T. Zachariah.)

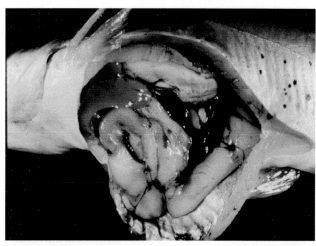

FIGURE 8-8 Fish showing brown blood color (methemoglobinemia) that is typical of nitrite poisoning. (Courtesy Ron Thune.)

ECDYSIS. Ecdysis usually occurs when Theraphosidae spiders (tarantulas) are dorsally recumbent or on their side (Figure 8-7).[12] The animal may have their legs in a flexed position, showing very little if any movement. The animal should not be handled when ecdysis is occurring since the underlying soft tissue is susceptible to trauma. Some clients become concerned that the animal may be dead, as most spiders die in an "upright" position with their legs flexed under the body.[12] The process usually is completed within several hours; therefore, animals found in this position for an extended period (days) should be evaluated for signs of life.

Fish

As with other exotic animal species, fish are susceptible to both dietary and environmental causes of neurologic disease. It can be argued that fish require much more oversight in maintaining a healthy environment because of overcrowding and toxicities that may be associated with poor water quality. There are many different fish species that are both farm raised and kept in aquariums. On a per-animal basis, fish are the most popular animal maintained as "pets." With the popularity of aquarium fish, there are many products at both local and national pet stores that cater to this interest. The fish owner must be aware of the fish that they purchase and the size of the environment in which the animal will be living. Many fish species are aggressive and require larger tanks to reduce stress associated with mixed population. Also, too many fish within an aquarium may contaminate the environment with biologic waste and uneaten food, increasing the possibility of water toxicoses. It is also extremely important that each species of tropical fish receives a complete diet and that enough food is fed to ensure that all animals receive an adequate nutritional offering. If an inadequate diet is being fed or not all fish are receiving an appropriate amount to meet their minimum daily nutritional requirements, nutritional deficiencies will arise. Common nutritional deficiencies in fish that lead to neurologic disease signs (e.g., abnormal swimming motion) include thiamine, niacin, biotin, and pyridoxine.[39]

Environmental Abnormalities

It is obvious to even the novice aquarium owner that dirty water can cause abnormal behaviors in fish. In some conditions, the water may appear "clean" but in fact is problematic to the health of the animals. Ammonia toxicity or "new tank syndrome" occurs when the pH of the water rises above 7.0.[39] The fish become listless and are reluctant to move; this is one of the most deadly and common problems fish owners encounter. To prevent ammonia toxicity, owners are encouraged to follow a routine maintenance schedule in which the water pH and ammonia are tested, fish population density is monitored, and the proper function of pumps and biological filters is checked. Carbon dioxide (CO_2) toxicity will occur when concentrations reach levels >20 mg/L water.[39] When fish appear lethargic and nonresponsive, it is recommended to again test the pH of the water for increased CO_2 levels. An increased concentration of CO_2 will cause the water pH to decrease. As the aquarium water is aerated, the CO_2 levels will decrease and cause a corresponding rise in the pH of the water.

Nitrite poisoning will also cause fish to become anorectic, listless, disoriented, and circled (curl from head to tail) (Figure 8-8). As with other adverse environmental conditions, overcrowding and poor tank maintenance will cause a continuous rise in nitrite levels until the fish are unable to properly function. Routine aquarium care, water changes, and testing will help reduce the incidence of nitrite poisoning. Fish appear to tolerate nitrite concentrations <0.5 mg/L water.[40]

Bacterial Encephalitis

Although rare, *Streptococcus* spp. encephalitis has been reported in rainbow sharks, rosy barbs, danios, tetras, and cichlids.[39] The pathophysiology of this bacterial infection is similar to that in other animals susceptible to infectious encephalitis. Exposure of the fish to the pathogenic bacterium can occur within the aquatic environment or through live food.[39] Fish diagnosed with streptococcal encephalitis will exhibit clinical signs that affect normal swimming and movement within the

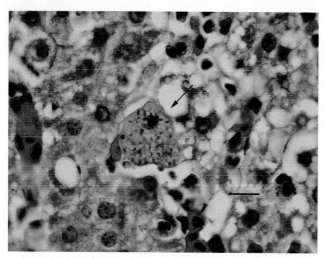

FIGURE 8-9 Liver of a leopard shark. Microsporidian spores are present in the cytoplasm of a melanomacrophage *(Arrow)*, Hematoxylin and Eosin. Bar = 20 μm (photo courtesy of Michael Garner, Northwest ZooPath).

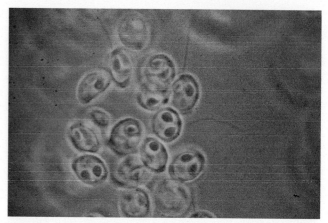

FIGURE 8-10 *Myxobolus cerebralis,* an organism that causes whirling disease in fish. (Courtesy Ron Thune.)

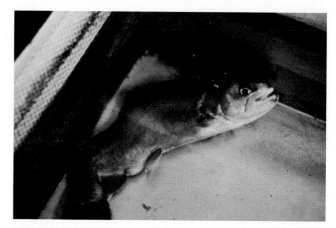

FIGURE 8-11 Fish with clinical signs of whirling disease. (Courtesy Ron Thune.)

water, appearing disoriented and lethargic. Culture and sensitivity of the diseased fish during a pathological examination may help identify the organism and determine an effective antibiotic treatment.

Neurologic Disease Caused by Parasites

Pleistophora hyphessobryconis is a microsporidium parasite (primitive fungus) that causes abnormal swimming in aquarium fish (Figure 8-9). This microsporidium infection is usually associated with neon tetras and therefore has been termed "neon tetra disease"; however, angelfish and zebrafish, among other freshwater aquarium fish, are susceptible.[39] Muscle damage by the parasite causes the abnormal swimming movement and there is no treatment once an individual has been infected. Histopathological examination of diseased muscle tissue (which may appear marbled/necrotic) from infected fish will confirm a diagnosis of the presence of *Pleistophora hyphessobryconis*.[40] Parasite (fungal) spores are also easily identified in wet mounts of infected tissue.[40] Recommended treatment is to remove all fish exhibiting clinical disease signs from the aquarium.[40]

Myxosporidian infections in freshwater fish are most often identified and highly pathogenic to wild populations and those farmed in highly intensive outdoor fishponds.[40] Myxosporidia are protozoan parasites that have an indirect life cycle and primarily use annelids as an intermediate host. Pathologically, these protozoa are often host and tissue specific. In captive environments, infected animals cannot expose other fish to the organism unless the intermediate host is present. Although noninfectious without the intermediate host, the diseased animals should be separated from the apparently healthy fish due to irreversible tissue damage that adversely affects their appearance and ability to swim.[40]

Myxobolus cerebralis is the organism that causes whirling disease in salmonids (Figure 8-10). When fingerling fish are exposed and infected with *Myxobolus cerebralis*, the developing cartilage of the vertebral column and skull are permanently damaged, resulting in skeletal deformities.[40] Common clinical disease signs in young fish include rapid tail-chasing behavior (e.g., whirling) when startled; hence, the name "whirling disease" (Figure 8-11).[40] *Myxobolus cerebralis* is also called "blacktail" because the tail and peduncle may darken when fish become infected.[40] Whirling disease may not be fatal if the fish is able to adapt to the skeletal deformities; however, the recovered fish are considered disease carriers. Moreover, the skeletal deformities that developed at a younger age never resolve. A presumptive diagnosis of whirling disease can be made by detection of spores from skulls of infected fish. To obtain a definitive diagnosis, histopathological examination of infected tissue or serologic testing is required. There is no treatment, and prevention is recommended by purchasing disease-free fish stock and maintaining an environment free of the intermediate host.[40] The intermediate host for *Myxobolus cerebralis* infections in fish is the tubifex worm (*Tubifex tubifex*).

Amphibians

When an amphibian patient is presented with neurologic clinical disease signs, a number of basic facts must be recognized. First, amphibians as a group contain many different and varied species. The life cycle of the amphibian is divided into 2 distinct anatomic forms that require the animal to live in an aquatic environment as a juvenile and terrestrially as an adult. As the animal goes through this growth transition, the

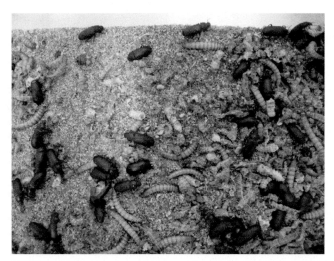

FIGURE 8-12 When used as the sole dietary source, crickets and mealworms will provide nutrition for amphibian species but will not provide adequate calcium concentrations required for normal bone structure.

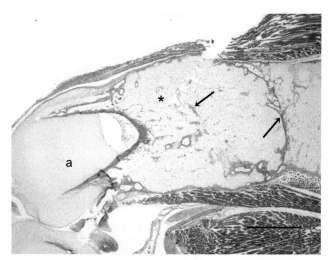

FIGURE 8-13 Asian horn frog, distal femur at stifle articulation (a), metabolic bone disease. Note widened metaphyseal region due to cartilagenous metaplasia (*), and attenuated medullary bone trabeculae (arrows). Hematoxylin and Eosin, bar = 300 μm (photo courtesy of Michael Garner, Northwest ZooPath).

diet required for adequate health in many species completely differs from the aquatic juvenile to the terrestrial adult. There are a few amphibian species (e.g., caecilians, newts) that live in aquatic environments for their entire life. However, the diet for the juvenile and adult phases of these aquatic species also varies. With the complexity and variation in an amphibian's natural diet, it is extremely difficult for owners to exactly match the nutritional requirements of the animals under their care. Consequently, the diets fed to captive amphibians are dependent on commercially available products that are nutritionally incomplete; primarily, mealworms and crickets (Figure 8-12). Many of the commercially available insects have low calcium content and often an inverse calcium to phosphorus (Ca:P) ratio.[41,42] Although pet owners will often "gut load" insects with calcium-impregnated food and "dust" the prey with a vitamin/mineral supplement, this has little effect on significantly improving the nutritional quality of the diet. It is rare that owners understand the specific environmental requirements for adult amphibian species, much less be able provide such an enclosure to ensure a healthy existence. Owners of one or more amphibian species are required to educate themselves on the nutritional and environmental requirements of their pets. With this knowledge, it is imperative that significant time and effort are invested to procure the necessary diet and maintain an appropriate clean living environment. The time and effort required to properly house and feed captive amphibian species are often more than people anticipate, which can lead to diseases associated with malnutrition and improper husbandry. There are very few infectious diseases that cause neurologic disease in amphibian species. Most amphibians that are presented to veterinary hospitals with neurologic problems are diagnosed with specific nutritional deficiencies or toxicities and diseases associated with being housed in an improper environment.

Metabolic Bone Disease

One of the most common disease conditions in captive amphibians related to an improper diet is metabolic bone

disease (MBD) (Figure 8-13). Diets low in calcium or with an inverse Ca:P ratio, low in vitamin D₃, or high in phosphorus are the primary contributors to the development of MBD.[42] There are other variables that may contribute to the development and/or severity of disease, such as the ability of an amphibian to process vitamin D₃ through access to an ultraviolet (UV) light source or sunlight and elevated concentrations of vitamin A that interfere with vitamin D metabolism.[41] However, the significance of either the processing of vitamin D₃ or hypovitaminosis A to the disease pathophysiology of MBD has not yet been established for a specific species or amphibians in general.[42] Based on metabolic interactions of vitamins, minerals, and UV light in other groups of animals (e.g., reptiles), one may hypothesize that in amphibians these interactions would differ between orders. Again, one may improve the low or imbalanced calcium in insects used as food or prey (e.g., mealworms, crickets, waxworms) by feeding the insects/worms a mineral-impregnated food or "dusting" with a supplement.[43] However, while buying the food supplement for the prey and then dusting the insects does increase the commitment an owner has for the captive amphibian, even when performed properly this rarely compensates for the nutritional deficiencies of the commercially available worms (Figure 8-14). This thus explains the common presentation of captive amphibian species, including anurans, caudates, and caecilians, with MBD.[41] Common clinical signs associated with MBD in amphibians include subcutaneous edema, skeletal deformities (e.g., folding long bone fractures, vertebra, mandibular), lack of cortical bone density, abnormal posture and locomotion, and muscle tetany.[41]

A definitive diagnosis can be made for MBD through nutritional information obtained from the owner, corresponding clinical signs, and radiographic evidence of poor cortical bone density. Treatment should focus on calcium and vitamin D₃ supplementation.[44] Parenteral calcium should only be provided intramuscularly (IM) with the initial injection, never

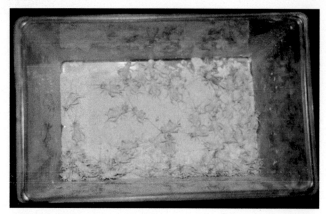

FIGURE 8-14 Dusting crickets with a calcium supplement will help improve the nutritional composition of the prey. However, the dust does not remain on the crickets. The inverse Ca:P ratio of many insects makes it necessary to look for other commercial food options to provide the necessary nutrition for captive amphibian species.

intravenously (IV), and then transitioned to oral supplementation or topical administration through soaking, depending on species or animal's stage of development.[41] There are commercially available oral calcium supplements that include vitamins and magnesium (Repashy Calcium Plus, Repashy Ventures Inc., San Marcos, CA). These complete calcium supplements can be administered by the owner at home for prolonged periods of time as the animal recovers and used as a nutritional supplement to improve the overall nutritional intake of the animal.

Vitamin B Deficiency

As with other vertebrate species, vitamin B_1 (thiamine) deficiency in amphibian species causes neurologic clinical signs (e.g., paralysis, peripheral nerve demyelination).[42] Other neurologic and associated musculoskeletal clinical signs of vitamin B deficiency, specifically thiamine, include hind limb paresis/paralysis and scoliosis in captive anuran species.[41] Animals fed diets deficient in vitamin B_1 and prey items that contain thiaminase (e.g., fish, invertebrates) are predisposed to this condition. Treatment and prevention of vitamin B/thiamine deficiency is usually effective through topical, oral, or feed supplementation.[45] In severe cases, parenteral IM supplementation can be used for an initial treatment.[45]

Toxicity

Amphibians live in a moist aquatic/semiaquatic environment for part or most of their lives. Their skin is highly permeable, therefore making them extremely susceptible to toxic exposure in a contaminated closed captive environment. As with fish, increased levels of nitrogenous wastes in the form of ammonia and nitrites will cause neurologic disease signs and death to amphibians. Water ammonia levels should be <0.02 parts per million (ppm) and nitrite levels <0.1 ppm.[34] To prevent ammonia and nitrite toxicity, water quality should be checked on a regular basis and water changed routinely. Treatment for toxicity includes a water change, monitoring/cleaning the filtration system, and review of animal densities within the habitat.[41] Although chronic low-level ammonia

toxicity may not cause overt clinical disease, it does lead to overall poor health and immunosuppression.[41]

Amphibians may be exposed to commercial pesticides through environmental contamination, overspray of captive habitats, or food items (e.g., dead insects). Common commercial pesticides that may cause neurologic signs in amphibians include organophosphates, carbamates, organochlorines, rotenone, and pyrethroids.[41] Tremors, seizures, reduced righting reflex and locomotor activity, and abnormal posture and behavior are typical neurologic signs associated with pesticide toxicity.[41] It is important to obtain a thorough history from the owner to identify the specific toxin that may be associated with the presenting condition. Supportive care and dilution or removal of a pesticide from the skin surface or gastrointestinal (GI) tract will increase the chance for patient recovery. Exposure to high concentrations of a pesticide or prolonged contact is often lethal or, if treated, provides a poor prognosis for recovery.[41]

Heavy metal toxicosis has been diagnosed in amphibians exhibiting neurologic signs.[46] Exposure can occur through ingestion or possibly absorption through the skin. Heavy metals that have caused clinical illness and death include copper, lead, aluminum, mercury, zinc, cadmium, arsenic, silver, manganese, molybdenum, and antimony.[41] The source of many amphibian heavy metal toxicosis cases has been wire used for enclosures and piping used for plumbing.[47] Clinical signs associated with heavy metal toxicosis in amphibians are similar to those in other animals: ataxia, disorientation, and paralysis or paresis. Treatment begins with a diagnosis and identifying the toxin source, after which chelation therapy is initiated. Supportive care is usually required to stabilize the patient and decrease the recovery period. Once the source of the heavy metal is identified, it should be removed from the animal's enclosure. Prevention of heavy metal toxicosis is achieved by avoiding the use of wire for the enclosure or metal for plumbing.[47]

Cleaning agents and disinfectants, especially those that contain high concentrations of chlorine, ammonia, and other volatile compounds, may cause neurologic signs and death to amphibian species.[41] Owners must be educated about the ease with which chemicals are absorbed through the skin of amphibians and remove all evidence of the cleaning agent from the enclosure before placing the animal inside. Concurrent skin lesions with neurologic signs and a recent history of cleaning the patient's enclosure are strong evidence that exposure to cleaning chemicals may be the underlying cause of the disease condition.

Chytridiomycosis

Batrachochytrium dendrobatidis (Bd) is a chytrid fungus that infects amphibians and the only fungus of its type known to have pathologic consequences in a vertebrate species (Figure 8-15).[48,49] The fungus was first recognized as a worldwide threat to wild amphibian populations in the last decade of the 20th century, but subsequently was identified in diseased amphibian specimens from the 1930s.[48,49] Although first recognized as a disease threat to wild populations, chytridiomycosis is considered a pathogen for animals maintained in captive collections.[50]

Adult anurans appear most susceptible to chytridiomycosis, although other amphibian species have been diagnosed

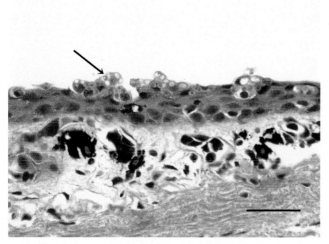

FIGURE 8-15 Tomato frog skin, chytridiomycosis. Note intracytoplasmic chytrid fungi in the superficial epidermis (arrow). The underlying dermis is edematous, with minimal lymphocytic inflammation. Hematoxylin and Eosin bar = 80 μm (photo courtesy of Michael Garner, Northwest ZooPath).

with the fungal infection (e.g., caudates).[41] Developing juvenile anurans (e.g., tadpoles) appear to be less susceptible to Bd but will develop a subclinical infection.[41] While primarily a disease of the epidermis (e.g., hyperkeratosis, dysecdysis, ulceration, cutaneous hemorrhage), neurologic signs including loss of righting reflex, abnormal posture, and a loss of fear when approached are also present.[41] Diagnosis of chytridiomycosis can be achieved through histological examination of keratinized epithelial cells, identification of scattered single chytrid thalli (sporangia), or evidence of small clusters of organism within the epidermal stratum corneum.[41] Most argyrophilic and argentophilic stains can be used to identify the chytrid sporangia, which have periodic acid-Schiff-positive walls.[41] Immunohistochemistry, polymerase chain reaction (PCR) testing of diseased skin samples, and fungal culture are other diagnostic tests that may be used to confirm Bd in an amphibian patient.[41,51] Successful treatment of captive frog species has been achieved using a medicated bath containing 0.01% itraconazole.[51] However, due to the ease of transmission of infective zoospores, prevention of exposure is recommended when obtaining animals for captive collections or relocating wild specimens.[41] If infected animals are identified, they should be separated from the rest of a collection and treated; exposed equipment and enclosures should also be disinfected. Prior to placing newly acquired amphibians into a collection, the animals should be quarantined for a minimum of 30 days. PCR testing of animals at the start and end of the quarantine period can minimize the likelihood of missing a positive Bd case.[41,52,53]

Other Disease Conditions

Although not specific to amphibian species, trauma, parasites, septicemia, and electrolyte imbalances are common disease presentations that may result in neurologic disease signs. Obtaining a thorough history from the owner, performing a complete external physical examination, and appropriate diagnostic testing will often identify the cause of the abnormal

neurologic presentation. Depending on the severity of the patient's condition, targeted medical treatment along with supportive care can lead to a positive outcome for the case.

Reptiles

Although there are neurologic disease conditions caused by inadequate nutrition and husbandry in captive reptile species, infectious disease is commonly diagnosed as the underlying source of the clinical signs. Diagnostic tests available to help diagnose diseases associated with neurologic clinical signs are helpful with many cases but may be inadequate due to the lack of basic research to generate accepted evaluation guidelines for the number of reptile species presented to veterinary practices. In certain instances, specifically for new or novel infectious diseases, the testing methodologies have yet to be validated on a large scale. Even with the limitations of diagnostic testing, pathological evaluation of affected tissue helps bolster the diagnostic capabilities for the practicing veterinarian when trying to identify a definitive cause of neurologic disease in a reptile patient.

Bacterial Diseases

As with other species, bacterial infections, whether localized or systemic, can result in neurologic disease conditions. Tremors, isolated to a certain area or involving the whole body, circling, ataxia, paresis/paralysis, and torticollis are all disease signs that may be caused by bacterial infections. Bacteria commonly isolated from reptile species that result in neurologic disease are Gram-negative organisms and include *Pseudomonas* spp., *Salmonella* spp., and *Mycoplasma* spp.[54,55] Although Gram-negative bacteria are most commonly isolated from reptile species in which neurologic disease clinical signs are present, other bacterial organisms may cause similar pathology and presentations (e.g., *Staphylococcus* spp., *Mycobacterium* spp.). It is not unusual for bacterial disease to initially affect the reptile patient in a body system apart from the nervous system such as the respiratory or GI tract. As the disease condition progresses, the animal becomes septic, with the infection then affecting some part of the nervous system. Cerebral lesions often cause animals to walk, without direction, in large circles, while brainstem, cerebellar, and vestibular lesions result in the animal walking in tight small circles.[56] Bacterial infections are a common cause of vestibular lesions and are often associated with torticollis. Abscesses are formed, in most cases, from a localized bacterial infection and may be found in the brain or bone. Osteomyelitis of the spine or long bones caused by a bacterial or fungal infection can cause bilateral or unilateral limb paresis/paralysis.[56] Treatment of reptile patients that are presented with neurologic clinical signs and diagnosed with bacterial infection is dependent on the location and severity of disease. Identification of the bacterial organism in a septic case is difficult, often due to the small size of the patient. Blood cultures may be possible in larger reptile patients but not possible in smaller individuals. Brain lesions are difficult to identify, and often require more advanced diagnostic imaging modalities, such as magnetic resonance imaging (MRI). Localized abscesses involving the spinal column or vestibular area may be identified and the affected tissue within the area of the lesion cultured.[56] Some bacterial disease conditions may be treated with antibiotic therapy alone, while others that involve abscesses will require

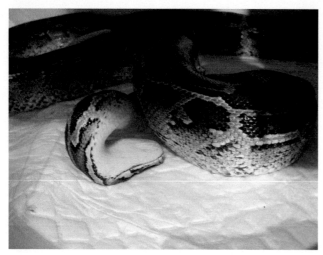

FIGURE 8-16 Snake with signs of neurologic disease, including the loss of its righting reflex (photo courtesy of Lionel Schilliger).

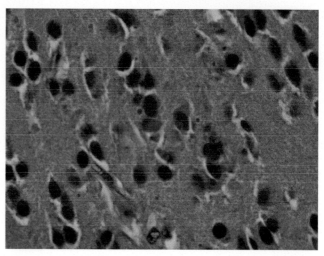

FIGURE 8-17 Brain of a red-tailed boa. Note the cytoplasmic inclusions typical of inclusion body disease. Hematoxylin and Eosin (photo courtesy of Michael Garner, Northwest ZooPath).

both surgery (if possible) and antimicrobial treatment. In all cases, supportive care must be provided as well as keeping an appropriate temperature zone within the animal's living environment to maintain the optimum healing metabolic rate and maximize the effectiveness of the antibiotic therapy.

Viral Diseases

OPHIDIAN PARAMYXOVIRUS. Snakes can be exposed to ophidian paramyxovirus (OPMV) through horizontal exposure to respiratory secretions from other infected animals or possibly mites *(Ophionyssus natricis)*.[54] OPMV not only affects the neurologic system of infected reptiles but also the respiratory and GI systems as well and is considered a disease primarily of the respiratory system.[57] Head tremors, stargazing, convulsions, and reduced righting reflexes, are neurologic signs that one may observe in infected animals (Figure 8-16). However, early in the disease process, the infection may be clinically inapparent, so the snake owner may not be able to determine that the animal is ill. In peracute cases, the viral infection may be so severe that an antibody response is not elicited.[5] The incubation period of OPMV in snakes has been determined to be from 6 to >10 weeks postexposure in acute cases; however, animals with chronic disease have been known to remain subclinical for up to 10 months.[57] With the chronic disease state, snakes may show nonspecific clinical signs, such as anorexia and regurgitation, for at least 7 months prior to developing any other overt clinical signs.[57] The immunocompromised state of the animal predisposes the individual to secondary bacterial and fungal infections of the respiratory and GI systems. Respiratory signs of OPMV include various degrees of dyspnea, while the GI system may have a gas-distended intestine. In affected reptile, torticollis is often present, as well as fetid feces, mucoid diarrhea, and severe protozoal infection.[57] One must remember to include OPMV as a top differential disease diagnosis, along with inclusion body disease (IBD), for snakes that are presented with severe neurologic signs. Although euthanasia is recommended for snakes definitively diagnosed with OPMV, antibiotic and anti-protozoal therapy will often extend the life of an infected

animal. However, infected snakes, even in treatment, will continue to shed the virus within the environment, posing a serious threat to other animals in the house and enclosure.

Antemortem diagnosis of OPMV is determined through clinical presentation and owner history and is historically confirmed using hemagglutination inhibition assay serologic titers of snakes.[57] Paired titers are obtained through serologic samples collected at least 8 weeks apart, since that is the time period usually required for seroconversion to take place.[57] Recently, an OPMV PCR test has been developed and is commercially available for antemortem testing, using either individual oral or cloacal swabs or a combined oral/cloacal swab.[54]

As stated, there is no specific treatment for OPMV and the recommended protocol for prevention is strict quarantine measures for new snakes brought into a collection. Quarantine requirements include isolation of all new animals for 60 to 90 days, testing of all snakes for OPMV on entrance and when released from quarantine, testing and treating for all parasites with 2 negative fecal samples prior to the animal leaving the quarantine area, and all other standard quarantine requirements.[57]

INCLUSION BODY DISEASE. Arguably, IBD is the most important viral disease identified in captive collections of boas and pythons.[58] Boa constrictors *(Boa constrictor constrictor)* and Burmese pythons *(Python molurus bivittatus)* are very common snakes maintained as pets, and subsequently have been diagnosed most often with IBD (Figure 8-17).[58] However, it is likely that all snakes of the family Boidae are susceptible to this disease. Although snakes within the family Boidae have been diagnosed with IBD, other snake species may serve as subclinical carriers or present with different clinical disease signs.[59] IBD was first recognized in the 1980s in collections of boid snakes maintained in different countries around the world.[51] Strong evidence of an underlying viral etiologic agent proved elusive until the recent identification of an arenavirus associated with IBD.[60]

Any boid snake that presents with acute onset of neurologic signs and that has a history of poor body condition

344444444444444444

should have IBD at the top of a differential disease diagnosis list. Neurologic signs consist of loss of righting reflex, head tremors, flaccid paralysis, ataxia, opisthotonos, and stargazing.[54,58] As with OPMV, IBD may initially present as a respiratory and/or GI disease along with poor body condition. Infected boa species often are presented with a history of regurgitation and chronic weight loss, while python species initially develop neurologic clinical signs. This disease appears to progress faster in pythons than in boas.[58] Susceptible snakes are believed to be exposed in a manner similar to OPMV, through respiratory secretions and (possibly) the snake mite.[58,61]

Historically, a diagnosis has been made through microscopic examination of biopsy tissue samples harvested from diseased snakes in an effort to detect typical intracytoplasmic inclusion bodies associated with IBD. Antemortem tissue samples commonly collected from patients are from the liver, kidney, and esophageal tonsil.[54] The white blood cells of infected patients, in particular the lymphocytes, may contain typical inclusion bodies and may be used for diagnostic purposes.[58] Postmortem samples include all of the major organ systems, brain, and spinal cord.[58] At this time, a PCR test is now available to test for arenavirus in a blood sample and/or esophageal swab collected from an animal believed to be infected with IBD.[54] There are no specific treatments for IBD-infected snakes. Treatment is supportive and should follow the same recommendations as those given for snakes infected with OPMV. Preventive measures against exposure of susceptible snake species to IBD within captive collections includes a strict quarantine protocol, testing the snakes prior to and just before release from quarantine, and euthanasia of infected animals.

AGAMID ATADENOVIRUS. An atadenovirus has been identified in commercial bearded dragon (*Pogona vitticeps*) collections.[62] In bearded dragons, the atadenovirus infection will retard growth as well as cause overt GI and neurological clinical signs.[54] Severely affected animals may die. As with many viral diseases, some infected animals may remain subclinical, thus becoming a serious management issue due to the potential for shedding the virus in clean facilities or enclosures. Naïve animals are exposed through horizontal transmission (i.e., fecal-oral). A PCR test is available for oral/cloacal swabs collected from suspect individuals or screening bearded dragons that may have subclinical infections.[54] The only methods to prevent exposure are to purchase noninfected animals and ensure strict quarantine prior to placement of new animals into a collection, with pre- and postquarantine testing. Infected animals exhibiting clinical signs carry a guarded prognosis and supportive treatment is recommended.

WEST NILE VIRUS. West Nile virus (WNV) is a vector-transmitted arbovirus in the family *Flaviviridae* that causes neurologic signs in reptiles and, in particular, crocodilian species.[63] Infected animals will exhibit neurological clinical signs (e.g., circling, ataxia, tremors, head tilt) and often death (Figure 8-18). A serious economic disease condition occurs in young infected farm-raised alligators (*Alligator mississippiensis*): skin lesions caused by a lymphohistiocytic proliferative syndrome that degrades hide quality (Figure 8-19).[64] Although infected with WNV, the young alligators may not exhibit overt clinical signs and will continue to grow without evidence of disease. When harvested, the hides of the affected animals

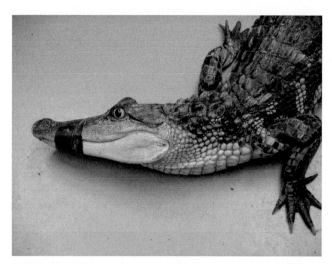

FIGURE 8-18 Alligator with clinical disease signs (head tilt and circling) of West Nile virus (photo courtesy of Javier Nevarez).

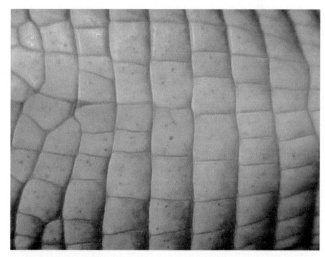

FIGURE 8-19 West Nile virus causes lesions in the skin that decrease the hide value of farm-raised animals (photo courtesy of Javier Nevarez).

will have numerous small defects that diminish the product value.

Diagnostic options for WNV in reptile species include PCR testing on collected tissue samples and serologic testing.[65] A WNV vaccine has been developed for crocodilian species and is commercially available. While the vaccine may be used as a preventive measure, infected animals should be euthanized due to the zoonotic nature of the virus.[54]

OTHER VIRAL DISEASES. A "paramyxo-like" virus was identified in rock rattlesnakes (*Crotalus lepidus*) as causing progressive clinical signs associated with the CNS (e.g., head tremors, loss of righting reflex, opisthotonos).[66] Since the initial report, this virus does not appear to cause significant disease in snake collections. However, because very little is known regarding exposure and infectivity, all snakes either purchased commercially or captured from the wild must be considered susceptible and subclinical carriers that may expose animals maintained in closed collections.

Although the significance is unknown at this time, reptile species are known to serve as reservoir hosts for Venezuelan equine encephalitis and western equine encephalitis.[67] At this time, disease associated with Togaviridae does not appear to be of clinical significance in captive reptile species.

Fungal Diseases

Disseminated or focal fungal infections (e.g., cryptococcosis, aspergillosis, candidiasis, zygomycosis) may cause neurologic clinical signs in reptile species.[55] As with other animal species, fungal infections in reptiles are difficult to treat and often result in death. A definitive diagnosis of a fungal infection, which is the underlying cause of overt neurologic signs, is often provided through postmortem examination of the animal.[54]

Parasitic Diseases

The primary parasites that cause neurologic signs in reptiles include protozoa and trematodes.[54] *Acanthamoeba* spp. is reported to infect animals, including reptiles, through exposure of the nasal mucosa.[67] The CNS is infected with the protozoal organism, which primarily causes a spasmodic opisthotonos that is intensified when the animal is stimulated.[67] *Acanthamoeba* meningoencephalitis is rarely diagnosed, and both animals and humans are thought to be infected through contaminated water supplies. A definitive diagnosis is primarily achieved through pathological examination of infected tissue. There is no recommended treatment at this time for *Acanthamoeba* spp. infection nor is antemortem diagnostic testing beneficial in most cases.

Other protozoal parasites reported to cause meningoencephalitis and associated neurologic signs in reptile species include *Nosema* spp., *Entamoeba* spp., *Encephalitozoon* spp., and *Toxoplasma* spp.[54,67] In exposed reptiles, species can become infected with toxoplasmosis through exposure to contaminated insects when their body temperatures are maintained at 37° C.[67] While successful treatment of toxoplasmosis has been achieved in mammalian species using clindamycin, no drug therapy has been specifically identified to use in infected reptile species. Clindamycin (5 mg/kg, orally [PO], q12 h) may be used to treat suspect or diagnosed cases of toxoplasmosis in reptile species, but the effectiveness of the drug has not been validated.[68] Microsporidiosis is a rising concern with captive bearded dragons. These primitive fungi, often referred to as parasites, can be found ante-mortem in fecal samples or from tissue biopsies. Fenbendazole (25 mg/kg, PO, q 24h) may be used to treat microsporidians (MA Mitchell, pers. comm.).

Toxins

Neurologic signs that are the result of toxin exposure are often observed in reptile patients and may be caused by a wide variety of products and compounds. All therapeutic agents should be considered toxins, and when a medication is prescribed, it is the veterinarian's responsibility to know the adverse side effects of the drug or antimicrobial agent and inform the owner. If any adverse side effects are noted, the treatment should immediately be discontinued and the clini-

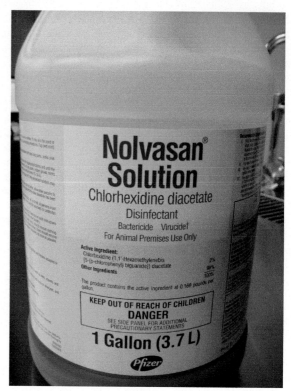

FIGURE 8-20 If not diluted, the antimicrobial agent chlorhexidine will cause neurologic signs when topically applied.

cian called to reassess the patient's condition and management of the disease condition.

THERAPEUTIC AND ANTIMICROBIAL AGENTS. Chlorhexidine solution (Chlorhexidine diacetate; Nolvasan solution, Zoetis, Florham Park, NJ), a cationic polybiguanide, is often recommended as a topical antimicrobial treatment for dermatological disease affecting reptile species (Figure 8-20). A 0.0024% dilute chlorhexidine is often safely used, but the stock 2% solution has been implicated in causing acute neurologic disease and death in reptile patients.[67] Clinical signs associated with chlorhexidine toxicity in snakes include acute loss of righting reflexes, reduced withdrawal reflexes in chelonians and lizards, and flaccid paralysis.[67] Chelonians have been reported to be extremely sensitive to this chemical agent, and in all species affected, patients usually die from severe neurologic and respiratory compromise.[67]

Insecticide products have been used for many years to treat and prevent exposure to ectoparasites. Any of the insecticide products used in the environment may cause toxicity to the animal due to the extreme sensitivity many reptile species have to these chemical compounds. Insecticide products in the form of powders, sprays, "no pest" strips, and baits can produce nonspecific neurologic clinical signs in captive reptile species.[69] Clinical signs described in reptiles with insecticide toxicity include torticollis, lack of a righting reflex, reduced withdrawal response, flaccid paralysis, circling, opisthotonos, and varying degrees of seizure activity.[67] Removal of the animal from the environment containing the insecticide product is the first step in treatment. Supportive care, including hydration therapy to dilute any circulating chemical

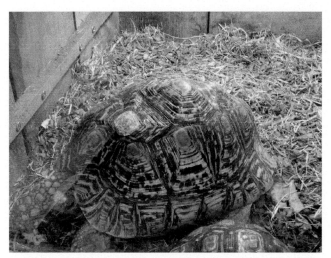

FIGURE 8-21 Leopard tortoises are very sensitive to ivermectin, an antiparasitic medication. Other chelonian species also have adverse reactions and exhibit neurologic signs when ivermectin is administered. Therefore, ivermectin should not be used to treat parasites in chelonian species.

metabolites and ensure adequate renal function during the toxic phase of the exposure, is critical for possible case resolution. Depending on class of insecticide and neurologic condition, respiratory support, utilizing oxygen and intermittent positive-pressure ventilation, may be required. As with all reptile patients that present with seizure activity, diazepam or midazolam may be used to treat this condition. Organophosphate or carbamate exposure often results in animals presenting with flaccid paralysis of their limbs, but they appear to be bright and alert. Organophosphate insecticides are acetylcholinesterase inhibitors that prevent the cessation of nerve conduction at the neuromuscular junction. Since the muscle is unable to rest, the muscle fatigue of the major muscle groups supporting the animal increases. The recommended treatment for organophosphate and carbamate toxicity is atropine.[69]

Ivermectin (Ivomec; Merial, Duluth, GA), a commonly used antiparasitic drug in all animal species, has been commercially available for use since the 1980s. The drug was produced from *Streptomyces avermitilis* and is a macrocyclic lactone that affects the gamma-aminobutyric acid (GABA) synapse to simulate excess release of GABA, an inhibitory neurotransmitter in nematodes.[70] Ivermectin is an effective antiparasitic medication in many animals because it does not cross the blood-brain barrier. However, it appears that in chelonians the drug either crosses the blood-brain barrier or GABA has an increased significance as a peripheral neurotransmitter. Regardless of the specific underlying cause, ivermectin causes general neuromuscular weakness in chelonians, and death usually occurs due to the paralysis of the respiratory musculature.[67] There are species variations regarding chelonian susceptibility to ivermectin intoxication, with leopard tortoises *(Stigmochelys pardalis)* being reported as extremely sensitive (Figure 8-21).[70] As with other intoxications, due to insecticides and other therapeutic agents, the primary treatment for ivermectin toxicosis is supportive, and because of the long-acting effect of the drug at the neurotransmitter site (7

days), support must be maintained for at least that period of time.[67] Moreover, the affected animal must be monitored and provided with adequate respiration and oxygen therapy due to the effect of the drug on the respiratory musculature. It is not uncommon for affected chelonians to be maintained on supportive ventilation during the treatment period. The prognosis for a chelonian patient with ivermectin toxicity is guarded to grave. For this reason, it is recommended that ivermectin never be administered to chelonian species.

Several antibiotic medications have been reported to cause neurologic signs in reptiles, including metronidazole, polymyxin B, and aminoglycosides.[71] However, there are possibly other antibiotic products that may cause neurologic signs, depending on species treated, dosage used, and condition of the patient. It is imperative that the veterinarian properly assesses the patient, if possible be aware of each product's use in the species being treated, and use the proper dosage while understanding the potential side effects. Torticollis, ataxia, lack of righting reflex, and paresis/paralysis are examples of clinical signs displayed by animals diagnosed with antibiotic toxicity. Doses of metronidazole >100 mg/kg in snakes have been linked to severe neurologic signs and death.[67] Reptile patients suffering from the toxic side effects of antibiotic therapy have responded to supportive care.

HEAVY METAL. Although uncommon, lead and zinc may cause intoxication in reptiles, leading to generalized neurologic signs including depression, ataxia, and paresis. Recommended diagnostic testing includes full-body radiographic images, assessment of lead and zinc blood concentrations, and a complete blood count (CBC). It is possible for animals to be diagnosed with lead toxicosis without evidence of metal objects in the GI system. Blood lead levels may be elevated if the animal ingests paint chips or microscopic particles in a tainted solution. The CBC will often indicate a nonregenerative anemia in chronically intoxicated patients. In cases of zinc toxicosis, metal is usually identified in the GI tract. If metallic object(s) are found in the GI tract, removal is recommended. Flexible endoscopy may be used on larger reptile patients, while a strong magnet glued to the end of a rubber feeding tube is effective in extracting magnetic objects, specifically those that are zinc plated. If manual removal is not possible, catharsis and gastric lavage are other options to consider.[67] The patient may exhibit clinical disease signs after the metal has been voided. Until the toxic metal levels are reduced and there are no identifiable foreign objects in the GI tract, the patient should be treated with calcium ethylenediaminetetraacetic acid (Ca EDTA) therapy (10 to 40 mg/kg, IM, q12 h).[67] Since lead is absorbed by and contained in osteoclasts, there is a real likelihood of rebound toxicity when those cells are resorbed by the body. The owners should be aware of this potential and ensure that blood lead levels are checked for 1 to 2 months after the initial presentation and treatment. Clinical neurologic signs associated with the rebound toxicity are similar to those described for the initial presentation.

MISCELLANEOUS TOXINS. There are many household products used for disinfecting reptile enclosures that if the animal ingests or is exposed, either topically or inhaled, may cause neurologic clinical signs. A thorough patient history, initiation of clinical signs, and suspect exposure are essential in making a definitive diagnosis. For many of the chemical compounds that a reptile may be exposed to, there are no diagnostic tests available for specific identification. Nicotine, naphthalene, paint solvents, and iodoforms are other household toxins that may cause neurologic signs including ataxia, seizures, torticollis, and loss of righting reflex.[69] Moreover, highly volatile wood chips (e.g., pine, cedar) that release aromatic organic compounds have been reported to cause a reversible ataxia in captive reptile species.[67]

Bearded dragons exhibited neurologic clinical signs including forceful head shaking, facial seizures, and mouth gaping after being fed fireflies from the genus *Photinus*.[72] *Photinus* spp. fireflies contain a steroidal pyrone called lucibufagins, and one insect is considered a fatal dose in bearded dragons.[72] Fireflies are not recommended as a food source for reptiles due to the inability of the owners to determine which fireflies are nontoxic and/or which reptile species can safely ingest fireflies.

Trauma

Pressure and pathology caused by disease conditions or blunt traumatic incidents to the brain, spinal cord, and/or peripheral nerves can cause neurologic disease conditions. Brain or spinal cord trauma may result in torticollis, ataxia, and seizure activity, while peripheral nerve damage in chelonians and lizards can cause paresis or paralysis of the affected limb(s). Bacterial and fungal abscesses or tumors can impinge on nerves, the spinal cord, and brain tissue, causing similar neurologic signs as described above. In snakes, a lytic proliferative spinal osteopathy has been described in many species of snakes, including boids.[73] Snakes diagnosed with spinal osteopathy may have overt spinal deformities, quivering, and torticollis.[73] Although no definitive underlying etiology has been determined for this disease process, a number of suspect causes have been suggested including a virus transmitted through feeder mice, a slow neoplasm, hypovitaminosis D, an immune-mediated disease, and septicemia.[67,73] Diagnosis can be confirmed through physical examination, palpation of the patient's vertebrae, and radiographic images that detail the skeletal pathology associated with the disease. The significant pathology of bone tissue with spinal osteopathy results in bony proliferation and ankylosis of the affected vertebrae.[67] Although blood cultures may aid in determining the specific bacteria (e.g., *Salmonella* spp.) involved with the disease process, patients are often too small for an appropriate volume of blood to be collected for this particular diagnostic test. Blood cultures, in general, often yield poor results when submitted for companion exotic patients. Vertebral biopsy with histopathology and culture should also be considered and can be diagnostic. When diagnosed with spinal osteopathy, prognosis is poor for a patient's condition, due to ingrowth of connective tissue and the lack of nerve fiber regeneration.[74] Treatment includes supportive care upon initial presentation, antibiotic therapy, and surgical debridement of severely lytic lesions affecting the vertebrae.[67]

Neoplasia

Spinal cord gliomas and pituitary adenomas have been reported in reptiles.[54] Brain and spinal cord tumors are rare in reptile species maintained in captivity but, when present, will cause ataxia, seizure activity, and loss of righting reflex.[54] A definitive diagnosis is usually made through postmortem examination, although advanced imaging (e.g., computed tomography [CT], MRI) through antemortem diagnostic assessment may provide evidence of a tumor.

Nutritional and Metabolic Diseases

Arguably, nutritional imbalances are the most common disease presentation of captive reptile species to veterinary clinics. Both nutritional and metabolic causes of disease conditions that result in neurologic clinical disease signs often have pathophysiologic commonalities. Treatment of the clinical condition, including neurologic problems, will often prevent collateral injury and stop progression of the disease process. The ability of the patient to respond to treatment is dependent on the severity and chronicity of the nutritional or metabolic imbalance.

Comparable to the condition of hypocalcemia that results in nutritional secondary hyperparathyroidism (NSHP) in amphibians, reptiles also develop this metabolic disease. Inadequate diets, low in dietary calcium and vitamin D_3 and high in phosphorus, often combined with inadequate ultraviolet B (UVB) lighting and low environmental temperatures, are reported as factors causing NSHP in reptiles.[54] Seizure activity, muscle fasciculations, ataxia, and generalized weakness are neurologic signs noted in animals diagnosed with NSHP. Diagnosis is based on the patient's history, physical examination, and radiographic images detailing the bone cortices (i.e., images are radiolucent, showing a lack of density). In cases of seizing patients, ionized calcium levels may be diminished. Recommended treatment includes calcium and magnesium supplementation, supportive care, and diazepam for seizure activity. Long-term therapy may include oral calcium and education of the owner on proper diet, supplementation, and environmental conditions for that particular species of reptile.

There are reports of hypovitaminosis E causing general weakness, ataxia, and paresis in a veiled chameleon (*Chamaeleo calyptratus*), green iguanas (*Iguana iguana*), and bearded dragons.[54,75,76] Diagnosis is centered on patient history, diet, and presenting clinical signs. A physical examination will aid in giving the veterinarian an overall assessment of the patient prior to developing a differential disease diagnosis list. Proper supplementation of vitamin E should help resolve the disease condition, along with educating the owner about proper nutrition and husbandry for the species being treated.

A hypoglycemic condition has been described in crocodilians that causes muscle fasciculations and loss of the righting reflex.[77] Although the underlying etiology and pathophysiology are unknown, affected animals improved after being administered oral glucose at a dose of 3 g/kg, and their environmental stressors were eliminated.[67,77]

Fish that are frozen and then thawed activate thiaminases, predisposing animals that were fed these fish to develop thiamine deficiency. Moreover, herbivorous reptile species fed plants that contain phytothiaminases may develop a vitamin B_1 deficiency. Muscle fasciculations, ataxia, seizures, and torticollis are neurologic signs reported in reptiles diagnosed with thiamine deficiency.[67] In chelonians, enophthalmos is the most obvious clinical sign of this nutritional deficiency.[67] Diagnosis is based on patient history, including diet fed and presenting clinical condition. Treatment with PO or subcutaneous (SC) vitamin B_1 supplementation (25 mg/kg/d) early in the disease process is effective in resolving the nutritional deficiency.[67] Prevention of vitamin B$_1$ deficiency in reptiles includes thiamine supplementation for animals fed frozen fish, herbivorous species potentially feeding on plants containing phytothiaminases, and animals receiving long-term antibiotic therapy.[67,77] Long-term antibiotic therapy has been proposed as a means to induce vitamin B$_1$ deficiency by reducing the population of GI microflora associated with production of thiamine.[77]

Raw infertile eggs, specifically containing albumin, also contain avidin, which has "antibiotin" activity.[67] In nature, egg-eating reptile species commonly eat fertile eggs and other small animals that contain biotin. In captive settings, the owners of egg-eating reptiles may provide a sole diet of unfertilized raw eggs, thereby inducing a biotin deficiency. Animals diagnosed with a biotin deficiency exhibit muscle fasciculations and generalized muscle weakness.[67] Effective treatment includes supplementation with vitamin B complex and dietary diversity that incorporates biotin into the diet.

Miscellaneous Neuropathies

Accumulation of cholesterol and macrophages in reptile species is called xanthomatosis.[67] Xanthomatosis is believed to be a condition brought about by hypercholesterolemia and hyperlipidemia.[67] The occurrence of xanthomas in the brain may result in hydrocephalus and concurrent neurologic signs (e.g., torticollis, loss of righting reflex, seizures).[54] Hyperuricemia, hypercholesterolemia, and hyperlipidemia are considered physiologic conditions that coincide with xanthoma formation and thought to be intensified by folliculogenesis, follicular degeneration, and yolk coelomitis.[67] Unfortunately, by the time neurologic signs become clinically evident, xanthomatosis treatment is ineffective. A definitive diagnosis is achieved through postmortem examination of the patient.[54]

A congenital neuropathic condition has been reported in newborn boa constrictors (*Boa constrictor*).[78] The condition routinely affects only the caudal aspect of the snake and does not appear to involve the brain or CNs.[78] The affected animals have difficulty moving, exhibit abnormal posture, and present with single to multiple coils of their spine.[78] When anesthetized, the coils can be straightened but recoil when the animal recovers.[54] This coiling syndrome results in death to newborns and chronic debilitation in juvenile animals.[78] At this time, no definitive cause for the coiling syndrome has been identified, although multiple leukocytic infiltrates are noted to surround the nerves and vessels within the perimysium, suggesting infection, inflammation, incubation, or neoplasia as possible etiologies.[78] There are no known treatments that resolve this condition.

Circling and torticollis have been observed in chelonian species emerging from brumation.[69] Suspected causes of these conditions include fatty liver syndrome or a bacterial infection forming microabscesses in the brain.[69] Although vitamin A supplementation is reported to improve the animal's overall condition, animals with torticollis do not appear to respond.[67]

Two circulatory disease conditions that may cause reptile patients to present with neurologic signs are visceral gout and granulocytic leukemia. The pathophysiology of gout on the nervous system is caused by circulatory anomalies and formation of tophi within nervous tissue.[67] Granulocytic leukemia has been reported to cause thrombus formation and infarction of the spinal cord in a gopher snake (*Pituophis melanoleucus*).[67]

Paralysis and ataxia are neurologic signs that one may expect to see when reptile patients are diagnosed with either of these circulatory disorders.

Birds

Neurologic disease is not one of the more common presentations for avian species to veterinary hospitals. However, birds do suffer from diseases that cause overt neurologic signs, and in many cases, the underlying cause and subsequent physical effects may be difficult to diagnose and treat. Knowledge of the diseases that affect the bird's brain, spinal cord, and peripheral nerves is important in being able to use the proper diagnostic techniques required to obtain a definitive diagnosis.

Bacterial Diseases

Listeria monocytogenes and *Mycobacterium* spp. infections can result in granulomas, abscessation in brain tissue, and/or preauditory sinus.[79,80] The bacterial granulomas/abscesses result in neurologic signs, including ataxia, depression, torticollis, and lateral recumbency. *Staphylococcus aureus*, *Enterococcus* spp., *Salmonella Typhimurium*, *Escherichia coli*, *Pasteurella* spp., and *Klebsiella* spp. are other bacterial isolates that may cause neurological signs consistent with encephalitis.[80] Lethargy, tremors, seizures, and opisthotonos have been observed in parrots infected with *Chlamydophila psittaci*, most notably in chronically infected birds.[81] It must be noted that it is extremely rare for birds to present with neurologic signs associated with avian chlamydiosis. Diagnosis of avian chlamydiosis is best achieved when the patient is exhibiting clinical signs. The diagnostic testing method of choice is an avian chlamydial panel: PCR testing of a combined conjunctival, choanal, and cloacal swab and whole blood plus serologic testing of immunoglobulin G (IgG) antibody titer. The treatment of choice for avian chlamydiosis is doxycycline. Although the recommended length of time for treating avian chlamydiosis is 45 days, results from experimentally inoculated cockatiels suggested that a 21-day treatment regimen using doxycycline and azithromycin was effective in clearing the infection.[82]

Viral Diseases

PARAMYXOVIRUSES. Paramyxoviruses (PMVs) containing at least 9 known serotypes are the causative agent of a number of the well-known diseases that produce neurological signs in parrots and other avian species.[79,83] Newcastle disease, PMV-1, is often associated with disease in poultry and pigeons, but other birds are extremely susceptible, including psittacine species.[54,84] Initially, clinical disease signs observed involve the GI tract (e.g., anorexia, vomiting, regurgitation) and respiratory system, followed shortly thereafter by neurologic conditions including depression, ataxia, torticollis, head tremors, leg/wing paralysis, and opisthotonos due to a nonsuppurative encephalitis.[79,84] If the bird survives the acute infection, chronic neurologic signs may persist for months.[79] There are different viral strains of PMV-1, and the different strains may not infect some avian groups or are not as pathogenic to the susceptible species.[54] Pigeon PMV-1 is not as pathogenic to pigeons as poultry strains are to chickens and parrots. PMV-1 causes high morbidity and mortality in chicken flocks, and exposure occurs through horizontal transmission (i.e., direct or indirect exposure to infected poultry or wild birds). Conversely, 70% of infected pigeons exhibiting neurologic signs will recover with supportive care unless significant tissue damage to the renal tissue occurs.[54] Parrots exposed to PMV-1 develop respiratory, GI, and neurologic signs.[54,79] Psittacine species, in particular Australian parakeets (*Melopsittacus undulatus*), are highly susceptible to PMV-1, and if infected have a high mortality rate.[54] Treatment is supportive and only effective in birds infected with a low pathogenic strain of PMV-1. Vaccination is recommended, where permitted, but selection of the proper vaccine product is essential. Poultry vaccines that contain certain lentogenic PMV strains have been reported to cause velogenic disease in raptors.[85] Vaccination for PMV-1 should never take place in unapproved areas or locations classified as PMV-1 "disease free." In disease-free locations, screening for PMV-1 takes place through evaluation of serum antibody titers, which may be elevated in vaccinated birds. Therefore, it would not be possible to determine whether the elevated PMV-1 serum titers are from natural infection or vaccination.

Other PMV serotypes that have been identified in psittacine species are PMV-2, -3, and -5.[83] Neurologic signs have been observed in passerine species (e.g., finches) infected with PMV-3, although subclinical infections may be present long before disease signs are obvious.[54] Depression, paralysis, muscle fasciculations, and torticollis are the abnormal disease conditions displayed by passerines infected with PMV-3.[54]

PSITTACINE PROVENTRICULAR DILATATION DISEASE. Psittacine proventricular dilatation disease (PDD), while primarily identified with the GI tract, has been reported to involve both the central and peripheral nervous systems.[79,86] The pathological find most consistent with PDD is a progressive lymphoplasmacytic ganglioneuritis.[54,79] As the disease name indicates, the body system most often affected by PDD is the GI system. Clinically, the entire GI tract becomes dysfunctional due to nerve pathology associated with the disease. The proventriculus loses muscle tone and becomes increasingly dilated (Figure 8-22). An enlarged proventriculus (diagnosed through radiographic images), cachexia, polyphagia, and delayed crop emptying (diagnosed through contrast imaging) are common clinical conditions associated with PDD in psittacine species.[54,86] Central or peripheral neuropathies occur most often in young birds (<1 year), especially in cockatoo species.[54,86]

Although no definitive cause of PDD has been determined at this time, a bornavirus has generated interest as being involved in the disease process.[87,88] Research is ongoing to determine whether the pathophysiologic connection to PDD is the bornavirus. Diagnostic options for PDD include PCR testing of blood and tissue samples and histopathological examination of crop biopsy samples. The crop biopsy samples should include at least one small blood vessel to ensure the presence of nerve tissue. The diagnostic sensitivity of crop biopsy samples has been reported to be as high as 70%, but the author believes that it is much less due to the inconsistent effect of PDD on neurons.[54] At this time, the recommended treatment for PDD is centered on nonsteroidal anti-inflammatory drug (NSAID) administration to reduce disease problems associated with neuritis. Although a number of NSAIDs have been used to treat PDD patients, including meloxicam and celecoxib, no consistent treatment response

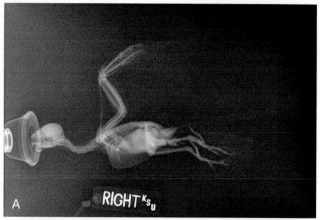

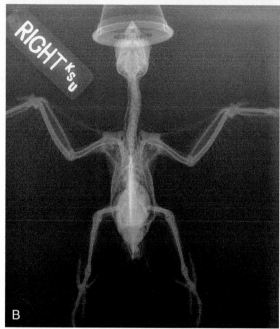

FIGURE 8-22 Radiographic images (*A*, lateral; *B*, dorsoventral) of a bird showing an enlarged proventriculus consistent with proventricular dilatation disease. This disease affects the neuromuscular junction of the gastrointestinal system and other body systems (photos courtesy of James Carpenter and Christine Higbie).

has been achieved. The goal of PDD treatment is to improve the patient's quality of life and extend its life expectancy postdiagnosis. However, regardless of treatment used, it appears that most birds do not respond to any treatment and slowly succumb to the disease.

TOGAVIRUS. Eastern, Western, and Venezuelan equine encephalitis virus, Highlands J virus, and avian viral serositis virus (AVSV) are classified as togaviruses. AVSV has been diagnosed in psittacine species and can develop into a focal cerebral meningitis, necrotizing encephalitis, and nonsuppurative encephalitis.[80] Both eclectus parrots and black palm cockatoos are reported to be susceptible to eastern equine encephalitis, and when infected develop muscle fasciculations, torticollis, and paralysis.[79] Cross protection of eastern equine encephalitis has been obtained in psittacine species using the equine vaccine.[79]

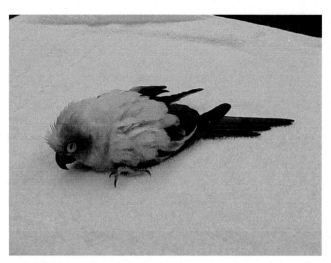

FIGURE 8-23 Sun conure (*Arainga solstitialis*) with WNV. Many bird species exhibit general neurologic signs when infected with WNV.

WEST NILE VIRUS. WNV has continued to spread its geographic range since 1937, when first identified in a human located in Uganda.[89] Mosquitoes are considered the major vector, with birds serving as the major vertebrate host.[54] Exposure can also occur through ingestion of infected bird carcasses or contaminated drinking water.[54] After a bird is inoculated with the WNV through experimental exposure or infected mosquitoes, a viremia develops and remains for ~2 to 7 days.[54,90] Clinical signs associated with the disease usually occur after the viremic phase, 12 to 18 days after exposure in certain avian species including red-tailed hawks (*Buteo jamaicensis*).[90] Ataxia, muscle fasciculations, torticollis, abnormal head posture, convulsions, inability to perch, and seizure activity are clinical signs that have been observed in birds diagnosed with WNV (Figure 8-23).[54,90] The severity of the disease process and ability to serve as an amplification host for the virus depends on the species of bird infected. Certain avian species (e.g., corvids, passerines) have been reported to be more effective in amplifying the virus within the environment due to maintaining higher viral concentrations for longer periods of time, relative to other birds.[54] There are noteworthy variations in susceptibility between avian species, with various raptor, psittacine, waterfowl, and passerine species having significantly more morbidity and mortality when infected with WVN than others within the same groups of birds.[54,91] To screen for the presence and concentration of virus within an environment, chickens and turkeys have been used as sentinel animals, due to their apparent reduced susceptibility to WNV, in surveillance programs by public health and mosquito abatement agencies in endemic areas.

General diagnostic testing is not very specific in determining whether a bird is infected with WNV, even when the animal exhibits clinical disease signs. Since the virus is present in large quantities in the oral and cloacal areas, swabs collected from these locations can be used early in the disease process for PCR testing.[54] Serologic testing for antibody titers may be used but is unreliable due to the inconsistent production of antibodies during the disease process and cross reactions with other *Flavivirus* that result in false positives.[54] A

definitive diagnosis of WNV can be achieved through tissue PCR, viral antigen detection, and/or viral isolation (brain tissue).[54,90]

Treatment is supportive and should include anti-inflammatory medication. The patient response to treatment will depend on the severity of the disease and ability of the animal to respond to the supportive care. Although not scientifically evaluated in many avian species, vaccination using the killed WNV vaccine (Fort Dodge Animal Health, Division of Wyeth, Fort Dodge, IA) is recommended for susceptible avian species.[90] The recommended vaccine protocol for susceptible species is 3 1-mL doses at 3-week intervals with annual boosters prior to warm weather and in the face of increased virus levels in the environment.[90]

REOVIRUS. African greys (*Psittacus erithacus*), Senegal parrots (*Poicephalus senegalus*), and cockatoos (*Cacatua* spp.) appear to be the most susceptible psittacines to reovirus infections.[79] Clinical signs noted in birds infected with reovirus include ataxia, depression, and anorexia. Paresis may occur secondary to vascular thrombosis of extremities, resulting in peripheral neuropathies.[79] Diagnosis of reovirus infection is based on histological examination of affected tissues and/or viral isolation.[79] Treatment is supportive and prevention is achieved through proper quarantine and purchasing birds from reputable vendors. There is currently no vaccine available to protect birds from reovirus infections.

AVIAN INFLUENZA. Avian influenza (AI) orthomyxovirus is a common disease condition that affects many avian species (e.g., poultry, psittacines, passerines, raptors, ratites, waterfowl) and is well established in many wild bird populations.[92] The pathogenicity of AI strains varies between avian species, with each strain classified by their outer membrane proteins. This viral organism is of extreme concern to poultry producers because of the ease of transmission and high morbidity and mortality associated with infection of highly pathogenic strains to which those species of birds are susceptible. AI is endemic in Anseriformes and Charadriiformes, which are considered index populations for the dissemination of the virus to new geographic locations.[54] Avian species, in which the virus strain is nonpathogenic, serve as subclinical hosts and will expose susceptible species to the virus. Many body systems are affected when a bird is infected with AI and clinical signs of disease may be found in the GI, respiratory, and nervous systems. Neurologic signs noted in ill birds include depression, incoordination, ataxia, and weakness.[54,79] If AI is suspected in wild bird patients, euthanasia is recommended, as is viral identification of the specific AI strain to test for poultry susceptibility. For antemortem diagnosis, serum antibody and PCR testing are available from collected blood and swab samples.[54] Supportive care is recommended for treatment, although in most cases, euthanasia is the preferred option due to the ease of transmission and pathogenic nature of the virus to other birds within the facility. Quarantine and enforced biosecurity measures are to be employed for birds being treated for AI and should remain in place until 2 consecutive negative PCR and viral isolation test results are obtained, taken at least 3 weeks apart.[54,93]

GALLID HERPESVIRUS. Marek's disease affects chickens, turkeys, and Japanese quail and is caused by gallid herpesvirus 1. The oncogenic herpesvirus is extremely contagious and difficult to control because it can be maintained within a population as a subclinical infection. The lymphoproliferative clinical disease affects the nervous system and results in neoplastic mononuclear cell infiltrates of peripheral nerves.[94]

Affected birds will exhibit unilateral leg lameness, paresis/ paralysis, wing drop, and opisthotonos.[54] Treatment is uniformly ineffective; therefore, vaccination of 1-day-old chicks prior to viral exposure is recommended.

Fungal Diseases

Fungal infections are rarely involved as an underlying cause of neurologic signs of disease in birds. However, *Aspergillus* spp. can cause granulomas that can invade or compress internal organs and peripheral nerves.[79] Generalized aspergillosis infections can also develop into secondary cerebral infections and toxin-induced peripheral neuropathies.[79,95] To reduce the incidence of aspergillosis infections in birds, it is vital to maintain the animals in an environment where there is reduced exposure to the fungal organism. Reduced exposure is especially significant for species that have an increased susceptibility (e.g., African grey) and immunocompromised individuals (e.g., sick, old, young). Hepatic encephalopathies caused by mycotoxin-induced hepatitis, usually from exposure to tainted food, can cause generalized nonspecific neurological signs and are very difficult to diagnose. It is an owner's responsibility to procure quality food and provide the storage facilities required to prevent the growth of organisms that produce mycotoxins.

Granuloma formation affecting the CNS, due to disseminated *Cryptococcus* spp. infection, will cause neurologic disease signs in birds.[96] Infected birds may also present with dyspnea, sinusitis, and ocular and nasal discharge.[54] Paralysis and reduced muscular activity are clinical signs associated with neurologic disease caused by *Cryptococcus* spp. infections.[97] A definitive diagnosis is achieved through identification of organisms on collected respiratory samples.[54] However, for CNS cases of cryptococcosis, necropsy examination of the patient may be the only option. Serious consideration should be given when treatment is elected due to the fact that *Cryptococcus* spp. is considered a zoonotic organism.[54] Fluconazole is the antifungal treatment of choice for birds exhibiting CNS disease signs, because this drug can cross the blood-brain barrier.[96] Additionally, amphotericin B, itraconazole, and voriconazole can be used for *Cryptococcus* infections affecting the respiratory system.[54] Unfortunately, curative treatment is uniformly elusive for avian cryptococcosis infections.[54]

Parasitic Diseases

Neurologic disease signs can be caused by *Sarcocystis* spp. and *Filaroides* spp.[79] Although uncommon, the effect of the parasitic infection will often lead to debilitating neurological conditions (e.g., torticollis, wing and leg paresis and/or paralysis, ataxia, circling, and muscle tremors).[79] Coccidian parasites, *Sarcocystis* spp. in particular, are known to cause disease in psittacines, passerines, doves, and pigeons (Figure 8-24).[98,99] There is a general belief that psittacine species from Australia, Africa, and Asia are more susceptible than those native to Central and South America.[54] Regrettably, it is generalizations regarding disease epidemiology that often lead veterinarians away from developing an appropriate differential disease diagnostic list to properly work up and ultimately treat the case. Macaws, parrot species from the new world, succumb to

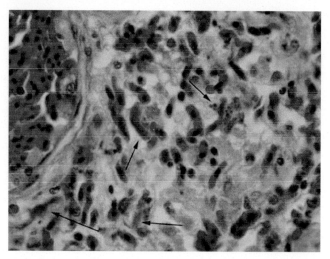

FIGURE 8-24 Lung of a lorikeet. Numerous *Sarcocystis* schizonts in various stages of maturation *(arrows)* are present in the endothelial cells lining the capillaries. Hematoxylin and Eosin (photo courtesy of Michael Garner, Northwest ZooPath).

Sarcocystis spp. infections, as do birds from Australia, Africa, and Asia. It is imperative that the clinician uses the information from the provided history, clinical presentation, and physical examination to determine a plan of action to determine a diagnosis. Although there may be species predilections to disease processes, very few people know what variables have been involved in establishing these often anecdotal proclamations. Consequently, if a group of birds is susceptible to a disease process, all species that comprise that group of birds should be considered "at risk" unless there is valid scientific evidence to the contrary. Birds are exposed to the *Sarcocystis* spp. organism through direct contact with the mammalian definitive host (e.g., Virginia opossum [*Didelphis virginiana*]) and/or indirectly through paratenic hosts (e.g., cockroaches) that come into contact with the contaminated feces of the mammalian host.[54] Infected birds may be presented with nonspecific clinical signs that include depression, a constant monotone vocalization, and subcutaneous hemorrhages along with neurologic signs (e.g., ataxia, torticollis). Antemortem diagnosis through skeletal muscle biopsies and serological antigen testing, and successful treatment for birds infected with *Sarcocystis* spp., are often difficult since many of the patients are severely ill when first presented to a veterinary hospital due to the chronic subclinical nature of the disease process. If other birds within an aviary have previously been positively identified with sarcocystosis, this will help direct the veterinarian toward diagnostic testing and initial treatment options. Positive identification of *Sarcocystis* spp. protozoal cysts in muscle and organ (e.g., muscle, heart, liver, brain, meninges) tissue with concurrent inflammation will provide a definitive diagnosis and usually occurs through postmortem examination. Successful treatment of birds infected with *Sarcocystis* spp. is rarely achieved due to the multiple life-cycle stages of the organism, including encystation; nevertheless, depending on severity of infection, some improvement in the patient's physical condition may be noted. Historically, trimethoprim-sulfa has been a treatment of choice for avian sarcocystosis, but a therapeutic cocktail that included

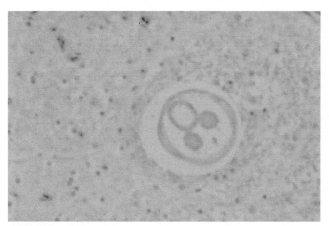

FIGURE 8-25 *Chandlerella quiscali* organism in emu brain tissue.

diclazuril, pyrimethamine, and trimethoprim sulfamethoxazole was reported to be a successful treatment regimen in a confirmed case in a pied pigeon *(Ducula bicolor bicolor)*.[100] The recommended preventive measures are quarantine, thorough history (i.e., did cage mate die of unknown causes?), physical examination, and diagnostic testing of birds obtained from areas in which *Sarcocystis* spp. are endemic. To prevent exposure of birds within an aviary, avoidance of the definitive mammalian hosts (e.g., Virginia opossum), paratenic hosts (e.g., cockroaches), and infected fecal material is essential and required.

Visceral larval migration of nematode species *Chandlerella quiscali* and *Baylisascaris procyonis* affect many avian species, resulting in mild to severe neurologic signs (e.g., ataxia, torticollis, abnormal neck position, weakness, death).[54,79,80,101–103] The life cycle of *Chandlerella quiscali* and *Baylisascaris procyonis* is different in birds, but the final effects of the larval migration through the brain and spinal cord are similar. Birds, in particular, ratites (e.g., emus), are exposed through the bite of small arthropod vectors (e.g., *Culicoides* spp.), after which the developing parasite migrates through the brain and spinal cord of the abnormal host (Figure 8-25).[101] Birds are exposed to the *B. procyonis* parasite through contact with contaminated raccoon feces. When birds are presented with nonspecific neurologic disease signs, history of potential exposure to raccoons, raccoon feces, and in the case of ratites, *Culicoides* spp., should be determined. Antemortem diagnostic testing for visceral larval migrans is relatively nonexistent at this time. A definitive diagnosis for both *B. procyonis* and *C. quiscali* is made through histological examination of infected neural tissue.[101–103] Observed within infected brain tissue sections are sections of the parasite, migration tracts, and inflammatory and neuronal degeneration.[79,80] Once neurologic signs appear, treatment using antiparasitic and antiinflammatory medications is consistently unrewarding. Preventive measures are the key to reducing the incidence of parasitic infections that cause visceral larval migration in avian nervous tissue. For *B. procyonis*, birds should not have contact with raccoons or raccoon feces. This is significantly easier than preventing exposure to the biting gnats that transmit *C. quiscali* in ratite species. If practicable, monthly treatment with an antiparasitic medication may be used for species susceptible to *C. quiscali*.[101]

Atoxoplasmosis is a disease condition, caused by *Isospora serini*, is commonly diagnosed in canaries and, to a lesser extent, other passerines.[54] Hepatomegaly and splenomegaly are the most common disease conditions associated with atoxoplasmosis, but nonspecific neurologic signs may also be observed. Depression and ataxia are the neurologic signs most often noted in juvenile birds that appear to be most susceptible to this protozoan parasite. Young birds that are immunocompromised are exposed by the infected parents that shed the organism when stressed while raising their young. As the juvenile birds continue to grow, the disease develops into a clinical illness with clinical signs including the bird becoming fluffed and depressed, and many die. Postmortem examination of a bird that is dying or has died with disease signs consistent with atoxoplasmosis is the most rapid method for determining a definitive diagnosis. Although sulfachloropyrazine and other sulfa-based antibiotics have been reported to be effective in treating passerines diagnosed with atoxoplasmosis, complete resolution of the infection may not be possible, resulting in the development of a subclinical carrier within the breeding flock. During treatment, environmental heat is necessary to aid in the bird's ability to overcome the infection. The supplemental heat should be applied to one corner of the cage, with perches placed nearby to allow the birds to move toward and away from the thermal source as needed.

Although rarely diagnosed, *Toxoplasma gondii* can infect birds, resulting in a disease condition affecting muscle, nerves, and respiratory tissue.[54,104] Birds are exposed to the organism through infected feces of the definitive host, the domestic cat. While there are antemortem testing options available to determine serologic antibody titers, the results are not specific in evaluating for clinical illness. Many avian species (e.g., waterfowl, raptors) maintain and have elevated serum antibody titers to *T. gondii* without developing overt illness.[104] As with other protozoal infections, postmortem evaluation of infected tissue is the best diagnostic method to determine a definitive diagnosis. Microscopic examination of brain and ocular tissue will reveal pseudocysts in birds exhibiting clinical signs associated with the disease.[54] Trimethoprim-sulfadiazine has been recommended to treat birds infected with *T. gondii*, with results indicating a possible reduction in mortality.[54] However, complete resolution of the disease through antibiotic treatment appears to be difficult and a positive therapeutic response is rarely achieved.[54]

Toxins

Birds are susceptible to a number of environmental toxins that will result in neurologic disease signs. Household disinfectants, paints, paint thinner, volatile organic solutions (e.g., gas), and air fresheners in the form of candles or "plug in" devices have been suspected, based on cause and effect, to result in neurologic disease signs and death. There has been scientific reports that have verified the toxic effects of Teflon, with affected birds becoming depressed, ataxic, and dying.[105] Atmospheric toxins will almost always cause respiratory disease, but pathology associated with the tissue insult can result in either direct secondary neurologic conditions or primary nervous signs due to the absorbed toxin(s). The avian respiratory system is much more sensitive and efficient in function than the mammalian model. To take a conservative

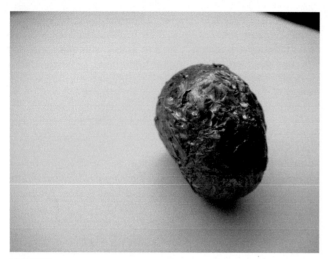

FIGURE 8-26 Lead will cause generalized neurologic signs in avian species. This lead fishing weight was chewed on by a parrot that died of lead toxicity.

approach toward prevention of toxic exposure and concurrent neurologic disease and death, birds should be protected from breathing noxious fumes from any source.

HEAVY METAL TOXICOSIS. One of the top differential disease diagnoses to consider when a bird is presented to a veterinary hospital with neurologic signs is heavy metal toxicosis. The primary metals of concern for avian patients are lead, zinc, and copper, although more unusual metals (e.g., cadmium, mercury) may cause similar neurologic signs. The primary route of metal exposure is ingestion and absorption through the GI tract. Furthermore, if a metallic fragment is located in or near a mobile joint, there may be enough vascular absorption to cause clinical signs of toxicity. There are many sources of metal within a house as well as the environment for birds to ingest; therefore, all species are susceptible to this disease condition. Parrot species are even more susceptible to metal exposure because of their curiosity and ability to break open electronic devices to which they have access and ingest parts of the circuit board. Lead seals, fishing weights, coins, lead-headed nails, copper wire, tire weights, shotgun pellets, lead-impregnated paint chips, galvanized zinc coating on cage material, and pieces of cast-metal toys are examples of items that have caused heavy metal toxicosis in birds (Figure 8-26).

Ataxia, depression, muscle weakness, and seizure activity are clinical signs often noted in birds diagnosed with elevated blood metal concentrations. Diazepam or midazolam may be used to treat initial seizure activity associated with this disease process. Non-neurologic signs, depending on avian species affected, range from hematuria to regurgitation.[54] If there is radiographic evidence of metal in the GI tract, it should be removed. The metal particles can be removed using endoscopy in larger patients, magnets attached to the tip of a rubber feeding tube for magnetic items, gastric lavage, and laxatives. Even if one suspects heavy metal toxicosis, treatment may be started using a chelating agent such as Ca EDTA, dimercaptosuccinic acid, or D-penicillamine. The chelation treatment of choice for birds is IM administration using Ca EDTA,

following the instructions in an exotic animal formulary for optimum effect, and reducing adverse side effects.[106] If possible, blood should be collected prior to initiating chelation therapy and submitted for metal concentrations, CBC, and a plasma biochemistry panel. In cases of chronic metal toxicosis, patients develop a hypochromic nonregenerative anemia.[54] Although the chelation therapy will reduce circulating concentrations of metal in the blood, it is not until the metallic pieces leave the GI tract that the treatment is complete. To remove metallic items from the GI tract, laxatives (e.g., peanut butter, mineral oil, psyllium) have been used with inconsistent results. A study that investigated the ability of different laxatives to remove metal particles from the ventriculus of budgerigars found that grit was the most rapid and effective.[107] Radiographic images are required to determine when the metal has finally passed through the GI tract. Chelation therapy must be continued until blood concentrations of the metal in question return to normal. Once zinc is no longer within the GI tract and no clinical disease signs are noted, chelation therapy can be discontinued, since zinc is a nutrient required by the bird. Lead is absorbed by the bone cells, and when these cells die and are resorbed by the body, a possible "rebound" toxicity may occur. The owners need to be aware of this phenomenon and blood lead concentrations must be evaluated once monthly for at least 2 months after the initial treatment was discontinued.[108] Prevention is based on owners keeping their birds away from metal items that they may ingest. It is impossible to prevent wildlife exposure, but public education may reduce the amount of metal items deposited into the environment that birds may ingest.

ORGANOPHOSPHATES/CARBAMATES. The exposure and physiologic effects of organophosphate/carbamate (OP/C) toxicity in avian species is similar to that described in reptiles. These compounds are used globally as insecticides and when ingested by birds cause an inhibition of acetylcholinesterase at the neuromuscular synapse, resulting in hyperactivity of the muscles. This hyperactivity of the muscles causes fatigue in such a manner that the bird cannot use its rear legs but is otherwise bright and alert. Birds appear to be more sensitive to OP/C than mammals. Clinical signs of OP/C toxicity in birds are rear limb paralysis, ataxia, muscle fasciculations, bradycardia, and diarrhea.[54,109] There are reports of certain OP formulations causing demyelination of nerve fibers and also causing paralysis in affected birds.[54,109] A diagnosis of OP/C toxicity is determined through historical assessment, presenting signs, clinical examination, and evaluation of blood acetylcholinesterase levels.[110] Similar to other neurologic diseases, diazepam or midazolam can be administered to birds that present with seizures.

THERAPEUTIC AGENTS. Any number of therapeutic agents, including antibiotic, antiparasitic, and antifungal, may cause nonspecific neurologic signs associated with toxicity. This is similar to all animals treated, and it is very important for the veterinarian to understand the adverse side effects associated with drug usage in the avian patient. Chloroquine, when administered to penguins at a dose of 25 mg/kg, PO, q24 h for 5 months, was reported to cause neuronal storage disease.[111] Chloroquine, used to treat avian malaria (*Plasmodium* spp.), is known to initiate neuronal storage disease in mammals; therefore, it was thought to be the underlying cause of the disease in the penguins.[111]

Trauma

Traumatic injuries should always be considered when an avian patient presents with nonspecific neurologic signs such as paralysis, paresis, ataxia, torticollis, and/or muscle fasciculations. Although owners will often provide historical accounts of the bird flying into objects (e.g., ceiling fans, sliding glass doors, windows), there may be more involved injuries that result in peripheral neurologic damage including bone fragments, brachial/pelvic nerve avulsion, or egg impingement on the ischiatic nerve.[79] Trauma that results in clinical neurologic signs can occur through predator attacks, gunshot wounds, vehicle collisions, cage-mate attacks, and cage trauma (i.e., body part getting caught in cage). An osprey presented to the author's hospital, apparently functional with no obvious recognition of its surroundings. The bird would face the back of the cage when perching but would not move from this abnormal position. No obvious abnormalities were noted on the external physical examination. When full-body radiographic images were taken, a single shotgun pellet was found in the middle of the osprey's brain, having traveled between the rami of the mandible, through the choanal slit, and into the brain. Radiographic images are often useful to detect fractures and eggs that may be causing peripheral neurological deficits. Rare vertebral luxation in avian patients does occur, especially in wildlife species involved in severe traumatic events such as collisions with moving vehicles. In cases where severe trauma is suspected, full-body radiographic images are required to determine the extent of injury. The most common location for vertebral luxation in birds is at the notarium and synsacrum, which can result in rear limb and tail paralysis.[112]

Traumatic CNS injuries require fluid and anti-inflammatory therapy and, if necessary, mannitol and furosemide.[79] For hens that appear to be egg bound, the patient should be assessed and treatment initiated. Limb fractures must be stabilized as soon as possible to prevent secondary vascular and nerve damage to the affected extremity.[79]

Neoplasia

In avian species, neoplasms are occasionally diagnosed, affecting the central or peripheral nervous systems. Unfortunately, for many of these cases, it is difficult to diagnose tumors in birds that only present with neurologic disease signs. General clinical diagnostic protocol usually requires the veterinarian to rule out other potential diagnoses before a brain tumor becomes the working diagnosis. Diagnosing tumors, especially CNS neoplasms, is clinically more difficult in avian species because of their size and the expense of advanced imaging techniques (e.g., CT, MRI).[79]

Budgerigars are the psittacine species most commonly affected by tumors of the nervous system.[79] Tumor types that have been identified with the CNS in birds include astrocytomas, glioblastomas, oligodendrogliomas, choroid plexus papillomas, neuroblastomas, ganglioneuromas, hemangiosarcomas, teratomas, lymphosarcomas, meningiomas, and pituitary adenomas.[80,113] Unfortunately, if a CNS neoplasm diagnosis is confirmed, there is little hope for treatment and resolution.[79] One of the most common CNS neoplasms diagnosed in avian patients are pituitary gland adenomas; they have been reported in budgerigars, cockatiels (*Nymphicus hollandicus*), and African grey parrots.[54] Budgerigars presenting

with pituitary gland adenomas exhibit ataxia, inability to perch, torticollis, and head pressing.

Neoplasia may also be the cause of birds presenting with unilateral leg lameness. Although trauma must be included as a differential disease diagnosis along with Marek's disease in chickens, trauma and Marek's disease are less likely to cause unilateral leg lameness in parrot species, in particular budgerigars, than a peripheral neuropathy resulting from ischiatic and/or pudendal nerve compression from an adrenal, gonadal, or renal neoplasm.[80] The most common tumor types that cause ischiatic and/or pudendal nerve compression are renal adenocarcinomas, ovarian or testicular tumors, adrenal tumors, and embryonal nephromas.[79] Schwannomas and malignant schwannomas have also been identified as tumor types that cause peripheral neuropathies in birds.[79]

Sertoli cell tumors and seminomas are the testicular tumors most often diagnosed in birds, with an interstitial cell tumor, lymphosarcoma, undifferentiated sarcoma, and teratoma also being described.[54,114] Cere color change in male budgerigars from blue to brown or a pinkish color has historically been reported in birds diagnosed with functional Sertoli cell testicular tumors.[54] Peripheral neuropathies associated with tumor growth may be treated with surgery and/or chemotherapy.[79] As with any cancer treatment, the bird's owner must be informed of the tumor type, prognosis, validation of treatment protocol in avian species, and quality of life anticipated after treatment.[79] Extremely difficult complete surgical removal of testicular neoplasms has been attempted in budgerigars, with about 50% of the patients surviving the surgical procedure.[114] Other treatment techniques suggested for avian testicular tumors are chemotherapy using carboplatin, radiation therapy, and laser ablation of the tumor.[54] At the present time, there are no scientifically validated protocols for the suggested therapeutic options to treat avian testicular tumors. Leuprolide acetate and deslorelin implants have been used as hormonal therapy to treat testicular tumors diagnosed in budgerigars.[54] The hormonal therapy has resulted in apparent clinical response in some cases.[54]

Nutritional and Metabolic Diseases

HYPOCALCEMIA. Hypocalcemia may be the most common metabolic disease diagnosed in birds. Clinical disease signs associated with hypocalcemia include seizures, muscle fasciculations, weakness, and long bone defects in chicks.[79] Unfortunately, it is often difficult to diagnose early-onset hypocalcemia because serum/plasma calcium concentrations are often within normal range.[79] Affected birds may have total blood calcium concentrations <2.0 mmol/L.[79] Total calcium measurements are imprecise, not only because they vary with the amount of calcium within the bird but also with albumin concentrations, as most of the calcium is protein bound.[79] Consequently, ionized calcium concentrations are preferred to assess physiologically available calcium to the animal.[115] The normal range of ionized calcium concentrations in the African grey parrot has been established to be 0.96 to 1.22 mmol/L, and any measurement <0.75 mmol/L is considered suspicious.[79] Birds exhibiting clinical signs of hypocalcemic tetany have ionized calcium concentrations <0.6 mmol/L and low vitamin D_3 levels.[79] A recent report has suggested that hypomagnesemia may induce or exacerbate clinical hypocalcemia in psittacine species.[116] There have been a number of

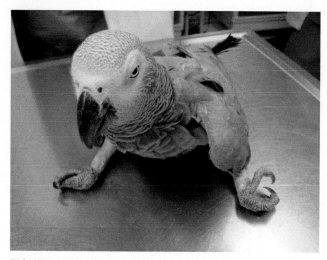

FIGURE 8-27 African grey with seizure activity due to hypocalcemia that may be complicated by a lack of vitamin D_3 and hypomagnesemia.

studies in chickens that have validated the effects of hypomagnesemia inducing and exacerbating clinical hypocalcemia (Figure 8-27).[116]

The underlying cause of hypocalcemia in avian species centers on the inability of the bird to maintain serum calcium concentrations because their diet does not contain the proper amounts of calcium, magnesium, and/or vitamin D_3, or they live in an environment that lacks sunlight.[86] Renal and/or parathyroid disease may affect calcium metabolism in the body, while drug therapy (e.g., tetracyclines) will chelate calcium into a metabolically inactive state.[86]

Treatment varies but is based on the underlying cause of the hypocalcemic condition.[79] Supportive therapy, treatment of seizures if present, and calcium, magnesium, and vitamin D_3 supplementation should be administered.[79] Owners should be informed of recommendations to prevent hypocalcemia in their bird, which includes a nutritionally complete diet, exposure to a UVB light source (280 to 315 nm) for 4 hours/day, access to calcium source (e.g., cuttlebone, mineral block), and calcium supplementation until cortical bone density is restored.[54]

RENAL DISEASE. Physiologic consequences of renal disease in birds can result in neurologic disease signs. When seizure activity and depression are observed in an avian patient, end-stage renal failure is present.[117] The pathophysiology of renal-induced neuropathy is believed to be uricemic/uremic toxins or impaired excretion of other substances produced by the body (e.g., parathyroid hormone, gastrin).[79,117]

HYPOGLYCEMIA. In birds, especially juvenile patients, malnutrition, hepatic disease, endocrine disorders, septicemia, renal disease, malabsorption, and neoplasia all may cause hypoglycemia.[79,80] Depression, ataxia, and seizures are most often observed when avian patients become hypoglycemic.[79] Blood glucose concentrations in birds normally range from 275 to 325 mg/dL, but when this analyte falls below 150 mg/dL, a clinical diagnosis of hypoglycemia can be made and treatment initiated.[54] Recommended treatment for birds diagnosed with hypoglycemia is IV or PO products that contain glucose or dextrose.[54] Once treatment is initiated, the bird should show an immediate response. If there are complicating disease factors (e.g., endocrine, hepatic) associated with the hypoglycemic condition, the hypoglycemic condition will not resolve with simple administration of glucose or dextrose.[54,79] In cases that are recalcitrant to glucose therapy, further diagnostic testing is required to determine the underlying cause of the low blood glucose concentrations. Conversely, there has been a published report describing a hyperglycemic syndrome in northern goshawks (*Accipiter gentilis*) that causes seizure activity.[118]

VITAMIN E/SELENIUM DEFICIENCY. Encephalomalacia, caused by vitamin E and selenium deficiency, is a disease condition that affects the brain tissue accompanied by muscular dystrophy and/or exudative diathesis.[79] Nonspecific nervous signs that include ataxia, weakness, torticollis, opisthotonos, and muscle fasciculations are observed in affected avian patients.[79] A definitive or strongly suspected diagnosis of vitamin E/selenium deficiency in an avian patient is attained through a history, presenting clinical disease signs, testing vitamin E/selenium blood concentrations, response to therapy or postmortem examination of gross lesions, and histopathological evaluation of brain/muscle tissue.[79] Gross lesions affecting the brain of diseased birds are characterized by extensive hemorrhage and edema, while histopathologic evaluation of cerebellar tissue reveals necrosis and degeneration of neurons, petechial hemorrhage, and edema.[119]

VITAMIN B DEFICIENCY. Vitamin B_1 or thiamine deficiency is rare but can occur in avian species. Opisthotonos, ataxia, and/or paresis are neurologic signs often noted in birds with thiamine deficiency.[79] As described for reptiles, frozen fish used for food exposes birds to thiaminases and may induce a thiamine deficiency.[54] Although an uncommon diagnosis, knowledge of the patient's diet, again through information obtained from the owner, will help guide the veterinarian toward a treatment plan. Rapid response to thiamine treatment in a suspected case will help confirm a diagnosis of hypovitaminosis B_1.[120] Moreover, it has been suggested that all avian patients that are presented with neurologic signs be treated with a vitamin B complex that contains thiamin.[79]

Riboflavin or vitamin B_2 deficiency is most often diagnosed in young birds (7 to 20 days old) that are presented with curled toes, paralysis, and generalized weakness.[79] Treatment for riboflavin deficiency is vitamin B–complex injections, which are also recommended for vitamin B_6 (pyridoxine) deficiency, whereby the bird exhibits seizure activity and/or a nervous jerky walk.[79]

HYPERCHOLESTEROLEMIA/HYPERLIPIDEMIA. Hypercholesterolemia/hyperlipidemia is most often observed in prolific egg-laying hens and obese birds fed a high-fat diet.[54] A presumptive diagnosis can be made through plasma chemical analysis that indicates elevated concentrations of triglycerides and cholesterol. The gross appearance of a centrifuged blood sample will be "milky" red, with an opaque plasma component.[54] Birds diagnosed with hypercholesterolemia/hyperlipidemia may develop cholesterol corneal plaques. Moreover, emboli within smaller blood vessels (i.e., especially the brain) may result in tissue ischemia that is observed as "stroke"-like neurologic signs (e.g., seizure activity, unilateral paralysis).[54] Diagnostic testing for affected brain tissue is best achieved through MRI. Fluid therapy along with supportive care, antiseizure therapy, and dietary and reproductive

TABLE 8-7

Treatment Options for Liver Disease

Immunosuppressants	Antifibrotics	Hepatoprotectants
Glucocorticoids	Colchicine Prevention of fibrosis	Ursodiol Shifts bile acid profile to less toxic form
Azathioprine Alternative to glucocorticoid use		Vitamin E antioxidant
		S-Adenosylmethionine Precursor of antioxidant glutathione
		Milk thistle, silymarin Antioxidant, anti-inflammatory

management will often improve a patient's condition and reduce the risk of further disease complications.[54] Although there have been recommendations for use of statin therapeutic agents in avian patients with hypercholesterolemia/hyperlipidemia, only one pharmacokinetic study has been performed in an avian species, with the results indicating inconsistent therapeutic concentrations obtained through oral administration of pimobendan.[121] At this time, with the current statin products available, it does not appear that treatment is effective in birds.

ATHEROSCLEROSIS. Avian species are susceptible to atherosclerosis lesions, which are accumulations of lipid, calcium, and inflammatory tissue within the intimal lining of blood vessels.[122] When atherosclerotic lesions restrict the blood flow in major vessels leaving the heart and within the brain, neurologic signs may occur such as ataxia, seizure activity, and rear limb paresis. Although antemortem diagnosis is not practicable at this time, a presumptive diagnosis can be made through history, physical examination, radiographic imaging, age, and species of patient.[122] Supportive treatment for avian patients diagnosed with atherosclerosis should be initiated along with antiseizure medication and dietary management.[122-124]

HEPATIC ENCEPHALOPATHY. Hepatic encephalopathy is an enigmatic disease process in which affected birds will present with one or more of the following clinical signs: seizures, ataxia, paresis, depression, anorexia, and proprioceptive deficits.[94] Although in other animals portosystemic shunts may contribute to the disease process, in birds hepatic encephalopathy is primarily the result of hepatic disease adversely affecting brain and brainstem function.[79,94] Pathophysiological theories for hepatic encephalopathy in birds are increased concentrations of neurotoxins (e.g., ammonia), alterations of monoamine neurotransmitters as a result of disturbed aromatic amino acid metabolism, alterations in amino acid neurotransmitters, GABA glutamate, and increased cerebral concentrations of endogenous benzodiazepine-like substances.[79,80,94] A definitive diagnosis is difficult to achieve and a presumptive diagnosis is often based on ruling out other disease conditions. Generalized treatment of liver disease has expanded with the use of a number of products that not only protect the liver but also improve function (Table 8-7).[79,125,126]

Mammals

There are a number of neurologic disease conditions diagnosed in small exotic mammals commonly maintained as companion animals. Neurological diseases detailed in this section affect ferrets, rabbits, rodents, hedgehogs, and sugar gliders. Some species of small mammals may not be specifically discussed (e.g., prairie dog), but the information provided will also be applicable to these patients. Where one animal or group of animals is more susceptible to a disease, condition, or syndrome, this differentiation is emphasized. Clinical disease signs associated with neurological disease in exotic small mammals do not differ from those described previously in other animal groups: torticollis, seizures, muscle fatigue and fasciculations, paralysis, and paresis. As with all clinical disease presentations, it is important to obtain a thorough patient history, practice keen observation of presenting overt disease signs, and perform a complete physical examination. Subsequently, the veterinarian should be able to develop a differential disease diagnosis list (Tables 8-8, 8-9, and 8-10).

Bacterial Diseases

Otitis interna should be considered a top differential disease diagnosis when rabbits and guinea pigs present with vestibular signs (e.g., torticollis, nystagmus, ataxia, rolling). *Pasteurella multocida* has long been the primary bacterium behind this disease process, but increasingly, veterinarians are recognizing that other bacterial organisms (e.g., *Staphylococcus aureus, Streptococcus* spp., *Bordetella bronchiseptica, Pseudomonas aeruginosa, Escherichia coli, Proteus mirabilis*) are just as likely to be the underlying cause of otitis interna.[127] *Mycoplasma pulmonis* and *Streptococcus pneumonia* have been isolated from mice and rats diagnosed with bacterial otitis media/interna.[128] Animals that are presented with neurologic signs consistent with otitis interna often have concurrent respiratory disease signs. It is generally accepted that the primary pathway of pathogenic bacteria into the middle/inner ear is through the nasal sinuses into the auditory or eustachian tubes.[128] Although extremely rare, inoculation of the middle ear may occur due to the rupture of the tympanic membrane as a result of severe otitis externa. The bacterial infection can spread to the brain, which results in progressively more severe clinical signs including seizures and death. Basic diagnostic techniques are required to select the most appropriate diagnostic tests to obtain a definitive diagnosis and knowledge about the extent of the disease process. Basic radiographic images may help confirm a diagnosis, but advanced imaging techniques, especially CT, are recommended for a detailed evaluation of the affected area and will be required by most surgeons for total ear canal ablation (TECA) surgery (Figure 8-28). Obtaining bacterial

TABLE 8-8

Differential Disease Diagnoses for Rabbits Presented with Neurologic Signs

Clinical Sign and Associated Differential Diagnoses		
Torticollis	**Paresis/Paralysis**	**Seizures**
Central vestibular disease	Vertebral fracture/luxation	Bacterial encephalitis
Bacterial infection	Spondylosis/spondylitis	Encephalitozoonosis
Encephalitozoonosis	Spinal abscess	Herpes viral encephalitis
Toxoplasmosis	Spinal neoplasia	Lead toxicity
Herpes simplex virus 1	Osteoarthritis	Fipronil toxicity
Cerebrovascular accident	Intervertebral disc protrusion	Pyrethrin/permithrin toxicity
Cerebral larval migrans	Encephalitozoonosis	Heat stroke
Trauma	Toxoplasmosis	Pregnancy toxemia
Toxins (heavy metal)	Splay leg	Hypocalcemia
Neoplasia	Hypovitaminosis A	Hypoxia
Rabies	Neoplasia	Azotemia
Peripheral vestibular disease		Electrolyte imbalance
• Bacterial otitis media/interna		Neoplasia
• Toxins (aminoglycosides)		Brain abscess
• Neoplasia		Cerebral larval migrans
		Hypovitaminosis A
		Hereditary ataxia
		Idiopathic epilepsy (blue-eyed white rabbits)
		Rabies

Meredith AL, Richardson J. Neurologic diseases of rabbits and rodents. *J Exot Pet Med.* 2015;24:21-33.

TABLE 8-9

Differential Disease Diagnoses for Rodents Presented with Neurologic Signs

Clinical Signs and Associated Differential Diagnoses		
Torticollis	**Paresis/Paralysis**	**Seizures**
Central vestibular disease	Traumatic spinal injuries	Epilepsy (G, C, D)
Bacterial infection	Lymphocytic choriomeningitis	Heat stress
• *Listeria* spp. (C)	Radiculoneuropathy (R)	Mites *(Trixascarus caviae)* (GP)
• *Clostridium piliforme* (M, R, H, G)	Streptomycin toxicity (G)	Human herpes simplex 1 virus (C)
Encephalitozoonosis	Aminoglycoside antibiotics	Lead toxicity
Toxoplasmosis (C)	Theiler's meningoencephalitis (M)	Lymphocytic choriomeningitis virus
Degenerative changes		Rabies
Visceral larval migrans		Pregnancy toxemia/ketoacidosis
• *Baylisascaris procyonis* (C)		Hypocalcemia (GP)
Trauma		
Toxins		
• Gentamicin (GP)		
Neoplasia		
• Pituitary adenoma (R)		
• Glioblastoma (H)		
• Astrocytoma (H)		
Rabies		
Peripheral vestibular disease		
• Bacterial otitis media/interna		
• *Bordetella bronchiseptica* (GP)		
• *Streptococcus zooepidemicus* (GP)		
• *Streptococcus pneumonia* (R)		
• *Mycoplasma pulmonis* (M, R)		

C, Chinchilla; *G,* gerbil; *GP,* guinea pig; *H,* hamster; *M,* mouse; *R,* rat.
Meredith AL, Richardson J. Neurologic diseases of rabbits and rodents. *J Exot Pet Med.* 2015;24:21-33.

TABLE 8-10

Neurologic Signs Associated with Vestibular, CNS, and Spinal Lesions in Small Mammal Patients

Disease	Clinical Signs
Vestibular	• Nystagmus, Horner's syndrome, facial paralysis • Ipsilateral paresis/paralysis: ear, eyelids, lips, and nares • Corneal ulceration • Ipsilateral strabismus with peripheral vestibular disease

CNS (brain)	• Ataxia, hypermetria, hemiparesis with proprioceptive deficits
	• Torticollis, circling, rolling
	• Behavioral changes
	• Circling
	  • Wide
	    • Cerebral or thalamic disease
	  • Tight
	    • Brainstem
	• Postural deficits
	  • Ipsilateral
	    • Brainstem disease
	  • Contralateral
	    • Thalamic or cerebral disease
	• UMN
	  • Affect all limbs or forelimbs and hind limbs on same side
	• Hemiparesis
	  • Contralateral
	    • Cerebral
	  • Ipsilateral
	    • Brainstem
	• CN deficits
	  • Brainstem disease
	• Seizures
	  • Disease affecting cerebral cortex

Spinal cord	• Lesion caudal to T2
	  • Only rear legs affected
	• Lesion cranial to T2
	  • All legs affected
	• UMN signs affect all limbs
	  • Lesion C1-C5
	• LMN signs in front legs with UMN in rear legs
	  • Lesion C6-T2
	• Front legs normal with UMN in rear legs
	  • Lesion T3-L3
	• Front legs normal with LMN in rear legs and bladder and tail
	  • Lesion L4, caudal

CN, Cranial nerve; *LMN,* lateral motor neuron; *UMN,* upper motor neuron.
Meredith AL, Richardson J. Neurologic diseases of rabbits and rodents. *J Exot Pet Med.* 2015;24:21-33.

isolates of the organism(s) involved in the infection is difficult. Deep aural or nasal swabbing, performed while the patient is under general anesthesia, yields the best chance for isolating the inciting bacteria.[127,128] Treatment resolution of the infection is correlated with the severity of the disease process. If otitis media/interna has been diagnosed in a rabbit or guinea

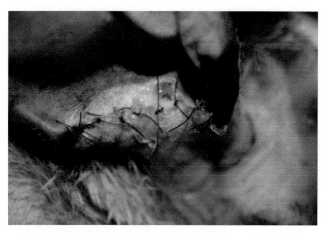

FIGURE 8-28 TECA surgery in a rabbit to treat middle/inner ear disease (photo courtesy of Greg Rich).

pig, long-term antibiotic therapy at elevated dosages is recommended. Enrofloxacin and other fluoroquinolones are the antibiotics of choice and may be administered at a dose of up to 20 mg/kg, PO, q12 h, for 4 to 6 weeks.[127] Resolution of clinical signs, especially torticollis, is variable and should not be considered essential in determining whether the animal has been successfully treated. Pet owners have to be informed that in most cases involving torticollis, some resolution of the head tilt should be expected but not a complete return to normal position. Also, when any rabbit or rodent is prescribed oral antibiotics, the owners should observe for any adverse GI signs (e.g., anorexia, diarrhea) and depression. If one or more of the adverse side effects is noted, the antibiotic therapy should be discontinued and the veterinarian called to reassess the case treatment plan. The prognosis is poor for rabbits that present with severe clinical signs such as torticollis and rolling. For rabbits, if the tympanic bulla becomes filled with inspissated necrotic cellular debris, TECA and ostectomy of the tympanic bulla are often indicated.[129]

Staphylococcus spp. and *Pasteurella multocida* are bacteria that have been identified as causing suppurative encephalomyelitis in rabbits through possible hematogenous inoculation.[128] As previously stated in the section describing otitis media/interna, severe ear infections can spread into the brain and are considered the primary method of exposure of brain tissue to pathogenic bacteria.[127]

Listeria monocytogenes and *Clostridium piliforme* (Tyzzer's disease) have been reported to cause neurologic disease in rodent species.[128] Encephalitis-induced ataxia and seizures have been observed in chinchillas diagnosed with listeriosis.[128] Mice, rats, hamsters, and gerbils develop torticollis, ataxia, and convulsions as a result of *Clostridium piliforme* infection.[130] Tyzzer's disease is most often diagnosed in animals maintained in laboratory settings.[130] Treatment of rodents diagnosed with either listeriosis or Tyzzer's disease is uniformly ineffective.[128]

Viral Diseases

RABIES. One of the most important viral diseases of small exotic mammals is rabies, a zoonotic virus that will cause death in both humans and animals. Vaccination is recommended for all veterinarians and workers who treat animals

TABLE 8-11	
American Ferret Association Recommended Vaccination Schedule	
Rabies	**Distemper**
IMRAB 3 (Merial, Inc., Athens, GA)	Nobivac Puppy DPv (Merck Animal Health, Millsboro, DE)
SC vaccination at 12 wk of age and annually thereafter	For healthy kits ≤14 wk of age from mothers whose vaccination history is unknown, incomplete, or outdated *or* for kits that have unknown, incomplete, or no vaccination history: a series of 3 vaccinations, 3 wk apart, with annual boosters thereafter
	For healthy ferrets >14 wk of age that have unknown, incomplete, outdated, or no vaccination history: a series of 2 vaccinations, 3 weeks apart, with annual boosters thereafter

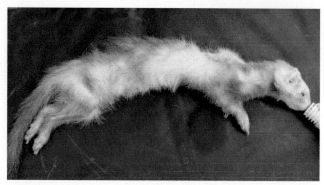

FIGURE 8-29 Ferrets often present moribund when infected with canine distemper virus.

that are susceptible. Ferrets, rabbits, and guinea pigs are susceptible, with published reports of clinical disease and death.[131,132] The nervous system is the primary target of the virus, with clinical signs described as hyperactivity, depression, ataxia, and posterior paresis.[128] The incubation period of the rabies virus in experimentally inoculated ferrets was 28 to 33 days, with the virus isolated in 63% of the salivary glands and 47% in the saliva of the subject animals.[132] In rabbits and guinea pigs, rabies has been diagnosed primarily in areas where the raccoon variant of the rabies virus is endemic.[127] However, any ferret, rabbit, or rodent that is not vaccinated and is exhibiting neurologic signs consistent with rabies infection should be considered suspect. An adult wild gray squirrel was presented to a wildlife hospital in south Louisiana viciously attacking its cage. The animal was euthanized and a full necropsy procedure was performed confirming that the animal was infected with the skunk variant form of rabies. Early signs of rabies in rabbits are nonspecific, after which the animal's clinical disease condition progresses to paralysis/paresis of the legs and possibly head tremors.[127] There is no treatment for animals diagnosed with rabies; therefore, vaccination to prevent the disease is recommended. Prevention also includes protection against predators, if housed outdoors, to reduce the chance of exposure to infected wildlife. There is no vaccine approved for rabbits or rodents, but a killed vaccine (IMRAB 3, Merial, Athens, GA) is approved for annual vaccination of ferrets (Table 8-11).

CANINE DISTEMPER. Ferrets are extremely sensitive to the canine distemper virus (CDV). As a species, ferrets that become infected with CDV experience a high morbidity and almost 100% mortality (Figure 8-29).[133] There may be an acute phase of the disease process that produces generalized disease signs associated with a viral infection (e.g., respiratory, GI, dermatologic), which then progresses to a neurotropic condition. The neurotropic phase of the disease is the presentation that many veterinarians are familiar with: hypersalivation, muscle fasciculations, and seizure activity.[133] Supportive treatment will provide comfort to the patient but will not prevent death in the

majority of cases. Vaccination is recommended to protect animals from CDV infection (see Table 8-11).

ALEUTIAN DISEASE. Aleutian disease virus (ADV) is a parvovirus that affects the nervous system of ferrets. The animals are first exposed through contact with infected animals and their waste (e.g., feces, urine). Mild ataxia, ascending paresis, muscle tremors, and quadriplegia are clinical signs often observed in ferrets diagnosed with ADV.[134] The incubation period of the disease following exposure ranges from 1 to 90 days.[134] Samples collected from suspect animals for PCR and enzyme-linked immunosorbent assay (ELISA) diagnostic tests may aid in confirming a diagnosis of ADV. A definitive diagnosis can be accomplished through postmortem examination of brain and spinal cord tissue sections that exhibit perivascular cuffing with lymphocytes and occasionally plasma cells exhibiting nonsuppurative meningitis, astrocytosis, mononuclear cell infiltration, and focal malacia.[134,135] ADV is rarely diagnosed in domestic ferrets, but veterinarians should be aware of this neurologic disease. There is no vaccination and treatment; supportive care may be effective, but subclinical infection may persist.[135]

HERPES SIMPLEX VIRUS. Rabbits and chinchillas have developed neurologic signs resulting from infection with human herpes simplex virus (HSV).[129,130] In the case descriptions, clinical disease signs involved both the ocular and nervous system.[136,137] Diagnosed as meningoencephalitis in rabbits and nonsuppurative meningitis/polioencephalitis in guinea pigs, these disease conditions led to ataxia and seizures.[136,137] There is no treatment available for rabbits and rodents diagnosed with HSV; therefore, euthanasia is recommended. A definitive diagnosis is achieved through postmortem examination of brain tissue supported by immunohistochemistry and in-situ hybridization or PCR investigation.[128] Infected rabbits can transmit the virus to susceptible cohorts, but the real concern for the single pet owner is exposure of the rabbit or rodent through close human contact when the active clinical disease condition of HSV (i.e., cold sores on the lips or around the mouth) is present.[128]

LYMPHOCYTIC CHORIOMENINGITIS VIRUS. An arenavirus, lymphocytic choriomeningitis virus (LCMV), can cause meningitis in all rodents, with disease signs ranging from subclinical infection to hind limb paralysis and death.[128] More important to veterinarians and pet owners is the fact that LCMV is a zoonotic disease. Although rare, humans can become infected through exposure to infected wild mice or pet animals.[138] Women can transmit the virus to their fetuses; therefore, reduced exposure during pregnancy and for immunocompromised individuals is recommended.[138] No treatment is recommended and preventive measures to reduce possible viral exposure of pet animals should be followed by all owners. Rodents are exposed to LCMV through horizontal (i.e., contaminated urine, feces, and saliva) and vertical transmission.[128]

THEILER'S MURINE ENCEPHALOMYELITIS VIRUS. Theiler's murine encephalomyelitis virus (TMEV) causes a demyelinating CNS disease similar to multiple sclerosis is humans.[128] Although, rare there was a significant seroprevalence of TMEV in mice purchased from pet stores in Germany.[128] This mouse virus has a range of disease presentations in infected animals, from subclinical to severe neurologic signs (e.g., paralysis, seizures), and death associated with encephalomyelitis.[128]

Parasitic Diseases

TRIXACARUS CAVIAE. *Trixacarus caviae* causes a severe dermatitis in guinea pigs. As with many mite infestations, *T. caviae* will cause pruritis; in many cases it is so severe that the animal will seizure.[139] Concurrent clinical signs that may help determine the cause of the seizure-like presentation include dermal excoriation, alopecia, and secondary bacterial/fungal dermatitis.[139] Treatment includes regular cleaning of the animal's environment, removal of cage toys, antiparasitic medication (Advantage Multi, Bayer HealthCare, Shawnee, KS), and NSAIDs.

TOXOPLASMA GONDII. Rabbits exhibiting neurologic signs (e.g., head tremor, rear limb paralysis, ataxia) as a result of *Toxoplasma gondii* infection are uncommon.[127] For most rabbits infected with *T. gondii*, the animal has a subclinical and latent infection.[127] As early as 7 days postexposure, rabbits can start to develop overt clinical signs as a result of toxoplasmosis.[127] Rodents are also susceptible to toxoplasmosis and will present with ataxic, cachexic, and respiratory disease signs.[130] Postmortem examination of animals infected with *T. gondii* may reveal a granulomatous meningoencephalitis along with foci of necrosis and tachyzoites in skeletal muscle, heart, lung, and lymph nodes.[127] In rabbits and rodents, diagnosis can be achieved through serologic testing and observation of the organism in periodic acid-Schiff/Giemsa-stained tissue sections.[127,128] Treatment may be attempted on diseased animals using trimethoprim-sulfamethoxazole and pyrimethamine or doxycycline.[127,128] Preventing exposure is achieved by keeping animals away from areas that may be contaminated by cat feces. *Toxoplasma gondii* is considered a zoonotic organism, but the magnitude of rabbit and rodent involvement in human exposure is unknown.

LARVAL MIGRANS. Although most often reported in North America, cerebrospinal nematodiasis, as a result of *Baylisascaris procyonis* or *Baylisascaris columnaris*, has been identified in small mammals housed in zoo collections close to raccoons in Germany, Ireland, and Japan.[130] Exposure and infection in rabbits and rodents (e.g., chinchillas, woodchucks) are similar to that described for birds. Raccoons infected with the *Baylisascaris* spp. roundworms defecate in and around food and environments in which rabbits and rodents live, and the parasite eggs are then ingested by the paratenic host. The ingested eggs, which may remain infective within the feces for

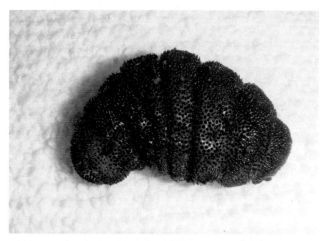

FIGURE 8-30 *Cuterebra* removed from the subdermal tissue of a rabbit.

≥1 year, release larvae in the GI tract that then migrate to the brain, causing a severe inflammatory response.[130] Torticollis, paralysis, seizures, and muscle fasciculations are clinical neurologic signs diagnosed in rabbits and rodents infected with *Baylisascaris* spp. Affected animals may show a slight improvement of clinical neurologic signs before the disease becomes more intense.[130] Moreover, cerebrospinal nematodiasis will cause rabbits to "sway and fall" more prominently than exhibited in other neurologic conditions.[130] Oxibendazole (60 mg/kg, PO, q24 h) is the recommended treatment and may decrease clinical neurologic signs.[127] However, discontinuing the antiparasitic treatment may cause a recurrence of disease signs. Total resolution of the disease and associated clinical signs should not be expected. Prevention is best achieved by keeping rabbits and rodents away from areas and food that may be contaminated with raccoon feces.

CUTEREBRA SPP. Botfly larvae of *Cuterebra* spp. are usually diagnosed in rabbits as subcutaneous parasite infestations (Figure 8-30). However, *Cuterebra* spp. can have aberrant migration through the ear canals and cerebrospinal tissue.[140] When aberrant migration occurs through the cerebrospinal tissue of rabbits, neurologic signs consistent with those noted for cerebrospinal nematodiasis occur.[140]

ENCEPHALITOZOON CUNICULI. Encephalitozoonosis in rabbits and rodents is caused by an obligate intracellular parasite, *Encephalitozoon cuniculi*. Although *E. cunculi* is not commonly diagnosed in rodents, mice from German pet shops had a seroprevalence of 10.7% for this parasite.[128] The significance of *E. cunculi* infection in rodent species is not known at this time, although evidence indicates that this parasite has been identified in both laboratory and wild rodents.[127] Conversely, encephalitozoonosis is a common disease in companion rabbits and widespread in rabbit populations.[128] Rabbits are exposed through ingestion of urine-contaminated food and water, inhalation of infected spores, and vertical transmission.[128] *Encephalitozoon* spores can remain infective under optimum environmental conditions for up to 1 month but are easy to kill using common disinfectants.[127]

Once an animal ingests the infective spores, replication takes place in the intestinal epithelium. Macrophages then transport infective spores to the liver, kidney, CNS, lungs, and

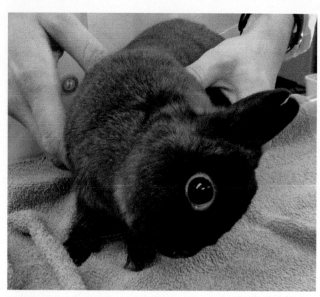

FIGURE 8-31 Rabbit with torticollis, a common clinical presentation when animal is infected with *Encephalitozoon cuniculi*.

heart.[127] In these target organs, inflammation and granuloma formation will occur due to the release of *E. cuniculi* spores from infected cells.[127] Neurologic signs associated with encephalitozoonosis are torticollis, paralysis, seizures, hind limb paresis, and tremors (Figure 8-31). Antemortem testing is available through indirect ELISA, measuring rabbit serum antibody titers.[128] A positive antibody titer will confirm exposure but not infection; therefore, a presumptive diagnosis can be achieved with associated clinical signs typical of encephalitozoonosis.[128] Positive *E. cuniculi* titers have been detected in rabbits without any overt clinical signs of the disease. Elevated antibody titers can be detected 3 to 4 weeks following exposure and infection and reach their highest level at 6 to 9 weeks.[127] Unfortunately, interpretation of *E. cuniculi* titers in rabbits can be difficult if the animal is immunocompromised and does not mount an antibody response to the organism. Rabbits may have a subclinical infection for many years, because their immune system suppresses replication of *E. cuniculi* spores and, when stressed, overt clinical disease develops. Microscopic examination of brain and renal tissue will often reveal granulomatous changes consistent with encephalitozoonosis in infected animals. To confirm an *E. cuniculi* infection through histopathologic examination of tissue samples, Ziehl-Neelsen and acid-fast trichrome stains should be used to identify the organism.[127] While diagnostic tests such as PCR, serum/plasma protein electrophoresis, cerebrospinal fluid analysis, and renal biopsy have been used to help diagnose encephalitozoonosis in rabbits, these tests are nonspecific or unreliable.[127,128] Treatment is based on prevention of spore formation and reducing inflammation associated with the disease process (Table 8-12).

Encephalitozoonosis is endemic in the pet rabbit population.[128] Although it is possible to establish an *E. cuniculi*-free rabbit colony, it is highly unlikely that rabbits sold as companion animals are obtained from these facilities. It is important to know the serologic antibody titers of pet rabbits, especially when owners are immunocompromised, because of the zoonotic nature of this organism.[127]

Toxins

DRUGS. Rabbits can develop neurologic signs, in particular seizure activity, following the topical administration of pyrethrin/permethrin or fipronil. There also are a number of antibiotics that are toxic to rodent species and result in neurologic signs (Table 8-13). For both rabbits and rodents, treatment is supportive, with fluid therapy and diazepam (for seizure control) recommended.[127] Animals that are presented with drug toxicity can recover with aggressive treatment, but the prognosis is guarded.

LEAD. Rabbits and rodents are primarily exposed to lead through ingesting paint that contains this metal. Ataxia, torticollis, and seizures are the most common clinical signs associated with lead toxicity in rabbits and rodent species. As with other animals, radiographic imaging may help diagnose larger metal particles but is not that effective in detecting lead from ingested paint chips. Measuring blood lead concentrations (elevated if >10 µg/dL) is the best method for making a definitive diagnosis of lead toxicosis.[127] Animals that present with seizure activity can be treated with diazepam or midazolam. For rabbits, the suggested treatment regimen is CaEDTA, 30 mg/kg, SC, q12 h for 5 to 7 days.[127] Recommended treatment for rodents was Ca EDTA at 30 mg/kg, SC, q12 h for 5 days.[127] Depending on the severity and chronicity of the lead toxicosis, a nonregenerative anemia may be present. Moreover, following the initial success of treatment, owners must be informed of a rebound effect of lead toxicosis due to lead uptake in bone released upon osteoclastic death.

Trauma

Injury can result in bone and muscle damage that will cause small exotic mammals to be presented with neurologic clinical signs. Blunt trauma to the head may result in brain concussion and pathology that can progress to seizure activity. Leg fractures may be observed as paresis/paralysis of the affected limb. Spinal injury as a consequence of trauma may cause inactivity in the rear limbs and is noted in a number of small animal species. Although a very infrequent presentation, intervertebral disc disease can also occur in animals, in which the vertebral disc protrudes and the nuclear tissue from the lumbar vertebra impinges on the spinal cord. This has been diagnosed in rabbits, ferrets, hedgehogs, and a prairie dog.[141-143] Rabbits are particularly susceptible to lumbar vertebral fractures or luxations because of their powerful rear leg muscles and tendency to kick when being held without proper support of the body. If a rabbit's spinal cord is damaged, both upper and lower motor neurons are affected, with possible complications affecting the ability to defecate, urinate, and have skin sensation posterior to the affected area, along with varying degrees of rear limb paresis/paralysis.[128] The most common location of spinal fracture in rabbits is the lumbosacral area (L6 to L7).[127] A definitive diagnosis in small exotic mammal patients that are presented with spinal trauma caused by vertebral fractures/luxations or intervertebral disc disease can be made by obtaining a history of the presenting condition, radiographic images, myelography, assessing clinical signs, and using advanced imaging techniques. Advanced imaging techniques including CT and MRI will allow better

TABLE 8-12

Treatment Options for Rabbits Diagnosed with Encephalitozoonosis[127,128]

Antibiotic/Antiparasitic	Comments
Albendazole 30 mg/kg orally q24h for 30 days	Possible side effects: pancytopenia, pyrexia, death Recommend serial complete blood counts to assess patient's health during treatment
Fenbendazole 20 mg/kg orally q24h for 30 days	
Oxibendazole 30 mg/kg orally q24h for 7-14 days then 15 mg/kg orally q24h for 30-60 days	Bone marrow suppression reported. Recommend serial CBCs during treatment. Recurrence of disease has been reported once treatment discontinued, thus long term therapy 15-30 mg/kg orally q24h has been recommended.
Fenbendazole 20 mg/kg orally q24h for 28 days *and* Trimethoprim-sulfamethoxazole 15-30 mg/kg orally q12h 7-10 days *or* Enrofloxacin 10 mg/kg orally q12h 7-10 days	

Anti-Inflammatory	Comments
Dexamethasone 0.1-0.2 mg/kg subcutaneous once every 2 days	Should be used for a very short time and with caution due to its immunosuppressive effects

Treating Neurologic Signs	Comments
Diazepam 0.5 mg/kg subcutaneous, intramuscular, or intravenous	To treat patients that present with severe torticollis, rolling
Midazolam 0.07-0.22 mg/kg intramuscular or intravenous	To treat patients that present with severe torticollis, rolling
Prochlorpherazine 0.2-0.5 mg/kg orally q8h	Dopamine antagonists acting on vestibular pathways
Meclizine 12.5-25 mg/kg orally q8h	

Antiemetic	Comments
Metoclopramide 0.5 mg/kg orally or subcutaneous q8h	To reduce nausea in patients with severe torticollis and/or rolling. The feeling of nausea is unknown in rabbits.

BID, Twice a day; *CBC,* complete blood count; *IM,* intramuscularly; *IV,* intravenously; *PO,* orally; *SC,* subcutaneously.
Meredith AL, Richardson J. Neurologic diseases of rabbits and rodents. *J Exot Pet Med.* 2015;24:21-33.
Fisher PG, Carpenter JW. Rabbit neurologic and musculoskeletal diseases. In: Quesenberry KE, Carpenter JW, eds. *Ferrets, Rabbits, and Rodents: Clinical Medicine and Surgery.* 3rd ed. St. Louis, MO: Elsevier/Saunders; 2012:245-256.

TABLE 8-13

Antibiotic Drugs That Cause Neurologic Toxicosis in Rodent Species

Antibiotic Drug	Rodent Species	Comment
Neomycin-streptomycin	Gerbils	Flaccid paralysis shortly after administration
Streptomycin	Mice, hamsters, guinea pigs	
Aminogylcosides	Guinea pigs, chinchillas	Flaccid paralysis, coma
Metronidazole	Chinchillas	Vestibular disease

Fisher PG, Carpenter JW. Rabbit neurologic and musculoskeletal diseases. In: Quesenberry KE, Carpenter JW, eds. *Ferrets, Rabbits, and Rodents: Clinical Medicine and Surgery.* 3rd ed. St. Louis, MO: Elsevier/Saunders; 2012:245-256.

assessment of vertebral fractures and/or vertebral luxations and the severity of the spinal cord trauma. Making a definitive diagnosis and evaluating the magnitude of injury are important when providing a prognosis for the owner. However, with spinal trauma, it is often difficult to determine how well the patient will respond to treatment, and the owner should always be made aware of the uncertainty as it relates to the effectiveness of medical therapy in these cases. It is also important for owners to understand the real possibility of further trauma to the spinal cord, thereby worsening the presenting condition due to the instability of the vertebral bodies at the injury site. Veterinarians and veterinary technicians/nurses alike should handle all small mammal patients that present with spinal trauma with extreme care to prevent further injury. Moreover, treatment should focus on preventing secondary tissue damage associated with the spinal injury and begin as soon as a diagnosis is made. Recommended treatment for spinal injuries in rabbits and other small exotic mammals includes fluid therapy, analgesia, anti-inflammatory medication (e.g., NSAIDs, opioids), and supplemental oxygen. The use of glucocorticoid therapy in cases of spinal injury is controversial at this time. There are reports in dogs and humans that glucocorticoids administered within 8 hours of spinal injury had no beneficial effect on the patient's condition.[128] The return to function of affected limbs and bodily functions is dependent on the severity of the spinal injury. For rabbits that present with minor rear limb paresis, many recover but the area that was affected should be considered a potential location for further injury. Animals that have difficulty urinating may be administered diazepam (0.2 to 0.5 mg/kg, PO) to relax the external urethral sphincter when manually expressing the bladder.[128] For rabbits that are able to defecate and urinate but unable to use the rear legs, wheeled carts have been employed as a means for the animal to maneuver around its environment and maintain a good quality of life. If the rabbit owner is willing to have the rabbit or other small exotic animal treated, they should be informed on the extensive care required for the animal to maintain a good quality of life. A recent case of intervertebral disc impingement on a young prairie dog was successfully diagnosed using advanced imaging techniques and treated through surgical intervention, a hemilaminectomy. The prairie dog presented with an inability to urinate and bilateral rear limb paralysis. After the surgical procedure, the animal regained its ability to walk and urinate.

Splay Leg

The developmental abnormality of abduction of the rear limbs, or splay leg, may occur in young rabbits (shortly after birth through 2 to 3 mo of age) or older rabbits that have trouble moving in their environment.[127] For young rabbits, splay leg has often been attributed to a smooth slippery floor or possible genetic predisposition.[127] Whatever the underlying cause, fast-growing rabbits can develop joint and long bone anomalies due to the improper position of the legs. The skeletal or joint abnormalities become increasingly difficult to treat the longer the rabbit is affected by this condition. Placing the affected leg into a more normal abducted position using splints and/or hobbles may improve the splay leg problem, but perfection should never be the end goal.[128] The splints or hobbles must be checked and reapplied on a regular basis during this rapid growth phase to prevent stricture of the vasculature supplying the distal leg tissue by the splint/hobble bandage material. Quality of life is the objective when treating leg abnormalities and emphasizing the treatment goal to the owner will often prevent disappointment when the patient's improvement plateaus.

Splay leg will also occur in geriatric rabbit patients due to inactivity and muscle atrophy. The abnormal position in older rabbits may cause osteoarthritis, thereby exacerbating the condition. Encouraging the patient to exercise and treating with anti-inflammatory drugs may improve the splay leg condition in older rabbits.

Neoplasia

FERRETS. Cervical chordomas, tumors that develop in the spinal cord, form from remnants of the notochord.[144] Ferrets that are diagnosed usually are presented showing clinical signs of ataxia and posterior limb paresis. Surgical resection of a cervical chordoma has been attempted with some success, although tumor recurrence is possible.[144]

A ferret presented with hind limb paresis and proprioceptive deficits was diagnosed with spinal T-cell lymphoma.[145] The patient was diagnosed through advanced imaging (e.g., CT, ultrasound) of the spinal cord and an ultrasound-guided biopsy of the tissue mass.[145] The treatment response to lymphoma is often related to the age of the animal on presentation, with animals <3 years old being less receptive to immunosuppressive prednisolone therapy. The presence of a leukocytosis and/or lymphocytosis is inconsistent in ferrets that are diagnosed with lymphoma, but if noted may help direct the veterinarian toward this disease condition.

Fibrosarcoma has also been diagnosed in ferrets that present with hind limb paresis.[127] In one study, surgical resection of the tissue mass from the area where it impinged on the spinal cord was helpful in providing some improvement in the patient's condition. However, metastasis occurred as well as regrowth of the tumor at the primary location.[127]

RABBITS. Rabbits have been diagnosed with a number of tumors that cause neurologic signs, including pituitary adenoma, teratoma, and ependymoma.[128] Lymphoma is the neoplastic disease most often diagnosed in pet rabbits.[128] Diagnosis of rabbit CNS tumors is similar to that employed for ferret tumors, and treatment is uniformly ineffective. A rabbit presented with a possible cholesteatoma within the inner ear canal, which was diagnosed using CT. A successful surgical technique has been used for dogs diagnosed with cholesteatoma, with the result of total removal of the tumor and no recurrence of growth.

RODENTS. The most common CNS tumor diagnosed in older rats is pituitary adenoma. Clinical signs observed in affected rats are ataxia, depression, head pressing, and torticollis. Diagnosis is made by ruling out possible differential diagnoses of other disease processes that can cause similar neurologic signs. Cabergoline has been used with some success to control the signs of pituitary tumors in rats. Currently, there is no treatment for rodents diagnosed with aural polyps, papillomas, and cholesteatomas. Older gerbils have been diagnosed with these tumor types affecting the middle ear canal, resulting in clinical signs of torticollis.[128] Guinea pigs have also been diagnosed with aural polyps and present with similar clinical signs.[128]

Miscellaneous Diseases

VITAMIN A DEFICIENCY Paralysis, seizures, and circling are clinical neurologic signs that have been noted in rabbits with hypovitaminosis A. Diagnosis is determined through dietary history and treatment response to vitamin A supplementation. Hypovitaminosis A in pregnant female rabbits has been associated with their young being born with hydrocephalus.[128]

MISCELLANEOUS FERRET DISEASES. The following diseases have been reported in ferrets that have presented with neurologic signs: acquired autoimmune myasthenia gravis, pseudohypoparathyroidism, and eosinophilic granulomatous infiltrate in the choroid plexus.[127] A ferret diagnosed with neuronal vacuolation presented with seizures and ataxia.[146] The clinical neurologic signs reported in these disease processes ranged from flaccid rear limb paralysis to seizure activity.[127] Prednisolone administered at immunosuppressive doses in combination with pyridostigmine bromine is the treatment of choice for myasthenia gravis. The ferret with pseudohypoparathyroidism was successfully treated with lifelong supplemental vitamin D and calcium therapy.[127]

PREGNANCY TOXEMIA. Ataxia and seizure activity along with death have been reported in rabbits, ferrets, chinchillas, and guinea pigs diagnosed with pregnancy toxemia.[128] Pregnancy toxemia and associated ketoacidosis has been identified in pregnant and pseudopregnant animals as well as those that are anorexic.[128] Pregnancy toxemia is diagnosed more often in obese pregnant animals that become anorexic.[128] Treatment should be immediate, with supportive care and fluid therapy (lactated Ringer's solution with 5% glucose). To reduce the incidence of pregnancy toxemia in rabbits, a high-energy diet is recommended late in the gestation period.

EPILEPSY. Chinchillas, degus, and blue-eyed white rabbits have been diagnosed with idiopathic epilepsy, and this disease condition may affect other small exotic mammals.[128] Prognosis is poor for animals diagnosed with idiopathic epilepsy. Treatment response with phenobarbital provided variable results.[128]

There is a spontaneous epileptiform condition in specific inbred lines of gerbils that results in seizure activity.[147] It is believed that gerbils that suffer from this disease condition do not produce cerebral glutamine synthetase, which is required to convert glutamate to glutamine.[147] In affected animals, seizure activity usually begins at 2 to 3 months of age and continues until ~6 months of age, after which they "grow out" of the disease.[147] There is no treatment recommended; however, phenytoin and primidone have been used.[128] In susceptible animals, prevention of the condition through frequent handling during the first 3 weeks of the animal's life has been advocated.[128]

HEAT STROKE. Rabbits and chinchillas are extremely susceptible to heat stroke, and if affected will present with ataxia, depression, and seizure activity due to ischemia and edema of the brain.[128] The prognosis is extremely guarded in small mammals that present with heat stroke and depends on the animal's body temperature upon presentation and length of time affected. Recommended treatment centers on reducing the patient's body temperature, controlling seizure activity, and administering mannitol to reduce cerebral edema.[128]

DEMYELINATING PARALYSIS. Demyelinating paralysis, also known as wobbly hedgehog syndrome (WHS), is a progressive paralysis that has been reported to occur in ~10% of North American hedgehogs.[148] Affected animals may not be able to form into a "ball" and then become progressively ataxic, finally developing seizure activity along with muscle atrophy and tremors.[148] The disease process, from initial clinical signs until death, is usually between 18 and 25 months.[148] Young animals <2 years of age are often diagnosed and confirmation is through histopathological evaluation of affected brain tissue and spinal cord.[148] At this time, there is no effective treatment for animals diagnosed with WHS, and euthanasia is recommended for animals that become severely affected by the disease.

SPECIFIC DIAGNOSTICS

Neurologic disorders that affect animals are often difficult to diagnose; therefore, selecting the proper treatment regimen is challenging as is determining a prognosis for recovery. It is always important to gain a thorough history of the patient and presenting disease process from the owner along with a complete external physical examination. Basic diagnostic testing, when and if possible, to gain a baseline evaluation of the patient's condition may also be helpful for better insight into the underlying cause of the neurologic signs observed.

Invertebrates and Fish

For invertebrates and fish, one is limited regarding a consistent medically accepted method to examine patients that present with neurologic disease. In most invertebrate and fish neurologic cases, a complete history of the animal's environment (including addition of new animals), care, nutrition, and disease condition are the primary sources of information to determine a disease diagnosis. Observation of the animal within its environment, assessment of food provided, and evaluation of abnormal neurologic signs are important for developing a differential disease diagnosis list that centers on nervous disorders. In multianimal enclosures, tanks, and ponds, the quickest means of determining a definitive disease diagnosis is through pathological examination of diseased animals. Animals that are exhibiting clinical signs that have caused significant morbidity and/or death are preferred over dead animals for necropsy submission. Live animal(s) that are to be submitted for necropsy should be euthanized immediately prior to placement in ice and shipped overnight to a pathology service that has expertise in invertebrates or fish.

Reptiles and Amphibians

Specific external neurologic examination protocols have been published for amphibian and reptile species.[149] Assessing the CNs of both amphibian and reptile species is important when patients present with clinical neurologic signs involving the head and cervical area. CN deficits can often be localized depending on the specific nerve(s) affected (Tables 8-2 and 8-3). A thorough patient history and physical examination are required for the amphibian or reptile patient that has been presented with neurologic signs as previously described. Table 8-14 outlines a specific guide to examine the amphibian or reptile patient.[149]

Once an external neurologic examination has been completed and a differential disease diagnosis list has been established, specific diagnostic tests can be prioritized to confirm a definitive diagnosis. Imaging, including radiography and advanced modalities (e.g., CT, MRI, ultrasound), serologic testing to determine antibody response to pathogens, PCR testing, and toxicology evaluations are available to diagnose neurologic disease in amphibian and reptile species.[150] Diagnostic tests recommended for specific neurologic diseases are found in the disease section of this chapter.

Birds

Specific external neurologic examination protocols have been published for avian species.[149] Assessing the CNs of avian species is important when patients present with clinical neurologic signs involving the head and cervical area. CN deficits can often be localized depending on the specific nerve(s) affected (Table 8-4). A thorough patient history and physical examination is required for a bird presented with neurologic

TABLE 8-14
Neurologic Examination Protocol for Amphibian or Reptile Patients

Distance observation
- Assess posture and symmetry: head, facial features, body
- Demeanor
- Alertness and cognizance to environment
- Snakes/monitors: presence or absence of tongue flicking

Assess hearing
- Loud noise to stimulate animal
- Normal amphibian/reptile may not respond

Assess vision/alertness
- Approach patient and observe for response
- Unilateral blindness may result in animal turning toward examiner with its functioning eye

Assess coordination, muscle tone, strength of grip
- If possible, observe patient climbing or walking

Assess responsiveness
- Menace reflex: Ensure air turbulence is not generated, i.e., one eye should be covered while the other is "menaced"
- Use a food item, especially for insectivore species, to generate response; olfactory effect may hinder specific ocular assessment

Assess PLR
- Shine bright light in each eye
- Consensual response should not be expected

Assess balance, strength, grip
- Rotate and maneuver in different directions with hand/perch while animal grasping
- Move snakes hand to hand

Assess body symmetry, muscle mass, tone
- Palpate body and limbs (where present)

Assess withdrawal response and pain perception
- Extend each limb and pinch toes/foot
- Extend each limb and allow to retract to normal position

Assess palpebral reflex
- With cotton-tipped applicator, lightly touch medial canthus
- Not possible in species without eyelids (e.g., snakes, geckos)

Assess facial sensation
- With mosquito forceps, pinch skin around face/head

Assess jaw tone and oral secretions
- Open mouth
- In oral cavity, observe glottis and tongue for symmetry and normal function

Assess oculocephalic reflex
- Move head from side to side while maintaining head in horizontal plane
- In healthy patients, nystagmus observed with the fast phase in direction of head movement

Assess muscle mass and tone of neck and spine
- Palpate along neck and spine

Assess muscle tone of vent
- Pinch vent with mosquito forceps
- Normal animals: vent sphincter constricts and tail moves from side to side

Assess righting reflex
- Roll patient on right and left sides to see response toward normal position

Assess placing reflex
- Without restricting limb movement, bring each foot in turn toward examination table or perch (e.g., chameleons)

Assess compensatory limb movements
- With patient in normal standing posture, hold limbs on one side against body wall and push patient in lateral direction, away from side with limbs restrained; repeat on opposite side
- Place one foot on exam table; perform hopping test on standing leg by maneuvering patient's body to change center of gravity laterally, medially, forward, and backward

Evaluate speed at which foot returns to normal position
- Support body but have patient stand on table
- Knuckle toes of one foot then release
- Place card under foot then slide lateral

Assess cutaneous pain sensation
- Pinch skin along either side of dorsal midline
- Slowly assess in craniocaudal position
- Reptiles lack panniculus reflex

PLR, Pupillary light response.
Data from Hunt C. Neurologic examination and diagnostic testing in birds and reptiles. *J Exot Pet Med.* 2015;24:34-51.

signs. Table 8-15 outlines a specific neurologic examination guide for avian patients.[149]

Once an external neurologic examination has been completed and a differential disease diagnosis list has been established specific diagnostic tests can be prioritized to confirm a definitive diagnosis. Imaging, including radiography and advanced modalities (e.g., CT, MRI, ultrasound), serologic testing to determine antibody response to pathogens, PCR testing, and toxicology evaluations are available to diagnose neurologic disease in avian species.[150] Diagnostic tests recommended for specific neurologic diseases are found in the disease section of this chapter.

Mammals

Small exotic mammals that are presented with neurologic signs should go through an examination process similar to that described for reptiles and birds.[151,152] It is very important to obtain a thorough history from the owner regarding the animal's history and current medical problems. An observational evaluation of the patient, preferably from a distance, is important to determine the animal's condition and abnormal clinical signs that occur without the influence of stress or handling. If possible, a "hands-on" physical examination, including a neurologic examination, is essential to assess the patient's condition to formulate a differential disease diagnosis list. A suggested neurologic examination protocol for small exotic mammals is listed in Table 8-16.

Once the differential disease diagnosis list has been organized, based on the history, presenting clinical signs, and physical and neurologic examination, diagnostic testing is required. The primary objective at this time is to confirm the top differential diagnosis and gain an understanding of the

TABLE 8-15

Neurologic Examination Protocol for Avian Patients

Distance observation
- Assess posture and symmetry: head, facial features, body
- Demeanor
- Alertness and cognizance to environment

Assess hearing
- Loud noise to stimulate bird

Assess vision/alertness
- Approach patient and observe for response
- Unilateral blindness may result in animal turning toward examiner with its functioning eye

Assess coordination, muscle tone, strength of grip
- Encourage bird to step up onto and off perch or hand

Assess responsiveness
- Menace reflex: Ensure air turbulence is not generated; one eye should be covered while other is "menaced"
- Throw cotton ball in bird's field of vision
- Show favorite food item, especially for raptors and corvid species

Assess PLR
- Shine bright light in each eye and assess PLR
- No consensual response in birds

Assess balance, strength, grip
- Rotate and maneuver hand, perch, and gloved hand in different directions while bird is perching

Assess body symmetry, muscle mass, tone
- Palpate body and limbs

Assess withdrawal response and pain perception
- Extend each limb and pinch toes/foot
- Extend each limb and allow to retract to normal position

Assess palpebral reflex
- With cotton-tipped applicator, lightly touch medial canthus

Assess facial sensation
- With mosquito forceps, pinch skin around face/head

Assess jaw tone and oral secretions
- Open mouth
- In oral cavity, observe glottis and tongue for symmetry and normal function

Assess oculocephalic reflex
- Move head from side to side while maintaining head in horizontal plane
- In healthy patients, nystagmus is observed with the fast phase in direction of head movement

Assess muscle mass and tone of neck/spine
- Palpate along neck and spine

Assess muscle tone of vent
- Pinch vent with mosquito forceps
- Normal animals: Vent sphincter constricts and tail moves from side to side

Assess withdrawal/pain response
- Extend each wing individually and pinch wing tip
- Observe how quickly bird retracts wing into normal resting position

Placing reflex
- Restrain bird holding shoulders and wings against body with legs unrestricted
- Bring feet toward examination table or perch

Assess compensatory limb movements
- Place one foot on exam table
- Perform hopping test on standing leg by maneuvering patient's body to change center of gravity laterally, medially, forward, and backward

Evaluate speed with which foot returns to normal position
- Support body, but have patient stand on table
- Knuckle toes of one foot, then release
- Place card under foot, then slide laterally

Assess cutaneous pain sensation
- Pinch skin along either side of dorsal midline
- Slowly assess in a craniocaudal position
- Birds lack panniculus reflex

Data from Hunt C. Neurologic examination and diagnostic testing in birds and reptiles. *J Exot Pet Med.* 2015;24:34-51.

patient's overall condition based on parameters gained from a CBC and serum chemistry panel. It is in the best interest of the patient, veterinarian, and pet owner that the fewest tests possible are performed to gain the information needed to confirm the diagnosis and adequately treat the patient.

There are neurologic disease presentations where infectious organisms may be the underlying cause of the presenting problem(s). Samples collected for microbiological culture may be submitted from animals in which vestibular disease or CSF infection is suspected. Samples for microbiological culture are best collected through endoscopic- or ultrasonographic-guided fine-needle aspirates.[151] Moreover, ultrasonography- and CT-guided fine-needle aspirates can be used for both diagnostic and assessment purposes of suspected inflammatory, infectious, and neoplastic disease. A 20- or 22-gauge needle is best when collecting a CSF sample for analysis and/or culture. The CSF sample should be collected prior to administration of contrast agents and acquired from a location caudal to the suspected lesion (e.g., cisterna magna,

lumbar subarachnoid space) to increase the chances of successful test results.[151] Collection of CSF from larger small exotic mammals is similar to the procedure used for dogs and cats, and reference values are available.[152,153] Endoscopic examination can be used for the external ear canal, especially in rabbits with severe external otitis, to evaluate the condition of the tympanic membrane. To aid in visualization of a debris-filled external ear canal, warm saline can be infused through the diagnostic sheath to flush the canal during the examination.[151] For larger patients, a rigid 2.7-mm endoscopic is appropriate for examination of the external ear canal, while a 1.9-mm endoscopic is an option for smaller exotic mammals.[151]

Although there is limited applicability of ultrasound evaluation for small exotic patients, the tympanic bulla may be examined using this imaging modality.[154] Conventional radiographic imaging and advanced imaging modalities (e.g., CT, MRI) are very helpful in detecting disease conditions that affect an animal's nervous system (Figure 8-32 and Table 8-17).

TABLE 8-16
Neurologic Examination of Small Exotic Mammals

General observation of mental status
- Allow animal to move freely while observing attitude, alertness, and responsiveness to surrounding environment
- Assess facial symmetry
- Determine whether limbs are positioned properly, paralysis and/or paresis is present, and animal's ability to walk

Palpate bone, joints, muscles

Assess postural reactions on nonslip mat
- Conscious proprioception/positioning: While in normal standing position, flex each paw to make contact between its dorsal surface and nonslip surface
  - Place card under each paw and slide laterally
  - Animal's paw should immediately return to normal position
- Wheelbarrow
  - Hold animal by rear limbs and push forward; animal should place its front legs in coordinated manner
- Hopping
  - While holding animal by rear legs off mat, lift 1 front leg off mat surface so that entire weight is supported by contralateral limb; move animal laterally and evaluate reaction; repeat for all limbs.
- Hemistanding/walking
  - Assess lateral movement while holding thoracic and pelvic limbs from 1 side of animal off mat
- Placing reactions
  - Support animal off mat by placing your hands under body
    - Cover patient's eyes with 1 hand and bring carpal area of both thoracic limbs in contact with table edge.
    - Immediate placement of paws in normal weight-bearing position is normal response
    - Repeat, allowing animal to see table
    - Difficult to assess with rear limbs
- Righting reactions
  - Hold animal on its side
  - Release and assess ability to rise and assume normal standing position

Assessment of spinal reflexes, useful in localizing LMN or UMN lesion
- If possible, hold patient in lateral recumbency; technician may be required to assist in restraint of limbs or head
- Back should be supported
- Use reflex hammer or mosquito forceps for testing purposes
- Responses recorded as absent (0), depressed (+1), normal (+2), exaggerated (+3), or exaggerated with clonus (+4)

- Patellar reflex
  - Hold one pelvic limb under femur
    - Maintain stifle in flexed position without restricting leg movement
    - Gently tap patellar ligament with reflex hammer or handle of mosquito forceps
    - Stifle joint should extend in reflex movement when patellar ligament is tapped
- Biceps reflex
  - Difficult to elicit and interpret
  - Support cranial and proximal portion of animal's elbow by placing index finger at level of insertion of biceps and brachialis tendons
  - Use reflex hammer to gently hit finger to elicit contraction of biceps muscle and flexion of elbow
- Triceps reflex
  - Difficult to elicit and interpret
  - Support flexed thoracic limb, holding under elbow without restricting movement
  - Use reflex hammer or handle of mosquito forceps to gently tap point of insertion of triceps brachii muscle tendon to stimulate elbow extension
- Withdrawal reflex
  - Pinch the toe or skin between toes
  - Normal withdrawal reflex: animal retracts stimulated limb
- Perineal reflex
  - Use tip of mosquito forceps to gently stroke perineum
  - Normal function: anal sphincter muscle contracts

Assessing CNs
- Menace response
  - Make threating gesture toward eye without generating air turbulence
- PLR
- While head is still, observe eye position
- Evaluate jaw tone
- Palpebral reflex
  - Lightly touch medial canthus of eye with cotton-tipped applicator to elicit "blink" response
- Corneal reflex
  - Lightly touch cornea with moistened cotton-tipped applicator
- Hearing
  - Make loud noise and observe for response

Assessment of superficial cutaneous pain
- Panniculus reflex
- Gently pinch or pull skin along patient's dorsal surface, cranial to caudal

CNs, Caudal nerves; *LMN;* lower motor neuron; *PLR*, pupillary light reflex; *UMN*, upper motor neuron.
Platt SR, Dennis PM, McSherry IJ, et al. Composition of the cerebrospinal fluid in clinically normal adult ferrets. *Am J Vet Res.* 2004;65:758-760.

A diagnostic test that may be used when animals are presented with neuromuscular signs is electromyography and assessment of nerve conduction velocity. Although many practices do not have access to electromyography, this should not dissuade one from investigating the possibility of its use. Neurologic disease is difficult to diagnose and being able to utilize the necessary means to identify the underlying cause will improve the veterinarian's ability to establish a definitive diagnosis, understand the pathophysiologic processes involved in the clinical presentation, and communicate a prognosis to the owner.

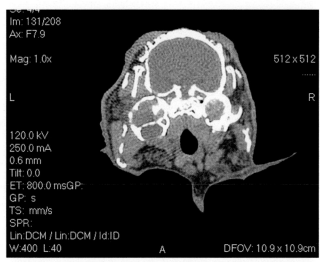

Se: 4/4
Im: 131/208
Ax: F7.9

Mag: 1.0x   512 x 512

L   R

120.0 kV
250.0 mA
0.6 mm
Tilt: 0.0
ET: 800.0 msGP:
GP: s
TS: mm/s
SPR:
Lin:DCM / Lin:DCM / Id:ID
W:400 L:40   A   DFOV: 10.9 x 10.9cm

FIGURE 8-32 Computed tomography is required to adequately assess bulla disease in rabbits (photo courtesy of Christine Higbie).

TABLE 8-17

Imaging in Small Exotic Mammals That Present with Neurologic Signs

Modality	Diagnostic Applications
Conventional radiographic imaging	• Traumatic, lytic proliferative lesions • Vertebral luxations/fractures, congenital abnormalities, discospondylitis, neoplasia
Myelography	• Iohexol (0.25-0.5 mL/kg) • Inject in subarachnoid space • Examine spinal cord • Identify expansile or compressive lesions
Computed tomography	• Vestibular disease: essential for evaluation prior to TECA surgery • Musculoskeletal • Skull, spinal cord

Magnetic resonance imaging	• Identification of disease pathology affecting soft tissue structures
	• Recommended in rabbits with CNS disease
	  • Soft tissue masses, inflammatory, edematous soft tissue pathology
	    • Granulomas
	    • Tumors

CNS, Central nervous system; *TECA*, total ear canal ablation.
Mancinelli E. Neurologic examination and diagnostic testing in rabbits, ferrets, and rodents. *J Exot Pet Med.* 2015;24:52-64.
Whittington JK, Bennel AR. Clinical technique: myelography in rabbits. *J Exot Pet Med.* 2011;20(3):217-221.[155]

Pathological diagnosis can be achieved through nerve, neuromuscular, and/or muscle biopsy. Unfortunately, with many neurologic case presentations, postmortem analysis is the ultimate diagnostic test. Both gross examination and histopathological assessment of collected tissue specimens often leads to a definitive disease diagnosis. Postmortem specimens are often submitted for testing of infectious disease causes, as

appropriate for the history, clinical presentation of the patient, and veterinarian's assessment of the case. Therefore, it is extremely important that the veterinarian submitting the tissue specimens or animal for biopsy and/or postmortem examination to the pathology service provide all pertinent information and request testing to allow for an appropriate and focused evaluation.

SUMMARY

Neurologic disease is arguably the most difficult case presentations a veterinarian will see in practice. For successful diagnosis, it is important to know and understand the underlying anatomy and physiology of the animal's nervous system. With a foundation in anatomy and physiology, the ability to assess, comprehend, and identify the pathophysiology of disease processes and conditions is easier. Diagnosing neurologic disease is often difficult and requires advanced and expensive imaging modalities. Owners of companion animals must understand the commitment required for diagnosis and treatment of neurologic disease before embarking on this tenuous journey. Ultimately, the diagnosis may give an explanation but treatment may not be possible (e.g., in the case of a brain tumor). Also, for invertebrates there may not be diagnostic testing methodologies available or treatment knowledge if a diagnosis is obtained. Thus, patients that are presented with neurologic disease require significant communication with the owner to inform them of the diagnostic and treatment limitations, difficulties, and expense so that they can make educated decisions regarding their animal's care.

REFERENCES

1. Bodri MS. Turbellarians. In: Lewbart GA, ed. *Invertebrate Medicine.* 2nd ed. Ames, IA: Blackwell Publishing; 2006:53-64.
2. Kotikova EA. Comparative characterization of the nervous system of the Turbellaria. *Hydrobiologia.* 1986;132:89-92.
3. Blair KA, Anderson PAV. Properties of voltage activated ionic currents in cells from the brains of the triclad cells from the brains of the triclad flatworm *Bdelloura candida. J Exp Bio.* 1993;185:267-286.
4. Raffia RB, Valdez JM. Cocaine withdrawal in *Planaria. Eur J Pharmacol.* 2001;430:143-145.
5. Scimeca JM. Cephalopods. In: Lewbart GA, ed. *Invertebrate Medicine.* 2nd ed. Ames, IA: Blackwell Pub; 2006:79-89.
6. Wells MJ. *Octopus: Physiology and Behavior of an Advanced Vertebrate Behavior of an Advanced Vertebrate.* London, UK: Chapman & Hall; 1978:417.
7. Boyle PR, Mangold K, Froesch D. The mandibular movements of *Octopus vulgaris. J Zoolo.* 1979;188:53-67.
8. Babu KS. Anatomy of the CNS of arachnids. *Zool Jahrb Anat.* 1965;82:1-154.
9. Babu KS. Certain histological and anatomic features of the CNS of a large Indian spider, *Poecilotheria. Am Zoolo.* 1969;9:113-119.
10. Bullock TH, Horridge GA. *Structure and Function in the Nervous System of Invertebrates.* San Francisco: WH Freeman; 1965.
11. Maynard DM. Organization of neuropile. *Am Zoolo.* 1962;2:79-96.
12. Pizzi R. Spiders. In: Lewbart G, ed. *Invertebrate Medicine.* Ames, IA: Wiley Blackwell; 2012:201.
13. Bernstein JJ. Anatomy and physiology of the central nervous system. In: Hoar WS, Randall DJ, eds. *Fish Physiology.* Vol 4. San Diego, CA: Academic Press; 1971:5-70.
14. Bleckmann H, Zelic R. Lateral line system of fish. *Integ Zool.* 2009;4:13-25.

15. Oksche A, Ueck M. The nervous system. In: Lofts B, ed. *Physiology of the Amphia*. Vol 3. New York, NY: Academic Press; 1976: 312-404.

16. Noble GK. *The Biology of Amphibia*. New York, NY: McGraw-Hill Book Company; 1931.

17. Kemali M, Braitenberg V. *Atlas of the Frog's Brain*. Berlin, Germany: Springer-Verlag; 1969.

18. Winkelmann E, Marx I. Experimentalle untersuchungen über die mikroskopischen und submikroskopischen veränderungen im telencephalon von *Ambystoma mexicanum* nach resection des riechorgans. *Z Mikrosk Anat Forsch*. 1969;81:71-95.

19. Kirsche K, Kirsche W. Experimental study on the influence of olfactory nerve regeneration on forebrain regeneration of *Ambystoma mexicanum*. *J Hirnforsch*. 1964;7:315-333.

20. Schönheit B, Rehmer H. Regeneration des durchtrennten rückenmarkes bei *Pleurodeles waltli. Z Mikrosk-Anut Forsch*. 1967;77: 453-528.

21. Herrick CJ. *The Brain of the Tiger Salamander*. Chicago, IL: University of Chicago Press; 1948.

22. Duellman WE, Trueb L. *Biology of Amphibians*. Baltimore, MD: Johns Hopkins University Press; 1994:393-395.

23. Wyneken J. Reptilian neurology anatomy and function. *Vet Clin North Am Exot Anim Pract*. 2007;10:837-853.

24. Belekhova MG. Neurophysiology of the forebrain. In: Gans C, Northcut RG, Ulinski P, eds. *Biology of Reptilia*. Vol 10. Neurology B. Chicago, IL: University of Chicago Press; 1979: 287-332.

25. Kardona K. *Vertebrates: Comparative Anatomy, Function, Evolution*. 4th ed. Boston MA: WCB/McGraw-Hill; 2005.

26. Larsell O. The cerebellum of reptiles: chelonians and alligator. *J Comp Neurol*. 1932;56:59-94.

27. Huxley TH. *A Manual of the Anatomy of Vertebrate Animals*. New York, NY: Appleton and Company; 1881.

28. Demski LS. Terminal, nerve complex. *Acta Anat*. 1993;148(2-3): 81-95.

29. Griffin EB. Functional interpretation of spinal anatomy in vertebrate paleontology. In: Thomason JJ, ed. *Functional Morphology in Vertebrate Paleontology*. Cambridge, UK: Cambridge University Press; 1993:235-248.

30. Tully TN. Neurology and ophthalmology. In: Harcout-Brown N, Chitty J, eds. *BSAVA Manual of Psittacine Birds*. 2nd ed. Gloucester, UK: BSAVA Publishing; 2005:234-235.

31. Orosz SE. Principles of avian clinical neuroanatomy. *Sem Avian Exot Pet Med*. 1996;5:127-139.

32. King AS, McClelland J. *Birds, Their Structure and Function*. 2nd ed. Bath, UK: Bailliere, Tindall; 1993:237-314.

33. Pessacq-Asenjo TP. The nerve endings of the glycogen body of embryonic and avian spinal cord: on the existence of two different varieties of nerve fibers. *Growth*. 1984;48:385-390.

34. Osofsky A, LeCouteur RA, Vernau KM. Functional neuroanatomy of the domestic rabbit *(Oryctolagus cuniculus)*. *Vet Clin North Am Exot Anim Pract*. 2007;10:713-730.

35. Wingerd B, Stein G. *Rabbit Dissection Manual*. 1st ed. Baltimore, MD: The Johns Hopkins University Press; 1985.

36. Butler A. *Comparative Vertebrate Evolution and Adaption*. 2nd ed. Hoboken, NJ: Wiley Interscience; 2005.

37. Oliver J Jr, Lorenz M. *Handbook of Veterinary Neurology*. 2nd ed. Philadelphia, PA: W.B. Saunders; 1993.

38. Foelix RF. *Biology of Spiders*. 2nd ed. Cambridge MA: Harvard University Press; 1996:330.

39. Francis-Floyd R: Merck Manual for Pet Health. <http://www.merckmanuals.com/pethealth/exotic_pets/fish/disorders_and_diseases_of_fish.html?qt=exotic%20pets%20fish%20disorders&alt=sh>; Accessed December 28, 2014.

40. Francis-Floyd R: <http://www.merckmanuals.com/pethealth/exotic_pets/fish/introduction_to_fish.html?qt=exotic%20and%20laboratory%20animals&alt=sh>; 2014 Accessed December 28.

41. Densmore CL, Green DE. Diseases of amphibians. *ILAR J*. 2007; 48(3):235-254.

42. Wright KM, Whitaker BR. Nutritional disorders. In: Wright KM, Whitaker BR, eds. *Amphibian Medicine and Captive Husbandry*. Malabar, FL: Krieger Publishing; 2001:73-87.

43. Barker D, Fitzpatrick MP, Dierenfeld ES. Nutrient composition of selected whole invertebrates. *Zoo Biol*. 1998;17:123-134.

44. Wright KM. Overview of amphibian medicine. In: Mader DR, ed. *Reptile Medicine and Surgery*. 2nd ed. St. Louis, MO: Saunders/Elsevier; 2006:941-971.

45. Crawshaw G. Anurans (Anura Salientia): frogs, toads. In: Fowler ME, Miller RE, eds. *Zoo and Wild Animal Medicine*. 5th ed. St. Louis, MO: Saunders/Elsevier; 2003:22-33.

46. Blaustein AR, Romansic JM, Kiesecker JM, et al. Ultraviolet radiation, toxic chemicals, and amphibian population declines. *Divers Distrib*. 2003;9:123-140.

47. Browne RK, Odum RA, Herman T, et al. Facility design and associated services for the study of amphibians. *ILAR J*. 2007;48: 188-202.

48. Berger L, Speare R, Daszak P, et al. Chytridiomycosis causes amphibian mortality associated with population declines on the rainforest of Australia and Central America. *Proc Natl Acad Sci*. 1998;95:9031-9036.

49. Weldon C, du Preez LH, Hyatt AD, et al. Origin of the amphibian chytrid fungus. *Emerg Infect Dis*. 2004;10:2100-2105.

50. Parker JM, Mikaelian I, Hahn N, et al. Clinical diagnosis and treatment of epidermal chytridiomycosis in African clawed frogs *(Xenopus tropicalis)*. *Comp Med*. 2002;52:265-268.

51. Annis SL, Dastoor FP, Ziel H, et al. A DNA-based assay identifies *Batrachochytrium dendrobatidis* in amphibians. *J Wildl Dis*. 2004; 40:420-428.

52. Pessier AP. An overview of amphibian skin disease. *Sem Avian Exot Pet Med*. 2002;11:162-174.

53. Johnson ML, Speare R. Survival of *Batrachochytrium dendrobatidis* in water. Quarantine and disease control implication. *Emerg Infec Dis*. 2003;9:922-925.

54. Headly J, Kubiak M. Neurologic disease of birds and reptiles. *J Exot Pet Med*. 2015;23-29.

55. Keeble E. Neurology. In: Girling SJ, Raiti P, eds. *Manual of Reptiles*. 2nd ed. Gloucester, UK: BSAVA Publishing; 2004:273-288.

56. Done L. Neurologic disorders. In: Mader D, ed. *Reptile Medicine and Surgery*. 2nd ed. St. Louis, MO: Saunders/Elsevier; 2006:852-857.

57. Bronson E, Cranfield MR. Paramyxovirus. In: Mader D, ed. *Reptile Medicine and Surgery*. 2nd ed. St. Louis, MO: Saunders/Elsevier; 2006:858-861.

58. Schumacher J, Mader D, eds. *Inclusion Body Disease Virus*. St. Louis, MO: Saunders/Elsevier; 2006:836-840.

59. Jacobson ER, Klingenberg RJ, Homer BL, et al. Inclusion body disease roundtable discussion. *Bull Assoc Reptl Amph Vet*. 1999;9(2): 18-25.

60. Stenglein MD, Sanders C, Kister AL, et al. Identification, characterization and in vitro culture of highly divergent arenaviruses from boa constrictors and annulated tree boas: candidate etiological agents for snake inclusion body disease. *MBiol*. 2012;3(4):e00180-12.

61. Schumacher J, Jacobson ER, Homer BL, et al. Inclusion body disease roundtable discussion. *Bull Assoc Reptl Amph Vet*. 1999;9(2): 18-25.

62. Kubiak M. Detection of agamid adenovirus-1 in clinically healthy bearded dragons *(Pogona vitticeps)* in the UK. *Vet Rec*. 2013; 172:475.

63. Nevarez JG, Mitchell MA, Kim KY, et al. West Nile virus in alligators ranches from Louisiana. *J Herp Med Surg*. 2005;15(3):4-9.

64. Nevarez JG, Mitchell MA, Morgan T, et al. Association of West Nile virus with lymphohistiocytic proliferative cutaneous lesions in American alligators *(Alligator mississippiensis)* detected by RT-PCR. *J Zoo Wildl Med*. 2008;39:562-568.

65. Jacobson ER, Johnson AJ, Hernadez JA, et al. Validation and use of an indirect enzyme linked immunosorbent assay for detection of antibodies to West Nile virus in American Alligators (*Alligator mississippiensis*) in Florida. *J Wildl Dis*. 2005;41:107-114.

66. Jacobson ER, Gaskin JM, Simpson CF, et al. Paramyxo-like virus infection in a rock rattlesnake. *J Am Vet Med Assoc*. 1980;177(9): 795-799.

67. Bennett RA, Mehler SJ. Neurology. In: Mader D, ed. *Reptile Medicine and Surgery*. 2nd ed. St. Louis, MO: Saunders/Elsevier; 2006: 239-250.

68. Carpenter JW, Mashima TY, Puppier DJ. Antimicrobial agents used in reptiles. In: Carpenter JW, Mashima TY, Puppier DJ, eds. *Exotic Animal Formulary*. 2nd ed. Philadelphia, PA: W.B. Saunders; 2001.

69. Lawton MPC. Neurologic disease. In: Benyon PH, ed. *Manual of Reptiles*. Gloucestershire, UK: BSAVA Publishing; 1992.

70. Teave JA, Bush M. Toxicity and efficacy of ivermectin in chelonians. *J Am Vet Med Assoc*. 1983;193(11):1195-1197.

71. Kolmstetter CM, Frazier D, Cox S, et al. Pharmacokinetics of metronidazole in the green iguana (*Iguana iguana*). *Bull Assoc Reptl Amph Vet*. 1998;8(3):4-7.

72. Glor R, Means C, Weintraub MJH, et al. Two cases of firefly toxicosis in bearded dragons (*Pogona vitticeps*). *Proc ARAV*. 1999;27-29.

73. Isaza R, Gardner M, Jacobson E. Proliferative osteoarthritis and osteoarthrosis in 15 snakes. *J Zoo Wildl Med*. 2000;31(1): 20-27.

74. Peary GM. A non-surgical technique for stabilizing multiple spinal fractures in a gopher snake. *VM/SAC*. 1977;72:1055.

75. Farnsworth RJ, Brannian RE, Fletcher KC, et al. A vitamin E-seleninum responsive condition in a green iguana. *J Zoo Anim Med*. 1986;17:42-43.

76. Cole GA, Rao DB, Steinberg H, et al. Suspected vitamin E and selenium deficiency in a veiled chameleon (*Chamaeleo calyptratus*). *J Herp Med Surg*. 2008;18:113-116.

77. Frye FL. Feeding and nutritional diseases. In: Fowler ME, ed. *Zoo and Wild Animal Medicine*. 2nd ed. Philadelphia, PA: W.B. Saunders; 1986.

78. Fitzgerald SD, Janovitz EB, Burnside T, et al. A caudal coiling syndrome associated with lymphocytic epaxial perineuritis in newborn boa constrictors. *J Zoo Wildl Med*. 1990;21(4):485-489.

79. Tully TN. Neurology and ophthalmology. In: Harcout-Brown JN, Chitty J, eds. *BSAVA Manual of Psittacine Birds*. 2nd ed. Gloucester, UK: BSAVA Publishing; 2005:236-239.

80. Jones MP, Orosz SE. Overview of avian neurology and neurological diseases. *Sem Avian Exot Pet Med*. 1996;5:150-164.

81. Gerlach H. Chlamydia. In: Richie BW, Harrison GJ, Harrison LR, eds. *Avian Medicine: Principles and Application*. Lake Worth, FL: Wingers Publishing; 1994:984-986.

82. Guzman DSM, Diaz-Figueroa O, Tully TN, et al. Evaluating 21-day doxycycline and azithromycin treatments for experimental *Chlamydophila psittaci* infection in cockatiels (*Nymphicus hollandicus*). *J Avian Med Surg*. 2010;24:35-45.

83. Alexander DJ. Taxonomy and nomenclature of avian paramyxoviruses. *Avian Path*. 1987;16:547-552.

84. De Herdt P, Passmans F. Pigeons. In: Tully TN, Dorrestein GM, Jones AK, eds. *Handbook of Avian Medicine*. 2nd ed. Oxford, UK: Elsevier; 2009:350-376.

85. Redig PT, Criz-Martinez C. Raptors. In: Tully TN, Dorrestein GM, Jones AK, eds. *Handbook of Avian Medicine*. 2nd ed. Oxford, UK: Elsevier; 2009:209-242.

86. Ritchie BW, ed. *Avian Viruses-Function and Control*. Lake Worth, FL: Wingers Publishing; 2003.

87. Kistler A, Gancz A, Clubb S, et al. Recovery of divergent avian bornaviruses from cases of proventricular dilatation disease: identification of a candidate etiologic agent. *Viro J*. 2008;5:88.

88. Honkavuori K, Shivaprasad H, Williams B, et al. Novel bornaviruses psittacine birds with proventricular dilatation disease. *Emerg Infect Dis*. 2008;14(12):1883-1886.

89. Smithburn KC, Hughes TP, Burke AW, et al. A neurotropic virus isolated from the blood of a native from Uganda. *Am J Trop Med*. 1940;20:471-472.

90. Redig PR, Tully TN, Ritchie BW, et al. Effect of WNV DNA-plasmid vaccination on response to live virus challenge in red-tailed hawks (*Buteo jamaicensis*). *Am J Vet Res*. 2011;72: 1065-1070.

91. Swayne DE, Beck JR, Smith CS. Fatal encephalitis and myocarditis in young domestic geese (*Anser anser domesticus*) caused by West Nile virus. *Emerg Infect Dis*. 2001;7:751-753.

92. Perkins LE, Swayne DE. Varied pathogenicity of Hong Kong-origin H5N1 avian influenza virus in four passerine species and budgerigars. *Vet Pathol*. 2003;40:14-24.

93. Hawkins MG, Crossley BM, Osofsky A, et al. Avian influenza A virus subtype H5N2 in a red-lored Amazon parrot. *J Am Vet Med Assoc*. 2006;228:236-241.

94. Bennett RA. Neurology. In: Richie BW, Harrison GJ, Harrison LR, eds. *Avian Medicine: Principles and Applications*. Lake Worth, FL: Wingers Publishing; 1994:723-747.

95. Greenacre CB, Latimer KS, Ritchie BW. Leg paresis in a black palm cockatoo (*Probosciger aterrimus*) caused by aspergillosis. *J Zoo Wildl Med*. 1992;23(1):122-126.

96. Velasco MC. Candidiasis and cryptococcosis in birds. *J Exot Pet Med*. 2000;9(2):75-81.

97. Oglesby BL. Mycotic diseases. In: Altman RB, Clubb SL, Dorrestein GM, eds. *Avian Medicine and Surgery*. Philadelphia, PA: W.B. Saunders; 1997:322-323.

98. Siegal-Willott JL, Pollock CG, Carpenter JW, et al. Encephalitis caused by *Sarcocystis falcatula*-like organisms in a white cockatoo (*Cacatua alba*). *J Avian Med Surg*. 2005;19(1):19-24.

99. Godoy SN, De Paula CD, Silvino Cubas Z, et al. Occurrence of *Sarcocystis falcatula* in captive psittacine birds in Brazil. *J Avian Med Surg*. 2009;23(1):18-23.

100. Sutherland-Smith M, Morris P. Combination therapy using trimethoprim-sulfamethoxazole, pyrimethamine, and diclazuril to treat sarcocystosis in a pied imperial pigeon (*Ducula bicolor bicolor*). *J Avian Med Surg*. 2004;18(3):151-154.

101. Law JM, Tully TN, Stewart TB. Verminous encephalitis apparently caused by the filarioid nematode *Chandlerella quiscali* in emus (*Dromaius novaehollandiae*). *Avian Dis*. 1993;37(2):597-601.

102. Diab SS, Uzal FA, Giannitti F, et al. Cerebrospinal nematodiasis outbreak in an urban outdoor aviary of cockatiels (*Nymphicus hollandicus*) in southern California. *J Vet Diagn Invest*. 2012;24:994-999.

103. Armstrong DC, Montali RJ, Doster AR, et al. Cerebrospinal nematodiasis in macaws due to *Baylisascaris procyonis*. *J Zoo Wildl Med*. 1989;20:354-359.

104. Dorrestein GM. Passerines. In: Tully TN, Dorrestein GM, Jones AK, eds. *Handbook of Avian Medicine*. 2nd ed. Oxford, UK: Elsevier; 2009:169-200.

105. Griffth FD, Stephens SS, Tayfun FO. Exposure of Japanese quail and parakeets to the pyrolysis products of fry pans coated with Teflon® and common cooking oils. *Am Indust Hygiene Assoc J*. 1973;34:176-178.

106. Carpenter JW, ed. *Exotic Animal Formulary*. 4th ed. St. Louis, MO: Elsevier/Saunders; 2012.

107. Lupu C, Robins S. Comparison of treatment protocols for removing metallic foreign objects from the ventriculus of budgerigars (*Melopsittacus undulatus*). *J Avian Med Surg*. 2009;23:186-193.

108. Kubiak M, Forbes N. Veterinary care of raptors: musculoskeletal problems. *In Pract*. 2011;33:50-57.

109. Hill EF. Avian toxicology of anticholinesterases. In: Ballantynem TC, Marrs TC, eds. *Clinical and Experimental Toxicology of Organophosphates and Carbamates*. Oxford, UK: Butterworth Heinemann; 1992:272-294.

110. Tully TN Jr, Osofsky A, Jowett PL, et al. Acetylcholinesterase concentration in heparinized blood of Hispaniolan Amazon parrots (*Amazona ventralis*). *J Zoo Wildl Med*. 2003;34(4):411-413.

111. Wunschumann A, Armien A, Wallace R, et al. Neuronal storage disease in a group of captive Humboldt penguins *(Sphenis humboldti). Vet Pathol.* 2006;43:1029-1033.

112. Grioni A. Tibiotarsal fracture and neurologic problems of a black-eared kite *(Milvus migrans). Vet Clin North Am Exot Anim Pract.* 2006;9:533-538.

113. Moulton JE, ed. *Tumors in Domestic Animals.* 3rd ed. Berkley, CA: University of California Press; 1990.

114. Reavill D, Echols MS, Schmidt R: Testicular tumors of 54 birds and therapy of 6 cases. *Proc Assoc Avian Vet.* 2014;2014:335-337.

115. Stanford M. Calcium metabolism in grey parrots: the effects of husbandry. Diploma of Fellowship Thesis: Royal College of Veterinary Surgeons Library, 2005.

116. Kirchgessner MS, Tully TN, Nevarez J, et al. Magnesium therapy in a hypocalcemic African grey parrot *(Psittacus erithricus). J Avian Med Surg.* 2012;26:17-21.

117. Lumeij JT. Nephrology. In: Ritchie BW, Harrison GJ, Harrison LR, eds. *Avian Medicine: Principles and Application.* Lake Worth, FL: Wingers Publishing; 1994:538-555.

118. Forbes NA. Differential diagnosis and treatment fitting in raptors with particular attention to the previously unreported condition of stress induced hyperglycemia in northern goshawks *(Accipiter gentilis). Isr J Vet Med.* 1996;51:183-188.

119. Klein DR, Novilla MN, Watkins KL. Nutritional encephalomalacia in turkeys: diagnosis and growth performance. *Avian Dis.* 1994;38(3):653-659.

120. Chitty J. Raptors: nutrition. In: Chitty J, Lierz M, eds. *BSAVA Manual of Raptors, Pigeons, and Passerine Birds.* Gloucester, UK: BSAVA Publishing; 2008:190-201.

121. Sanchez-Migallon Guzman D, Beaufrere H, Kukanich B, et al. Pharmacokinetics of single oral dose of pimobendan in Hispaniolan Amazon parrots *(Amazona ventralis). J Avian Med Surg.* 2014;26: 95-101.

122. Beaufrere H. Avian atherosclerosis: Parrots and beyond. *J Exotic Pet Med.* 2013;22:336-347.

123. Beaufrere H, Holder KA, Bauer R, et al. Intermittent claudication-like syndrome secondary to atherosclerosis in a yellow-naped Amazon parrot *(Amazona ochrocephala auropalliata). J Avian Med Surg.* 2011;25(4):266-276.

124. Beaufrere H, Nevarez J, Gaschen L, et al. Diagnosis of presumed acute ischemic stroke and associated seizure management in a Congo African grey parrot. *J Am Vet Med Assoc.* 2011;239(1):122-128.

125. Grizzle J, Hadley TL, Rotein DS, et al. Effects of dietary milk thistle on blood parameters, liver pathology, and hepatobiliary scientigraphy in White Carneaux pigeons *(Columbia livia)* challenged with B₁ aflatoxin. *J Avian Med Surg.* 2009;23(2):114-124.

126. Hochleithner M, Hochleithner C, Harrison LD. Evaluating and treating liver. In: Harrison GJ, Lightfoot T, eds. *Clinical Avian Medicine.* Vol 2. Palm Beach, FL: Spix Publishing; 2006:441-449.

127. Fisher PG, Carpenter JW. Rabbit neurologic and musculoskeletal diseases. In: Quesenberry KE, Carpenter JW, eds. *Ferrets, Rabbits, and Rodents: Clinical Medicine and Surgery.* 3rd ed. St. Louis, MO: Elsevier/Saunders; 2012:245-256.

128. Meredith AL, Richardson J. Neurologic diseases of rabbits and rodents. *J Exot Pet Med.* 2015;24:21-33.

129. Capello V. Surgical treatment of otitis externa and media in pet rabbits. *Exot CVM.* 2004;6:15-21.

130. Hollamby S. Rodents: neurological and musculoskeletal disorders. In: Keeble E, Meredith A, eds. *BSAVA Manual of Rodents and Ferrets.* Gloucester, UK: BSAVA Publishing; 2009:161-168.

131. Eidson M, Matthews SD, Willsey SD, et al. Rabies virus infection in a pet guinea pig and seven pet rabbits. *J Am Vet Med Assoc.* 2005;227:932-935.

132. Niezgoda M, Briggs DJ, Shadduck J, et al. Pathogenesis of experimentally induced rabies in domestic ferrets. *Am J Vet Res.* 1997;58: 1327-1331.

133. Fox JG, Pearson RC, Gorham JR. Viral diseases. In: Fox JG, ed. *Biology and Diseases of the Ferret.* 2nd ed. Baltimore, MD: Lippincott Williams and Wilkens; 1998:335-374.

134. Une Y, Wakimoto Y, Nakano Y, et al. Spontaneous Aleutian disease in a ferret. *J Vet Med Sci.* 2000;62:553-555.

135. Welchman Dde B, Oxenham M, Done SH. Aleutian disease in domestic ferrets, diagnostic findings and survey results. *Vet Rec.* 1993;132:479-484.

136. Muller K, Fuchs W, Heblinski N, et al. Naturally occurring herpes simplex encephalitis in a domestic rabbit *(Oryctolagus cuniculus). Vet Pathol.* 1997;34:44-47.

137. Wohlsein P, Thiele H, Fehr M, et al. Spontaneous human herpes virus type I infection in a chinchilla *(Chinchilla lanigera* f. dom). *Acta Neuro Path.* 1983;59:63-69.

138. Deibel R, Woodall JP, Decher WJ, et al. Lymphocytic choriomeningitis virus in man: serologic evidence of association with pet hamsters. *JAMA.* 1975;232:501-504.

139. Flecknell P. Guinea pigs. In: Meredith A, Redrobe S, eds. *BSAVA Manual of Exotic Pets.* 4th ed. Gloucester, UK: BSAVA Publishing; 2002:52-64.

140. Hendrix CM, Cox NR, Clemons-Chevis CL, et al. Aberrant intracranial myiasis caused by larval *Cuterebra* infection. *Comp Cont Ed Pract Vet.* 1989;11:550-559.

141. Baxter JS. Posterior paralysis in a rabbit. *J Small Anim Pract.* 1975; 16:267-271.

142. Lu D, Lamb CR, Patterson Kane JC, et al. Treatment of a prolapsed intervertebral disk in a ferret. *J Small Anim Pract.* 2004;45:501-505.

143. Raymond JT, Aguilar R, Dunker F, et al. Intervertebral disc disease in African hedgehogs *(Atelerix albiventris):* four cases. *J Exot Pet Med.* 2009;18:220-223.

144. Williams BH, Eighmy JJ, Berbert MH, et al. Cervical chordoma in two ferrets *(Mustela putorius furo). Vet Pathol.* 1993;30(2):204-206.

145. Hanley CS, Wilson GH, Frank P, et al. T-cell lymphoma in the lumbar spine of a domestic ferret *(Mustela putorius furo). Vet Rec.* 2004;155:329-332.

146. Hamir AN, Miller JM, Yeager MJ. Neuronal vacuolation in an adult ferret. *Can Vet J.* 2007;48(4):389-391.

147. Laming PR, Cosby SL, O'Neill JK. Seizures in the Mongolian gerbil are related to a deficiency in cerebral glutamine synthetase. *Comp Biochem Physiol C.* 1989;94(2):399-404.

148. Graesser D, Spraker TR, Dressen P, et al. Wobbly hedgehog syndrome in African pygmy hedgehogs *(Atelerix* spp.). *J Exotic Pet Med.* 2006;15(1):59-65.

149. Hunt C. Neurologic examination and diagnostic testing in birds and reptiles. *J Exot Pet Med.* 2015;24:34-51.

150. Knipe MG. Principles of neurological imaging of exotic animal species. *Vet Clin North Am Exot Anim Pract.* 2007;10:893-907.

151. Mancinelli E. Neurologic examination and diagnostic testing in rabbits, ferrets, and rodents. *J Exot Pet Med.* 2015;24:52-64.

152. Jass A, Matiasek K, Henke J, et al. Analysis of cerebrospinal fluid in healthy rabbits and rabbits with clinically suspected encephalitis. *Vet Rec.* 2008;162(19):618-622.

153. Platt SR, Dennis PM, McSherry LJ, et al. Composition of the cerebrospinal fluid in clinically normal adult ferrets. *Am J Vet Res.* 2004;65(6):758-760.

154. King AM, Hall J, Cranfield F, et al. Anatomy and ultrasonographic appearance of the tympanic bulla and associated structures in the rabbit. *Vet J.* 2007;173(3):512-521.

155. Whittington JK, Bennel AR. Clinical technique: myelography in rabbits. *J Exot Pet Med.* 2011;20(3):217-221.

156. Dammann P, Hilken G, Hueber B, et al. Infectious microorganisms in mice *(Mus musculus)* purchased from commercial pet shops in Germany. *Lab Anim.* 2011;45:271-275.

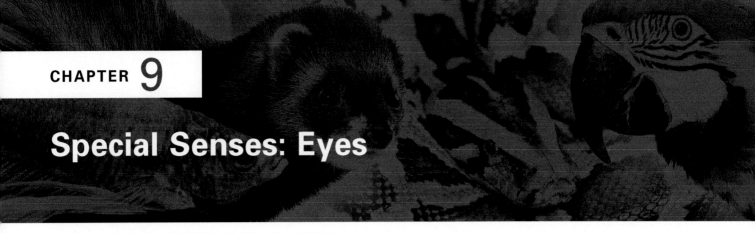

CHAPTER 9

Special Senses: Eyes

Amber Labelle, DVM, MS, DACVO

INTRODUCTION

The eyes represent an essential organ system that is not extensively evaluated during most routine physical examination. While it is not uncommon for the eyes to be examined, many clinicians perform only a cursory exam. A thorough ophthalmic examination provides the veterinarian not only insight into that system but also information about other systems in the patient (e.g., sepsis, hypertension). Exotic pets can develop many of the same ophthalmic disease conditions noted in domestic species, although loss of vision in exotic pets, especially prey species (e.g., rabbits and rodents), can have negative impacts on the animal's overall welfare and long-term quality of life. For this reason, it is important that veterinarians perform thorough ophthalmic examinations and learn to recognize the different ophthalmic diseases encountered in exotic pets. The purpose of this chapter is to review the ophthalmic anatomy and disease conditions commonly reported in exotic pets, as well as potential treatments.

ANATOMY

Invertebrates

The diversity of invertebrate eyes is truly astounding. From the simple eye, which contains only one lens, to the compound eye, which contains multiple lenses, invertebrates display an anatomical array unmatched in the natural world. Those interested in a detailed analysis of invertebrate ocular anatomy are encouraged to read the excellent text *Evolution's Witness* by Ivan R. Schwab. While these anatomical variations are fascinating, they are unfortunately of little clinical utility to the practicing clinician. Ocular disease of invertebrates is poorly described in veterinary medicine, and experienced practitioners are encouraged to share their experiences to build the collective knowledge base.

Fish

The anatomy of the piscine eye is adapted for vision under water, with the majority of the refractive (focusing) power in the lens rather than in the cornea. The globe is a compressed ellipse with a flattened cornea, shallow anterior chamber, and rounded posterior segment. Most fish (particularly teleosts, the bony fish) lack eyelids and have a complete bony orbit. The anterior sclera may contain cartilage or bony ossicles. The cornea is avascular and thicker in freshwater than that of marine fish. Pupil shape is generally round but may vary and is frequently immobile, lacking a normal pupillary light reflex. The iris may be covered by an argentea, which contains chromophores that give the iris characteristic iridescence. The lens is almost perfectly round and protrudes through the pupil into the anterior chamber (Figure 9-1). The lens is supported by the suspensory ligament dorsally and the retractor lentis muscle ventrally, which may be continuous with the falciform process (also known as the tunica vasculosa retinae). The choroidal gland (also called the choroidal rete) is a vascular structure located within the choroid. The choroidal gland is proposed to play a thermoregulatory or nutritional role in ocular health. Some fish have a falciform process overlying the retina and optic nerve. Conversely, elasmobranchs (cartilaginous fish) have an avascular retina and are dependent on the choroid for vascular supply. The choroidal gland communicates with an accessory gill, termed the pseudobranch, which is believed to play a role in concentrating oxygen in the choroidal gland. Rod-cone ratios are variable across species, and some species may possess a fibrous tapetum.

Amphibians

The ocular anatomy of amphibians is as diverse as amphibian species themselves (Figure 9-2). Ocular structures change with developmental stages. Most amphibians lack eyelids in their adult stages; however, a fold of conjunctiva ventral to the globe may act as a false eyelid, particularly when the globe is retracted. Amphibians possess a harderian gland and nasolacrimal system. The cornea is highly curved, unlike fish, and is similar to that of mammals in the adult stages. Iris color is variable but often iridescent due to the presence of guanine crystals in the iris stroma. The shape of the constricted pupil is highly variable, although the pupillary aperture is generally round when dilated to its maximum extent. The iris connects to a rudimentary ciliary body and protractor lentis muscles, which also arise from the peripheral cornea. These protractor lentis muscles provide for lens movement and accommodation. The lens is round and located posterior to the iris.

The retina is avascular and atapetal. Retinal blood supply is provided by the underlying choroid and, in anurans, by a vascular vitreal membrane that lies on the surface of the retina. The retina contains four or more types of photoreceptors, compared to the typical three found in the mammalian retina. Cartilage is present in the sclera of most amphibians, although some may have bony ossicles or lack cartilage altogether. The retractor bulbi muscle is responsible for posterior

435

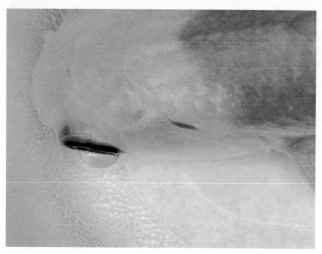

FIGURE 9-1 The normal left eye of a goldfish. Note the clear, spherical lens protruding through the pupil into the anterior chamber.

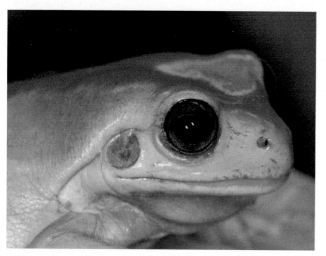

FIGURE 9-2 The normal right eye of a White's tree frog.

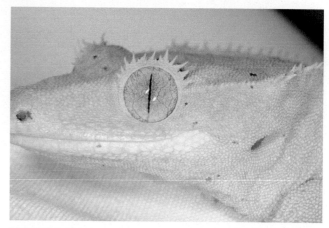

FIGURE 9-3 The normal left eye of a crested gecko. Note the pupil shape in photopic conditions.

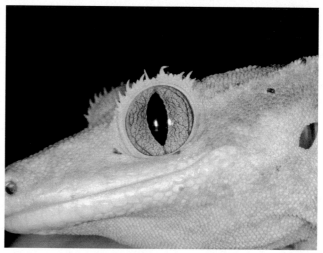

FIGURE 9-4 The normal left eye of a crested gecko. Note the pupil shape in scotopic conditions and the difference from the example shown in Figure 9-3.

retraction of the globe. During swallowing, the retraction of the globe depresses a thin membrane between the orbit and oral cavity, facilitating the movement of the food bolus into the pharynx. Normal globe size, structure, and retractor bulbi muscle function are essential for normal feeding in anurans. The two orbits are not separated by an orbital septum.

Reptiles

Reptiles have remarkably similar eyes despite the diversity present within this class, with the exception of snakes. Mobile eyelids are present in most species, with the notable exception of some geckos (non-Eublepharidae species) and all snakes. Snakes and ablepharine geckos have a transparent, fused eyelid-like structure termed the spectacle. This spectacle, which covers the cornea, is shed with the skin during ecdysis. Some reptiles have transparent eyelids. Harderian and orbital glands that produce lubricating fluid for the ocular surface are present in nonsnake species. The nasolacrimal duct is present in most species but notably absent in chelonians. The cornea is similar to the mammalian cornea. The pupil shape varies by species, and striated muscle is present in the iris, giving the reptile voluntary control over pupil size (Figures 9-3 and 9-4). Mydriatic ophthalmic products are not effective in reptiles because they can voluntarily control the dilation of their pupil. The lens is flatter than that found in fish and amphibians. Many reptile species have exceptionally large accommodative ranges. Some reptiles have an annular pad at the lens equator that connects directly to the ciliary body. The retina is avascular and dependent on the choroid for blood supply. Some species have a conus papillaris that covers the optic nerve head and extends into the vitreous. Vitreal hyaloid vessels may also nourish the retina in some reptiles. Most reptiles are atapetal, and the ratio of rods to cones varies widely by species. Foveas are present in some lizard species while cartilage or ossicles are present in the sclera of most reptiles.

Birds

Birds have three distinct globe shapes: flat, globose, and tubular. The unique tubular globe is found in owls, whereas most psittacines have flat or globose globes. Birds have mobile upper, lower, and third eyelids. The third eyelid is nearly transparent with fine, branching vessels. Its movement is controlled by the quadratus and pyramidalis muscles, which are innervated by cranial nerve IV. The lower eyelid is typically more mobile than the upper lid. A cartilaginous tarsal plate is present in the lower eyelid. Birds do not have meibomian glands but do have lacrimal and harderian glands. The cornea is similar to that of mammals, and similar to the reptile, both striated and smooth muscle are present in the iris. The lens has an annular pad at its equator, and the ciliary body is adhered directly to the lens without zonules. The retina is avascular and atapetal, relying on the choroid for blood supply. A vascular pecten, analogous to the reptilian conus papillaris, overlies the optic nerve head. Birds may have none or more than one fovea and have variable concentrations of rods and cones. Both cartilage and ossicles are present in the sclera.

Mammals

The mammalian globe is the anatomic reference for all lower species. The globe is round and lacks cartilage or bone in the sclera. The upper, lower, and third eyelids are all mobile. Among mammals, only primates lack a third eyelid. The ocular surface is lubricated by secretions of the meibomian glands located at the eyelid margin. Mucous produced by the conjunctival goblet cells, and the lacrimal glands of the third eyelid and orbit also lubricate the globe. The cornea has five layers: the precorneal tear film, epithelium, stroma, Descemet membrane, and endothelium. Zonules connect the lens to the ciliary body. The iris color and pupil shape vary by species, with the retinal vascular pattern ranging from paurangiotic to holangiotic to merangiotic. The presence of a tapetum is variable, as is the ratio of rods to cones.

DISEASES, DIAGNOSTICS, AND TREATMENTS

Invertebrates

Little information is available regarding the prevalence, diagnosis, and treatment of ocular diseases in invertebrates.[1] However, because of the similarities in the basic structures of invertebrate eyes and those in the more evolved vertebrates, veterinarians can use the standard ophthalmologic approach to manage eye cases in invertebrates. Veterinarians are encouraged to publish their experiences in order to add to the body of medical knowledge and enhance the veterinary community's ability to provide care for invertebrate pets.

Trauma is presumed to be the most common cause of ocular disease in most species. Regeneration of traumatized eyestalks is reported in paenid prawns *(Penaeus monodon)*.[2] Giant spiders are commonly kept as pets, and trauma associated with a fall, even over a relatively short distance, may result in ocular injury. Since the ocular surface is continuous with the exoskeleton in many invertebrates, external parasites and infectious agents affecting the exoskeleton may also affect the eye.

When developing a treatment plan for invertebrates one must take into account the fact that some drugs can have a direct negative impact on the invertebrate. For example, copper sulfate, a common drug used to treat parasites in aquatic

systems for fish and amphibians, can be fatal to invertebrates. The author recommends reviewing the mechanism of action of any therapeutic agent prior to treating an invertebrate.

Fish

Corneal Ulcers

Corneal ulcers are common in captive fish and frequently occur due to mechanical trauma, although chemical trauma is possible. Primary infections of the cornea is uncommon, but any epithelial defect places the cornea at risk for secondary infection with bacteria or fungi. Ulcers are classified by their depth: superficial with only loss of epithelium, deep with loss of stroma, and descemetocele, in which all stroma has been lost with subsequent exposure of Descemet membrane. Ulcers can also be described by their size, presence of cellular infiltrate or malacia, and location in the cornea. Accurate classification of the ulcer is paramount to development of a therapeutic plan. Given the speed with which the cornea can succumb to secondary infection, prompt assessment and treatment of any corneal ulcer is advised. This is especially important for fish because of the large number of opportunistic microbial pathogens in the aquatic environment.

While a corneal ulcer may appear as a distinct defect in the cornea surface, it may also appear as focal or diffuse corneal edema. In a healthy cornea, the epithelium acts as in impenetrable barrier to the fish's aqueous environment. A defect in this barrier results in the rapid and severe accumulation of fluid in the cornea, visible as edema. Fish may guard the affected eye, turning away from the observer. A complete ophthalmic examination should be performed on an anesthetized fish, using a bright focal light source such as a Finoff transilluminator. Instillation of fluorescein sodium solution to the ocular surface should be performed in all cases of corneal opacity. Positive fluorescein retention by the cornea confirms the diagnosis of corneal ulceration. A descemetocele is recognized by its distinctive lack of fluorescein retention in the basin of the ulcer, as Descemet membrane does not bind fluorescein dye. It is important to remember that the use of buffered tricaine for rinsing fluorescein stain away from the cornea after application may cause false-negative results when assessing retention of the staining solution, while the use of unbuffered tricaine as an anesthetic agent may cause corneal ulceration.[3] Plain saline solution should be used to rinse away any excessive fluorescein stain from the ocular surface to avoid false-negative results. Samples should be collected for bacterial and fungal culture/sensitivity and cytology (Table 9-1).

If the ulcer is superficial (involving only loss of epithelium), treatment can include daily immersion in 0.017 g/L furazone green bath (Dyna-Pet, Campbell, CA), an antimicrobial agent comprised of monofuracin, furalizodone, and methylene blue, until the ulcer is resolved.[4] Adding 5 g/L (part per thousand, ppt) rock or aquarium salt to a freshwater aquarium is another effective treatment for these cases. Flooding the ocular surface with a broad-spectrum antibiotic preparation (such as neomycin-polymyxin-gramicidin or a fluoroquinolone such as ofloxacin 0.3%) for 30 to 60 seconds at the time of diagnosis is a useful adjunctive therapy. For deeper ulcers, a tissue glue patch can be applied to stabilize the ocular surface. The fish should be anesthetized and placed in lateral recumbency with the affected eye up; then, the ocular surface is flooded with antibiotics, as described above. The ocular surface is then

TABLE 9-1

Published Reference Values for Ophthalmic Diagnostic Tests

Species	Specific Species	IOP (mmHg)	Method	Reference	STT (mm/min)	Reference	Conjunctival Flora	Reference	PRT	Reference
Rabbit		15-23, mean 18	Rebound/applanation	Vet Ophth 2011 Pereira	0-11.2	AJVR 1990 Abrams	*Staphylococcus, Micrococcus, Bacillus, Stomatococcus, Neisseria, Streptococcus, Moraxella*	Vet Rec 2011 Cooper		
Ferret		mean 14.5 +/- 3.27	Applanation	Vet Ophth 2006 Montiani-Ferreira	5.32 +/- 1.32	Vet Ophth 2006 Montiani-Ferreira	*Staphylococcus, Corynebacterium*	Vet Ophth 2006 Montiani-Ferreira		
Rat	Norwegian brown rat	20.8 +/- 1.8	Rebound	IOVS 2009 Morrison						
		28.5 +/- 0.2	Applanation	IOVS 2009 Morrison						
Mouse	CD-1 mice	11.7-13.2	Rebound	J Ocular Pharm Ther 2008 Johnson						
	C57BL/6	12.3 +/- 0.62	Applanation	Exp Eye Res 2004 Reitsamer						
Guinea pig	Various	16.5 +/- 3.2	Applanation	Vet Ophth 2002 Williams	3.8 +/- 1.3	Vet Ophth 2002 Williams				
	Duncan-Hartley				0.36 +/- 1.09	Vet Ophth 2007 Trost			16 +/- 4.7 per 15 seconds	Vet Ophth 2007 Trost
	Various	18.27 +/- 4.55	Applanation	JAVMA 2008 Coster	3	JAVMA 2008 Coster	*Corynebacterium,* alpha-hemolytic *Streptococcus, Staphylococcus epidermidis, Micrococcus, Streptococcus,* Gram-negative rods, *Myroides*	JAVMA 2008 Coster	21.26 +/- 4.19	JAVMA 2008 Coster
Chinchilla		17.71 +/- 4.17	Applanation	Vet Ophth 2010 Lima	1.07 +/- 0.54	Vet Ophth 2010 Lima	*Streptococcus, Staphylococcus aureus,* coagulase-negative *Staphylococcus*	Vet Ophth 2010 Lima		
		2.9 +/- 1.8	Rebound	Vet Ophth 2010 Muller					14.6 +/- 3.5	Vet Ophth 2010 Muller

TABLE 9-1

Published Reference Values for Ophthalmic Diagnostic Tests—cont'd

Species	Specific Species	IOP (mmHg)	Method	Reference	STT (mm/min)	Reference	Conjunctival Flora	Reference	PRT	Reference
Hedgehog	Long-eared hedgehog (Hemiechinus auritus)	18.2 +/- 4.0 males		Vet Ophth 2012 Ghaffari	2.2 +/- 1.2 males	Vet Ophth 2012 Ghaffari				
	Long-eared hedgehog (Hemiechinus auritus)	22.0 +/- 3.2 females		Vet Ophth 2012 Ghaffari	1.3 +/- 1.1	Vet Ophth 2012 Ghaffari				
Fish	Japanese koi (Cyprinus carpio)	4.9	Rebound	Vet Ophth 2007 Lynch						
	Channel catfish (Ictalurus punctatus)	<5	Applanation	Vet Comp Ophth 1996 McLaughlin						
Reptiles	Red-eared slider (Trachemys scripta elegans)	9-58, median 31.5	Applanation	JHMS 2013 Labelle						
	Red-eared slider (Trachemys scripta elegans)	6.1 +/- 2.3	Rebound	JHMS 2013 Labelle						
	Loggerhead sea turtle (Caretta caretta)	4-9, median 5	Applanation	Vet Rec Chittick 2001						
	Red-footed tortoise (Geochelone carbonaria)	15.3 +/- 8.8	Applanation	J Zoo Wildl Med Selmi 2001						
	Yellow-footed tortoise (Geochelone denticulata)	14.2 +/- 1.2	Applanation	Vet Ophthalmol Selmi 2003						
	Hermann's tortoise (Testudo hermanni)	15.7 +/- 0.2	Applanation	Am J Vet Res Selleri 2012						

IOP, Intraocular pressure; PRT, perception response time; STT, Schirmer tear test.

carefully dried using cotton-tipped applicators to absorb all moisture and remove any surface debris. Canned air applied directly over the corneal surface may be useful for rapid drying. A thin layer of *n*-butyl cyanoacrylate tissue adhesive can then be applied to the ulcer bed through a 25-17 gauge needle attached to an appropriate sized syringe. Using a 25- to 27-g needle through a 1-cc syringe to the ulcer bed. The glue must be allowed to dry completely prior to returning the fish to the tank.[4] The glue typically remains for 5 to 10 days. Daily monitoring in the tank is important to assess healing.

As with most teleost diseases, maintaining excellent water quality is imperative to encourage healing in cases of corneal ulceration. Additional methods of decreasing microbial burden in the tank, such as ultraviolet (UV) sterilization or water additives, should be considered. It is also important to consider that caustic water additives may be a cause of chemical irritation and corneal ulceration. Maintenance of pH and water parameters is essential for ocular health.

Nonulcerative Keratitis

A variety of parasites have been reported to attach to or develop within the cornea of wild and aquacultured fish, leading to nonulcerative keratitis. Reports of parasitic nonulcerative keratitis are uncommon in aquarium fish as most parasites require an intermediate host for development that is absent in the aquarium environment. Clinical signs include corneal opacity and corneal vascularization without ulceration. Histopathology is the gold standard for identification of these parasites.[5] Vitamin A, thiamin, and riboflavin deficiency in aquacultured fish can be associated with nonulcerative and ulcerative keratitis; however, improvements in dietary management of these fish have reduced the incidence of nutritional deficiencies.[6,7] Exposure to excessive UV radiation may also result in keratitis.[8] Treatment of nonulcerative keratitis is aimed at identifying and eliminating the underlying cause of disease. Once corneal opacification has occurred, it is irreversible in many cases, but clinical and histopathologic examination of affected fish is key to successfully treating the remaining fish.

Cataract

Cataract is defined as opacification of the lens resulting from disruption of normal lens fiber integrity and arrangement. The lens anomaly causes impairment of vision by distorting light rays as they pass through the lens, with complete blindness resulting when the cataract occupies the entire lens. Cataract can be identified on clinical examination as a white opacity, present within the pupil, that obscures the view of the retina. The lens opacity can be classified by size, location, shape, and etiology. Many etiologies for cataract development have been well described in fish, particularly commercially farmed and wild fish. Aquarium fish are affected by cataracts less than their commercial or free-living counterparts. Reported causes of cataract in farmed and wild fish include exposure to UV radiation, dietary imbalances, change in water osmolarity, environmental pollutants, and genetics.[7,9-14]

A unique feature of cataract in fish is the high prevalence of parasite-associated lens pathology, a finding that is uncommon in mammals. The trematode parasite *Diplostomum*, also known as the eye fluke, frequently affects freshwater and marine fish.[15] Snails act as an intermediate host, releasing

motile cercariae that penetrate fish skin. The cercariae can be identified in virtually any organ, but the eye is preferred site of infection. Within the lens, the parasite develops to its metacercariae form and causes cataract formation. When large numbers of parasites are present, lens capsule rupture and endophthalmitis (inflammation of the anterior and posterior segments of the eye) may occur. When the fish is eaten by a bird, the parasite matures to its final adult stage within the avian gut, eventually releasing eggs into the water where by the snail intermediate host is exposed and becomes infected.

Treatment of trematode-associated cataract consists of cestocide treatment and reducing local parasite burden. In order to prevent the transmission of the parasite in at-risk aquariums, removal of all snails is recommended.[16] A single, 2-hour medicated bath with 2 mg/L praziquantel (Droncit, Bayer Animal Health, Shawnee Mission, KS) is reported to be effective in killing some but not all metacercariae.[17] Unfortunately, dead parasites are often more inflammatory to body tissues than live parasites, and treatment with parasiticides does not reduce the resulting inflammatory response. Where cataracts are associated with lens capsule rupture, severe uveitis, or a decreased ability of the fish to find food and lead a reasonable quality of life, surgical removal of the cataract is recommended. Successful lens extraction via phacoemulsification for removal of blinding cataracts has been reported in the gulf sturgeon (*Acipenser oxyrinchus desotoi*).[18] Referral to a board-certified veterinary ophthalmologist is recommended for any lens-extraction procedure. Where surgical lens extraction is not an option, and the fish is unable to successfully find food and navigate its environment, euthanasia is a humane treatment option.

Uveitis

The uveal tract is the vascular tunic of the eye, and in fish, consists of the iris, choroid, choroidal rete (also known as the choroidal gland), and falciform process (also known as the tunica vasculosa retinae). Inflammation of these vascular structures is termed uveitis. Inflammation of the anterior (iris) and posterior (choroid, choroidal rete, falciform process) uvea is termed endophthalmitis. When inflammation involves the entire uveal tract and extends into the sclera/orbit, it is termed panophthalmitis (Figure 9-5). Classic clinical signs of uveitis include rubiosis iridis (a red appearance to the iris), aqueous flare, hypopyon, hyphema, posterior synechiae (adhesions between the iris and the anterior lens capsule), and vision loss. Fundoscopy is challenging but possible in fish and is the best way to clinically diagnose lesions of the retina/posterior uvea. Causes of uveitis are varied and include corneal disease (such as ulcerative keratitis), trauma, infectious agents, sepsis, and environmental toxins. Infectious agents may invade the eye directly or through a hematogenous route. When clinical signs of uveitis are identified, a complete ophthalmic examination and systemic workup are warranted to identify the underlying cause. Treatment depends on the underlying cause of uveitis; however, maintaining excellent water quality and enforcing strict quarantine of all new fish are always recommended.

Retinal Disease

Fortunately, retinal disease is rare in fish, particularly aquarium fish. Impaired vision is the first sign of retinal disease; however, descriptions of retinal disease in fish are largely

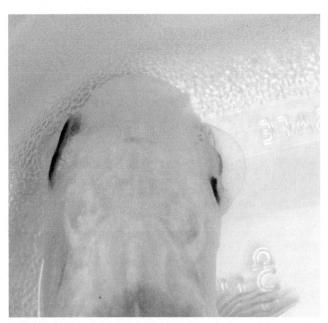

FIGURE 9-5 The right eye of a goldfish. The cataractous lens is posteriorly subluxated and the anterior chamber is deep. Chronic uveitis was suspected as the underlying cause.

based on histopathologic findings. Inflammation of the choroid as part of uveitis may lead to secondary inflammation of the retina, or the retina may be primarily affected. Causes of retinal disease are varied and include genetics, toxins, infectious agents, systemic diseases, dietary imbalances, and gas bubble disease (see below). Treatment is aimed at identification and correction of the underlying cause of retinal disease.

Exophthalmos

Exophthalmos is the cranial displacement of the globe from the orbit. A space-occupying mass is the most common cause of exophthalmos. Dramatic exophthalmos can result from minor orbital lesions in fish because the orbit tightly conforms to the globe, leaving little room for diseased tissue. It is important to differentiate exophthalmos from buphthalmos. Buphthalmos is an increase in the size of the globe and results from intraocular disease such as glaucoma or gas bubble disease. Measuring the vertical and horizontal corneal diameters and comparing with those of the normal contralateral eye or a normal conspecific helps differentiate buphthalmos (where eye size is increased) from exophthalmos (where eye size is normal). Exophthalmos may be associated with other ocular disease. Since fish do not have eyelids and live in aqueous environments, exophthalmos does not result in exposure of the cornea, as it does in birds or mammals; however, an exophthalmic globe is more likely to be inadvertently traumatized. Corneal ulcers, uveitis, hyphema, lens displacement, retinopathy, and blindness may all be observed concurrently with exophthalmos.

Exophthalmos can be associated with infectious organisms, dietary imbalances, retrobulbar neoplasia, and trauma. Perhaps the most common cause of both exophthalmos and buphthalmos in fish is gas bubble disease (GBD). GBD is a well-recognized disease affecting free-living, farmed, and aquarium fish. GBD results from immersion of the fish in water

supersaturated with atmospheric gases, where the total pressure of the gases in the water is greater than that of the ambient atmospheric pressure. Supersaturation may occur where water is pumped into the tank from a deep well is infused with leaking air or when water flowing into the tank produces bubbles of atmospheric gas via the Venturi effect. Additional factors that may contribute to the pathogenesis of GBD include elevated water temperature, increased water depth, increased tank illumination, concurrent infectious disease, environmental toxins, stress, and species susceptibility.

When fish reside in supersaturated water, gas bubbles can accumulate within any organ, but the globe and orbit, gills, kidney, skin, and gastrointestinal tract seem to be frequently affected. Gas accumulation in the orbit and choroidal rete can lead to exophthalmos. Gas accumulation in the globe leads to multiple ocular abnormalities, including buphthalmos, corneal edema, vascularization and fibrosis, lens subluxation or luxation, free intraocular gas bubbles, retinal degeneration, and vision loss. Chronic GBD may be associated with endophthalmitis, cataract, anterior synechiae, rupture of the globe, and phthisis bulbi.[19,20] Diagnosis of GBD is generally made during clinical examination, but histopathology of affected globes can confirm the diagnosis.

Successful treatment of aquarium fish with GBD on a consistent basis has not been reported, although addressing water quality and aeration is key to preventing other fish in the aquarium from becoming affected. A tensiometer can be used to measure the partial pressures of dissolved gases within aquarium water. The aquarium water source and all piping should be carefully inspected, as should flow of water into and out of the aquarium. One report suggests that fish can maintain a good quality of life if carefully managed despite limited vision associated with GBD.[20]

Amphibians

Ocular disease in amphibians is poorly represented in the peer-reviewed literature. When a clinician is presented an amphibian with ocular disease, careful attention should be paid to husbandry, including temperature and humidity. Optimal housing is essential for ocular surface and skin health of captive amphibians. The eyelid skin may be affected by infectious organisms, including bacteria, viruses, and fungi, just as skin in other nonocular locations. When treating amphibians, care should be used if topical therapy is applied. Medications that are safe for the skin may be irritating or ulcerative to the cornea.

Corneal Ulcers

Corneal ulcers can be diagnosed with the application of fluorescein stain and treated with broad-spectrum topical antibiotics. The absorbent and permeable skin of amphibians makes drug selection considerations more challenging. Unfortunately, no pharmacokinetic data are available for topical ophthalmic antibiotics in amphibians, and drug concentrations in ophthalmic formulations may result in systemic toxicity. Great care should be taken when selecting drugs for ophthalmic disease in amphibians. Common ophthalmic antibiotics used in amphibians include neomycin-polymyxin-gramicidin, tetracyclines, and fluoroquinolones. Antibiotic selection should be based on microbial culture and antibiotic sensitivity.

Corneal Lipidosis

The most frequently described ophthalmic condition affecting amphibians is corneal lipidosis of frogs, particularly Cuban tree frogs *(Osteopilus septentrionalis).*[21-23] High-cholesterol diets are significantly associated with a higher prevalence of corneal lipidosis. Commercially available insects may have a higher fat content than wild-type insects, so dietary lipid content may be elevated even when a seemingly appropriate diet is being fed.[24] Affected frogs show white, crystalline corneal opacification (lipid) associated with variable vascularization and ulceration. The crystalline opacification typically begins perilimbally and progresses toward the axial cornea. Once present, the corneal lipidosis is irreversible. Corneal ulceration may result from epithelial instability. Treatment with topical antibiotics when the cornea is ulcerated is warranted. Although some authors have proposed treatment with topical corticosteroids, this has the potential to exacerbate corneal degeneration.[24] Systemic nonsteroidal anti-inflammatories may be used for analgesia. Systemic administration of vitamin A is unlikely to influence disease outcome.[24] Some authors state that careful dietary management may stabilize the disease and slow or prevent progression. The loss of vision associated with corneal lipidosis may interfere with normal predation and thermoregulatory behaviors resulting in considerable stress for the affected animal.[24] Prevention via dietary management is recommended.

Uveitis

As in other species, uveitis can be an ocular manifestation of systemic disease in amphibians, particularly septicemia (Figure 9-6).[25-28] Keratitis may accompany uveitis.[29] Identification of corneal edema, intraocular fibrin, or hypopyon should prompt thorough physical examination and further systemic workup. Treatment (e.g., broad-spectrum antibiotics, nonsteroidal anti-inflammatories) should focus on systemic disease.

Reptiles

Congenital and Developmental Diseases

A recent report summarized cases of congenital and developmental ocular diseases of reptiles and hypothesized the progressive stages from which the defects arose.[30] Overall, congenital and developmental ocular diseases are uncommon but may also be underreported. Environmental temperatures may influence the incidence of congenital disease, stressing the importance of appropriate husbandry during reproductive phases and incubation.

Hypovitaminosis A

Chelonians are particularly susceptible to hypovitaminosis A, but other reptiles may also be affected.[31,32] Dramatic periocular swelling that may force the eyelids to close is the most prominent clinical sign (Figure 9-7). The swelling results from squamous metaplasia of orbital glands with subsequent obstruction of the draining ducts, duct rupture, and blepharoconjunctivitis. Young, rapidly growing chelonians fed vitamin A deficient diets are most frequently affected. Wild-caught specimens that do not adapt to captivity are also commonly affected. Parenteral administration of vitamin A may reverse the ocular clinical signs; however, dietary modification is also advised.[33] Typical dosing is 1500 IU/kg vitamin A, administered via an intramuscular injection. Repeat dosages may be given but are generally not necessary if fed an adequate diet. It is important not to overdose a chelonian with parenteral vitamin A, as it can lead to hypervitaminosis A. Affected animals may slough their skin, creating a larger problem than the original hypovitaminosis A. It is also important to note that hypoviatminosis A may be one of the most misdiagnosed diseases of captive chelonians. Since the 1970s, it has been common dogma to treat all chelonians with periocular disease and nasal discharge with parenteral vitamin A. However, infectious diseases (e.g., mycoplasmosis, herpesvirus, and ranavirus) are also common causes for similar clinical signs, therefore it is important for the veterinarian to broaden his or her differential diagnosis list when managing these cases.

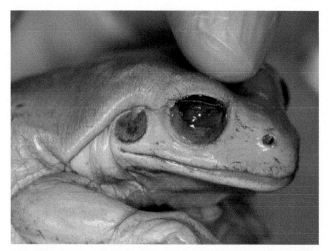

FIGURE 9-6 Keratoconjunctivitis and uveitis in a White's tree frog of unknown etiology.

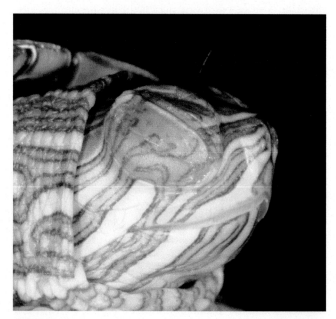

FIGURE 9-7 The right eye of a young red-eared slider turtle with hypovitaminosis A. Note the dramatic periocular swelling.

Conjunctivitis

Conjunctivitis is a nonspecific clinical sign that may result from a variety of ocular insults.[33] Conjunctivitis may be the result of concurrent ocular disease, dietary deficiencies (particularly vitamin A), environmental toxins/irritants, infectious diseases, and foreign material. Conjunctivitis results in hyperemia or redness of the conjunctiva with variable edema, termed chemosis (Figures 9-8 and 9-9). A thorough ophthalmic and physical examination is warranted in all patients with conjunctivitis. Cytology and culture/sensitivity may be useful in determining disease etiology and treatment goals. Conjunctivitis may be challenging to treat in chameleons due to their unique eyelid conformation.[34] A blunt-tipped nasolacrimal lavage cannula can be placed within the palpebral fissure with gentle pressure applied to close the lids to lavage the ocular surface. If the chameleon is held in a head-down position, the resultant solution may be collected from the oral cavity for cytology.[35]

Eyelid/Periocular/Orbital Masses

Periocular masses have a multitude of causes that require a thorough ocular examination and diagnostic workup to diagnose and formulate an effective treatment plan. Masses of the adnexa result in impaired lid function and exposure keratitis. Orbital masses can cause periocular swelling and changes in globe position, including exophthalmos and strabismus. Infectious agents and environmental toxins can be associated with ulcerative or proliferative lesions of the eyelids in a variety of reptile species.[33,36] Herpesvirus is a cause of fibropapillomatous masses in green sea turtles and other chelonians, while poxvirus is implicated in caimans.[37,38] Neoplasia of the eyelids is infrequently reported, with squamous cell carcinoma being the most commonly described neoplasm (Figure 9-10).[39–42]

Cytology, culture/sensitivity, and biopsy are useful tools for determining etiopathogenesis and treatment of eyelid lesions. Periocular and orbital masses may be infectious, neoplastic, vascular, or developmental.[34,39,43–45] Establishment of surgical drainage, culture, and biopsy is useful for determining prognosis and treatment strategies.[46] Advanced imaging may prove useful for determining the extent of the lesion.[47,48]

Spectacular Disease in Snakes

The spectacle is an ocular structure unique to reptiles, and disease of the spectacle is the most common ophthalmic disorder in snakes.[33] The spectacle is shed as part of the normal ecdysis. Failure of normal shedding, or dysecdysis, may result in a retained spectacle. A retained spectacle gives the surface of the eye a cloudy and wrinkled appearance (Figures 9-11 and 9-12). Dysecdysis is most often a function of poor husbandry, and a retained spectacle is often treated with changes in housing and management. Adequate ambient humidity (desert species: 30% to 50%, temperate species: 50% to 70%, tropical species: 70% to 90%) and adequate access to "furniture" to rub on within the enclosure are essential for normal ecdysis. Once changes in housing and the animal's environmental conditions are made, the next ecdysis results in shedding of the retained spectacle. Alternatively, topical therapy with 20% *N*-acetylcysteine may help dislodge the retained spectacle. Surgical removal of the spectacle is not generally recommended as the underlying cornea is easily traumatized, and exposure keratitis with corneal perforation can result.

Keratocanthoma is an important but rarely reported differential diagnosis for retained spectacle.[49] A keratocanthoma would be more opaque and have an increased proliferative appearance than the typical retained spectacle, which helps the clinician differentiate these two conditions.

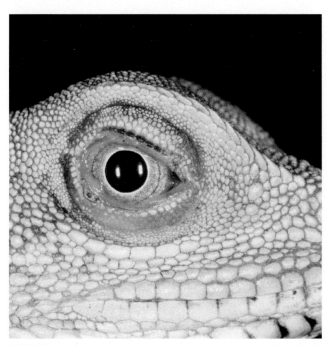

FIGURE 9-8 The right eye of a Chinese water dragon. Note the chemosis, conjunctival hyperemia, and mucoid ocular discharge.

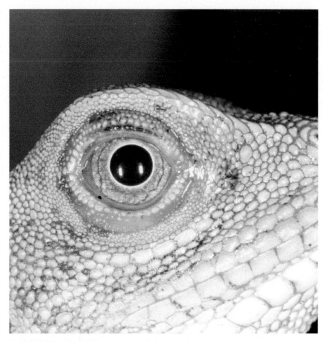

FIGURE 9-9 The same patient as in Figure 9-8, post treatment. The conjunctivitis is resolved.

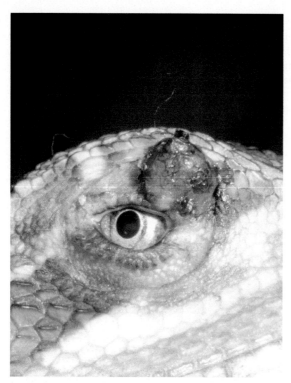

FIGURE 9-10 The right eye of a bearded dragon. A 1-cm ulcerated mass is present on the upper eyelid. Histopathology confirmed squamous cell carcinoma. Debulking and cryoablation were curative.

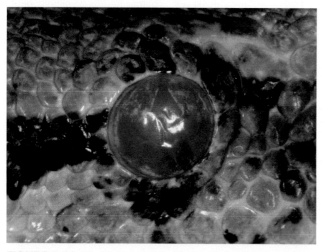

FIGURE 9-11 The right eye of a boa constrictor. A retained spectacle is present. Note the opaque, wrinkled appearance of the spectacle.

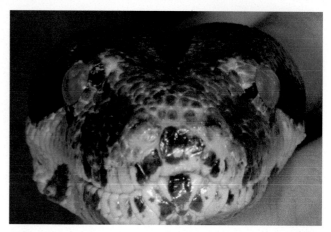

FIGURE 9-12 The same patient as in Figure 9-11. Note that retained spectacles are present bilaterally.

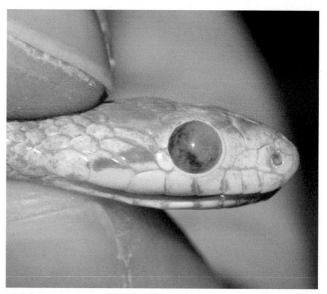

FIGURE 9-13 The right eye of a corn snake. A subspectacular abscess is present. Note the yellow-red exudate present in the subspectacular space.

Beneath the spectacle is the subspectacular space. It communicates with the oral cavity via the lacrimal duct. Purulent debris may accumulate in the subspectacular space, leading to a subspectacular abscess (Figure 9-13). Clinically, the eye appears opaque with yellow, tan, white, or reddish flocculent material filling the subspectacular space and precluding intraocular examination. Affected snakes are functionally blind with severe abscesses. Opacification of the subspectacular space may give the globe a falsely enlarged appearance, termed pseudobuphthalmos or hydrobuphthalmos.

Subspectacular abscesses are thought to result from one of three mechanisms. First, infection within the oral cavity may ascend through the lacrimal duct. Alternately, infection may hematogenously seed the subspectacular space. Finally, penetrating trauma to the spectacle may inoculate infectious organisms into the subspectacular space. In all cases of subspectacular abscessation, a thorough examination of the oral cavity and spectacle itself should be performed. Cytology, culture, or biopsy of any oral lesion is warranted.

As with abscesses in other sites, identification of the underlying cause and surgically establishing drainage are essential for resolution of subspectacular abscesses.[33,50] A partial spectaculectomy can be performed under general anesthesia to allow evacuation of the abscess material. To perform a partial

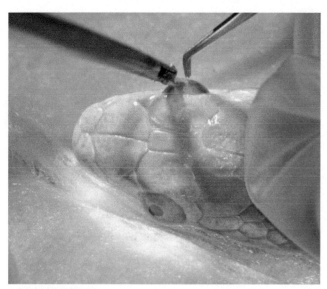

FIGURE 9-14 The same patient as in Figure 9-13. The snake is anesthetized and a pair of iris scissors is used to sharply incise the spectacle.

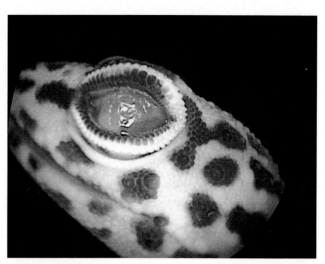

FIGURE 9-16 The left eye of a leopard gecko. A retained eye cap is present. Note the yellow-tan, dry cellular debris present in the palpebral fissure.

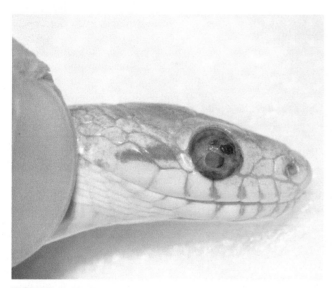

FIGURE 9-15 The postoperative appearance of the same patient as in Figures 9-13 and 9-14. Note the approximately 30-degree wedge resection of the ventral spectacle. The abscess material has been evacuated from the subspectacular space.

spectaculectomy one should use a sharp-tipped instrument to make a 30-degree, wedge-shaped incision in the ventral spectacular surface (Figures 9-14 and 9-15). If the abscess material is caseous, it may need to be gently removed from the subspectacular space using a small toothed forceps. Retrieved abscess fluid or inspissated debris should be submitted for bacterial and fungal culture. The subspectacular space can be gently lavaged using a 27- to 30-g cannula through which dilute povidone iodine solution is applied. Systemic treatment with antibiotic or anti-inflammatory drugs may be warranted if other organ systems are affected. Topical antibiotic ointments can be applied 3 to 4 times a day to keep the ocular

surface moist and treat infection. Eventually, the spectacle will epithelialize, closing the defect.

Obstruction of the lacrimal duct can also result in normal glandular secretions accumulating in the subspectacular space. This may also create the impression of an enlarged globe, or pseudobuphthalmos.[33] Unlike a subspectacular abscess, lacrimal duct obstruction typically results in translucent or mildly flocculent fluid accumulating in the subspectacular space. Oral examination is indicated. Treatment of oral cavity disease and restoration of normal lacrimal duct patency will often resolve the ocular signs. Nonsteroidal anti-inflammatory agents (meloxicam, 0.2 to 0.4 mg/kg, per os, once daily) may be used to help reduce the inflammation within the lacrimal duct. Establishment of an alternate drainage pathway via conjunctivorhinostomy has been reported.[51]

Retained Eye Caps in Geckos
While members of the subfamily Eublepharidae have true eyelids, most geckos have a spectacle similar to that of snakes. Spectacular disease is uncommon in geckos, but a unique syndrome termed retained eye caps is diagnosed in geckos with eyelids. Failure to shed the conjunctival lining underneath the eyelids results in the accumulation of cell debris in the palpebral fissure (Figure 9-16). Poor husbandry and nutrition are implicated in the disease pathogenesis. Retained eye caps are treated by careful removal with a small, toothed forceps. If presented late in the course of disease, animals can develop permanent visual impairment. Hand feeding blind geckos can be a successful method of managing these animals long term.

Ulcerative Keratitis
Ulcerative keratitis may occur in reptiles as in other species. Trauma, environmental toxins and irritants, pathogens, and exposure may contribute to the pathogenesis. Excessive exposure to UV light as part of an inappropriate lighting system may also contribute to corneal ulceration.[52] Application of fluorescein stain to the ocular surface is the definitive

diagnostic tool. Cytology of the ocular surface and culture/ sensitivity are indicated. Corneal ulcers should be treated with broad-spectrum antibiotics or based on culture and sensitivity results. Medication should be delivered 3 to 4 times per day to ensure the best treatment response.

Uveitis

Uveitis is infrequently reported in reptiles. It may be an ocular manifestation of systemic disease or the result of intraocular extension of corneal disease.[33,53,54] Uveitis can be associated with sepsis; however, intraocular infectious organisms may not be present. Clinical signs of uveitis often include corneal edema, aqueous flare, and hypopyon. Periocular swelling and blepharospasm are variable conditions associated with this disease. A complete physical examination is indicated in every reptilian patient that is presented with evidence of uveitis. Topical (flurbiprofen, 1 drop inthe affected eye, 3 to 4 times daily) and systemic anti-inflammatory medications (meloxicam, 0.2 to 0.4 mg/kg once daily) are warranted to treat uveitis diagnosed in reptile species.

Cataracts

As described above, cataract is defined as opacification of the lens resulting from disruption of normal lens fiber integrity and arrangement. The lens opacity causes impairment of vision by distorting light rays as they pass through the lens, with complete blindness resulting when the cataract occupies the entire lens. Cataract can be identified on clinical examination as a white opacity present within the pupil that obscures the view of the retina and are classified by size, location, shape, and etiology. Cataracts are becoming a more common finding in captive reptiles as husbandry methods improve and animals live longer. Reptiles that utilize olfaction to hunt (e.g., snakes) can thrive in captivity with cataracts. Successful cataract surgery has been reported in reptiles.[55-57] Cataract surgery is indicated for patients whose quality of life is impacted by vision loss resulting from cataract; however, the size of the eyes of small reptiles may preclude these patients from being good surgical candidates. Consultation with a board-certified ophthalmologist is recommended to determine the potential for surgical success with a particular case.

Glaucoma

There are no reports of glaucoma of reptiles, but normal intraocular pressure (IOP) ranges are available for several chelonian species (see Table 9-1).[58-62] Chelonian IOP is influenced by body position, so consistency should be used when performing serial tonometry measurements.[58] Ideally, the same tonometer and same method of restraint would be used at every examination to ensure the greatest level of measurement comparability. If glaucoma is suspected in a reptile case, standard treatments used for mammals are recommended (see Rabbits).

Birds

Eyelid Disease

Cryptophthalmos is the term for severe scarring of the eyelid such that the palpebral fissure is significantly narrowed (Figure 9-17). Only a few millimeters of cornea may be visible. Previously described in cockatiels, it can theoretically occur after blepharitis or trauma of the eyelids in any

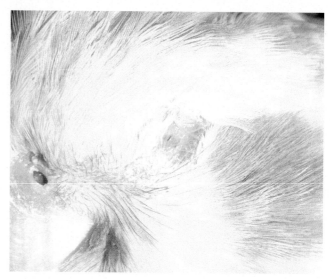

FIGURE 9-17 The left eye of a cockatiel. Cryptophthalmos is present. Note the severe narrowing of the palpebral fissure.

species.[63] Surgical correction often fails as the cicatrix recurs.[63] Affected birds may be visually impaired but do not appear uncomfortable.

Avian poxvirus is the most common infectious cause of blepharitis in birds. Affected birds may develop blepharoedema, proliferative blister-like eyelid lesions, or ulcerative eyelid lesions.[64] Conjunctivitis might be identified concurrently, and if the eyelid margin is involved, keratitis may be present. Self-trauma may exacerbate the blepharitis. Careful daily cleaning of the eyelids, prevention of self-trauma, and adequate nutrition help support recovery in these birds.

Knemidokoptes pilae is a mite that is frequently associated with foot and leg lesions; however, the periocular skin and eyelids can also be affected. The classic appearance is a proliferative, scaly tissue that appears near the base of the beak and extends toward the eyelids. Systemic ivermectin (0.2 mg/kg per os or intramuscularly) is recommended to successfully treat *Knemidokoptes pilae*.

Conjunctivitis

Conjunctivitis is a nonspecific clinical sign that results from a variety of etiologies. Clinical signs include conjunctival hyperemia, chemosis, ocular discharge that may range in character from serous to mucoid to mucopurulent, periocular alopecia, and periocular depigmentation. Trauma is a common cause of conjunctivitis in pet birds, including lacerations of the third eyelid and is often inflicted by cage mates.[65] Primary repair of such defects is recommended.[66] Absorbable 6-0 to 8-0 suture is necessary to close the palpebral conjunctival surface only; full-thickness sutures should not be placed as they may result in corneal ulceration. The third eyelid should be carefully inspected for evidence of any foreign material implanted at the time of trauma. Foreign material, including feedstuffs, may also be a cause of conjunctivitis in birds.[67] Well-meaning handlers may inadvertently contaminate the ocular surface with slurries or liquid food formulations. Conjunctival foreign bodies may require use of magnification to identify the offensive material.

Parasites are a frequent cause of avian conjunctivitis.[67] *Oxyspirura* spp. nematodes can be identified on the bulbar conjunctival surface with the aid of magnification. *Philophthalmus gralli* and *Thelazia* sp. may be identified in the conjunctival fornix. Conjunctivitis associated with *Cryptosporidium* spp. is typically associated with sinusitis and rhinitis. Toxoplasmosis has been associated with conjunctivitis and endophthalmitis. Treatment of conjunctival parasites includes removal of visible parasites and topical or systemic administration of avermectin dewormers.

Bacterial conjunctivitis is common in birds.[67] Upper respiratory tract disease may accompany ocular disease. Since normal ocular flora can vary significantly between avian species interpretation of culture results requires knowledge of the normal bacterial population for the bird being examined. The most common ocular pathogens include *Citrobacter* spp., *Escherichia coli*, *Klebsiella* spp., *Pseudomonas* spp., and *Staphylococcus* spp.[67] Cytology of the conjunctiva may be useful in guiding antibiotic selection; however, culture and sensitivity are recommended in all cases. When gram-positive bacteria are identified on the initial cytologic evaluation, a triple-antibiotic solution is an excellent treatment choice; gram-negative bacteria would be more effectively treated with a topical fluoroquinolone or aminoglycoside. If respiratory signs are noted, concurrent administration of systemic antibiotics is indicated.

Chlamydia psittaci does cause conjunctivitis, especially in cockatiels. Due to the zoonotic potential of the disease, *Chalmydia psittaci* should be considered a differential disease diagnosis in cases of avian conjunctivitis. The role of *Mycoplasma* spp. as a primary pathogen in avian conjunctivitis is somewhat controversial; previously believed to be a secondary pathogen, *Mycoplasma* spp. is now considered a primary cause of ocular disease in birds.[68] Concurrent respiratory disease is common. Mycoplasmosis is difficult to definitively diagnose as the fastidious organism is challenging to culture. House finches are thought to be particularly susceptible to *Mycoplasma* spp. (Figures 9-18 and 9-19).[69–71] If concurrent respiratory signs are detected, systemic treatment is warranted along with topical fluoroquinolone or tetracycline ophthalmic formulations.[72]

While fungal organisms may be part of the normal avian conjunctival flora, they may also act as opportunistic pathogens.[67] Fungal conjunctivitis may also involve the cornea (termed keratoconjunctivitis) and/or the paranasal sinuses. Newer triazole antifungals such as voriconazole 1% have been used in cases of equine mycotic keratoconjunctivitis.[73] Systemic administration of voriconazole has been reported to be a safe treatment in several avian species; thus, topical administration of voriconazole may be appropriate for susceptible filamentous fungi associated with conjunctivitis in birds.[74,75]

Conjunctivitis has been described in peach-faced lovebirds (*Agapornis roseicollis*), mynah birds (*Acridotheres tristis*), and cockatiels (*Nymphicus hollandicus*); however, it should be assumed that all species of Psittaciformes are susceptible to developing conjunctivitis.[67] Further investigation into these clinical cases is needed to define disease etiopathogenesis and more consistently design effective treatment strategies.

Environmental irritants, including elevated ammonia and particulate matter, may increase susceptibility to infectious conjunctivitis.[76] Ensuring that the patient lives in a clean environment is essential for disease resolution in such cases.

Corneal Disease
Corneal ulceration in birds most often results from traumatic injury to the eye and is treated similarly to other species (see discussion of corneal ulceration in Corneal Disease, under Rabbits), below) (Figure 9-20). Careful examination of the environment should be performed to eliminate any potential

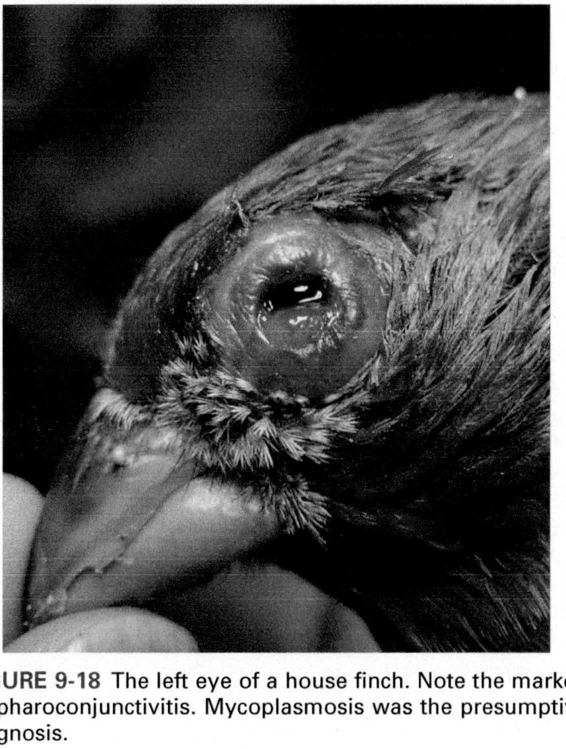

FIGURE 9-18 The left eye of a house finch. Note the marked blepharoconjunctivitis. Mycoplasmosis was the presumptive diagnosis.

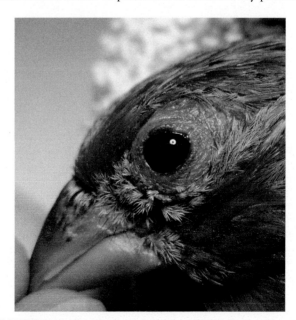

FIGURE 9-19 The same patient as in Figure 9-18. Note the complete resolution of blepharoconjunctivitis posttreatment.

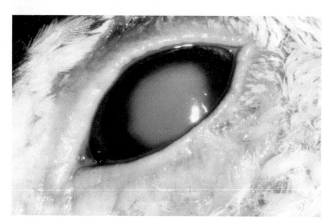

FIGURE 9-20 The left eye of a wood duck. Note the fluorescein-positive, superficial corneal ulcer.

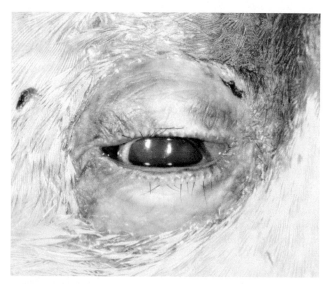

FIGURE 9-21 The right eye of a Pionus parrot. Note the severe periocular swelling and bruising, chemosis, and conjunctival hyperemia. Trauma was suspected as the underlying etiology.

sources of injury. Cage mates are a possible source of trauma, and if appropriate, flock dynamics should be carefully considered (Figure 9-21).

Uveal/Retinal Disease

Uveitis may be a consequence of trauma or ocular manifestation of systemic disease in birds. Clinical signs of uveitis include blepharospasm, corneal edema, and aqueous flare in acute presentations, and iridal hyperpigmentation, posterior synechiae, and cataract in chronic cases. Trauma is a well-recognized cause of intraocular inflammation, hyphema, vitreal hemorrhage, and retinal detachment in raptors; the effects of trauma are less frequently documented in pet birds.[77] Systemic sepsis has been reported as a cause of uveitis in a lovebird.[78] A complete physical exam should be performed in all birds with uveitis. Administration of systemic anti-inflammatory medication (meloxicam, 0.2 to 1.0 mg/kg, once to twice daily; safety levels may vary among species, and signs of side effects [e.g., anorexia, gastric ulcers, melena, and renal

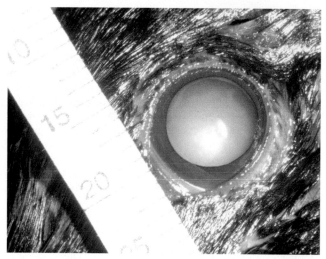

FIGURE 9-22 The left eye of a mallard duck. A mature cataract is present.

disease] should be monitored) is essential for the treatment of uveitis. When topical anti-inflammatory agents are administered concurrently, consideration should be given to the total daily dose that small patients are receiving.

Cataract

As with other species there are a number of underlying etiologic disease causes for cataract formation in birds. Cataract is defined as opacification of the lens resulting from disruption of normal lens fiber integrity and arrangement. The lens opacity causes impairment of vision by distorting light rays as they pass through the lens, with complete blindness resulting when the cataract occupies the entire lens. Cataract can be identified on clinical examination as a white opacity present within the pupil that obscures the view of the retina and classified by size, location, shape, and etiology. Cataract surgery has been reported in wild but not pet birds (Figure 9-22).[79-81] Phacoemulsification is the technique of choice for removal of cataractous lens material; however, the minimum incision size of 3.2 mm renders the technique difficult or impossible to perform in very small eyes. Surgery may still be possible via alternate techniques, including irrigation/desiccation or extracapsular lens extraction.[82-84]

Mammals

Rabbits

EYELID DISEASE. Blepharitis is commonly identified in domesticated rabbits[85] and can be a primary disease condition associated with an infectious process or secondary to nasolacrimal duct obstruction. Clinical signs of blepharitis include edema and erythema of the eyelid skin, often associated with serous or mucoid ocular discharge. Rabbit syphilis caused by *Treponema paraluiscuniculi* is associated with ulcerative blepharitis and mucopurulent ocular discharge.[86] Affected rabbits may show ulceration of the mucocutaneous junctions of the urogenital, nasal, and perioral skin. Diagnosis may include serology in conjunction with dark-field microscopy of scrapings from affected lesions.[86] Recommended treatment includes parenteral penicillin, 42,000 IU/kg, subcutaneously, every 7

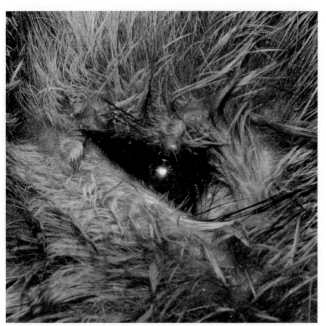

FIGURE 9-23 The right eye of a house rabbit. Blepharitis and entropion of the upper and lower eyelids are present.

days for 2 to 6 weeks.[87] All affected rabbits and those in contact with affected rabbits should be treated.

Several viruses can be associated with mass lesions on the eyelids of rabbits, including myxoma virus, shope fibroma virus, shope papillomavirus, and poxvirus. Myxoma virus and shope fibroma virus are associated with firm, discrete nodules within the eyelid skin, whereas shope papillomavirus typically produces proliferative warty lesions of the eyelid skin.[88,89] Poxvirus lesions are typically macules and papules with crusts and occasionally ulceration.[90] Myxomatosis is typically associated with ocular discharge and severe systemic disease, including pyrexia, anorexia, and lethargy. Treatment for all viral lesions is supportive, although the prognosis for myxomatosis may be very poor in some rabbit breeds.

Entropion is a condition caused by malpositioning of the eyelids such that the haired eyelid skin contacts the corneal surface, resulting in ocular surface irritation and keratitis. Entropion may be congenital or secondary to chronic blepharitis (Figure 9-23). It is important to differentiate primary anatomic entropion from secondary spastic entropion. If application of a topical anesthetic solution eliminates the patient's blepharospasm and entropion, then the entropion is spastic. If the entropion persists despite topical anesthesia, then the entropion is anatomic. Treatment of secondary entropion includes addressing the primary ocular surface disease (usually a corneal ulceration) and may involve temporary surgical tacking of the eyelids in an everted position in order to relieve the mechanical abrasion of the cornea by the eyelids. Permanent surgical corrections should not be performed in cases of secondary (spastic) entropion, as resolution of the painful ocular surface disease is expected to resolve the eyelid malposition. Primary anatomic entropion does require surgical correction.[91] Procedures commonly utilized in canine patients are also appropriate for rabbits.[92]

NASOLACRIMAL DISEASE. The function of the nasolacrimal duct is to drain tears from the ocular surface. The length of the rabbit nasolacrimal duct is particularly tortuous from the single inferior ocular puncta to the nasal cavity, with several abrupt changes in diameter, a small nasal opening, and robust epithelium that leave it predisposed to obstruction.[93,94] Of note is its proximity to the roots of the molar and incisor teeth, locations in which the duct also makes dramatic changes in direction.[93,94] The duct may be obstructed extraluminally by impingement of nearby structures (proliferative bone) or intraluminally by inflammatory debris. Dental disease has been described as the most common cause of nasolacrimal duct obstruction in rabbits, although rhinitis has also been implicated.[95] Primary bacterial infection is the second most common cause, with *Pasteurella multocida* and *Staphylococcus aureus* reported as pathogens. While other organisms have been cultured from ocular or nasal exudates, their role as primary pathogens is unclear. Clinical signs of nasolacrimal duct obstruction include ocular discharge that can range in character from serous to creamy white to yellow and caseous. Secondary disease conditions such as blepharitis and periocular dermatitis, including alopecia, erythema, and excoriations, may occur while corneal ulceration can develop due to self-trauma.

The diagnostic workup for a rabbit with ocular discharge begins with a complete ophthalmic examination (including Schirmer tear test, tonometry, and fluorescein staining) to rule out other causes of blepharoconjunctivitis or tear hypersecretion, followed by a complete physical and oral examination. Sedation or anesthesia may be required for a thorough dental examination. Prior to the instillation of any topical solution, a culture of the ocular discharge should be obtained. The inferiorly positioned ocular puncta can be cannulated using a 23- to 27-g intravenous catheter or metal lavage catheter, after administering a topical anesthetic agent and sterile saline lavaged through the nasolacrimal duct. Adding fluorescein sodium to the lavage solution may aid in visualization of the fluid at the nares. Following successful lavage, treatment with a topical antibiotic-corticosteroid solution every 12 hours for 7 to 14 days is recommended. Culture results will guide modification of antibiotic therapy if necessary.

Resistance to lavage pressure is consistent with nasolacrimal duct obstruction. Therapy using topical and systemic antibiotic and anti-inflammatory agents (e.g., meloxicam, 1 mg/kg, per os, once daily) is recommended. Lavage attempts can be repeated after a course of medical therapy. Imaging of the nasolacrimal duct, indicated when obstruction is persistent, has traditionally consisted of skull radiographs with the intraluminal administration of radiopaque agents to delineate the nasolacrimal duct.[94] Advanced imaging techniques for the rabbit skull have been reported, including the use of computed tomography (CT) for rabbits with dental disease.[96-99] Identifying and addressing the underlying cause of nasolacrimal duct obstruction is imperative to disease resolution.

CONJUNCTIVAL DISEASE. Given the intimate anatomical association of the conjunctiva, nasolacrimal system, and eyelids, conjunctivitis may be associated with nasolacrimal duct obstruction, dacryocystitis, or blepharitis. Clinical signs can mimic those of nasolacrimal disease and include blepharospasm, serous to mucoid to mucopurulent ocular discharge, conjunctival hyperemia, chemosis, and blepharitis. Periocular

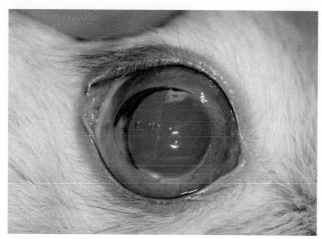

FIGURE 9-24 The right eye of a dwarf rabbit. Conjunctival overgrowth is present. Note the conjunctiva circumferentially encroaching onto the corneal surface.

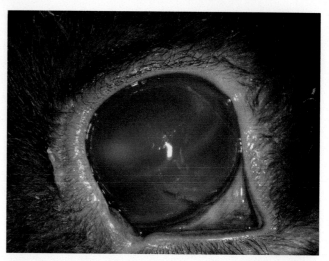

FIGURE 9-25 The left eye of a dwarf rabbit. A deep laceration is present in the ventral cornea. Diffuse corneal edema, a superficial axial corneal ulcer, and hypopyon are also present. Trauma was suspected as the underlying cause.

dermatitis can develop with chronic ocular discharge. Diagnosis of conjunctivitis is based on clinical examination and ruling out nasolacrimal duct obstruction and other ocular conditions (e.g., corneal ulceration, uveitis, glaucoma). Culture of the affected conjunctiva should be interpreted with knowledge of normal rabbit conjunctival flora (see Table 9-1). *Staphylococcus* spp. may be associated with multicentric disease or localized conjunctivitis.[100-102] Use of autogenous vaccine has been reported.[103] Conjunctivitis may also be associated with environmental irritants such as dust/particulate matter, overhead hay racks, and high ammonia levels.[104] Removal of the environmental irritant should result in resolution of conjunctivitis.

Conjunctival overgrowth is most frequently reported in dwarf rabbits, although other rabbit breeds may be affected.[105-108] Other names for the disease include epicorneal membrane, pseudopterygium, circumferential conjunctival hyperplasia, conjunctival centripetalization, or aberrant conjunctival stricture. Clinically, the lesion appears as a conjunctival membrane overlying, but not adhered to, the cornea extending from the limbus toward the axial (central) cornea 360 degrees around the ocular surface (Figure 9-24). The underlying cornea is normal, and intraocular abnormalities are not associated with the condition. Vision loss can occur as the opaque conjunctiva progresses toward the center of the visual axis. Once thought to be a model of pterygium formation in humans, the two diseases have been shown to have limited similarities.[107] Collagen dysplasia is the major histologic feature of conjunctival overgrowth. Etiopathogenesis remains unknown for conjunctival overgrowth in rabbits.

Medical therapy of conjunctival overgrowth is not recommended as a monotherapy.[109] While the aberrant conjunctival membrane can be excised, rapid recurrence of the lesion can be expected.[109] Successful treatment of conjunctival overgrowth has been reported when surgical excision is followed by topical corticosteroid and cyclosporine A therapy; the highest published success rates are associated with incising and suturing the conjunctiva into the fornix.[107,109] This technique involves incising the conjunctival membrane from its axial margin toward the limbus in four to six locations

and then suturing the axial margin into the adjacent fornix with 6-0 or 7-0 nonabsorbable suture.[109] The sutures are passed through the skin such that the knots lie on the skin surface. Postoperatively, the rabbit is treated with a broad-spectrum antibiotic-corticosteroid ophthalmic preparation (e.g., neomycin-polymyxin-gramicidin-dexamethasone) every 12 hours for 3 weeks. Sutures may be removed after 3 weeks.

CORNEAL DISEASE. Corneal ulceration is the most common disease of the rabbit cornea.[110] A corneal abrasion is any corneal wound that does not completely remove the epithelium, whereas ulceration results in complete loss of the epithelium. Corneal ulcers can be divided into two major categories: superficial (resulting from loss of epithelium only) and deep (loss of epithelium and stroma). A descemetocele is a deep ulcer resulting from loss of all the corneal stroma with exposure of Descemet membrane. Clinical signs of corneal ulceration include blepharospasm, epiphora, conjunctival hyperemia, corneal opacity, visible defect in the corneal surface, and corneal vascularization. Anterior uveitis (miosis, aqueous flare, iris hyperemia) may be present secondarily. Diagnosis of a corneal ulcer requires the application of water-soluble sodium fluorescein solution to the ocular surface, followed by gentle rinsing with a saline eyewash solution. Where the hydrophobic corneal epithelium is missing, leaving the hydrophilic stroma exposed, fluorescein dye will bind with characteristic yellow-green fluorescence. A cobalt-blue filtered light source can be used to enhance this fluorescence.

The cause of corneal ulceration is frequently unknown, but trauma is suspected to be the most common cause (Figure 9-25).[110] Trauma should be considered a diagnosis of exclusion. Other important differential diagnoses of corneal ulceration include trichiasis (face hairs touching the cornea), entropion, chronic blepharitis, eyelid masses (such as those caused by myxoma virus or poxvirus), chronic dacryocystitis, embedded foreign body, and keratoconjunctivitis sicca (KCS). Several diseases may lead to exposure of the ocular surface and cause corneal ulceration, including facial nerve paralysis, which impairs the ability to blink; chronic glaucoma leading to buphthalmos; and exophthalmos associated with orbital disease (including orbital abscesses). A careful ocular and systemic examination can rule out many of these causes, leaving a presumptive diagnosis of trauma.

Application of fluorescein to the cornea should be performed in all cases to confirm the diagnosis of corneal ulceration. Cytology and culture/sensitivity of the ulcer bed should be performed in all cases where the ulcer is deep, any white or yellow corneal stromal infiltrate or corneal malacia is present, and in all cases of nonhealing ulcers. Two slides should be prepared for cytologic examination: one to be stained to examine cellular morphology and one for Gram staining to examine microorganism morphology. Lack of visible microorganisms on cytology does not rule out infection, particularly in deep corneal ulcers and those with visible cellular infiltrate.

Treatment of corneal ulcers is based on their clinical appearance and the presence of any complicating factors. If an underlying cause for the ulcer can be identified (e.g., a buphthalmic, glaucomatous globe leading to exposure keratitis), that cause must be addressed as part of therapy for the ulcer. Failure to recognize complicating factors may lead to a prolonged course of healing, or worse, corneal perforation and loss of the globe. Trichiasis can be managed by careful trimming of facial hairs. Entropion may require surgical correction (if primary anatomic entropion) or temporary eversion of the eyelids (if secondary spastic entropion). Blepharitis or eyelid masses may need to be treated with systemic antibiotic and anti-inflammatory agents and the cornea treated with a lubricating gel or ointment to provide additional protection of the cornea from mechanical abrasion by the eyelids. Treatment of dacryocystitis is discussed in the preceding section. The conjunctiva, particularly the bulbar surface of the third eyelid, should be carefully examined with magnification for any foreign material. A Schirmer tear test can be performed to rule out KCS (see Table 9-1). A palpebral reflex, performed by gently touching the medial and then lateral canthus (cranial nerve V) and observing a brisk blinking response (cranial nerve VII) should be performed in all patients to ensure adequate protection of the cornea by the eyelids (see Chapter 8 for more information on causes and treatment of facial nerve paralysis).

Tonometry should be performed in all painful eyes with corneal ulcers where corneal perforation is not imminent and elevated IOP confirms the diagnosis of glaucoma (see Table 9-1). The clinician should be mindful that a buphthalmic, chronically glaucomatous globe may have a normal IOP and that other clinical signs of glaucoma should be observed to confirm the diagnosis (see Glaucoma below). The underlying cause of any exophthalmos needs to be addressed to correct exposure associated with an exophthalmic globe (see Orbital Disease below).

The goals of treating a simple ulcer with no underlying cause are twofold: preventing infection and controlling pain. A broad-spectrum antibiotic solution should be administered into the affected eye every 8 hours. The ideal antibiotic would be broad spectrum and bactericidal and have minimal epithelial toxicity. Triple antibiotic solution (neomycin-polymyxin-gramicidin) is ideal. Use of an aminoglycoside solution (gentamicin, tobramycin) as a monotherapy should be avoided

since this class of drug has minimal gram-positive coverage, but could be combined with another drug class such as a cephalosporin. Cefazolin 5% solution can be easily compounded in the clinic for ophthalmic use using commercially available intravenous preparations. Solutions are preferable to ointments as they cause less matting of the periocular hair and less grooming behavior, leading to ingestion of ointment. Pain control can be achieved in some cases with 1% topical atropine solution, which provides cycloplegia and relief from painful ciliary body spasm. Some rabbits have atropinase in their iris, which rapidly degrades atropine, negating its effects. Atropinase levels can vary with gender and season, but given its low cost and minimal toxicity, atropine is useful in most patients, although response to therapy may be variable.[111] Other treatment strategies for providing analgesia include the administration of topical preservative-free 0.5% to 1% morphine every 8 to 12 hours, administration of systemic nonsteroidal anti-inflammatory agents (e.g., 0.2 to 1.0 mg/kg, per os, every 24 hours), and bandage contact lens placement.[112–114] Complete resolution should be expected in 3 to 7 days.

Treatment of deep ulcers, infected ulcers, or ulcers with keratomalacia requires more aggressive therapy than that for a simple, superficial ulcer (Figure 9-26). The goal of treating a deep/infected/melting ulcer is elimination of infectious organisms, inhibition of proteolytic/collagenolytic enzymes that contribute to malacia, and support for the prolonged wound healing process. Ulcers with stromal loss may heal by epithelialization alone, leaving a thin area of cornea known as a facet, which is inherently weaker than normal-thickness cornea. Corneal ulcers with stromal loss should be allowed to vascularize, as blood vessels provide support for the tissue remodeling process. Any ulcer with >50% stromal loss is a

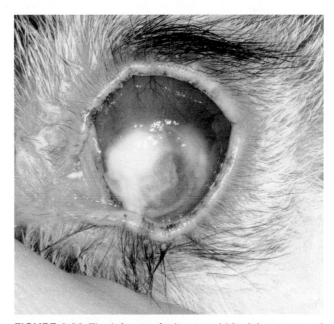

FIGURE 9-26 The left eye of a house rabbit. A large corneal ulcer with dense, white stromal infiltrate and malacia is present in the central cornea. Corneal vascularization has extended to the margin of the lesion. *Pseudomonas* was cultured from the ulcer bed.

candidate for surgical stabilization. Referral to a board-certified veterinary ophthalmologist is strongly recommended in cases where severe corneal ulceration has been diagnosed.

Corneal cytology and culture/sensitivity are very useful for guiding treatment decisions in cases of deep/infected/melting ulcers. In the absence of visible microorganisms on cytological evaluation and prior to receiving culture results, starting treatment with a fluoroquinolone antibiotic solution (ciprofloxacin 0.3%, ofloxacin 0.3%, levofloxacin 0.5%, or moxifloxacin 0.5%) every 2 to 4 hours is indicated. Fluoroquinolones have the advantage of being highly potent, bactericidal, and broad spectrum. Keratomalacia can be treated with autologous serum every 2 to 4 hours, which can be prepared by harvesting whole blood from the patient, placed into a sterile collection tube, and centrifuged to separate the serum. Harvested serum should be stored in a sterile, refrigerated container (a syringe is ideal, although the needle should be removed for administration of a single drop to the ocular surface). Other agents that can be used to inhibit proteolytic/collagenolytic enzymes include EDTA 1% solution and topical tetracycline ointment. Secondary uveitis which is frequently diagnosed in cases of deep/infected/melting ulcers should be treated with topical atropine 1% solution every 12 hours and systemic nonsteroidal anti-inflammatory medication. A recheck examination is recommended within 24 to 48 hours of initiating therapy to ensure that healing is progressing as planned. With resolution of cellular stromal infiltrate and/or malacia, the frequency of therapy can be decreased. Topical antibiotic agents should be continued until all cellular infiltrate has resolved and the cornea is fluorescein negative. Corneal perforation, should it occur, is an indication for enucleation.

Indolent (nonhealing) corneal ulcers in rabbits can be frustrating to treat and may take weeks to resolve. The hallmark of an indolent ulcer is a superficial corneal ulcer that has nonadherent epithelial flaps at its margins. Signs of ocular pain are quite variable in these cases, with some rabbits showing minimal ocular discomfort and others extreme blepharospasm. Corneal vascularization may also be quite variable, with more chronic cases developing increased vascularization. Corneal cytology is recommended to rule out infection prior to treatment. Debridement with a dry cotton-tipped applicator, grid keratotomy, and multiple punctate keratotomy are possible interventions.[110] When intervention is necessary, the author's practice has experienced the most success through the application of cyanoacrylate glue to the corneal surface (Figure 9-27).[115] After carefully drying the ocular surface with cotton-tipped applicators, a small amount of cyanoacrylate glue is applied to the center of the ulcer and gently brushed with a 25-g needle tip to cover the corneal surface. The lids should be firmly restrained until the glue has completely dried. Positioning the cornea horizontally during the application process facilitates accurate glue placement. Topical antibiotic therapy should be continued after glue application. The glue will gradually slough over 1 to 4 weeks. Glue application can be repeated if necessary.

LENS DISEASE. Cataract is any opacity of the lens and can be classified by their size, shape, location within the lens, etiology, and age of the patient at onset. Cataract is a common ocular abnormality in laboratory rabbits where a genetic predisposition is suspected, and the frequency may be

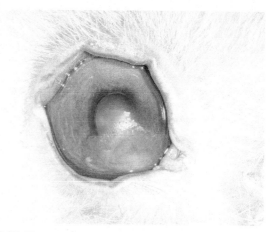

FIGURE 9-27 The right eye of a dwarf rabbit. Cyanoacrylate tissue glue has been applied to the ulcer bed and is visible as a refractile opacity overlying the ulcerated cornea. An immature cataract is also present.

underreported in pet rabbits.[85,116,117] Regardless of cause, once a cataract progresses to causing significant visual impairment, surgical intervention is the only way to restore vision to the patient. Phacoemulsification for the surgical removal of spontaneous cataracts has been reported in pet rabbits.[118] Cataracts can be associated with significant lens-induced uveitis, and treatment with a topical nonsteroidal anti-inflammatory solution (e.g., diclofenac 0.1% solution, flurbiprofen 0.03% solution) is recommended to prevent the onset of secondary glaucoma. Prompt referral to a board-certified veterinary ophthalmologist is recommended for evaluation when owners are interested in pursuing cataract surgery.

Encephalitozoon cuniculi is a microsporidial fungal parasite associated with neurologic, ocular, and renal disease of rabbits. Young dwarf rabbits are more frequently affected than other breeds of rabbit, but no sex predilection has been identified.[119] The ocular clinical signs of *E. cuniculi* include tan to yellow to white masses in the iris associated with rubiosis iridis, aqueous flare, ocular hypotension, keratitic precipitates, focal or diffuse cataract, lens capsule rupture, blepharospasm, serous ocular discharge, and secondary glaucoma (Figures 9-28 and 9-29). The iris masses represent a focal pyogranulomatous response to a ruptured lens capsule adjacent to an area of cataractous lens containing parasite spores. The inflammation associated with spontaneous rupture of the lens capsule is termed phacoclastic uveitis.[120]

Evaluation of a rabbit with suspected ocular *E. cuniculi* should include a complete physical examination and neurologic examination.[119] *E. cuniculi* is an important differential diagnosis for cataract in any dwarf rabbit, but the classic signs of white masses in the anterior chamber associated with cataract in any breed of rabbit should prompt investigation for *E. cuniculi*. The combination of an enzyme-linked immunosorbent assay (ELISA) and protein electrophoresis of patient serum has recently been demonstrated to be more sensitive and specific for confirming the diagnosis of *E. cuniculi* infection; however, identification of microsporidial spores in tissue remains the gold standard for diagnosis.[121,122] Polymerase chain reaction (PCR) testing of fluid obtained during the

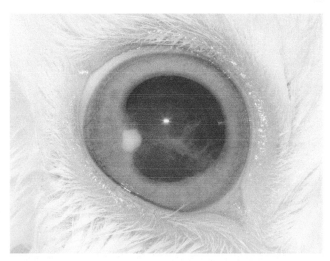

FIGURE 9-28 The right eye of a dwarf rabbit with *E. cuniculi.* Note the focal white granuloma in the iris/lens, iritis, and immature cataract.

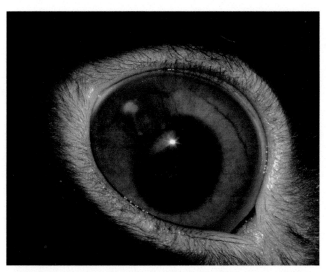

FIGURE 9-29 The right eye of a dwarf rabbit with *E. cuniculi.* Note the focal tan/white granuloma in the iris and lens that is also visible in the pupillary aperture and the severe iritis.

course of phacoemulsification can be examined directly for evidence of *E. cuniculi* organisms or submitted for PCR.[123,124]

Treatment of rabbits with *E. cuniculi* ocular lesions varies with the severity of the lesion. In cases of focal cataract without lens capsule rupture or uveitis, topical nonsteroidal anti-inflammatory drugs such as flurbiprofen 0.03% or diclofenac 0.1% solution every 12 to 24 hours are recommended. Once lens capsule rupture occurs, phacoemulsification to remove the lens material is the treatment of choice.[123] If phacoemulsification is not an option, medical therapy including topical corticosteroids (prednisolone acetate 1% suspension) every 8 to 24 hours should be initiated until any active uveitis is controlled. The rabbit may then be maintained on topical nonsteroidal anti-inflammatory agents. The development of secondary glaucoma may occur, and enucleation is advised in all cases of secondary glaucoma or cases of refrac-

tory phacoclastic uveitis. Additional therapy includes fenbendazole, 20 mg/kg, per os, every 24 hours for 28 days.[119]

GLAUCOMA. Although rabbits are an important laboratory model for glaucoma in humans and the disease been extensively studied as part of the development of new therapies, little information is available regarding the treatment of glaucoma in pet rabbits. Tonometry is essential for the diagnosis of glaucoma. Use of both applanation and rebound tonometry has been reported in the rabbit, with a range of normal IOP values of 15 to 23 mmHg and a mean of 18 mmHg. New Zealand white rabbits are affected by a hereditary form of glaucoma that results in buphthalmos at <6 months of age, and it is this form of glaucoma that most information regarding this disease in rabbits is available.[125,126] Medical therapy has not been reported to be successful New Zealand white rabbits diagnosed with glaucoma. While no epidemiological studies of glaucoma in pet rabbits are available, the most likely cause of increased IOP in rabbits is secondary to chronic intraocular inflammation. Rabbits with phacoclastic uveitis associated with *E. cuniculi* are particularly susceptible to developing glaucoma. Treatment of secondary glaucoma can be very frustrating and unrewarding for the patient and veterinarian. Recommended therapies include topical carbonic anhydrase inhibitors such as dorzolamide 2% or brinzolamide 1% solution every 8 to 12 hours or the beta blocker timolol 0.5% solution every 8 to 12 hours.[127] Caution must be used with the ocular administration of beta-blockers in small patients, careful monitoring for cardiorespiratory side effects such as bradycardia or bronchospasm. Additional therapies include the topical prostaglandin analogs lantanoprost 0.005% solution or travaprost 0.004% solution every 12 to 24 hours.[128]

ORBITAL DISEASE. The rabbit orbit is a frequent site of disease. Orbital diseases generally cause cranial displacement of the globe in the orbit, known as exophthalmos. Exophthalmos must be differentiated from buphthalmos, an enlargement of the globe. Exophthalmic globes will have a normal horizontal corneal diameter, whereas the horizontal corneal diameter of a buphthalmic globe will be increased. Measuring both globes for comparison is useful. Infrequent signs of orbital disease in rabbits include elevation of the third eyelid, strabismus, and enophthalmos.

Exophthalmos may be bilateral or unilateral. Bilateral exophthalmos can be iatrogenic from overzealous restraint, with subsequent engorgement of the large retrobulbar venous plexus, but is expected to resolve when restraint is discontinued. Space-occupying neoplasms of the thorax and mediastinum may also lead to inconsistent presentations of bilateral exophthalmos, with thymoma being most commonly reported.[129,130] While systemic treatment is being pursued, it is important to protect the corneas from exposure keratitis resulting from the exophthalmos with frequent (every 4 to 6 hours) application of artificial tears gel or ointment.

Unilateral exophthalmos is associated most often with orbital abscesses and dental disease has been implicated as the primary underlying cause. Other infrequent causes of unilateral exophthalmos include orbital neoplasia, parasitic cysts, vascular malformations, myositis, hematoma, mucocele, granuloma, or other infectious diseases. Treatment of orbital abscesses has been reported, but the prognosis is generally considered poor without aggressive treatment.[131] Bacteria commonly cultured from dental-associated abscesses include *Fusobacterium* spp., *Prevotella* spp., *Peptostreptococcus* spp., *Streptococcus* spp., *Actinomyces* spp., and *Arcanobacterium* spp.[132] Antibiotic therapy alone is unsuccessful in resolving orbital abscesses, therefore surgical drainage is required, including complete removal of the abscess capsule. Direct surgical access to the orbit via a lateral approach and endoscopic approaches have been reported.[133–135] Instillation of antibiotic agents directly into the orbit may be useful after all abscess material has been removed.[133] Alternately, enucleation with debridement of the orbit can be performed. When enucleating the rabbit globe, great care must be taken to avoid penetrating the venous plexus posterior to the globe, which can result in life-threatening hemorrhage.[136] Profound hemorrhage also occurs when excising the third eyelid, consequently beginning closure of the periocular skin prior to removing the third eyelid and its associated glands may be prudent and aid in hemostasis.[136]

Ferrets

CONJUNCTIVAL DISEASE. Conjunctivitis in ferrets is most often an ocular manifestation of systemic disease. Ferrets are highly susceptible to canine distemper virus (CDV), and the initial signs of disease may be ocular.[137] Intially chemosis, conjunctival hyperemia, and a mucopurulent ocular discharge develop, with the discharge accumulating and crusting the eyelids shut. Secondary blepharitis, corneal ulceration, and KCS may subsequently develop during the disease process. Treatment is only supportive and based on clinical disease signs, as CDV disease is highly fatal, with the canine strain of virus having a shorter survival time than the ferret strain. Vaccination of all ferrets for CDV is highly recommended. A recent report suggests that vitamin A supplementation of 30 mg per os daily is useful in reducing the severity of clinical signs of CDV when supplementation begins at time of exposure. Ferrets are susceptible to infection with human influenza virus, which also produces conjunctivitis and serous ocular discharge.[138] Conversely, no ocular signs are observed with experimental infection with avian influenza.[139]

Mycobacterium genavense has been reported as a cause of conjunctivitis in two ferrets.[140] Both ferrets were suspected to have disseminated disease, but the initial presenting complaint was profound conjunctival swelling involving the third eyelids (unilateral in one case and bilateral in the second case). Treatment was considered successful, although one ferret died 4 months post treatment of renal disease and the second ferret died 10 months post treatment of a suspected ovarian neoplasm. The relationship between *M. genavense* and death is unknown in these cases. Treatment consisted of rifampin 30 mg per os every 24 hours, clofazimine 12.5 mg per os every 24 hours, and clarithromycin 31.25 mg per os every 24 hours for 3 months in the case that died 4 months post treatment and rifampin 14 mg per os every 24 hours for 4 weeks in the case that died 10 months post treatment.

CATARACT. Hereditary cataracts have been reported in laboratory ferrets, and presumably, the prevalence in the pet ferret population is underreported.[141] Congenital vascular remnants associated with the tunica vasculosis lentis and hyaloid artery systems, which are essential for the embryologic development of the lens but regress in order to maintain lens transparency, have also been reported in association with

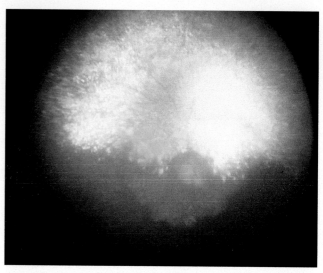

FIGURE 9-30 The fundus of a ferret with retinal degeneration. Note the severe, diffuse tapetal hyperreflectivity and marked vascular attenuation.

cataract in ferrets.[142] There are no published articles in the peer-reviewed literature that describe cataract surgery to restore vision in ferrets.

RETINAL DEGENERATION. Retinal degeneration is purportedly a common disease of ferrets according to one author; however, others have noted that the funduscopic appearance of the ferret retina can be quite variable, making a diagnosis of retinal degeneration more challenging to confirm (Figure 9-30).[143,144] Electrophysiologic studies of retinal degeneration in ferrets have not been performed nor has heritability been confirmed.

Mice/Rats

Ocular disorders are infrequently reported in pet rats and mice.[145] While some ocular diseases are well documented in laboratory rodents, they may not be commonly diagnosed in pet rodents.[146]

CHROMODACRYORRHEA. The rodent harderian gland secretes porphyrin that is incorporated into the tear film. Parasympathetic innervation controls porphyrin secretion; thus, any event associated with increased parasympathetic stimulation can also be associated with excessive release of porphyrin-laden tears.[147] The staining of periocular skin with these porphyrin-laden tears is termed chromodacryorrhea. Porphyrins have a characteristic red-brown appearance, which can easily be confused with blood. Porphyrins have a unique fluorescence under UV light, providing the practitioner with an easy method to differentiate porphyrin from blood.[148] When chromodacryorrhea is identified, the patient should be carefully examined for any evidence of systemic disease or chronic stress.

SIALODACRYOADENITIS VIRUS. Sialodacryoadenitis (SDA) virus is a highly contagious coronavirus that is spread via aerosol transmission, direct contact, or fomites. Sialodacryoadenitis virus infection results in unilateral or bilateral inflammation of the harderian gland, blepharospasm, photophobia, conjunctivitis, chromodacryorrhea, and, in some cases, self-mutilation leading to corneal ulceration and blepharitis.[149]

The viral infection is typically self-limiting and does not require treatment; however, some rats may persistently shed the organism.[150] Isolation protocols should be observed when introducing new rats into a household to prevent spread of SDA.

CONJUNCTIVITIS. Conjunctivitis is a frequent ocular disease of rats and mice. Environmental irritants including poor ventilation and dusty bedding material are thought to play a major role in the development of conjunctivitis and may predispose the affected tissue to infectious organisms. *Mycoplasma pulmonis* is the most common infectious disease associated with conjunctivitis and upper respiratory infection in rats. All captive rats should be considered positive. The disease typically manifests when an animal is stressed (e.g., cage-mate aggression, concurrent disease). Conjunctivitis and chromodacryorrhea are common presenting signs of mycoplasmosis. Over time the infection becomes more severe, eventually leading to pulmonary disease. A single animal in a group of rats can show signs, while others are clinically normal. Diagnostic tests including serology and PCR are available, but most clinicians skip the tests and pursue treatment due to its ubiquitous nature. Topical and systemic antibiotic therapy with broad-spectrum drugs is warranted. Typically, doxycycline (5.0 mg/kg, per os, twice daily), enrofloxacin (5.0 to 10.0 mg/kg, per os, twice daily), or a combination of the drugs are used to control the disease. Treatment is typically prescribed for 14 days but may need to be extended based on the rat's response. Macrolides (e.g., azithromycin) have also been used in some cases when the infection becomes refractory to the other antibiotics. Improved husbandry is key to managing and resolving clinical signs.

CORNEAL DYSTROPHY/DEGENERATION. Corneal lipid dystrophy/calcium degeneration has been reported in several laboratory rat species, although it has not been described in pet animals.[151,152] Environmental irritants have been implicated as a cause, although genetic factors are also thought to be involved. No treatment is required for most cases, as the white corneal opacities are not associated with any ocular discomfort or visual impairment.

Guinea Pigs

CONJUNCTIVITIS. Conjunctivitis caused by *Chlamydia caviae* (previously known as *Chlamydia psittaci*, the guinea pig inclusion conjunctivitis strain) is most common in laboratory colonies but has also been reported in pet guinea pigs.[153,154] Young animals are more likely to be affected and may also show concurrent respiratory disease. Ocular signs include conjunctivitis with chemosis and yellow or white ocular discharge. The diagnosis may be confirmed by conjunctival cytology and the observation of intracytoplasmic elementary and reticular bodies in the conjunctival epithelium. PCR testing may be more sensitive and specific and also allows for speciation of the organism.[153] Treatment for conjunctivitis caused by *Chlamydia caviae* includes topical tetracycline ophthalmic ointment every 8 hours for 10 to 14 days. Oral tetracyclines may also be useful.

FATTY EYE/PEA EYE. Subconjunctival fat deposition visible bilaterally in the lower lateral conjunctival fornix of guinea pigs has been colloquially termed pea eye or fatty eye. The condition is seen most often in obese guinea pigs[155] (Figures 9-31 and 9-32). Pea eye is not associated with any ocular discomfort and needs no treatment in most cases. If

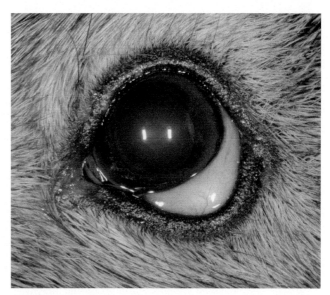

FIGURE 9-31 The left eye of a guinea pig with "pea eye." Note the ectropion of the lower lid associated with subconjunctival fat prolapse.

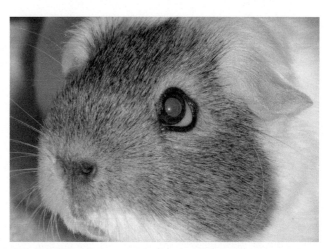

FIGURE 9-32 The same patient as in Figure 9-31. Note the marked deviation of the lower lid. The guinea pig is markedly overconditioned.

eyelid closure is impaired by the conjunctival protuberance, artificial tears gel or ointment administered every 6 to 12 hours is warranted. Weight loss is likely to be helpful in resolving the condition.

HETEROTOPIC BONE FORMATION. Heterotopic bone formation (also known as osseous choristoma) is a condition unique to the guinea pig that results in new bone formation in the ciliary body that can be visible as a white, crystalline opacity at the limbus.[155-158] The underlying cause remains unknown, although glaucoma has been proposed as an etiology by some authors, while others have found no evidence of glaucoma in clinically affected guinea pigs.[155,159] The role of ascorbic acid metabolism by the guinea pig in disease pathogenesis of the ciliary body also remains unknown. Visual deficits and ocular discomfort are not reported in affected animals; thus, no treatment is recommended.

CATARACT. Cataract is reported to be the most common ocular anomaly affecting pet guinea pigs.[155] Diabetes mellitus and hereditary etiologies have been proposed, as has insufficient dietary ascorbic acid; however, recent studies suggest that supplementing dietary ascorbic acid does not prevent cataracts associated with UV light exposure.[160] Further investigation is warranted into the apparently high prevalence of cataracts in pet guinea pigs. Cataract surgery to restore vision in guinea pigs blinded by cataract has not been reported.

Hedgehogs

PROPTOSIS/EXOPHTHALMOS. The shallow orbit of the hedgehog leaves the globe of this species vulnerable to displacement from the orbit. Exophthalmos occurs secondarily to space-occupying orbital lesions, including neoplasms, cellulitis, and foreign bodies. Proptosis is the cranial displacement of the globe from the orbit with entrapment of the eyelids caudal to the globe. Overconditioned hedgehogs with excessive orbital fat may be at more risk for traumatic proptosis.[161] The visual prognosis for proptosed brachycephalic canine eyes is poor, and a similar prognosis is expected in hedgehogs.[161,162] An acutely proptosed globe can be replaced under general anesthesia, and a temporary tarsorrhaphy placed to close the lid and prevent reproptosis using 5-0 or 6-0 nonabsorbable suture. Postoperative care includes topical and systemic antibiotics and systemic analgesics. If the globe is ruptured or the proptosis is chronic, enucleation is recommended.

REFERENCES

1. Williams DL. Biology and pathology of the invertebrate eye. *Vet Clin Exot Anim.* 2002;5:407-415.
2. Desai UM, Achuthankutty CT. Complete regeneration of ablated eyestalk in penaeid prawn. *Curr Sci.* 2000;79:1602-1603.
3. Davis MW, Stephenson J, Noga EJ. The effect of tricaine on use of the fluorescein test for detecting skin and corneal ulcers in fish. *J Aquat Anim Health.* 2008;20:86-95.
4. Williams CR, Whitaker BR. The evaluation and treatment of common ocular disorders in teleosts. *Sem Avian Exotic Pet Med.* 1997;6:160-169.
5. Shariff M. The histopathology of the eye of the big head carp, *Aristichthys noblis* (Richardson), infested with Lernaea piscinae Harding, 1950. *J Fish Dis.* 1950;4:161-168.
6. Hughes SG. Nutritional eye diseases in salmonids: a review. *Prog Fish Cult.* 1985;47:81-85.
7. Hughes SG. Biomicroscopic and histologic pathology of the eye in riboflavin deficient rainbow trout (*Salmo gairdneri*). *Cornell Vet.* 1981;71:269-279.
8. Mayer SJ. Stratospheric ozone depletion and animal health. *Vet Rec.* 1992;131:120-122.
9. Siezen RJ. Reversible osmotic cataracts in spiny dogfish (*Squalus acanthias*) eye lens. *Exp Eye Res.* 1998;46:987-990.
10. Waagbo R, Hamre K, Bjerkas E, et al. Cataract formation in Atlantic salmon, *Salmo salar* L., smolt relative to dietary pro- and antioxidants and lipid level. *J Fish Dis.* 2003;26:213-229.
11. Leclercq E, Taylor JF, Fison D, et al. Comparative seawater performance and deformity prevalence in out-of-season diploid and triploid Atlantic salmon (*Salmo salar*) post-smolts. *Comp Biochem Physiol A Mol Integr Physiol.* 2011;158:116-125.
12. Liakonis KM, Waagbo R, Foss A, et al. Effects of chronic and periodic exposures to ammonia on the eye health in juvenile Atlantic halibut (*Hippoglossus hippoglossus*). *Fish Physiol Biochem.* 2012;38:421-430.
13. Zigman S, Rafferty NS, Scholz DL, et al. The effects of near-UV radiation on elasmobranch lens cytoskeletal actin. *Exp Eye Res.* 1992;55:193-201.
14. Breck O, Bjerkas E, Campbell P, et al. Histidine nutrition and genotype affect cataract development in Atlantic salmon, *Salmo salar* L. *J Fish Dis.* 2005;28:357-371.
15. Chappell LH. The biology of diplostomatid eyeflukes of fishes. *J Helminthol.* 1995;69:97-101.
16. Jurk I. Ophthalmic disease of fish. *Vet Clin North Am Exot Anim Pract.* 2002;5:243-260.
17. Plumb JA, Rogers WA. Effect of droncit (praziquantel) on yellow grubs (*Clinostomum marginatum*) and eye flukes (*Diplostomum spathaceum*) in channel catfish. *J Aquat Anim Health.* 1990;2:204-206.
18. Bakal RS, Hickson BH, Gilger BC, et al. Surgical removal of cataracts due to *Diplostomum* species in Gulf sturgeon (*Acipenser oxyrinchus desotoi*). *J Zoo Wildl Med.* 2005;36:504-508.
19. Speare DJ. Histopathology and ultrastructure of ocular lesions associated with gas bubble disease in salmonids. *J Comp Pathol.* 1990;103:421-432.
20. Grahn BH, Sangster C, Breaux C, et al. Case report: clinical and pathologic manifestations of gas bubble disease in captive fish. *J Exotic Pet Med.* 2007;16:104-112.
21. Carpenter JL, Bachrach A Jr, Albert DM, et al. Xanthomatous keratitis, disseminated xanthomatosis, and atherosclerosis in Cuban tree frogs. *Vet Pathol.* 1986;23:337-339.
22. Russell WC, Edwards DL Jr, Stair EL, et al. Corneal lipidosis, disseminated xanthomatosis, and hypercholesterolemia in Cuban tree frogs (*Osteopilus septentrionalis*). *J Zoo Wildl Med.* 1990;21:99-104.
23. Shilton CM, Smith DA, Crawshaw GJ, et al. Corneal lipid deposition in Cuban tree frogs (*Osteopilus septentrionalis*) and its relationship to serum lipids: an experimental study. *J Zoo Wildl Med.* 2001;32:305-319.
24. Wright K. Cholesterol, corneal lipidosis, and xanthomatosis in amphibians. *Vet Clin North Am Exot Anim Pract.* 2003;6:155-167.
25. Brooks DE, Jacobson ER, Wolf ED, et al. Panophthalmitis and otitis interna in fire-bellied toads. *J Am Vet Med Assoc.* 1983;183:1198-1201.
26. Glorioso JC, Amborski RL, Amborski GF, et al. Microbiological studies on septicemic bullfrogs (*Rana catesbeiana*). *Am J Vet Res.* 1974;35:1241-1245.
27. Mauel MJ, Miller DL, Frazier KS, et al. Bacterial pathogens isolated from cultured bullfrogs (*Rana castesbeiana*). *J Vet Diagn Invest.* 2002;14:431-433.
28. Olson ME, Gard S, Brown M, et al. *Flavobacterium indologenes* infection in leopard frogs. *J Am Vet Med Assoc.* 1992;201:1766-1770.
29. Imai DM, Nadler SA, Brenner D, et al. Rhabditid nematode-associated ophthalmitis and meningoencephalomyelitis in captive Asian horned frogs (*Megophrys montana*). *J Vet Diagn Invest.* 2009;21:568-573.
30. Sabater M, Perez M. Congenital ocular and adnexal disorders in reptiles. *Vet Ophthalmol.* 2013;16:47-55.
31. Wallach JD. Environmental and nutritional diseases of captive reptiles. *J Am Vet Med Assoc.* 1971;159:1632-1643.
32. Elkan E, Zwart P. The ocular disease of young terrapins caused by vitamin A deficiency. *Pathol Vet.* 1967;4:201-222.
33. Millichamp NJ, Jacobson ER, Wolf ED. Diseases of the eye and ocular adnexae in reptiles. *J Am Vet Med Assoc.* 1983;183:1205-1212.
34. Coke RL, Couillard NK. Ocular biology and diseases of Old World chameleons. *Vet Clin North Am Exot Anim Pract.* 2002;5:275-285.
35. Coke RL, Carpenter JW. Use of ocular/nasolacrimal flushes for treating periocular swelling in old world chameleons. *Exotic DVM.* 2001;3(5):14-15.
36. Tangredi BP, Evans RH. Organochlorine pesticides associated with ocular, nasal, or otic infection in the eastern box turtle (*Terrapene carolina carolina*). *J Zoo Wildl Med.* 1997;28:97-100.

37. Coberley SS, Herbst LH, Ehrhart LM, et al. Survey of Florida green turtles for exposure to a disease-associated herpesvirus. *Dis Aquat Organ.* 2001;47:159-167.

38. Jacobson ER, Popp JA, Shields RP, et al. Poxlike skin lesions in captive caimans. *J Am Vet Med Assoc.* 1979;175:937-940.

39. Abou-Madi N, Kern TJ. Squamous cell carcinoma associated with a periorbital mass in a veiled chameleon *(Chamaeleo calyptratus). Vet Ophthalmol.* 2002;5:217-220.

40. Ardente AJ, Christian LS, Borst LB, et al. Clinical challenge. Squamous cell carcinoma. *J Zoo Wildl Med.* 2011;42:770-773.

41. Emerson JA, Walling BE, Whittington JK, et al. Pathology in practice. Squamous cell carcinoma (SCC) of the skin of the upper right eyelid. *J Am Vet Med Assoc.* 2012;240:1175-1177.

42. Hannon DE, Garner MM, Reavill DR. Squamous cell carcinomas in inland bearded dragons *(Pogona vitticeps). J Herp Med Surg.* 2011;21:101-106.

43. Allgoewer I, Gobel T, Stockhaus C, et al. Dacryops in a red-eared slider *(Chrysemys scripta elegans):* case report. *Vet Ophthalmol.* 2002;5:231-234.

44. Schumacher J, Pellicane CP, Heard DJ, et al. Periorbital abscess in a three-horned chameleon *(Chamaeleo jacksonii). Vet Comp Ophthalmol.* 1996;6:30-33.

45. Whittaker CJG, Schumacher J, Bennett RA, et al. Orbital varix in a green iguana *(Iguana iguana). Vet Comp Ophthalmol.* 1997;7:101-104.

46. Mayer J, Pizzirani S, DeSena R. Bilateral exophthalmos in an adult iguana *(Iguana iguana)* caused by an orbital abscess. *J Herp Med Surg.* 2010;20:5-10.

47. Banzato T, Russo E, Di Toma A, et al. Evaluation of radiographic, computed tomographic, and cadaveric anatomy of the head of boa constrictors. *Am J Vet Res.* 2011;72:1592-1599.

48. Banzato T, Selleri P, Veladiano IA, et al. Comparative evaluation of the cadaveric, radiographic and computed tomographic anatomy of the heads of green iguana *(Iguana iguana)*, common tegu *(Tupinambis merianae)* and bearded dragon *(Pogona vitticeps). BMC Vet Res.* 2012; 8:53.

49. Hardon T, Fledelius B, Heegaard S. Keratoacanthoma of the spectacle in a boa constrictor. *Vet Ophthalmol.* 2007;10:320-322.

50. Maas AK, Paul-Murphy J, Kumaresan-Lampman S, et al. Spectacle wound healing in the royal python *(Python regius). J Herp Med Surg.* 2010;20:29-36.

51. Millichamp NJ, Jacobson ER, Dziezyc J. Conjunctivoralostomy for treatment of an occluded lacrimal duct in a blood python. *J Am Vet Med Assoc.* 1986;189:1136-1138.

52. Gardiner DW, Baines FM, Pandher K. Photodermatitis and photokeratoconjunctivitis in a ball python *(Python regius)* and a blue-tongue skink *(Tiliqua* spp.). *J Zoo Wildl Med.* 2009;40:757-766.

53. Bonney CH, Hartfiel DA, Schmidt RE. *Klebsiella pneumoniae* infection with secondary hypopyon in tokay gecko lizards. *J Am Vet Med Assoc.* 1978;173:1115-1116.

54. Tomson FN, McDonald SE, Wolf ED. Hypopyon in a tortoise. *J Am Vet Med Assoc.* 1976;169:942.

55. Colitz CM, Lewbart G, Davidson MG. Phacoemulsification in an adult Savannah monitor lizard. *Vet Ophthalmol.* 2002;5:207-209.

56. Kelly TR, Walton W, Nadelstein B, et al. Phacoemulsification of bilateral cataracts in a loggerhead sea turtle *(Caretta caretta). Vet Rec.* 2005;156:774-777.

57. Myers G, Webb T, Corbett CR, et al. Phacoemulsification for removal of bilateral cataracts in a black water monitor *(Varanus salvator macromaculatus). J Herp Med Surg.* 2011;21:96-100.

58. Chittick B, Harms C. Intraocular pressure of juvenile loggerhead sea turtles *(Caretta caretta)* held in different positions. *Vet Rec.* 2001;149:587-589.

59. Labelle AL, Steele KA, Breaux CB, et al. Tonometry and corneal aesthesiometry in the red-eared slider turtle *(Trachemys scripta elegans). J Herp Med Surg.* 2012;22(1–2):30-35.

60. Selleri P, Di Girolamo N, Andreani V, et al. Evaluation of intraocular pressure in conscious Hermann's tortoises *(Testudo hermanni)* by means of rebound tonometry. *Am J Vet Res.* 2012;73:1807-1812.

61. Selmi AL, Mendes GM, MacManus C. Tonometry in adult yellow-footed tortoises *(Geochelone denticulata). Vet Ophthalmol.* 2003;6:305-307.

62. Selmi AL, Mendes GM, McManus C, et al. Intraocular pressure determination in clinically normal red-footed tortoise *(Geochelone carbonaria). J Zoo Wildl Med.* 2002;33:58-61.

63. Buyukmihci NC, Murphy CJ, Paul-Murphy J, et al. Eyelid malformation in four cockatiels. *J Am Vet Med Assoc.* 1990;196:1490-1492.

64. McDonald SE, Lowenstine LJ, Ardans AA. Avian pox in blue-fronted Amazon parrots. *J Am Vet Med Assoc.* 1981;179:1218-1222.

65. Kern TJ, Paul-Murphy J, Murphy CJ, et al. Disorders of the third eyelid in birds: 17 cases. *J Avian Med Surg.* 1996;10:12-18.

66. Stuhr CM, Murphy CJ, Schoster J, et al. Surgical repair of third eyelid lacerations in three birds. *J Avian Med Surg.* 1999;13:201-206.

67. Abrams GA, Paul-Murphy J, Murphy CJ. Conjunctivitis in birds. *Vet Clin North Am Exot Anim Pract.* 2002;5:287-309.

68. Luttrell MP, Stallknecht DE, Fischer JR, et al. Natural *Mycoplasma gallisepticum* infection in a captive flock of house finches. *J Wildl Dis.* 1998;34:289-296.

69. Hartup BK, Mohammed HO, Kollias GV, et al. Risk factors associated with mycoplasmal conjunctivitis in house finches. *J Wildl Dis.* 1998;34:281-288.

70. Luttrell MP, Fischer JR, Stallknecht DE, et al. Field investigation of *Mycoplasma gallisepticum* infections in house finches *(Carpodacus mexicanus)* from Maryland and Georgia. *Avian Dis.* 1996;40: 335-341.

71. Ley DH, Berkhoff JE, McLaren JM. *Mycoplasma gallisepticum* isolated from house finches *(Carpodacus mexicanus)* with conjunctivitis. *Avian Dis.* 1996;40:480-483.

72. Wellehan JF, Zens MS, Calsamiglia M, et al. Diagnosis and treatment of conjunctivitis in house finches associated with mycoplasmosis in Minnesota. *J Wildl Dis.* 2001;37:245-251.

73. Clode AB, Davis JL, Salmon J, et al. Evaluation of concentration of voriconazole in aqueous humor after topical and oral administration in horses. *Am J Vet Res.* 2006;67:296-301.

74. Sanchez-Migallon Guzman D, Flammer K, Papich MG, et al. Pharmacokinetics of voriconazole after oral administration of single and multiple doses in Hispaniolan Amazon parrots *(Amazona ventralis). Am J Vet Res.* 2010;71:460-467.

75. Burhenne J, Haefeli WE, Hess M, et al. Pharmacokinetics, tissue concentrations, and safety of the antifungal agent voriconazole in chickens. *J Avian Med Surg.* 2008;22:199-207.

76. Murakami S, Miyama M, Ogawa A, et al. Occurrence of conjunctivitis, sinusitis and upper region tracheitis in Japanese quail *(Coturnix coturnix japonica)*, possibly caused by *Mycoplasma gallisepticum* accompanied by *Cryptosporidium* sp. infection. *Avian Pathol.* 2002;31:363-370.

77. Labelle AL, Whittington JK, Breaux CB, et al. Clinical utility of a complete diagnostic protocol for the ocular evaluation of free-living raptors. *Vet Ophthalmol.* 2012;15:5-17.

78. Bounous DI, Schaeffer DO, Roy A. Coagulase-negative *Staphylococcus* sp. septicemia in a lovebird. *J Am Vet Med Assoc.* 1989;195: 1120-1122.

79. Carter RT, Murphy CJ, Stuhr CM, et al. Bilateral phacoemulsification and intraocular lens implantation in a great horned owl. *J Am Vet Med Assoc.* 2007;230:559-561.

80. Kern TJ, Murphy CJ, Riis RC. Lens extraction by phacoemulsification in two raptors. *J Am Vet Med Assoc.* 1984;185:1403-1406.

81. Wilson D, Pettifer GR. Anesthesia case of the month. Mallard undergoing phacoemulsification of a cataract. *J Am Vet Med Assoc.* 2004;225:685-688.

82. Brooks DE, Murphy CJ, Quesenberry KE, et al. Surgical correction of a luxated cataractous lens in a barred owl. *J Am Vet Med Assoc.* 1983;183:1298-1299.

83. Moore CP, Pickett JP, Beehler B. Extracapsular extraction of senile cataract in an Andean condor. *J Am Vet Med Assoc.* 1985;187: 1211-1213.

84. Van Niekerk WH, Petrick SW. Unilateral lentectomy in a black-shouldered kite. *J S Afr Vet Assoc.* 1990;61:124-125.

85. Jeong MB, Kim NR, Yi NY, et al. Spontaneous ophthalmic diseases in 586 New Zealand white rabbits. *Exp Anim.* 2005;54: 395-403.

86. Cunliffe-Beamer TL, Fox RR. Venereal spirochetosis of rabbits: description and diagnosis. *Lab Anim Sci.* 1981;31:366-371.

87. Cunliffe-Beamer TL, Fox RR. Venereal spirochetosis of rabbits: eradication. *Lab Anim Sci.* 1981;31:379-381.

88. Rivers TM. Infectious myxomatosis of rabbits: observations on the pathological changes induced by virus myxamatosum (Sanarelli). *J Exp Med.* 1930;51:965-976.

89. Shope RE, Hurst EW. Infectious papillomatosis of rabbits: with a note on histopathology. *J Exp Med.* 1933;58:607-624.

90. Greene HS. Rabbit pox: I. Clinical manifestations and course of disease. *J Exp Med.* 1934;60:427-440.

91. Fox JG, Shalev M, Beaucage CM, et al. Congenital entropion in a litter of rabbits. *Lab Anim Sci.* 1979;29:509-511.

92. Gelatt KN, Whitely RD. Surgery of the eyelids. In: Gelatt KN, Gelatt JP, eds. *Veterinary Ophthalmic Surgery.* Edinburgh: Saunders; 2011:89-137.

93. Burling K, Murphy CJ, da Silva Curiel J, et al. Anatomy of the rabbit nasolacrimal duct and its clinical implications. *Prog Vet and Comp Ophthalmol.* 1991;1:33-40.

94. Marini RP, Foltz CJ, Kersten D, et al. Microbiologic, radiographic, and anatomic study of the nasolacrimal duct apparatus in the rabbit *(Oryctolagus cuniculus).* *Lab Anim Sci.* 1996;46:656-662.

95. Florin M, Rusanen E, Haessig M, et al. Clinical presentation, treatment, and outcome of dacryocystitis in rabbits: a retrospective study of 28 cases (2003-2007). *Vet Ophthalmol.* 2009;12:350-356.

96. Van Caelenberg AI, De Rycke LM, Hermans K, et al. Computed tomography and cross-sectional anatomy of the head in healthy rabbits. *Am J Vet Res.* 2010;71:293-303.

97. Van Caelenberg AI, De Rycke LM, Hermans K, et al. Comparison of radiography and CT to identify changes in the skulls of four rabbits with dental disease. *J Vet Dent.* 2011;28:172-181.

98. Van Caelenberg AI, De Rycke LM, Hermans K, et al. Low-field magnetic resonance imaging and cross-sectional anatomy of the rabbit head. *Vet J.* 2011;188:83-91.

99. De Rycke LM, Boone MN, Van Caelenberg AI, et al. Micro-computed tomography of the head and dentition in cadavers of clinically normal rabbits. *Am J Vet Res.* 2012;73:227-232.

100. Bhambani BD. A case report of conjunctivitis and dermonecrosis in rabbit due to *Staphylococcus aureus. Indian Vet J.* 1966;43:555-558.

101. Snyder SB, Fox JG, Campbell LH, et al. Disseminated staphylococcal disease in laboratory rabbits *(Oryctolagus cuniculus). Lab Anim Sci.* 1976;26:86-88.

102. Millichamp NJ, Collins BR. Blepharoconjunctivitis associated with *Staphylococcus aureus* in a rabbit. *J Am Vet Med Assoc.* 1986;189: 1153-1154.

103. Hinton M. Treatment of purulent staphylococcal conjunctivitis in rabbits with autogenous vaccine. *Lab Anim.* 1977;11:163-164.

104. Buckley P, Lowman DM. Chronic non-infective conjunctivitis in rabbits. *Lab Anim.* 1979;13:69-73.

105. Donnelly TM, Fisher PG, Lackner PA. Epicorneal membrane on the eye of a Rex rabbit. *Lab Anim (NY).* 2002;31:23-25.

106. Matros LE, Ansari MM, Van Pelt CS. Eye anomaly in a dwarf rabbit. *Avian Exotic Pract.* 1986;3:13-14.

107. Roze M, Ridings B, Lagadic M. Comparative morphology of epicorneal conjunctival membranes in rabbits and human pterygium. *Vet Ophthalmol.* 2001;4:171-174.

108. Arnbjer J. Pseudopterygium in a pygmy rabbit. *Vet Med Small Anim Clin.* 1979;74:737-738.

109. Allgoewer I, Malho P, Schulze H, et al. Aberrant conjunctival stricture and overgrowth in the rabbit. *Vet Ophthalmol.* 2008;11: 18-22.

110. Andrew SE. Corneal diseases of rabbits. *Vet Clin North Am Exot Anim Pract.* 2002;5:341-356.

111. Liebenberg SP, Linn JM. Seasonal and sexual influences on rabbit atropinesterase. *Lab Anim.* 1980;14:297-300.

112. Stiles J, Honda CN, Krohne SG, et al. Effect of topical administration of 1% morphine sulfate solution on signs of pain and corneal wound healing in dogs. *Am J Vet Res.* 2003;64:813-818.

113. Simsek NA, Ay GM, Tugal-Tutkun I, et al. An experimental study on the effect of collagen shields and therapeutic contact lenses on corneal wound healing. *Cornea.* 1996;15:612-616.

114. Carpenter JW, Pollock CG, Koch DE, et al. Single- and multiple-dose pharmacokinetics of meloxicam after oral administration to the rabbit *(Oryctolagus cuniculus). J Zoo Wildl Med.* 2009;40:601-606.

115. Bromberg NM. Cyanoacrylate tissue adhesive for treatment of refractory corneal ulceration. *Vet Ophthalmol.* 2002;5:55-60.

116. Holve DL, Mundwiler KE, Pritt SL. Incidence of spontaneous ocular lesions in laboratory rabbits. *Comp Med.* 2011;61:436-440.

117. Munger RJ, Langevin N, Podval J. Spontaneous cataracts in laboratory rabbits. *Vet Ophthalmol.* 2002;5:177-181.

118. Keller RL, Hendrix DV, Greenacre C. Shope fibroma virus keratitis and spontaneous cataracts in a domestic rabbit. *Vet Ophthalmol.* 2007;10:190-195.

119. Kunzel F, Joachim A. Encephalitozoonosis in rabbits. *Parasitol Res.* 2010;106:299-309.

120. Wolfer J, Grahn B, Wilcock B, et al. Phacoclastic uveitis in the rabbit. *Prog Vet Comp Ophthalmol.* 1993;3:92-97.

121. Giordano C, Weigt A, Vercelli A, et al. Immunohistochemical identification of *Encephalitozoon cuniculi* in phacoclastic uveitis in four rabbits. *Vet Ophthalmol.* 2005;8:271-275.

122. Cray C, Arcia G, Schneider R, et al. Evaluation of the usefulness of an ELISA and protein electrophoresis in the diagnosis of *Encephalitozoon cuniculi* infection in rabbits. *Am J Vet Res.* 2009;70:478-482.

123. Felchle LM, Sigler RL. Phacoemulsification for the management of *Encephalitozoon cuniculi*-induced phacoclastic uveitis in a rabbit. *Vet Ophthalmol.* 2002;5:211-215.

124. Kunzel F, Gruber A, Tichy A, et al. Clinical symptoms and diagnosis of encephalitozoonosis in pet rabbits. *Vet Parasitol.* 2008;151: 115-124.

125. Hanna BL, Sawin PB, Sheppard LB. Recessive buphthalmos in the rabbit. *Genetics.* 1962;47:519-529.

126. Tesluk GC, Peiffer RL, Brown D. A clinical and pathological study of inherited glaucoma in New Zealand white rabbits. *Lab Anim.* 1982;16:234-239.

127. Percicot CL, Schnell CR, Debon C, et al. Continuous intraocular pressure measurement by telemetry in alpha-chymotrypsin-induced glaucoma model in the rabbit: effects of timolol, dorzolamide, and epinephrine. *J Pharmacol Toxicol Methods.* 1996;36:223-228.

128. Gupta SK, Agarwal R, Galpalli ND, et al. Comparative efficacy of pilocarpine, timolol and latanoprost in experimental models of glaucoma. *Methods Find Exp Clin Pharmacol.* 2007;29:665-671.

129. Vernau KM, Grahn BH, Clarke-Scott HA, et al. Thymoma in a geriatric rabbit with hypercalcemia and periodic exophthalmos. *J Am Vet Med Assoc.* 1995;206:820-822.

130. Kunzel F, Hittmair KM, Hassan J, et al. Thymomas in rabbits: clinical evaluation, diagnosis, and treatment. *J Am Anim Hosp Assoc.* 2012;48:97-104.

131. Harcourt-Brown F. Diagnosis, treatment and prognosis of dental disease in pet rabbits. *In Pract.* 1997;19:414-421.

132. Tyrrell KL, Citron DM, Jenkins JR, et al. Periodontal bacteria in rabbit mandibular and maxillary abscesses. *J Clin Microbiol.* 2002;40:1044-1047.

133. Visigalli G, Cappelletti A, Nuvoli S. A surgical approach to retrobulbar abscessation in a pet dwarf rabbit. *Exotic DVM.* 2008;10(1):11-14.
134. Ward ML. Diagnosis and management of a retrobulbar abscess of periapical origin in a domestic rabbit. *Vet Clin North Am Exot Anim Pract.* 2006;9:657-665.
135. Martinez-Jimenez D, Hernandez-Divers SJ, Dietrich UM, et al. Endosurgical treatment of a retrobulbar abscess in a rabbit. *J Am Vet Med Assoc.* 2007;230:868-872.
136. Holmberg BJ. Enucleation of exotic pets. *J Exotic Pet Med.* 2007;16:88-94.
137. Davidson MG. Canine distemper virus infection in the domestic ferret. *Compen Cont Ed.* 1986;8:448-453.
138. Barnard DL. Animal models for the study of influenza pathogenesis and therapy. *Antiviral Res.* 2009;82:A110-A122.
139. Zitzow LA, Rowe T, Morken T, et al. Pathogenesis of avian influenza A (H5N1) viruses in ferrets. *J Virol.* 2002;76:4420-4429.
140. Lucas J, Lucas A, Furber H, et al. *Mycobacterium genavense* infection in two aged ferrets with conjunctival lesions. *Aust Vet J.* 2000;78:685-689.
141. Miller PE, Marlar AB, Dubielzig RR. Cataracts in a laboratory colony of ferrets. *Lab Anim Sci.* 1993;43:562-568.
142. Lipsitz L, Ramsey DT, Render JA, et al. Persistent fetal intraocular vasculature in the European ferret *(Mustela putorius):* clinical and histological aspects. *Vet Ophthalmol.* 2001;4:29-33.
143. Kawasaki T. Retinal atrophy in the ferret. *J Sm Exotic Anim Med.* 1992;1:137.
144. Miller PE. Ferret ophthalmology. *Sem Avian Exotic Pet Med.* 1997;6:146-151.
145. Beaumont SL. Ocular disorders of pet mice and rats. *Vet Clin North Am Exot Anim Pract.* 2002;5:311-324.
146. Williams DL. Ocular disease in rats: a review. *Vet Ophthalmol.* 2002;5:183-191.
147. Harkness JE, Ridgway MD. Chromodacryorrhea in laboratory rats *(Rattus norvegicus):* etiologic considerations. *Lab Anim Sci.* 1980;30:841-844.
148. Donnelly TM. What's your diagnosis? Blood-caked staining around the eyes in Sprague-Dawley rats. *Lab Anim.* 1997;26:17-18.
149. Weisbroth SH, Peress N. Ophthalmic lesions and dacryoadenitis: a naturally occurring aspect of sialodacryoadenitis virus infection of the laboratory rat. *Lab Anim Sci.* 1977;27:466-473.
150. Hanna PE, Percy DH, Paturzo F, et al. Sialodacryoadenitis in the rat: effects of immunosuppression on the course of the disease. *Am J Vet Res.* 1984;45:2077-2083.
151. Bellhorn RW, Korte GE, Abrutyn D. Spontaneous corneal degeneration in the rat. *Lab Anim Sci.* 1988;38:46-50.
152. Van Winkle TJ, Balk MW. Spontaneous corneal opacities in laboratory mice. *Lab Anim Sci.* 1986;36:248-255.
153. Strik NI, Alleman AR, Wellehan JF. Conjunctival swab cytology from a guinea pig: it's elementary! *Vet Clin Pathol.* 2005;34:169-171.
154. Deeb BJ, DiGiacomo RF, Wang SP. Guinea pig inclusion conjunctivitis (GPIC) in a commercial colony. *Lab Anim.* 1989;23:103-106.
155. Williams D, Sullivan A. Ocular disease in the guinea pig (*Cavia porcellus*): a survey of 1000 animals. *Vet Ophthalmol.* 2010;13(suppl):54-62.
156. Brooks DE, McCracken MD, Collins BR. Heterotopic bone formation in the ciliary body of an aged guinea pig. *Lab Anim Sci.* 1990;40:88-90.
157. Donnelly TM, Brown C, Donnelly TM. Heterotopic bone in the eyes of a guinea pig: osseous choristoma of the ciliary body. *Lab Anim (NY).* 2002;31:23-25.
158. Griffith JW, Sassani JW, Bowman TA, et al. Osseous choristoma of the ciliary body in guinea pigs. *Vet Pathol.* 1988;25:100-102.
159. Schaffer EH, Pfleghaar S. [Secondary open angle glaucoma from osseous choristoma of the ciliary body in guinea pigs]. *Tierarztl Prax.* 1995;23:410-414.
160. Mody VC, Kakar M, Elfving A, et al. Drinking water supplementation with ascorbate is not protective against UVR-B-induced cataract in the guinea pig. *Acta Ophthalmol.* 2008;86:188-195.
161. Wheler CL, Grahn BH, Pocknell AM. Unilateral proptosis and orbital cellulitis in eight African hedgehogs (*Atelerix albiventris*). *J Zoo Wildl Med.* 2001;32:236-241.
162. Gilger BC, Hamilton HL, Wilkie DA, et al. Traumatic ocular proptoses in dogs and cats: 84 cases (1980-1993). *J Am Vet Med Assoc.* 1995;206:1186-1190.

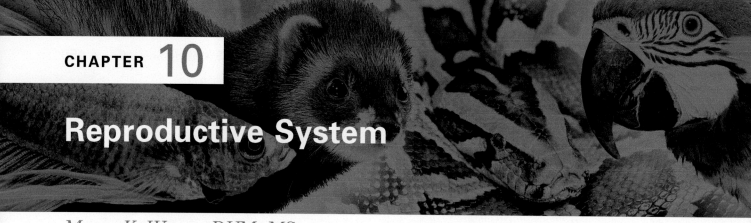

CHAPTER 10

Reproductive System

Megan K. Watson, DVM, MS

INTRODUCTION

Reproductive medicine in exotic pets may present a challenge to the practitioner due to the extreme diversity among species. Reproductive anatomy and physiology vary greatly across taxa. For example, in terms of physiologic processes of reproduction, exotic animals maintained in captivity may range from asexual reproduction, to egg laying, to live bearing. They possess different accessory sex glands and different numbers of functional gonads. They may have no distinct external reproductive characteristics, minimal differences only known to the educated eye, or may be similar to the more familiar dog or cat. The reproductive system often plays a primary role in presenting complaints of owners and disease presentations of exotic pet species. Owners may range from active breeders to first-time owners of a particular species. Many exotic pet species are not routinely spayed or neutered for various reasons such as cost, lack of client education, or possible complications of an elective procedure in some species. For these reasons, as in small animal medicine, reproductive system knowledge is utilized on a daily basis to perform sex determination, manage complex disease conditions and chronic reproductive conditions, and assist in breeding different species of exotic animals. Possessing a firm grasp on the comparative anatomy and physiology of each species contributes to the assessment of individual disease processes. As a compounding factor, reproductive disease is often multifactorial and may not always present as the primary disease process or complaint. This chapter addresses sex identification and basic comparative anatomy and physiology across exotic pet species. It also reviews common reproductive disease conditions presented to the veterinarian, diagnostic methods related to reproductive diseases among species, current treatments for reproductive disease, and common surgical procedures.

ANATOMY AND PHYSIOLOGY

Invertebrates

Among exotic pet species, invertebrates are an extremely diverse and captivating group. Knowledge about the biology of invertebrates is vast; however, veterinary medical knowledge for this group is still limited. This chapter focuses pri-

marily on invertebrates commonly encountered in the pet trade and their associated reproductive issues. Theraphosidae (giant spiders or tarantulas) are the most common spiders sold through the pet trade and likely the most common family encountered by veterinarians accepting invertebrate patients. Sex determination is important, as females may live over 20 years and males only 6 to 18 months. Sexing is fairly straightforward in adult males. All males will have a thickening of the distal tarsal pedipalp. This is due to the pear-shaped palpal organ. The majority of male theraphosids will also have visible spurs on the tibia of the first pair of legs. The most accurate method for sex determination is examination of the shed skin under stereomicroscopy for the presence of paired spermathecae in females. This is considered the gold standard and is provided by most hobbyist associations with memberships.[1]

Fish

Each species of fish has internal and external reproductive variations that allow it to thrive in its particular environmental niche. For example, most species have two distinct sexes, but others are hermaphroditic (e.g., clownfish [*Amphiprion* spp., *Premnas* spp.] are sequential hermaphrodites). Some species only reproduce once in their lifetime (e.g., salmonids), while many others have seasonal reproductive activity. Most fish rely on external fertilization to reproduce, although some use internal fertilization (e.g., guppies, *Poecelia* spp.) and some undergo self-fertilization.[2] The fish reproductive system is entirely separate from its urinary system. Fish have paired gonads internally, with extremely limited differentiation between sexes externally (i.e., few fish are sexually dimorphic). Sex differentiation via secondary sex characteristics is seen in elasmobranchs, as the males possess external claspers. These are modifications of the medial edge of the pelvic fins and are used by males to attach to the females during breeding. Common species of fish treated by the veterinarians include koi, carp, and goldfish, which are all members of the freshwater fish family Cyprinidae. These particular fish are oviparous and use external fertilization to reproduce.[3]

In females, the ovaries are long and generally paired, although they may also be partially fused. The ovarian tissue develops a beaded texture and enlarges as the oocytes develop. The reproductive organs may be difficult to identify in sexually immature fish and may simply be thin ribbon-like structures ventral to the swim bladder.[4] When a fish is reproductively active, the ovaries may take up a large percentage of the coelomic cavity, causing coelomic distension. Ova are expelled into the coelomic cavity where they accumulate and pass through oviducts at the genital pore. After ovulation, any oocytes left behind are reabsorbed.[5] Females possess two openings cranial to the anal fin, with the most cranial being the vent where gastrointestinal waste and urine exit and the caudal opening being the reproductive portal.[3]

Males possess long testes that are made of branching seminiferous tubules that produce spermatozoa. The spermatozoa are expelled into a deferent duct that carries them to the genital pore.[5] Some fish species have paired gonads, whereas others may have a single fused gonad. In the goldfish, the testes fuse posteriorly to form a Y-shaped organ. The sex of a fish can be determined post mortem by performing a wet mount on the reproductive tissues to examine for sperm or ova.

Amphibians

Amphibians are another diverse class of vertebrates and include the anurans (frogs and toads), urodelans (newts and salamanders), and caecilians. Sexual dimorphism is seen in many amphibians, although it is lacking in most caecilians. The most common form of sexual dimorphism is body size, which occurs in >90% of amphibians. Recently, more species have been found to exhibit sexual dichromatism (females and males differ in color). Two forms of dichromatism exist: dynamic (temporary change during breeding season) and ontogenetic (permanent change at onset of sexual maturity).[6] The presence of spines, tubercles, or tusks can also be used to determine sex in some species.[7,8] For example, some male anurans and newts develop nuptial pads on their digits as their testicular hormones rise. These pads enable the male to keep in contact with the female despite moving currents.[8]

In all amphibians, the gonads are paired and the gametes travel to the cloaca. The majority of caecilians are viviparous, while the majority of salamanders and anurans are oviparous. Salamander testes are lobed, and additional lobes develop with each breeding season. Male salamanders produce a gelatinous structure known as a spermatophore, which is taken into the cloaca of the female. The spermatophore is not deposited through true internal fertilization since males do not possess an intromittent organ.[7] Female newts and salamanders possess a spermatheca, which is a site for storage of sperm at the dorsal aspect of the cloaca.[9] After collecting the sperm packets, the female salamander may store viable sperm for extended periods of time (sometimes years) to fertilize eggs as they pass through the oviduct. In females, the follicles are surrounded by a thin membranous ovisac, which ruptures when ovulation occurs. Like salamanders, most frogs and toads do not possess an intromittent organ. Therefore, external fertilization is the primary reproductive strategy for these animals. The Bidder's organ is a remnant of ovarian tissue found on the testes of adult bufonids; under certain conditions (e.g., reduction in female population), these animals can switch sexes.[9] Anurans primarily rely on oviposition next to a water source. Parental care is exhibited with some amphibians; however, traits vary widely among species. A few species of caecilians, approximately 10% of anurans and most salamanders, exhibit some form of parental care.[8]

Reptiles

Reptiles are an extremely variable and diverse group of animals that demonstrate marked differences in reproductive anatomy and physiology, even within taxa. This chapter's primary focus is snakes, lizards, and chelonians and only briefly covers crocodilians, which are rarely presented to the exotic pet practitioner. It is important to have a basic understanding of reptile breeding and reproduction when seeing reptile patients, as there is a significant interest in hobby and larger-scale reptile breeding, along with pet ownership. Reptiles do not always possess external genitalia or secondary sex characteristics, making sex determination difficult. Unlike amphibians, all reptiles reproduce by internal fertilization. Most reptiles lay eggs and are referred to as oviparous. Oviparous females bearing young, producing eggs or follicles, are referred to as gravid. However, some female reptiles, most commonly snakes, bear live young. These are generally referred to as viviparous.

Sexual dimorphism is observed in a number of different reptiles. Some lizards (e.g., chameleons) display obvious signs of sexual dimorphism. For example, male Jackson's chameleons (*Chamaeleo jacksonii*) possess horns while females do not. Femoral pores, which are pores located along midline of the ventral thigh, may also be an indication of sex in certain species. Generally, male lizards such as the bearded dragon (*Pogona vitticeps*) and the green iguana (*Iguana iguana*) possess large, prominent femoral pores, which may be spiked in the case of iguanas. It should be noted that these femoral pores are also present in females; however, they are much smaller in size. Male iguanas also have a large dewlap (fold of skin) located under their chin. Male snakes and lizards have 2 copulatory organs, the hemipenes. These structures are located on the cranioventral aspect of the base of the tail, caudal to the vent. In some species of lizards, the hemipenes are visualized as bulges. Sometimes, these bulges also change the appearance of the base of the tail, causing it to be thickened or enlarged (Figure 10-1). Each hemipenis is an invagination from the cloacal wall. The hemipenes are maintained in the tail by a retractor muscle. During copulation, only one of the hemipenes is everted into the female's cloaca. Sperm travels along a groove on the outside of the everted hemipenis. The hemipenes serve a single function, transporting sperm, and are not involved in the excretion of urine. In some species, hemipenal casts may develop outside of breeding season, which may interfere with copulation during normal breeding. The casts are formed from previously shed skin, sperm, and other exudates (e.g., smegma). These casts should be removed prior to the onset of the breeding season.[10]

Lizards have a cloaca, which is the common space where waste (e.g., urine and feces) is collected and expelled from the body. There are three main components of the cloaca: the coprodeum, urodeum, and proctodeum. The reproductive tract is connected to the urodeum. The ureter is not associated with the hemipenes and exits via the cloaca. Females have a bircornuate reproductive system with paired ovaries. Ovarian size (i.e., follicle size) increases with breeding season and decreases out of breeding season. This is important to consider because ovariectomies are easier to perform during the breeding season when the mesovarium is stretched. Female lizards have the ability to produce and lay eggs in the absence

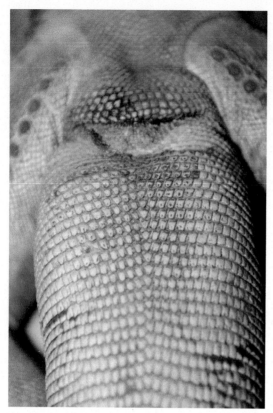

FIGURE 10-1 Photograph of the hemipenal bulges and prominent femoral pores of a male green iguana.

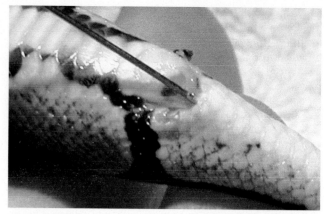

FIGURE 10-2 The technique for probing a snake is noted in this photograph. The tip of the blunt probe is inserted in the vent in a caudal direction to determine the presence/absence of a hemipenis.

of a male (similar to a chicken); however, these eggs will not be fertile or hatch. The oviducts are where albumin is produced and the shell created. In general, most lizard eggs have thin, flexible shells.[11] Female lizards do not possess a true uterus. As in the males, the terminus of the reproductive tract empties into the cloaca. In some iguanid lizards, spermatozoa may survive in the epithelial folds of the caudal oviduct and fertilize up to two clutches.

Few snakes are sexually dimorphic; therefore, they can be difficult to sex from external cues alone. In snakes that do have secondary sex characteristics, tail size and the presence of spurs may be helpful. Typically, the tail of the male snake is thicker caudal to the vent due to the presence of the paired hemipenes. The female tail may appear thinner in some species; however, this may be difficult to discern in species with shorter tails. Boid snakes (pythons and boas) have vestigial hind limbs called spurs on the lateral aspects of the cloaca. Spurs in the males are generally larger and used for tactile stimulation of the female.[12] As in other reptiles, secondary sex characteristics are subjective and do not always prove true. The most common and effective technique used to sex snakes is cloacal probing which involves placing a slender, blunt instrument (usually a stainless steel metal probe) into the vent and probing caudally until resistance is met (Figure 10-2). In males, the probe freely inserts and enters the inverted hemipenis. In females, resistance is commonly met shortly after insertion, although in some cases the probe may extend into a short blind sac (diverticulum). After the probe meets resistance, it should be marked at the level of the cloaca with a

finger. The probe should then be removed and measured against the scales. Generally, the probe will extend past four scales in length for males and less than four scales for females. Internally, the gonads are located in the cranial aspect of the caudal third of the body, just cranial to the kidneys. The right gonad is cranial to the left gonad. As in lizards, a hemipene will engorge and evaginate for copulation. All fertilization occurs internally.[13] Male snake anatomy is similar to lizards, with the exception of the epididymis being reportedly absent in snakes. Snakes may also develop hemipenal casts or plugs, which must be removed prior to breeding season.[10] Cloacal examination is important in snakes to evaluate a patient for possible cloacitis, impactions (scent gland, fecal or urate), or other issues.

Most chelonians are sexually dimorphic, although its anatomic variation may not always be apparent in sexually immature juveniles. Males have a cloacal phallus; however, it should be kept in mind that females can develop clitoral hyperplasia resulting in a penis-like protrusion from the cloaca, as the clitoris is the homolog to the penis and is in the same location.[14] Males typically have longer, broader tails than females. The distance between the vent and the caudal edge of the plastron is also longer in males than females. In most terrestrial species, males have a concave plastron to aid in mounting the female. However, it should be noted that these characteristics described above for sexing chelonians are guidelines and do not apply to all species or even within species. In eastern box turtles (*Terrapene carolina carolina*) males typically develop red-colored irises whereas females have yellow-brown irises. Male gopher tortoises (*Gopherus polyphemus*) develop large mental glands in their mandibles. Male red-eared slider turtles (*Trachemys scripta elegans*) typically have longer claws on their front legs that are used to stimulate the females. Desert tortoise (*Gopherus agassizii*) males have more prominent mental glands, and their gular scutes are elongated and more prominent than the females. Elongated gular scutes are also seen in other tortoises (e.g., African spurred tortoise, *Centrochelys sulcata*). As previously discussed, in many of the species that display sexual dimorphism or possess secondary sex characteristics, the differences may not be evident in juveniles. The animal may have to reach sexual maturity before one can determine its sex based on these characteristics alone. Imaging modalities such as radiographs, computed tomography (CT) scans, or ultrasound can be used to aid in sex determination in chelonians; however, these options can be costly and may not be viable in small or juvenile chelonians. Endoscopy is beneficial for determining the sex of juvenile chelonians. A coelioscopic approach can be performed to visualize the gonads and take diagnostic samples if necessary.

All chelonians are oviparous and slow to sexually mature. They become reproductively active based on size rather than age.[14] In the female chelonian, two ovaries are present in the coelomic cavity, and are suspended from the dorsal coelomic membrane. Chelonians have paired oviducts that transport ova to the urodeum of the cloaca. Females of certain species are capable of storing sperm for 4 to 6 years. Internal fertilization is thought to occur within the oviduct, after ovulation.[15] Calcification of the egg occurs in the caudal portion of the oviduct. As the ova pass through the glandular segment of the uterus, albumin is secreted around the ova, and the shell membranes are laid down in the isthmus,[16] which is the intermediate segment of the uterus. The most distal aspect of the uterus deposits the calcium. The oviducts enter the urodeum, located within the cloaca. Shelled eggs can be held in the oviducts prior to oviposition.[14] The eggs may be retained in the oviduct from 9 days to 6 months, depending on the species.[10] The egg shells of chelonians vary from soft and flexible to hard and brittle. Breeding season and control are poorly understood. Environmental factors such as rainfall, humidity, food supply, and photoperiod all play important roles in the reproductive physiology of chelonians.[15] Ovarian size can vary greatly with the reproductive cycle.[14] Female chelonians rely on finding an ideal nesting site. During oviposition, females excavate a nest site with their hind limbs. They then deposit the eggs and cover the nest. In general, eggs are deposited in a protected, remote site and are left to hatch without maternal care. The eggshell consists of an external mineral layer and an internal fibrous layer. When laying, some species will deposit so-called ghost eggs without embryos to allow for proper aeration and spacing within the nest. Dystocia may result when females cannot find a suitable nesting site.

Male chelonians have paired testes located in the dorsal coelomic cavity just cranioventral to the kidneys. The testes can fluctuate in size throughout the season. As in mammals, sperm is transported through the epididymis to the vas deferens. Unlike mammals, sperm is then deposited in the urodeum of the cloaca. Ventral to the opening of the vas deferens is the bulbous urethralis and the beginning of the phallus, which contains the corpora cavernosa that engorges during erection. The corpora fibrosa directs the phallus ventral and cranial at full erection.[14] Male chelonians have a single phallus that originates from the floor of the proctodeum. The chelonian phallus differs from the mammalian penis in that it is not involved in urination (no urethra).

Birds

The reproductive system of a bird is entirely internal, with no external genitalia present across species. Birds that are not sexually dimorphic can be sexed by DNA analysis of blood from commercial test kits (Antech Diagnostics, Irvine, CA, http://www.antechdiagnostics.com; Avian Biotech,

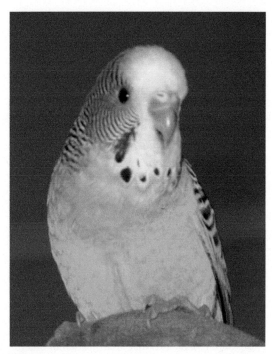

FIGURE 10-3 A male budgerigar is depicted in this photograph. Note the blue cere distinguishing the sex. (Photo courtesy of Matthew S. Johnston.)

Tallahassee, FL, http://www.avianbiotech.com) or by endoscopic examination. Some psittacines such as the eclectus parrot *(Eclectus roratus)* possess secondary sex characteristics that are sexually dimorphic. Females are purple and red with a black beak, whereas males are green and yellow with a "candy corn"–colored beak. In budgerigars *(Melopsittacus undulatus)*, the cere is typically blue in males and grayer (whiter) in females (Figure 10-3). When they are engaged in reproductive activity, the cere of the female budgerigar turns brown and is thickened (hyperplastic). Wild-type grey cockatiels *(Nymphicus hollandicus)* can be sexed by the presence of bars on the tail and primary flight feathers of females and a bright orange cheek patch on males.

Much like reptiles, all birds have a cloaca, and it is composed of a coprodeum, urodeum, and proctodeum, as mentioned above. The cloaca serves the same purpose in birds as in reptiles, and the reproductive tract is similarly connected to the urodeum. The urodeum contains the openings of the ureters and the genital ducts.[17] The reproductive tract of all female psittacines is located on the left side of the coelom. The right ovary and oviduct normally regress prior to hatching in psittacines; however, in some species, such as raptors, these organs may be vestigial remnants or, in rare cases, functional after hatching. The reproductive tract of an adult female bird has a functional left ovary that is connected to the urodeum via the associated oviduct. The ovary is located cranial to the left kidney and caudal to the adrenal gland. The oviduct is made up of five sections: the infundibulum, magnum, isthmus, uterus (shell gland), and vagina.[18] During the breeding season, the oviduct takes up much of the left coelom.[19] The ovary contains follicles that vary in size. Peristalsis transports the ovum from the cranial oviduct to the uterus, where smooth muscle contractions move the ovum toward the sperm. A vaginal sphincter is located at the junction between the uterus and the vagina, which is where sperm is stored.[20] The uterus is the site for the formation of the shell of the egg.[20] Oviduct transit time varies across species but is generally 24 hours in the chicken and most companion birds. It usually takes 48 hours to fully form an egg, and 80% of that time is spent in the uterus (shell gland) acquiring calcium to fully form the shell.[21]

Unlike female birds, the male reproductive organs are paired and located on both the right and left sides of the coelom. The testes are located ventral to the cranial border of the kidney. Sperm formation occurs in the seminiferous and straight tubules of the testis. Mature spermatozoa travel through the rete testis, the epididymis, the epididymal duct, and the ductus deferens.[20] The ductus deferens connects the testes to the urodeum, where sperm is stored. The last few millimeters of the ductus deferens protrude into the urodeum and form a papilla. Birds do not possess accessory sex glands. Most companion birds do not have a protruding phallus, and copulation involves eversion of the cloacal wall to expose the slightly raised papilla to transfer the semen to the orifice of the oviduct.[19] Waterfowl are an exception to this rule. In this group, males have a phallus that is comprised of erectile lymphatic tissue with an external groove (seminal groove) used to transport semen. The phallus of waterfowl is purely reproductive in function and may be amputated if necessary (e.g., traumatic injury).[22]

It is important to obtain an understanding of the basics of the reproductive cycle in birds in order to successfully manage reproductive disease in the group. The reproductive cycle of psittacines is complex and not fully elucidated; therefore, we often extrapolate our approach from what is known for Galliformes (e.g., chickens). As in all vertebrates, the reproductive system is regulated by the hypothalamus-pituitary-gonadal axis. In response to environmental triggers and other internal factors, the hypothalamus produces gonadotropin-releasing hormone (GnRH), which then stimulates the pituitary gland to produce luteinizing hormone (LH) and follicle-stimulating hormone (FSH). LH increases in concentration with lengthening photoperiod.[23] A study observing mating behaviors of cockatiels found that LH concentrations were significantly elevated in conjunction with lengthened photoperiod and mate and nest box access.[24] LH and FSH are in charge of regulating gonadal function and producing androgens and estrogens. The role of FSH in avian reproduction remains unclear.[23] Estrogens are responsible for secondary sex characteristics, stimulation of medullary bone production, and a number of products used to form the egg.[23] These steroids provide feedback regulation to the hypothalamus, which controls GnRH production and release.[25] LH also stimulates progesterone production, although both estrogens and progesterone must first prime the pituitary and hypothalamus. When progesterone increases, there is a preovulatory LH surge. The release of prostaglandin (PG) $F_{2\alpha}$ (PGF$_{2\alpha}$) coincides with shell gland contractions. Both PGF$_{2\alpha}$ and PGE$_2$ increase smooth muscle contractions in the connective tissue of the follicle, which cause the follicle to rupture. The ratio of PGF$_{2\alpha}$ to PGE$_2$ changes with the transition of midsequence oviposition and terminal oviposition; PGF$_{2\alpha}$ is most prominent at midsequence oviposition, while PGE$_2$

concentration is higher at terminal oviposition. After oviposition, parathyroid-hormone-related protein concentration in the shell gland increases, which may lead to increased blood flow to the shell gland while the egg is present and membranes are deposited on the egg surface. It also may serve as a signal for deposition of calcium. PGF$_{2\alpha}$ binds at the shell gland receptor sites to cause a mobilization of calcium, which in turn causes shell gland muscle contractions. Binding sites for PGE$_2$ predominate in the vagina and are thought to be present to block binding of PGF$_{2\alpha}$. This is thought to allow for relaxation of the uterovaginal sphincter and vagina. This also suggests that PGF$_{2\alpha}$ has no ability to relax the uterovaginal sphincter.

Mammals

Rodents

Generally, small rodents, including mice (*Mus musculus*), rats (*Rattus norvegicus*), hamsters (*Mesocricetus* spp.; *Phodopus* spp.), Mongolian gerbils (*Meriones unguiculatus*), and degus (*Octodon degus*), have similar reproductive anatomy. All of them are polyestrous, spontaneous ovulators. Rodents are prolific breeders. Reproductive problems in terms of breeding are minimal. Sex determination of rodents can be reliably made by anogenital distance, defined as the distance between the anus and genital papilla. This distance is greater in males than females. Also, the genital papilla is usually more prominent, with a round opening in the males.[26] There are also specific species characteristics. For example, male mice are typically twice the size of a female mouse. All male rodents have testicles that are relatively large for their body size and usually descended into a scrotum with an open inguinal ring.[27] Specifically when performing surgical procedures such as castration, it should be kept in mind that all rodents and rabbits have open inguinal rings. These testes can be directed from the abdomen, through the inguinal canal, and into the scrotum by applying pressure to the caudal abdomen or holding the animal vertically. Also, male rats, gerbils, and mice have no teat development. In female mice, teats develop at 9 to 13 days.[28] All female rodents have a bicornuate uterus with a uterine body. The body is generally short, with a single cervix. The mesovarium is short and the oviducts encircle the ovaries.

Mice have a relatively short average life span (~2 years) and thus become reproductively active early in life. Although not outwardly apparent, mice exhibit sexual dimorphism in splenic size. The spleen is 50% larger in males than females.[28] An unusual characteristic of female reproductive anatomy is that they possess paired clitoral glands. They have extensive mammary glands consisting of three pairs of thoracic and two pairs of inguinal glands. These reach from the ventral midline to over the flank and thorax and extend cranially to include part of the neck. Age of onset of puberty in females is 28 to 40 days, and females may begin initiating breeding ~50 days old. Their estrus cycle is short, 5 to 6 days, and gestation is 19 to 21 days.[29]

The female rat has six pairs of mammary glands. Like mice, their mammary tissue is extensive and is located from the cervical region to the inguinal region and includes the shoulders and flank dorsally. Their reproductive cycle is extremely sensitive to light. As little as 3 days of constant light can lead to persistent estrus, hyperestrogenism, polycystic ovaries, and endometrial hyperplasia.[30] The reproductive system of male rats is highly developed and has several accessory glands, including a pair of vesicular glands, a bulbourethral gland, and a prostate.

Female hamsters have a duplex uterus, therefore their uterine horns do not fuse and they have two cervices that connect the uterine horns to the vagina. Male hamsters have a fat pad in the inguinal canal that tends to keep the testes in the scrotum. Due to their fat pad, male hamsters have a rounded perineal profile when compared to females.[26] Both males and females have glands on either side of the flank that is usually covered with hair. These flank glands are more prominent in intact males. The flank glands are sebaceous in nature and produce secretions in response to androgen stimulation and to mark territory.[28,30] Unique to rodents, the male hamster has an os penis (penile bone) consisting of two distal lateral prongs and a dorsal prong.[30] Mating is confirmed by the presence of a copulatory plug within the vagina or on the cage floor. Female hamsters are generally larger than males and produce a large amount of vaginal discharge after ovulation, which is often mistaken by owners as abnormal discharge. Female hamsters also have paired vaginal pouches that collect leukocytes, making it difficult to interpret vaginal cytology as an indicator of the stage of estrus. Hamsters have the shortest gestation of all small mammals, ranging from 6 to 19 days.

Ferrets

Most ferrets in the United States are born at breeding facilities where they are spayed or castrated before 6 weeks of age. In the intact male ferret, or hob, the male reproductive anatomy is similar to the dog, with a palpable os penis. Ferrets are easy to sex because the prepuce in males is located on the ventral abdomen, and, unlike the dog, the os penis has a J-shaped tip and lies dorsal to the urethra. The testicles are located ventral to the anus, much like a cat. The only reproductive accessory gland present in the male ferret is the prostate gland. It is important to note that the prostate surrounds the urethra at the base of the bladder and, when enlarged, has a tendency to cause urethral obstruction. Each ductus deferens opens into the urethra at the level of the prostate.[31] Neutered male ferrets are referred to as gibs.

The reproductive anatomy of a jill, or intact female ferret, is similar to other carnivores and the dog. The vulva is located in the perineal region ventral to the anus. It consists of the vestibule, clitoris, and labia. In anestrus females, the vulva is a small slit opening. Paired ovaries are located caudal to the kidneys. The ovaries are attached to the body wall with a suspensory ligament. They are connected to the uterine horns caudally via the proper ligament.[32] There are two long, slender uterine horns that fuse to form a short uterine body with a single cervix. The urethral orifice lies cranial to the clitoral fossa on the ventral floor of the vagina. Ferrets in estrus exhibit a red and swollen vulva that may express a thick vaginal discharge. Jills are generally sexually mature at 6 to 12 months of age. They are induced ovulators and will remain in estrus if they are not bred. If not induced, a jill can develop life-threatening estrogen-induced pancytopenia. Ferrets are long-day breeders. In the wild, the ferret breeding season is from March to August, although artificial lighting in captivity may induce a year-round breeding state for intact animals.

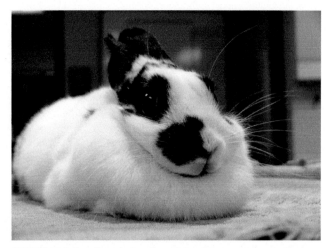

FIGURE 10-4 A female intact rabbit with a prominent dewlap. (Photo courtesy of Matthew S. Johnston.)

Gestation length is 42 days, and litters of 5 to 10 kits are common.[32,33] A spayed female ferret is known as a sprite.

Rabbits

Sexing rabbits, especially young rabbits, can be a challenge to the inexperienced practitioner or pet owner. The scrotal sacs do not develop in the male rabbit until approximately 3 months of age.[28] Female and male rabbits also have a similar anogenital distance. Sexing can be achieved by stretching the perineum, lifting the tail, and applying slight pressure to the slit located cranial to the anus. In males, the penis will be everted and is retromingent, meaning it is directed caudally, similar to a cat. The orifice will be circular in shape in males, whereas in females, the vulva will be more slit-like. One should always remember that female rabbits have a vaginal papilla that can be mistaken for a penis.[34] Although rabbits are not considered sexually dimorphic, one characteristic that can make intact rabbits look sexually dimorphic is the dewlap under the neck in female rabbits[28] (Figure 10-4). The dewlap will regress in size in spayed females or never develop if the rabbit is spayed early in life. Intact female rabbits use the dewlap as a source of fur to create a nest prior to parturition.

Unlike other placental mammals, male rabbits, or bucks, have two hairless scrotal sacs cranial to the penis on either side of the anus (Figure 10-5). This is similar to marsupials, whose penis is also located caudal to the testicles. The testes and epididymis descend into the sacs at about 12 weeks of age, therefore in young rabbits of this age, the scrotal sacs will not be visible or developed. Often, neutered males are sold as females or vice versa. It is always good practice to consciously sex the rabbit during a new patient examination to prevent future disease and possible unwanted breeding. Similar to rodents, the inguinal canals of rabbits remain open after the development of the scrotal sacs. Because of this, the testicles can be freely retracted into the abdominal cavity throughout life. This should be considered during castration in terms of postoperative monitoring. The testes may be guided into the scrotal sacs by applying gentle pressure to the caudal abdomen. Bucks do not have a glans or os penis, but they have white inguinal glands located to the side of the penis. These open by a single duct into folds of skin near the penis and produce

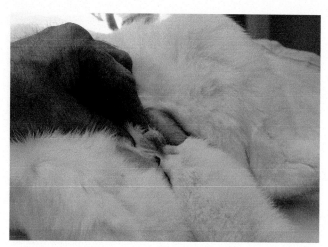

FIGURE 10-5 External male genitalia of a rabbit. The testicles are manually being descended into the hairless scrotal sacs on either side of the penis. (Photo courtesy of Matthew S. Johnston.)

a sebaceous odorous secretion associated with sexual attraction. Rabbits also possess ampullary, vesicular, prostatic, and bulbourethral glands as accessory sex glands that are rarely affected by disease processes.[30]

When compared with domestic mammals, several variations exist in the reproductive tract of rabbits. The reproductive tract of a doe (female rabbit) lacks a uterine body. Each of the uteri has a cervix and a separate opening into the vagina. The vagina is long and flaccid. The anatomy differs from rodents where the vagina exits through the vulvar cleft, which is external to the body and separate from the urethral exit. Rabbits have a common urogenital opening and the vagina ends just caudal to the pubic bone. The urethra opens along the proximal portion of the deep vaginal vestibule,[35] causing urine to pool in the vagina prior to urination. The mesometrium, or broad ligament, is a location for fat storage, which makes visualization of uterine vessels difficult during an ovariohysterectomy (OHE). Associated uterine vessels may be quite large in older female rabbits. Females have four sets of mammary glands located in the axillary, thoracic, abdominal, and inguinal regions. The best indication for sexual receptivity is lordosis, which is defined as a reverse arching or flattening of the back, raising of the pelvis in response to attempts of the buck's mounting, or chin rubbing. Also, the vulva may appear reddened and swollen. Does generally reach sexual maturity at 4 to 6 months of age, while bucks may reach sexual maturity at a slightly earlier age of 3 to 4 months. The average gestation period of a rabbit is 31 days. Like cats and ferrets, rabbits are induced ovulators and have no estrous cycle. Ovulation occurs 10 to 14 hours after copulation. Ten to 14 days after copulation, the does may be palpated for evidence of fetuses. Fetal bone structure will be radiographically evident in the last trimester of the pregnancy, or ~20 days.[34]

Hedgehogs

Hedgehogs (*Atelerix albiventris*) are unusual among exotic pet mammals kept as pets in the United States due to the fact they are classified as insectivores. Insectivores have novel features of the reproductive system that are not yet fully understood

and have yet to be studied in detail.[36] Hedgehogs are easily sexed when they are not "balled up". Unfortunately, general anesthesia is required on many hedgehog patients to facilitate a thorough physical examination. Similar to the ferret, the male hedgehog has a prepuce that is located on the midventral abdomen. In female hedgehogs, the vulva is located close to the anus. The anogenital distance of females is short compared to males, much like in rodents. Female hedgehogs have a large, long vagina that is always patent, unlike other small mammals that may only be receptive at certain periods of the estrous cycle (e.g., chinchillas [*Chinchilla lanigera*] and guinea pigs [*Cavia porcellus*]). In the abdominal cavity, the vagina is flanked by fan-shaped glands similar to the Cowper's gland in the male; these should not be confused as a mass on examination. Female hedgehogs have a bicornuate uterus with no uterine body and a single cervix.[36] The ovaries are located in a tough peritoneal capsule. The urethral opening is located in the distal portion of the vagina, several millimeters cranial to the vulva.[37] Hedgehogs have 3 pairs of mammary glands. Females reach sexual maturity at ~6 to 8 months of age. They are polyestrous and there is some evidence that they may be induced ovulators, given the fact they have been found to ovulate after an injection of human chorionic gonadotropin (hCG).[36] Female hedgehogs also may experience pseudopregnancy with sterile mating.[36] The gestation time of hedgehogs is 32 to 37 days. The most straightforward diagnostic test to determine pregnancy in a female hedgehog is evidence of weight gain. A weight gain of 50 g in a 2- to 3-week period after being with a male is indicative of pregnancy.[37] Young hedgehogs are known as pups or hoglets. Females may desert or kill their young in response to human contact, which should be minimized post pregnancy.

The male hedgehog penis has a prominent glans with lateral horns, giving it the appearance of a snail head.[36] Male hedgehogs do not have a scrotum, but the testicles can be palpated in the para-anal recesses, which are surrounded by fat. The reproductive accessory glands of the male hedgehog are quite extensive and consist of multilobed seminal vesicles, paired prostate glands, bulbourethral glands, and Cowper's glands.[37]

Hystricomorph Rodents

Hystricomorph rodents, such as guinea pigs, chinchillas, and degus, are so named because of the increased size of their infraorbital sinuses; however, they also possess unique reproductive characteristics in comparison to other rodents. In general, offspring of hystricomorph rodents are precocious, so they are born able to stand with their eyes open and teeth already present.

GUINEA PIGS. Both male and female guinea pig external genitalia consist of a Y-shaped depression in the perineal tissues, with the branches of the Y surrounding the urethral opening. In the female, these branches form the urogenital opening, which contains a U-shaped vulva and makes up the vaginal orifice. Females have a well-developed clitoris, which may be extruded through the urethral orifice. This may be mistaken for a penis. In males, the penis can be manually extended from the cup of the Y shape by placing pressure on either side of the prepuce.[38] In general, adult female guinea pigs are approximately 200 to 250 g smaller than the average adult male guinea pig.

Female guinea pigs, or sows, have paired uterine horns with a short uterine body. A single cervix opens to the vagina. A unique characteristic they possess is a vaginal closure membrane, which is only open at estrus, approximately day 26 to 27 of gestation, until parturition.[39,40] Female guinea pigs are nonseasonally polyestrous with spontaneous ovulation. The typical guinea pig estrous cycle lasts 15 to 17 days.[39] During ovulation, the vaginal membrane is open for 2 to 3 days but closes after ovulation.[30] Their gestation period spans an average of 68 days, which is extended when compared to other rodents. Young females reach puberty at 2 months of age. During estrus, the perineal color changes from a dull color to a deep red. Also during estrus, the female guinea pig produces Kurloff cells. These are large, mononuclear, granular lymphocytes that contain large intracytoplasmic inclusions. During estrogen stimulation, Kurloff cells are highly concentrated within the placenta. They may also be seen in peripheral blood smears, especially during estrus.[28]

Impending parturition is not always apparent since sows do not exhibit nesting behavior. In reproductively active females, the pubic symphysis is not fused. Palpating a gap within the symphysis may be indicative of impending parturition. Generally, separation is noted 2 days prior to parturition. Normal parturition is rapid, with only a few minutes in between births. Indications of dystocia include a depressed sow, bloody vaginal discharge, and an extended period of time between individual births.[39]

Male guinea pigs, also known as boars, have accessory sex glands including vesicular glands, a prostate gland, coagulating glands, and bulbourethral glands. These accessory glands contribute to forming a copulatory plug that will remain in the female tract after copulation. This prevents a second ejaculate from reaching fertilization. The copulatory plug remains in the female's tract until closure of the vaginal membrane. Discovery of a copulatory plug in the enclosure provides evidence of successful copulation. The seminal vesicles, or vesicular glands, are long, coiled, blind sacs, located ventral to the ureters. They are similar in appearance to the uterus and should not be mistaken for uterine horns.[28] Like rabbits, the testes are located in open inguinal canals; however, unlike rabbits and more typical to rodents, guinea pigs do not have a scrotum. Also unlike rabbits, but similar to ferrets and dogs, guinea pigs possess an os penis, which is located in a pouch. Two horned styles, or spicules, are everted from the pouch[40] and project externally during erection. Young male guinea pigs reach puberty at ~3 months of age.

CHINCHILLAS. The recommended method to externally sex a chinchilla is by measuring the anogenital distance which is shorter in females. Females have a long urinary papilla where the urethral orifice is located and can be mistaken for a penis. The vaginal orifice may not be readily noted since it is only open during estrus or birth. Female chinchillas are typically larger than males.[28]

Unlike guinea pigs and more like rabbits, female chinchillas have two uterine horns and two cervices. They have 3 pairs of mammary glands. Like guinea pigs, a vaginal membrane closes the vulva, except during estrus and parturition. Chinchillas (both male and female) reach sexual maturity at ~8 months. Also similar to guinea pigs, chinchillas are nonseasonally polyestrous and are spontaneous ovulators. During estrus, the perineum turns a deep shade of red. Expulsion of the copulatory plug by the female is a sign that mating has occurred. Pregnancy may be detected by palpation of the developing fetuses at 90 days. Gestation length is, on average, 111 to 114 days, which is likely the longest of all small exotic pet mammals. Chinchillas and guinea pigs are placentophagic, which describes animals that consume the placenta after birth. Blood on the nose and paws is an indication that the placenta has passed and the birthing process is complete.

Similar to guinea pigs and other rodents, male chinchillas do not have a scrotum. The testes are contained entirely in the inguinal canal, which is open, and therefore the testes can be withdrawn into the abdomen. A unique feature of male chinchillas is that they possess two small sacs next to the anus (postanal sacs) wherein the caudal epididymis can drop; these resemble the nonpendulous scrotum of a cat. Identical to guinea pigs, chinhillas also possess well-developed accessory sex glands. The vesicular gland provides the bulk of secretions involved in the copulatory plug. Chinchillas also have an os penis.

Marsupials

Sugar gliders (*Petaurus breviceps*) are one of the most popular marsupials kept as a companion exotic mammal in the United States. Sexing is straightforward in intact sugar gliders. Male sugar gliders have a pendulous scrotum originating from a stalk on the midventral abdomen. In general, marsupials differ from placental mammals with the presence of marsupial bones and pouches (marsupium). They also have a cloaca, which is similar to birds and reptiles. The cloaca is the site for exit of the reproductive, urinary, and gastrointestinal tracts. Due to the presence of the cloaca, cloacal temperatures will be significantly lower than a true rectal temperature. The sugar glider does not have marsupial bones, but does have a pouch. Intact males will develop a frontal scent gland on the dorsal skull and upper chest that may appear as a hairless area but should not be confused for alopecia. The male may be noted to rub the scent gland on a female's chest.

Other reproductive anatomy of the sugar glider differs considerably from that of the exotic companion mammals that has been described. Female sugar gliders are typically smaller than males. The female's reproductive tract consists of two equal halves. Each half is composed of a proximal component: ovary, oviduct, uteri, and vagina. There are two lateral and median vaginal canals forming the distal half. The median canal is short and the lateral canals are long. All marsupials give birth via the median vaginal canal. The three vaginal canals join and form a urogenital sinus that ends in the cloaca. Female marsupials also possess paracloacal glands that are more pronounced in males. Each pouch in a female sugar glider contains two mammae. Females reach sexual maturity at 8 to 12 months of age, are seasonally polyestrous, average a 29 day estrous cycle, and have a 15–17 day gestation length. A typical litter size is two joeys. The fetus is born early in gestation in an amniotic sac through the urogenital opening into the cloaca. It then breaks free from the sac and makes its way from the cloacal opening up to the pouch where it attaches to a teat. After a joey has entered the pouch, it will typically stay there for 70 to 74 days.[40] Often, the dam will lick this pathway. Generally, one dominant male will breed with all the mature females in the colony. After the joeys have been deposited in the pouch, they will stay there until they

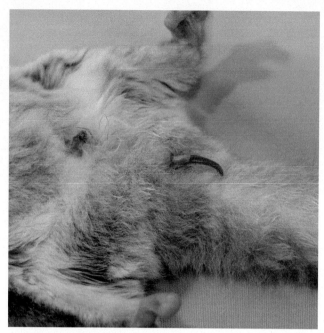

FIGURE 10-6 The forked penis of a sugar glider. (Photo courtesy of Matthew S. Johnston.)

outgrow the pouch. Joeys will then remain in the nest until they are weaned, which is ~110 to 120 days of age.[40]

Sugar glider males have a forked penis that lies on the ventrum of the cloacal floor (Figure 10-6). Males urinate from the proximal portion of the penis, not through the forked component. They have an external prepenile, pendulous scrotum on the midventrum. The scrotum is attached to the body wall via a long, narrow stalk. The permanently descended paired testes and epididymides located within the scrotum are ellipsoid. They are connected by vasa defentia to the prostatic portion of the urethra. This is comprised of a large prostate gland that constricts in the cranial third. Male sugar gliders also have two pairs of multilobed bulbourethral glands (Cowper's glands) that lie dorsal and lateral to the rectum[41] and three paracloacal glands.[42]

DISEASES ASSOCIATED WITH THE REPRODUCTIVE SYSTEM

Invertebrates

Reproductive diseases are uncommon in invertebrates. In most cases, the most tenuous situations result from typical mating behaviors and harm inflicted from their own species. It should be kept in mind that when breeding spiders, improper mating (e.g., time) may result in the death of the male. If the female is not receptive or the reproductive process is not performed properly, the female will often kill the male.

In breeding situations, females allowed to retain their egg sac are also at risk to cannibalize the egg sac if disturbed. Another common problem in captivity is fungal overgrowth of egg sacs. This may be due to environmental factors such as excessive moisture in the substrate, improper hygiene, and waste accumulation. If detected, the sac should be removed

from the female and opened. The eggs may then be sorted and the healthy eggs should be separated from the affected eggs. Problems may also occur in gravid females when they fail to lay all of their eggs.

Fish

Generally, reproductive diseases of captive fish are rare, with neoplasia being the most represented in the literature. Testicular and ovarian neoplasia has been described in koi and carp and should be a differential diagnosis for coelomic distension in a koi.[3] Testicular adenomas are common reproductive tumors found in goldfish and carp.[43] Other potential tumors include seminomas, dysgerminomas, teratomas, and Sertoli cell tumors.[2] Stress has also been associated with impaired reproductive function in cultured species, likely due to elevated cortisol concentrations.

Tissue coccidiosis is an uncommon problem in most fish, but has been known to cause serious reproductive disease as well. The infective stage, the sporozoite, is ingested and then penetrates the intestinal wall to reach the site of infection, ultimately forming an oocyst.[43] Infection sites can include reproductive organs in both males and females, causing parasitic castration in some species. A diagnosis may be made by identifying oocysts on a wet mount from affected tissue or histopathology. There are few published studies regarding treatment, but ponazuril, a coccidiocide, and monensin or sulfadimidine, coccidiostats, may be effective.[43]

Dystocia, or egg retention, can occur when captive fish are not exposed to normal temperature, light, or water quality, as they typically rely on these environmental cues to stimulate ovulation. It can be difficult to decide when to treat a fish for dystocia. Prolonged periods of a distended abdomen into late summer and early fall should be an indication of a problem. Noninvasive screening such as ultrasound may be helpful in determining whether the distended abdomen is due to eggs or another issue (e.g., ovarian cancer). Medical treatment with hCG at 20 IU/kg intramuscularly (IM) may be considered.[3] Often, these eggs can be manually stripped; however, after initial stripping, the fish often fail to lay properly in the future and require additional intervention. Ovarian prolapse may be a concurrent problem associated with dystocia, which will require surgical removal of the necrotic tissue present.

Amphibians

True reproductive disorders in amphibians are fairly rare. Successful reproduction in amphibians involves numerous stages of development including ovulation, spermiation, fertilization, oviposition, embryonic development, and metamorphosis. A problem at any of these stages can lead to reproductive failure. One of the most common problems observed in gravid female amphibians is a failure to lay some, or all, of their eggs. This can happen from stress during or before oviposition, unrelated illness, or a lack of appropriate environmental or physiologic stimuli for release. Unrelated illness may include infectious causes or neoplasia. Some reproductively active dendrobatid and hylid frogs will accumulate large amounts of fluid in the coelomic and subcutaneous tissues, which is typically a transudate in nature. Generally, as the fluid builds up, egg production declines. Affected females can be treated palliatively by removing fluid via aspiration. Soaking the frog in a hypertonic solution (e.g., sodium chloride) may remove fluid from the animal as well. The specific etiology associated with the fluid accumulation is unknown, but it has been speculated that it may be related to reproductive issues.

Cloacal prolapse may occur secondary to neoplasia, granulomatous disease, heavy parasite load, toxicosis, nutritional disorders, trauma, or gastrointestinal obstruction. Cloacal prolapse may occur in conjunction with a rectal, oviductal, or bladder prolapse. Often, the affected tissue will swell in the water and become edematous, taking on the appearance of a fluid filled balloon. In order to reduce the prolapse, the frog should be placed in a hypertonic solution. This will remove fluid from the prolapsed tissue thus improving one's chance of reducing the tissue. Radiographs, ultrasound, and blood ionized calcium concentrations may be used to determine an underlying cause of the prolapse (e.g., foreign body, nutritional secondary hyperparathyroidism). Prognosis for recovery depends on diagnosing the inciting cause of the prolapse as well as the response to treatment. Tissue that has become desiccated or devitalized may need to be removed, resulting in a poor prognosis.[9]

In cases of hypovitaminosis A, secondary reproductive disease may be observed in amphibian species. Hypovitaminosis A is often manifested as low reproductive success due to low fertilization rates, low egg numbers, early death of larvae, and failure of larvae to complete metamorphosis. Hypovitaminosis A specifically causes squamous metaplasia of mucus-secreting epithelial cells. Many affected amphibians are subclinical for the classic signs of hypovitaminosis A, such as short tongue syndrome (i.e., cannot withdraw prey into the mouth). Another classic sign would include white raised lesions in the periorbital area.[9] A thorough review of the patient's history and dietary testing should be performed to assess for hypovitaminosis A.

Reptiles

As is true for amphibian and reptile diseases involving other body systems, the majority of the reproductive diseases encountered in captive reptiles are often associated with improper husbandry. This is not true for all cases of reproductive disorders diagnosed in reptile species. Reproductive disease is commonly diagnosed in pet reptiles and will vary depending on species due to the vast diversity of animals in this class.

Follicular stasis is a common reproductive problem encountered in captive lizards. Follicular stasis, also known as preovulatory egg binding, needs to be distinguished from dystocia, which is defined in oviparous animals as postovulatory egg binding. Follicular stasis is characterized as a static condition of ovarian follicle development. Predisposing factors of preovulatory egg binding may include inappropriate husbandry (e.g., temperature, substrate, photoperiod) or poor nutrition. Clinical signs may be vague (e.g., lethargy and anorexia), with the most notable finding being a full or distended coelomic cavity.[44] Treatment options may include benign neglect, since follicles may be reabsorbed; correcting husbandry deficiencies; and surgery. In some cases, these follicles may rupture, leading to a more serious yolk coelomitis. Coelomic exploratory surgery and ovariectomy are the treatments of choice in suspected follicular stasis cases, especially in large lizards (e.g., green iguana).

In cases of dystocia, the follicles have (appropriately) ovulated into the oviduct, but the eggs are retained and not laid. It has been reported that dystocia occurs in ~10% of all captive reptiles. Snakes, chelonians, and lizards can all present for dystocia. There are two types of dystocias: obstructive and nonobstructive. In cases of obstructive dystocia, the reptile is unable to pass eggs through the oviduct and/or cloaca. Reasons for this include misshapen eggs or maternal abnormalities such as previous trauma or malformation of the pelvis or stenosis, oviductal stricture, or a space-occupying mass such as a cystic calculi, abscess, or fecolith.[16] Predisposing factors for reptiles diagnosed with dystocia include environmental or husbandry-related issues such as a lack of appropriate nesting sites, inadequate temperature, inappropriate humidity or photoperiod, or metabolic bone disease. Reptile patients with prolonged dystocia may exhibit clinical signs that are similar to secondary nutritional hyperparathyroidism, such as weakness and muscle tremors.

Dystocia in a chelonian is defined as "a failure to deposit eggs within a time considered usual for the species concerned" and is also referred to as egg retention.[14] This can be variable and subjective. Little is known about normal egg production and retention times among species. There are many likely etiologies for retained eggs in a chelonian. Inadequate nesting sites due to competition, interspecies aggression, or inappropriate environmental conditions are major causes for dystocia in chelonian species. Retained eggs can also occur secondarily to a specific disease process (e.g., hypocalcemia, hypokalemia, dehydration, systemic illness) or improper husbandry conditions (e.g., diet, lighting, temperature, humidity). In most cases of retained eggs, the cause is associated with a primary reproductive disease: oversized or misshapen eggs, infection, ectopic eggs, or endocrinopathy. The clinical signs may not become apparent until there are secondary concerns such as egg yolk coelomitis and straining or prolapse of oviductal structures. Retained eggs can also lead to infectious salpingitis and/or urinary or colonic obstruction due to the large size of the eggs. Clinical signs in affected animals include abnormal posture, hind limb paresis, anorexia, lethargy, straining, malodorous cloacal discharge, fecal or urinary retention, and cloacal organ prolapse. Often retained eggs are an incidental finding on routine radiographic studies and may not be the cause of a disease condition. On physical examination, eggs may be palpated in the inguinal region but should be distinguished from cystic calculi.

Cloacal prolapse can occur in all reptiles and should always be considered an emergency. In most cases the abnormal tissue is not readily identified by owners, but once noted the tissue should be covered and kept moist when transporting the animal to the clinic. Many reproductive structures may prolapse through the cloaca, including the phallus in chelonians and crocodilians, hemipenes in snakes and lizards, or the oviduct. Nonreproductive tract organs may also prolapse, including the gastrointestinal tract and urinary tract. Risk factors for cloacal prolapse include high reproductive output, hypocalcemia, and poor husbandry.[45] It should be noted that cloacal prolapse is a clinical sign, not a disease. Prolapse is often secondary to another issue that may cause straining, such as cystic calculi or gastrointestinal disease. Initial diagnostics should be performed to determine the primary cause of the prolapse. As in amphibians, radiographs may be helpful in assessing the bone density and any other space-occupying masses that may be causing secondary straining and prolapse. Hypocalcemia due to nutritional deficiency or reproductive depletion can reduce the ability of smooth muscle to contract, resulting in constipation and subsequent straining.

Male lizards and snakes may present with hemipenal prolapse. Underlying causes of himipenal prolapse include trauma, infection, or excessive breeding. In snakes, hemipenal prolapse is most often diagnosed in sexually mature, actively breeding boa constrictors (*Boa constrictor*) and ball pythons (*Python regius*). In lizards, it is more commonly associated with trauma following some form of excitement (e.g., lizard was startled and prolapsed its hemipenis) or nutritional secondary hyperparathyroidism (e.g., spinal abnormalities and neurologic damage). Iatrogenic trauma associated with probing an animal can also lead to hemipenal prolapse. The risk of hemipenal prolapse increases for snakes bred on particulate substrates. Prolapse may also occur if animals are physically separated before copulation is complete. The prolapsed hemipenis will appear as a solid tissue mass with no lumen protruding from the vent. Abscessation of the hemipenis may occur in snakes that have been used to breed a large number of females. Lizards with vitamin A deficiency may develop hemipenal plugs secondary to squamous metaplasia. In cases of a suspected infection, bacterial culture should be performed to guide treatment. It is important to clean the prolapsed hemipenis (warm sterile saline) and assess the tissue. If there is necrosis, hemipenal amputation is warranted. If the tissue is still viable, lavaging with a hypertonic solution (e.g., 50% dextrose) will reduce the associated edema and size of the tissue allowing for easier replacement with the aid of a lubricant. Placing two stay sutures in the vent will help prevent recurrence; the 2 sutures can remain in place for 5 to 10 days. It is important to confirm that the vent remain patent before discharging the animal. Figure 10-7 illustrates bilaterally necrosed hemipenes in a green iguana. In lizards with hemipenal plugs, removal of the adhered material is necessary. To prevent hemipenal prolapse, breeding males should not be placed with a large number of females. Also, it is recommended that the breeding environment

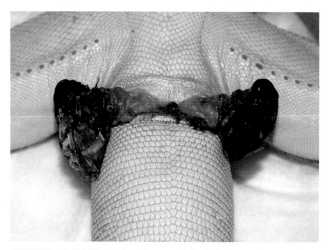

FIGURE 10-7 Bilateral prolapse of the hemipenes with hemipenal necrosis in an iguana. (Photo courtesy of Matthew S. Johnston.)

be cleaned regularly and be free of particulate substrate. Adequate nutrition is also necessary to prevent hemipenal plugs secondary to hypovitaminosis A and nutritional secondary hyperparathyroidism.[12]

Phallus prolapse may occur for a number of reasons in chelonians and crocodilians. Structural changes associated with nutritional secondary hyperparathyroidism may cause the shell or skin to grow abnormally, eventually exposing the cloaca and leading to a prolapse of the phallus. Phallus prolapse may also occur secondary to other systemic illness, neurologic dysfunction, excessive libido, trauma during breeding, infection, or straining from gastrointestinal disease or cystic calculi. Young growing chelonians may prolapse their phallus secondary to single pets mounting inappropriate objects or excessive breeding.

In snakes, lizards, and chelonians, the oviduct or shell gland may prolapse secondary to dystocia. Oviductal tissue can be identified in a prolapse by its longitudinal striations versus the smooth surface of the lumen of the colon. In most cases, the oviduct is too damaged to be manually replaced, in which case surgery will be required for removal. Many times, ova are still retained within the oviduct. Often, this condition is secondary to other illness. Indicators of cloacal disease in snakes may include passing of blood or discharge from the vent, straining, or obvious swelling around the vent or cloaca. Endoscopy may be used to evaluate the cloaca and samples collected for culture, biopsy, and/or cytology.[10] If the cause of the prolapse is not identified and corrected, recurrence is probable.

Reproductive tumors are rarely reported in reptiles; however, ovarian tumors reported in green iguanas include teratoma, dysgerminoma, adenocarcinoma, and a granulosa cell tumor. The granulosa cell tumor was diagnosed in a green iguana after failure to remove all ovarian tissue during a previous ovariosalpingectomy. It has been suggested that ovariectomy should be considered as an alternative to removing the oviduct, because if any ovarian tissue remains, it can regrow with subsequent folliculogenesis. Without the oviduct, normal oviposition is not possible and secondary complications will arise if the ovarian tissue is not completely excised.[46] A granulosa cell tumor has also been reported in a privately owned garter snake. The snake passed blood after periods of mating and ultimately experienced weight loss and weakness prior to death.[47]

Dystocia is much more common than follicular stasis in snakes. The predisposing factors for dystocia in snakes are similar to those for both chelonians and lizards, including inappropriate temperature and/or humidity, no nest site, inappropriate nesting substrate, malnutrition, and environmental stress. Many snakes require a covered box of damp moss or vermiculite for nesting. Poor body condition of the female may also contribute to dystocia. Presenting complaints may include visible coelomic swellings or nonspecific complaints of anorexia and lethargy; however, snakes may also be clinically normal. Although physical examination may reveal palpable masses indicative of eggs, it may be difficult to distinguish abnormal, retained eggs from normal eggs.[16] The eggs may be distributed throughout the lower third of the body or located in the cloaca. Radiography or ultrasonography may be used to confirm the number of eggs and any abnormalities in egg shape or size. In live-bearing snakes, ultrasound can be useful for determining whether fetuses the developing embryos are alive.

Birds

Reproductive disorders are one of the most common disease presentations of birds, regardless of whether owners are actively involved in maintaining the animal for breeding or it is simply a companion animal with or without a mate. Nutritional disorders may result in dysfunction of the reproductive tract. Vitamin E deficiency has been linked to perihatchling death due to underdevelopment of the pipping muscle.[22]

Chronic egg laying is a common problem observed in pet female birds. Excessive egg laying over a prolonged period of time may occur in any species of reproductively active hens; however, it is most commonly seen in finches, canaries, budgies, lovebirds, and cockatiels. Chronic egg laying occurs when a hen lays repeated clutches without regard to the presence of a normal mate or breeding season. Abnormal laying behavior occurs when hens lay more than two or three clutches per year; moreover chronic egg layers often lay more than the average two to four eggs per clutch.[20] Chronic egg laying is a presentation of an overactive reproductive tract that otherwise has normal function. This is a serious metabolic drain that will eventually exhaust the reproductive tract and also cause the patient to become immunocompromised. The metabolic drain on calcium stores also predisposes the bird to dystocia, yolk peritonitis, salpingitis, metritis, nutritional depletion, and osteoporosis. When the bird's calcium stores are depleted, eggs can become abnormally soft and thin shelled. These underdeveloped eggs can become impacted and contribute to the dystocia or obstruction in the oviduct.[20] If the underdeveloped eggs rupture, they can cause secondary oviductal adhesions or salpingitis. Predisposing factors may include increased artificial photoperiod, unbalanced or inadequate diet, presence of nesting materials, and presence of a perceived mate with associated inappropriate behavior (e.g., human cohabitant, cage furniture, toys). A thorough history should be obtained to identify environmental cues or issues that may be primary underlying factors associated with abnormal egg-laying behavior, specifically focusing on social interactions, environment, and diet. Initial diagnostics may reveal a leukocytosis characterized by a heterophilia and monocytosis due to chronic inflammation and possible secondary infection. Biochemistry results may reveal hypercalcemia or hypocalcemia depending on the reproductive status of the bird, hypercholesterolemia, and hyperglobulinemia.[48] Chronic egg laying is a concern, not only because of the increased risk of dystocia, but also as a chronic drain on calcium stores. Hypocalcemia can manifest itself as muscle fasciculations or seizures in affected birds.

Dystocia, commonly referred to as egg binding, is a common disease presentation of pet birds. When eggs fail to pass through the oviduct at a normal rate this is considered dysotcia. "Egg binding" can be characterized as a mechanical obstruction of the caudal oviduct, vaginal-cloacal junction, or cloaca. Dystocia may occur because an egg cannot pass due to its large size or is adhered to the oviductal mucosa, the oviduct is not functioning properly, or the oviduct has prolapsed with the egg still in the reproductive tract. There are many suspected etiologies for dystocia in pet birds, including muscle dysfunction caused by nutritional deficiencies such as

calcium, selenium, or vitamin E; misshapen or malformed eggs; excessive egg production; prior damage to the oviduct; obesity; minimal exercise; genetic abnormalities; age of the bird; tumors; infection of the reproductive tract; and stress factors such as environment changes (e.g., surroundings, temperature, social dynamic).[20,49–51] Smaller birds, such as budgerigars, canaries, lovebirds, and cockatiels, are most commonly affected. Dystocia should be considered an emergency presentation with the patient being assessed and stabilized immediately. The space-occupying effect of the egg can result in shock, circulatory disorders, and nerve paralysis secondary to the compression of pelvic and renal vasculature. Pressure necrosis from the egg can lead to the rupture of the oviductal wall, resulting in secondary coelomitis. Presenting clinical signs may include depression, fluffed feathers, open-mouth breathing, widened stance, decreased droppings or droppings primarily containing water, and ultimately a distended coelomic cavity with a palpable egg. Open-mouth breathing may be observed due to the retained egg acting as a space-occupying mass in the coelom, reducing the amount of available air sac space. If there is increased water content in the droppings, it may be because the rectum cannot resorb water due to a cloacal obstruction. Paresis of the left leg may occur secondarily to the egg compressing the sciatic nerve. The owner may have observed the bird straining to defecate or pass an egg along with persistent tail wagging. Winking of the vent may also be noted.

Follicular stasis may occur in birds and is defined as the formation of mature follicles on the ovary that fail to ovulate into the oviduct.[52] This condition is also known as cystic ovarian disease or preovulatory egg binding, similar to what was described in reptiles. Affected birds often present with nonspecific clinical disease signs, such as depression and inappetence. On physical examination, poor body condition along with distension of the caudal coelom may be noted. Many of the results from hematologic diagnostic tests (e.g. complete blood count, plasma chemistry panel) are similar to those associated with cases of chronic egg laying. Prognosis for birds diagnosed with follicular stasis is guarded for return to reproduction.

Cloacal prolapse may include prolapse of the oviduct, ureter, intestines, cloacal tissue, or phallus in certain species.[20] Causes of repeated cloacal prolapses may include neoplasia of the cloaca, oviduct, or uterus; cloacitis; ureteral obstruction; gastrointestinal foreign body; constipation; parasitism; or often, another concurrent reproductive disorder. A prolapse of the oviduct can be grossly differentiated from a cloacal prolapse by the corrugated appearance of the oviductal mucosa. An oviductal prolapse will often contain an egg (Figure 10-8). Cloacal prolapse is often secondary to another clinical disease, therefore a complete diagnostic workup should be performed to identify the inciting cause. In some cases, the etiology of the prolapse may never be identified.[53]

Coelomitis may occur due to a number of different reproductive diseases, including cystic ovarian disease, salpingitis, metritis, cystic hyperplasia, oviductal rupture, neoplasia, or an associated septicemia.[54] Reproductive-associated coelomitis can directly result from ectopic ovulation or egg yolk coelomitis. Egg yolk coelomitis transpires when egg yolk material is released into the coelomic cavity. It can develop into either an aseptic or septic condition. Egg yolk coelomitis is a serious

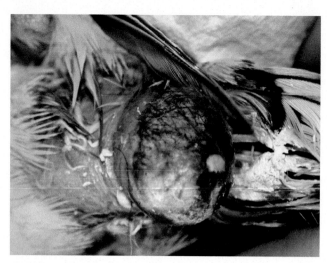

FIGURE 10-8 Oviductal prolapse with an egg in a female budgerigar. (Photo courtesy of Matthew S. Johnston.)

condition with a poor to grave prognosis, depending on how quickly the condition is detected and treated. It remains the most common fatal reproductive condition in captive birds. Acute signs of egg yolk coelomitis include decreased or a cessation of egg production, depression, anorexia, and a recent history of broodiness or egg laying. Abdominal swelling and ascites are common chronic clinical signs while respiratory distress may develop as a result of the decreased air sac space.[55] Complete blood count (CBC) and plasma biochemistry testing will often reveal a leukocytosis, hypercholesterolemia, and hypercalcemia. Cytologic examination of the coelomic fluid can be used to distinguish septic versus aseptic inflammation, and the fluid can also be analyzed for cell count, protein concentration, and bacterial or fungal culture and antibiotic sensitivity. Yolk material may also be identified on cytology. Treatment should include analgesic and anti-inflammatory medications, along with antibiotics if the bird is septic. In some cases, it may be necessary to surgically explore the coelom to remove foreign egg material or treat the underlying cause. Coelomocentesis may also be a helpful palliative treatment to reduce the volume of coelomic fluid and increase available air sac space.[25]

Ovarian and oviductal cancers are the most common tumor types found in the reproductive tract of captive birds. Neoplasia of the reproductive tract is most commonly reported in budgerigars. Ovarian tumors can enlarge to up to one-third of a bird's body weight, causing organ displacement. Ovarian tumors can invade renal tissue and cause compression of the sciatic nerve, which causes a left limb paresis.[56] The most common clinical sign in affected birds is dyspnea, which is secondary to abdominal organ enlargement and associated decrease in air sac space. Other clinical signs include abdominal distension, ascites, depression, inappetence, and chronic reproductive behavior. Secondary sex characteristics, such as the color of the cere, may also change in affected budgerigars.[20,49] Radiographic evidence of a mass in the area of the ovary may be indicative of a mass originating from the kidney or the ovary, as the ovary is located just cranial to the kidney, and it is difficult to distinguish these two organs from each other in a radiographic image. Functional ovarian tumors can

cause polyostotic hyperostosis (increased medullary bone density), which is best appreciated on radiographs and similar to what is observed in reproductively active hens.[57] Documented tumors of the reproductive tract of birds include adenocarcinoma, hemangiosarcoma, leiomyosarcoma, leiomyoma, adenoma, and carcinomatosis.[58,59] Cystadenoma and cystadenocarcinoma can also present with a left-sided lameness due to pressure on the lumbar plexus. These masses are large and have multiple cystic spaces. Surgical removal is indicated; however, it is difficult to achieve complete resection.[52]

Salpingitis (inflammation, or infection of the oviduct) and metritis (inflammation, or infection of the uterus) can occur in a bird for a number of different reasons. As previously mentioned, these can occur secondary to dystocia and ruptured eggs, as a result of an ascending infection, (e.g., from the gastrointestinal tract) or due to inflammation from surrounding tissues (e.g., air sacculitis). Salpingitis can cause a chronic condition and has been associated with the development of a large mass in the coelomic cavity.[60] Clinical signs are as previously described for dystocia and include subtle changes in breathing and activity level or appearance of the droppings. Salpingitis may also lead to dystocia of the oviduct by affecting motility.

Orchitis, or inflammation of the testis, in male birds is most often associated with infection. Clinical signs in affected birds may be vague (e.g., depression, inappetence) and only noted in breeding birds because of poor reproductive success.[54] Orchitis may occur as a result of an ascending infection, bacterial dissemination from associated organs, or hematogenous spread. Orchitis can be caused by a variety of different bacteria including *Escherichia coli*, *Salmonella* spp., and *Chlamydophila psittaci* in sexually active males. The latter may cause orchitis or epididymitis following a general systemic infection. Orchitis can lead to sterility, even with treatment. Enlarged testicles may be visible on radiographs; however, one should note that avian testes are normally enlarged during the breeding season. Diagnosis is often confirmed after obtaining a testicular biopsy via coelioscopy[25] and performing cytology, bacterial culture and antibiotic sensitivity testing, and histopathology.

Testicular neoplasia is not common in captive birds. However, when present, much like ovarian cancer, it appears to occur most commonly in male budgerigars. Owners often first note changes in the secondary sex characteristics of affected birds, such as a color change of the cere in the case of budgerigars. A change in behavior may also be observed, such as increased aggression.[20] Testicular tumors, like ovarian tumors, can have a presentation similar to that of renal cancer. As in female birds, reproductive tumors in males may result in unilateral paresis or paralysis of the leg, abdominal distension, or cyanosis of the pelvic limbs.[54] Seminomas and Sertoli and interstitial cell tumors have been diagnosed in birds.[52]

As with other species that possess a cloaca, such as lizards and tortoises, cloacal disease can affect both sexes in birds. Disease includes cloacitis due to bacterial or fungal infection, inflammation, cancer, or prolapse. Cloacoliths can develop into large concretions and, in some cases, cause obstruction of the cloaca, resulting in urinary and fecal obstruction. Clinical signs may include tenesmus, hematochezia, decreased dropping size or production, soiling/staining of the vent, change in posture, prolapse, lethargy, anorexia, or an inability to lay eggs. On external examination of the vent, size, symmetry, and tone should be evaluated. Internal examination should also be performed. To perform an examination of the cloacal mucosa, the tissue should be everted. In order to evert cloacal mucosa, a lubricated swab should be gently inserted into the cloaca and then gently retracted. The mucosa may then be examined for health, ulceration, lesions, or possible masses. Swabs may be collected for bacterial or fungal cultures as well as cloacal cytology. Owners should be informed that the bird might have a small amount of blood in their droppings 24 to 48 hours after the cloacal examination.

A cloacal examination should always be performed on New World psittacines (e.g., macaws, *Ara* spp.; Amazon parrots, *Amazona* spp.). These birds have a predisposition to develop cloacal papillomas in both sexes. However, this does not exclude Old World psittacines from being affected, as cases have been reported in African greys *(Psittacus erithacus)* and cockatoos *(Cacatua* spp.).[61,62] During cloacal eversion, small, raised lesions may be noted on the wall of the cloaca, along with discoloration of the mucosa. Although there is still some debate, a herpesvirus has been proposed as the underlying etiologic agent. A herpesvirus has been isolated from cloacal papillomas of African greys[61] and multiple New World parrots.[63,64] Papillomavirus has also been isolated from papilloma lesions in African grey parrots, but it does not appear to be responsible for the development of lesions in unrelated birds.[65] There have also been documented cases where neither a papillomavirus nor a herpesvirus was isolated from a papilloma lesion.[62] In severe cases, the papillomas may become large enough to cause tenesmus and obstruction. Associated inflammation and straining can lead to subsequent cloacal prolapse.[54] In cases where large papillomatous lesions are adversely affecting the patient's health, surgical removal may be required. Removal is a palliative treatment and will not cure the disease. Pet owners should be aware that regrowth is highly likely. Scarring and subsequent stricture formation may also occur after surgical removal. Although the exact correlation is unknown, cloacal papillomatosis has been diagnosed in birds (e.g., Amazon parrots, macaws) with concurrent biliary, hepatic, intestinal, and pancreatic carcinomas.[66-69] Papillomas are fairly benign; however, they can spread cranially throughout the gastrointestinal tract which results in more serious side effects. At this time there is no known treatment that will slow the progression or development of papilloma growths; however, anecdotally, an antiviral medication may help to curb the progression of the disease. Lysine has also been recommended for treatment, although its efficacy is unknown. Papillomas should not be the only differential disease diagnosis for a cloacal mass. Cloacal fibrosarcoma,[70] carcinoma, and leiomyoma/sarcoma have all been documented in pet birds.

As previously mentioned, poor nutrition and hypovitaminosis can lead to a variety of reproductive disorders. The most common vitamin deficiencies related to reproductive disease in birds is A and D. Birds offered a seed-only diet are more susceptible to developing hypovitaminosis A. Vitamin A deficiency can manifest in the reproductive tract as poor egg laying and decreased sexual activity. Hypovitaminosis D, which can contribute to a hypocalcemic condition is linked to the development of thin-shelled, soft eggs and an increased rate of early embryonic death.[71]

Mammals

Rodents

Neoplasia is one of the most common disease conditions diagnosed in mice and rats. However, the presentation and pathophysiology associated with cancer in these two species differ. In mice, mammary tumor formation has been shown to have a viral etiology. The mouse mammary tumor virus is passed placentally and through milk.[30] Mammary adenocarcinomas and fibrosarcomas are the most common tumors found in mice. Most mammary tumors in mice and gerbils are malignant and frequently have either ulcerated or metastasized by the time of initial diagnosis. These tumors have a tendency to be invasive and difficult to surgically remove. Mass removal does not prolong survival time in affected mice due to the malignant nature of the cancer. Early ovariectomy does not appear to limit the development of this cancer in mice, possibly because the etiologic agent is a virus.

The most common tumor in rats, a subcutaneous fibroadenoma, also targets mammary tissue. Females have an increased risk for developing mammary tumors with age, specifically after 14 months of age. Males have an increased risk as well, after 16 months, although the incidence of disease is much lower in males than females.[72] An incidence of 2% to 16% has been reported in male rats.[73] Hormones, primarily estrogen and prolactin, are thought to play a role in the development of these tumors.[30] Mammary gland development occurs during puberty under the influence of estrogen. Early neutering is recommended as a preventive measure to reduce the incidence of mammary tumors in rats. Ovariectomy of young female rats has been shown to decrease the potential for the development of mammary neoplasia.[74] By neutering a rat before it reaches sexual maturity, the estrogen influence during mammary growth is removed, essentially, limiting the growth of mammary tissue. There is also an increased risk of mammary cancer in rats that have a prolactin-secreting pituitary tumor. In contrast to mouse mammary gland tumors, these are benign tumors. Affected rats present with well-circumscribed, mobile, firm, subcutaneous masses that can be located at any location within the extensive mammary tissue. The tumors grow rapidly and can reach extremely large sizes, eventually affecting the rat's mobility and quality of life (Figure 10-9). When the tumors grow to large sizes, they also tend to ulcerate and become painful. Ulceration also predisposes rats to secondary infections that could lead to death. Standard surgical protocols are followed for removal of rat mammary tumors.

Urethral plugs are a normal finding in healthy, intact male rats, gerbils, hamsters, mice, and guinea pigs.[75] However, urethral plugs have been associated with urethral obstruction in rats and mice.[76] When a urethral obstruction occurs the plug may be manually removed via catheterization. Urethral plugs are composed of proteins from the seminal vesicles mixed with vesiculase from the coagulating glands, which then congeal to form the plug.[77,78] The size of the plug decreases after castration.

Rodents are prolific breeders and generally do not have many issues associated with breeding or parturition. In mice, the most common problems encountered are uterine

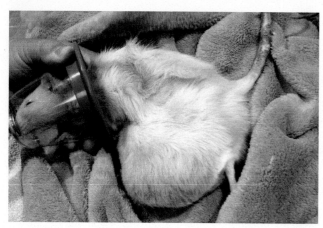

FIGURE 10-9 Large mammary tumor in a rat. (Photo courtesy of Matthew S. Johnston.)

and/or vaginal prolapse after parturition. Treatment includes replacing the tissue into a normal anatomical position and placing a purse-string suture around the vaginal orifice.[79] In rats, focal mammary abscesses are more common than diffuse mastitis. *Pasteurella pneumotropica* and *Staphylococcus aureus* are most commonly isolated from rat mammary abscesses.[28] Female hamsters normally secrete a copious amount of white, milky discharge at the end of their 4 day estrous cycle. The discharge will fill the vagina and often can be extruded in a thread-like fashion. The discharge is often mistaken by owners as pus or an indication of infection, but it is a normal phenomenon.[79]

Cannibalism accounts for a significant amount of mortality in preweanling hamsters, with up to a 97.5% mortality rate being noted in preweanling hamsters in a group-housed laboratory setting.[80] Cold temperatures and low body weights may contribute to death in young hamsters.[81,82] Owners should be advised to leave the mother hamster an ample amount of food and avoid disturbing her for 1 to 2 weeks after birth. A lean diet may also be a predisposing factor to cannibalism; therefore, pregnant female hamsters should be provided with additional caloric intake (including fresh fruit, greens, moist mash, dried milk) prior to parturition. Having noted this, some breeding facilities that provide these conditions still see a high rate of cannibalism. It is unknown whether cannibalism of young occurs because the mother is eliminating sick or weak offspring or it is associated with some other stress in the environment.[80]

There is a high incidence of ovarian disease in female Mongolian gerbils that are ≥2 years of age. Ovarian cysts and neoplasia are the 2 most common types of ovarian disease diagnosed in this species. Presenting complaints may include abdominal distension, bilateral alopecia, weight loss, decreased appetite, decreased litter size, and infertility. On physical examination, enlarged ovaries may be palpated. The respiratory effort of affected gerbils may be increased secondary to chest compression from large ovarian cysts. Cystic disease in gerbils is very similar to that of guinea pigs, which is discussed later. Granulosa cell tumors are the most common ovarian tumor to affect gerbils. An OHE is the treatment of choice for both diseases. Large blood-filled cysts may be associated with granulosa cell tumors. Aspiration of these cysts or removal may lead to hypovolemic shock.[83]

Ferrets

Primary reproductive tract disorders of ferrets are discussed in this chapter; however, it should be kept in mind that these diseases are becoming less common in the United States. The majority of the pet population of domestic ferrets in the United States is obtained from commercial breeding farms where the animals are neutered or spayed at or before 6 weeks of age. However, secondary disease syndromes, such as adrenal gland disease, are often diagnosed as a result of this practice. In contrast to small animals, such as dogs, where adrenal gland disease typically affects the zona glomerulosa and fasciculata layers, adrenocortical disease in ferrets affects the deepest cortical layer of the adrenal gland, the zona reticularis. The zona reticularis is the layer that is responsible for androgen production, including estradiol, 17α-hydroxyprogesterone, androstenedione, and dehydroepiandrosterone sulfate. Overproduction of these androgenic hormones in females may be clinically manifested as a swollen vulva and in males may result in prostatic cysts, prostatomegaly, and secondary urethral obstruction. In both males and females, adrenal gland disease will commonly result in alopecia, pruritis, and muscle atrophy due to excessive hormonal production.[84]

In intact female ferrets (jills) that have not mated, prolonged estrus may result in bone marrow toxicity from chronic elevations of estrogen.[33] This is also known as hyperestrogenism, estrogen toxicity, or postestrus anemia. Ferrets are one of the animals most susceptible to the toxic effects of estrogen. Since ferrets are induced ovulators, intact jills will remain in estrus if not bred. Normally, breeding will induce ovulation allowing for pregnancy or pseudopregnancy.[85] Elevated estrogen concentrations due to prolonged estrus is most common in young (<1 to 2 years of age) jills, whereas clinical signs of prolonged estrus in ferrets >2 years of age are often secondary to adrenal gland disease. Adrenal gland disease rarely leads to clinical hyperestrogenism. Hyperestrogenism may occur when intact jills are housed in artificial lighting environments with prolonged photoperiods over 12 hours, are not bred, and therefore remain in estrus throughout the year. Clinical signs will typically become apparent when the jill is in estrus for >1 month. Other causes of hyperestrogenism include structural abnormalities such as a cystic ovary or an ovarian remnant. In two cases, alopecia was found to be due to excessive hormone production via tumor formation in an ovarian remnant.[86] Hyperestrogenism is a serious disease condition in ferrets and can result in bone marrow suppression and hypoplasia of all cell lines. As previously mentioned, initial clinical signs may be similar to adrenal gland disease or estrus (e.g., swollen vulva and bilateral alopecia). As the disease progresses, other clinical signs may develop, including anorexia, lethargy, a systolic heart murmur secondary to the anemia, petechial and ecchymotic hemorrhages, pale mucous membranes, and melena. Early CBC results may show a neutrophilia and thrombocytosis; however, by the time the disease is detected, CBC results will commonly show a nonregenerative anemia, neutropenia, thrombocytopenia, and hematocrit of <20%.[85] Similar to other small mammals, the risk of spontaneous bleeding occurs when the platelet count is <20,000 cells/mL.

The most common cause of death in these cases is hemorrhage secondary to thrombocytopenia.[33] The prognosis is often correlated to the degree of anemia present. A hematocrit of >25% is associated with a fair to good prognosis after performing an OHE, whereas a hematocrit of <15% is associated with a guarded to grave prognosis.[85] This disease can be prevented by spaying all intact jills not intended for breeding purposes. If being used for breeding, jills should not be in estrus for >2 to 4 weeks. Jills may either be housed outside or in a controlled artificial lighting environment to prevent prolonged reproductive stimulation.

In pregnant jills, diseases such as dystocia, pregnancy toxemia, agalactia, and mastitis may occur. In domestic ferrets, dystocia is relatively uncommon; however, it is defined as labor lasting longer than 12 to 24 hours or whenever difficulty during labor is observed.[85] Pregnancy toxemia is diagnosed in jills and usually occurs during the last 10 days of gestation.[87] As with rabbits, primiparous jills are more likely to be affected. Also, jills are more likely to be affected if they are carrying >10 kits. Proper nutritional support during pregnancy is necessary, as toxemia is almost always associated with inadequate nutrition or fasting.

Pseudopregnancy may occur after ovulation if failure of implantation occurs. When pseudopregnancy occurs, the physical changes associated with pregnancy are evident. Jills may experience weight gain, nesting behavior, and development of mammary tissue. The main physical difference between pseudopregnancy and pregnancy occurs 1.5 weeks prior to "whelping," when pseudopregnant jills develop a full hair coat. Pregnant jills lose their hair coat and develop hairless rings around their nipples prior to whelping. Reduced light intensity prior to breeding may increase the likelihood of a pseudopregnancy. Also, ensure that hobs are mature and fertile prior to breeding. After "whelping," pseudopregnant jills will return to a normal estrus.

Pyometra, hydrometra, and mucometra should be considered as differentials for a fluid-filled uterus in a ferret. Pyometra may occur as a result of ascending bacteria from the vagina.[85] Stump pyometra is occasionally diagnosed secondary to adrenocortical disease due to excess sex steroid production.[88] Pyometra in jills may also occur in conjunction with hyperestrogenism. Treatment for pyometra includes OHE and appropriate antibiotic and fluid therapy. Hydrometra is the accumulation of aseptic fluid in the uterus and occurs as a result of a persistent corpora lutea. Predisposing factors for hydrometra are not always identified; however, it is often associated with an ovarian tumor.[85,86]

Neoplasia of the ferret female reproductive tract is a relatively common finding. Ovarian tumors are often an incidental finding when performing an OHE. A retrospective study found ovarian leiomyoma as the most common reproductive tumor in jills.[89] In spayed females, tumors may also occur in the ovarian pedicle remnant. Generally, an OHE is the treatment of choice and usually curative. Metastasis is not commonly seen with reproductive tumors in ferrets.

Mastitis may occur in ferrets and may be characterized as acute or chronic. Acute mastitis may occur immediately after whelping or after the third week of nursing when kits become more aggressive feeders due to peak milk production. This can cause excess stress to the jill or cause the kits to physically injure the teats. Acute mastitis can become severe and

gangrenous within just a few hours. Chronic mastitis may develop secondary to acute mastitis or also 3 weeks after whelping. In contrast to acute mastitis where the clinical signs are dramatic, clinical signs associated with chronic mastitis may be subtle. The glands may be firm and appear to be full of milk; however, the glandular tissue will have been replaced by fibrotic tissue and will not be painful or discolored. The most obvious problem encountered in chronic mastitis cases will be the poor condition of the kits, as they may continue to grow in size, but not weight, as a result of the inadequate nutrition. Systemic antibiotics should be used to treat both chronic and acute mastitis. It may be helpful to culture the milk prior to starting antibiotic therapy. In severe cases of gangrenous acute mastitis, surgical excision may be required.

Prostatic disease is the most common reproductive disorder in both neutered and intact males, with the highest incidence occurring in middle-aged (3 to 4-years-old) to older neutered animals. Enlargement of the prostate can lead to urinary tract disease. In some cases, the prostatomegaly may result in complete urinary obstruction due to compression of the urethra. Presenting complaints associated with the patient's condition may include lower urinary tract signs such as pollakiuria, stranguria, hematuria, or anuria.[85] Owners may confuse stranguria as constipation. Affected animals may excessively lick at their prepuce, leading to redness and irritation. Ferrets with prostatic abscesses or prostatitis may be pyrexic, anorexic, and lethargic. In cases of urethral obstruction, the ferret may be lethargic and depressed due to azotemia. On physical examination, prostatomegaly may be palpable as a fluctuant structure located dorsal to the bladder.

Frequently clinical signs of adrenal gland disease such as alopecia, pruritis, and increased sexual behavior may accompany lower urinary tract disease signs. Often, prostatomegaly, prostatic cysts, prostatitis, and prostatic abscesses are noted in conjunction with adrenal gland disease.[90] Adrenal gland disease is thought to be common in the United States because ferrets are neutered or spayed at a young age. Outside of the United States, hobs are not routinely castrated until several months of age, therefore adrenal disease is relatively uncommon. A retrospective study in The Netherlands, where ferrets are neutered at an older age, suggested that age at neutering may be associated with the development of hyperadrenocorticism.[91] It is postulated that adrenal tumors develop secondary to chronic stimulation by LH. Although the exact mechanism is unknown, elevated circulating androgenic hormones are thought to stimulate production of prostatic glandular tissue. This can lead to the development of sterile prostatic cysts.[85] The prostatic glandular tissue may be infiltrated and become cystic and inflamed, which creates an environment conducive to bacterial prostatitis. Bacterial prostatitis and/or prostatic cysts may also cause urinary semiblockage and urine stasis due to prostatomegaly, promoting bacterial growth in the urine and subsequent migration into prostatic tissue. Often, the prostatitis can mimic a bacterial cystitis due to the communication with the bladder. Prostatitis may also results in a thick white or yellow discharge from the penis that may or may not be associated with urination.

Rabbits

One of the most common reproductive diseases seen in rabbits is uterine adenocarcinoma. It is the most common neoplasia of female rabbits.[92] Age has been shown to be the most important risk factor for this cancer. In intact does >3 years of age, the incidence of uterine adenocarcinomas may approach 80%.[93] Spaying rabbits at a young age will prevent the occurrence of this cancer. The incidence of uterine adenocarcinomas has greatly decreased in the United States due to education regarding the importance of spaying female animals. Veterinarians treating exotic small mammals should be aware that client education is an important tool for prevention. In cases where educated owners do not elect preventive OHE surgery, the importance of biannual examinations of intact female rabbits after the age of 3 should be stressed for early detection of this tumor.[94] It is strongly recommended that female rabbits be spayed before 2 years of age to prevent the development of uterine adenocarcinomas. Also, if a rabbit is spayed before 1 year of age, there will be significantly less intra-abdominal fat present thereby improving exposure during the surgical procedure. With uterine adenocarcinoma, the endometrium undergoes progressive changes, invades the myometrium (which can extend through the uterine wall to the peritoneal cavity), and eventually spreads hematogenously to the lungs, liver, and brain. If caught early, the disease may appear as endometrial hyperplasia[95] but can progress to uterine adenoma and eventually uterine adenocarcinoma. Clinical signs for all stages of uterine tumor development are similar. Often, the owner's presenting complaint for their rabbit will be hematuria or a serosanguinous vaginal discharge; however, other common complaints include swollen abdomen or suspected pregnancy. Clinical signs in breeding does can include reduced fertility, small litters, abortion, or stillbirth. On physical exam, it may be possible to palpate an enlarged uterine horn or nodular mass in the abdomen. This cancer may also be associated with fluid accumulation in the abdomen. An inflammatory leukogram may be noted on a CBC. In rabbits, often the first sign of inflammation is thrombocytosis.[93] An OHE is curative if the disease has not yet metastasized; however, it is possible that microscopic disease could be present and would not be detected with standard diagnostic testing (e.g., radiographs or ultrasound). The tumor is generally slow growing, although it can spread via local and hematogenous routes.[96] The most common site for metastasis is the lung(s). Rabbits without evidence of pulmonary metastases at the time of surgery should be rechecked later because early metastases may have not been (radiographically) apparent.[94,95] Mammary adenocarcinoma may also be associated with uterine adenocarcinoma.[95] A thorough palpation and examination of the mammary tissue should be performed prior to surgery.

As mentioned previously, uterine disease in rabbits may occur on a continuum, as in humans. Endometrial changes may start with polyp formation but progress to cystic hyperplasia, adenomatous hyperplasia, and finally adenocarcinoma. However, there are some reports that suggest that there is no association between cystic hyperplasia and adenocarcinoma. Regardless, all of these changes are associated with aging. Clinical signs of endometrial hyperplasia can mimic that of adenocarcinoma and may include intermittent hematuria, lethargy, or anemia. Concurrent development of cystic mammary glands and ovaries may also be observed. Often, a tubular mass may be palpated in the caudal abdomen. As in the case of adenocarcinoma, OHE is the treatment of choice.[94]

Pyometra and endometritis are other common reproductive disorders in female rabbits. Similar to other small mammals, clinical signs commonly include vaginal discharge, anorexia, lethargy, and a possible distended abdomen. Pyometra is usually reported shortly after a rabbit delivers her young.[97] In breeding does, early endometritis may be subtle. A rabbit may appear clinically normal but may have a recent history of parturition and subsequent infertility. On physical examination, a large, doughy uterus may be palpated. If noted, extra care should be taken when palpating the doe, as the uterine walls can become extremely thin and friable in cases of endometritis. Ultrasound is an important diagnostic tool that can be used to differentiate a fluid-filled uterus from a uterine mass, polyp, or cystic changes. Cytology and culture of vaginal discharge may also be an important tool in identifying a bacterial etiology or inflammation. Abdominal exploratory surgery along with an OHE is the treatment and procedure of choice to confirm a diagnosis and remove the diseased tissue. Tissues should be submitted for histopathology, as pyometra may occur secondary to uterine adenocarcinoma. A culture should be taken intraoperatively. *Pasteurella multocida* and *Staphylococcus aureus* are the most common pathogens isolated in rabbit pyometra and endometritis cases. Venereal transmission of pathogenic bacteria can occur between infected bucks and does. Postpartum metritis in does can also occur secondary to hypervitaminosis A. For cases with mild endometritis, treatment with antibiotics, fluid, and anti-inflammatory therapy may be sufficient; however, one should remember that due to the caseous nature of the rabbit inflammatory processes (i.e., abscesses), this may be insufficient and OHE will be required.

Other less common reproductive abnormalities of the female rabbit include uterine torsion, extrauterine pregnancies, and dystocia.[98,99] Extrauterine pregnancies have been documented, and extrauterine or abdominal pregnancies most commonly occur secondary to fetal implantation originating in the uterus.[100] Due to trauma or decreased viability of uterine tissue, the fetus enters the abdominal cavity through a perforation in the uterus. Primary extrauterine pregnancies are less common and occur when a fertilized ovum fails to travel the normal route and instead is passed into the abdominal cavity.[101] Ectopic pregnancies have been reported in rabbits with apparently normal intact reproductive tracts and also with evidence of a ruptured vaginal wall.[102] Affected rabbits present for failure of parturition and will have a palpable mass in the abdomen. The most common outcome of an extrauterine pregnancy is fetal mummification but, in most cases, will not clinically affect the rabbit and may only be an incidental finding on necropsy.

While dystocia is rare in rabbits, it is important to be aware of normal gestation and parturition parameters when counseling clients. Gestation in rabbits averages 31 to 32 days but can last anywhere from 28 to 36 days. Normally, delivery of all young is complete within 30 minutes of onset. Normal litter size may vary from 4 to 12 animals. Similar to other mammals, predisposing factors for dystocia include obesity, small pelvic canal diameter, abnormally large fetuses, or uterine inertia. Clinical signs of dystocia may include persistent straining or abnormal vaginal discharge that has a bloody to brownish-green consistency. It is recommended to take radiographs before initiating therapy to determine whether the delivery problem is primarily mechanical or physiologic. If the fetuses are determined to be too large to pass through the pelvic canal, medical therapy may be initiated. If not, surgery is required.

Endometrial venous aneurysms may occur in conjunction with the changes in the uterus noted during progression to uterine adenocarcinoma. These aneurisms may cause episodic bleeding, which manifests clinically as hematuria. Cylindrical-shaped clots may form in the uteri and pass into the urine. In rabbits with this condition, multiple blood-filled endometrial veins rupture into the lumen of the uterus.[103] The blood loss may lead to a significant anemia, or if severe enough, fatal exsanguination. Treatment includes stabilizing the patient and performing an OHE.

Pseudopregnancy can occur in breeding rabbits or individually housed rabbits that are not bred. Affected animals may initiate normal nesting behaviors and show signs of mammary development. This condition is often self-limiting, although it may lead to hydrometra or pyometra. Pseudopregnancy in rabbits generally lasts 16 to 17 days. The specific cause of pseudopregnancy in the rabbit is unknown. An OHE is the treatment of choice.[94,97]

Pregnancy toxemia may also occur in does and is commonly diagnosed during the last week of pregnancy. Around that time, does also start exhibiting nesting behavior, pulling the hair from their hip and dewlap area and decreasing their food intake. The hair pulling may lead to hairball formation secondary to inappetence and gastrointestinal ileus. Similar to other animals, obese rabbits frequently are predisposed to pregnancy toxemia, although the exact causes leading to pregnancy toxemia are unknown. There appears to be a predilection for this disease in the Dutch and Polish breeds.[119] Progression of the disease may be acute or chronic. In severe cases, the rabbit may be dyspneic and have ketotic breath. The urine of affected does becomes acidic, giving it a clear color (i.e., reduced calcium carbonate crystals). Hepatic changes, such as hepatic lipidosis, may occur in some does. Evaluating hepatic enzyme activities may be helpful in determining the condition of the patient's liver. Pregnancy toxicity carries a grave prognosis despite intensive supportive care with fluid therapy, nutritional support, and/or analgesia. For this disease, prevention is key. Rabbits should be encouraged to continue eating and avoid fasting or stress during late pregnancy. Although not typically recommended, alfalfa hay and pellets may be fed to increase caloric intake until after the young are weaned.[94]

Infections of the reproductive tract can occur in both bucks and does. Orchitis, epididymitis, and metritis are most common.[104] Orchitis and epididymitis may develop via venereal transmission and are typically caused by a bacterial infection. In exotic pet mammals, mastitis most commonly affects guinea pigs, rabbits, and rats. Rabbits may develop a unique cystic mastitis that typically occurs in nonbreeding does >3 years of age.[105] Cystic mastitis may cause does to exhibit signs of pseudopregnancy and often occurs concurrently with cystic endometrial hyperplasia. Affected rabbits present with swollen mammary glands. Since cystic mastitis typically occurs along with uterine disease, clinical signs associated with uterine disease, such as hematuria, may also be reported. On physical examination, it may be possible to express a serosanguinous fluid from the mammary glands. Bacterial mastitis should be ruled out via fine-needle aspiration (FNA), cytology, and bacterial culture. An OHE is the recommended treatment for cystic mastitis. If the OHE is not curative, removal of the affected mammary gland(s) should be considered. If left untreated, cystic mastitis may progress to benign and eventually malignant neoplasia.[105]

Inflammation and infections may occur acutely during lactation due to teat trauma by the young (with milk serving as a nidus for bacterial growth through the teat canal) or bacteria entering through the bloodstream. Predisposing factors for bacterial mastitis include abrasive bedding, unsanitary conditions, and mammary impaction. Clinical signs of mastitis in rabbits include enlargement of the affected glands, a purulent-to-bloody discharge from the teat(s), pyrexia, anorexia, depression, increased thirst, and death of the neonates. The affected glands may also be hyperemic, cyanotic, warm, and painful. The skin over the mammary glands is initially pink to red but will eventually become blue to purple. This is why the mastitis in rabbits is commonly referred to as blue breast.[101] In rabbits, the most common bacterial pathogens isolated in mastitis cases are *Staphylococcus aureus*,[106,107] *Pasteurella* spp., and *Streptococcus* spp. Parenteral penicillin is the treatment of choice for this disease, unless culture and antibiotic sensitivity testing suggest otherwise. It is important to note that penicillin should never be given orally (PO), as it can cause a life-threatening bacterial dysbiosis. Supportive care including fluid therapy, assisted feeding, analgesia, and warm compresses is also recommended.[28] Fostering young from an affected doe to a healthy doe is not recommended due to the possible risk of disease transmission. Young rabbits should be removed from affected does to prevent bacterial enteritis or starvation.

Venereal spirochetosis is caused by *Treponema paraluiscuniculi*, which is also known as rabbit syphilis, treponematosis, or vent disease. This is a sexually transmitted disease of rabbits that is passed during direct and venereal contact. It is not a zoonotic disease. Both males and females can be affected. Lesions appear on the skin of the perineum and genitalia. Initially, erythema may be noted on the prepuce or vulva, but the lesions can soon progress to edema, vesicles, ulcerations, and a dry scaliness of the tissues. Autoinfection can lead to proliferative facial lesions around the chin, lips, nostrils, and eyelids (Figure 10-10). These lesions are likely painful and can lead to excessive grooming and nasal discharge, with subsequent ulceration of the tissue. Rabbit syphilis can develop into an epidemic in a rabbitry that results in decreased conception rates, increased incidence of metritis, retention of the placenta, and increased neonatal deaths. The distribution of the lesions is generally sufficient to make a presumptive diagnosis; however, lesions on the face may initially be mistaken for dermatophyte or bacterial dermatitis lesions. A definitive diagnosis can be obtained through skin biopsy and silver staining of the tissue.[28,94] The skin biopsy and cytology also may be examined via fluorescent antibody dark-field microscopy. Both of these techniques require visualization of spirochetes from active lesions, which may or may not be present. Microhemagglutination tests and other serologic tests may be used to screen and verify infected animals in a large rabbitry setting. Carrier bucks are often subclinical carriers until they are stressed, although examination may reveal a star-shaped scar on the scrotum. The recommended treatment protocol

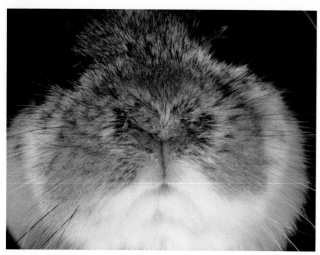

FIGURE 10-10 Nasal lesions associated with venereal spiro-chetosis (syphilis).

for rabbit syphilis consists of three weekly injections of par-enteral penicillin (procaine or G benzathine) at 50,000 U/kg to all exposed animals.[108] Response to treatment will confirm the diagnosis. Breeding facilities are the most at risk, and it may be wise to consider a closed breeding colony to prevent the spread of this pathogen.

Testicular neoplasia is rarely reported in rabbits; however, in a necropsy review of 100 laboratory rabbits, the prevalence of this disease was >20%.[92] Frequently, these tumors are benign and restricted to the testicle itself. There have been reports of seminomas, interstitial cell tumors, or granular cell tumors in rabbits.[93,109] Orchidectomy is recommended and curative if the tumor is confined to the testes.

Failure of one or both of the testicles to descend in bucks by 4 months of age is defined as cryptorchidism. True crypt-orchids may not show development of the scrotal sacs. Affected bucks will have an intact sexual drive, but their fertil-ity is impaired. Due to the assumptions that cryptorchidism may be hereditary and places the animal at a higher risk for developing testicular neoplasia, castration is recommended. Castration may be performed via a standard midline abdomi-nal approach. If the age of the rabbit is in question, it may be prudent to delay castration a few weeks past the assumed age to prevent unnecessary abdominal surgery.[94]

Hedgehogs

Primary reproductive disease in female hedgehogs may be detected first as hemorrhagic vaginal discharge or hematuria. Primary disease differentials for reproductive disease in female hedgehogs include uterine neoplasia or endometrial polyps, with endometrial venous aneurysms being a secondary concern. Owners may mistake hemorrhagic vaginal discharge for hematuria or vice versa.[110] Similar to rabbits, uterine neoplasia may cause hematuria, and a tissue mass may be palpable in the abdomen. Uterine cancers documented in hedgehogs include adenosarcoma, endometrial stromal sarcoma, adenoleiomyosarcoma, spindle cell tumor, and ade-noleiomyoma.[111,112] Radiographs may confirm the presence of a uterine mass (Figure 10-11). In hedgehogs, uterine neopla-sia typically has a low grade of malignancy; therefore, an

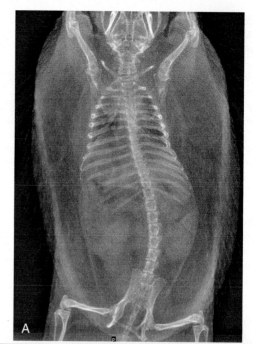

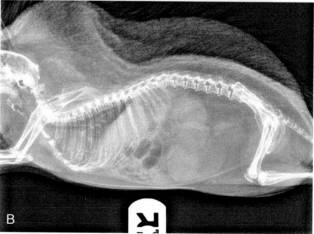

FIGURE 10-11 *A,* Ventro-dorsal radiographic image of a female intact hedgehog with a uterine mass. *B,* Lateral radio-graphic image of a female intact hedgehog with a uterine mass. (Images courtesy of Matthew S. Johnston.)

OHE may be curative.[112] Other primary reproductive disor-ders or diseases associated with parturition in hedgehogs are uncommon. Agalactia can occur and is usually noted by a failure of the young to thrive within 72 hours after birth. Although uncommon, dystocia may also occur and treatment includes stabilization and performing a subsequent caesarean section, similar to other small mammals.

Guinea Pigs

Reproductive disease is fairly common in guinea pigs, with the most common diseases being cystic ovaries, dystocia, and pregnancy toxemia. Approximately 76% of intact female guinea pigs develop cystic ovaries.[113] Cystic ovaries are also common in gerbils, as previously noted. Ovarian cysts have a clear fluid and increase in prevalence and size as a guinea pig

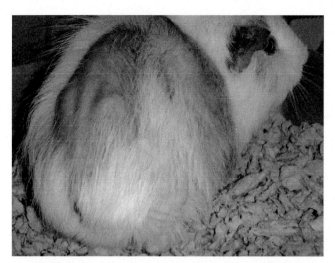

FIGURE 10-12 Dorsal/bilateral alopecia of a guinea pig with ovarian cysts. (Photo courtesy of Matthew S. Johnston.)

ages[114]; they also seem to be a normal component of the cyclic guinea pig ovary.[115] Most of the time, both ovaries are affected and the cysts are nonfunctional. If only one ovary is affected, it is typically the right ovary; the reason for this is unknown. Clinical signs may include abdominal distension, occasional anorexia, lethargy, and depression. Hormonally functional cysts, or follicular cysts, can result in bilaterally symmetric hair loss in the area of the flank (Figure 10-12). The cysts can grow large enough to be palpated. Ultimately, the cysts lead to compromised reproductive performance and secondary reproductive issues such as cystic endometrial hyperplasia, mucometra, endometritis, and fibroleiomyomas.[116] Diagnosis is difficult to obtain via radiographs because of the similar opacity between cysts, neoplasia, and trichobezoars. Abdominal ultrasound is recommended because it is the best diagnostic test for identifying and characterizing follicular cysts.[117] There are two different types of ovarian cysts that develop in guinea pigs, and they can only be identified on histopathology. Serous cysts, or cystic rete ovarii, are the most common. These are incapable of steroidogenesis and do not seem to respond to surges of LH. On the contrary, follicular cysts form when preovulatory follicles fail to ovulate. Follicular cysts are also diagnosed in horses and cattle, where they are considered follicular structures that lack a functional corpus luteum.[116]

Dystocia is one of the most common reproductive issues in guinea pigs. Guinea pigs are unique when compared to rabbits and other rodents due to the fact that the pubic symphysis does not fuse in a young, reproductively active female guinea pig. During the last week of pregnancy, the hormone relaxin is released from the pituitary gland and endometrium. This hormone causes the fibrocartilage of the pubic symphysis to disintegrate, allowing for separation of the symphysis. If the sow does not give birth before she is 7 to 8 months old, the symphysis will fuse permanently, predisposing the animal to dystocia. In some cases, guinea pigs bred for the first time after 8 months will undergo normal parturition. If the date of conception is known, the guinea pig should be examined on day 60. At this time, the pubic symphysis can be palpated to

determine whether it has separated. If the symphysis has separated, it is likely that the guinea pig will deliver her piglets without complication. If not, it is likely that the symphysis will not separate by day 65, in which case a caesarean section should be performed at the first onset of signs of parturition. Inadequate concentrations of vitamin C in the diet, obesity, uterine inertia, and abnormally large piglets will also increase the likelihood for dystocia in guinea pigs. During normal parturition, all piglets should be delivered within 30 minutes. If the female is straining for >20 minutes or fails to give birth after 2 hours, dystocia should be considered.[40] Clinical signs of dystocia include unproductive contractions and straining along with bloody or greenish-brown vulvar discharge. Pressure from the gravid uterus may also lead to hind limb paresis. On physical examination, the cervix should be dilated ~2.5 to 3 cm.

Leiomyoma is the most common cancer associated with the guinea pig reproductive tract. In one study, cystic rete ovarii were present in 100% of cases with leiomyomas.[118] This disease correlation was suspected to be associated with a hormonal imbalance, but has yet to be confirmed. Clinical signs of female guinea pig reproductive neoplasia may include hemorrhagic vaginal discharge, abdominal distension, and abdominal pain. Mammary gland tumors may also occur in guinea pigs, with both males and females affected.

As previously noted, pregnancy toxemia can occur in rabbits, guinea pigs, and hamsters.[28] However, pregnancy toxemia is diagnosed more often in guinea pigs than rabbits.[101] Regardless of the species, the clinical signs and predisposing factors are similar. Prevention of pregnancy toxemia in guinea pigs consists of providing balanced diets to prevent obesity, encouraging exercise, avoiding stress, and offering prompt treatment to affected animals. Pregnant animals should not be subjected to changes in diet or other stressors, such as travel. Pregnancy toxemia typically occurs in guinea pigs during the last 2 weeks of gestation or the week following parturition. Pregnancy toxemia typically occurs in rabbits during the last week of gestation, although it can also occur post partum.[28] Pregnancy toxemia is more common in multiparous animals than primiparous animals; it can also occur in pseudopregnant animals. Two different forms of pregnancy toxemia are reported: fasting/metabolic and toxic/circulatory.[40] The metabolic form stems from a negative energy balance and metabolism of fat due to increased energy demands from fetal growth; it is commonly referred to as pregnancy ketosis. Obese animals are more at risk for fasting/metabolic form of the disease. The toxic or circulatory form, also referred to as preeclampsia, is due to uteroplacental ischemia. This occurs in very large sows during late pregnancy when the gravid uterus compresses the aorta, resulting in ischemia and disseminated intravascular coagulopathy. For these cases, emergency cesarean with or without an OHE is required to save the sow; this condition carries a grave prognosis. Clinical signs for both forms of pregnancy toxemia have an acute onset and include lethargy, anorexia, and subsequent dyspnea. Affected animals may also be depressed, have an acetone odor on the breath, and decreased urine production due to acidosis.[120] Blood and urine samples often reveal the sows to be hypoglycemic, ketonemic, proteinuric, and aciduric. Hypertension and elevated creatinine are other disease conditions associated with the circulatory form.[28] Treatment for guinea pig patients diagnosed with pregnancy toxemia includes nutritional support and correction of electrolyte imbalances; however, sows typically do not respond well and the prognosis is guarded to grave. Unfortunately, death occurs rapidly in pregnancy toxemia cases, often within hours following the onset of clinical signs. Abortion, ataxia, seizures, and coma may precede death in severe cases.

Vaginitis, orchitis, and scrotal plugs may also affect guinea pigs. Poor environmental conditions, such as wet, soiled bedding, in combination with inguinal sebaceous secretions, can lead to substrate material becoming adhered to the external genitalia, predisposing animals to secondary bacterial infections. In boars, orchitis and epididymitis may occur from sexual transmission, bite wounds, and hematogenous spread of a bacterial pathogen. The most common bacterial isolates in genital infection cases are *Bordetella bronchiseptica* and *Streptococcus* spp. Boars that are treated and recover after appropriate antibiotic therapy may serve as subclinical carriers; therefore, it may be prudent to remove these animals the breeding population.

Pyometra and endometritis can be induced by the aforementioned ovarian cysts or normal ovarian activity. After the animal has been stabilized, an OHE is recommended. Uterine and/or vaginal prolapse are commonly associated with parturition; however, these conditions can occur due to another disease process. Upon presentation, tissue may be noted as protruding from the vulva after parturition. Depending on how long the tissue has been prolapsed, the sow may be stable or could also be systemically compromised. A complete physical examination should be performed to determine the status of the sow, and supportive care initiated prior to correcting the prolapse. If necrosis is noted, an OHE is recommended.

Mastitis in guinea pigs has a similar presentation as described in rabbits. Clinical signs in affected guinea pigs are often followed by maternal neglect and death of the sow. In guinea pigs, mastitis frequently speads to all mammary glands. The most common pathogens isolated in cases of guinea pig mastitis are *Streptococcus* spp. and *Escherichia coli*.[121]

Chinchillas

Despite the similarities in the reproductive anatomy and behaviors of guinea pigs and chinchillas, primary reproductive disease in chinchillas is rare. Female chinchillas housed in a breeding situation can become aggressive toward unsuitable males. Female animals may attempt to deny males through urinating, kicking, or biting. These bite wounds can progress to abscesses, so it is important to monitor the males closely during the breeding season. *Staphylococcus* spp. is most commonly isolated from the abscesses.

Endometritis and pyometra may occur in chinchillas, as in other mammals, although they are uncommon. Affected animals may present for vaginal discharge exhibiting signs of lethargy and anorexia. Definitive treatment for pyometra in any mammal is an OHE. Special care should be taken not to spill uterine contents into the abdominal cavity when performing an OHE. Prior to closure, the abdomen should be lavaged with copious amounts sterile saline. Again, unlike guinea pigs, dystocia is fairly uncommon in chinchillas; however, surgical intervention is required for animals exhibiting signs of labor >4 hours.

Fur ring occurs in male chinchillas when fur accumulates around the base of the penis and forms a restrictive ring. This can progress to cause paraphimosis and/or inflammation to the penis. Balanoposthitis, the term used to describe an inflammatory condition of the prepuce and glans penis, can occur secondary to retention of fur with or without smegma.[122] Acute balanoposthitis can also develop as part of a systemic *Pseudomonas aeruginosa* infection, whereas chronic balanoposthitis may present as a preputial abscess, preventing extrusion of the penis. Clinical signs associated with fur ring includes excessive grooming, straining to urinate, pollakiuria, lethargy, and inappetence. In severe cases, fur ring may progress to urethral obstruction, causing an enlarged urinary bladder or infection and damage to the penis. The most common cause is fur retained from a female after copulation, although it can also occur in males housed without females. Treatment simply requires the removal of the restrictive fur ring, which may require sedation or anesthesia. The glans penis should be cleaned with warmed saline and a dilute betadine solution to minimize irritation to the surface of the penis. In cases where paraphimosis has occurred, a thorough examination should be performed to examine the penis for bite wounds or evidence of infection. A lubricant can be used to aid in replacing the penis into the prepuce. A hypertonic solution (e.g., 50% dextrose) can also be used to reduce penile edema if needed.[123] Prognosis is guarded to grave if the prepuce or glans penis has evidence of necrosis. Recurrence of fur ring is possible; therefore, pet owners should be educated as to how to monitor their pet to identify this condition before it becomes a problem. Penile disorders may also be an incidental finding at the time of physical examination. Penile paralysis may occurs secondary to exhaustion if a male is housed with several females. Penile paralysis is not associated with fur ring, edema, or physical damage to the penis.

Sugar Gliders

Primary reproductive issues are rare in sugar gliders, although self-mutilation of the reproductive anatomy may occur in solitary or stressed animals. Self-mutilation is more common in males and often involves the mutilation of the penis and/or scrotum. Since male sugar gliders do not urinate out of the distal portion of their penis, amputation may be considered if the trauma has occurred at the forked portion of the penis. Castration is also a possible treatment for males that are exhibiting mutilation of their pendulous scrotum, as it may be related to sexual frustration.[42]

It is important to inspect the pouch of the female sugar glider during a routine examination. A saline-moistened cotton swab can be used to facilitate the examination. If abnormal secretions or malodorous substances are found, cultures are recommended. Infections can occur in both the pouch wall and mammary gland. The pouch may be cleaned with a dilute chlorhexidine solution. It is important to remember that if the female is housed with an intact male, joeys may be present.[124] Joeys attached to a teat should never be detached, as this can result in a failure to thrive. In cases where reproductive failure is noted, the stress level of the dam's environment should be evaluated and addressed. Due to the presence of a cloaca in these animals, infection of the reproductive tract may occur as an extension of infections already present in the gastrointestinal or urinary tracts.

SPECIFIC DIAGNOSTICS

Invertebrates

Diagnostic testing opportunities are limited or not warranted in cases of invertebrate reproductive disease. Many of the issues encountered are husbandry related and can be approached by collecting a thorough history and correcting any deficiencies. In large-scale breeding programs of invertebrates where reproductive activity is not ideal, necropsy and assessment of the reproductive systems of representative animals may be helpful. Abnormal egg sacs may be cultured for fungal or bacterial infections to rule out environmental contamination.

Fish

Diagnostic imaging can be used in fish to assess reproductive activity. In the case of elasmobranchs, ultrasound may be used to confirm a pregnancy and viability of the pups. Ultrasound may also be useful in teleosts to assess the size and condition of the ovaries or testes and confirm the sex of an individual patient. Endoscopy and gonadal biopsy (if necessary) can also be used to determine the sex of a fish that is not sexually dimorphic. Histopathology and microbiological culture can be used to confirm the presence of infectious agents in the reproductive tract or eggs. Although not routinely available, hormone profiles may be performed to assess the reproductive activity of fish and determine the best time for breeding.

Amphibians

Much like fish, diagnostic imaging is acceptable when assessing the sex and gonads of amphibian patients. Coelomocentesis can be used in conjunction with cytology and culture to characterize potential problems with the reproductive tract. The value of necropsy and histopathology cannot be overstated for large-scale amphibian breeding programs when reproductive failure is noted. Necropsy and histopathology are often the quickest way to confirm a diagnosis and determine a method for treatment.

Reptiles

Diagnostic imaging is also an invaluable tool for assessing the reproductive system of reptiles. Radiographs, ultrasound, CT, and endoscopy may be used to determine sex in nonsexually dimorphic species and identify specific disease processes affecting the reproductive system.

Radiographs can be used to confirm the sex of a nondimorphic reptile and if there are developed follicles (ova) or mineralized eggs. This is most practical in lizards, although mineralized eggs can be observed in snakes and chelonians. Radiographs have also been used to confirm the sex of a male reptile by demonstrating the mineralized outline of the hemipenes. This diagnostic imaging technique is most often used to monitor lizards. Ultrasound is also an applicable diagnostic technique to characterize the sex of snakes, lizards, and chelonians. The advantage of ultrasound over radiographs is that it can be used to identify female reptiles both during (well-developed follicles) and out of (poorly developed follicles) the breeding season. CT also has an advantage over radiographs because it can be used to identify different viscera (soft tissue structures), including the gonads. Finally,

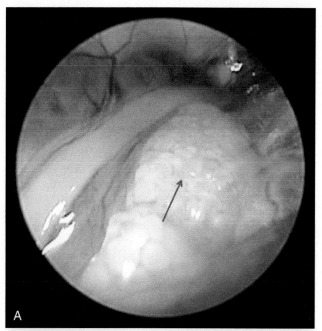
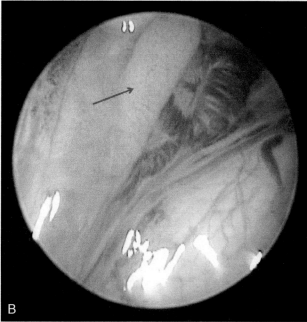

FIGURE 10-13 *A,* Sex determination in a juvenile Blanding's turtle using endoscopy. This animal is a female. *Arrow,* Ovary. *B,* Sex determination in a juvenile Blanding's turtle using endoscopy. This animal is a male. *Arrow,* Testicle.

endoscopy is effective in not only visualizing the gonads but also when collecting biopsy samples to confirm the sex through histopathology (Figure 10-13). This is most beneficial in neonatal animals when gross differences between the gonads may not be obvious.

Radiographs are a first-order diagnostic test to pursue when reproductive disease (e.g., follicular stasis, dystocia, ovarian cancer) is suspected in reptiles. One of the most common reasons to use radiographic imaging in these situations is for suspected cases of follicular stasis, especially in lizards. Multiple round (grape-like clusters), soft tissue opacities within the coelomic cavity in a confirmed female reptile is a strong indication that the animal is reproductively active. Additional historical information, such as time of year (e.g., breeding season) and anorexia and loss of body condition (e.g., muscle atrophy), add to the likelihood that the radiographic signs are associated with follicular stasis and not just reproductive activity. A pneumocoelomogram (infusing air into the coelom) may be used to highlight follicles if they cannot be identified on a plain survey radiograph. In smaller lizards (e.g., geckos), masses may be directly visualized via transillumination of the coelom. Radiographs are also useful diagnostic tools in cases of dystocia (i.e., mineralized eggs in shell gland that for some reason are not oviposited). The radiographs allow the clinician to evaluate egg number, size, and shape to determine whether the case should be managed medically (e.g., using oxytocin and husbandry changes if eggs should be able to pass) or surgically (e.g., egg is too large to pass, misshapen, or in abnormal direction and requires surgical intervention). Radiographs can also be used in reproductively active reptiles to assess their general bone health. The amount of calcium and energy required for shell development can be costly to a reptile, especially one that is provided borderline nutrition and husbandry. Abnormal radiographic signs such as thin long bone cortices (e.g., humerus and femur) and/or pathologic fractures may direct the clinician toward a diagnosis of nutritional secondary hyperparathyroidism. It is important to correct the dietary and husbandry deficiencies in these cases and provide supplemental calcium (e.g., calcium glubionate, 1 mL/kg, PO, once or twice daily [SID-BID]) and supportive care (e.g., fluids and nutritional support).

Ultrasound is another useful tool for confirming the presence of follicular stasis or reproductive disease (e.g., ovarian cancer), especially in chelonians and snakes, where radiographic imaging may be less rewarding. An added benefit to this diagnostic test is that it can be used to collect FNA samples for cytology and histopathology from the reproductive tract or from free fluid in the coelom (e.g., coelomitis).

CT provides a greater level of detail over both radiographs and ultrasound. In some cases, CT is the preferred method because radiographs provide little detail (e.g., in chelonians because of their shell), or the ultrasound provides too narrow a window into the coelom (e.g., in larger tortoises). Figure 10-14 represents a Russian tortoise (*Testudo horsfieldii*) that presented for follicular stasis. A diagnosis could not be made from the radiographs (Figure 10-14, *A*) but was obvious after CT (Figure 10-14, *B*). An exploratory surgery confirmed that this tortoise had follicular stasis, so an ovariectomy was performed. CT can also be used to screen for possible cancer in the reproductive tract using contrast studies.

As noted previously, endoscopy provides direct visualization of the reproductive tract. In addition to being able to determine the sex of an animal, it can be used to visualize pathologic conditions in the reproductive tract. Collecting specimens for culture and histopathology can be achieved without performing a more aggressive coeliotomy, thus decreasing the pain and healing time associated with the procedure.

Both the CBC and biochemistry profiles should be performed in cases where reproductive disease is suspected to ascertain both the patient's overall condition and treatment

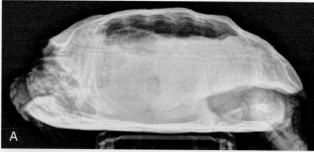

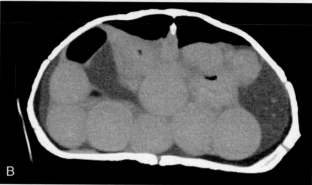

FIGURE 10-14 *A,* Lateral radiographic image of a Russian tortoise presented for follicular stasis. It is not possible from this image to confirm a diagnosis. *B,* Computed tomography scan of the same Russian tortoise as in *A.* Note the numerous echogenic follicles on the ovaries.

options for stabilization. Hematology can be a useful tool for characterizing the reproductive status of female reptiles, with gravid females maintaining higher concentrations of calcium, phosphorus, total protein, cholesterol, and albumin compared to nongravid females and males.[125] These changes in biochemistry profiles coincide with the mobilization of the proteins and minerals necessary for egg development. When follicular stasis or dystocia occurs, animals may become dehydrated and hemoconcentrated. Heterophilia with or without toxic changes and monocytosis may also be present and are suggestive of inflammation (e.g., cancer) or infection. Although not widely used, blood hormone assays can also be used to determine where reptiles are in their reproductive cycle and identify potential disease conditions (e.g., ovarian cancer).

Cytologic evaluation of a coelomic effusion or discharge from the reproductive tract can be used to diagnose active reproductive disease such as salpingitis or yolk coelomitis. Bacterial culture should also be pursued in these cases if cytology suggests infection is present.

Birds

As with reptiles, imaging is an important diagnostic tool for assessing dystocia. On radiographs, polyostotic hyperostosis, an increase in deposition of medullary bone, may be observed and affirms that calcium is being mobilized and the hen is in a laying state. Polyostotic hyperostosis has been reported in a variety of species including ducks, chicken, pigeons, and psittacines. Hens normally produce a large amount of endosteal bone in the humerus and femur during laying periods.

Cases of polyostotic hyperostosis are commonly seen in the skull, sternum, vertebrae, and sacrum in the parakeet. Lesions in males have only been documented with estrogen-secreting tumors. For these reasons, polyostotic hyperostosis is related to an excess of estrogen, and with most cases no ovarian abnormalities are observed.[126] Also, polyostotic hyperostosis detected in a bird without a recent history of reproductive activity may be indicative of an ongoing elevation in estrogen secondary to another disease process. Hyperostotic hyperostosis of the sternum has been reported in association with an oviductal adenocarcinoma in a female cockatiel.[57]

If an egg is palpated on physical examination, radiography can provide more information regarding its location and size (Figure 10-15). It also may be possible to visualize the position of the egg in the coelom. If the egg can be palpated, it is typically located in the distal oviduct. Eggs may not be visible radiographically if they are soft shelled or not fully formed. Other differential disease diagnoses to consider for a distended coelomic cavity include a mass (e.g., hepatic or renal) or abnormal ovary, which may also be detected through radiographic imaging. In cases of follicular stasis, radiographs may identify a soft tissue density cranial to the left kidney. Ascites is a common finding in these cases. Ultrasound or endoscopy may be used to definitively diagnose fluid-filled cyst-like structures in the area of the ovary. The follicles may be aspirated, or they may be removed via salpingohysterectomy and partial ovariectomy.

Although ultrasound is not usually a productive diagnostic tool in birds due to their significant air sac system and bone structure (e.g., large keel and ribs), it may be used to confirm the presence of an egg if it is not readily palpable, possibly identify the origin of a large space-occupying mass that may be reducing air sac space, or differentiate kidney and reproductive disease after abnormalities are observed in radiographic images.[49] Often it is not possible to visualize normal kidney and reproductive tissue via ultrasound; however, ultrasound may be used to identify developing follicles, renal neoplasia, cysts, and egg binding.[127] Developing follicles may be observed as focal round areas with echogenic content, which is the yolk. Ultrasound may also be used to confirm the presence and location of coelomic fluid present secondary to a yolk coelomitis.

Endoscopy of the reproductive tract of birds is an important tool for imaging and subsequent sexing. Endoscopy has also been used for orchidectomy and salpingohysterectomy in pigeons.[128] The size of the patient and the size of the available endoscope should also be considered prior to a procedure. Before DNA sexing, endoscopy was the definitive diagnostic method used to sex birds. General anesthesia is necessary for endoscopy in birds. The bird should be placed in right lateral recumbency. The most common entry site is located where the caudal border of the ribs, synsacrum, and greater trochanter of the femur meet. The right legs should be extended caudally with the left leg brought forward and secured to the neck with nonadhesive bandage material (e.g., vetwrap) for the procedure. A small incision should be made on the left caudal aspect of the body, the muscle dissected, the endoscope inserted, and the ovary or testicle identified to sex the birds. Endoscopy can also be used to assess the reproductive tract and collect biopsies in cases where disease is suspected. One should remember that endoscopy should not be performed in

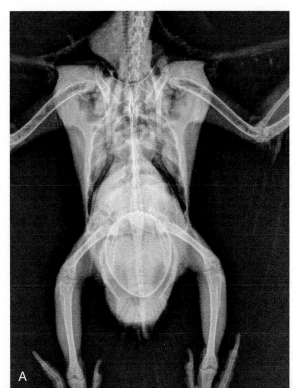

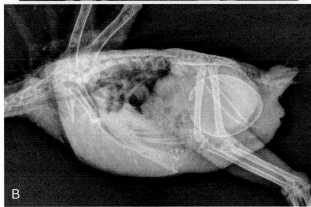

FIGURE 10-15 *A,* Ventro-dorsal radiographic image of an eclectus parrot with dystocia. Note the mineral opacity of the shell in the coelomic cavity. *B,* Lateral radiographic image of an eclectus parrot with dystocia. Note the mineral opacity of the shell in the coelomic cavity. (Images courtesy of Matthew S. Johnston.)

cases of coelomic effusion, due to the risk of drowning the patient after penetrating an air sac space.

Mammals

Diagnostic testing in mammals is similar across species, therefore methods used for dogs and cats should be considered for exotic pet mammals. When performing an OHE in any animal other than one that is healthy, the tissue should always be submitted for histopathologic evaluation. Hematologic testing (CBC/biochemistry profile) may be used to assess the overall systemic health of a patient prior to anesthesia; these tests may also aid in determining a prognosis for a severely compromised animal. Radiographs are often sufficient to obtain a diagnosis of a mass associated with the reproductive tract. However, ultrasound may be used to further differentiate the mass effect from fluid-filled structures and guide sample collection (e.g., FNA). Specific variations are briefly discussed below.

In cases of prostatic disease in ferrets, it may be difficult to distinguish between a prostatitis and cystitis using urinalysis and urine culture alone. A diagnosis for these cases requires a complete workup including whole-body radiographs, ultrasound, CBC, blood biochemistry profile, and urinalysis. A CBC may reveal evidence of inflammation in a prostatitis case while urinalysis results may provide evidence of a concurrent bacterial cystitis, although this could occur without any evidence of infection or inflammation in the urine. Ultrasound is the best diagnostic tool for evaluating the prostate and to determine whether there are any fluid-filled cysts in the prostate, which in the case of prostatic abscesses or prostatitis often contain hyperechoic sediment. Ultrasound-guided aspirates may be used to collect samples of fluid from the cysts for diagnostic purposes. The collected fluid should be submitted for cytology, microbiologic culture, and antibiotic sensitivity testing.

Radiographs can be used to identify a uterine mass in a rabbit. In these cases, it is routine to observe a large mass(es) displacing the surrounding viscera and a redistribution of fat, with a large amount of fat surrounding the uterine horns, but the animal will have an overall thin body condition (Figure 10-16). Ultrasound can be used to confirm that the structures are a solid mass versus cysts, pyometra, or hydrometra. Pulmonary metastases may be detected using radiography, although CT scans are a more sensitive screening tool and can be used with contrast to provide greater detail. The recommended treatment for uterine masses is an OHE, unless pulmonary metastasis is noted. When performing the OHE, it is common to observe multiple nodules along the uteri with abnormal tissue present. Figure 10-17 shows the gross appearance of a uterine adenocarcinoma while performing an OHE. Tissues removed during surgery should be submitted for histopathology to confirm the diagnosis.

TREATMENT

Reptiles

Dystocia in reptiles may not be an emergency and can often be corrected with husbandry changes or medical management. It should be noted that treatment is only warranted when a true dystocia has been diagnosed. The status of the patient should always be considered, and in apparently healthy animals, immediate intervention may not be necessary. The first step to treating dystocia is to provide an adequate habitat. Overcrowding should be corrected and the animals provided with a proper nesting substrate. The nesting substrate should be deep enough, preferably 1 to 2 times the length of the animal, for the reptile to excavate an appropriate sized nest chamber; the nesting area should be 4 to 5 times larger than the female reptile.

If the animal is clinically compromised (e.g., lethargic and dehydrated), it should be placed in a heated environment and rehydrated. It may also be efficacious to lube the cloaca

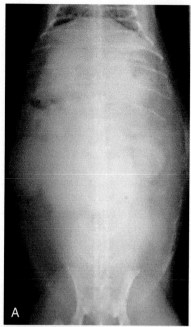
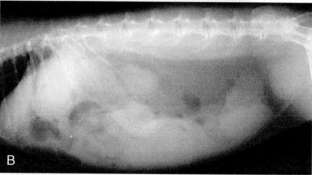

FIGURE 10-16 *A,* Ventro-dorsal radiographic image of a rabbit with a uterine mass. Note the mass effect in the caudal ventral abdominal cavity with increased soft tissue and surrounding fat opacity. *B,* Lateral radiographic image of a rabbit with a uterine mass. (Images courtesy of Matthew S. Johnston.)

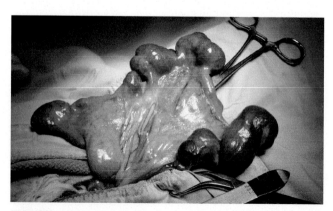

FIGURE 10-17 Intraoperative view of the uterine horns during OHE to remove a uterine mass. Noted the enlarged, hyperemic appearance to the uterine horn on the right side. (Photo courtesy of Matthew S. Johnston.)

prior to placing the animal in a heated, quiet place. If the animal is clinically dehydrated, it should be rehydrated first to ensure proper fluid homeostasis in the reproductive tract. Fluids can be administered intracoelomically, intravenously, or intraosseously; however, care should be exercised with the intracoelomic route because of the presence of the enlarged reproductive tract and eggs. If the animal is hypocalcemic, calcium gluconate (50 to 100 mg/kg) may be administered to aid in oviductal contractions. If these treatment measures fail to result in oviposition, oxytocin (5 to 20 IU/kg) IM is recommended in cases of nonobstructive dystocia. Multiple doses of oxytocin (2 to 4) may be necessary to stimulate oviposition. Beta-blockers (e.g., atenolol) have been reported to potentiate the effects of oxytocin.[10] Medical treatment for dystocia, using oxytocin, has proven effective in turtles but has generated variable results in lizards.[16] If the patient with dystocia is refractory to oxytocin, another treatment option is percutaneous ovocentesis. This procedure was done successfully in a leopard gecko (*Eublepharis macularius*).[129] Ovocentesis allowed the eggs to shrink to a size enabling the gecko to pass contracted structures within 36 hours. This technique should only be attempted in species that have soft-shelled eggs and should never be attempted with hard-shelled eggs due to the risk of rupture and leakage of egg contents into the coelomic cavity. If conservative management is unsuccessful and the animal is showing signs of increased debilitation, or if abnormally shaped eggs are present, more aggressive surgical treatment (e.g., OHE or salpingotomy) is required.

In snakes, medical management of dystocia may be attempted but typically is not successful. There is a small window of opportunity for medical management in this group. If obvious straining is observed, oxytocin may be administered within 48 to 72 hours IM.[12] Dosing may be repeated in 6 to 12 hours. If two to three doses have been administered with no response, it is likely that medical management will not be successful and manual manipulation or surgical treatment is required.[12] If the ova have been retained for more than several days, they can degenerate and break down, resulting in salpingitis and adhesion within the oviducts. In cases where the oviducts have adhesions, administration of oxytocin may result in torsion, tearing, or rupture.[12] Eggs may be digitally manipulated toward the cloaca, but this should be performed with caution due to the risk of oviductal tears and follicle rupture. It is recommended to first anesthetize the patient before digital manipulation is attempted. Only gentle pressure should be used, as eggs may have adhered to the oviduct. Since snake eggs are generally soft shelled and will collapse once emptied, ovocentesis may be performed externally to remove the contents of the egg(s). Ovocentesis is performed by isolating the egg to the lateral body wall and prepping the area in a sterile manner. A large-bore needle (16 to 18 gauge) is then inserted between the scales at the level of the first row of lateral scales and the contents aspirated. In most cases, the snake will pass the eggs on her own; however, if they are not passed within 12 to 24 hours, a coeliotomy will be required to remove the eggs.[12]

To perform a coeliotomy in a snake, the initial incision should be made between the first and second rows of lateral scales. The coelom can then be entered ventrally through the rectus abdominis muscles. This approach avoids irritation of the incision site after the snake recovers. When planning

surgery to remove the gonads of a snake, ultrasound may be used to locate the gonads; typically, the gonads are one-third the length of the snake cranial to the vent.[130] In cases where the oviduct has prolapsed and is devitalized, surgical removal of the oviduct and the ipsilateral ovary should be performed to avoid potential future ovulation complications and coelomitis.[12] Due to the elongated nature of snake ovaries, multiple incisions may be required to remove the entire ovary.

Orchidectomy and vasectomy are rarely indicated for reptile species. Castration may be performed in male iguanas in an attempt to decrease aggression with the greatest success being achieved prior to the patient's reaching maturity.[11]

Ovariectomy is more commonly performed to prevent future reproductive problems or as a treatment for current disease. To perform an ovariectomy in a lizard, a paramedian incision should be made to avoid the ventral abdominal vein. Once the ovaries are visualized, all vessels within the mesovarium, or ovarian ligament, should be ligated. In iguanas, ovarian tissue is diffuse and closely associated with the vena cava and adrenal gland.[46] The right ovary is attached to the vena cava by a thin membrane, which contains several short vessels, while the right adrenal gland is closely associated with the opposite side of the vena cava.[11] Special care should be taken to place all ligatures distal to the adrenal gland. In iguanas, this gland is a pale pink color and tubular in appearance.[44] Surgical hemoclips are preferred for ligating ovarian vessels for their ease and speed of application. After ligatures are applied, the vessels on the ovarian side may be severed and the ovary removed.[11] The left ovary is attached to a branch of the renal vein by the left adrenal gland, therefore care should be taken to avoid removing the left adrenal gland. On the left side, vessels are ligated between the adrenal gland and the ovary.[11] One then carefully removes the entirety of ovarian tissue, as remnants have the ability to regrow and develop folliculogenesis or become diseased. It is not necessary or recommended to remove the oviducts if they are normal. After ligating the associated vessels and removing the ovaries, the body wall may be sutured in a simple continuous fashion. When closing the skin, an everting, horizontal mattress pattern should be used to allow for proper healing, as reptile skin tends to invert. The placement of everting sutures will help prevent dysecdysis issues in the future. Reptile skin heals slowly, consequently it is recommended to keep sutures in place for 40 to 45 days following the surgical procedure.

In cases of postovulatory follicular stasis, the oviducts will be filled with eggs and should be obvious upon approach. A bilateral ovariosalpingectomy can be performed in these cases if the pet owner does not care about the breeding status of the reptile, while a salpingotomy should be performed to remove the eggs if the owner wants the animal to breed again. Ovariosalpingectomies are not routinely performed in snakes due to the extensive length of their reproductive tract. Instead, an ovariectomy and salpingotomy are surgical options to prevent further reproductive activity and remove any postfollicular eggs, respectively. For salpingectomies, the oviducts should be ligated close to their insertion at the cloaca.[130] In snakes, multiple coeliotomy and salpingotomy incisions may be necessary.

In cases of hemipenal prolapse (lizards and snakes) and subsequent necrosis, amputation must be performed. Anesthesia (local or general) is necessary to successfully reduce or amputate the affected hemipenis. To perform a hemipenal amputation, the hemipenis should be fully everted and clamped at the base. The base is then ligated with two trans-fixation sutures using an absorbable monofilament material.[11] The hemipenis should be transected distal to the ligature, and the stump replaced back into the base of the tail. If only one hemipenis is removed, the animal will still retain its ability to breed.[10] In animals with excessive necrosis and infection, multiple surgeries may be necessary to remove all of the affected tissue.

In cases of penile prolapse (chelonians and crocodilians), the tissue should first be inspected to determine whether it is viable. If the tissue appears viable, the phallus should be cleaned and returned to the cloaca. Hypertonic solutions such as 50% dextrose may be used to help reduce edema, shrink the phallus, easing one's ability to reduce the affected tissue. Two simple interrupted sutures placed through the pericloacal scales will help prevent recurrence. It is important to space the sutures so that they allow passage of feces and urine but not allow reprolapse of the phallus. Alternatively, a purse-string suture may be placed around the cloaca and maintained in place for 3 to 4 weeks. Before the patient is released from the veterinary hospital, it is important to ensure feces and urine can pass through the vent with the purse-string suture in place. If the tissue is nonviable, the phallus may be amputated without concern of affecting the urinary system; however, breeding will be affected.[10] The procedure to amputate the phallus of a reptile is similar to that described for hemipenal amputation.

There are several different methods that may be used to approach the treatment of a cloacal prolapse. If the prolapse cannot be manually reduced, the vent opening may be slightly enlarged by incising the scales (laterally) on either side of the vent. Once reduced, a purse-string suture or two transcloacal sutures may be placed to prevent a recurrence of the prolapse.[131] In cases of oviductal prolapse, surrounding tissues are often affected, and manual reduction of the oviduct is not possible. An oviductal prolapse will often require a coeliotomy and subsequent removal of the affected reproductive tract tissue.

Birds

The goal for treatment of chronic egg laying in birds is complete cessation of egg laying. Treatment via medical management may include injections of leuprolide acetate (Lupron; TAP Pharmaceuticals, Inc., Deerfield, IL). This is a GnRH agonist that is used to control laying behavior and egg production by decreasing production of LH.[20] Leuprolide binds to the GnRH receptors in the pituitary, inhibiting the synthesis of LH and FSH by negative feedback.[132,133] This negative feedback mechanism reduces estrogen and androgen production, decreasing egg production. Studies performed in the cockatiel suggest that Lupron can inhibit egg laying for 19 to 28 days.[18,134] Published studies suggest wide ranges of doses (100 to 800 µg/kg) and varying frequencies of administration, which must be adjusted according to brooding and egg-laying behavior. It is also recommended to remove any materials in the cage that are perceived as nesting substrate as well as any toys or mirrors that may stimulate sexual activity. Owners that are perceived as a mate by the bird should be instructed to avoid inappropriate behaviors such as petting the pelvis, dorsum, or cloacal region or kissing the beak.

Another environmental alteration that can be made to halt egg laying includes limiting the bird's photoperiod to no more than 10 hours per day. Cockatiels are indeterminate layers, meaning that removal of an egg may stimulate the bird to lay additional eggs. Owners should be advised not to remove eggs after they are laid. Surgery is another option for birds that are uncontrolled egg layers. Salpingohysterectomy can prevent recurrence; however, it is not without risk in smaller birds such as lovebirds, cockatiels, and parakeets. Removal of the ovary is not recommended in psittacines because of the high risk of bleeding and exsanguination. Consequently, it is possible, but not likely, that internal ovulation can occur post salpingohysterectomy.

Treatment for dystocia in birds begins with initial stabilization, which should include supplemental heat (incubator heated to 85° F to 90° F), intramuscular calcium, selenium, and vitamins A, E, and D_3. More compromised patients may require nutritional supplementation via gavage feeding and intravenous or intraosseus fluid therapy. Often, this supportive care, along with a lubricant being placed around the egg if it is visible in the vent, will be enough to allow the bird to pass the egg. If not, once the patient is stabilized, assistance in removing the egg may be required. A PGE_2 gel has been shown to relax the vaginal sphincter and increase oviductal contractions. Prepidil (Pharmacia and Upjohn Co., New York, NY) is commercially available and can be applied topically to the cloaca at a dose of 0.02 to 0.2 mg/kg.[135] Previous recommendations may have included $PGF_{2\alpha}$, which causes shell gland contractions. For this reason, it is generally contraindicated and should not be administered in cases of dystocia, as it does not relax the vaginal sphincter and can cause unwanted side effects such as hypertension, bronchoconstriction, and uterine rupture, as in mammals. Another synthetic analog of PGE_1, misoprostol, may be effective when crushed and mixed with a lubricant and applied topically to the cloaca. In human medicine, misoprostol is used for cervical ripening because of its biological effects within the cervix, including remodeling of extracellular collagen, increasing water content, and changing the extracellular matrix to cause softening, effacement, and dilatation of the cervix.[136] Much like $PGF_{2\alpha}$, oxytocin targets the uterus and does not relax the uterovaginal sphincter. Its use is contraindicated if the uterovaginal sphincter is not dilated and if uterine or oviductal mucosal adhesions are present. If hormonal therapy does not result in oviposition, the next step is digital pressure. Digital pressure is only advised if the egg is visible in the cloaca and can be manipulated transcloacally. Ovocentesis is contraindicated in eggs with a hard shell, as the egg can break and result in shell fragments entering the coelomic cavity and causing a secondary coelomitis. Soft-shelled eggs will easily collapse and are candidates for ovocentesis; however, if the composition of the egg is in question, ovocentesis should be avoided. Surgical intervention is warranted if the egg cannot be removed using the less invasive techniques.

In birds, surgery involving the reproductive tract has been described as difficult and high risk; however, it is possible to reduce risk by having a firm understanding of the avian reproductive anatomy. A left lateral coeliotomy is a recommended approach to access the female reproductive tract. It is essential to understand the blood supply to the reproductive tract and have proper hemostasis options during surgery, as blood loss in birds can result in serious consequences. When a bird is reproductively active, the blood supply to the ovary and oviduct is significant.[137] Two procedures can be performed on the avian reproductive tract: an ovariectomy or a salpingohysterectomy. Ovariectomies are difficult in birds due to the position of the ovary relative to the surrounding vasculature. It can be difficult to successfully ligate the ovarian artery, which increases the risk of fatal exsanguination. An ovariectomy should only be considered in cases that directly affect the ovary (e.g., ovarian neoplasia), and the owner should be informed of the significant risk associated with the procedure. Due to the high risk associated with an ovariectomy procedure, the salpingohysterectomy is the preferred method to control chronic egg laying and/or dystocia in birds that cannot be medically managed. It is important to remember that a salpingohysterectomy may not stop unwanted breeding and sexual behaviors because the procedure does not involve removing the ovary. While in most cases removal of the oviduct and uterus will suppress ovulation, there may be some patients that continue ovulation. A procedure has been described for performing a salpingohysterectomy endoscopically in cockatiels and suggests that with experience it can be performed safely in small birds by veterinarians familiar with endoscopy and avian anatomy.[138]

There are different methods for correcting a cloacal prolapse in birds, depending on the inciting cause. When presented with a cloacal prolapse, the tissue should be flushed and cleaned, kept moist with warm saline, and covered with a sterile lubricant. A prolapse may be replaced manually using a cotton-tipped applicator, lubricant, and inward pressure. After the prolapse has been reduced, two vent sutures or a purse-string suture should be placed using monofilament sutures. In cases of recurrent prolapse, a cloacopexy may be necessary while patients diagnosed with a prolapse secondary to papillomatosis, removal and debulking of the papillomas is often required. Cloacotomy has been described to remove severe cloacal papillomas in a macaw. This procedure is similar to an episiotomy in mammals. The cloacotomy is performed by first making a ventral midline incision through the skin, sphincter muscle, and cloaca. This provides visibility of the entire cloacal mucosa and will allow a more accurate determination of the margins of the masses. It is important to preserve the ureteral papillae and rectal opening. Complications include stricture and incontinence if the sphincter muscle is disrupted. Radiographs or CT scans are recommended during the initial workup of a cloacal papilloma case, prior to surgery, because of the suspected relationship between papillomas and bile duct carcinoma.[139]

In cases of dystocia where the coelom must be explored for the removal of an egg, a salpingohysterectomy may be indicated. In cases of yolk coelomitis, organs may be adhered to one another and should be carefully dissected to free the egg and/or oviduct. In cases of coelomic effusion, copious lavage should be performed to minimize the risk of postoperative infection.

Mammals

An OHE is typically performed in exotic small mammals for elective sterilization, following caesarean section to treat dystocia, removal of cancerous reproductive tissues, and other reproductive tract diseases, such as pyometra and cystic

ovaries. OHE procedures in exotic small mammals are similar to those described for the dog or the cat, with a few exceptions. It is important to take the anatomy of each individual exotic mammal species into consideration when performing an OHE. As described earlier in the chapter, not all exotic small mammal reproductive anatomy is the same. For example, it should be known prior to starting an OHE, whether the animal has two cervices, a uterus, or easily accessible ovaries.

Rabbits are routinely presented to veterinarians for elective OHE. To prepare a rabbit for an OHE, the entire abdomen should be clipped and aseptically cleaned from the xiphoid to just caudal to the pubis. For optimum exposure of the ovaries and vagina, the incision should be made in the middle third of the abdomen between the umbilicus and the pubis. Special care should be used when entering the abdominal cavity, as the cecum, bladder, or intestines are frequently lying just beneath the body wall. These organs are easily nicked with an aggressive approach. After entering the abdomen and isolating the reproductive tract, it is common to see a large amount of fat, which is typical of the mesometrium. This fat may be exteriorized to locate the uteri on either side. A spay hook should not be used in the rabbit, due to ease of identification of the uterine horns and risk of damage to the cecum with coarse manipulation.[140] Once a uterine horn is located, it can be followed cranially to identify the ovary. The ovary is small, yellow, and bean shaped. The ovarian artery can be ligated with one to two circumferential ligatures. This procedure should be repeated for the opposite side. The mesometrium, or broad ligament, is typically a primary site for fat storage; great care should be observed to avoid large vessels when the mesometrium is manually dissected. The uterine blood vessels are located in the broad ligament just lateral to the vagina and may be well developed. The surgeon should carefully locate and ligate or cauterize the uterine vessels. Moreover, the bladder should not be mistaken for the flaccid, distensible vagina. Since rabbits have two cervices, there are two approaches that can be utilized when removing the uteri. One approach is to ligate each uterus just cranial to the cervices. Since retrofilling of the vaginal vault occurs during micturition or expression of the urinary bladder, care is observed to tie off the cervix tightly to avoid leakage of urine into the abdomen.[38] Another technique involves placing a transfixation ligature caudal to both cervices in the cranial vagina. The vagina is then incised and removed cranial to the ligature, removing both ovaries, uteri, cervices, and the cranial portion of the vagina. The uterine vessels may be included in the ligature if not individually ligated. The latter technique is commonly used in cases of pyometra or uterine neoplasia. When using the latter technique, extra care is required to prevent damage to the urethra, which enters the proximal vaginal vestibule. Careful attention by the surgeon is required to avoid the ureters and caudal vesicular artery, which is a branch of the uterine artery. Closure is routine, although it is important to avoid incorporating vital organs when closing the body wall.[34] Possible postoperative complications include intestinal adhesions due to a fibrin clot, ligation of a ureter, or leakage of urine from the vaginal stump.

The approach to an OHE in a hystricomorph rodent, such as a guinea pig, chinchilla, or degu, is similar to that for a rabbit. The ovaries are supported by a mesovarium, which originates near the caudal pole of the kidney. The mesovarium is short in these species, making it difficult to exteriorize the ovary. The abdominal incision may be extended cranially to avoid tearing the friable ligaments. A "window" should be made through the mesovarium, and ligatures may be placed around the ovarian vessels. The suspensory ligament, mesovarium, and ovarian vessels are then transected distal to the ligatures. A final ligature may be placed around the uterine body, so the the uterus and ovaries are removed as a single unit.

In a case of dystocia in a rabbit, medical management may be initiated before surgical intervention takes place. Prior to administration of oxytocin, calcium glubionate should be given PO if uterine inertia is suspected. Oxytocin may be provided (1 to 3 IU, IM) to encourage uterine contractions. If the doe does not respond to medical management, caesarean section should be performed. In these cases, the primary goal of the caesarean section should be saving the doe, as the litter may not survive. Caesarian sections are most often needed for guinea pig dystocias. In a guinea pig, the width of the cervix should first be palpated. If the space is adequate and one suspects that dystocia is associated with uterine inertia, injectable calcium may be supplemented, followed by administration of oxytocin (0.2 IU/kg, IM). If dystocia is caused by a physical obstruction, such as a fused pubic symphysis or enlarged or malpositioned feti, a caesarean section is indicated but carries a poor prognosis. A less common cause for dystocia is ectopic pregnancy,[141,142] in which case caesarean section would also be indicated for treatment.

When performing a caesarean section, a longitudinal incision into the dorsal or ventral uterus is required. The incision may be closed with an absorbable monofilament suture in a simple continuous fashion. An OHE may also be performed on a gravid uterus to both retrieve young and prevent future pregnancy.

For guinea pigs with cystic ovaries, there are different treatment recommendations. Although the exact mechanism is unknown, cystic ovaries are often diagnosed in conjunction with uterine disease (e.g., leiomyoma, cystic endometrial hyperplasia, and endometritis), and for that reason, an OHE is the treatment of choice.[27] In cases where surgery is not an option, palliative drainage via ultrasound-guided FNA may be performed. Unfortunately, cysts may refill. Medical management may be used to induce leutinization of follicular cysts, including treatment with GnRH or hCG hormone. If the cysts are nonfunctional, medical management may not be successful.[143] Ovariectomy may be indicated in guinea pigs with cystic ovaries. Special care should be taken when manipulating cystic ovarian tissue on removal to avoid rupture. Surgical treatment for nonfunctional cysts may be pursued if the size of the cyst is adversely affecting the patient (i.e., decreased activity level, inappetence, pain). Figure 10-18 shows the gross appearance of large cystic ovaries in the process of being surgically removed from the patient.

Uterine or vaginal prolapse associated with parturition or other disease process requires treatment. First, the prolapsed tissue should be cleaned and assessed. If the tissue is viable, 50% dextrose or another hypertonic solution may be applied to the tissue to reduce edema and ease replacement. When replacing the uterine horn into the abdomen, the tissue must be replaced in the correct anatomical location to prevent

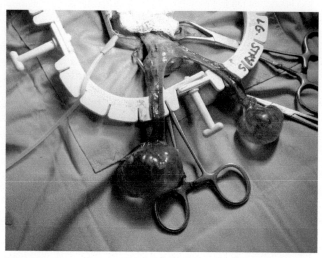

FIGURE 10-18 Cystic ovaries in a guinea pig viewed during OHE. (Photo courtesy of Matthew S. Johnston.)

recurrence. A blunt probe (e.g., cotton-tipped applicator) may be used to replace the tissue into the midabdomen. If the sow reprolapses, an OHE should be immediately performed. A purse-string suture should not be used to keep the uterus in place, because it is possible that the uterine tissue could be retained in the vagina and cause a urinary obstruction. If the tissue is not viable at examination, an OHE should be performed with the prognosis being guarded to grave in these cases. Surgical laparotomy carries a higher risk of postsurgical complications in guinea pigs than other rodent species.[144]

In most rodents, including rats, an ovariectomy will control reproduction because the uterus rapidly involutes and very rarely causes clinical problems post ovariectomy.[145] Ovariectomized rats have a significantly lowered incidence of pituitary tumors compared to intact females.[27] Ovariectomized rats are also less likely to develop mammary neoplasia later in life. A technique that has been described for dorsal ovariectomy in rodents is advantageous over the typical OHE and/or abdominal approach because it avoids the need to manipulate the gastrointestinal tract and therefore decreases the risks and complications associated with dehiscence.[146] The ovaries are located just caudal to the kidneys in a large fat pad. The uterine horn wraps around the ovary, and the vessels are not well developed. The ovarian ligament is long, leading to ease of visualizing the ovary.[147] The ovaries may be approached via one of two skin incisions: one on the dorsal aspect of each side of the body or through a medially placed incision. After making a small skin incision caudal to the ribs and ventral to the epaxial muscles, a hemostat can be used to penetrate the body wall. After the retroperitoneal space has been entered, the ovarian tissue will be exteriorized. Generally, a fat deposit is identified first and can be exteriorized, leading to exteriorization of the ovary. The vessels may be ligated using a circumferential ligature or hemoclips. In most cases, the body wall is not closed and a single skin staple placed for closure. The procedure may be repeated for the other side. Complications include hemorrhage via the renal vessels or postoperative dehiscence.

When mammary tumors are present in rats, mass removal is recommended. Surgical removal of the tumor is straightforward, but due to the extensive nature of mammary tissue in rats, it can be difficult to obtain adequate margins, and the masses frequently regrow. Moreover surgical removal may not prolong the patient's survival time. Abnormal tissue removed during surgery should be submitted for histopathology, as a small percentage of rat mammary masses are adenocarcinomas.

Expeditious removal of the mass during the surgical procedure is required. These masses are routinely easy to remove, and only minimal margins are required. If the mass is benign and not ulcerated or penetrated during removal, the skin can be preserved, allowing for routine closure of the surgical site. If the skin is ulcerated and/or the mass is malignant, the skin should be removed along with the tumor. The surgical site may be closed in one or two layers. To decrease dead space, it is recommended to tack the subcutaneous layer to deeper tissue (e.g., body wall) during closure. If the patient is unstable under anesthesia, one layer closure utilizing skin stapling is adequate.[27] More staples than normal, may be placed to reduce the incidence of incision site trauma by the patient. It should be kept in mind that rodents will commonly chew at their incision site, particularly if tension has been applied or there is other associated tissue irritation. To avoid further irritation and bruising, the remaining skin should never be gripped with forceps or other instrumentation. Without concurrent or subsequent neutering, the mass is likely to return. Ovariectomy or orchidectomy and mass removal are recommended to remove hormonal stimulation and prevent regrowth of the tumor.

Medical management of rat mammary tumors has been attempted; however, none of the treatments has proven effective. Cabergoline, a prolactin inhibitor by way of dopamine receptor agonism, can be administered to suppress prolactin at the level of the pituitary. It has been used in the palliative treatment of a pituitary adenoma and was shown to reduced the size of a pituitary tumor. Although not yet investigated, this drug may be helpful in rats that have mammary tumor development secondary to the pituitary tumor.[148] Due to the invasive nature and cost of surgery, many clients do not pursue early-age OHE. Since deslorelin, a GnRH agonist, has been shown to down-regulate and suppress levels of gonadotropins and sex hormones in other species, it is being investigated for contraception in rats. Studies suggest that it may be effective, but no studies have yet looked at a correlation between deslorelin implants and their effects on possibly reducing or eliminating mammary tumors.[149]

For many exotic small mammal species, orchidectomy is indicated to prevent reproduction, decrease undesirable sexual behavior, and reduce the likelihood for reproductive disease (e.g., testicular neoplasia, orchitis). If testicular neoplasia is present (e.g. Leydig cell tumor, Sertoli cell tumor, seminoma), in almost all cases an orchidectomy will be curative because these tumor types generally have a low metastatic rate. There has been no documented evidence that aggressive, undesirable behaviors will resolve after orchidectomy in rodents, as they may have become learned behaviors post puberty.

The procedure for orchidectomy in rats, mice, hamsters, gerbils, and rabbits is similar and follows the scrotal approach to orchidectomy in a cat. While the testicles can be retracted into the abdomen in all of these species, they can be easily pushed into the scrotum by applying pressure to the caudal abdomen. In rodents, there is a large amount of fat that surrounds the testicle, typically preventing herniation of abdominal contents despite the presence of an open inguinal ring. It is recommended to perform a closed castration to prevent herniation through the inguinal canal. The scrotum should be clipped and aseptically prepared. A 0.5- to 1.0-cm incision is made in a dorsal-to-ventral line as dorsally as possible in each scrotum. In a closed castration, special care should be taken to avoid incising the vaginal tunic. In order to do this, gently pry the scrotum from the vaginal tunic with the aid of dry gauze. This will also break down the ligament of the tail of the epididymis, which is necessary to exteriorize the testicle and isolate the spermatic cord. It is advised to avoid clamping the cord to avoid tearing the tunic or testicular vessels. Place one to two encircling ligatures of a 4-0 absorbable suture distal to the epididymal fat, and transect the cord. If an open castration is performed, allow the testicle to be exteriorized through the tunic. Break down the ligament of the tail of the epididymis, so the testicle is free from the tunic and scrotum. Ligate the spermatic cord, consisting of the testicular artery and vein, and ductus deferens, as close to the testicles as possible. The tunic can be left open or ligated closed. Each scrotal incision may heal by second intention, or be closed with a tissue adhesive. Sexual activity usually ceases in 1 to 2 weeks; however, it may persist for several weeks following the surgical procedure. Since viable sperm will still be present in the ductus deferens, it is recommended to keep males and females separate for several weeks following the procedure.[27]

It is recommended to neuter male rabbits after 3 months of age. Neutering will often prevent or truncate unwanted behaviors such as urine spraying, marking, or humping. For pain control, it is recommended to perform an intratesticular block with lidocaine for local analgesia prior to the procedure. The neutering procedure begins with a single ~1 cm in length incision longitudinally in the scrotum. A closed castration technique is recommended for young rabbits (<6 months of age), since the inguinal canal is open. Caution is observed when incising through the scrotum, to avoid opening the vaginal tunic during a closed castration. To complete the removal of the testicle, one to two circumferential sutures can be placed around the tunic. If the tunic is compromised, the ligament of the testicle should be broken down to expose the testicle and spermatic cord. The spermatic cord is then ligated and transected, as described for rodents. Always make sure to inspect the testicle after removal, to ensure removal of all relevant tissue. In older rabbits, the vaginal tunic and ligament of the testicle may be tightly adhered to the scrotum, and significant tissue damage may be incurred by manually breaking down the tunic. In these cases, open castration may be performed to minimize tissue trauma. It is not necessary to close the inguinal canal, as the inguinal fat pad should prevent herniation; however, herniation is a postoperative risk of surgical castration in a rabbit. A thin rabbit with minimal fat stores may be predisposed to herniation, due to the decreased size of the inguinal fat pads. Failure of the ligatures may also occur postoperatively, consequently the rabbit should be observed for any evidence of postoperative bleeding. The incisions are routinely kept open and heal by second intention, for less risk of postoperative complications, although tissue adhesive can also be used to close the scrotum.

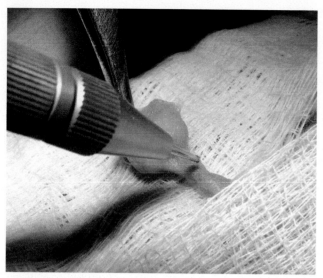

FIGURE 10-19 Use of a CO_2 laser to castrate a sugar glider. The laser is used to sever the scrotal stalk. (Photo courtesy of Matthew S. Johnston.)

Sugar gliders are routinely neutered to curb aggressive behavior and fighting, along with routine sterilization. Complications arise when sugar gliders self-mutilate or overgroom the surgical site following surgery, despite variations in closure. A recent technique has been described for castration of sugar gliders that involves severing the scrotal stalk midway between the testicles and the body wall with a CO_2 laser (Figure 10-19).[150] Preoperatively, the testicles are provided local analgesia via a lidocaine block. The site is surgically prepared using standard techniques. The CO_2 laser quickly severs the scrotal stalk, leaving no open wound to manage or close. Ultimately, the remainder of the stalk will regress after the procedure. This procedure is quick and has had no reports of postoperative self-mutilation.

In ferrets, treatment of hyperestrogenism consists of removing the source of the excess estrogen, which typically requires an OHE. Prior to surgery, the ferret should be stabilized; this may include blood transfusions. Since ferrets do not have blood groups, multiple transfusions can be administered, as needed. It may be possible to end estrus in a ferret by stimulating ovulation. In mild cases, this may be achieved via breeding. In moderate to severe cases, medical management can be attempted via injections of hCG (100 IU, IM) or GnRH (20 µg/kg, IM or subcutaneously [SC]).[151] Both of the treatment options may be repeated in 1 to 2 weeks if signs of estrus persist. As previously described, although it is unknown why ferrets in the United States develop adrenal disease, many of the disease conditions may be managed with a GnRH analog by down-regulation of GnRH receptors at the pituitary, similar to birds. Leuprolide acetate has been shown to reduce circulating concentrations of plasma estradiol, 17α-hydroxyprogesterone, androstenedione, and dehydroepiandrosterone. It also was shown to reduce, and in some cases eliminate, clinical signs associated with disease. Medical management of adrenal gland disease may result in resolution of an enlarged, swollen vulva. However, all clinical signs eventually recurred.[84] Another GnRH analog, deslorelin acetate,

has proven effective in eliminating clinical signs and decreasing hormone concentrations for extended periods of time. Recently, a deslorelin implant (Suprelorin F; Virbac Animal Health, Fort Worth, TX) became available in the United States that is approved for use in ferrets. Each implant is reported to last up to 1 year in reducing or eliminating clinical signs.

Melatonin is thought to be involved in the regulation of GnRH and possibly prolactin secretion. Melatonin has been administered to minks in an effort to stimulate molting by increasing melatonin concentrations and decreasing the amount of prolactin produced; this resulted in a thicker coat. In ferrets, it has been used to manage clinical signs associated with adrenal gland disease and has been shown to be effective in decreasing clinical signs for approximately 8 months when administered PO.[152]

Surgical management of adrenal gland disease via adrenalectomy is a viable treatment option. The procedure is similar to that described for dogs. An adrenalectomy is also a treatment option for prostatic disease in the ferret, as hyperplasia, cysts, and abscesses of the prostate are typically secondary to adrenal gland disease. Surgical debulking and/or aspiration of large, space-occupying prostatic cysts can take place during the adrenalectomy. Postoperatively, the prostate may shrink in size; however, problems may not completely resolve. Medical management may also be an option for treating prostate disease. An antiandrogen agent, flutamide (10 mg/kg, PO, q12 to 24 h), has been advocated and used anecdotally for the medical management of prostatomegaly, although currently no studies have been performed to scientifically evaluate its efficacy. Other antiandrogen agents to consider include finasteride (5 mg/kg, PO, q24 h) or bicalutamide (5 mg/kg, PO, q24 hr); these drugs may be used in conjunction with leuprolide to medically manage prostatomegaly.[85]

The recommended treatment for prostatitis or prostatic cysts is antibiotic agents that are known to penetrate the prostatic capsule, such as fluoroquinolones or potentiated sulfonamides. Antibiotic therapy to treat prostatitis or prostatic cysts is prolonged and should be continued for 4 to 6 weeks. Antibiotic therapy alone may not be sufficient to treat infections, and surgical management including omentalization or marsupialization may be necessary. Culture of the prostatic fluid and urine should be repeated 2 to 4 weeks after completion of antibiotic therapy to ensure a successful resolution of the infectious process.

REFERENCES

1. Pizzi R. Spiders. In: Lewbart GA, ed. *Invertebrate Medicine*. 1st ed. Ames, IA: Blackwell; 2006.
2. Leatherland JF. Endocrine and reproductive systems, including their interaction with the immune system. In: Woo PT, Leatherland JF, Bruno DW, eds. *Fish Diseases and Disorders*, Volume 2. 2nd ed. Non-infectious Disorders. Cambridge, MA: CAB International; 2011.
3. Lewbart GA. Reproductive medicine in koi (*Cyprinus carpio*). *Vet Clin North Am Exot Anim Pract*. 2002;5:637-648.
4. Noga EJ. Postmortem techniques. In: Noga EG, ed. *Fish Disease: Diagnosis and Treatment*. Ames, IA: Blackwell; 2000.
5. Stoskopf MK. *Fish Medicine*. Philadelphia, PA: W.B. Saunders Company; 1993.

6. Bell RC, Zamudio KR. Sexual dichromatism in frogs: natural selection, sexual selection and unexpected diversity. *Proc Biol Sci.* 2012;279(1748):4687-4693.
7. Mylniczenko N. Amphibians. In: Mitchell MA, Tully TN, eds. *Manual of Exotic Pet Practice.* St. Louis, MO: Saunders; 2011.
8. Wright KM. Anatomy for the clinician. In: Wright KM, Whitaker BR, eds. *Amphibian Medicine and Captive Husbandry.* Malabar, FL: Krieger; 2001.
9. Whitaker BR. Reproduction. In: Wright KM, Whitaker BR, eds. *Amphibian Medicine and Captive Husbandry.* Malabar, FL: Krieger; 2001.
10. Sykes JM. Updates and practical approaches to reproductive disorders in reptiles. *Vet Clin North Am Exot Anim Pract.* 2010;13:349-373.
11. Funk RS. Lizard reproductive medicine and surgery. *Vet Clin North Am Exot Anim Pract.* 2002;5:579-613.
12. Stahl SJ. Veterinary management of snake reproduction. *Vet Clin North Am Exot Anim Pract.* 2002;5:615-636.
13. Mitchell MA. Snakes. In: Mitchell MA, Tully TN, eds. *Manual of Exotic Pet Practice.* St. Louis, MO: Saunders; 2011.
14. Innis CJ, Boyer TH. Chelonian reproductive disorders. *Vet Clin North Am Exot Anim Pract.* 2002;5:555-578, vi.
15. McArthur S. Anatomy and physiology; reproductive system. In: McArthur S, Wilkinson R, Meyer J, et al., eds. *Medicine and Surgery of Tortoises and Turtles.* Oxford, England: Blackwell Science; 2004.
16. Denardo D. Reproductive biology. In: Mader DR, ed. *Reptile Medicine and Surgery.* Philadelphia, PA: W.B. Saunders; 1996.
17. Ritzman TK: Cloacal disease and disorders in the avian patient. *Proc Eur AAV/ECAMS.* 2005;327-332.
18. Pollock CG, Orosz SE. Avian reproductive anatomy, physiology and endocrinology. *Vet Clin North Am Exot Anim Pract.* 2002;5:441-474.
19. Joyner KL. Theriogenology. In: Ritchie BW, Harrison GJ, Harrison LR, eds. *Avian Medicine: Principles and Application.* Delray Beach, FL: Wingers Publishing, Inc.; 2004.
20. Hadley TL. Management of common psittacine reproductive disorders in clinical practice. *Vet Clin North Am Exot Anim Pract.* 2010;13:429-438.
21. Tully TN. Birds. In: Mitchell MA, Tully TN, eds. *Manual of Exotic Pet Practice.* St. Louis: Saunders; 2011.
22. Macwhirter P. Basic anatomy, physiology, and nutrition. In: Tully TN, Dorrestein GM, Jones AK, eds. *Handbook of Avian Medicine.* 2nd ed. Edinburgh: Saunders Elsevier; 2009.
23. Hudelson KS. A review of the mechanisms of avian reproduction and their clinical applications. *Sem Avian Exot Pet Med.* 1996;5:189-198.
24. Shields KM, Yamamoto JT, Millam JR. Reproductive behavior and LH levels of cockatiels *(Nymphicus hollandicus)* associated with photostimulation, nest-box presentation, and degree of mate access. *Horm Behav.* 1989;23:68-82.
25. Crosta L, Gerlach H, Bürkle M, et al. Physiology, diagnosis, and diseases of the avian reproductive tract. *Vet Clin North Am Exot Anim Pract.* 2003;6:57-83.
26. Lennox AM, Bauck L. Small rodents: basic anatomy, physiology, husbandry, and clinical techniques. In: Quesenberry KE, Carpenter JW, eds. *Ferrets, Rabbits, and Rodents. Clinical Medicine and Surgery.* 3rd ed. St. Louis, MO: W.B. Saunders; 2011.
27. Bennett RA. Small rodents: soft tissue surgery. In: Quesenberry KE, Carpenter JW, eds. *Ferrets, Rabbits, and Rodents. Clinical Medicine and Surgery.* 3rd ed. St. Louis, MO: W.B. Saunders; 2011.
28. Harkness J. Biology and husbandry. In: Harkness J, Turner PV, VandeWoulde S, et al., eds. *Biology and Medicine of Rabbits and Rodents.* 5th ed. Ames, IA: Wiley-Blackwell; 2010.
29. Tully TN. Mice and rats. In: Mitchell MA, Tully TN, eds. *Manual of Exotic Pet Practice.* St. Louis, MO: Saunders; 2011.
30. Noakes DE, Parkinson TJ, England GCW, eds. *Arthur's Veterinary Reproduction and Obstetrics.* London: Elsevier Health Sciences; 2009.
31. Capello V, Lennox A. Gross and surgical anatomy of the reproductive tract of selected exotic pet mammals. *Proc AAV.* 2006;19-28.
32. Powers LV, Brown SA. Ferrets: basic anatomy, physiology, and husbandry. In: Quesenberry KE, Carpenter JW, eds. *Ferrets, Rabbits, and Rodents. Clinical Medicine and Surgery.* 3rd ed. St. Louis, MO: W.B. Saunders; 2011.
33. Orcutt CJ. Ferret urogenital diseases. *Vet Clin North Am Exot Anim Pract.* 2003;6:113-138.
34. Bishop CR. Reproductive medicine of rabbits and rodents. *Vet Clin North Am Exot Anim Pract.* 2002;5:507-535, vi.
35. Vella D, Donnelly TM. Rabbits: basic anatomy, physiology, and husbandry. In: Quesenberry KE, Carpenter JW, eds. *Ferrets, Rabbits, and Rodents. Clinical Medicine and Surgery.* 3rd ed. St. Louis, MO: W.B. Saunders; 2011.
36. Bedford JM, Mock OB, Nagdas SK, et al. Reproductive characteristics of the African pygmy hedgehog, *Atelerix albiventris. J Reprod Fertil.* 2000;120:143-150.
37. Ivey E, Carpenter JW. African hedgehogs. In: Quesenberry KE, Carpenter JW, eds. *Ferrets, Rabbits, and Rodents. Clinical Medicine and Surgery.* 3rd ed. St. Louis, MO: W.B. Saunders; 2011.
38. Brower M. Practitioner's guide to pocket pet and rabbit theriogenology. *Theriogenology.* 2006;66:618-623.
39. Quesenberry KE, Donnelly TM, Mans C. Biology, husbandry, and clinical techniques of guinea pigs and chinchillas. In: Quesenberry KE, Carpenter JW, eds. *Ferrets, Rabbits, and Rodents. Clinical Medicine and Surgery.* 3rd ed. St. Louis, MO: W.B. Saunders; 2011.
40. Donnelly TM, Brown CJ. Guinea pig and chinchilla care and husbandry. *Vet Clin North Am Exot Anim Pract.* 2004;7:351-373, vii.
41. Johnson-Delaney CA. Reproductive medicine of companion marsupials. *Vet Clin North Am Exot Anim Pract.* 2002;5:537-553.
42. Ness RD, Johnson-Delaney CA. Sugar gliders. In: Quesenberry KE, Carpenter JW, eds. *Ferrets, Rabbits, and Rodents. Clinical Medicine and Surgery.* 3rd ed. St. Louis, MO: W.B. Saunders; 2011.
43. Noga EJ. Problems 55 through 72. In: Noga EJ, ed. *Fish Disease: Diagnosis and Treatment.* Ames, IA: Blackwell Publishing; 2000.
44. Backues K, Ramsay E. Ovariectomy for treatment of follicular stasis in lizards. *J Zoo Wildl Med.* 1994;25:111-116.
45. Lock BA. Cloacal prolapse. In: Mayer J, Donnelly TM, eds. *Clinical Veterinary Advisor: Birds and Exotic Pets.* St. Louis, MO: Saunders; 2013.
46. Cruz Cardona JA, Conley KJ, Wellehan JF, et al. Incomplete ovariosalpingectomy and subsequent malignant granulosa cell tumor in a female green iguana *(Iguana iguana). J Am Vet Med Assoc.* 2011;239:237-242.
47. Onderka DK, Zwart P. Granulosa cell tumor in a garter snake *(Thamnophis sirtalis). J Wildl Dis.* 1978;14:218-221.
48. Kirchgessner M. Birds: chronic egg laying. In: Mayer J, Donnelly TM, eds. *Clinical Veterinary Advisor: Birds and Exotic Pets.* St. Louis, MO: Saunders; 2013.
49. Bowles HL. Reproductive diseases of pet bird species. *Vet Clin North Am Exot Anim Pract.* 2002;5:489-506, v.
50. Clayton LA, Ritzman TK. Egg binding in a cockatiel *(Nymphicus hollandicus). Vet Clin North Am Exot Anim Pract.* 2006;9:511-518.
51. Harrison GJ, Lightfoot TL, eds. *Clinical Avian Medicine.* Palm Beach, FL: Spix Publishing; 2006.
52. Rodriguez Barbon A. Birds: follicular stasis. In: Mayer J, Donnelly TM, eds. *Clinical Veterinary Advisor: Birds and Exotic Pets.* St. Louis, MO: Saunders; 2013.
53. Sanchez-Migallon Guzman D. Birds: cloacal prolapse. In: Mayer J, Donnelly TM, eds. *Clinical Veterinary Advisor: Birds and Exotic Pets.* St. Louis, MO: Saunders; 2013.
54. Rosen LB. Avian reproductive disorders. *J Exot Pet Med.* 2012;21:124-131.
55. Romagnano A. Avian obstetrics. *Sem Avian Exot Pet Med.* 1996;5:180-188.
56. Kumbalek SL, Hanley CS, Matheson JS, et al. What is your diagnosis? *J Am Vet Med Assoc.* 2006;229:1567-1568.

57. Carleton RE, Garner MM. Oviductal adenocarcinoma with osseous and myeloid metaplasia associated with sternal hyperostosis in a cockatiel (*Nymphicus hollandicus*). *J Avian Med Surg.* 2002;16:309-313.

58. Mickley K, Buote M, Kiupel M, et al. Ovarian hemangiosarcoma in an orange-winged Amazon parrot (*Amazona amazonica*). *J Avian Med Surg.* 2009;23:29-35.

59. Antinoff N, Hoefer HL, Rosenthal KL, et al. Smooth muscle neoplasia of suspected oviductal origin in the cloaca of a blue-fronted Amazon parrot (*Amazona aestiva*). *J Avian Med Surg.* 1997;11:268-272.

60. Degernes LA. Abdominal mass due to chronic salpingitis in an African grey parrot (*Psittacus erithacus*). *Vet Radiol Ultrasound.* 1993;35:24-28.

61. Styles DK, Tomaszewski EK, Phalen DN. A novel psittacid herpesvirus found in African grey parrots (*Psittacus erithacus erithacus*). *Avian Pathol.* 2005;34:150-154.

62. Gartrell BD, Morgan KJ, Howe L, et al. Cloacal papillomatosis in the absence of herpesvirus and papillomavirus in a sulphur-crested cockatoo (*Cacatua galerita*). *NZ Vet J.* 2009;57:241-243.

63. Styles DK, Tomaszewski EK, Jaeger LA, et al. Psittacid herpesviruses associated with mucosal papillomas in neotropical parrots. *Virology.* 2004;325:24-35.

64. Goodwin M, McGee ED. Herpes-like virus associated with a cloacal papilloma in an orange-fronted conure (*Aratinga canicularis*). *J Assoc Avian Vet.* 1993;7:23-25.

65. Latimer KS, Niagro FD, Rakich PM, et al. Investigation of parrot papillomavirus in cloacal and oral papillomas of psittacine birds. *Vet Clin Pathol.* 1997;26:158-163.

66. Shaw SN. Papillomas. In: Mayer J, Donnelly TM, eds. *Clinical Veterinary Advisor: Birds and Exotic Pets.* St. Louis, MO: Saunders; 2013.

67. Hillyer EV, Moroff S, Hoefer H, et al. Bile duct carcinoma in two out of ten Amazon parrots with cloacal papillomas. *J Assoc Avian Vet.* 1991;5:91-95.

68. Kennedy EA, Sattler-Augustin S, Mahler J, et al. Oropharyngeal and cloacal papillomas in two macaws (*Ara* spp.) with neoplasia with hepatic metastasis. *J Avian Med Surg.* 2013;10:89-95.

69. Gibbons PM, Busch MD, Tell LA, et al. Internal papillomatosis with intrahepatic cholangiocarcinoma and gastrointestinal adenocarcinoma in a peach-fronted conure (*Aratinga aurea*). *Avian Dis.* 2002;46:1062-1069.

70. Palmieri C, Cusinato I, Avallone G, et al. Cloacal fibrosarcoma in a canary (*Serinus canaria*). *J Avian Med Surg.* 2011;25:277-280.

71. Jankowski GR. Birds: hypovitaminosis. In: Mayer J, Donnelly TM, eds. *Clinical Veterinary Advisor: Birds and Exotic Pets.* St. Louis, MO: Saunders; 2013.

72. Goya R, Lu J, Meites J. Gonadal function in aging rats and its relation to pituitary and mammary pathology. *Mech Ageing Dev.* 1990;56:77-88.

73. Wyre NR, Donnelly TM. Small mammals, rats: mammary and pituitary tumors. In: Mayer J, Donnelly TM, eds. *Clinical Veterinary Advisor: Birds and Exotic Pets.* St. Louis, MO: Saunders; 2013.

74. Hotchkiss CE. Effect of surgical removal of subcutaneous tumors on survival of rats. *J Am Vet Med Assoc.* 1995;206(10):1575-1579.

75. Kunstýr I, Küpper W, Weisser H, et al. Urethral plug—a new secondary male sex characteristic in rat and other rodents. *Lab Anim.* 1982;16:151-155.

76. Lejnieks DV. Urethral plug in a rat (*Rattus norvegicus*). *J Exot Pet Med.* 2007;16:183-185.

77. Bradshaw B, Wolfe H. Coagulation proteins in the seminal vesicle and coagulating gland of the mouse. *Biol Reprod.* 1977;16:292-297.

78. Carballada R, Esponda P. Role of fluid from seminal vesicles and coagulating glands in sperm transport into the uterus and fertility in rats. *J Reprod Fertil.* 1992;95:639-648.

79. Brown C, Donnelly TM. Disease problems of small rodents. In: Quesenberry KE, Carpenter JW, eds. *Ferrets, Rabbits, and Rodents. Clinical Medicine and Surgery.* 3rd ed. St. Louis, MO: W.B. Saunders; 2011.

80. Renshaw H, Van Hoosier G, Amend N. A survey of naturally occurring diseases of the Syrian hamster. *Lab Anim.* 1975;9:179-191.

81. Schneider JE, Wade GN. Effects of maternal diet, body weight and body composition on infanticide in Syrian hamsters. *Physiol Behav.* 1989;46:815-821.

82. Schneider JE, Wade GN. Effects of ambient temperature and body fat content on maternal litter reduction in Syrian hamsters. *Physiol Behav.* 1991;49:135-139.

83. Latney L, Donnelly TM. Small mammals: gerbils: ovarian disease. In: Mayer J, Donnelly TM, eds. *Clinical Veterinary Advisor: Birds and Exotic Pets.* St. Louis, MO: Saunders; 2013.

84. Wagner RA, Bailey EM, Schneider JF, et al. Leuprolide acetate treatment of adrenocortical disease in ferrets. *J Am Vet Med Assoc.* 2001;218:1272-1274.

85. Pollock CG. Ferrets: disorders of the urinary and reproductive systems. In: Quesenberry KE, Carpenter JW, eds. *Ferrets, Rabbits, and Rodents. Clinical Medicine and Surgery.* 3rd ed. St. Louis, MO: W.B. Saunders; 2011.

86. Patterson MM, Rogers AB, Schrenzel MD, et al. Alopecia attributed to neoplastic ovarian tissue in two ferrets. *Comp Med.* 2003;53:213-217.

87. Dalrymple EF. Pregnancy toxemia in a ferret. *Can Vet J.* 2004;45:150-152.

88. Martínez-Jiménez D, Chary P, Barron HW. Cystic endometrial hyperplasia-pyometra complex in two female ferrets (*Mustela putorius furo*). *J Exot Pet Med.* 2009;18:62-70.

89. Li X, Fox JG, Padrid PA. Neoplastic diseases in ferrets: 574 cases (1968-1997). *J Am Vet Med Assoc.* 1998;212:1402-1406.

90. Coleman GD, Chavez MA, Williams BH. Cystic prostatic disease associated with adrenocortical lesions in the ferret (*Mustela putorius furo*). *Vet Pathol.* 1998;35:547-549.

91. Shoemaker NJ, Schuurmans M, Moorman H, et al. Correlation between age at neutering and age at onset of hyperadrenocorticism in ferrets. *J Am Vet Med Assoc.* 2000;216:195-197.

92. Weisbroth SH. Neoplastic diseases. In: Manning PJ, Ringler DH, Newcomer CE, eds. *The Biology of the Laboratory Rabbit.* 2nd ed. San Diego, CA: Academic Press, Inc.; 1994.

93. Heatley JJ, Smith AN. Spontaneous neoplasms of lagomorphs. *Vet Clin North Am Exot Anim Pract.* 2004;7:561-577, v.

94. Klaphake E, Paul-Murphy J. Rabbits: disorders of the reproductive and urinary systems. In: Quesenberry KE, Carpenter JW, eds. *Ferrets, Rabbits, and Rodents. Clinical Medicine and Surgery.* 3rd ed. St. Louis, MO: W.B. Saunders; 2011.

95. Walter B, Poth T, Böhmer E, et al. Uterine disorders in 59 rabbits. *Vet Rec.* 2010;166:230-233.

96. Raftery A. Letter: uterine adenocarcinoma in pet rabbits. *Vet Rec.* 1998;142(25):704.

97. Vennen K, Mitchell MA. Rabbits. In: Mitchell MA, Tully TN, eds. *Manual of Exotic Pet Practice.* St. Louis, MO: Saunders; 2011.

98. Sebesteny A. A case of torsion of the uterus in a rabbit. *Lab Anim Sci.* 1972;6:357-358.

99. Segura Gil P, Peris Palau B, Martínez Martínez J, et al. Abdominal pregnancies in farm rabbits. *Theriogenology.* 2004;62:642-651.

100. Eales NB. Abdominal pregnancy in animals, with an account of a case of multiple ectopic gestation in a rabbit. *J Anat.* 1932;67:108-117.

101. Bergdall VK, Dysko RC. Metabolic, traumatic, mycotic, and miscellaneous disease. In: Manning PJ, Ringler DH, Newcomer CE, eds. *The Biology of the Laboratory Rabbit.* 2nd ed. San Diego, CA: Academic Press; 1994.

102. Jacobson HA, Kibbe DP, Kirkpatrick RL. Ectopic fetuses in two cottontail rabbits. *J Wildl Dis.* 1975;11:540-542.

103. Bray MV, Weir EC, Brownstein DG, et al. Endometrial venous aneurysms in three New Zealand White rabbits. *Lab Anim Sci.* 1992;42(4):360-362.

104. DeLong D, Manning PJ. Bacterial diseases. In: Manning PJ, Ringler DH, Newcomer CE, eds. *The Biology of the Laboratory Rabbit.* 2nd ed. San Diego, CA: Academic Press; 1994.

105. Bingley M, Vella D. Rabbits: mammary gland disorders. In: Mayer J, Donnelly TM, eds. *Clinical Veterinary Advisor: Birds and Exotic Pets.* St. Louis, MO: Saunders; 2013.

106. Adlam C, Thorley C, Ward P, et al. Natural and experimental staphylococcal mastitis in rabbits. *J Comp Pathol.* 1976;86:581-593.

107. Viana D, Selva L, Callanan JJ, et al. Strains of *Staphylococcus aureus* and pathology associated with chronic suppurative mastitis in rabbits. *Vet J.* 2011;190:403-407.

108. DiGiacomo RF, Lukehart SA, Talburt CD, et al. Clinical course and treatment of venereal spirochaetosis in New Zealand White rabbits. *Br J Vener Dis.* 1984;60:214-218.

109. Alexandre N, Branco S, Soares TF, et al. Bilateral testicular seminoma in a rabbit *(Oryctolagus cuniculus). J Exot Pet Med.* 2010;19:304-308.

110. Phillips ID, Taylor JJ, Allen AL. Endometrial polyps in two African pygmy hedgehogs. *Can Vet J.* 2005;46:524-527.

111. Done L, Deem S, Fiorello C. Surgical and medical management of a uterine spindle cell tumor in an African hedgehog *(Atelerix albiventris). J Zoo Wildl Med.* 2007;38:601-603.

112. Mikaelian I, Reavill D. Spontaneous proliferative lesions and tumors of the uterus of captive African hedgehogs *(Atelerix albiventris). J Zoo Wildl Med.* 2004;35:216-220.

113. Keller LSF, Griffith JW, Lang CM. Reproductive failure associated with cystic rete ovarii in guinea pigs. *Vet Pathol.* 1987;24:335-339.

114. Nielsen T, Holt S, Ruelokke M, et al. Ovarian cysts in guinea pigs: influence of age and reproductive status on prevalence and size. *J Small Anim Pract.* 2003;44:257-260.

115. Shi F, Petroff BK, Herath CB, et al. Serous cysts are a benign component of the cyclic ovary in the guinea pig with an incidence dependent upon inhibin bioactivity. *J Vet Med Sci.* 2002;64:129-135.

116. Donnelly TM, Richardson VCG. Small mammals: guinea pigs: ovarian cysts. In: Mayer J, Donnelly TM, eds. *Clinical Veterinary Advisor: Birds and Exotic Pets.* St. Louis, MO: Saunders; 2013.

117. Beregi A, Zorn S, Felkai F. Ultrasonic diagnosis of ovarian cysts in ten guinea pigs. *Vet Radiol Ultrasound.* 1999;40:74-76.

118. Field JK, Griffith JW, Lang CM. Spontaneous reproductive tract leiomyomas in aged guinea pigs. *J Comp Path.* 1989;101:287-294.

119. Greene HSN. Toxemia of pregnancy in the rabbit. II. Etiological considerations with especial reference to hereditary factors. *J Exp Med.* 1937;1937:369-388.

120. Greene HSN. Toxemia of pregnancy in the rabbit I. Clinical manifestations and pathology. *J Exp Med.* 1937;65:809-835.

121. Kinkler RJ, Wagner JE, Doyle RE, et al. Bacterial mastitis in guinea pigs. *Lab Anim Sci.* 1976;26:214-217.

122. Mans C. Small mammals: chinchillas: penile disorders. In: Mayer J, Donnelly TM, eds. *Clinical Veterinary Advisor: Birds and Exotic Pets.* St. Louis, MO: Saunders; 2013.

123. Mans C, Donnelly TM. Disease problems in chinchillas. In: Quesenberry KE, Carpenter JW, eds. *Ferrets, Rabbits, and Rodents. Clinical Medicine and Surgery.* 3rd ed. St. Louis, MO: W.B. Saunders; 2011.

124. Carboni D, Tully TN. Marsupials. In: Mitchell MA, Tully TN, eds. *Manual of Exotic Pet Practice.* St. Louis, MO: Saunders; 2011.

125. Harr KE, Alleman R, Dennis PM, et al. Morphologic and cytochemical characteristics of blood cells and hematologic and plasma biochemical reference ranges in green iguanas. *J Am Vet Med Assoc.* 2001;218:915-921.

126. Schlumberger HG. Polyostotic hyperostosis in the female parakeet. *Am J Pathol.* 1959;35:1-23.

127. Krautwald-Junghanns ME, Pees M. Imaging techniques. In: Tully TN, Dorrestein GM, Jones AK, eds. *Handbook of Avian Medicine.* 2nd ed. Edinburgh: Saunders Elsevier; 2009.

128. Hernandez-Divers SJ, Stahl SJ, Wilson GH, et al. Endoscopic orchidectomy and salpingohysterectomy of pigeons *(Columba livia):* an avian model for minimally invasive endosurgery. *J Avian Med Surg.* 2007;21:22-37.

129. Hall AJ, Lewbart GA. Treatment of dystocia in a leopard gecko *(Eublepharis macularius)* by percutaneous ovocentesis. *Vet Rec.* 2006;158:737-739.

130. Alworth LC, Hernandez SM, Divers SJ. Laboratory reptile surgery: principles and techniques. *J Am Assoc Lab Anim Sci.* 2011;50:11-26.

131. Mader DR, Bennett RA, Funk RS. Surgery. In: Mader DR, ed. *Reptile Medicine and Surgery.* Philadelphia, PA: W.B. Saunders; 1996.

132. Mitchell MA. Leuprolide acetate. *Sem Avian Exot Pet Med.* 2005;14:153-155.

133. Ottinger MA, Wu J, Pelican K. Neuroendocrine regulation of reproduction in birds and clinical applications of GnRH analogues in birds and mammals. *Sem Avian Exot Pet Med.* 2002;11:71-79.

134. Millam JR, Finney HL. Leuprolide acetate can reversibly prevent egg laying in cockatiels *(Nymphicus hollandicus). Zoo Biol.* 1994;13:149-155.

135. Carpenter JW. *Exotic Animal Formulary.* 4th ed. St. Louis, MO: W.B. Saunders; 2013.

136. Hawkins JS, Wing DA. Current pharmacotherapy options for labor induction. *Expert Opin Pharmacother.* 2012;13:2005-2014.

137. Echols MS. Surgery of the avian reproductive tract. *Sem Avian Exot Pet Med.* 2002;11:177-195.

138. Pye GW, Bennett RA, Plunske R, et al. Endoscopic salpingohysterectomy of juvenile cockatiels *(Nymphicus hollandicus). J Avian Med Surg.* 2001;15:90-94.

139. Dvorak L, Bennett RA, Cranor K, et al. Cloacotomy for excision of cloacal papillomas in a Catalina macaw. *J Avian Med Surg.* 1998;12:11-15.

140. Jenkins JR. Rabbits: soft tissue surgery. In: Quesenberry KE, Carpenter JW, eds. *Ferrets, Rabbits, and Rodents. Clinical Medicine and Surgery.* 3rd ed. St. Louis, MO: W.B. Saunders; 2011.

141. Martinho F. Dystocia caused by ectopic pregnancy in a guinea pig *(Cavia porcellus). Vet Clin North Am Exot Anim Pract.* 2006;9:713-716.

142. Hong CC, Armstrong ML. Ectopic pregnancy in 2 guinea-pigs. *Lab Anim.* 1978;12:243-244.

143. Hawkins MG, Bishop CR. Disease problems of guinea pigs. In: Quesenberry KE, Carpenter JW, eds. *Ferrets, Rabbits, and Rodents. Clinical Medicine and Surgery.* 3rd ed. St. Louis, MO: W.B. Saunders; 2011.

144. Evans BA. Small mammals: guinea pigs: uterine and vaginal disorders. In: Mayer J, Donnelly TM, eds. *Clinical Veterinary Advisor: Birds and Exotic Pets.* St. Louis, MO: Saunders; 2013.

145. Olson ME, Bruce J. Ovariectomy, ovariohysterectomy and orchidectomy in rodents and rabbits. *Can Vet J.* 1986;27:523-527.

146. Stout Steele M, Bennett RA. Clinical technique: dorsal ovariectomy in rodents. *J Exot Pet Med.* 2011;220:222-226.

147. Mayer J: Surgical techniques for spaying rabbits and rat. *Proc NAVC.* 2008;1854-1855.

148. Mayer J, Sato A, Kiupel M, et al. Extralabel use of cabergoline in the treatment of a pituitary adenoma in a rat. *J Am Vet Med Assoc.* 2011;239:3-7.

149. Grosset C, Peters S, Peron F, et al. Contraceptive effect and potential side-effects of deslorelin acetate implants in rats *(Rattus norvegicus):* preliminary observations. *Can J Vet Res.* 2012;76:209-214.

150. Morges MA, Grant KR, MacPhail CM, et al. A novel technique for orchiectomy and scrotal ablation in the sugar glider *(Petaurus breviceps). J Zoo Wildl Med.* 2009;40:204-206.

151. Wolf TM. Ferrets. In: Mitchell MA, Tully TN, eds. *Manual of Exotic Pet Practice.* St. Louis, MO: Saunders; 2011.

152. Ramer JC, Benson KG, Morrisey JK, et al. Effects of melatonin administration on the clinical course of adrenocortical disease in domestic ferrets. *J Am Vet Med Assoc.* 2006;229:1743-1748.

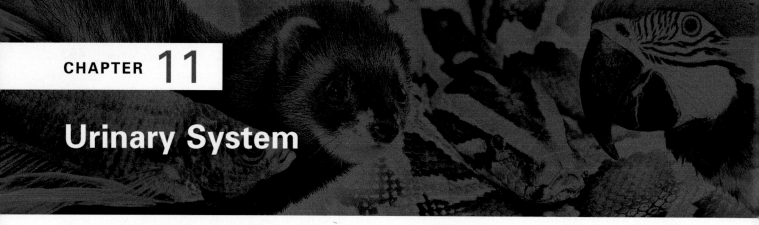

CHAPTER 11

Urinary System

James G. Johnson III, DVM • João Brandão, LMV, MS • Sean M. Perry, DVM •
Mark A. Mitchell, DVM, MS, PhD, DECZM (Herpetology)

INTRODUCTION

Excretion of metabolic wastes from an organism is fundamental to life and is accomplished in an effort to maintain homeostasis within the environment and prevent pathologic accumulation of waste products. Waste products expelled through the excretory system predominantly consist of inorganic salts and nitrogenous wastes. Nitrogen intake is essential for life because it is a major element of amino acids that are the building blocks of proteins necessary for physiological processes. Nitrogenous wastes are produced as a result of nutrient consumption by organisms for production of energy. They consist of ammonia, urea, or uric acid, depending on the species, and are the by products of proteins and amino acids in the liver.[1,2] Unlike carbohydrates and fats, protein and amino acids derived from protein degredation cannot be stored in the body, hence, excess amino acids are further reduced to ammonia and excreted or converted to uric acid or urea in the liver.[3]

Ammonia is the most toxic of the nitrogenous wastes and accumulation can lead to acid-base imbalances and interference with ion transport in cells, especially those of involving the central nervous system.[4] Urea is less toxic than ammonia; however, high concentrations can cause destabilizing effects on cellular macromolecules such as proteins.[4] In high concentrations, uric acid can precipitate out of solution into tissues due to its low aqueous solubility. Nitrogenous wastes, such as ammonia, may also have beneficial functions, including acid-base regulation during chronic acidosis; increased ammonia excretion in the kidneys increases the net acid excretion, maintaining the blood pH closer to normal.[3]

The excretory system is also important for water regulation and electrolyte balance in the body.[2] Both invertebrates and vertebrates use their excretory system, or some derivative, to maintain fluid homeostasis by regulating the amount of fluid and electrolytes excreted by the body. This becomes especially important for captive exotic animals when husbandry conditions are less than ideal. Animals that are fed diets that are deficient in moisture or electrolytes may be predisposed to dehydration and compartmental fluid shifts. If left uncorrected, these problems can lead to chronic renal failure.

The excretory or urinary system of most mammalian species can be divided into the upper and lower urinary tracts

that direct urine, the liquid by-product of urinary excretion, to the cloaca or urogenital sinus.[2] The upper urinary tract is comprised of the kidneys and ureters, while the lower urinary tract consists of the urinary bladder and urethra. Many non-mammalian urinary systems lack a urinary bladder and urethra, or the urinary bladder is a simple outpouching of the cloaca and not connected in sequence with the rest of the urinary tract. Since the urinary system is highly variable across species, the exotic animal practitioner should pay careful attention to variations in urinary anatomy and physiology by taxon when evaluating dysfunction and disease of the urinary system in a patient. Diseases of the urinary system, whether primary or secondary to other systemic diseases, account for a considerable amount of morbidity and mortality in exotic animals. Compared to domestic dogs and cats, where knowledge of excretory function is widespread within the veterinary profession due to similarities in renal physiology, caveats and differences exist among exotic species that cannot be directly extrapolated from domestic animal practice, namely, birds, reptiles, amphibians, fish, and invertebrates. These variations can be directly attributed to the natural history of each species, owing in part to environment and habitat differences that may affect fluid balance and modulation of metabolic wastes (Figure 11-1). For example, the excretory system of a fish that inhabits an aquatic environment has evolved very differently from that of terrestrial animals, and even among fish, variations exist depending on the salinity of the environment.

ANATOMY AND PHYSIOLOGY

Invertebrates

The invertebrate urinary system is rudimentary compared to even the most primitive vertebrate counterpart and varies greatly among taxa. Most aquatic invertebrates excrete nitrogenous wastes in the form of ammonia through the gills via passive diffusion or sodium-ammonia exchange.[1] Although crustaceans such as crabs are both terrestrial and aquatic, they still are primarily ammonotelic, therefore various mechanisms must accommodate the two different environments that they inhabit. The excretory organs of crabs are paired modified glandular coelomoducts. The glandular coelomoducts are located immediately caudal to the eyes and are composed of a terminal coelomic end sac, an excretory tubule,

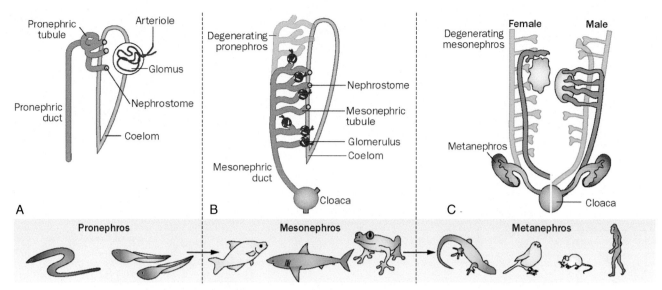

FIGURE 11-1 The kidney through evolution, as it proceeded through a series of successive phases, each marked by the development of a more advanced kidney: the pronephros, mesonephros, and metanephros. *A,* The pronephros is the most immature form of kidney; it represents the first stage of kidney development in most animal species but became functional only in ancient fish, such as lampreys or hagfish, or during the larval stage of amphibians. *B,* The mesonephros, the functional mature kidney in most fish and amphibians, represents the second stage of kidney development in most animal species. It is made up of an increased number of nephrons, usually dozens to hundreds. *C,* The metanephros represents the last stage of kidney development after degeneration of the pronephros and mesonephros in reptiles, birds, and mammals, where it persists as the definitive adult kidney; it consists of a substantially increased number of nephrons, usually from thousands to millions. (From Romagnani P, Lasagni L, Remuzzi G. Renal progenitors: an evolutionary conserved strategy for kidney regeneration. *Nat Rev Nephrol.* 2013;9:137-146. Figure 1, p. 139.)

and a bladder that opens to the environment.[5] It is across the wall of the end sac that ultrafiltration of dissolved solutes (e.g., ammonia) occurs.[5] In insects, such as cockroaches, the Malpighian tubules serve as the primary excretory organ.[5] The Malpighian tubules consist of blind-ended structures of ectodermal origin that empty into the alimentary tract and lie at the junction of the midgut and hindgut.[5,6] The Malpighian tubules actively absorb water, salts, amino acids, and nitrogenous products from the blood by osmotic forces, producing an isosmotic filtrate into the tubular lumen.[5,6] Water and certain dissolved solutes can be reabsorbed at the proximal end of the tubule and in the colon.[5] In addition to the Malpighian tubules, urate cells within the fat body of insects function to store insoluble urates and uric acid in the body.[5] Arachnids also have Malpighian tubules; however, they are of mesodermal origin and produce guanine as the end product, a substance that is related to uric acid.[5] Arachnids also have coxal glands that open at the base of the legs, which are coelomoduct derivatives that consist of a coelomic end sac and straight tubule.[5] Silk glands in arachnids are modified coxal glands that secrete proteinaceous silk stored in the lumen.[5]

Fish

Vertebrate kidneys consist of paired compact masses of tubules that conduct urine to the cloaca or distal urinary tract.[2] The

most primitive renal anatomy of vertebrates is found in fish, whose aglomerular kidneys are located along the ventral aspect of the vertebral column and can function in both hematopoiesis and excretion, depending on the species.[2,7] The kidneys of fish arise from the pronephros in the anterior nephric ridge, which is transient in most larval fish and later degenerates, contributing its tubules to an extended mesonephric kidney termed the opisthonephros.[2] The pronephros, or cranial kidney, of teleost fish is responsible for hematopoiesis, while the mesonephros, or caudal kidney, is where excretion of fluids occurs because it consists of nephrons that drain into the mesonephric duct.[8] In elasmobranchs, the cranial kidney degenerates and hematopoiesis occurs in the epigonal organ; thus, the kidney is composed only of the mesonephros that drains through archinephric ducts to the cloaca.[8] Most fish possess a glomerulus in their nephron, where filtrates from capillary blood are transferred into Bowman's space and the nephron; however, some species of fish (e.g., seahorses, pipefish, frogfish) lack a glomerulus (Figure 11-2).[1] While arterial blood flows into the glomeruli from the aorta and renal arteries, venous blood to the tubules arrives via the caudal vein of the tail that divides into right and left branches and acts as a portal system into each kidney.[1] However, in some species of fish, blood from the caudal vein flows directly back to the heart, and the renal tubules are supplied by branches of vessels from the flank musculature.[1]

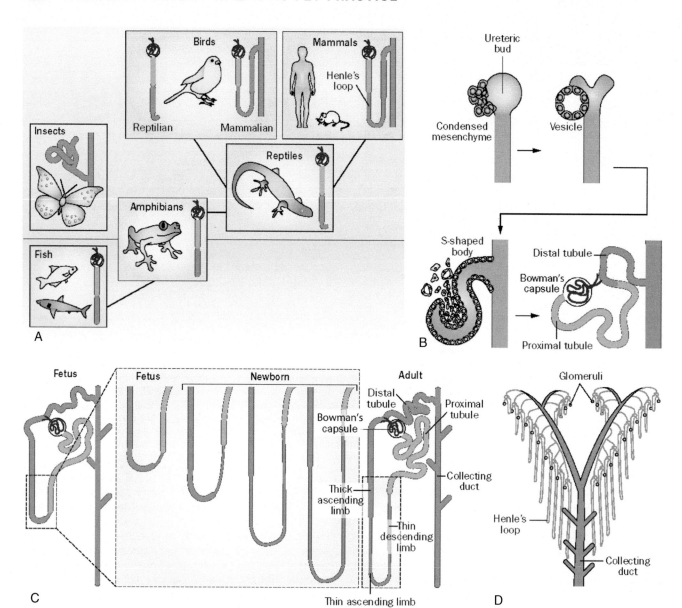

FIGURE 11-2 The nephron: an evolutionary link. *A,* Nephrons, the basic functional unit of the kidney, are quite similar across phyletic groups. In general, in vertebrates, they consist of a corpuscle, the filtering unit, which is connected through a neck to a tubule that can be divided into a proximal tubule, an intermediate segment and a distal tubule that connects to an excretion unit. Avian and mammalian kidneys show a major modification to the basic structure of the nephron—Henle's loop—which enabled urine to be concentrated. Bird kidneys contain two types of nephrons: nephrons with Henle's loop ("mammalian type") and nephrons without Henle's loop ("reptilian type"). By contrast, all nephrons in mammals display Henle's loop, although the lengths of these loops differ both within and between species. Even in insects, which are invertebrates, the renal system is recognizable as an analogue of the vertebrate renal tubule. *B,* Phases of nephron development in all animals. The metanephric mesenchyme condenses around the ureteric bud and is induced to convert into epithelium and generates in sequence a vesicle and an S-shaped body. Then, the S-shaped body becomes invaded by blood vessels at one extremity and elongates and segmentates at the other, thus generating the whole nephron. This sequence of events is similar during development across all animal species. *C,* In birds and mammals, after nephron development has completed and concomitant with the development of the renal papilla in the newborn, the thin ascending limb of Henle's loops is generated as an outgrowth from the S3 segment of the proximal tubule and from the distal tubule anlage of the nephron. *D,* The pattern of nephron distribution along the collecting ducts in adult mammalian kidney, and its characteristic pyramid shape. (From Romagnani P, Lasagni L, Remuzzi G. Renal progenitors: an evolutionary conserved strategy for kidney regeneration. *Nat Rev Nephrol.* 2013;9:137-146. Figure 2a, p. 140.)

Fish are primarily ammonotelic, meaning that they excrete nitrogenous waste through the kidneys and their gills in the form of ammonia, which is highly soluble in water.[2] Some fish species are also ureotelic; these animals primarily excrete urea after arginine and purine breakdown.[4] However, nitrogenous waste excretion can vary, even in a single species such as the African lungfish (*Protopterus* sp.), which excretes ammonia while swimming in bodies of water and converts the ammonia into less toxic urea that can accumulate safely in the body during drought.[2] In addition to excretion of nitrogenous wastes, kidneys of fish are uniquely designed to compensate for fluctuations of water and ions in and out of the body, depending on the salinity of the environment. Freshwater fish are typically hyperosmotic to their environment and constantly battle an inward absorption of water, whereas saltwater fish are typically hyposmotic to their environment and constantly battle an outward loss of water.[2,7] Hence, the kidneys of freshwater fish are designed to excrete large quantities of dilute urine, ~10 times the volume of marine fishes.[2] Several exceptions exist among fish, such as sharks, skates, and rays, which have tissue fluid that is osmotically similar to their environment due to high circulating levels of urea.[2,7] Elasmobranchs are unique in that they are predominantly ureotelic, producing urea in the liver via a urea-ornithine pathway, reabsorbing urea in the kidneys and excreting urea in largest quantities through the gills.[4] This adaptation varies with environment such that freshwater elasmobranchs have been shown to have a 70% lower plasma-urea concentration.[4] Additionally, compared to marine teleosts that excrete sodium and chloride through the gills, elasmobranchs possess a rectal gland that serves as the primary site of excess salt excretion.[9]

Fish share the same endocrine control over the urinary system as found in higher vertebrates, although fewer hormones contribute to overall osmoregulatory function, and other organ systems related to osmoregulation are linked to renal osmoregulation, such as the branchial arch and gill epithelium.[1] Fish have a neurohypophysis, similar to higher vertebrates, that secretes hormones (e.g., arginine, vasotocin, and isotocin) into circulation; these hormones have diuretic and antidiuretic effects on the fish.[1] Angiotensin II is the product of the renin-angiotensin-aldosterone system in fish and sharks, similar to other vertebrates, and functions in fluid homeostasis by increasing systemic blood pressure and drinking behavior and decreasing the glomerular filtration rate (GFR).[1] Natriuretic peptides may also affect renal function and are synthesized and released by heart chamber enlargement during increased blood volume or increased sodium concentrations and osmolality.[1] Natriuretic peptides are likely more important in marine fish than freshwater fish, since salt significantly contributes to fluid volume.[1]

Amphibians

Amphibians have paired mesonephric kidneys (see Figure 11-1).[7,10] The larval amphibian kidney also begins as a transient pronephros that becomes a larval mesonephros and at metamorphosis is replaced with an opisthonephros, as in fish.[2] Nephrons in the amphibian opisthonephros lack a loop of Henle and as a result are unable to concentrate urine beyond the osmolarity of their plasma (see Figure 11-2).[3,7,10] The nephrons are divided into proximal and distal regions prior to

joining urinary ducts.[2] In aquatic species, the proximal region is very long and the distal segment is very short, while in terrestrial species, the proximal segment is short and the distal segment long.[1] Caecilian kidneys are relatively unchanged from their embryonic form, and similar to other aquatic animal renal anatomy, the kidneys extend the length of the coelomic cavity.[11] Urine passes from the urinary ducts into the cloaca and is subsequently directed to the urinary bladder, an embryonic outpouching of the cloaca.[10] Amphibians excrete ammonia, urea, and uric acid, depending on the ecology of the species.[10] Ammonia is excreted by larval and aquatic adult amphibians, while terrestrial species excrete either urea or uric acid.[10] Waxy tree frogs (*Phyllomedusa sauvagii*) are commonly kept as pets and are an example of a frog that excretes uric acid as a means of water conservation.[12] In addition, African clawed frogs (*Xenopus laevis*) can alternate between ammonotelism and ureotelism depending on water availability.[10]

In addition to the kidneys, the urinary bladder and skin also contribute to body fluid homeostasis. Fluid can evaporate through the skin of amphibians, causing marked water loss. Terrestrial amphibians are more tolerant of water loss, occasionally as much as 50% in some species.[1] Angiotensin II can stimulate water absorption across the skin, similar to how it induces oral drinking in other vertebrates.[1] The ventral surface of skin, known as the "drinking patch," is an important source of water intake for anurans, accounting for up to 80% of the water they require to maintain fluid homeostasis. Water absorption through the gastrointestinal tract is generally considered minimal, except in certain species (e.g., waxy tree frogs).[12] Hence, oral fluids are of little value for a dehydrated terrestrial amphibian, and soaking the animal in an electrolyte-balanced fluid is preferred. Aquatic amphibians also can absorb fluid across their skin in a hyposmotic freshwater environment and as a result must conserve plasma solutes and excrete copious amounts of dilute urine.[12] The urinary bladder of amphibians plays a significant role in water storage for amphibians, conserving large volumes of dilute urine that can be later used during periods of drought or low water availability.[1] Permeability of the bladder epithelium to water is controlled by arginine vasotocin.

Reptiles

The amniote kidney is evolutionarily the most advanced. The most rudimentary amniote kidney is found in reptile species, which begins as an embryonic mesonephros and is the first to be completely replaced by the posterior metanephros (see Figure 11-1). The metanephros is composed of metanephric tubules that drain into the metanephric duct, also termed the ureter.[2] Reptilian nephrons have a glomerulus with a rudimentary juxtaglomerular apparatus, long convoluted tubule, short intermediate segment, and short distal tubule, but lack a loop of Henle.[1,10] The distal tubule can vary in length, with reptiles that inhabit more arid environments possessing longer distal tubules to increase fluid reabsorption.[1] Reptilian kidneys lack a renal pelvis and pyramids and are asymmetrically situated in dorsal coelom.[10] Among the reptiles, only chelonians and certain species of lizards have urinary bladders that, similar to amphibians, are an outpouching of the cloaca, connected by a short urethra, and not in sequence between the ureters and the bladder.[10] Hence, urine is refluxed from the cloaca into the urinary bladder, or into the distal colon in species that lack a urinary bladder, for water reabsorption.[13]

Since reptiles lack a loop of Henle, they cannot concentrate urine beyond their plasma osmolarity.[10] Terrestrial reptiles excrete nitrogenous waste as uric acid through the renal tubules rather than the glomerulus.[10] Uric acid is poorly soluble in water and precipitates from solution in the bladder with sodium, potassium, or ammonium salts.[2,10] With the formation of uric acid, nitrogenous waste is excreted with minimal water loss, and fluid can be reabsorbed in the colon, cloaca, or urinary bladder. In addition, the urinary bladder actively absorbs sodium and secretes potassium and urates.[10,14,15] Water is also conserved in reptiles by reducing the GFR in response to arginine vasotocin, which constricts afferent glomerular arterioles and decreases the excretion of salts and nitrogenous wastes.[10] However, this may increase salt concentrations in the body, so some reptiles are equipped with salt glands (e.g., periorbital or within nares) to actively excrete excess sodium and potassium.[10] Reptiles also possess a well-developed renin-angiotensin system for fluid preservation that can decrease the GFR. During reduction of GFR and afferent glomerular perfusion, blood flow is still supplied to the renal tubules from the renal-portal veins, preventing tubular necrosis.[10] The renal-portal system also drains blood from the caudal half of the body through the kidneys into the caudal vena cava. The effect of this circulatory characteristic on first-pass effect following drug administration in the caudal half of the body is not fully understood; however, there currently is enough scientific evidence to recommend administration of drugs, that undergo tubular excretion, in the cranial half of the body.[16,17]

Birds

The avian kidney is derived from the same embryologic origins as the reptilian kidney; however, the avian kidney is the first to develop loops of Henle, which are a standard characteristic structure in mammals (see Figures 11-1 and 11-2).[2] While there is no corticomedullary definition in avian kidneys, nephrons are classified as cortical or medullary.[10] Cortical nephrons comprise ~90% of the nephrons in the avian kidney and are most reminiscent of reptilian nephrons in that they lack a loop of Henle.[10] Medullary nephrons are less numerous in the avian kidney but are still located in the cortical region and are more reminiscent of mammalian nephrons because they possess a loop of Henle that courses into the medullary region.[10,18] Nephron loops in the kidney enable animals to concentrate their urine above the plasma osmolality to preserve body fluid.[2] Although the GFR of the individual avian nephron is much lower than that of mammalian nephrons, avian kidneys contain many more nephrons than do mammals.[1] The avian nephron also possesses a juxtaglomerular apparatus that releases renin to convert angiotensin I to angiotensin II, resulting in sodium absorption, potassium excretion, and decreased GFR; all of this is mediated by aldosterone.[1] Birds also possess atrial natriuretic peptide to increase sodium and water excretion.[1]

The avian kidney is arranged in three lobes: cranial, middle, and caudal.[10] There is some variation in this arrangement, in that certain species, such as passerines and hornbills, have two portions instead of three.[10] Regardless, avian kidneys are

relatively large structures in the retroperitoneum that are located in the renal fossa of the ventral synsacrum and can extend from the caudal synsacrum to the lungs. These organs are intimately associated with nerves and vessels of the lumbar and sacral plexuses, which often pass through the renal parenchyma.[10] Bird kidneys lack a renal pelvis, and urine is carried in collecting ducts that connect to branches of the ureters that run along the ventral surface of each kidney.[10] The terminus of the ureter is within the dorsal wall of the urodeum, where it deposits urine that can be retrograded into the colon and rectum for fluid reabsorption, similar to many reptile species.[10] However, some species of birds (e.g., ostrich) possess a rectocoprodeal sphincter that prevents water from refluxing into the colon, allowing the coprodeum to function in a manner similar to a bladder.[1] As a result, ostriches can pass either fecal droppings or solely urine.[1] Renal perfusion is provided by caudal renal arteries that provide blood flow to the glomeruli and by the caudal renal-portal vein that, similar to reptiles, perfuses renal tubules and serves as the primary route of uric acid excretion.[10] Blood flow into the renal-portal veins is controlled by valves that allow blood flow through the kidneys in a hydrated bird and close to shunt blood to the heart and brain in dehydrated birds.[19]

Similar to terrestrial reptiles, birds primarily excrete nitrogenous waste in the form of uric acid. Ammonia is first converted to amino acids, which later follow the purine synthetic pathway that produces uric acid.[1] This process requires more energy to perform than the mammalian urea cycle; however, uric acid, which is 40,000 times more insoluble than urea, cannot be reabsorbed in the cloaca in the adult nor in the allantois within the egg.[1] This is of benefit for an avian embryo, if urea were to be generated in the egg, it would get reabsorbed back into the embryonic blood and reach potentially toxic concentrations.[1] Arginine in birds can still be degraded by arginase into urea; however, the highest concentrations of arginase occur in the kidney, rather than the liver, and are inhibited by adenosine triphosphate during energy abundance.[1] Since the protein found in the urine of birds that is used to maintain uric acid in suspension does not contribute to osmotic pressure, sodium, potassium, and chloride predominate the urine osmolality, making urine specific gravity measurements erroneous in birds.[1] Urine may also be refluxed into the colon for additional water reabsorption, further confounding urine specific gravity measurements.[1]

Mammals

Similar to other amniotes, the mammalian kidney is derived from the embryonic mesonephros that is completely replaced by the metanephros, whose tubules become well differentiated into proximal, intermediate, and distal (see Figure 11-1).[2] The mammalian kidney is the most advanced, with marked corticomedullary definition and each nephron containing an elongated intermediate renal tubule between the proximal and distal convoluted tubules, termed the loop of Henle.[2] The loop of Henle descends from the renal cortex into the medulla, turns sharply, and returns to the cortex (see Figure 11-2). This design, by actively pumping electrolytes into the interstitium, creates a solute concentration gradient that favors water reabsorption in the collecting ducts, allowing mammals to concentrate their urine for water conservation adapted for terrestrial life.[2]

The GFR in mammals is often preserved by neuroendocrine control, despite alterations in systemic blood pressure.[1] The proximal convoluted tubule serves to reabsorb most of filtered ions and water in comparable amounts so as not to change the filtrate tonicity.[1] The epithelium in the thin, descending limb of the loop of Henle is permeable to water, which is passively absorbed due to an increasing concentration gradient in the interstitial fluid toward the renal medulla.[1] Electrolytes are pumped out of the filtrate in the ascending limb of the loop of Henle, contributing to this concentration gradient.[1] Urea is passively reabsorbed by carrier-mediated diffusion in the distal convoluted tubule, which also contributes to the concentration gradient, and electrolytes are continually reabsorbed in the distal convoluted tubule as well.[1] The final conduits of the filtrate, the distal convoluted tubule and collecting ducts, are selectively permeable to water and modulated by the renin-angiotensin-aldosterone system, antidiuretic hormone, and natriuretic peptides. Angiotensin II increases aldosterone and antidiuretic hormone, resulting in thirst and systemic vasoconstriction to increase blood pressure.[1] Aldosterone causes increased water reabsorption by increasing sodium reabsorption through principal cells in the distal nephron.[1] Water is also reabsorbed in the distal nephron through aquaporin channels, whose up-regulated production and insertion in the membranes of the principal cells are stimulated by antidiuretic hormone.[1] These processes are countered by natriuretic peptides, such as atrial natriuretic peptide, which produces sodium and water loss in the filtrate in response to higher blood volume and pressure.

Mammalian kidneys are adapted to varying environments by the number of juxtamedullary nephrons and the length of the loops of Henle.[1] Longer loops of Henle, more nephrons along the medulla, and longer renal papillae are characteristics of animals with the highest concentrating ability for water preservation, such as those that inhabit arid terrestrial or high salinity aquatic environments.[1] Hence, the ratio of the renal medulla to cortex is a direct measure of the length of the loops of Henle for any mammalian species. For example, humans have far fewer nephrons along the medulla than other species; however, we have a larger renal cortex compared to our medulla.[1] The ratio of the renal medulla to cortex in humans is approximately 5, in cats it is 8, and in some desert-dwelling mammals, it is as high as 20.[1]

Despite similarities in the physiologic function of the mammalian nephron, variation in renal anatomy and physiology exists among mammals. The kidney can have a variety of shapes among mammals, with most possessing the typical "kidney bean" shape with one renal papilla. However, the classic exception to the single papilla kidney is that of a cow, whose kidney is arranged in distinct lobules that, despite the separations between lobules, possess a continuous cortical layer and multiple renal papillae. The most striking anatomical difference from other mammals is that of marine mammals and bears, whose kidneys are termed reniculate or multilobed, with each renule (lobe) having all of the typical anatomy of a metanephric kidney.[20]

Rabbits are unique among mammals in that although their kidneys appear grossly similar to most other mammals, they have marked variation in function. Within the rabbit kidney, not all glomeruli may be active at once, and very well-hydrated rabbits can recruit dormant glomeruli to increase diuresis without increasing renal plasma flow and individual GFR.[10] Rabbits also lack the carbonic anhydrase found in other mammalian kidneys that functions in the conversion of carbon dioxide and bicarbonate, which would normally acidify urine.[10] In lieu of this and the abundant bicarbonate produced by bacterial fermentation in the gut, rabbits can generate high circulating bicarbonate and excrete the compound through the kidneys, resulting in a more exaggerated urine alkalinity than other herbivorous mammals, including rodents.[10] Only low circulating bicarbonate stimulates an ammonium buffering system in the kidney, which is normally stimulated in other mammals by high acid load, making rabbits susceptible to acid-base imbalances such as acidemia.[10]

Mammalian nitrogenous waste produced from protein breakdown is principally excreted in the form of urea. Urea is generated from the oxidation of amino acids or ammonia in the liver via the urea cycle at an energetic cost. Urea excretion appears to be adapted for terrestrial life and aids in water conservation. The energetic cost of producing urea, as opposed to uric acid, is rewarded by the fact that urea requires 10 times less water for excretion than uric acid.[3] Urea is also less toxic than ammonia, so increased serum concentrations can be better tolerated during times of dehydration or decreased excretion due to renal disease.[3] Hence, elevated serum urea measured as blood urea nitrogen (BUN) can be used to quantify levels of dehydration or decreased renal excretion, possibly due to renal dysfunction in mammalian patients.

DISEASES OF THE URINARY SYSTEM

Fish

Fish can present to the clinician with several nonspecific problems related to renal disease. Clinical signs that can be caused by primary renal disease in fish include lethargy, anorexia, weight loss, emaciation, alterations in skin color, coelomic distension, ascites, and sudden death.

Infectious Diseases

BACTERIAL DISEASES. Bacterial diseases are common in ornamental fish. The majority of infections are associated with Gram-negative bacteria, although acid-fast bacteria (e.g., *Mycobacterium* spp.) are also frequently identified as the underlying cause of disease. In most cases, skin lesions are present, and sampling these sites can help confirm a specific diagnosis (see Chapter 2). However, bacterial sepsis, in which the infection is only internal, also occurs. For these cases, the kidney is a common site of infection. Samples can be collected antemortem or postmortem (see diagnostic section) for microbiologic culture and histopathology. Histopathology may also be invaluable for evaluating kidney samples for other infectious diseases (e.g., viral). While not well studied in ornamental fish, several viruses that can infect the kidney are important pathogens of fish (e.g., koi herpesvirus; see Chapter 2).

PARASITIC DISEASES. *Hoferellus carassii* is a myxozoan parasite that infects goldfish. Infections associated with this parasite typically become problematic in ponds during late summer or fall. Commonly called "kidney bloater," affected fish develop severe abdominal swelling and ascites. *H. carassii* directly infects the kidney, leading to severe renal hypertrophy. An antemortem diagnosis can be determined from a renal

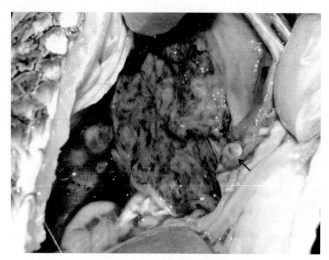

FIGURE 11-3 Renal adenocarcinoma in an oscar fish. Note the mottled appearance of the kidney and localized metastases *(arrow)*.

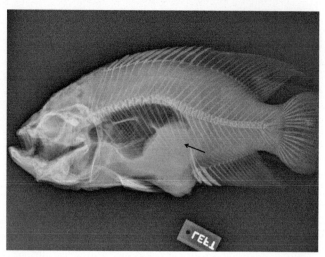

FIGURE 11-4 Radiographic image of an oscar fish showing a large soft tissue mass *(arrow)*. This was confirmed to be an adenocarcinoma at necropsy.

biopsy or by collecting urine and looking for the spores. Postmortem examination will reveal a grossly distended kidney, while microscopic examination will provide evidence of spores and distended tubules. There is no treatment. Culling all exposed fish, disinfecting the pond, and restocking are recommended when there is high mortality associated with the parasite infection.

Noninfectious Diseases

NEOPLASIA. As ornamental fish live for a relatively long period of time, the incidence of renal neoplasia is increased. Nephroblastoma and adenocarcinoma are two types of cancers reported in teleosts. Nephroblastoma is commonly associated with salmonids, while adenocarcinoma is diagnosed more often in ornamental fish (i.e., renal adenocarcinoma is a cancer commonly seen in adult oscar fish [*Astronotus ocellatus*]) (Figure 11-3). Affected fish present for depression, weight loss, and lethargy. Diagnostic imaging (Figure 11-4) with fine-needle aspirate or biopsy can be used to confirm the presence of the neoplasm. Unfortunately, these tumors metastasize locally and can be quite invasive. The prognosis for these fish is grave.

HEAVY METAL. Copper is commonly used to manage algae in ponds and treat parasitic diseases in ponds and aquariums. Most of the copper products commercially available are chelated products. Thus, they are bound to a carrier and released over time to ensure effective treatment. However, the concentrations of these products can vary in the water column based on pH and alkalinity. In some cases, copper concentrations can reach toxic levels for fish. Affected fish become immunosuppressed and more susceptible to infections. The kidney is internal organ in which copper can accumulate. A diagnosis can be determined by obtaining a detailed history of previous copper treatment and by measuring copper concentrations in the water. Removing fish from the system and performing a full water and substrate exchange can help to reduce copper levels in the aquarium or pond. Resins are also commercially available that can be added to a filter to help remove copper from the water.

Amphibians

Amphibians can present to the clinician with several nonspecific problems related to renal disease. Clinical signs associated with primary renal disease in amphibians include lethargy, hyporexia, anorexia, weight loss, emaciation, alterations in skin color and texture, coelomic distension, ascites, changes in urine output (anuria to polyuria), and sudden death.

Infectious Diseases

BACTERIAL DISEASES. Bacteria are ubiquitous within the environment of most amphibians, and there is a high risk for opportunistic infections in captive animals that live in closed systems. Epithelial disease, injury, and trauma are common in amphibians and can quickly lead to septicemia and nephritis. Bacterial infections that have been reported to cause nephritis in amphibians include *Pseudomonas* spp., *Aeromonas* spp., *Salmonella* spp., *Acinetobacter* spp., *Proteus* spp., *Flavobacterium* spp., and *Chlamydophila psittaci*.[21-23] *Leptospira interrogans* has been detected in anurans using serology and culture; however, no pathologic lesions have been observed in frogs. *Streptococcus* spp. have been isolated on postmortem culture from an American bullfrog (*Rana catesbeiana*). When bacterial diseases are suspected in an amphibian case, gram-negative organisms should be ruled out first.

Mycobacterium spp. are acid-fast bacteria that are considered secondary pathogens in amphibians. Mycobacterial species documented to infect amphibians include *Mycobacterium xenopei*, *M. chelonae*, *M. ranae*, and *M. ranicola*.[23] Immunocompromised amphibians appear to be more susceptible to infection, and many of these cases are related to poor husbandry. Lesions are typically dermal in origin; however, chronic disease often leads to the dissemination of the mycobacteria infection into other organs, including the kidneys. In chronic cases, lesions can develop over months, and death is due to multiorgan dysfunction and failure.[24] Mycobacterial infections in amphibians also pose a risk to humans because of potential zoonosis.

FUNGAL DISEASES. Mucormycosis and zygomycosis are fungal infections caused my *Mucor* spp. and *Rhizopus* spp. that are thought to infect Australian anurans and cane toads (*Bufo marinus*). Chromomycosis, which is attributed to the genera *Cladosporium*, *Fonsecaea*, and *Phialophora*, affects numerous amphibian species. Most fungal diseases develop through a similar disease pattern in all amphibian species. Dermal nodules containing the fungi invade the vasculature and spread hematogenously to internal organs, including the kidneys, leading to generalized organ dysfunction.[25,26]

PARASITIC DISEASES. Parasitic infections can vary from nonpathologic to fully disseminated disease. Ciliated protozoa consistent with *Entamoeba ranarum* have been recovered from the kidneys of amphibians with pathologic suppurative tubular nephritis, whereas *Trichodina urincola* has been recovered from the urinary bladder, skin, and gills of multiple anuran and caudate species with no pathologic lesions reported.[27] A coccidian parasite, *Isospora lieberkuehni*, has been (rarely) associated with renal disease and tubular nephritis but is not considered to be a significant pathogen of amphibians.[28]

Renal nematodes have been reported in clawed frogs (*Xenopus laevis*). These animals presented for anorexia and color change. Subcutaneous nematodes were discovered, in addition to a migratory nematode present in the kidney (Bowman's space) on histologic examination.[29] Clinical signs of trematode infestations are similar to what is described above; however, death can occur due to ureteral or renal tubular obstruction because of the type of organism. Monogenean trematodes, especially *Polystoma* spp., have been recovered from multiple organs without causing pathologic lesions. Many digenean trematodes (e.g., *Alaria* spp., *Echinostoma* spp.) use amphibians as intermediate hosts, while other trematodes, such as *Gorgodera amplicava*, use amphibians as final hosts. *G. amplicava* develops and matures in the mesonephros and is a common finding in the urinary bladder of anurans and salamanders.[27] Metacercarial cysts from *Clinostomum* spp., *Diplostomum* spp., and *Manidostomum* spp. induce granuloma formation in the kidneys and other internal organs. Additionally, flukes are observed as white nodules in the kidneys or bladder.

A few myxozoan parasites have been described in the kidneys of amphibians. *Leptotheca ohlmacheri* is a common finding in the renal tubules; however, it causes no apparent pathologic lesions.[30,31] *Chlormyxum* spp., another myxozoan parasite, has been associated with a suppurative interstitial nephritis, resulting in renal tubular dilation and necrosis.[32] Polycystic renal disease in African hyperoliid frogs (*Hyperolius marmoratus*) is thought to be caused by *Hoferellus* sp., another genus of myxozoan parasites.[33]

VIRAL DISEASES. Viruses have been isolated from amphibians and are associated with renal disease and pathology. Ranaviruses, both type III and I (frog virus 3), have been found to cause edema, dermal hemorrhages, and necrosis in multiple organs, including the kidneys. Bohle iridovirus leads to fatal viral hemorrhagic septicemia and nephritis. Luckè herpesvirus, or ranid herpesvirus, has been found to induce renal carcinomas in northern leopard frogs.[11]

Noninfectious Diseases

NEOPLASIA. Renal carcinomas occur spontaneously in northern leopard frogs (*Rana pipiens*) and are associated with Luckè herpesvirus or ranid herpesvirus-1. The neoplasm develops in the mesonephros, where the neoplastic cells metastasize to the liver, adipose, and urinary bladder.[34] The tumor is often diagnosed on necropsy because few animals show overt signs of disease until the cancer has disseminated. Affected frogs present with coelomic distension, lethargy, and death due to renal failure or emaciation.[34] Additionally, renal cell carcinomas have been described without viral association. Nephroblastoma, lipomas, myeloid leukemia, paracloacal transitional cell carcinoma, and lymphocytic hyperplasia have all been reported in amphibians.[11,35]

DEHYDRATION. Amphibians are prone to dehydration and desiccation. Any amphibian that is maintained with improper husbandry can be affected. Toads and other terrestrial amphibians may be more resistant to dehydration and can return to a normal hydrated state within 24 hours after access to water. Desert-adapted anurans can regain 30% of their body mass per hour when going through a rehydration process.[36] Urine production typically returns to normal once an animal regains its normal hydration status.

NUTRITIONAL DISEASES. Nutritional disorders are common in captive amphibians due to inappropriate husbandry and limited information on each species' nutritional requirements. Inappropriate nutrition can lead to the development of renal/urogenital disease or progression of kidney disease, as in other species. Leopard frog tadpoles fed diets high in oxalates (e.g., spinach, kale) have been shown to develop oxalate calculi in their kidneys.[28] A waxy frog (*Phyllomedusa sauvagii*) was reported to develop hydrocoelom, subcutaneous edema, and lethargy after being fed silver queen, *Aglaonema roebelenii*, an oxalate-producing plant. This diet was suspected to cause renal insufficiency. Postmortem evaluation of the kidneys revealed oxalate crystals.[37] Additionally, high-protein diets can also contribute to the development of uric acid crystals and gout. As with other species, high-protein diets should be avoided if kidney disease is suspected.[11]

TOXINS. The highly permeable nature of amphibian skin predisposes these animals to absorb contaminants or toxins present within their environment; some of which can induce acute kidney injury. The authors cannot stress enough how important water quality is to amphibians, as inappropriate water parameters (e.g., abnormal temperature, pH, hardness, and alkalinity) can increase toxin absorption.

Polyvinyl chloride (PVC)-associated toxicosis has been reported in poison dart frogs exposed to a newly established habitat where PVC glue was not allowed to cure. Improper curing allowed the compound to dissolve in the water, which resulted in the frogs developing acute renal failure. Additionally, heavy metals, such as copper, zinc, and lead, have been reported to adversely effect renal function in many amphibian species and should be considered when evidence of renal toxicosis is present.[28]

Reptiles

Renal disease in reptiles has been associated with a number of different pathologic conditions, including interstitial nephritis, glomerulonephritis, pyelonephritis, glomerulosclerosis, tubulonephrosis, amyloidosis, renal edema, bacterial nephritis, and cancer (tubular adenoma and renal adenocarcinoma).[38,39] Ultimately, to determine a specific cause of the renal disease, biopsies and histopathology are required. In addition, microbiological culture or polymerase chain reaction (PCR) testing may be necessary to confirm the presence of a specific pathogen. The histopathological assessment of submitted renal samples can be used to guide the clinician when selecting advanced diagnostic tests.

Infectious Diseases

Bacterial, fungal, viral, and parasitic infections can adversely affect the kidneys. In cases of bacterial, fungal, and viral infections, renal disease is typically secondary to the systemic spread of the primary illness. The most common bacteria isolated from reptile kidneys are gram-negative in origin. Examples of bacterial organisms that are frequently isolated from diseased renal tissue include *Salmonella* spp., *Citrobacter* spp., *Pseudomonas* spp., and *Aeromonas* spp. Fungal infections caused by primitive fungal pathogens (e.g., microsporidians) are not uncommon in bearded dragons. Viruses that may infect the kidneys of reptiles include *Atadenovirus* (e.g., bearded dragons), *Herpesvirus* (e.g., chelonians), and *Arenavirus* (e.g., snakes). If an infectious disease is suspected, a biopsy with histopathological assessment and PCR/culture are required to confirm the presence of disease. Antimicrobial isolation and sensitivity testing is recommended when bacterial infections are suspected. Parasitic diseases of the kidneys may be associated with protozoal, trematode, and nematode infections. Large numbers of active protozoa (e.g., *Entamoeba invadens*) or trematodes (e.g., monogenean infections of the urinary bladder of freshwater turtles; *Styphlordora* spp. in snakes) and nematode eggs in the feces/urine may be the first indicators of renal parasitism. Treatment for protozoa, trematodes, and nematodes can typically be managed with metronidazole (25 to 50 mg/kg by mouth [PO], once daily [SID], for 5 to 7 d), praziquantel (5-8 mg/kg, subcutaneously [SC], once, repeated in 14 d), and fenbendazole (25 to 50 mg/kg PO, SID, 5 to 7 d), respectively.

Noninfectious Diseases

NEOPLASIA. Neoplasms involving the reptile urinary system are not commonly reported; however, cases of adenoma, adenocarcinoma, and carcinoma have been diagnosed in lizards, snakes, and chelonians.[40] Affected reptiles may present with a history of lethargy, depression, and weight loss. A complete diagnostic workup, including hematology and biochemistries, urinalysis, and diagnostic imaging with biopsy, should be performed to assess the general health of the reptile and confirm a diagnosis. A unilateral nephrectomy may be performed in snakes and chelonians to remove a neoplastic kidney; however, this procedure would be difficult in a lizard with intrapelvic kidneys.

NUTRITIONAL DISEASES. Renal disease in captive reptiles is commonly associated with nutritional disorders. Feeding herbivorous reptiles high-protein diets, especially those composed of animal-based proteins, can lead to tubulonephrosis and glomerulonephrosis. Antemortem biopsies of the kidneys (see diagnostic section) can be used to help confirm the presence of these degenerative disorders. Unfortunately, in many of these cases, the disease is widespread at the time of diagnosis, and the prognosis is guarded to grave. A thorough nutritional history, that includes the diet provided and what the animal eats, can be used to guide the clinician since many of the affected animals are fed or have direct access to domestic pet food (e.g., dog, and cat).

Renal secondary hyperparathyroidism is less common than nutritional secondary hyperparathyroidism but does occur in reptiles. Chronic renal disease can lead to the accumulation of phosphorus, loss of calcium, and reduction in vitamin D synthesis. As a result, the elevated phosphorus binds to available calcium, forming calcium phosphate and further reducing serum calcium concentrations. This stimulates the parathyroid glands to secrete parathyroid hormone in an attempt to correct the low serum calcium concentrations. Unfortunately, these cases can be very difficult to manage. Treatment should focus on the provision of intravenous (IV) or intraosseous (IO) fluid therapy to correct renal dysfunction, phosphate binders to reduce phosphorus absorption, oral calcium treatment, and UVB exposure to increase vitamin D synthesis.

Calculi may form in all locations of the excretory system of reptiles, including the kidneys, ureters, urethra, urinary bladder, and cloaca (in reptiles without urinary bladders). Nutritional (e.g., hypovitaminosis A, high oxalates, high protein) and infectious (e.g., bacterial) diseases are commonly associated with calculi formation. Ultimately, to confirm a specific etiology, the calculus must be analyzed. The clinical signs associated with calculi in the excretory system depend on the location and size of the calculus or calculi. In certain cases, cystic calculi are an incidental finding identified during a physical or radiographic examination. In cases where calculus is causing a problem, anorexia, dehydration, decreased urine output or anuria, decreased fecal output, cloacal prolapse, hematuria/hematochezia, or unilateral/bilateral rear leg lameness may be noted. Calculi located within the urinary bladder or cloaca of lizards, snakes (cloaca only), and chelonians are often palpated during a physical examination. Radiographs can be used to confirm the presence of these calculi; these images can also be used to identify calculi elsewhere in the excretory system (e.g., kidneys, ureters). Calculi in reptiles are frequently composed of urates, including uric acid dehydrate, ammonium urates, sodium urates, calcium urates, and potassium urates.[41] Hematologic testing and urinalysis are typically unrewarding in these cases; however, they do have value in assessing the overall health of the patient and assist with anesthetic and surgical planning for calculi removal. The surgical approach to remove the calculi depends on their location. Cloacoliths in snakes, lizards (e.g., bearded dragons), and chelonians can often be removed through the cloaca with lubricants and endoscopy. Cystic calculi in lizards can be approached through a paramedian ventral incision (Figure 11-5), while a plastronotomy or prefemoral incision surgical options for a chelonian depending on the location and size of the calculi. General anesthesia and aseptic techniques are required to perform these surgical procedures. The approach for a cystotomy in a reptile is similar to that in mammals, although the urinary bladder wall of reptiles is thinner than in mammals. The coelomic cavity should be packed off to minimize leakage into the coelom (Figure 11-6). Aspirating urine from a reptile urinary bladder can be difficult due to the presence thick urates. Subsequently, stay sutures should be placed into the urinary bladder to maintain the location of the incision and limit urine contamination of the coelom (Figure 11-7). The incision into the bladder should be made in a

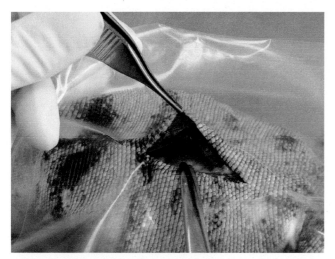

FIGURE 11-5 A paramedian incision in a spiny-tailed iguana. This approach ensures that the surgeon will not accidently lacerate the ventral abdominal vein.

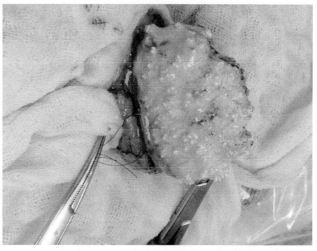

FIGURE 11-8 The incision should be large enough to remove the cystic calculi without damaging the urinary bladder.

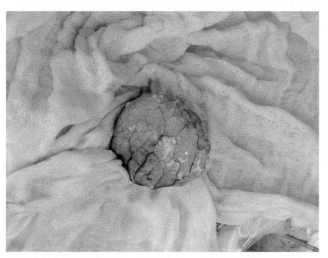

FIGURE 11-6 The coelomic cavity is packed off to minimize the likelihood of contamination during a cystotomy.

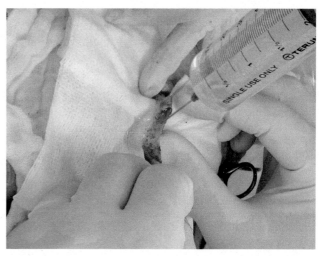

FIGURE 11-9 The urinary bladder should be irrigated with saline to remove any debris.

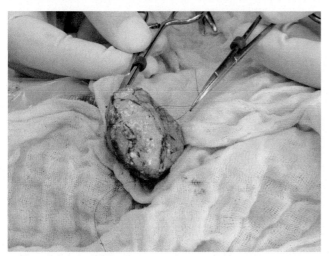

FIGURE 11-7 Stay sutures should be placed in the urinary bladder to maintain control of the incision and limit urine leakage.

relatively avascular area to minimize hemorrhage. The calculi should be removed, the urinary bladder irrigated with saline, and the bladder wall closed with a two-layer closure (e.g., Lembert and Cushing) (Figures 11-8 and 11-9). Saline can be injected into the urinary bladder to evaluate the integrity of the incision. Closure of the body wall (e.g., simple continuous suture pattern) and skin (e.g., horizontal mattress suture pattern) is routine. Skin sutures should remain in place for 4 to 6 weeks.

Gout is a common condition noted in reptile patients and can occur in a variety of forms, including articular, periarticular, and visceral. Gout is most frequently diagnosed in humans and primates, and is considered the most common form of inflammatory arthritis reported in humans.[42] Fortunately, gout is noted far less often in domestic animal patients.[43] Therefore, our knowledge of the pathophysiology and treatment of this condition in reptiles relies heavily on extrapolation of the human medical literature.[43] Uric acid formation is the result of protein breakdown into purines, primarily

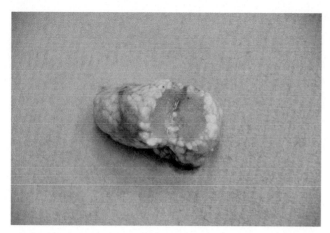

FIGURE 11-10 Renal gout in a blue-tongued skink (*Tiliqua* sp.). The renal cortex is markedly obscured by extensive deposition of uric acid tophi that appear as pale tan to white nodules.

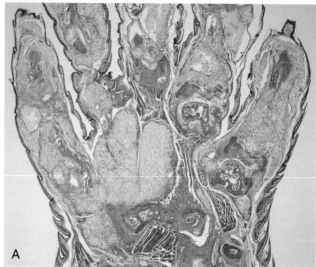

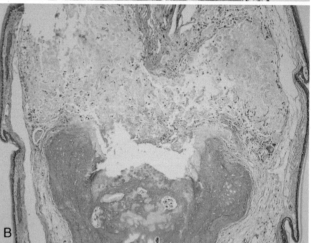

FIGURE 11-11 *(A)* Reptile manus; *(B)* interphalangeal joint. Joint spaces and periarticular connective tissue have small to large accumulations of irregular, pale eosinophilic to colorless acellular material (urates) and surrounding and admixed low to moderate numbers of macrophages. Destruction of articular cartilage and subchondral bone is evident in the interphalangeal joint. (Photo courtesy of Michael Kinsel and the University of Illinois Zoological Pathology Program, Maywood, Illinois.)

adenine and guanine, which are further degraded to xanthine and then into uric acid by the enzyme xanthine oxidase.[43,44] Reptiles that form uric acid clear this compound from the blood through the renal tubules.[43] Uric acid is poorly water soluble and precipitates at low concentrations, therefore when uric acid concentrations are elevated in the blood or body fluids, the uric acid precipitates into insoluble crystals of monosodium urate that are deposited in various tissues, including synovial fluid, periarticular tissues, and other internal organs (Figures 11-10, 11-11, and 11-12).[43,44]

Primary gout is related to the overproduction of uric acid, while secondary gout occurs when hyperuricemia is caused by other diseases or the effect of drugs on uric acid excretion.[43] Increased uric acid production can be the result of inherited enzyme defects in humans as well as excessive intake of inappropriate protein diets, such as a herbivorous reptile consuming a diet that contains large amounts of animal protein.[43,45] Hyperuricemia in humans has been shown to occur secondary to the use of thiazide diuretics, cyclosporine, low-dose aspirin, metabolic syndrome, obesity, renal insufficiency, hypertension, heart failure, organ transplant, and cytotoxic events that can result in tissue breakdown.[44] Environmental factors such as decreased temperatures and dehydration have been implicated in the development of secondary gout in reptiles due to their cumulative effect in reducing renal perfusion and tubular excretion of uric acid.[43]

Diagnosing gout in reptiles is achieved by taking a detailed history, performing a thorough physical examination, and the selection of appropriate diagnostic tests. Animals with a history of inappropriate temperature, humidity, nutrition, or water availability may be at higher risk for developing the disease. Patients with articular or periarticular gout may present with various soft tissue swellings at or near the joints or with visible white to tan subcutaneous plaques at those locations. Radiographs may show lytic lesions associated with the joints as well as mineral opacities in the kidneys and urinary bladder if monosodium urates/calcium complexes are present.[43] Ultrasound can also be used to evaluate the internal organs and soft tissues for the presence of monosodium urate crystal deposition in cases of visceral gout.[46] Laboratory

evaluation may show elevated uric acid levels in the blood; however, clinical gout can occur with normal blood uric acid levels.[43] Definitive antemortem diagnosis of gout is achieved by demonstrating monosodium urate crystals in or around the joints or in affected tissues with the crystals being refractile when viewed through a polarizing lens filter (Figure 11-13).[43,47]

Treatment of gout in humans is multimodal and aimed at relieving the pain and inflammation associated with the disease process as well as lowering uric acid concentrations, if necessary.[45] Nonsteroidal anti-inflammatory drugs and colchicine, which has anti-inflammatory properties, are the primary modalities of treatment for acute gout; however, glucocorticoids and corticotropin have also been used less frequently.[44] In humans, there is evidence that urate crystals

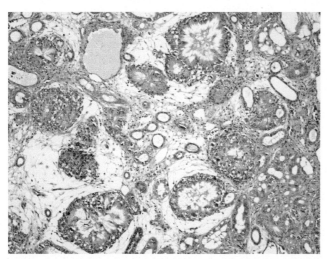

FIGURE 11-12 Reptile kidney. Obscuring many tubules are stellate accumulations of colorless material and surrounding aggregates of macrophages and rare heterophils (gout tophi). The interstitium is edematous and has rare, widely scattered macrophages and lymphocytes. (Photo courtesy of Michael Kinsel and the University of Illinois Zoological Pathology Program, Maywood, Illinois.)

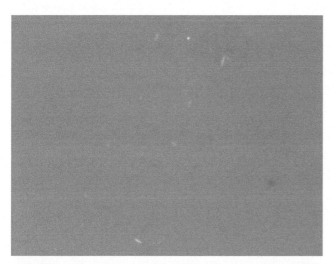

FIGURE 11-13 Aspirate cytology from the soft tissue swelling of the digit (polarizing filter) of a bearded dragon (Pogona vitticeps). Numerous tan, birefringent, needle-shaped crystals are present within the background. These are consistent with monosodium urate crystals. (From Johnson JG, Hulesch J, Schnelle A, et al. Diagnostic challenge. *J Exotic Pet Med.* 2014;23:113-116, Figure 4, p. 115.)

stimulate the release of interleukin-1β, so newer treatments involving the use of interleukin-1β antagonists such as anakinra, rilonacept, and canakinumab are currently being investigated.[45] Xanthine oxidase inhibitors, uricosuric agents, and uricase agents are commonly used to lower uric acid concentrations in humans with chronic hyperuricemia.[44] Xanthine oxidase inhibitors (e.g., allopurinol, febuxostat) block the synthesis of uric acid from xanthine.[44] Uricosuric drugs (e.g., probenecid, sulfinpyrazone) block the reabsorption of

uric acid from the renal tubules; however, they are contraindicated in patients with nephroliths and are generally ineffective in patients that have been diagnosed with renal insufficiency.[44] Uricase agents (e.g., pegloticase) convert uric acid into allantoin, which is more soluble and easily excreted; however, uricase agents are used primarily in humans who are refractory to conventional gout treatments.[44] Although several of these treatments are now the standard of care in human medicine, their use in reptile medicine has not been determined.[43] The prognosis for persistent or severe gout in reptiles is poor, but therapy should be directed at slowing disease progression and controlling pain and inflammation.[43] In reptiles, the conventional treatment for gout includes antiinflammatory therapy (meloxicam 0.2 to 0.5 mg/kg, PO, SID) and the use of xanthine oxidase inhibitors (e.g., allopurinol). By the time articular gout is diagnosed, it is likely that the damage to the joint is permanent; therefore, therapy to decrease the progression of the disease and control the pain and inflammation is essential. Dosages of allopurinol vary but range from 10 to 20 mg/kg, PO, every 24 hours in most species; 25 mg/kg PO every 24 hours for green iguanas (Iguana iguana); to 50 mg/kg, PO, every 24 hours for 30 days and then every 72 hours for chelonian species.[43,48] Probenecid has also been used at 250 mg/kg, PO, every 12 hours but should be used with caution when a combination protocol with allopurinol is prescribed.[43,48] Fluid support is also strongly recommended (maintenance: 10 to 30 mL/kg/d, plus correcting dehydration). In addition to medical therapy, appropriate environmental and husbandry practices are required such as correcting any dietary or environmental temperature deficiencies and ensuring that the reptile has free access to fresh clean water.[43]

Birds

Avian renal disease is common in psittacines, although this disease condition is often only possible when significant pathology to the renal tissue has occurred.[49] From 1988 to 1989, renal tissue was collected during 605 necropsies performed at the Schubot Exotic Bird Health Center of the College of Veterinary Medicine at Texas A&M University, and 37% of all birds examined had pathologic renal changes.[50] Antemortem diagnosis of renal disease is challenging due to associated nonspecific clinical signs and the fact that birds often succumb to the disease prior to making a definitive diagnosis or pursuing any treatment.[50] As with other groups of animals, clinical signs of renal disease in birds may include lethargy, weakness, crop stasis, vomiting, polyuria, polydipsia, lameness, muscle atrophy, deposition of urates in joints, feather-damaging behavior or self-mutilation over the synsacrum, and changes in urate character.[49] Many types of renal diseases have been described and may include congenital, infectious (bacterial, fungal, parasitic, viral), noninfectious, idiopathic, inflammatory, toxic, and neoplastic.[51]

Infectious Diseases

BACTERIAL DISEASES. Bacterial infections affecting the kidneys and the urinary tract often enter the kidney by ascending the ureters or hematogenous spread.[19,51] Some investigators have suggested that the majority of bacterial renal disease cases are associated with a multisystemic disease processes.[52] Renal lesions associated with bacterial infections include granulomas, interstitial nephritis, nephrosis, and glomeru-lopathies.[52] Although not commonly reported, it is said that 50% of avian nephritis cases were associated with bacterial disease.[49] Physiologically, the exposure of distal ureters to gastrointestinal contents is usually protected by folds of the urodeum.[53] Nevertheless, the ureters may be exposed to gastrointestinal tract bacteria that allow infection to develop in the excretory system. When colitis is diagnosed, infectious agents, toxins, and inflammatory products can gain access to the kidneys if blood flowing from the colon is diverted into the renal vasculature.[49] It has been suggested that the renal-portal system also creates the potential for exposure of renal tissue to microbial or toxic agents from the alimentary tract.[49]

The prevalence of renal disease associated with bacterial infections in birds has not been reported; however, bacterial pathogens that have been isolated from the kidneys of birds include *Staphylococcus* spp., *Streptococcus* spp., *Listeria* spp., *Escherichia coli*, *Klebsiella* spp., *Salmonella* spp., *Yersinia* spp., *Proteus* spp., *Citrobacter* spp., *Edwardsiella* spp., *Enterobacter* spp., *Morganella* spp., *Providencia* spp., *Serratia* spp., *Pasteurella* spp., *Pseudomonas* spp., *Mycobacterium* spp., and *Chlamydophila psittaci*.[52,54-56] Staphylococci and streptococci have been reported as causative agents of renal disease in finches and canaries.[49] Septicemia caused by *E. coli* often targets avian renal tissue, although clinical signs of renal involvement may or may not be present.[57] Renal disease associated with salmonellosis in pigeons will often result in the patient presenting with polyuria and polydipsia accompanied by a decreased albumin/globulin ratio, increased creatinine and haptoglobin concentrations, and decreased chloride concentration in the plasma.[56] Urinalysis from these birds may show a low urinary density as well as erythrocytes and leukocytes. Following a water deprivation test in 3 infected birds, urine production decreased and plasma-urea concentration increased.[56] Ascending *Salmonella* spp. infections have also been reported in some birds diagnosed with ulcerative cloacitis.[49] *Mycobacterium avium* and *Chlamydophila psittaci* infections can cause pathology of the kidneys, but these diseases are usually secondary to widespread systemic illness. However, there have been reports of *C. psittaci* infections only affecting the kidneys in psittacines.[49] Chlamydial nephritis is poorly documented, but in a survey of 23 birds infected with avian chlamydiosis, 35% had renal congestion, bile pigment nephrosis, and glomerulopathy.[12] Interestingly, *C. psittaci* could not be detected in the renal tissues of these birds.[58] *C. psittaci* has also been associated with necrosis of renal tissue in birds.[59]

In ostriches, where urine is voided independently of the feces, 89% (n = 35) of the samples had measureable nitrite concentrations.[60] The most common source of nitrite in the urine was hypothesized to be related to the nitrate-reducing bacteria found as normal microflora of the urinary tract.[60]

FUNGAL DISEASES. Fungal infections affecting the kidneys are commonly associated with an extension of a fungal airsacculitis or systemic infection (fungal thrombosis); however, the kidney is rarely involved in either disease condition.[49] Unless the kidney is severely affected, renal function is not typically compromised with these infections.[49] If renal function is affected due to a mycotic infection, the bird usually has other signs of systemic fungal disease, such as weight loss, labored or open-mouth breathing, voice change, or decreased vocalizations.[49] Aspergillosis of the lower respiratory tract

(e.g., caudal air sacs) often leads to clinical signs associated with the gastrointestinal tract and other organs (e.g., kidneys, liver) because of the anatomical relationship of the air sacs and the coelomic cavity.[61] In the case of a black palm cockatoo (*Probosciger aterrimus*) with a 10-month-old history of anorexia, weight loss, episodic depression, muscular tremors, and bilateral leg paresis, a greenish-white proliferative cavitating mass was detected on the left abdominal air sac.[62] This mass extended into the left kidney and caused inflammation and necrosis of the kidney and sacral plexus (including the ischiatic nerve).[62] The mass was identified as a granuloma caused by *Aspergillus* sp.[62] The uric acid concentration of the bird was reported to be slightly elevated, but no other renal deficiencies were found. Fungal nephritis has been reported in a gray-headed albatross (*Diomedea chrysostoma*).[63] The fungus was identified as a member of the *Aspergillus flavus-oryzae* group.[63] Renal infections have also been reported in disseminated *Aspergillus flavus* cases involving broiler breeder pullets.[64]

Microsporidians, a diverse and ubiquitous group of eukaryotic single-celled organisms, are obligate intracellular parasites that infect a wide range of vertebrate and invertebrate hosts.[65] Microsporidians are currently considered a true fungi that descended from a zygomycete ancestor.[66] The most common microsporidian affecting birds is *Encephalitozoon hellem*, although *Encephalitozoon cuniculi*, *Encephalitozoon intestinalis*, and *Enterocytozoon bieneusi* have also been reported.[67-69] The species of microsporidians that were detected in 196 fecal specimens from birds within the families of Psittacidae, Emberizidae, Icteridae, and Columbidae included *E. hellem* (16.3%), *E. bieneusi* (5.6%), *E. intestinalis* (1.5%), and *E. cuniculi* (1%). Fecal specimens randomly collected from captive exotic birds (orders: Psittaciformes, Passeriformes, and Columbiformes) housed at Bohemian pet stores, avian breeders, and avian keepers in the Czech Republic were screened for the presence of human pathogenic microsporidians by PCR testing.[70] Single-species infection was detected in 36 birds (12.5%) for *E. bieneusi*, 36 birds (12.5%) for *E. cuniculi*, and 18 birds (6.3%) for *E. hellem*.[70] Co-infections were also reported.[70] In feral pigeons (*Columba livia*) from Murcia, Spain, 12 were positive for only *E. bieneusi* (9.7%), 5 for *E. intestinalis* (4%), and 1 for *E. hellem* (0.8%).[71] Co-infections were detected in eight additional pigeons: *E. bieneusi* and *E. hellem* were detected in six animals (4.8%), *E. bieneusi* was associated with *E. intestinalis* in one case (0.8%), while *E. hellem* and *E. intestinalis* coexisted in one pigeon.[71] Among captive pet and breeding parrots (species not specified) in South Korea, 8/51 (15.7%) were positive for *E. hellem*, while 1/51 (2%) was positive for both *E. hellem* and *E. cuniculi*.[72] *E. cuniculi* has also been identified in wild birds in Slovakia, including great cormorants (*Phalacrocorax carbo*) (17/40, 42.5%), a great crested grebe (*Podiceps cristatus*) (1/5, 20%), and a white stork (*Ciconia ciconia*) (1/2, 50%).[73] *E. hellem* is primarily found in the liver, intestine, and kidney, but it has also been identified in the eyes, lungs, and spleen of infected birds.[65] *E. hellem* infection in one eclectus parrot (*Eclectus roratus*) led to the prominent distension (2 to 4 times the normal diameter) of renal tubules due to the presence of microsporidians and cellular debris.[74] A cellular inflammatory reaction to the organism was considered rare.[74] In general, it is believed that these common parasites, which cause minimal tissue damage, are found in the kidneys of birds that died from other diseases.[67] *E. cuniculi* has been diagnosed in the kidneys of chickens *(Gallus gallus)*.[75] *E. bieneusi* was first detected in chickens housed at a poultry abattoir in Germany.[76] Since then, *E. bieneusi* has been reported in captive falcons in the United Arab Emirates and pigeons in Spain, the United States, and The Netherlands.[77] In Portugal, 5/39 (12.8%) caged pet birds from the orders Psittaciformes and Passeriformes, and 19/44 (43.2%) free-range pigeons, were infected with genotype Peru 6–like and the zoonotic genotype Peru 6 of *E. bieneusi*.[77] Although there is a paucity of published information regarding avian cases of *E. intestinalis* it has been identified in domestic geese and feral pigeons.[70,71,78–80] Table 11-1 provides a summary of the species of microsporidians found in birds.

It is important to consider that *E. bieneusi* and the *Encephalitozoon* spp. (*E. cuniculi*, *E. intestinalis*, and *E. hellem*) are the four major microsporidian species associated with human infections.[77] Thus, birds may serve as a significant source of environmental contamination and exposure for humans.[69] The prevalence of microsporidian infections in waterfowl (8.6%) was significantly higher than the prevalence of microsporidian infections in other birds (1.1%); waterfowl fecal droppings contained significantly more spores (mean, 3.6×10^5 spores/g) than nonaquatic bird droppings (mean, 4.4×10^4 spores/g); and the presence of microsporidian spores of species known to infect humans in fecal samples was statistically associated with the aquatic status of the avian host.[78]

PARASITIC DISEASES. Renal coccidians, especially *Eimeria* spp., are renal parasites of particular importance due to the significant tissue damage associated with infections (Table 11-2).[94] Although many host species harbor both renal and intestinal coccidia, the species of *Eimeria* that infect kidney tissue are distinct and different from those that target the intestinal tract.[95] Currently, there is limited knowledge regarding the life cycles of renal coccidians; however, these organisms appear to have a direct life cycle, similar to their intestinal counterparts.[94] Sporozoites of renal *Eimeria* sp. invade and develop in renal epithelial cells. The unsporulated oocysts are passed into the ureters and voided, with excreta from the cloaca.[95] Most reports of renal coccidiosis involve birds with subclinical illness or birds that show minor physiological or pathological changes due to the parasite;[94] however, infected young and immunocompromised birds are more likely to exhibit clinical signs associated with renal coccidiosis.[94] A definitive diagnosis of renal coccidiosis can be determined through postmortem examination of infected birds that have succumbed to the disease. Gross evidence of renal pathology is often absent, but tubular necrosis, coccidians in the tubular epithelial cells or free in the lumen, along with inflammatory cells and necrotic debris are common histopathologic findings.[50,51]

Although rare, cryptosporidial infection of the kidney has been reported in birds.[96] In a retrospective study of cryptosporidial infections in zoo and pet birds, no renal cryptosporidium was diagnosed or reported.[97] However, in a black-throated finch *(Poephila cincta)* with cryptosporidiosis, the kidneys were extremely large, with numerous protozoans in the lumen and attached to the epithelium of the tubules.[98] Other authors also suggest that necrotic cells can be detected within the tubular lumen and that an interstitial infiltrate of mononuclear cells and heterophils may also be present.[96]

Renal cryptosporidiosis has also been reported in a gray jungle fowl *(Gallus sonneratii)*.[99] During the postmortem examination the kidneys of the bird were described as enlarged and pale.[99] Microscopically, the ureteral branch and collecting duct epithelium in the jungle fowl was hyperplastic,[99,100] and developmental stages of *Cryptosporidium* sp. were accompanied by heterophils along with sloughed and degenerating (and regenerating) tubular epithelial cells.[99,100] In commercial poultry, two layer houses experienced an increased incidence of visceral gout associated with cryptosporidiosis, with an average daily mortality 1% to 2% higher than expected; however, egg production was within normal limits.[101] Numerous developing stages of *Cryptosporidium* sp. were observed on the apical surface of epithelial cells lining renal collecting tubules and ureters of the birds.[101]

Interstitial nephritis and a predominately lymphoplasmacytic infiltrate are disease conditions that are identified in birds with systemic sarcosporidial infections.[96] In a retrospective study of sarcosporidiosis infection in birds from Brazil, the lungs were the primary organs affected, but pathologic changes were also observed in the liver, spleen, kidneys, intestines, and skeletal muscles.[102] In budgerigars *(Melopsittacus undulatus)* that were experimentally infected with sarcosporidiosis, merogony occurred primarily in the pulmonary capillaries and venular and venous endothelia; however, significant burdens were also detected in the kidneys (glomerular endothelial cells).[103] Renal lesions, including tubular hydropic changes, increased tubular lysosomes, and tubular necrosis, were identified more often than meronts in the kidneys.[103] A novel fatal *Sarcocystis*-associated encephalitis and myositis has been reported in racing pigeons. Although organisms were difficult to identify affected birds had induced lymphohistiocytic interstitial nephritis and eosinophilic and lymphocytic glomerulonephritis in the kidneys.[96,104]

Schizonts of *Leukocytozoon* spp. and *Plasmodium* spp. have been identified in avian renal tissue.[96,105] Raptors often are infected with *Leukocytozoon toddi*.[105] *Plasmodium gallinaceum* and *Plasmodium durae* may partially or completely block capillaries, leading to leakage of plasma proteins, edema, and hemorrhage.[106] These lesions may occur in the heart, lungs, renal glomeruli, and brain.[106] Sporozoites of *Haemoproteus* spp. develop into schizonts within various tissues, including the vascular endothelium, lungs, liver, kidneys, spleen, heart, and skeletal muscle.[105] In passerines, *Haemoproteus* spp. may be observed in the kidneys, with accompanying lymphoplasmacytic interstitial nephritis.[107] Lymphoplasmacytic heterophilic interstitial nephritis has also been diagnosed in passerines, along with tubulointerstitial nephritis, tubular degeneration, and necrosis.[107]

Renal trematodes have been reported in multiple species of birds, including Columbiformes, Passeriformes, Anseriformes, Stercorariidae, Piciformes, Psittaciformes, and Galliformes.[108] Trematodes may be an incidental finding or lead to clinical renal disease in certain avian species, primarily waterfowl.[96] The renal trematode *Renicola thapari* has been reported in blue-footed boobies *(Sula nebouxii)* and brown pelicans *(Pelecanus occidentalis)*.[109] This parasite occurs in pairs and encysts at the apex of the renal collecting ducts. Interestingly, these parasites induce no gross pathology.[109] Trematodes belonging to the family Eucotylidae, including *Paratanaisia* spp., are parasites of the kidney and ureter and

TABLE 11-1

Microsporidians Found in Birds

Fungi	Target Species	Renal Involvement	References
Encephalitozoon cuniculi	Gyrfalcon (Falco rusticolus)	Not reported	68
	Chicken (Gallus gallus)	Not reported (only abstract available)	81
	Chicken	Present in the kidney (only abstract available)	75
	Cockatiel (Nymphicus hollandicus)	Identified in feces, no necropsy	82
	Multiple captive species (Psittaciformes, Passeriformes, and Columbiformes)	Identified in feces	70
	Great cormorant (Phalacrocorax carbo), great crested grebe (Podiceps cristatus), white stork (Ciconia ciconia)	Identified in feces	73
Encephalitozoon hellem	Peach-faced (Agapornis roseicollis), masked (Agapornis personatus), and Fischer's (Agapornis fischeri) lovebirds	Clinically normal, but organisms found in the kidney	67,83
	Eclectus parrot (Eclectus roratus)	Histopathology: many renal tubules prominently distended from two to four times normal diameter with microsporidial organisms and cellular debris; cellular inflammatory reaction to organism was rare	74
	Ostrich (Struthio camelus)	Not reported	84
	Anna's hummingbird (Calypte anna)	Enteric disease with voluminous pale feces	85
	Black-chinned hummingbird (Archilochus alexandri) and Allen's hummingbird (Selasporus sasin)	Fecal shedding	85
	Gouldian finch (Erythrura gouldiae)	Not reported	86
	Lovebird (Agapornis sp.)	Renal impression: smear revealed presence of organisms	87
	Lovebirds (Agapornis roseicollis, A. personata, A. fischeri)	Presence in the feces, PBFD PCR-positive birds were more likely to shed microsporidians	88
Consistent with E. hellem (no DNA identification)	Tricolored parrot finch (Erythrura tricolor)	No renal involvement but presence of diffuse granulomatous inflammation in the perirenal air sacs	89
	Mallard duck (Anas platyrhynchos), Greylag goose (Anser anser), mute swan (Cygnus olor), carrion crow (Corvus corone), budgerigar (Melopsittacus undulatus), Nicobar pigeon (Caloenas nicobarica), black swan (Cygnus atratus), black-necked swan (Cygnus melanocoryphus), coscoroba swan (Coscoroba coscoroba), black-crowned crane (Balearica pavonina)	Fecal identification	78
	Blue-fronted parrot (Amazona aestiva), mealy parrot (Amazona farinose), peach-fronted parakeet (Aratinga aurea), blue-and-gold macaw (Ara ararauna), scaly headed parrot (Pionus maximiliani), blue-headed parrot (Pionus menstruus), grassland yellow finch (Sicalis luteola), saffron finch (Sicalis flaveola), double-collared seedeater (Sporophila caerulescens), Chopi blackbird (Gnorimopsar chopi), pigeon (Columba livia)	Identification in feces	79

TABLE 11-1

Microsporidians Found in Birds—cont'd

Fungi	Target Species	Renal Involvement	References
Encephalitozoon intestinalis	Domestic goose *(Anser anser domestica)*	Identified in feces	78
Enterocytozoon bienusi	*Falco* sp.	Yellowish plaques on intestines (17/24), liver (15/24), and/or kidneys (10/24); kidneys showed multifocal, severe, diffuse degeneration with pyogranulomatous inflammation; most renal tubuli contained protein cylinders	90
	Lovebird *(Agapornis* sp.), cockatiel, African grey parrot *(Psittacus erithacus),* star finch *(Bathilda ruficauda),* pigeon	Identified in feces, no histopathology	69
	Pigeon	Identified in feces	69,71,91–93
	Chicken	Identified in feces	76
	Blue-fronted parrot, budgerigars *(Melopsittacus undulates),* saffron finch, pigeon		79

PBFD, Psittacine beak and feather disease; *PCR,* polymerase chain reaction.

TABLE 11-2

Species of *Eimeria* Reported in Avian Species

Host Species	Renal *Eimeria* Species	References
Ducks	Eimeria boschadis, Eimeria somatariae,* Eimeria mulardi, Eimeria spp.	123–126
Geese	Eimeria truncate,* Eimeria sp.	94,127–129
Swans	Eimeria christianseni	94
Gulls	Eimeria wobeseri, Eimeria goelandi, Eimeria renicola	94,130
Cormorants	Eimeria auritusi,* Eimeria spp.	94,131,132
Loons	Eimeria gaviae	94,133
Puffins	Eimeria fracterculae	94,134
Shearwaters	Eimeria serventyi,* Eimeria spp.	94,95
Penguins	Eimeria spp.*	95
Kiwi	Eimeria spp.	135

*Represent pathogenic effects in certain species of birds.

can infect several bird species.[110] *Paratanaisia bragai* has been associated with renal infections in domestic pigeons, with prevalence rates ranging from 25% to 40%.[111,112] In turkeys *(Meleagris gallopavo),* the prevalence of these parasites can be as high as 20%. Histologic findings in affected turkeys may include significant distension of the collecting ducts and several flukes within the lumen of these structures.[113] It has been suggested that the geographical distribution of this parasite was restricted to the American continent and the Philippines; however, *Paratanaisia* spp. has been recorded from the right kidney of a cattle egret *(Bubulcus ibis)* in the Nile Delta, Egypt. The egret was found to have marked emaciation.[114]

Necropsy findings of the egret revealed marked enlargement and brownish discoloration of the kidneys, and on microscopic examination, marked dilatation of the renal tubules with hyperplasia of the epithelium was observed due to the presence of the trematode.[114] The renal trematode *Paratanaisia bragai* has been diagnosed in ring-necked pheasants *(Phasianus colchicus). Paratanaisia bragai* alters renal morphology in ring-necked pheasants by dilating the renal ducts and causing local inflammation, despite failing to induce gross pathology.[109] Renal trematodes can also cause disease in psittacines. An adult female blue-and-gold macaw *(Ara ararauna),* an adult female blue-winged macaw *(Propyrrhura maracana),* and an adult male white-eared parakeet *(Pyrrhura leucotis)* with trematode infestations presented for severe dehydration and cachexia.[110] Necropsies of the 3 birds revealed that the kidneys were enlarged and had brown-yellowish discoloration and irregular cortical surfaces.[110] On the cut surface, there was a brown-yellowish material and visible parasites flowing out of the parenchyma.[110] Histologically, there was an interstitial, multifocal to coalescent, lymphoplasmacytic infiltrate with low numbers of epithelioid macrophages and a few heterophils, characterizing a granulomatous nephritis.[110] Adult worms and eggs were observed within dilated tubules and the renal pelvis. In the blue-and-gold macaw, parasite eggs were located interstitially and associated with an intense localized granulomatous reaction.[110]

Tanaisia bragai is a trematode that has been associated with renal collecting duct obstruction and has been reported in Passeriformes, chickens, pigeons, and penguins.[59] In a captive population of Puerto Rican plain pigeons *(Patagioenas inornata),* histopathological examination revealed an interstitial infiltrate of inflammatory cells within renal tubules that was composed of heterophils and limited numbers of eosinophils.[115] In addition, there were numerous flukes within the renal collecting ducts.[115] In one study, 15.7% of the pigeons sampled in Rio de Janeiro, Brazil, were infested by *Tamerlanea bragai*; the flukes were found in the kidneys and ureters.[116] The cortical renal tissue is rarely invaded, but the urinary tubes can be enormously dilated and filled with amorphous and crystallized debris.[116] This parasite has also been reported in captive collections in the United Kingdom. A total of 8 animals comprised of multiple avian species (red bird of paradise, *Paraisaea rubra*; Socorro dove, *Zenaida graysoni*; Mindanao bleeding-heart dove, *Gallicolumba crinigera*; laughing dove, *Strepopelia senegalensis*; and emerald dove, *Chalcophaps indica*) have been diagnosed with *P. bragai*. A known intermediate snail host, *Allopeas clavulinum*, was present in the enclosures but there was no direct evidence of trematode infection.[117]

Renicola heroni infects the kidneys of the giant heron (*Ardea goliath*) and induces degenerative changes, necrosis, and vasculitis of the renal blood vessels.[118] Metacercariae of *Renicola* spp. have been recovered from the pyloric ceca and mesenteries of sardines and other small fish, consequently piscivorous birds become infected by ingestion of these intermediate hosts.[109]

The flukes are found in the collecting tubules in the medullary cone, causing tubule dilation with minimal to no inflammation.[96] Severe infections result in obstruction of the tubules, variable inflammation, and necrosis and secondary dilatation proximal to the block.[96] Cestodes can also cause renal disease. *Cloacotaenia* sp. inhabits the ureter or the tubular area that transports wastes from the kidneys to the cloaca in certain waterfowl species.[94] Although this condition may not be a common clinical condition, high or increasing prevalence in some wild populations has been reported.[119,120] Schistosomiasis is common in waterfowl.[96] and is associated with intravascular trematodes belonging to the family Schistosomatidae.[121] Larval forms invade the skin of waterfowl during swimming, and on maturation, eggs that are laid in the bloodstream lodge as emboli, pass through the vessel wall and interstitial tissues, and are extruded through the enteric mucosa into the gut lumen.[121] The adult flukes in vessels and the granulomas surrounding egg emboli are readily identified through microscopic examination of infected tissue.[121] Although the inflammatory response is usually minimal for adults and migrating larval forms, eggs elicit severe granulomatous inflammation when restricting blood flow in small veins or slowly migrating through tissues.[121] *Bilharziella* spp. and *Trichobilharzia* spp. are commonly associated with renal disease.[122]

VIRAL DISEASES. Many different types of viruses can infect avian kidneys, causing a multitude of secondary disease conditions ranging from minimal inflammation to renal tumors.[136] However, the level of renal disease associated with most viral infections in birds is not clinically significant and frequently are incidental postmortem findings. Several viral infections can produce polyuria, although none is characterized by polyuria or renal disease alone.[52] Renal damage secondary to viral infections is highlighted in Table 11-3.

Among viral infections, polyomavirus infection often results in clinically relevant renal disease. Since first being detected in 1981, avian polyomavirus has been known to cause acute and chronic diseases in several bird species.[137] Avian polyomavirus infection in nestling budgerigars frequently results in a generalized disease that is grossly characterized by discoloration of the abdominal skin, ascites, and various degrees of spleen and liver enlargement.[138] Histologically, inclusion bodies with karyomegaly can be identified in tissue obtained from multiple organs.[138] Viral inclusions can be differentiated from those of adenovirus by their tinctorial properties.[96] Recently, histopathologic examination of tissues collected from a fledgling budgerigar revealed, confluent hepatic necrosis and hemorrhages under the epicardium, in the myocardium, and in the kidney interstitium.[139] Live nestlings are typically stunted, have distended abdomens and feather dystrophy, and possibly develop intention tremors.[140] A percentage of nestlings survive avian polyoma virus outbreaks with only feather dystrophy.[140]

Overall, in nonbudgerigar species, clinical signs associated with avian polyoma virus infection are nonspecific and are of 24 to 48 hours' in duration. These nonspecific clinical disease signs include delayed crop emptying; weakness with a lack of vigor, pallor, yellow urates; renal failure; bleeding from feather follicles or subcutaneous bruising; and hemorrhage into the intestinal lumen.[141] In hand-fed nestling parrots, sudden death with little or no prodromal period is common, but clinical signs, when they occur, last <24 hours and include weakness, pallor, subcutaneous hemorrhage, prolonged bleeding times, anorexia, dehydration, inappetence, and crop stasis.[140] Due to hepatic necrosis, plasma concentrations of the alanine aminotransferase may be elevated.[140] In chicks that survive the acute disease form, generalized edema and ascites commonly develop (potentially) secondary to hypoproteinemia due to liver necrosis and/or the result of progressive glomerular damage.[140] Nestling cockatoos infected with a genetic variant of polyomavirus have slow development, fail to gain weight, and become severely dyspneic prior to death.[140] Dyspnea is a result of severe diffuse interstitial pneumonia and pulmonary edema.[140] A distinct disease course found in older psittacines is characterized by sudden death accompanied by a membranous glomerulopathy caused by the deposition of dense aggregates of immune complexes.[96,137] Up to 70% of these birds will develop secondary glomerulopathy.[96] Interstitial nonsuppurative inflammation and mesangial cell necrosis may be noted in psittacine birds with avian polyomavirus disease.[49]

In Gouldian finches (*Erythrura gouldiae*), chronic renal disease with glomerular sclerosis has been reported in birds with acute polyomavirus infection.[49] Inclusion bodies in the renal tubular epithelial cells associated with small interstitial foci of lymphocytes were also found in these finches.[142] Gouldian finches with polyomavirus infection may have both renal tubular epithelial and mesangial karyomegaly with intranuclear inclusion bodies.[96]

Goose hemorrhagic polyomavirus causes acute death with poor or no premonitory signs and lesions, including ascites, subcutaneous edema, nephritis, and intestinal hemorrhages.[143]

Infectious bronchitis virus is known to have a tropism for renal cells, but paramyxovirus, reovirus, or herpesvirus may also affect the kidney.[59]

All nine serotypes of avian paramyxoviruses are part of the genus *Avulavirus*, subfamily Paramyxovirinae, family Paramyxoviridae, order Mononegavirales, but all isolates of Newcastle disease virus (NDV) belong to serotype 1 (APMV-1); therefore, NDV is synonymous with APMV-1.[144] NDV typically causes lesions in one or more of four organs or body

TABLE 11-3

Viruses Associated with Renal Disease in Birds

		Renal Lesion		
Virus	**Species**	**Gross**	**Microscopic**	**References**
Adenovirus	Various species	Swollen kidneys	Basophilic intranuclear inclusion bodies, usually minimal, ranging from mild interstitial mononuclear cell infiltration to tubular epithelial cell vacuolation and necrosis; scattered tubular epithelial cells have karyomegalic nuclei containing large, darkly eosinophilic, or basophilic inclusion bodies	51,148
Alphavirus	Chukar partridge (*Alectoris chukar*)	Renal distention with presence of urates		148
Alphavirus	Guinea fowl	Swollen kidneys		148
Alphavirus	Turkeys		Renal necrosis	148
Astrovirus	Chickens and turkeys	Swollen congested kidneys		148
Avian leukosis/sarcoma virus	Chickens	Solid tumors: myeloblastosis: grayish tumors; nephroblastomas: enlarged, encapsulated, cystic masses; renal adenomas and carcinomas: discrete or diffuse nodules	Accumulation of neoplastic lymphocytes	148
Poxvirus	Canada goose (*Branta canadensis*)	Shrunken and necrotic, dry and firm	Large, well-demarcated areas of necrosis, margins of which are separated from the more normal tissue by a thin fibrous tissue layer; at least one organizing venous thrombus could be seen at the periphery of the necrotic area; amyloidosis also detected	149
Coronavirus	Ostrich (*Struthio camelus*)	Necrotic-appearing kidneys		148
Coronavirus	Gallinaceous	Visceral gout and renomegaly		148
Coronavirus (infectious bronchitis virus)	Chickens	Gout, polyuria, rarely renal congestion; some strains cause renal enlargement		148
Eastern equine encephalitis virus	Chickens	Pale and distended kidneys		148
Eastern equine encephalitis virus	Gouldian finch (*Erythrura gouldiae*)	Pale kidneys		148
Eastern equine encephalitis virus	Cranes	Visceral gout	Renal inflammation and necrosis	148
Influenza A virus	Ratites	Swollen, pale kidneys with ureters filled with greenish urates		148
Marek's disease	Various species	Formation of lymphoid tumors		148
Pacheco's disease	Various species	Usually acute with no lesions, possibly enlarged kidneys	Uncommonly have inclusion bodies in the renal tubular epithelium	96,148

Continued

TABLE 11-3

Viruses Associated with Renal Disease in Birds—cont'd

Virus	Species	Renal Lesion		References
		Gross	Microscopic	
Parakeet herpesvirus	Bourke's parrot (Neopsephotus bourkii)		Herpesvirus-like particles within intranuclear inclusion bodies in the kidneys	148
Paramyxovirus	Pigeon (Columba livia)		Interstitial lymphoplasmacytic nephritis and tubular necrosis with granular and hyaline casts present in the tubules	51
Paramyxovirus (Newcastle disease)	Cormorant and pigeon		Nonsuppurative nephritis consisting of multiple small areas of infiltration of renal parenchyma with lymphocytes and plasma cells; small foci of necrosis of renal tubule cells observed in association with the inflammatory cells	145
Picornavirus (avian nephritis virus)	Chickens	Renal discoloration	Insterstitial lymphocytic infiltration; degeneration of epithelial cells of proximal convoluted tubules	148,150
Pigeon herpesvirus	Pigeon	Potential secondary renal infections	Renal necrosis	148
Polyomavirus	Budgerigar (Melopsittacus undulatus)		Renal necrosis, virus microscopic identification in the kidneys as well as inclusion bodies; renal tubular epithelial cells may have karyomegaly, with affected nuclei containing clear or amophophilic, slightly granular inclusion bodies	51,148
Polyomavirus	Psittacines (nonbudgerigars)	Pale swollen kidneys, commonly secondary glomerulopathy	Membranous glomerulopathy, potential inclusion bodies; intranuclear inclusion bodies and accompanying karyomegaly commonly seen in mesangial cells; glomeruli appear swollen	51,148
Reovirus	African grey parrot (Psittacus erithacus)	Swollen kidneys	Kidney necrosis; nonsuppurative inflammation may be present in renal interstitium	51,148
Reticuloendotheliosis virus	Pheasants	Grayish-white nodules		148
Reticuloendotheliosis virus	Turkeys	Neoplasia formation		148
West Nile virus			Variable; lymphocytic interstitial nephritis	51
Western equine encephalitis virus	Emu (Dromaius novaehollandiae)	Renal swelling and inflammation	Inflammation and necrosis	148

systems, including the central nervous system, kidneys, alimentary tract, and respiratory system.[145] NDV pathogenic to wild bird species appears to affect the central nervous system and kidneys most often or causes generalized, rapidly fatal disease accompanied by few recognizable gross or histological lesions.[145] Nonsuppurative nephritis, consisting of multiple small areas of renal parenchymal infiltrates consisting of lymphocytes and plasma cells, has been a common disease

condition associated with NDV in cormorants and pigeons.[145] Small foci of necrosis of renal tubule cells have been observed concomitantly with the inflammatory cells.[145] In chickens experimentally inoculated with Newcastle disease, extensive zones of necrosis were detected 5 days postinoculation in several organs, including the gastrointestinal tract, liver, kidney, pancreas, and bone marrow.[146] In Columbiformes (pigeons and doves) and some Passeriformes, the kidneys appear to be chronically infected, leading to long-lasting NDV exposure via renal excretion.[146,147]

If an infectious process is suspected or confirmed, treatment should be based on diagnostic test results (e.g., culture and antimicrobial sensitivity testing). While culture and sensitivity are pending, empirical broad-spectrum antibiotic agents or antibiotic medication that provides excellent therapeutic levels within the renal tissue should be initiated. Antibiotic drugs suggested for bacterial nephritis include cephalosporins (mainly third generation), β-lactams (e.g., amoxicillin, amoxicillin/clavulanate, piperacillin), and fluoroquinolones.[58,136] In mammals, the diagnosis of a bacterial renal/urinary infection is often achieved by testing a sterile urine sample collected by cystocentesis. Unfortunately, this is not possible in birds due to significant anatomical differences regarding the urinary anatomy. However, one can culture tissue samples obtained from a renal biopsy.[151] The prognosis for birds with bacterial nephritis is guarded to grave. A blood culture may be able to identify the cause of sepsis and bacterial nephritis.[58] Some authors suggest that blood-borne bacteria lodge in the glomeruli, with the infection extending into the interstitium.[151] These cases may result in false-negative blood cultures.

Fungal infections that involve renal tissue (e.g., aspergillosis) should be treated promptly with antifungal medications. Submitting a sample for culture is highly recommended because the treatment options can vary depending on the fungal organism involved. Antifungal sensitivity tests are available in specialty laboratories; however, they are not commonly performed and can be expensive.

Parasitic diseases associated with the kidneys are typically diagnosed from a fecal sample or renal biopsy. Treatment of these conditions should be based on the classification of the parasite, with ponazuril being used for coccidia, praziquantel for trematodes, and benzamidazoles for nematodes. It is important to consider that toxicity associated with certain pharmaceuticals (e.g., fenbendazole) has been reported in some avian species.[152]

Noninfectious Diseases

NEOPLASIA. Although kidney neoplasms have been reported in several bird species, renal tumors in budgerigars constitute a remarkably high proportion of all tumors in this species.[51,153] Renal carcinoma is the most common tumor of the kidney; however, adenoma, nephroblastoma, cystadenoma, fibrosarcoma, lymphosarcoma, and other neoplasms have also been reported in avian species.[51,96] Of 74 budgerigars, most of which clinically exhibited unilateral leg lameness as the predominant sign of disease, 47 (63.5%) had renal cancer.[153] In a retrospective study of 1203 budgerigars, 16.1% had cancer; of this 16.1%, 23.2% were renal, 22.7% lipomas, 18% gonadal tumors, and 13.4% liver tumors.[58,153] In a few cases, the latter neoplasms were also associated with renal tumors.[153] In wild Australian birds, renal adenocarcinomas were identified in 28 animals, of which 25 (89%) were in budgerigars.[154] Among a total of 473 tumors in multiple avian orders, 28 (5.9%) were affecting the kidney; of those, 17 were malignant and 11 were benign.[155] Among 220 psittacine neoplastic biopsy submissions, renal adenocarcinoma accounted for 2.7% of cases, with the majority of cases (4/6) affecting budgerigars.[155] It has been suggested that the high prevalence

of renal tumors in budgerigars could be associated with avian leukosis sarcoma virus, but contradicting reports exist.[148,153] In one study, the presence of a retrovirus has been suggested to be related to renal tumors, but the enzyme-linked immunosorbent assay (ELISA) tests for avian leukosis sarcoma virus p27 and virus isolation were negative.[156] In another study, no evidence of retroviral involvement was detected.[157]

Renal adenocarcinoma sometimes causes osteolysis and sclerosis of the ileum and synsacrum and potentially infiltrates nearby muscle and other surrounding tissues.[153] Distant metastasis (e.g., skin, lung, liver, and oviduct) involving renal adenocarcinomas rarely occurs.[58] The most common clinical sign of renal neoplasia is unilateral or bilateral lameness or paralysis due to compression of the lumbar and sacral nerve plexi as they pass through or lie dorsal to the kidney, respectively, or from tumor growth into and adjacent to the synsacrum.[96] Similar clinical signs have been reported in a northern pintail (*Anas acuta*) with polycystic renal disease.[158] If a large coelomic mass exists, dyspnea and tail bobbing may be associated with increased respiratory effort.[159] Other intracoelomic masses can lead to similar clinical signs, in particular, reproductive hyperplasia, dystocia or neoplasia, pheochromocytomas, or other intracoelomic neoplasias.[160] Dyspnea, lameness, and lethargy was reported in a Pekin duck (*Anas platyrhynchos domesticus*) with bilateral mixed germ cell–sex cord–stromal testicular tumors.[161] The clinical signs associated with bilateral mixed germ cell–sex cord–stromal testicular tumors can be attributed to the mass effect of the tumor displacing and compressing the coelomic organs.[161] Although pheochromocytomas are rare in birds, they have been reported in a Nicobar pigeon, a budgerigar, and a chicken.[162–164] In the case of the Nicobar pigeon diagnosed with a pheochromocytoma, intermittent lameness was reported[162] and attributed to osteoarthritis in the left tarsometatarsal joint; however, compression of the sciatic nerve due to a mass effect caused by the enlarged adrenal could have induced or contributed to the lameness as well. Pheochromocytoma metastasis has also been reported in a budgerigar.[164] In addition, one of the authors (J.B.) is aware of a case of a pheochromocytoma in a cockatiel, which presented with similar clinical signs (e.g., lameness, dyspnea) to that of a renal adenocarcinoma.

As a general concept, cancer treatment should focus on tumor eradication and may require several different forms of medical management, used together or sequentially.[165] Surgery, radiotherapy, and photodynamic therapy are used to treat localized tumors, while chemotherapy and biological response modification are effective for metastatic disease.[165] This concept is not specific to birds and most likely cannot be adapted to avian species. In birds, unless renal cancer is contained and pedunculated, surgical removal is virtually impossible because of limited access to the respective renal arteries and the short length of the renal artery to the aorta, which makes ligation or hemostasis difficult if not impossible.[165] Palliative treatment is selected more often for the management of renal tumors in birds, including the use of analgesics and corticosteroids (e.g., methylprednisolone).[58] Carboplatin (5 mg/kg, IV) has been used to treat renal adenocarcinoma in a budgerigar.[166] Although the bird's limb use improved, the mass continued to develop.[166]

DEHYDRATION. Dehydration is a common finding in avian patients suffering from illness and may be a significant contributor to the development of renal disease. As uric acid secretion decreases, urates may precipitate in renal tubules and ureters, leading to impaction and subsequent renal failure.[58] It is suggested that any bird presented in critical condition can be assumed to be dehydrated.[167] In the case of severe and persistent dehydration, increased water reabsorption occurs and there is a subsequent reduction in urine output.[58] As in other animals, dehydration in birds occurs when water losses exceed water intake.[168] Nevertheless, some species of birds, mainly those originating from dry environments, are able to tolerate water deprivation with minimal consequences. Species that originate from areas where water is not abundant tend to usually have lower water intake demands.[169] For example, a budgerigar with an average weight of 30 g requires 5% of its body weight in water per day, whereas a common house sparrow *(Passer domesticus)* requires ~30%.[169] Daily requirements vary with species, bird size, and environmental temperature.[169] The general range of renal output in birds is between 100 and 200 mL/kg/d; however, in dehydrated birds, renal output can decrease to 25 mL/kg/d.[19,167] In an experiment where house sparrows were dehydrated for 30 h, body weight decreased by 12%, plasma osmolarity increased, GFR declined from 7.7 to 3.5 mL/h, and urine flow rate declined from 0.2 to 0.03 mL/h.[170] The rate of water loss in the excreta of hydrated sparrows was 0.2 mL/h, while in dehydrated birds, it was 0.04 mL/h.[170] Although healthy birds may be able to tolerate dehydration with minor consequences, in the case of a diseased bird, dehydration may have severe consequences. Severe or persistent dehydration increases resorption of water, causing a subsequent reduction in urine flow.[58]

In mammals, dehydration is commonly classified according to the type of fluid lost from the body and the tonicity of the remaining body fluids. Pure water loss and loss of hypotonic fluid result in hypertonic dehydration, while loss of fluid with the same osmolality as that of extracellular fluids (ECFs) results in isotonic dehydration.[168] In the case of hypertonic dehydration, the tonicity of the remaining body fluids is increased, while in isotonic dehydration, the remaining body fluids are unchanged in tonicity.[168] Loss of hypertonic fluid or loss of isotonic fluid with water replacement results in hypotonic dehydration because the remaining body fluids become hypotonic.[168] Such classification has not been scientifically validated in birds; however, it is thought that changes associated with dehydration are expected to be similar to that reported in mammals.

During dehydration, there is decreased urine flow, leading to sludging of urate crystals within the tubules. As uric acid concentrations increase in the blood and exceed the solubility of plasma, uric acid precipitation can occur, thus increasing the possibility of gout development.[49] Ureteral obstructions (urolithiasis) are rare but can form due to urates or calcium salts, neoplasia, inflammatory processes, and cloacal prolapse.[59] Bilateral obstructions lead to visceral gout, while unilateral obstructions are associated with atrophy of the affected kidney and hypertrophy of the contralateral organ.[59] Urolithiasis has been reported in a double yellow-headed Amazon parrot *(Amazona oratrix)*, a lesser seed finch *(Sporophila angolensis)*, Galliformes, and a Magellanic penguin *(Spheniscus magellanicus)*.[171-174]

Treatment options are limited, and the prognosis is guarded.[59] Fluid therapy can be administered in an attempt to

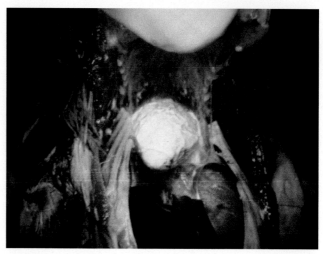

FIGURE 11-14 Pericardial visceral gout in an eclectus parrot *(Eclectus roratus).* (Photo courtesy of Paul Welch of Forest Trails Animal Hospital, Tulsa, Oklahoma.)

dissolve the blockage, but in cases of complete obstruction, aggressive fluid therapy is contraindicated.[59] One case of urolithiasis in a Magellanic penguin *(Spheniscus magellanicus)*, the urolith was disintegrated using extracorporeal shockwave lithotripsy.[171] A case of urolithiasis in a 21-year-old double yellow-headed Amazon parrot was resolved by ureterotomy.[172] It is said that surgical removal of ureteroliths may be an effective treatment for this uncommon condition, but it is complicated by certain anatomic features of birds and may result in ureteral stricture.[172] Vitamin A supplementation should also be considered for these cases, as squamous metaplasia may play a role in the formation of the calculi. Urolithiasis and visceral gout are important causes of renal failure in pullets and caged laying hens, but in companion birds, these conditions are rarely reported.[58] Other investigators suggest that gout is more a sign of renal failure than a distinct disease.[59] Visceral gout is defined as the accumulation of uric acid tophi on serosal surfaces of the pericardium (Figure 11-14), liver capsule, air sacs, and within the kidney but may be found in any tissue, whereas urolithiasis is simply the presence of urinary tract calculi.[58] Articular gout is defined as urate deposits within joints urate deposits are absent in other areas of the body and does not appear to be associated with elevated blood uric acid concentrations or primary kidney disease.[151] The etiologies of visceral gout in birds are diverse and may include nutritional and husbandry-related issues (e.g., water deprivation, excesses of trace elements, high-calcium and -protein diets, hypovitaminosis A, sodium bicarbonate supplementation), toxins (e.g., mycotoxins [oosporein and ochratoxin A], heavy metals, nephrotoxic medications [diclofenac and allopurinol]), and infectious causes (e.g., viral infections [nephropathogenic infectious bronchitis virus, avian nephritis virus, and hemorrhagic polyomavirus] and bacterial infections [*Brachyspira alvinipulli* and *Pasteurella multocida*]).[175] Experimentally, visceral gout has been induced in chickens fed excessive dietary calcium and a diet deficient in vitamin A, administered various nephrotoxic agents, and following ureteral ligation and urolithiasis. It has been suggested that gout may only occur under unusual circumstances, such as deficiency of vitamin A.[136]

If gout is suspected, fluid therapy is usually the first line of treatment. Although fluid therapy may decrease the hyperuricemic condition, it may have little effect on visceral gout. Allopurinol is a potent inhibitor of xanthine oxidoreductase and has been widely used for the treatment of gout and hyperuricemia in humans.[176] Allopurinol is widely recommended for the treatment of gout; however, treatment effectiveness and side effects may vary among avian species.[177] Anecdotal reports of its use in psittacines and passerines (dose ranges from 10 to 30 mg/kg, PO, q24 h to q8 h, and 300 to 830 mg/L of drinking water) have been reported.[178] Allopurinol dosed at 40 to 50 mg/kg, PO, q8 h to ethanol-fed turkey poults was found to reduce their plasma uric acid concentrations.[179] In chickens, allopurinol at 25 and 50 mg/kg reduced plasma uric acid concentrations over time, but no differences were detected between the two doses.[176] The results of this study did suggest that allopurinol dosed at 50 mg/kg may cause nephropathy and renal failure in chickens, which would explain the reduced feed intake and growth observed in that group of birds.[176] In another study involving chickens, allopurinol dosed at 25 mg/kg was also found to significantly decrease plasma uric acid concentrations;[180] however, reduced weight gain was noted in this group of birds. The investigators suggested that the lower plasma uric acid concentrations may have been related to the lower protein diet provided to the treatment group.[180] Allopurinol (50 mg/kg, PO, SID) administered to red-tailed hawks caused slight, but significantly elevated, plasma uric acid concentrations compared to controls and vomiting in the majority of treated birds.[177] Toxicity was suspected to be related to allopurinol.[177] A follow-up study evaluating red-tailed hawks given allopurinol at 25 mg/kg, PO, SID found that the lower dose did not produce toxic effects; however, the dose failed to cause a significant effect on plasma uric acid concentrations.[181] Based on these studies, it appears that in some species there is a risk of toxicity associated with the use of allopurinol. Another drug that has received some attention is urate oxidase (uricase). Humans and, in all probability, birds do not have a functional uricase gene and excrete uric acid as the end product of purine metabolism.[182] From a theoretical point of view, and based on experiences in human medicine, one can expect that urate oxidase (uricase) has uricolytic potential in birds.[182] Uricase used in red-tailed hawks (200 and 100 U/kg, IM, SID) and pigeons (200 and 600 U/kg, IM, SID) caused a significant postprandial suppression of plasma uric acid concentrations.[182] The ability of urate oxidase to prevent postprandial hyperuricemia in red-tailed hawks and reduce plasma uric acid concentrations to undetectable levels shows a great potential of this drug for use in treating avian hyperuricemia.[182] Another medication that has been used in human medicine for the treatment of gout, and has been considered a potential treatment of avian gout, is colchicine, which reduces uric acid concentrations by reverse inhibition of xanthine dehydrogenase.[49] An anecdotal avian dose of 0.01 to 0.04 mg/kg, PO, q12 to 24 h has been suggested for colchicine.[12] Unfortunately, colchicine has been found to exacerbate gout in some avian cases, therefore clinicians would need to closely monitor patients.[58] Other authors have suggested only using colchicine until clinical signs associated with hyperuricemia and/or histologic fibrosis

normalize; although it can also be used in conjunction with allopurinol.[136] In turkeys diagnosed with articular gout, colchicine administered at does as high as 0.18 mg/kg for 7 d failed to influence uric acid concentrations or the clinical course of the disease condition.[183] The use of low-dose aspirin (0.5 to 1 mg/kg, PO, q12 to 24 h) has also been reported as a treatment for gout, but the beneficial effects of low-dose or specific nonsteroidal anti-inflammatory drug (NSAID) therapies have not been studied in birds with renal disease.[184]

AMYLOIDOSIS. Amyloidosis includes a group of disease entities that share a common characteristic of an abnormal extracellular deposition and accumulation of protein and protein derivate.[185] Amyloidosis can be classified as a conformational disease because pathologic protein aggregation is due to folding instability and predisposition for variable conformation.[186] This protein misfolding disorder (protein conversion in a structure that differs from the native state) occurs with any pathological state related to the accumulation of extracellular amyloid deposits in which soluble proteins accumulate as insoluble amyloid fibrils.[187,188] Amyloidosis was first identified in birds in 1867 and is best described in waterfowl.[121,189–194] Spontaneous amyloidosis is occasionally detected in free-ranging birds, but it is a common finding in captive birds.[195,196] Anseriformes (mainly Anatidae and Anserinae), Gruiformes (particularly Gruidae), and Phoenicopteriformes have the highest incidence of amyloid disease.[194] Age and stress of captivity are predisposing factors to the development of amyloidosis in birds.[194] In domestic poultry, susceptibility varies with species, but chronic infections (e.g., bumblefoot) and stress are predisposing factors.[194] Physical stress and glucocorticoid production due to stress enhance the synthesis of serum amyloid A (SAA).[197]

Amyloidosis can affect the liver, spleen, kidneys, and small intestine.[194] In the kidneys, amyloid can affect the renal arteries and arterioles, glomerular basement membrane, and basement membrane of the tubules.[151] Renal amyloidosis often occurs in Anseriformes in conjunction with amyloid development in other organs (e.g., liver) and secondary to chronic inflammation.[19] In a retrospective study measuring the prevalence of amyloid in the kidneys of zoo birds, amyloid was detected in 49% of 275 analyzed organs.[191] In captive trumpeter swans, 11/31 birds had evidence of amyloidosis and 6/11 had renal amyloidosis.[121] In most cases, the renal pathology is associated with a generalized amyloidosis, which causes severe glomerular damage and results in nephrotic syndrome and gout.[59] In ducks, renal amyloidosis can lead to massive proteinuria and nephrotic syndrome due to severe glomerular damage.[19] Vascular deposition is also commonly detected in the kidneys, where it was often associated with glomerular sclerosis.[191] Renal amyloidosis has been reported in a diamond firetail finch (*Stagnopleura bella*) with concurrent proventricular cryptosporidiosis; Japanese quail and a chukar partridge (*Alectoris chukar*) with systemic amyloidosis; a roseate flamingo (*Phoenicopterus ruber*) with septic airsacculitis, hemosiderosis, atherosclerosis, and systemic amyloidosis; a hooded merganser (*Lophodytes cucullatus*); a ring-necked dove and pigeons with mycobacteriosis; mallard and bobwhites fed lead shot; a Canada goose with poxvirus infection; and a guinea fowl with *Mycoplasma synoviae* infection.[136,149,198–206] Clinically, this may be recognized as ascites or edema of the feet and legs.[19] Despite having a good appetite, birds lose weight and appear lethargic.[59] Grossly, the kidneys may be enlarged, pale, and somewhat friable, while histologically, the amyloid is eosinophilic or amphophilic and may be deposited in glomerular or tubular basement membranes and the walls of renal arteries and arterioles.[51,96] When Congo red stain is applied to tissue sections, amyloid appears red-orange and bright green when examined under polarized light.[136]

Amyloidosis is often associated with chronic inflammatory conditions such as sepsis, gout, enteritis, and arthritis.[58] Considering that the underlying cause of amyloidosis is inflammation, control of condition is a necessity. One can attempt to reduce the inflammatory response associated with amyloidosis through the use of NSAIDs or potentially cortico steroids. However, the use of cortico steroids is questionable due to the risk of induced immunosuppression and secondary diseases (e.g., aspergillosis). Pododermatitis or bumblefoot, may be a significant source of inflammation in captive birds, particularly waterfowl.[189] In hunting falcons, the likelihood of developing amyloidosis is significantly increased in birds with bumblefoot and visceral gout.[207] Surgical or medical management of pododermatitis must be addressed in these cases. In small animals, colchicine has been used to block the synthesis and secretion of SAA and decrease the formation and increase the breakdown of collagen; therefore, colchicine should be considered for cases requiring treatment of amyloidosis and hepatic fibrosis, respectively.[136]

RENAL LIPIDOSIS. Deposition of lipid in renal tubules is an important problem of chicks, poults, and adult captive merlins (*Falco columbarius*) and has also been reported in budgerigars, a sulfur-crested cockatoo (*Cacatua galerita*), and sacred ibis.[58,208,209] First reported by Marthedal and Veiling (1958), renal lipidosis was at one time known as "pink disease" because one of the most striking autopsy features was the pink tinge of body fat and the very pale liver and kidneys.[210,211] Renal lipidosis has been correlated with high-fat or low-protein diets, starvation, biotin deficiency, and chronic liver disease (fatty liver).[58] This condition has been referred to as fatty liver–kidney syndrome. Poultry may exhibit acute onset of lethargy, followed by paralysis and death.[58] This condition generally affects broiler chicks between 3 and 5 weeks of age.[210] Acute death is common in merlins, with affected birds presenting in good flesh or slightly overweight.[58] A retrospective paper on morbidity and mortality in merlins found that fatty liver–kidney syndrome was the single largest cause of death.[208,212] Renal lipidosis has also been observed microscopically in houbara bustards (*Chlamydotis undulate*).[213]

Fatty liver–kidney disease is said to be prevalent in merlins.[208] This small raptor relies heavily on insects in its natural diet, and it is proposed that the high levels of fats contained in captive raptor foods, especially day-old chicks, may be responsible for the condition.[214] Providing an appropriate diet can possibly reduce the incidence of this disease condition.

RENAL CYSTS. Polycystic kidneys have been reported in birds but are usually an incidental finding. A captive 10-year-old female northern pintail (*Anas acuta*), with a history of unilateral lameness, was diagnosed at necropsy with polycystic disease of which the right kidney was most severely affected.[158] The lameness was attributed to pressure on the sacral nerve plexus, caused by the unusually large cyst arising from the right kidney.[158] There was no evidence of renal dysfunction

reported in the duck, and the plasma biochemistry values were within normal ranges. Thirty to 35 variably sized renal cysts have also been observed as an incidental finding during postmortem examination of one young adult female pigeon.[215] There was no evidence of adjacent organ invasion/compression or renal dysfunction noted in this study. Polycystic kidney disease has been mentioned but not described in a bald eagle.[151] In poultry, although cystic kidneys are sometimes encountered as a result of chronic nephritis, this condition appears to be rare.[210]

NUTRITIONAL DISEASES. Human foods can be a source of toxins for avian pets.[216] Dietary indiscretions, nutritional deficiencies, and toxicities have all been reported and can lead to renal disease. Feeding green onions (*Allium ascalonicum*) to white Chinese geese (*Threskiornis spinicollis*) was found to increase mortalities in two different flocks.[217] Accumulation of hemosiderin in hepatocytes, Kupffer cells, macrophages, and renal tubules, as well as moderate to severe hepatic necrosis, vacuolation of hepatocytes, splenitis, and renal tubular nephrosis, were reported.[217] Anemia was also reported in geese fed green onions under experimental conditions; however, Heinz bodies were not a consistent finding.[217] Renal damage secondary to garlic (*Allium sativum*) ingestion has also been reported in a dusky-headed conure (*Aratinga weddellii*).[218] The bird presented for anorexia and lethargy but died shortly thereafter.[218] At necropsy, half a clove of garlic and chicken were found in the crop.[218] Histopathologic findings included hemoglobinuric nephrosis and hepatosplenic erythrophagocytosis, which were strongly suggestive of an acute hemolytic event.[218] The toxic components of chocolate are theobromine and caffeine, both methylxanthines.[216] In mammals, renal adenosine receptor inhibition from chocolate toxicity results in decreased kidney function and polyuria.[216] Reports of chocolate toxicity in captive birds are rare and anecdotal.[216,219] It has been suggested that birds are less likely to eat toxic quantities of chocolate but they may also be more sensitive to its effects; all reported clinical cases have resulted in the patient's death.[216,219] A wild adult male kea (*Nestor notabilis*) was found to have died acutely with only 20 g of chocolate in its crop.[220] A conservative estimate of the dose of methylxanthines ingested by the bird was 250 mg/kg theobromine, 20 mg/kg caffeine, and 3 mg/kg theophylline.[220] Histopathological examination revealed acute degenerative changes to hepatocytes, renal tubules, and cerebrocortical neurons.[220] Although anecdotal, chocolate toxicity has been reported in a captive African grey parrot (*Psittacus erithacus*) and a myna bird (*Gracula religiosa*); the grey parrot died due to hepatic, pulmonary, and renal congestion after eating a chocolate doughnut.[221,222] Coast live oak (*Quercus agrifolia*) has been reported to be toxic to a double-wattled cassowary (*Casuarius casuarius*). Severe diarrhea, anorexia, and polydipsia were noted antemortem, while penile prolapse, severe enteritis, and renal swelling with subcapsular urate deposits were reported postmortem.[223] Three geese that presented for ethylene glycol intoxication were found to have severe degeneration of renal tubular epithelium and congestion of the kidneys and liver.[224]

Many owners do not provide an appropriate diet to their pet birds, which may lead to acute or chronic deficiencies that predispose these animals to renal disease. The lack of appropriate vitamin supplementation is a common problem associated with nutritional disease development. Vitamin A is the vitamin that is most likely to be deficient in the diets of both captive and wild birds because the amount of this vitamin consumed in foodstuffs can be variable.[225] Vitamin A is critical for vision, cellular differentiation, immune function, and numerous other physiologic processes.[226] The two basic functions of vitamin A in cells are hormone-like regulatory actions of retinoic acid and photoreceptor actions of retinal.[225] The hormone-like action of vitamin A involves binding to nuclear and cytoplasmic receptors to induce regulation of cellular replication, differentiation, and preprogrammed cell death.[225] Hypovitaminosis A, among several other conditions, can also lead to renal disease.[136] Pet psittacines fed a seed-based diet are likely to have low vitamin A concentrations because seeds are deficient in this nutrient.[49] An association between renal disease and hypovitaminosis A can be made in pet birds.[49] Nephrosis and nephritis were diagnosed in poultry fed diets high in protein and calcium, containing urea, or deficient in vitamin A.[49] Vitamin A deficiency causes metaplastic changes of the ureters and collecting ducts as well as decreased secretions of mucus within the ureter that can ultimately lead to partial or complete ureteral obstruction and secondary hydronephrosis, hyperuricemia, and oliguric/anuric renal failure.[19,49,58,59,96] Secondary bacterial infections are also common.[96] In poultry, histological renal lesions secondary to hypovitaminosis A include dilatation and impaction of the collecting ducts in the medulla with cell debris, inflammatory cells, and urates and severe interstitial fibrosis and compression of other medullary components.[210] Hyperemia and areas of tubular degeneration and necrosis in the cortical tissue are frequently reported. Some tubules may be filled with mononuclear inflammatory cells, debris, urate crystals, hyaline casts, and interstitial tophi.

Vitamin D and its involvement in calcium homeostasis are described in depth in Chapter 6. This section focuses on dietary supplementation of vitamin D and its impact on the renal system. Birds are able to synthesize cholecalciferol in their skin from cholesterol but require an adequate amount of sunlight to do so.[225] Since most companion birds do not have sufficient UVB exposure to stimulate the photobiochemical conversion of vitamin D, they require a dietary source of vitamin D.[225] In general, birds are not able to convert D_2, the form available for cats and dogs, into vitamin D_3 for use in metabolism; instead, this form of vitamin D is excreted in the bile.[225] Hypervitaminosis due to the excessive supplementation of vitamin D in the diet or from exposure to cholecalciferol rodenticide baits causes an excessive calcium uptake from the intestines, mimicking hypercalcinosis.[227,228] It has been suggested that all bird species are susceptible to hypervitaminosis D.[136] Hypervitaminosis D and/or excessive dietary calcium often leads to hypercalcemia, soft tissue mineralization of the renal parenchyma, or nephrocalcinosis.[58,59] Ureteral concretions can cause postrenal failure.[59] Clinical signs of hypervitaminosis D in birds include hypercalcemia, anorexia, nausea, polyuria, polydipsia, demineralization of bones, disorientation, painful joints, and muscle weakness.[136] Vitamin D toxicity is exacerbated by high dietary levels of calcium and/or phosphorus.[227] Vitamin D toxicity has been induced in macaws at lower dietary levels (1000 IU/kg) than in other species, which suggests that vitamin D metabolism varies among psittacines.[216] Other researchers have suggested that dietary vitamin D concentrations ranging from 500 to 3300 IU/kg

did not result in metastatic mineralization with a low-calcium diet.[96] Vitamin D rodenticide drugs have also been reported to cause accidental mortality in birds housed at a zoological facility.[228] Although not reported in pet birds, poultry chickens receiving excessive vitamin D supplementation use the egg as an excretion vehicle that leads to embryonic death.[216] Susceptibility to cholecalciferol toxicity appears to be species specific. When fed 2000 mg/kg cholecalciferol, no mallard duck (*n* = 6) died, but 25% of the chickens (*n* = 4) and 75% of the canaries (*n* = 4) died.[229] In budgerigars, excessive dietary calcium was shown to be more toxic than hypervitaminosis D.[136] High-calcium diets did not produce renal calcinosis, but when dietary $CaCO_3$ content was raised to 14%, calcium deposits were observed histologically in the renal tubules and interstitium.[210] Hypercalcinosis secondary to excessive calcium supplementation has been reported in chickens, ostriches, and budgerigars.[227]

Renal disease including nephritis, renal calcification, and gout resulting from nutritional problems in birds have been associated with high calcium and vitamin D, low vitamin A, and high protein levels in the diet.[49] Excess dietary protein has also been correlated with increased production of uric acid, but even with very high levels of dietary protein (i.e., 80%), gout only develops in genetically susceptible individuals.[58] Nevertheless, it is still theorized that feeding high-protein diets, long term, can induce hyperuricemia in granivorous or nectivorous birds.[58]

Mycotoxins are toxic compounds produced by fungi.[230] In humans, mycotoxicosis can cause multiple organ damage, including renal disease.[231] The avian kidney has been shown to have a remarkable ability to maintain adequate function after mycotoxin challenge.[232] Only three nephrogenic mycotoxins, citrinin, ochratoxin A, and aflatoxin B_1, have been shown to alter avian renal function.[232] Citrinin is one of the most potent and well-known quinone methide mycotoxins, and *Penicillium citrinum* is a potent producer of citrinin.[233] Other citrinin-producing fungi include *Aspergillus niveus*, *A. niger*, *A. oryzae*, *Monascus ruber*, and *P. camemberti*.[233] In chickens, ducklings, and turkeys, citrinin is associated with hepatic and lymphoid necrosis as well as renal alterations.[233] At nonlethal doses, citrinin appears to have acute reversible effects on the distal portion of the nephron, possibly acting to inhibit water absorption.[230] Several species of fungi may produce mycotoxins known as ochratoxins A, B, and C.[234] Ochratoxin A is the most common mycotoxin and is primarily nephrotoxic, causing mortalities and renomegaly in ringneck pheasants (*Phasianus colchicus*) and immunosuppression in turkeys under laboratory conditions.[234] Ochratoxin A is more potent and less acute than citrinin but less site specific in that both proximal and distal tubules are damaged, resulting in severe loss of both fluids and electrolytes.[230] Aflatoxins are the best known toxic secondary metabolites and are a major group of polyketide-derived mycotoxins produced by three species of *Aspergillus*: *A. flavus*, *A. parasiticus*, and, rarely, *A. nomius*. These fungi have a cosmopolitan distribution.[233] Aflatoxicosis is responsible for significant economic losses in the poultry industry (e.g., ducklings, broilers, layers, turkeys, and quail).[235] Dosages and durations of exposure to aflatoxin B_1, that induced hepatotoxicity in birds, were also sufficient to cause nephrogenic effects, including increased urinary calcium excretion and decreased inorganic phosphate excretion.[230] In commercial broilers, aflatoxin B_1 has been shown to decrease plasma concentrations of 25-hydroxycholecalciferol and 1,25-dihydroxycholecalciferol; it may also decrease endogenous parathyroid hormone synthesis and renal sensitivity to parathyroid hormone.[230] Furthermore, exposure to aflatoxin B_1 may cause prolonged alterations in renal function (e.g., reduced GFR).[230] Liver and kidney damage reflect the toxic insults of aflatoxin and ochratoxin A, respectively; however, when provided in combination, the target organ was the kidney.[230] Although commercial poultry operations are commonly exposed to mycotoxins, wild birds can also ingest these toxins through contaminated feeders.[234,236,237] Mycotoxins have also been found in pet bird food.[238,239]

HEAVY METALS. Heavy metal toxicity is very well described in both wild and captive birds, and most cases are associated with lead or zinc exposure.[216,240,241] Renal disease may occur as a secondary condition due to heavy metal toxicity. Zinc-induced renal disease is nonspecific but may include the loss of renal architecture, apoptosis of individual cells, and acute tubular necrosis.[216] Lead-induced renal lesions can include proximal tubular necrosis and degeneration, visceral gout, and acid-fast intranuclear inclusion bodies.[136] Unlike mammals, renal damage does not occur in every patient diagnosed with heavy metal toxicosis; it has been suggested that in raptors, heavy metal toxicosis does not cause renal damage.[240,241] Various dietary concentrations of cadmium have been associated with renal tubular necrosis in adult mallard ducks and young Japanese quail within 4 weeks of hatching.[242] The kidney is a major reservoir of inorganic mercury in birds as well as mammals.[243] In renal tissue, mercury binds to metallothionein.[243] Mercury has been associated with necrosis of proximal tubular cells in birds.[243]

Other noninfectious renal diseases in birds may occur secondary to metabolic and hormonal-related diseases. These conditions are discussed in further detail in Chapter 6.

IATROGENIC. Drug-induced renal disease is primarily related to the use of NSAIDs and antibiotic medications. Among antibiotic agents, aminoglycosides may be the most problematic. Gentamicin has a narrow range between therapeutic and toxic tissue levels.[244] It has been suggested that the primary route of elimination and pharmacokinetic behavior of aminoglycosides in birds is similar to mammals; therefore, renal toxicity should also be a concern in birds.[244,245] Renal toxicity secondary to gentamicin administration has been reported in pigeons.[50] Aminoglycoside pharmacokinetic studies have been reported in blue-fronted Amazon parrots, budgerigars, cockatiels, chickens, turkeys, red-tailed hawks, great-horned owls, golden eagles, pigeons, Japanese quail.[246-257] Dosages obtained from these studies should be used as a guide to minimize the likelihood of inducing renal disease in birds.

In mammals, the most common adverse effects of NSAIDs involve the gastrointestinal tract, renal system, and coagulation pathway due to the effects on cyclooxygenase (COX) enzymes.[258] The most common adverse effect of NSAIDs reported in birds are associated with renal tissue and function.[258] Although several NSAIDs have been studied and shown to be safe in multiple avian species, certain species have been shown to be extremely sensitive to specific NSAIDs. Rapid population declines of the vultures *Gyps bengalensis*, *Gyps indicus*, and *Gyps tenuirostris* have been observed in India

and Pakistan. The decline of these vulture species has been correlated with the ingestion of domestic animal carcasses (e.g., cattle) that received a normal veterinary dose of diclofenac shortly before death.[259-261] Surveys at veterinary clinics indicated that diclofenac use in India began in 1994 and coincided with the onset of *Gyps* spp. declines.[262] Based on available data, diclofenac is considered to be toxic to all 8 *Gyps* species.[263] The tissues of cattle treated with diclofenac are a hazard to wild vultures, with the intestines, kidneys, and liver having the highest diclofenac concentrations.[264] Mortality rates reached catastrophic levels and complete extirpation of vulture colonies occurred in some areas of the Indian subcontinent.[265,266] Surveys in India from the 2000s were compared with initial surveys from the early 1990s and revealed that populations of *G. bengalensis* in 2007 had fallen to 0.1% of the early 1990 population numbers; populations of *G. indicus* and *G. tenuirostris* were found to have fallen to 3.2% of their earlier levels.[267] Severe, acute renal tubular necrosis and uric acid crystal formation in the kidneys and other tissues were common findings in animals that ingested diclofenac-contaminated carcasses.[268] The lack of fibrosis or other pathological changes associated with chronic renal disease were rarely noted thereby providing evidence of an acute disease process.[268] Several hypotheses have been proposed to explain the toxicity of diclofenac to vulture species, including impairment of renal physiology, differential toxicity to both proximal and distal kidney tubules via a mitochondrial cell death pathway, a combination of cell death from increased reactive oxygen species (ROS) interference with uric acid transport, and duration of exposure.[269] Both diclofenac and meloxicam are toxic to avian renal tubular epithelial cells following 12 h of exposure, due to an increase in production of ROS; however, when avian cultures were incubated with either drug for only 2 h, meloxicam showed no toxicity in contrast to diclofenac.[270] In addition, diclofenac decreased the transport of uric acid by interfering with the para-aminohippuric acid channel.[270]

With populations declining by ~50% annually, the long-term survival of *Gyps* vultures in South Asia required the removal of diclofenac as an NSAID for cattle and the establishment of captive populations for future restoration once the environment was free from contamination.[265] The governments of India, Pakistan, and Nepal took action in 2006 to prevent the veterinary use of diclofenac for domesticated livestock.[271] Long-billed vulture abundance, nest occupancy, and nest productivity declined 61%, 73%, and 95%, respectively, in the 3 years before the diclofenac ban and then increased 1 to 2 years after the ban by 55%, 52%, and 95%, respectively.[272] The decline of *G. bengalensis* in India has also slowed following the diclofenac ban, although recent information indicates that the elimination of diclofenac from the vultures' food supply is incomplete and remains available through some commercial sources.[267,273,274] Although there is no clear evidence that diclofenac is toxic to Egyptian vultures (*Neophron percnopterus*) or red-headed vultures (*Sarcogyps calvus*), since the diclofenac ban, the decline of these species has also apparently decreased.[275,276] Based on the evidence described above both species may have been adversely impacted by diclofenac and have benefited from the legal actions made against the use of diclofenac.[275,276] Although the ban of diclofenac on the Indian subcontinent is starting to show beneficial effects in the local vulture populations, the use of this drug in other regions of the world is concerning. Recently, the use of diclofenac has been authorized in Spain, where >95% of the European vulture population resides.[277]

The risk of NSAID toxicity for vultures may not be limited to diclofenac.[278] Ketoprofen has been associated with mortality events in an unreleasable Cape griffon vulture (*Gyps coprotheres*) and wild-caught African white-backed vultures (*G. africanus*); the birds received doses of 1.5 and 5 mg/kg, which are within the dosage range recommended for the clinical treatment of birds, and showed similar acute clinical signs described in birds with diclofenac toxicity.[279,280] Aceclofenac, a derivative of diclofenac with fewer gastrointestinal complications in humans and analgesic, antiarthritic, and antipyretic properties, has been hypothesized to be toxic also to vultures.[269] Such a hypothesis is based on the fact that aceclofenac is converted into diclofenac, and its metabolites have been found in all mammal species tested to date; there is a logical concern that these same pathways will be followed in livestock.[269] Therefore, the use of aceclofenac as a veterinary NSAID for treating livestock in South Asia, or other countries with any species of *Gyps* vultures, poses a high risk of toxicity to vultures scavenging on the carcasses of domestic ungulates that were dosed with aceclofenac prior to death.[269] Carprofen and flunixin meglumine have also been reported to be associated with mortalities in captive *Gyps* sp.,[281] and flunixin meglumine has recently been identified as a cause of death in a wild *G. fulvus*.[277] However, this should not be unexpected, as flunixin meglumine has been found to increase glomerular mesangial matrix synthesis after 3 to 7 days of treatment, and tubular necrosis was found in 6/8 (75%) budgerigars after 7 days of treatment.[282] Flunixin nephrotoxicity has also been reported in flamingos, cranes, and a northern bobwhite quail.[49] It is important to note that diclofenac, aceclofenac, ketoprofen, flunixin, and carprofen are all aryl alkanoic acid derivatives.[278] Two mortality events as a result of renal disease and gout associated with ibuprofen and phenylbutazone have also been reported in birds.[281]

Although not as significant as the decline noted in *Gyps* spp., diclofenac has also been found to be toxic to other wild birds. Two steppe eagles (*Aquila nipalensis*) showed evidence of acute toxicity secondary to diclofenac exposure, suggesting that diclofenac may be toxic to other accipitrid raptors.[283] As was previously mentioned, there is no clear evidence that diclofenac is toxic to Egyptian vultures or red-headed vultures, but population declines have been reported for these species during the same time period noted with the *Gyps* spp. Similar concerns have been voiced with bearded vultures (*Gypaetus barbatus*) in Nepal because of rapid population declines; however, this lacks scientific validation.[284]

Diclofenac has been tested in a New World vulture species (turkey vultures, *Cathartes aura*) and pied crows (*Corvus alba*), both of which were unaffected by the diclofenac (even at very high doses).[285,286] Chickens (*Gallus gallus domesticus*) were also tested and appear to only be susceptible at doses 50 to 100 times greater than that found to be toxic for the white-rumped vulture.[287] Chickens have been proposed to be a potential animal model for further studies to characterize the mechanism of toxicity of diclofenac. However chickens are not an appropriate model to simulate the dose–response relationship of the vulture to the other NSAIDs.[287]

The only NSAID found to be safe in *Gyps* spp. is meloxicam. Dosages of 0.5 and 2 mg/kg orally have been shown to be safe in Oriental white-backed vultures, long-billed vultures, Egyptian vultures, cattle egrets (*Bubulcus ibis*), house crows (*Corvus splendens*), large-billed crows (*Corvus machrorhynchos*), and common mynas (*Acridotheres tristis*).[288] Oral and intramuscular pharmacokinetics of meloxicam in Cape griffon vultures (*Gyps coprotheres*), as well as therapeutic drug monitoring in white-backed vultures, Egyptian vultures, and one lappet-faced vulture (*Torgos tracheliotos*), have also confirmed the safety of meloxicam in vultures. In all of these vulture species, meloxicam was characterized by a short half-life of elimination and rapid metabolism, which suggests that it is unlikely that the drug would accumulate in *Gyps* spp.[289] It has been hypothesized that other oxicam derivatives, such as piroxicam, lornoxicam, and tenoxicam, would also be safe in vultures, but further scientific validation is needed to confirm this belief.[278]

Another pharmaceutical agent with the potential risk for inducing renal disease is fenbendazole, commonly used to treat gastrointestinal parasites in birds (e.g., *Capillaria* spp.)[290–295] Although many *Capillaria* spp. cases remain subclinical, a disease process causing emaciation, depression, diarrhea, dysphagia, oral lesions (which can resemble trichomoniasis), and death may occur.[296] It is important to mention that fenbendazole toxicity has been reported in several avian species. Pigeons and doves treated with 50 and 100 mg/kg oral fenbendazole or albendazole experienced significant mortalities, with shorter survival times and higher weight loss noted when the 100 mg/kg dosage was used.[297] Eight/12 pigeons that were treated with fenbendazole at 30 mg/kg orally for 5 consecutive days developed anorexia, lethargy, and dehydration and died 2 days after the onset of the clinical signs.[298] Histopathology results of the birds that died from fenbendazole toxicity revealed acute hemorrhagic enteritis, diffuse lymphoplasmacytic enteritis, small intestinal crypt necrosis, periportal lymphoplasmacytic hepatitis, bile duct hyperplasia, and renal tubular necrosis.[298] Fenbendazole toxicity has also been reported in cockatiels, white-backed vultures, lappet-faced vultures, Marabou storks (*Leptoptilos crumeniferus*), and painted storks (*Mycteria leucocephala*).[299,300] It is hypothesized that the sensitivity to fenbendazole is due to species specificity, a dose related response, or higher tubulin affinity to benzimidazoles in comparison to mammals.[300]

Treatment options for renal disease in birds are limited. The prognosis for avian renal disease cases is often guarded to grave, in part due to the advanced stage of disease at the time of diagnosis but also because of limited treatment options available to clinicians. Most of the recommendations mentioned in this section are empirical and based in mammalian medicine since there is a lack of specific information regarding avian species. Overall, the best treatment option is to address the cause of renal disease. For example, if a bacterial infection is diagnosed as the cause of a nephropathy, adequate antimicrobial therapy is the best option. Nevertheless, supportive care and management of secondary and concurrent diseases is imperative.

As stated by Steinohrt, "five important questions must be addressed when formulating a fluid therapy plan for an avian patient: Is fluid therapy indicated? What type of fluid should be given? By what route should the fluids be given? How much and how rapidly should fluids be given? When should fluid therapy be discontinued?"[167]

Independent of the underlying cause of renal disease, fluid therapy is a hallmark for the treatment of nephropathy in any species. In most cases, fluid therapy will be beneficial, although the rate and route of administration may vary with the condition and severity of the disease. In the case of urolithiasis, fluid therapy can be tried in an attempt to dissolve the blockage, but in cases of complete obstruction, aggressive fluid therapy is contraindicated.[59]

The selection of a fluid product should be based on patient assessment and an electrolyte assessment of that individual. Based on that information, the fluid product and supplementation should then be selected. Knowledge of the plasma osmolality of a particular species or individual is of paramount importance when formulating the patient's fluid treatment plan, because most prepackaged fluids are specifically prepared for human patients.[301] Studies assessing the fluid osmolality of several species of birds have been reported.[301,302] Comparisons of osmolality values between mammals and psittacines suggest that plasma osmolality is slightly higher in parrots than in mammals, species-specific differences exist, and differences between reported values occur.[302] Overall, fluids with an osmolarity close to 300 to 320 mOsm/L, such as Normosol-R, Plasma-Lyte-R, Plasma-Lyte-A, and NaCl 0.9%, can be recommended in parrots for fluid replacement therapy when isotonic fluids are required.[302] As osmolality determination may not be readily available, formulations for the calculation of osmolarity have been suggested. In Hispaniolan Amazon parrots. The equation $(2 \times [Na^+ + K^+])$ + (uric acid concentration/16.8) + (glucose concentration/18) yielded values that had the highest agreement with the measured osmolality of parrots.[301]

The kidneys are responsible for maintaining homeostasis in the body; kidney failure typically leads to imbalances of fluid, electrolyte, and acid-base balance.[303] The goal of treatment is to correct these imbalances.[303] The acid-base balance can be influenced by a range of internal and external factors, including diet, environmental conditions, and metabolism.[304] Collectively, these factors constantly affect regulation of pH in blood and tissues.[304] Many of the final metabolites are acids that can be removed from the body by the kidneys and lungs.[304] In the case of a renal abnormality, the normal control of metabolite removal may be affected and this physiologic disorder must be corrected to regain normal function. For example, in the case of diabetes insipidus, hypernatremia is a common development.[305,306] In cases of hypernatremia, one should provide the patient with fluids to compensate for ongoing losses and (in hypotensive patients) volume deficits with the replacement fluid having a Na concentration close to that of the patient's serum (e.g., 0.9% saline).[307] Once fluid volume requirements have been met, replace the free water deficit with a hypotonic solution (e.g., 5% dextrose in water [D5W]).[307] Do not exceed changes in sodium levels of 1 mmol/h in acute cases or 0.5 mmol/h in chronic cases; thereby reducing the risk of cerebral edema.[307] In a case of presumptive diabetes insipidus secondary to head trauma in an umbrella cockatoo (*Cacatua alba*), severe hypernatremia occurred.[308] In this case, although unsuccessful, multiple intravenous fluids and desmopressin were administered.[308]

Although IV or IO fluid administration would be preferred in cases of moderate to severe dehydration, placement and maintenance of IV or IO catheters may be challenging in psittacines. In the authors' experience, most nonpsittacine species tend to tolerate intravenous catheters, but parrots, in the majority of cases bright and alert animals, are unlikely to tolerate catheters. Furthermore, in the event of damage to the intravenous line, hemorrhage may occur that has detrimental consequences for the patient. Intraosseous catheters do not pose such a threat but may predispose birds to infection. Intraosseous fluid administration has been shown to be a viable alternative to IV catheters in birds.[309] Oral administration is considered an excellent choice for animals with mild dehydration and also allows for the administration of hypertonic fluids. The subcutaneous route is convenient and practical and may be a reasonable option for maintenance fluids.[167] Most maintenance fluids cannot be given SC because of their hypotonicity.[302] The most appropriate route of fluid administration for an avian patient should be based on disease process, the patient's clinical status, and its temperament.[167]

Maintenance fluid therapy in birds is estimated to vary between 50 and 100 mL/kg/d.[302] In birds with chronic disease, hydration deficits usually do not rapid replacement; instead, the fluid deficit can be calculated and added to the daily maintenance requirements, with the total volume being administered over a 24- to 48-hour period.[167] Several conditions, including renal disease, may warrant a decrease in fluid replacement. In the case of an obstructive disease, rapid administration of fluids can induce hemodilution and increase the cardiac preload, leading to cardiovascular abnormalities. Nevertheless, a high fluid volume may be necessary to destroy the obstruction. In a case with a decreased GFR, fluids may be necessary to improve renal clearance and vascularization; however, if renal function is impaired, fluid may not be cleared from the body and cardiovascular abnormalities can occur. Volume overload is best prevented rather than treated, but diuretics (e.g., furosemide, mannitol) or renal vasodilators (e.g., dopamine) may be indicated if the animal is well hydrated and urine production is poor.[58]

Overall, fluid therapy should be discontinued when signs of overhydration develop. Signs include serous nasal discharge, tachypnea, dyspnea, ascites, cough, polyuria, tachycardia, shivering, and pulmonary edema.[167] However, when treating a renal disease case, discontinuing fluid therapy altogether may not be advisable. Instead, a reduction in the fluid rate and constant monitoring of cardiorespiratory function and blood biochemistries are recommended. In small animals, outpatient subcutaneous fluid therapy is an option when the initial crisis is controlled.[303] In avian cases, this may not be a viable option unless the client can be trained to safely administer the fluids.

Mammals

Rabbits

Urolithiasis is a common finding in pet rabbits. Calculi or sediment can be found anywhere in the urinary system, including the kidneys, ureters, urethra, and urinary bladder. Since rabbits can passively absorb calcium through the gastrointestinal tract without the presence of vitamin D and actively excrete calcium through the kidneys, they can generate high concentrations of calcium in both the blood and urine if offered high-calcium diets. In these cases, the calcium can build up to form sediment or calculi that partially or completely obstruct urine outflow through the urinary tract. Rabbits with urolithiasis may present for depression, lethargy, stranguria, hematuria, increased vocalization during urination, and bruxism. Radiographs and urinalysis can be used to diagnose the type, number, and location of calculi (or sediment) in the urinary system. Calcium oxalate crystals are the most common type of crystal associated with calculi and sediment in rabbits, although ammonium phosphate and calcium carbonate may occur. Hematology and biochemistry analyses can be performed to assess the overall health of the rabbit. Elevated BUN and creatinine concentrations can be used to confirm that a rabbit is azotemic and the possible existence of a postrenal obstruction. Elevated calcium concentrations may affirm the increased risk of crystalluria and stone formation. Urine samples (collected via cystocentesis or catheterization) should also be submitted for microbiologic culture, since bacterial infections can serve as a nidus for calculi formation.

Urolithiasis treatment should be based on the type and location of the calculi (or sediment). If urolithiasis is localized to the urinary bladder as sediment, providing fluid therapy to help "wash out" the sediment, altering the diet to reduce calcium concentrations (e.g., no alfalfa hay or pellets, no calcium oxalate–based greens), and providing potassium citrate (20 mg/kg, PO, twice daily [BID]) as an alkalinizing agent for the urine may be sufficient. If firm calculi are present, surgical correction is required. A nephrectomy should be performed in cases where renoliths or ureteroliths have resulted in hydronephrosis. Hematologic, biochemistry, and urinalysis data should be used to confirm that contralateral kidney function is normal. For calculi located in the urethra, a catheter can be inserted into the urethra and saline used to retropulse the calculi into the urinary bladder. A cystotomy can then be performed to remove the calculi; this technique is also recommended for calculi originally localized in the urinary bladder.

Chronic renal failure is typically a disease of older rabbits, whereas acute renal failure is a disease that can occur in a rabbit at any age and is typically associated with exposure to a nephrotoxin. Examples of nephrotoxins include aminoglycoside treatment (e.g., parenteral gentamicin) and tiletamine/zolazepam. Rabbits that present with renal failure may look similar to those diagnosed with urolithiasis. Affected animals are often depressed, lethargic, and anorexic. However, unlike urolithiasis cases, rabbits with renal failure are often polyuric, polydipsic, and dehydrated. A complete diagnostic workup should be performed on rabbits suspected to have renal failure, including hematologic and biochemistry testing, urinalysis, microbiologic culture, and diagnostic imaging (e.g., radiographs, ultrasound). Rabbits in renal failure are typically anemic, azotemic (elevated BUN and creatinine), hyperphosphatemic, and hyperkalemic. Rabbits may also become hypercalcemic; however, as the renal failure worsens, hypocalcemia may develop. Urine samples from renal failure cases are typically isosthenuric and positive for protein, blood, glucose, and renal casts. Gram-negative bacteria are most commonly isolated from the urinary tract of rabbits with renal failure. Ultimately, a fine-needle aspirate or biopsy of the kidney is required to confirm a specific etiology for renal failure. Ultrasound or endoscopy can be used to collect these samples. Common histopathologic findings often indicate that the chronic renal failure is attributed to nutritional disorders, such as high calcium and vitamin D diets, or infectious diseases (e.g., *Pasteurella multocida*, *E. coli*, *Pseudomonas aeruginosa*, *Encephalitozoon cuniculi*).

Treatment for renal failure should focus on preserving any remaining renal function. Initially, IV or IO fluids are administered to diurese the rabbit. It is important to closely monitor fluid delivery with acute renal failure cases, as it is possible to induce fluid overload. Specific treatments should focus on the final diagnosis. For example, an antibiotic should be prescribed for cases where a specific bacterial pathogen was isolated or fenbendazole (25 mg/kg, PO, SID) for a confirmed diagnosis of *E. cuniculi*. Correcting the diet is also necessary for patients that are diagnosed with renal failure. Alfalfa hay and pellets, calcium oxalate–rich plants, and high protein diets (e.g., pellets) should be avoided. Chronic renal failure cases in rabbits typically require life-long therapy, therefore clients should be educated on how to administer SC fluids in order to maintain the proper hydration status of their pet.

Renal cancer is uncommon in rabbits; however, cases of adenocarcinoma and lymphoma have been seen by one of the editors (M.A.M.). Renal cancer in rabbits is typically identified as an incidental finding during a routine examination or based on a history of hematuria. A definitive diagnosis can be achieved through the use ultrasound and biopsy sample collection with subsequent histological assessment of the collected specimens. A unilateral nephrectomy can be curative if the neoplasm has not metastasized.

Guinea Pigs

Calculi and sediment are common findings in the urinary system of older (>2 y) guinea pigs (Figure 11-15). The calculi may be found in the kidneys, ureters, urinary bladder, or urethra; sediment is most common in the urinary bladder but can also be found in the ureters and urethra. Complete obstructions in the ureters and kidneys can lead to hydronephrosis. The calculi and sediment are commonly composed of calcium oxalate crystals. Guinea pigs with calculi or

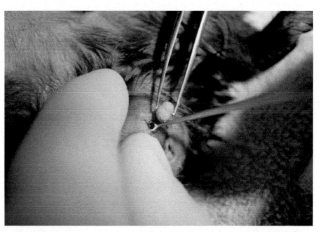

FIGURE 11-15 Removal of a urethral stone in a female guinea pig. In this case, the stone was located near the urethral orifice; therefore, direct removal was possible. In female guinea pigs, the urethral orifice is easily accessible and is located ventral to the vaginal orifice.

sediment in the urinary system may show no clinical signs or present for stranguria, hematuria, anuria, and increased vocalization during urination. Hematology, biochemistries, and a urinalysis should be performed to assess the general health of the guinea pig, while radiographs and ultrasound can be used to confirm the presence, location, and number of calculi. In nonobstructive cases (e.g., sediment), potassium citrate is recommended. Potassium citrate (20 mg/kg, PO, BID) is an alkaline salt that can help realkalinize the urine. In addition, fluid support, antibiotic therapy to control secondary infection, and lowering calcium concentrations in the diet (i.e., use timothy rather than alfalfa hay or pellets; increase hay and decrease pellets; and reduce calcium oxalate–rich plant matter in the diet) are recommended. For obstructive cases, surgery is required. A unilateral nephrectomy can be performed for cases of hydronephrosis, a ureterotomy for an obstruction in the ureter, and a cystotomy for cyctic calculi. The surgical approach for the procedures listed above is similar to that described for domestic pets.

Cystitis and urethritis can occur in both male and female guinea pigs. Urethritis is often more common in males and secondary to reproductive tract secretions (e.g., semen) congealing within the urethra. The clinical signs associated with cystitis and urethritis are similar to those described for urinary tract calculi, including stranguria, hematuria, anuria, and increased vocalization during urination. Most cases of cystitis in female guinea pigs are associated with a bacterial infection. *Staphylococcus pyogenes* is a common gram-positive isolate, while gram-negative isolates can include *E. coli*, *Klebsiella* spp., and *Pseudomonas* spp. Since both gram-positive and -negative bacteria have been associated with urinary tract disease in guinea pigs, samples should be collected via cystocentesis or urinary catheterization and submitted for microbiological culture and antibiotic sensitivity testing. Bacterial infections in the urinary bladder can serve as a nidus for sediment and calculi formation within the urinary bladder; therefore, radiographs are required to rule in/out their presence. Urine collected from cystocentesis or urethral catheterization should be submitted for urinalysis. The presence of bacteria and blood cells within the urine sample can be used to confirm a diagnosis of cystitis. Treatment for cystitis should focus on the selection of an appropriate antibiotic drug based on culture and sensitivity testing. Trimethoprim sulfa (24 mg/kg, PO, BID) or enrofloxacin (5 to 10 mg/kg, PO, BID) may be initially used while culture and sensitivity testing are pending.

Chinchillas

Urinary calculi are an occasional problem encountered in male chinchillas. Affected animals may present for anuria, straining to urinate, vocalizing while urinating, and hematuria. Calculus in the penis are often identified during the physical examination; however, in most cases, survey radiographs are required to visualize calculi in the urinary bladder or urethra. Surgery is required to remove an urethral or cystic calculus. The surgical approach to remove an urethral or cystic calculus for these cases is similar to that described for domestic mammals. When the calculus is located within the urethra of the penis, a cutdown to remove the calculus is possible (Avery Bennett, pers. comm.). The urethra and penis can be allowed to heal by second intention. Antibiotic medication (trimethoprim sulfadimethoxazole, 24 mg/kg, PO, BID or enrofloxacin 5 to 10 mg/kg, PO, BID for 10 to 14 d) and NSAIDs (meloxicam, 0.5 to 1 mg/kg, PO, SID-BID) are recommended for urinary calculi cases to reduce the likelihood of opportunistic infections. Stricture is a potential risk, and owners should be made aware of this, but one of the editors (M.A.M.) has not appreciated any complications in chinchillas that present and are treated for urinary calculi. The urinary calculi removed from chinchilla patients are typically comprised of calcium carbonate. To reduce the likelihood of recurrence, dietary changes are required. Alfalfa-based pellets and hay are higher in calcium than timothy-based pellets or hay. In addition, a urinalysis should be submitted and the results analyzed. If the pH is acidic, potassium citrate (20 mg/kg, PO, SID) should be considered as a treatment option.

Oxalate nephrocalcinosis has been reported in chinchillas.[310] Affected chinchillas were found to be weak and developed calcium oxalate crystals in their renal tubules. The specific etiology for this disease was not identified, but exposure to oxalic acid plants, moldy feed, and vitamin B deficiency were considered as differential disease diagnoses.

Ferrets

Anuria and stranguria are not uncommon presentations for male ferrets. The two most common causes for these disease problems are prostate disease and urolithiasis. Prostate disease can be a primary disease (e.g., bacterial prostatitis) or secondary disease (e.g., secondary to adrenal gland disease). The urethra of a ferret passes through the prostate, similar to dogs and humans; thus, any enlargement of the prostate can restrict urine flow through the urethra. This condition is discussed in detail in Chapters 6 and 10. Urolithiasis is typically a problem in ferrets fed inappropriate diets, although bacterial infections (e.g., urease-producing bacteria) can also lead to the formation of excretory calculi. Ferrets should be fed a meat-based, high-protein ferret diet. This ensures that the urine pH will remain acidic. Plant-based proteins can cause the urine to become alkaline, which predisposes ferrets to develop struvite (magnesium ammonium phosphate) calculi. Since dogs are omnivores, dog foods often have a higher percentage of plant proteins and should be avoided in ferrets. The calculi can be found at any location in the urinary system from the kidneys to the urethra, with urethral calculi being the most common diagnosis and frequently leading to an emergency presentation. In some cases, sediment forms in the urinary bladder. This is the type of disease (urinary sediment) is more common in female ferrets fed a diet high in plant-based proteins. In addition to stranguria and anuria, hematuria, depression, lethargy, and vocalization are common in ferrets diagnosed with urolithiasis. A complete blood count, biochemistry panel, and urinalysis (cystocentesis) should be submitted to assess the general health and physiologic state of a ferret with urolithiasis. Radiographic images and ultrasound can be used to determine where the calculi are located in the excretory system. Treatment should focus on stabilizing the ferret and correcting a complete obstruction in a timely manner. Passing a urethral catheter in a male ferret can be a challenge because of the small urethral opening and J-shaped os penis. Placing a few drops of lidocaine on the tip of the penis and instilling saline via a needle into the distal tip of the urethra may help facilitate the passage of a catheter. A 3.5 French red rubber tube or silicone urethral catheter should be used to catheterize the urethra. If this is not possible, a cystocentesis should be performed to prevent rupture of the urinary bladder and a cystotomy planned. Cystocentesis in ferrets is similar to cats. A 22- to 25-gauge needle attached to a 12- to 20-mL syringe can be used to collect the urine from a ferret. Ultrasound may be used to reduce the likelihood of inserting the needle through gastrointestinal structures and ensure the collection of a "clean" sample. Similar to dogs and cats, a cystotomy is required in cases where the calculi can be directed into the bladder to remove the mineral stones and limit the likelihood of the calculus reobstructing the urethra. If the calculi cannot be removed from the urethra, a perineal urethrostomy is required. The approach for both the cystotomy and urethrostomy procedures is similar to that described for cats. It is important to provide ferrets with a ferret-specific diet to decrease the likelihood of calculi reformation. If a bacterial infection was the cause of calculi formation, long-term antibiotic treatment (14 to 21 d), based on antibiotic sensitivity testing, is required to eliminate any remaining pathogens in the excretory system.

Cystitis can occur in both male and female ferrets but frequently is more common in females because of their short urethra. Most cases of cystitis in females are associated with a bacterial infection. While most true cystitis cases in males are also bacterial in origin, urolithiasis and prostatic disease (primary or secondary) are other causes of this disease condition that should be considered. Urinalysis and microbiological culture can be used to confirm the presence of a bacterial cystitis. The urine should be collected via a cystocentesis to minimize the likelihood of contamination. Radiographs and ultrasound should be performed in cases where urolithiasis or prostate disease is also suspected. Antimicrobial sensitivity testing should be performed for any bacterial isolates to determine the best treatment options.

Primary renal disease is an uncommon finding in ferrets; however, secondary disease associated with other systemic illnesses may affect the kidneys. Primary renal disease may be associated with cancer (e.g., lymphoma, adenocarcinoma), infectious diseases (e.g., Aleutian disease), inappropriate diets (e.g., high-protein diets in geriatric ferrets), and nephrotoxic drugs (e.g., aminoglycosides, ethylene glycol). Ferrets with chronic renal disease often present for lethargy, depression, dehydration, and weight loss; acute cases of renal failure will not have associated weight loss. As animals become uremic, oral ulcers develop. The diagnostic workup for these cases should follow recommendations for domestic mammals, including a complete blood count, plasma biochemistry profile, urinalysis, and radiographs/ultrasound. Common abnormalities found in cases of chronic renal disease include anemia, hypocalcemia, hyperphosphatemia, elevated BUN and creatinine, hyperkalemia, isosthenuria, and abnormal renal architecture. Ultrasound-guided biopsies of the kidney should be collected and submitted for histopathologic examination and microbiologic culture. Treatment is dependent on the specific etiology associated with the renal disease; if unconfirmed, supportive care (e.g., fluids and broad-spectrum antibiotics) should be pursued.

Renal cysts are not an uncommon finding in ferrets during a physical examination, ultrasound imaging, or necropsy. A 17-year study evaluating the prevalence of renal cysts in ferrets found that 69% (n = 37) of the animals were diagnosed with renal cysts, while 26% (n = 14) and 20% (n = 11) had primary and secondary polycystic disease, respectively.[311] Affected kidneys may have one to many cysts, and the size can vary from being extremely small (millimeters) to large (multiple centimeters). Renal cysts often change the topographical surface of the kidney, making it possible to palpate these abnormal structures during a physical examination. Any time the surface of a kidney palpates abnormally, ultrasound imaging should be performed to determine the number and sizes of the cysts as well as to rule out other disease (e.g., neoplasia). Ferrets diagnosed with renal cysts should have a complete medical evaluation to determine whether the renal cysts are associated with a reduction in renal function. Blood work (e.g., hematology, a plasma biochemistry profile), and an urinalysis can be performed to rule in or out any renal disease. Hyperphosphatemia and elevated BUN are common findings in ferrets with renal disease and renal cysts.[311] The specific etiology associated with renal cyst formation in ferrets is unknown at this time. Treatment should be focused on providing supportive care and protecting any remaining healthy renal tissue. In cases where the renal cysts have become large and painful, a unilateral nephrectomy may be required.

Hydronephrosis can occur in mammals as a result of any obstruction in the renal pelvis or ureter. Since ferrets are spayed at a young age, accidental ligation of the ureter and secondary hydronephrosis can occur.[312] One of the editors (M.A.M.) has diagnosed this condition in a young ferret. The animal was less than 1 year of age and the enlarged kidney was palpated during a routine examination. An ultrasound examination confirmed a diagnosis of unilateral hydronephrosis. Blood work and a urinalysis were performed to assess renal function. Since the ferret had apparently normal renal function, a unilateral nephrectomy was performed to remove the hydronephrotic kidney. The ferret had no post surgical complications associated with the kidney removal.

Excretory system cancer is uncommon in ferrets. Albeit rare, renal lymphoma, adenocarcinoma, and urinary bladder transitional cell carcinoma are the three most common excretory system cancers observed by one of the editors (M.A.M.). Ferrets with excretory system neoplasia do not typically present until the patient is in advanced stages of the disease, because the contralateral kidney appears to maintain overall renal function. Ferrets with excretory system cancer may present for weakness, lethargy, dehydration, an enlarged abdominal mass, anuria, dysuria, stranguria, or hematuria. Hematology and a plasma biochemistry panel, diagnostic imaging (e.g., radiographs, ultrasound), and fine-needle aspirates or biopsies with cytology and histopathology, respectively, can be used to confirm a diagnosis of cancer and determine how the ferret is managing the disease. If the neoplasm is localized to one kidney, a nephrectomy can be performed. The prognosis for metastatic disease is grave.

SPECIFIC DIAGNOSTIC TESTING

Fish

Renal Culture and Biopsy

ANTEMORTEM. Fine-needle aspirates or biopsies of the kidney can be collected using ultrasound or endoscopic imaging in fish. However, size and body condition play a role in the likelihood for success with these diagnostic imaging modalities. In small fish, localization of the kidney can be difficult with either method, unless there is significant renomegaly. In obese fish, it can be difficult to manipulate the endoscope. Samples collected antemortem can be submitted for microbiologic culture and/or histopathologic assessment.

POSTMORTEM. The kidney is considered the best site for collecting samples for microbiological testing. Postmortem sampling of the kidney can be done using a ventral or dorsal approach. For the ventral approach, sterile dissection is required. First, disinfect the ventral abdomen with alcohol or by searing the skin. Next, a scalpel blade is used to incise the ventral abdomen. Sterile instruments are then employed to gently displace the gastrointestinal tract, reproductive tract, and swim bladder. The kidney, dorsal to the swim bladder, appears as a thin and narrow red to brown tissue ventral to the vertebrae in small fish. In larger fish, the kidney may appear "thicker and meatier." A sterile swab can be inserted directly into the kidney or a biopsy of the kidney can be collected for culture. In some cases, the thin membrane overlying the kidney may need to be incised to gain access to the kidney. For the dorsal approach, the dorsal fin should be removed and the dorsal surface of the fish sterilized with alcohol or searing with flame. Next, sterile scissors should be used to cut through the dorsum of the fish. Due to anatomic variability among fish species, the authors prefer to make the approach at the caudal aspect of the dorsal fin. After cutting through the vertebrae the fish is then bent in half to expose the kidney for sample collection.

Amphibians and Reptiles

Anamnesis

A detailed anamnesis can be used to direct a clinician when treating amphibian and reptile renal disease cases. As with higher vertebrates, amphibians and reptiles can present for either acute or chronic renal disease. In the authors' experience, the majority of cases are associated with chronic disease. True acute renal disease cases typically have a recent history of an toxin exposure (e.g., aminoglycosides, ethylene glycol), whereas chronic renal disease cases are associated with poor husbandry conditions of an extended period of time.

Amphibians and reptiles presenting for renal disease are often lethargic, depressed, and dehydrated. In some species, such as green iguanas (*Iguana iguana*), a color change may be apparent; iguanas with renal disease may have a yellow to golden hue to their skin. Affected animals often produce little to no urine. Fecal material may not be produced or appear pasty because of the obstructive nature of the kidneys (i.e., renomegaly) within the pelvis. Many of these patients have a history of "less than adequate" husbandry conditions; low environmental temperature and humidity are common findings. Amphibians and reptiles that are not allowed to establish appropriate core temperatures on a daily basis can experience decreased metabolic rates, leading to poor growth and development. Low environmental humidity can result in dessication of captive amphibians and reptiles, which can ultimately lead to fluid homeostasis issues and renal disease. While reptiles, similar mammals and birds, derive much of their hydration through food, less than adequate captive diets (e.g., low moisture cereal diets) can lead to chronic dehydration. It is

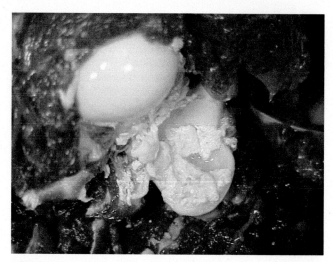

FIGURE 11-16 Coxofemoral articular gout in a sulcata tortoise. This animal was not provided any access to water.

important to provide all amphibians and reptiles with direct access to fresh, clean water daily. Some herpetoculturists recommend precluding some species, such as sulcata tortoises (*Centrochelys sulcata*), from water; however, differences in the moisture content of captive reptile diets can lead to serious dehydration and disease (e.g., gout) (Figure 11-16) when water is not provided to these reptiles. Inappropriate diets comprised of high proteins (purine based) and excessive oral vitamin D can also predispose a reptile to renal disease. Herbivorous reptiles (e.g., green iguanas) should only be offered a plant-based diet. While these animals will eat omnivorous foods (e.g., dog food) or carnivorous foods (e.g., cat foods), their bodies cannot process these inappropriate diets. The overwhelming amounts of protein obtained from these diets can lead to direct renal insult. Oral vitamin D can also contribute to reptile disease conditions. Oversupplementation via powdered supplements (e.g., dusting of insects) or other dietary components can lead to excessive levels of vitamin D being absorbed through the gastrointestinal tract. Once absorbed, the high vitamin D within the body can lead to excessive calcium absorption and dystrophic mineralization. Due to this risk, the preferred method for providing captive reptiles vitamin D is through exposure to UVB radiation. Vitamin D synthesized via UVB radiation has not been found to result in toxic accumulations of this steroid hormone. This has been attributed to the fact that several metabolites (e.g., tachysterol and lumisterol) produced during the photobiochemical synthesis of vitamin D can limit the amount of vitamin D synthesized.

Physical Examination

Amphibians and reptiles have evolved to mask their illness; however, with renal disease, especially renal failure, the animals have a difficult time masking the associated clinical signs of depression, lethargy, and dehydration. The body weight and condition of an amphibian and reptile patients should be measured and determined during the physical examination thereby providing useful information for characterizing acute versus chronic renal disease. Animals with a history of acute nephrotoxic exposure are often in good body condition and weight, whereas amphibians and reptiles with chronic renal disease are underweight and poor body condition as a result of the dehydration and muscle atrophy.

It is always important to perform a thorough and consistent physical examination on an amphibian and reptile, regardless of the presentation. Abnormal findings obtained through the physical examination of an amphibian or reptile with renal disease may include tacky and pale mucous membranes, delayed skin elasticity, sunken eyes in severe cases of dehydration from a loss of fluid in the retro-orbital fat pads, loss of muscle condition, muscle fasciculations or seizures secondary to hypocalcemia, renomegaly, and ascites or anasarca. Renomegaly is frequently diagnosed in reptiles with chronic renal disease. Enlarged kidneys may be palpated in snakes by inserting fingers, through the cloaca, ventrally into the coelomic cavity. The kidneys of a snake should be two-thirds to three-quarters body length from the head. In many of the lizard species presented to veterinarians, the kidneys are intrapelvic. With renomegaly, the cranial aspect of the kidney may protrude into the coelomic cavity. The cranial poles of the kidneys may be palpated by inserting fingers cranial to the rim of the pubis. It is difficult, if not impossible, to palpate the kidneys of chelonians. Cystic calculi in amphibians, lizards, and chelonians may be palpated during routine palpation of the coelomic cavity. Snakes and some species of lizards (e.g., bearded dragons) do not have urinary bladders; however, they can develop ureteroliths or cloacoliths that can be palpated during an examination. Ascites or anasarca may occur secondary to hypoalbuminea from protein loss through the kidneys.

Diagnostic Methods

Hematology and plasma biochemistry profiles can provide important insight into the physiologic state of an amphibian or reptile with renal disease. Anemia of chronic disease is not uncommon in amphibians and reptiles with renal disease. Hemoconcentration may also be evident in amphibians and reptiles with renal disease, especially if the animals are severely dehydrated. Total protein and total solid concentrations may be elevated as a result of dehydration or decreased due to protein loss through the kidneys. Leukocytosis is an uncommon finding because many of the animals with renal disease are presented with chronic illness. Monocytosis or azurophilia (in snakes) is often associated with renal disease in reptiles. Hyperuricemia (>10 mg/dL) is useful for assessing the potential for gout in a reptile, but a poor predictor for renal disease. Calcium homeostasis is often influenced by the adverse effects of renal disease in reptile species. Under normal conditions, the kidneys resorb calcium and excrete phosphorus. However, in reptiles suffering from renal disease, the kidneys cannot perform resorb calcium and excrete phosphorus. Measuring serum or plasma calcium and phosphorus concentrations are diagnostic options to evaluate renal function. Under normal conditions, the calcium : phosphorus ratio in reptiles is 1.5 : 1 to 3 : 1. When this ratio becomes inverted, it is highly suggestive of renal disease. In severe cases, the ratio can be 1 : 15. The prognosis for cases improves the closer the calcium : phosphorus ratio is to 1 : 1. In severe cases (e.g., 1 : 10 to 1 : 15), the prognosis for recovery is grave. Aspartate aminotransferase (AST) and creatine kinase (CK) may be elevated in reptiles with renal disease; however, the elevations of these enzymes are often associated with muscle atrophy therefore are not considered a renal-specific marker. The electrolytes sodium, chloride, and potassium may be altered by renal disease in reptiles. Hyperkalemia may be interpreted as the consequence of decreased renal function and associated inability to properly excrete potassium. Hypo- or hypernatremia and hypo- or hyperchloremia may occur depending on level of renal function and dehydration, respectively.

As a result of the limitations in diagnosing renal disease from hematologic and biochemistry data, other methods are required for evaluating renal function in reptiles. Measuring GFR is one diagnostic test that has proven to be useful for diagnosing renal disease in green iguanas.[313] The clearance of iohexol from the reptile body occurs almost entirely through the kidneys. Consequently this compound is used to measure GFR in reptile patients. An additional benefit gained with the use of iohexol to measure reptile GFR is that only blood samples have to be submitted, thereby negating the need to catheterize the excretory system to measure urine output. In the green iguana study, 75 mg/kg iohexol was administered IV after which blood samples were collected at 4, 8, and 24 hours, post treatment.[313] The iguana blood samples were transported on ice to the Diagnostic Center for Population and Animal Health at Michigan State University (East Lansing, MI) for testing. The average GFR for the iguanas was determined to be 16.6 ± 3.9 mL/kg/h. Additional studies in other reptile species are needed to determine baseline GFR values for use in assessing this renal function in a reptile patient.

URINALYSIS. Urinalysis is an important first-order diagnostic test for mammalian patients that are presented with excretory system problems. Unfortunately, it has become dogma that urinalysis is not valuable for reptiles. This primarily stems from the fact that reptiles lack a loop of Henle, do not concentrate urine, and the urine passes through the cloaca where it may become contaminated by fecal material. While recognizing these limitations as important, there are certainly other aspects of a urinalysis that can provide useful information to aid in assessing the overall health of a reptile with renal disease. Urine samples can be collected from reptiles using cystocentesis or catheterization. Cystocentesis is achieved in lizards using a ventral approach just cranial to the pelvis and in chelonians through the prefemoral fossa. Ultrasound imaging can be quite helpful when attempting urine collection by cystocentesis. To perform a cystocentesis in small reptiles a 5/8-inch 25-gauge needle is used while a 1- to 1.5-inch 22-gauge needle is adequate for larger animals. Direct passage of a red rubber or Tomcat catheter with or without endoscopic assistance is also appropriate for reptile urine collection. Endoscopy is also beneficial when trying to visualize and catheterize a ureter for direct urine collection.

The urine should be evaluated for color, turbidity, and specific gravity. In general, normal reptile urine is clear and colorless. Yellow pigmentation may be apparent with higher urate concentrations. Green pigmentation can be indicative of biliverdinuria, which occurs with cachexia and liver disease. Increased turbidity is associated with high urate discharge as well as inflammation and infections. In reptile species the urine specific gravity is typically hyposthenuric to isosthenuric; however, with renal disease, the specific gravity can increase as glucose and protein are lost. Urine pH in reptiles, much like mammals, is based on diet. Herbivores routinely have alkaline urine, while carnivores have acidic urine. Alterations in urine pH may be a sign that a disease condition is present. For example, alkaline urine in carnivores may be associated with an infection, while acidic pH in an herbivore indicates [?] is possibly due to being fed a high-protein diet. Zero to trace levels of protein and glucose are normal in reptile urine; higher levels may be indicators of renal disease or diabetes mellitus. Low numbers of erythrocytes and leukocytes may be observed in reptile urine, especially if contaminated samples are collected from the cloaca. It is important to evaluate all urinalysis parameters in light of the reptile's condition, where the sample was collected, and based on other diagnostic results (e.g., hematology and biochemistry data, diagnostic imaging, and histopathology).

Urine sediment should be included with the urinalysis evaluation. Collected urine should be centrifuged to increase the likelihood of concentrating material in the sample. The samples can be evaluated using the same techniques described for mammals (with or without sediment stains). Low numbers of blood cells, bacteria, epithelial cells, crystals, and renal casts are commonly found in reptile urine. The most common crystals identified are urate crystals and calcium oxalate crystals, although sodium urate, triple phosphate, leucine, cysteine, hippuric acid, cholesterol, and tyrosine crystals may be present.[314] As the numbers of cells, casts, and crystals rise, the likelihood of renal pathology also increases. It is important to consider the urine sediment results in combination with the rest of the urinalysis and diagnostic tests to build a complete picture of the health and condition of a reptile patient.

DIAGNOSTIC IMAGING. Radiographs, ultrasound, computed tomography (CT), and endoscopy are different forms of diagnostic imaging that can provide some insight into the excretory system of amphibians and reptiles. Radiographs are best suited for assessing mineralized calculi in the kidneys, ureters, urethra, urinary bladder, or cloaca and soft tissue mineralization, including severe cases of gout. The soft tissue opacity of the kidneys, and a lack of surrounding air or fat as in birds and mammals, respectively, can make the kidneys difficult to identify in reptiles on survey radiographs. One exception is in lizards that have intrapelvic kidneys. In cases of chronic renal disease, fibrosis increases the size of the kidneys, and the cranial pole of the organ may be observed extending out of the pelvis (Figure 11-17). In addition, obstruction of the pelvic canal may lead to an enlargement of the colon and urinary bladder as evacuation of fecal material and urine becomes more difficult. In cases where radiography is the only diagnostic imaging tool available, contrast-enhanced radiographs can be performed to improve visualization of the kidneys. Iohexol dosed at 800 to 1000 mg/kg has been used with success in reptiles for this purpose, with serial images taken at baseline, 0.5, 2, 5, 15, 20, and 60 minutes postinjection.[315]

In cases of suspected renomegaly, ultrasound imaging can be used to confirm the enlargement. An additional benefit of ultrasonograhy is that it can be used to direct fine-needle aspirate or biopsy sample collection of the kidney. Cytology and histopathology can then be performed to confirm the cause of the renomegaly.

Computed tomographic scans are also invaluable for assessing renal disease because they can provide important information on the entire excretory system. With other

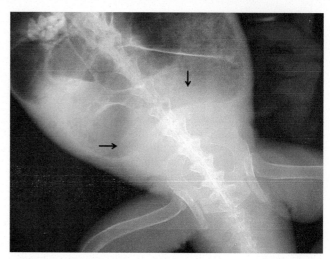

FIGURE 11-17 Dorso-ventral radiographic image of a green iguana with renal failure. The cranial poles of the kidney extend past the pelvis *(arrows).*

diagnostic modalities (e.g., endoscopy), it is not possible to completely visualize the entirety of the kidney, especially intrapelvic locations, nor is it possible to visualize the entire length or contents of the ureters, urethra, and urinary bladder. Contrast-enhanced CT scans can enable the clinician to re-create three-dimensional (3D) images of the entire excretory system. As facilities with CT imaging become more common in urban areas, veterinarians that treat companion exotic animals should consider using this diagnostic tool.

Endoscopy can be used to both visualize and collect biopsies from the excretory system. A distinct advantage of this modality is that it allows the clinician to observe the appearance, color, and topography of the kidneys. The authors prefer 1.9- and 2.7-mm rigid endoscopes. The recommended approach to the kidneys is through the flank or ventrum (paramedian to avoid ventral abdominal vein) in lizards, ventrum of snakes, and prefemoral fossae of chelonians. The examination should take place while the reptile patient is under general anesthesia using sterile techniques. Insufflation can increase the visualization of the excretory system, and while saline or carbon dioxide can be used, carbon dioxide is preferred. Closure is routine using a single everting horizontal mattress suture.

For clinicians who do not have access to endoscopy, renal biopsies collected from a cranial tail-cutdown technique or an exploratory coeliotomy. Sedation (alfaxalone; Jurox Ltd., Rutherford, New South Wales, Australia) and a local anesthetic (lidocaine, 2 to 3 mg/kg) may be used for the cranial tail cutdown technique. The cranial base of the tail should be disinfected using standard surgical preparation techniques. The approach will only provide access to one kidney, therefore if only one kidney is thought to be diseased, that side should be examined. The surgical approach is initiated with a small incision (1 to 2 cm) along the lateral processes of the caudal vertebrae at the base of the tail to access the kidney. Cranial and medial blunt dissection of the muscles at the base of the tail is performed to visualize the caudal pole of the kidney (Figure 11-18). When renal tissue is observed, biopsy samples are collected. Hemorrhage is typically controlled

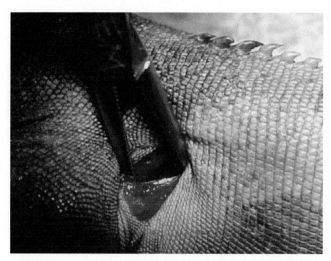

FIGURE 11-18 Cranial tail-cutdown technique to access the caudal kidney for a biopsy. Once the incision is made, blunt dissection can be done to gain access to the kidney.

with direct pressure using a sterile cotton-tipped applicator. Closure is routine by placing horizontal mattress sutures to close the initial skin incision.

An exploratory coeliotomy is another surgical technique used to examine the kidneys of a reptile. For lizards, a paramedian approach is recommended for the coeliotomy procedure. A plastronotomy is required to access the coelom of chelonians. A ventral approach can also be used for snakes, although the skin incision should be made between the first and second rows of the dorsal scales after which the incision site is rotated ventrally to access the coelom through the rectus abdominal muscles. The benefit of an exploratory coeliotomy is that it also provides the clinician with an opportunity to visualize other organ systems. This can be especially valuable in lizard and chelonian cases with cystic calculi.

Birds

Clinical Pathology

As for other species, renal function can be assessed using a multitude of diagnostics tests. Clinical pathology, in particular, plasma biochemistry and urinalysis, are the most common diagnostic tests used to assess kidney function. Clinical pathology is extremely useful and minimally invasive; however, certain limitations exist and it is important to acknowledge such limitations when interpreting the results.

As previously stated, assessing renal function in birds is challenging and often unrewarding. In comparison to their mammalian counterparts, plasma or serum marker assessment is not as worthwhile and may not truly correlate with actual renal function. Nevertheless, renal function assessment based on multiple tests including uric acid quantification is advisable.

Birds, as well as most reptiles, excrete nitrogenous wastes in the form of uric acid; therefore, measurement of plasma uric acid allows a basic assessment of uric acid concentration of in the blood. In chickens, uric acid, not urea, is produced as the main end product of nitrogen metabolism, with uric acid being the excretory vehicle for 80% of metabolized nitrogen.[316,317] Hyperuricemia is defined as "any plasma uric acid

concentration higher than the calculated limit of solubility of sodium urate in plasma"; the theoretical limit of solubility of sodium urate in birds is estimated to be 10.8 mg/dL (600 µmol/L).[136] It is believed that elevation of plasma uric acid above reference intervals may support a tentative diagnosis of renal disease.[52] However, due to active renal tubular secretion, blood uric acid concentrations are not notably affected by dehydration until GFR is decreased to the point that uric acid is not transported through the tubules, which may only occur in severe dehydration.[318] The concentration of uric acid can only increase with serious kidney damage (<30% functionality) or severe dehydration and is considered a late indicator of renal dysfunction.[319,320]

In general, a circulating uric acid concentration >15 mg/dL indicates renal impairment from a variety of causes such as nephrotoxic aminoglycoside antibiotics or lead toxicity, urinary tract obstruction, nephritis, nephrocalcinosis, and nephropathy associated with hypovitaminosis A.[319] Hyperuricemia has been correlated with tubular nephrosis and interstitial nephritis due to mycotoxicosis in chickens.[321] In dehydrated chickens, significantly increased serum uric acid concentrations at 48 h were frequently associated with mild dilatation of distal tubules and, less frequently, with mild dilatation of collecting ducts.[322] The renal toxin oosporein caused hyperuricemia, visceral and/or articular gout, and swollen pale kidneys in broiler chickens and turkeys.[323,324] Concentrations >10 to 15 mg/dL are considered elevated for most birds, with the exception of carnivorous birds that routinely have a significant elevation in blood uric acid following a protein meal.[151] Furthermore, quantification of circulating uric acid in pigeons did not correlate with the severity of histopathological findings of gentamicin-induced renal disease.[50] Mean serum concentrations of uric acid did not differ significantly in samples obtained from pigeons before and after gentamicin administration (6.500 and 6.130 mg/dL, respectively).[50] In red-tailed hawks receiving gentamicin of 10 mg/kg, IV, q12 h, uric acid concentrations increased significantly by day 4.[325] Changes in uric acid concentrations, clinical signs, and microscopic lesions suggested that a 10-mg/kg dose was toxic in red-tailed hawks.[325]

The main limitation of blood uric acid quantification is that the values can be influenced by several variables such as species, age, and diet.[319] In peregrine falcons (*Falco peregrinus*) (n = 5), uric acid had a marked postprandial increase.[326] Higher concentrations of uric acid were reached at 3 and 8 h, remained elevated for at least 16 h, and only returned to the original values by 24 h.[326] In black-footed penguins (n = 12), uric acid concentrations were significantly lower in the 4 to 6 h postprandial samples than in the 0 to 2 h postprandial samples.[317] Preprandial uric acid concentrations were <10 mg/dL, and 0 to 2 h postprandial concentrations were >13.4 mg/dL (mean concentration = 21.2 mg/dL).[317] Raptors and other carnivores have higher uric acid reference intervals, and marked postprandial increases may be observed; therefore, sampling of carnivorous birds should be performed after a 24 h fast.[318] Fasting hyperuricemia of >16.7 mg/dL (>1000 µmol/L) in peregrine falcons has been reported to be suggestive of renal failure.[327] In psittacines, it is said that uric acid changes secondary to high-protein diets did not show a positive correlation.[49] Indeed, in breeding parakeets, it has been shown that the levels of crude protein from 13% to 25% did not affect plasma uric acid concentrations.[328] However, in cockatiels, serum uric acid concentrations increased linearly with dietary protein levels, and uric acid was significantly greater in birds fed 70% crude protein compared to 11%, 20%, or 35% crude protein.[328] However, it was concluded that the hyperuricemia was due to dietary protein concentration and not renal disease.[328] Fasting also will decrease the likelihood of lipemia, which frequently is observed in postprandial samples.[318] Uric acid concentrations increased with age in ospreys (Pandion haliaetus).[329] This increase could be related to progressive maturation of renal function, a consequence of rapid growth, the amount of ingested protein, or individual nutritional status.[329] The osprey nestlings generally showed noticeably higher values of uric acid than Eurasian black vultures (Aegypius monachus), Iberian imperial eagles (Aquila adalberti), golden eagles (Aquila chrysaetos), Bonelli's eagles (Aquila fasciata), booted eagles (Hieraaetus pennatus), Swainson's hawks (Buteo swainsoni), Californian condors (Gymnogyps californianus), bald eagles (Haliaeetus leucocephalus), Egyptian vultures (Neophron percnopterus), and white-backed vultures (Pseudogyps africanus). In booted eagles (Hieraaetus pennatus) (n = 199), uric acid concentrations were higher in adults (n = 55) than nestling birds (n = 143), while adult males (n = 24) had higher uric acid concentrations than adult females (n = 28).[330] Overall, the highest uric acid concentrations were detected in nestling females (n = 63).[330] In adult captive collared scops owls (Otus lettia), significant differences in uric acid concentrations were detected between males (n = 20) and females (n = 17).[331] In the same study, no significant differences were detected between male (n = 22) and female (n = 15) adult captive crested serpent eagles (Spilornis cheela hoya).[331] In adult Japanese quail (n = 125 males and 151 females), no differences in uric acid concentrations were detected.[332] Uric acid concentrations in wild female goshawks (Accipiter gentilis) were similar to captive female goshawks, but male wild goshawks had higher concentrations than captive males.[333] It was hypothesized that males are under higher energy demands during the breeding season because they hunt for the female and the young; therefore, the higher uric acid concentrations were related to decreased body condition or food stress.[333] In pigeons, transport and handling stress led to a significant decrease in uric acid, although this is apparently without diagnostic relevance.[334] In chickens, it was demonstrated that transportation stress caused an increase in uric acid.[335]

Some investigators suggest that birds with suspected renal disease based on one single laboratory value of hyperuricemia should be given a total of 100 mL/kg subcutaneous isotonic fluids (SID or BID) for 2 days and then rechecked.[136,336] This method may allow the clinician to distinguish between true renal hyperuricemia and non-renal-related hyperuricemia.

Although the major nitrogenous waste product in birds is uric acid, creatinine and urea are also produced but at much lower values compared to mammals.[319] Furthermore, both BUN and creatinine levels may be below the minimum detectable limit of the assays in the laboratory.[318] Urea is present in very small amounts in avian plasma, and plasma concentrations have traditionally been considered an inappropriate parameter to evaluate renal function in birds.[337] Birds produce little creatinine from the precursor creatine.[151] Furthermore, the muscle metabolite creatinine appears to be

an insensitive renal marker because the dominant energy breakdown product of muscle metabolism in birds is creatine and because birds excrete creatine before it is converted to creatinine.[320,337] Creatinine is filtered, actively secreted, and, in the normal bird, may be reabsorbed.[151] Nevertheless, some attention has been given to these parameters over the years. Although elevations in BUN may be influenced by diet and hydration status, BUN can be used for prerenal assessments.[320] Blood urea nitrogen has little value in the detection of renal disease in most birds but is a sensitive indicator of hydration: In the dehydrated bird, up to 99% of BUN is reabsorbed.[58] In normal hydration conditions, 100% of filtered urea is excreted.[136] In 3 d water-deprived pigeons, the plasma-urea-nitrogen concentration increased by 6.5- to 15.3-fold, whereas uric acid concentration showed only a 1.4- to 2-fold increase, suggesting that urea may be useful to assess prerenal azotemia.[337] In 48 h water-deprived ostriches (n = 16), BUN doubled in value but uric acid remained similar.[338] Other factors might also influence BUN concentrations in birds. In peregrine falcons, BUN concentrations increased postprandially, with the highest concentrations reached at 8 h.[326] However, uric acid had a marked increase after food ingestion than BUN.[326] In black-footed penguins, postprandial uric acid was elevated but BUN was unaffected.[317] In cockatiels, serum urea concentrations increased with increasing dietary protein, in contrast with broiler chickens in which increased protein in the diet did not cause changes in BUN.[328,339] Sex has also been shown to influence BUN concentrations. In species with marked sexual dimorphism, such as ospreys, higher growth patterns in females, along with increased food demands during the second half of the nestling period, could explain the higher urea concentrations.[329] Red-tailed hawks with gentamicin-induced nephrotoxicity showed no significant change in BUN concentrations at 20 mg/kg, IV, q12 h for 2 d; however, at 10 mg/kg, IV, q12 h, BUN and uric acid concentrations were significantly increased by day 4.[325]

It is important to mention that the mean urea concentration in osprey nestlings was double the mean concentration of uric acid.[329] This higher contribution of urea to nitrogenous waste is a phenomenon that has already been observed to occur in other raptors and piscivorous species including storks, pelicans, and herons as a result of a diet rich in protein.[329] Interestingly, in piscivorous seabirds, urea concentrations are said to be low.[340]

Measurement of plasma creatinine concentrations serve as a crude assessment of the GFR in mammals, but in birds, plasma creatinine concentrations are routinely assessed because physiologic creatinine concentrations are below the detection limits of commonly used creatinine assays.[341] Clinically, creatinine concentrations may be elevated in pet birds fed high-protein diets; however, the relationship between creatine and creatinine in birds with renal disease is poorly understood, and differentiation does not appear to be clinically useful.[136] In water-deprived broiler chickens, plasma creatinine values were significantly higher at 24 h than at 6 h.[342] No significant differences in serum creatinine concentrations were detected between male and female Japanese quail.[332] In pigeons, only a 30% increase in blood creatinine concentrations were associated with dehydration.[337]

Due to the low sensitivity of the previously mentioned renal markers, several research studies investigated the use of other renal markers. Creatine and *N*-acetyl-β-D-glucosaminidase (NAG) were selected for study in the pigeon.[320] Results from this project revealed that NAG tissue concentrations were highest in the kidneys, while the greatest concentrations of creatine were found in the pectoral muscles.[320] After renal toxicity was induced through the administration of gentamicin, the pigeons' plasma creatine increased (>5 times) as did NAG (~6 times), which paralleled uric acid (>10 times).[320]

Although creatinine has little clinical relevance in birds, an exogenous creatinine clearance test may be useful to assess renal function. One study has evaluated the feasibility of performing and modeling exogenous plasma creatinine excretion in pigeons. Data revealed stringent elimination curves after IM or IV administration of exogenous creatinine at a dose of 50 mg/kg in pigeons.[341] However, this method has limitations because it is unclear as to whether exogenous creatinine clearance reflects the true GFR in birds. Further studies are warranted to investigate the usefulness of the exogenous creatinine clearance test.

In advanced renal disease, normocytic-normochromic anemia, hyperuricemia, uremia, and changes in plasma electrolytes, calcium, and phosphorus concentrations may be detected.[58] A simple and common test performed in birds is hematocrit. In cases of dehydration, hematocrit may be elevated due to hemoconcentration. In conscious, unrestrained, 4 to 5 d water-deprived Gambel's quail (*Callipepla gambelii*), hematocrit was 45.1% ± 5.3, while in normohydrated birds, hematocrit was significantly lower (35.1% ± 7.5).[343] Pigeons that endured, water deprivation for 24 to 48 h did not show significant changes in the hematocrit.[344] Nevertheless, many reasons for hematocrit alterations have been reported, including age, sex, reproductive status, altitude, energy and metabolism, season, parasitism, nutrition, and condition.[345]

As for the hematocrit, in cases of dehydration, total protein and total solid concentrations may increase. In 48 h water-deprived ostriches, hematocrit increased to 37% when compared with baseline hematocrit (hydrated animals).[338] In cases of renal failure, hypoproteinemia is said to be more common, but information associating plasma proteins with renal disease is limited, and different species may have dissimilar plasma protein concentrations under comparable disease conditions.[136] For example, a reduction in serum albumin concentrations may be used as an early and suitable indicator of the deleterious effect of mycotoxins in developing chickens.[346] Significant elevations of α_2 globulins are reported to be highly suggestive of acute nephritis; in these cases, most of the proteins are lost through the kidneys but the percentage of macroglobulins increases accordingly.[347,348] Pigeons experimentally infected with *Salmonella* were found to develop polyuria and become hypoalbuminemic.[56] In chickens with advanced tubular nephrosis and interstitial nephritis, hypoproteinemia was also reported; however, chickens with urolithiasis or those exposed to the fungal nephrotoxin (oosporein) did not become hypoproteinemic on a regular basis.[136] Hypoalbuminemia does not routinely occur in birds with renal failure, possibly because the disease process is not typically associated with glomerular disease (i.e., tubular nephritis or interstitial nephritis), the patient is in the early stages of glomerular disease, or birds just do not lose protein with glomerular disease.[336]

URINALYSIS. Biochemical and cytological sediment analysis of avian urine has been advocated as potentially useful in diagnosing avian renal disease.[136] In general, indications for urinalysis include persistent biochemical or radiographic abnormalities consistent with renal disease or persistent polyuria.[58] Causes of polyuria are extensive and nonspecific and include fluid therapy, renal disease, liver disease, gastrointestinal disease, diabetes mellitus, pituitary tumors, sepsis (with or without renal involvement), and psychogenic polydipsia.[58] Stress can also cause polyuria during examination.[49,58] Urinalysis may confirm renal disease well before renal dysfunction can be demonstrated in the plasma biochemical profile because with renal disease, intracellular enzymes are not released into the systemic circulation but may be voided in the urine.[327] Collection of an urine sample and accurate assessment of urinalysis results is problematic in birds because of the normal mixing of urine and feces in the cloaca, and due to intestinal reabsorption of water from urine. Therefore, urinalysis must be interpreted with care because protein, bacteria, inflammatory cells, and erythrocytes may originate from the gastrointestinal tract.[336] Some researchers suggest that a urinalysis is not diagnostic for renal disease in birds, because of fecal contamination and all other parameters included with a urinalysis are suspect due to fecal contamination therefore practically all parameters included with a urinalysis are suspect.[184] One of the exceptions to this mixing effect in the cloaca is the ostrich and, to a certain degree, other ratites. In all ratites, a strong rectal-coprodeal sphincter allows for separate defecation and voiding of urine; feces are stored in the rectum and urine in the proctodeum.[349,350] Studies have shown that the ostrich coprodeum is dissimilar to the mammalian bladder; furthermore, the abundance of goblet cells in the coprodeum results in a copious secretion of mucus that establishes a thick unstirred layer which provides osmotic protection.[351] A study assessing the lower intestine of wild ostriches found that urine, but not feces, was found in the coprodeum, and retrograde flow into the colon was not observed.[352] In ostriches, urine and feces were excreted separately, with urine voided first.[353] Anatomically, the terminal rectum has an unusual tunica muscularis externa and is clearly demarcated from the caudal part of the rectum proper by a semilunar fold, an abrupt thickening of the gut wall, and an increase gut capacity.[354] The cloaca had a distinct rectocoprodeal fold at the terminal rectum–cloaca junction with a well-formed sphincter muscle.[354] In rheas, a dilated pouch of the ureter stores urine.[355]

As previously mentioned because of the exposure of urine to fecal material in most birds, the diagnostic value of a urinalysis is questioned.[49] In polyuric birds, it is possible to collect a urinary sample relatively free of urates and overt fecal contamination.[327] Several techniques for collecting pure urine have been described, but they are not practical and are invasive. In one example, pigeons were placed on their backs and fastened to a board. A 1-mL syringe with the tip cut off and plunger removed was inserted into the cloaca.[356] This method allowed for the collection of 4 mL of urine and the cannula remained in the cloaca from 20 to 200 min.[356] In psittacines, snap-cap microtubes (300, 600, and 1500 μL) with small windows (3, 5, or 7 mm, respectively) were cut near the top of the tube at an ~90° angle on either the left or right side of the cap hinge.[357,358] The cap remained attached to the tube and was used to guide the insertion of the closed end of the tube into the cloaca and subsequently position and hold the window over the ureteral papilla for urine collection.[357,358] Other methods used for avian urine collection may be applied to small species such as sparrows, including the use of Foley catheters, micropipette tips, PE-240 tubes, and microcentrifuge tubes.[359-363] In poultry, several methods for pure urine collection have been described, but some of these methods are invasive and not clinically useful. For example, pure urine collection has been achieved by surgical colostomy; removing the colon from the cloaca allowed the animals to void pure urine.[364-366] Less invasive methods for collecting urine have also been described. The simplest method is to pipette liquid urine from a dropping, while avoiding the feces and urates. The sample can then be centrifuged to further separate any contaminants. Housing the bird on a nonabsorbable material (e.g., stainless steel cage with no paper bedding) can improve the probability of collecting a useful urine sample.

URINE BIOCHEMISTRIES. Both kidney biochemistries and urine enzyme concentrations can provide information regarding specific damage to renal tubules.[367] Reference ranges for urine chemistries in clinically normal falcons and farmed ostriches have been reported.[60,368,369]

In ostriches, several urine biochemistries changes were reported relative to the length of water deprivation.[369] Water deprivation caused significant urinary chemical changes in volume, osmolality, urea, uric acid, creatinine, sodium, chloride, potassium, and calcium.[369] In pigeons, urine creatine and NAG increased dramatically (~60 times and ~50 times, respectively) in response to gentamicin-induced renal disease.[320] In hens, serum NAG was significantly lower than urine NAG (0.11 to 0.14 mU/mg and 6.44 to 12.27 mU/mg, respectively).[367] Renal disease induced with 3 times the recommended amount of liquid vitamin D_3 supplement did not cause significant changes in urine NAG by 10 d, but by 40 d of supplementation, elevation of urine NAG was detected.[367] Both studies concluded that NAG, when measured in the urine, may be a valuable noninvasive renal marker.[320,367]

URINE SPECIFIC GRAVITY. Avian urine specific gravity is typically between 1.005 and 1.020 g/mL because birds have a decreased capacity for concentrating urine; only 10% to 30% of avian nephrons have loops of Henle.[49] Furthermore, the precipitate is not measured in the specific gravity of the urine supernatant; therefore, urine specific gravity is often lower in birds and reptiles than mammals.[318] In *Falco* spp., urinalysis testing was performed using voided liquid urine collected by aspirating the sample into a syringe and centrifuging. The supernatant was then analyzed by commercial dipstick and wet chemistry analyses for alkaline phosphatase, gamma-glutamyl transferase, glucose, chloride, and total protein concentrations.[368] In the study, 57% of the falcons had specific gravity equal to or greater than 1.020 g/mL.[368]

Urine osmolality and specific gravity, measured using a veterinary refractometer, has been reported in Hispaniolan Amazon parrots (*Amazona ventralis*).[370] Specific gravity and osmolality measurements were found to be highly correlated in the Hispaniolan Amazon parrots.[370] The use of the reference-canine scale to approximate the osmolality of parrot urine led to an overestimation of the true osmolality of the sample, and this error increased as the concentration of urine

increased.[370] Compared with the human-canine scale, the feline scale provides a closer approximation to urine osmolality of Hispaniolan Amazon parrots, although it still results in an overestimation of osmolality.[370] An equation to calculate the specific gravity results from a medical refractometer for Hispaniolan Amazon parrots has been proposed: $USG_{Hap} = 0.201 + 0.798 (USG_{ref})$.[370] In this equation, USG_{ref} represents the urine specific gravity measured from the bird's urine and USG_{Hap} represents the corrected specific gravity.

Pigeons experimentally infected with *Salmonella* were found to develop polyuria and produce hyposthenic urine (60% had density <1.007).[56] In two animals, urine osmolality values of 229 and 330 mOsmol/kg were recorded, which is higher than the normal upper range of 193 mOsmol/kg.[56] Plasma urea increased, but creatinine and uric acid concentrations remained within initial ranges.[56] In another study of experimentally inoculated pigeons, plasma concentrations of urea, uric acid, and creatine did not change, which may indicate that the clearance function of the kidney is not affected or kidney lesions are not always accompanied by biochemical plasma changes. Unfortunately, urinalysis was not performed as part of the study.[371] It is possible that urinalysis may provide a valuable diagnostic test to assess the renal function of pigeons with salmonellosis.

OSMOLALITY. Osmolality is another important aspect to the analysis of urine. Birds, like mammals, can produce hypertonic urine when body water must be conserved to maintain a stable blood plasma osmolality;[372] however, avian urine is typically isosmotic because of the predominance of reptilian-type nephrons in their kidneys. In normal birds, urine osmolality can be increased to a maximum of 2.0 to 2.5 times that of plasma osmolality, while in mammals it can increase fourfold.[136,372] Although clinical reference intervals of urine osmolality appear to be rarely reported, a significant amount of research regarding the effects of water deprivation and normal urine osmolality in multiple avian species has been reported.[373-375]

URINE COLOR. Urine color can provide important insight into the health of a bird. Under normal conditions, bird kidneys excrete a pasty white to yellow urate and a sparse, clear, and colorless watery urine.[52] However, pigments present in feces or newspaper can leach into urine and urates over time.[58] Avian species lack biliverdin reductase; thus, they do not form bilirubin as an end product of heme catabolism. Therefore, biliverdinuria is a common sequela to hepatic dysfunction.[151] In cases of liver disease, biliverdin accumulates in the bloodstream, surpassing the renal threshold, and is excreted in the urine. When this occurs, the urates and urine stain a lime-green to sulfur-yellow color.[151] Biliverdinuria is a common sign of hepatic disease associated with systemic infections (e.g., *Chlamydia psittaci*, Pacheco's disease, polyomavirus), hepatic lipidosis, increased red blood cell destruction (including immune-mediated hemolytic anemia), and lead toxicosis.[151,240,376,377] Prior to diagnosing biliverdinuria, one should evaluate whether fecal contamination is present by measuring urobilinogen using a urine dipstick.[318] Red urine may be observed with hematuria, hemoglobinuria, or myoglobinuria.[58] Hemoglobinuria has been reported in Amazon parrots (*Amazona* spp.) diagnosed with lead toxicosis; the birds produced dark red to pink urates. Hematuria has been associated with renal neoplasia, nephritis, and toxic nephropathy in birds. However, because blood can also originate from the intestinal or reproductive tracts, it is important to distinguish hemorrhage from these systems versus true hematuria.[58] Myoglobinuria may be associated with exertional myopathy and myoglobinuric syndrome.[378,379] Myoglobinuria secondary to capture myopathy or extensive muscle necrosis has been reported in ostriches and flamingos.[58]

URINE DIPSTICK. The pH of avian urine typically ranges from 6.0 to 8.0; however, the pH may be influenced by diet and cloacal contents. Urine is often more acidic in laying hens but is increased in alkalinity with bacterial metabolism.[58] In *Falco* spp., urine pH ranged from 5 to 7.[368] The majority of the animals had a pH of 7 (63%), followed by 6 (28%), and 5 (9%).[368] In pigeons (n = 61), urine pH was found to range from 5.5 to 6.9.[356]

Assuming there is no fecal contamination, normal avian urine should not contain detectable protein on a urine dipstick.[318] The urate precipitate is composed of uric acid, sodium, and/or potassium, and protein.[318] Any protein not reabsorbed in the proximal tubule is generally precipitated with uric acid; therefore, if only clear liquid urine is assessed, protein should not be present.[318] Most urine dipsticks are too insensitive to distinguish between moderate and severe proteinuria and may not properly detect protein in polyuric patients.[19]

Glucose concentrations in bird urine should be zero to trace.[58] Glucose is completely filterable and normally absorbed by the kidney; therefore, glucosuria can serve as an indicator that renal absorption is dysfunctional or that excessively high levels of glucose are being presented to the kidneys (e.g., diabetes mellitus).[19] It is not uncommon for diabetic birds to have urine glucose concentrations ranging from 3 to 4+ on a urine dipstick.[380,381] Ketonuria is also commonly present in cases of diabetes mellitus.[380-383] If diabetes mellitus is suspected and ketones are not measured, the urine should be rechecked in 48 h.[384] Glucosuria without hyperglycemia may be a sign of renal damage.[19] Nevertheless, a positive urine glucose test is an indicator of hyperglycemia. It should be noted that stress hyperglycemia can also cause up to 3+ glucosuria on a urine dipstick.[318]

Normal urine sediment is generally composed of uric acid precipitates and crystals, sloughed squamous epithelial cells, <3 white blood cells/40× field, <3 red blood cells/40× field, and low quantities of predominantly gram-positive bacteria.[384] Bacteria present in normal urine sediment samples are attributed to fecal contamination.[384]

Diagnostic Imaging

As for many disease conditions in birds, imaging is an important part of the clinical assessment of a patient and may provide significant complement to other diagnostic tests. Radiography is an important part of the diagnostic workup of urogenital disease in birds.[385] Other imaging techniques such as contrast radiography, ultrasonography, CT, and scintigraphy may also be useful for assessment of renal disease in birds. If morphologic information is needed, radiographs and ultrasonography are the imaging methods of choice, but if functional information is required, nuclear medicine is preferred.[386]

RADIOGRAPHY. Survey radiographs provide information regarding the size, location, and radiopacity of the kidneys.[19] Survey radiographic imaging of the abdomen has been considered the antemortem procedure of choice to identify malignant renal tumors in birds.[387] However, the avian kidney is difficult to evaluate radiographically because of its position within the synsacral fossa.[58] The synsacrum, formed by the fusion of the caudothoracic, lumbosacral, and caudal vertebrae with the pelvis, houses and protects the kidneys.[385] The kidneys are located in the synsacrum ventral renal fossae and are surrounded by the abdominal air sacs. Due to the presence of these air sacs, a rim of air is routinely observed dorsal to the kidneys. If this radiolucency is not present, it could suggest pathological swelling.[19] Renomegaly is detected more often in a lateral projection but can also be observed in the ventrodorsal projection (Figure 11-19).[58] Abnormalities commonly identified on survey radiographs include renal swelling, crystalline inclusions indicative of urate deposits, nephrocalcinosis, and gout.[19]

A generalized enlargement of the kidney(s) suggests diffuse renal disease or renal neoplasia.[151] Renal enlargement is often noted by the loss of the air space around the kidneys in psittacines, ventral displacement of the abdominal viscera beneath the kidneys, or enlargement of the kidneys.[388] Tumors developing in the caudal kidney may displace abdominal organs in a cranial and ventral direction, while tumors developing in the cranial and middle divisions of the kidneys tend to displace the intestinal mass caudally and ventrally and the ventriculus and liver cranially and ventrally.[151] Increased renal opacities can occur as a result of small kidney size, dehydration, and renal mineralization.[58] Birds with a prolonged negative calorie balance may develop smaller kidney shadows.[151] In severely dehydrated birds and birds with advanced kidney disease, extensive intratubular and, in the case of renal gout, extratubular urates may be detected through radiographic imaging.[151] Since uric acid calculi are usually radiolucent on radiographs, CT is considered a more sensitive test than radiography.[389] Improper positioning (e.g., lateral position is rotated) can artifactually change the appearance of the air-filled diverticulum surrounding the kidneys, making it more difficult to assess the kidneys.[136] An oblique view may be used to improve assessment of the kidneys because the renal silhouettes are superimposed on the lateral view of the coelom.[136] If differentiation is difficult, contrast radiography to demonstrate intestine or kidney is recommended.[59]

Contrast radiographic studies are useful not only for distinguishing the gastrointestinal tract from the renal silhouette but also for visualizing different renal structures. Excretory urography may be used to differentiate renal versus extrarenal abnormalities and to determine potential disturbances in the normal pattern of opacification of the renal parenchyma and collecting system.[390] Differentiation of the kidney and ureter from other structures, identifying an obstruction in the ureter, or demonstrating a functional disturbance in the renal system are examples in which excretory urography would be beneficial.[59] Radiopaque substances containing elements with large atomic numbers (e.g., barium, iodine) are commonly used to increase radiographic contrast.[391] Contrast media containing barium sulfate are limited to oral application (e.g., examination of the gastrointestinal tract), while water-soluble, iodine-based contrast media (e.g., iohexol) have broader application and can be administered IV.[391] In birds, rapid elimination of the contrast medium is common, although vein selection can have an effect on the clearance

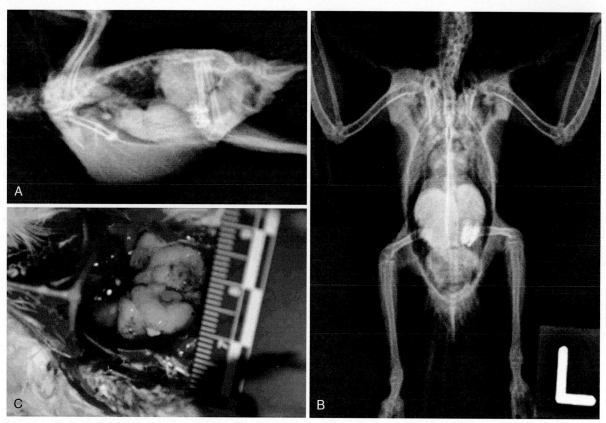

FIGURE 11-19 *(A)* Left lateral and *(B)* ventro-dorsal radiographic projections and *(C)* corresponding intracoelomic postmortem picture of a 20-year-old intact male cockatiel. The animal presented with a 1-week history of severe right hind leg lameness. On radiographs, an intracoelomic mass was detected on the renal-gonadal area. The intracoelomic mass was assessed via ultrasonography, but samples could not be collected due to lack of safe approach. On gross necropsy, an irregular, smooth-surfaced, off-white, multilobular mass extended from the cranial pole of the left kidney. Gonads and adrenal were obliterated and could not be identified. On histopathology, a testicular seminoma with renal, pulmonary, and sciatic nerve invasion as well as hepatic metastasis was diagnosed. In vivo renal function assessment based on blood work did not support abnormal renal function.

rate. For example, contrast is cleared more quickly when administered in the femoral vein than the ulnar vein.[59,391] In cases of renal dysfunction, a much slower elimination of the contrast agent may occur, leading to delayed filling of the ureters.[391] A lack of or reduced contrast within renal tissue is occasionally associated with renal cysts or tumors.[391] Many variables affect the nephrographic opacity, therefore the urogram cannot be used as a quantitative index of renal function.[385]

Iopamidol and iohexol (400 mg iodine/kg) are the preferred contrast agents to assess the kidneys.[59] Radiographs should be taken after intravenous administration of the contrast compound at 10 sec (to increase contrast of the heart, aorta, and pulmonary artery), 60 sec (imaging the kidneys and ureters), and 2 min (to highlight the entire cloaca).[392] Other investigators suggest that the first radiograph should be taken 30 sec after injection, because in most cases, the kidney will still be visible.[59] Multiple exposures (every 0.5 to 2 sec) are useful, especially for angiography, but require suitably equipped radiology units.[59] Fluoroscopy can be used to show

a real-time dynamic visualization of the urography; however, urography should not be performed in cases of severe renal dysfunction.[59]

Urography is useful for assessing renal morphology. Unfortunately, there are not many reports regarding the use of urography in avian medicine. Urography has been investigated in a limited number of avian species, including a ring-necked dove *(Streptopelia risoria)*, nanday conure *(Aratinga nenday)*, and orange-winged Amazon parrot *(Amazona amazonica)*.[390] Radiographic urography was also used for the postoperative assessment of an ureterolith removal in a male double yellow-headed Amazon parrot *(Amazona oratrix)*.[172] In Amazon parrot case, images were acquired at 1, 2, 7, and 10 min following intravenous injection of 400 mg/kg iohexol via the right medial metatarsal vein.[172]

ULTRASONOGRAPHY. In mammals, the greatest advantage of ultrasonography is its ability to provide superior assessment of internal renal parenchymal architecture.[393] Ultrasonography is superior to radiographic methods in assessing perinephric masses; detecting and localizing mineralization or nephroliths within/to the renal pelvis, pelvic diverticula, or cortex; and detecting renal masses, alterations of renal shape, and the presence of perirenal, subcapsular, or retroperitoneal fluid.[393] Sonographic examination also allows characterization of renal masses as solid or cystic and evaluation of adjacent organs for metastasis.[393] Unfortunately, in birds, ultrasonography may not be as useful, although there are examples where sonographic examination in birds can be diagnostic.[394] The presence of air sacs and the small space between the sternum and pubic bones can compromise the ultrasonographic exam.[385] End-fire mechanical sector scanners of high frequency, 7.5 and 10 MHz, provide the best images, although 5-MHz transducers may also be useful.[394] Some newer probes have a smaller-sized transducer ("hockey stick") and are useful for ultrasonographic examination of small birds. In one of the author's (J.B.) experience, this probe can be used in small birds; however, renal assessment continues to be difficult and limited in normal animals.

Studies investigating standard assessment of renal tissue in birds are limited. There are three standard acoustic windows for the avian urogenital tract: (1) the cranioventral approach, midabdominally directly behind the caudal margin of the sternum, (2) the caudo-ventral approach, which is situated between the pubic bones of the pelvis, and (3) the lateral approach via the flank directly behind the last rib.[394] Due to the small size of budgerigars, the approach to the coelomic cavity is limited to a window between the caudal margin of the sternum and the pubic bone of the pelvis (ventromedian approach).[395] In one study, the urogenital tracts of 386 pet birds (97 normal animals and 289 animals with clinical abnormalities) were assessed using transcutaneous ultrasonography.[394] The sonographic evaluation of the normal kidney was impossible because of its position along the vertebral column and the surrounding abdominal air.[394] In apparently healthy ostriches, the cranial renal lobe and the cranial part of the medial lobe could be assessed by placing the ultrasound probe in the mid-dorso-lateral area between the rib cage and the pelvic area.[396]

When the kidneys are enlarged because of neoplasia or renal cysts, if the liver or spleen is enlarged, or there is perihepatic or intraperitoneal fluid present, the kidneys may be visualized with ultrasonography.[397] Renal neoplasia is frequently accompanied by massive organ enlargement and complex parenchymal lesions, leading to secondary compression of the abdominal air sacs and displacement of the adjacent intestinal loops.[395] These anatomical changes make the neoplastic kidney easy to identify ultrasonographically as a round, nonhomogeneous structure through the ventromedian window.[395] In a study assessing renal neoplasia in budgerigars, ultrasonography did not allow a conclusive diagnosis in two birds due to their small size, but 11 birds (55%) were correctly diagnosed with systemic disease (liver disease, salpingitis, coelomitis) or neoplasia (gonadal or renal).[157] In another study, 29 renal disorders were diagnosed among 386 animals; inflammatory nephromegaly was identified in 11 animals; neoplasia in 12 animals; and cysts in 12 animals.[394] Sonographically, renal inflammation is most often described as hypoechoic with a reduced ability to image internal structures, while renal neoplasia frequently images as homogeneous hyperechoic tissue or nonhomogeneous parenchyma with focal necrosis.[398] Renal cysts often present as hyperechoic structures with smooth walls and hypoechoic contents.[398] In the case of renal crystallization or gout due to dehydration, hyperechoic nonhomogeneous reflections will be apparent if the kidney is enlarged.[398]

ADVANCED IMAGING. Computed tomography and magnetic resonance imaging (MRI) provide superior image quality compared to with traditional radiography. However, some researchers suggest that CT and MRI have limited value for evaluating bird kidneys because of costs and a lack of machine availability in most practices.[59] Although this may be true, CT is commonly used in mammalian medicine for this same purpose. In mammals, CT is most often used for the evaluation of ectopic ureters and surgical planning for large masses that involving the retroperitoneal space, adrenal glands, or kidneys.[399] Dynamic renal CT to estimate global and split renal function in pigs, dogs, and cats has been described.[399] Studies assessing normal anatomy of avian species through CT imaging are limited.[400-403]

Magnetic resonance imaging of the avian patient offers many advantages over conventional radiography and CT, including multiplanar imaging, no ionizing radiation, and improved soft tissue contrast resolution.[404] A limited number of publications have described normal structures of birds through MRI.[404] In a study assessing the use of MRI for sexing white-eyed parakeets (*Aratinga leucophthalma*), it was possible to visualize the birds' kidneys.[405] In another study investigating the use of MRI in pigeons by comparing the T1-weighted images of the kidneys with and without contrast media, it was apparent that distinct renal vasculature, as well as an increased signal intensity in the renal parenchyma, was visible after contrast media injection.[404] However, it was also noted that the contrast medium passed too quickly through the vasculature to be of diagnostic value.[404]

NUCLEAR SCINTIGRAPHY. Nuclear scintigraphy is a potentially valuable diagnostic test for assessing renal function in birds. Although it has been used multiple times in birds to determine renal function in research, nuclear scintigraphy has rarely been reported as a diagnostic option for clinical cases. Nuclear medicine scans detect and map the distribution of radiopharmaceuticals that have been administered to a patient in order to diagnose and monitor disease processes.[406] Quantitative determination of GFR is one of the most important indices of kidney function in dogs and cats in clinical and research settings, as it directly correlates to the number of functional nephrons.[50,386,407] Quantitative camera-based renal scintigraphy permits one to evaluate the function of each kidney and provides an objective index to monitor the progression or regression of renal impairment.[50] The gold standard for measuring GFR is inulin clearance.[386] Inulin is an ideal marker for measuring GFR since it is metabolically inert, is filtered by the glomerulus, and has no tubular secretion or absorption.[386] In birds, inulin clearance is not a viable option because it requires extensive anesthesia and cannulization of the ureter for extended periods of time to obtain urine that has not been contaminated with feces.[49]

Renal scintigraphy has been described in the chicken, pigeon, and cockatiel.[50,385,408] Different isotopes have been used, including 3H-inulin/kg and 14C-para-aminohippuric acid in chickens, and technetium-99m (^{99m}Tc)-dimercaptosuccinic acid (DMSA) and ^{99m}Tc-diethylenetriamine pentaacetic acid (DTPA) in pigeons and cockatiels.[50,385,408] Due to its short half-life (6 h) and ideal energy range (140 KeV), ^{99m}Tc is used most often for nuclear medicine scans.[385] While several ^{99m}Tc-labeled agents are available for renal imaging, DTPA is the preferred radionuclide for measuring GFR because it is non-toxic, not metabolized by the kidneys, not secreted or absorbed, and minimally (5%) protein bound.[385] Bird kidneys may be difficult to identify using this technology due to a low kidney to background ratio, but radiopharmaceutical accumulation in the cloaca is obvious.[399] In pigeons, ^{99m}Tc-DTPA can be used to evaluate renal function because it correlates well with renal histological grades. ^{99m}Tc-DMSA does not correlate well with histologic assessment but can be used to quantify changes in the size or shape of the kidneys or to document space-occupying lesions.[50]

ENDOSCOPY. Rigid endoscopy has been well investigated and is a common diagnostic test in avian medicine. The ability to exploit the air sac system of birds enables the endoscopist to visualize most, if not all, of the major organs of clinical interest, including the kidney, ureter, and cloaca.[409-411] Endoscopy allows for both the gross examination of the excretory system as well as the opportunity to collect biopsy samples for microscopic review. One important disadvantage of coelioscopy is related to the fact that the lateral approach through the caudothoracic and abdominal air sacs only allows for the visualization of one kidney.[410] In order to assess both kidneys, both sides of the body need to be examined, which will extend the anesthetic time.[410]

Patient positioning and the approach to a renal endoscopic exam are similar to the techniques described for a general coelioscopic examination.[409,411] Renal biopsies can be collected from the cranial, middle, or caudal divisions of the kidney.[409] Extra care is required when collecting samples from the cranial division of the kidney to avoid the cranial renal artery.[52] In general, there is no need to use scissors because the renal parenchyma is easily accessed.[409] Hemorrhage is not typically a concern with renal biopsies, with average postbiopsy hemorrhage lasting, on average, 67 sec (range: 10 to 172 sec).[410] A study evaluating renal biopsies in birds found that a majority (90%) of the samples could be histologically evaluated.[410]

Mammals

The diagnostic workup of an exotic mammal case for urinary tract disease should follow the same protocols outlined for amphibians, reptiles, and birds. An anamnesis and thorough physical examination should be accomplished first, this information often provides the clinician with enough evidence to determine that there is a problem associated with the urinary system. Follow-up diagnostic testing, including hematology, a plasma biochemistry panel, urinalysis, culture, diagnostic imaging, and histopathology, as outlined in the amphibian, reptile, and bird sections, can be submitted with results confirming the presence of urinary tract disease. Specific diagnostic tests for exotic small mammals can be found in the disease section.

TREATMENTS

Since diseases of the urinary system are caused by a variety of different etiologies, Tables 11-4 through 11-13 have been delineated by animal group, treatment method, and drug type to guide the veterinarian for managing these various disorders. Specific treatment options by disease are also located in the disease section of this chapter.

TABLE 11-5

Treatment Options for Fish

Medications	Dosage
*Antimicrobial Therapeutics**	
Ceftazidime	22 mg/kg IM, ICe, q72-96 h[415]
Ciprofloxacin	15 mg/kg, IM, IV, q24 h[416]
Enrofloxacin	5-10 mg/kg, q24 h, PO, SC, IM[417,418]
Renal Therapeutics	
Furosemide	2-5 mg/kg, IM, q12-72 h[419]

ICe, Intracoelomically; *IM*, intramuscularly; *IV*, intravenously; *PO*, by mouth; *SC*, subcutaneously.
*All infectious diseases of the urinary tract should be ideally treated with appropriate culture and sensitivities, rather than empirical antibiotics. These are several antibiotic choices that show good efficacy and penetration in urinary tract disease in small animal medicine.

TABLE 11-4

Treatment Options for Invertebrates

Medications	Dosage
*Antimicrobials**	
Ceftazidime	20 mg/kg, intracardiac, q72 h for 3 wk[412]
Enrofloxacin	5 mg/kg, IM, IV[413,414]
	10-20 mg/kg, PO, q24 h[413]

IM, Intramuscularly; *IV*, intravenously; *PO*, by mouth.
*All infectious diseases of the urinary tract should be ideally treated based on microbiologic culture and antibiotic sensitivity profiles, rather than empirical antibiotics. These are several antibiotic choices that show good efficacy and penetration in urinary tract disease in small animal medicine.

TABLE 11-6

Treatment Options for Amphibians

Medication	Dosage
*Antimicrobial Therapeutics**	
Ceftazidime	20 mg/kg, SC, IM, q72 h
Ciprofloxacin	10 mg/kg, PO, q24 h[420]
Enrofloxacin	5-10 mg/kg, q24 h, PO, SC, IM[420,421]
Renal Therapeutics	
Allopurinol	10 mg/kg, PO, q24 h[420]
Calcitonin	50 IU/kg, q7 d[420]
Calcium glubionate	1 mL/kg, PO, q24 h[420]
Calcium gluconate	100-200 mg/kg, SC[420]

IM, Intramuscularly; *PO*, by mouth; *SC*, subcutaneously.
*All infectious diseases of the urinary tract should be ideally treated with appropriate culture and sensitivities, rather than empirical antibiotics. These are several antibiotic choices that show good efficacy and penetration in urinary tract disease in small animal medicine.

TABLE 11-7

Treatment Options for Reptiles

Medications	Dosage
Antimicrobial Therapeutics*	
Amoxicillin	10 mg/kg, IM, q24 h[422]
	22 mg/kg, PO, q12-24 h[415,423]
Ceftazidime	20-40 mg/kg, SC, IM, IV, q48-72 h[424–426]
Ciprofloxacin	10 mg/kg, PO, q48 h[422]
Danofloxacin	6 mg/kg, SC, IM[427]
Enrofloxacin	5-10 mg/kg, q24 h, PO, SC, IM, ICe[428]
Renal Therapeutics	
Allopurinol	10-20 mg/kg, PO, q24 h[429–431]
Aluminum hydroxide	100 mg/kg, PO, q12-24 h[432]
Calcitonin	1.5 U/kg, SC, q8 h × 14-21 d, prn[433]
	50 U/kg, IM, repeat at 14 d[428,434]
Calcium glubionate	10 mg/kg, PO, q12-24 h, prn[435]
Calcium gluconate	100 mg/kg, SC, IM, ICe, q6-24 h[434,436]
Furosemide⁺	2-5 mg/kg, PO, IM, IV, q12-24 h[437,438]
Hydrochlorothiazide	1 mg/kg, q24-72 h[429]
Probenecid	250 mg/kg, PO, q12 h[439]
Miscellaneous Therapeutics	
Epoetin alfa (Epogen)	100 U/kg, SC, q72 h[440]

ICe, Intracoelomically; *IM,* intramuscularly; *IV,* intravenously; *PO,* by mouth; *prn,* as needed; *SC,* subcutaneously.

*All infectious diseases of the urinary tract should be ideally treated with appropriate culture and sensitivities, rather than empirical antibiotics. These are several antibiotic choices that show good efficacy and penetration in urinary tract disease in small animal medicine.

⁺Lower vertebrates do not possess a loop of Henle, so efficacy is questionable.

TABLE 11-8

Treatment Options for Birds

Medications	Dosage
Antimicrobial Therapeutics⁺	
Amoxicillin/clavulanate (Clavamox, Pfizer)	125 mg/kg, PO, q8-12 h[441,442]
Ceftazidime	50-100 mg/kg, IM, IV, q4-8 h[443,444]
Ciprofloxacin	15-20 mg/kg, PO, IM, q12 h[445]
Danofloxacin mesylate (A180)	5 mg/kg PO, IM, IV[445]
Enrofloxacin	15-30 mg/kg, q12-24 h, PO, IM, IV, SC[442,443,446]
Renal Therapeutics	
Aluminum hydroxide	30-90 mg/kg, PO, q12 h*
Allopurinol	10-15 mg/kg[447]
Calcitonin	4 U/kg, IM, q12 h, for 14 d[448]
Calcium glubionate	23 mg/kg, PO, q24 h[449]
Calcium gluconate (10%)	5-10 mg/kg, IV slowly to effect[450]
Colchicine	0.2 mg/kg, PO, q12 h[448]
Furosemide	0.1-2 mg/kg, PO, SC, IM, IV, q6-24 h[451]
Mannitol	0.25-2 mg/kg, q24 h, IV slow[448]
Urate oxidase (Uricozyme, Sanofi Winthrop)	100-200 U/kg, IM, q24 h[182]

IM, Intramuscularly; *IV,* intravenously; *PO,* by mouth; *SC,* subcutaneously.

*Rupiper DJ. pers. commun. 2004.

⁺All infectious diseases of the urinary tract should be ideally treated with appropriate culture and sensitivities, rather than empirical antibiotics. These are several antibiotic choices that show good efficacy and penetration in urinary tract disease in small animal medicine.

TABLE 11-9

Treatment Options for Mammals

Medications	Dosage
Antimicrobial Therapeutics*	
Amoxicillin	30 mg/kg PO, IM, divided q12-24 h × d (SG)[452,453]
	15 mg/kg, PO, SC, IM, q12 h (H)[454,455]
	20 mg/kg, PO, SC, q12 h (F)[456]
Amoxicillin/clavulanate (Clavamox, Pfizer)	12.5 mg/kg, PO, SC, divided q12-24 h (SG)[453,457]
	12.5 mg/kg, PO, q12 h (H, F)[453,458,459]
	20 mg/kg, PO, q12 h (Ro)[453]
Ampicillin	10 mg/kg, IM, q12 h (H)[454,455,460]
Ceftazidime	20-100 mg/kg, PO, SC, IM (Ro)[453,461]
	100 mg/kg, IM, q12 h (Ra)[462]
Ciprofloxacin	5-20 mg/kg, PO, q12 h (H)[453]
	5-20 mg/kg, q12-24 h (Ro)[453,463]
	10-20 mg/kg, PO, q12 h (Ra)[464]
	10-30 mg/kg, PO, q24 h (F)[465]
Enrofloxacin	10 mg/kg, PO, q12 h (SG)[453]
	2.5-5 mg/kg, PO, IM, q12-24 h (SG)[466]
	2.5-5 mg/kg, PO, IM, q12 h (H)[467]
	5-10 mg/kg, PO, SC, IM, q12 h (H, Ra, F)[455,459,468,469]
	5-20 mg/kg, PO, SC, IM, q12 h (Ro)[453,463,470,471]
Renal Therapeutics	
Aluminum hydroxide	100 mg/kg PO with each syringe feeding (H)[472]
	20-40 mg/animal, PO, prn (Ro)[473]
	30-60 mg/kg, PO, q8-12 h (Ra)[474]
Calcitonin	50-100 U/kg (SG)[475]
Calcium glubionate	150 mg/kg, PO, q24 h (SG)[452]
Calcium gluconate	100 mg/kg, SC, q12 h × 3-5 d; dilute in saline to 10 mg/mL (SG)[476]
	50 mg/kg, IM (H)[477]
	100 mg/kg, IM (Ro)[478]
Furosemide	1-4 mg/kg SC, IM, q6-8 h (SG)[466,479]
	1-5 mg/kg, PO, q12 h (SG)[466]
	2.5-5 mg/kg, PO, SC, IM, q8 h (H)[453,458]
	0.3-2 mg/kg, SC, IM, IV, prn (Ra)[480]
	1-4 mg/kg, PO, SC, IM, IV, q4-6 h, prn (Ra, F)[453,459,481]
Mannitol	0.5-1 g/kg, IV, over 20 min (F)[482]
Magnesium hydroxide	5-10 mg/kg, SC, IM, q12 h (Ro)[481,483]
Potassium citrate	4 mg/kg, PO (Ro)[484]
	10-30 mg/kg, PO, q12 h (Ro)[453]
	33 mg/kg, q8 h (Ra)[485]
Miscellaneous Therapeutics	
Epoetin alfa (Epogen)	100 U/kg, SC, q48-72 h (H)[477]
	50-150 U/kg, SC, q48-72 h (Ra)[474]
	50-150 U/kg, PO, IM, q48 h (F)[459]

F, Ferrets; *H,* hedgehogs; *IM,* intramuscularly; *IV,* intravenously; *PO,* by mouth; *prn,* as needed; *Ra,* rabbits; *Ro,* rodents; *SC,* subcutaneously; *SG,* sugar gliders.

*All infectious diseases of the urinary tract should be ideally treated with appropriate culture and sensitivities, rather than empirical antibiotics. These are several antibiotic choices that show good efficacy and penetration in urinary tract disease in small animal medicine.

TABLE 11-10

Fluid Requirements in Exotic Species

	Maintenance Requirements (mL/kg/d)	Blood Volumes/Shock Doses (mL/kg)
Invertebrates	15-25 mL/kg[486]	Hemolymph accounts for 20% of body weight in tarantulas[412]
Fish	1-3% body weight[487] 10-30 mL/kg, PO 20-60 mL/kg, IV, ICe	Unknown
Amphibians	2-5% body weight, ICe, q12 h[420]	Unknown
Reptiles	Replacement therapy estimated at 10-30 mL/kg/d[488]	Unknown
Birds	100-150 mL/kg/d; some passerines drink 250-300 mL/kg/d[489]	Fluid bolus for CPR 25 mL/kg[490]
Hedgehogs	50-100 mL/kg/d[487]	50-60 mL/kg[490]
Rodents[488,489]		
Gerbil	40-70 mL/kg/d	67 mL/kg
Guinea pig	100 mL/kg/d	75 mL/kg
Hamster	80-100 mL/kg/d	78 mL/kg
Mouse	150 mL/kg/d	79 mL/kg
Rat	100-120 mL/kg/d	64 mL/kg
Rabbits	50-100 mL/kg/d[491]	50-60 mL/kg[490]
Ferrets	75-100 mL/kg/d[466]	50-60 mL/kg[490] Blood volume reported at 60-80 mL[466]

CPR, Cardiopulmonary resuscitation; *ICe,* intracoelomically; *IV,* intravenously; *PO,* by mouth.

TABLE 11-11

Miscellaneous Fluids in Exotic Species

FISH		
Sodium acetate		40 mEq/L of IV fluids at 20-30 mL/kg/h, IV (elasmobranchs)[492]
Sodium chloride		1-3 g/L tank water[493]
Sodium bicarbonate		1 mEq/L of IV fluids[487]
AMPHIBIANS		
Amphibian Ringer's solution (ARS)	Formulation: 6.6 g NaCl, 0.15 g KCl, 0.15 g CaCl$_2$, NaHCO$_3$ in 1 L water[420]	Place animal in shallow ARS for 24 h, replace with fresh solution daily, slowly wean with more dilute solutions[420]
Dextrose 5% solution		Place animal in bath for up to 24 h, replace daily, and wean animal off, changing solution concentration gradually[420,494]
Hetastarch (6% in 0.9% NaCl)		*Bath not to exceed 1 h without reassessment
REPTILES		
Hetastarch (6% in 0.9% NaCl)		3-5 mL/kg, IV/IO slowly, bolus prn, not to exceed 20 mL/kg[496,497]
Reptile Ringer's	Formulations:	10 mL/kg, q24 h[495]
	1 part Normosol-R + 2 parts 2.5% dextrose in 0.45 NaCl[495]	
	1 part Normosol-R + 1 part 5% dextrose + 1 part 0.9% saline	20 mL/kg, q12 h[436]
Oxyglobin		3-5 mL/kg, slow IV or IO[496,497]
BIRDS AND MAMMALS		
Oxyglobin		5 mL/kg over several min[490] 2 mL/kg over 10-20 min[498]
Sodium bicarbonate		1 mEq/kg, IV, q15-30 min for max of 4 mEq/kg total dose[486,498]

IO, Intraosseously; *IV,* intravenously.
*Wright KM. pers. comm. 2011.

TABLE 11-12

Electrolyte Composition of Commonly Used Commercially Available Fluids

Fluid	Glucose (g/L)	Na⁺ (mEq/L)	CL⁻ (mEq/L)	K⁺ (mEq/L)	Ca²⁺ (mEq/L)	Mg²⁺ (mEq/L)	Buffer (mEq/L)	Osmolarity (mOsm/L)	Cal/L	pH
5% Dextrose	50	0	0	0	0	0	0	252	170	4.0
10% Dextrose	100	0	0	0	0	0	0	505	340	4.0
2.5% Dextrose in 0.45% NaCl	25	77	77	0	0	0	0	280	85	4.5
5% Dextrose in 0.45% NaCl	50	77	77	0	0	0	0	406	170	4.0
5% Dextrose in 0.9% NaCl	50	154	154	0	0	0	0	560	170	4.0
0.45% NaCl	0	77	77	0	0	0	0	154	0	5.0
0.9% NaCl	0	154	154	0	0	0	0	308	0	5.0
Ringer's lactate solution	0	130	109	4	3	0	28 (L)	272	9	6.5
Ringer's solution	0	147.5	156	4	4.5	0	0	310	0	5.5
Normosol-M in 5% dextrose	50	40	40	13	0	3	16(A)	364	175	5.5
Normosol-R	0	140	98	5	0	3	27(A)	296	18	6.4
Plasma-Lyte	0	140	103	10	5	3	47(A)	312	17	5.5

Adapted from Chew DJ, DiBartola SP. *Manual of Small Animal Nephrology and Urology.* New York: Churchill-Livingstone; 1986:308.
A, Acetate; *L,* lactate.

TABLE 11-13

Additives and Special Solutions

20% Mannitol	200 (M)	0	0	0	0	0	0	1099	—	—
7.5% NaHCO₃	0	893	0	0	0	0	893	1786	0	—
8.4% NaHCO₃	0	1000	0	0	0	0	1000 (B)	2000	0	—
10% CaCl₂	0	0	2720	0	1360	0	0	4080	0	—
14.9% KCl	0	0	2000	2000	0	0	0	4000	0	—
50% Dextrose	500	0	0	0	0	0	0	2780	1700	4.2

Adapted from Chew DJ, DiBartola SP. *Manual of Small Animal Nephrology and Urology.* New York: Churchill-Livingstone; 1986:308.[499]
B, Bicarbonate; *M,* mannitol.

REFERENCES

1. Holz PH, Raidal SR. Comparative renal anatomy of exotic species. *Vet Clin North Am Exot Anim Pract.* 2006;9:1-11.
2. Kardong KV. *Vertebrates: Comparative Anatomy, Function, Evolution.* Boston: McGraw-Hill; 2006.
3. Wright PA. Nitrogen excretion: three end products, many physiological roles. *J Exp Biol.* 1995;198:273-281.
4. Walsh PJ, Smith CP. Urea transport. In: Wright P, Anderson P, eds. *Fish Physiology.* San Diego: Academic Press; 2001:279-307.
5. Leake LD. *Comparative Histology. An Introduction to the Microscopic Structure of Animals.* London: Academic Press; 1975.
6. Bradley T. The excretory system: Structure and physiology. In: Kerkut GA, Gilbert LI, eds. *Comprehensive Insect Physiology, Biochemistry and Pharmacology.* Oxford: Pergamon Press; 1985:421-465.
7. Whiteside DP. Anatomy and physiology (Part 2: Vertebrates). In: Irwin MD, Cobaugh AM, eds. *Zookeeping: An Introduction to the Science and Technology.* Chicago: University of Chicago Press; 2013:116-130.
8. Stospkf MK. Anatomy. In: Stoskopf MK, ed. *Fish Medicine.* Philadelphia: Saunders; 1993:2-30.
9. Marshall WS, Grosell M. Ion transport, osmoregulation, and acid-base balance. In: Evans D, Claiborne JB, eds. *The Physiology of Fishes.* 3rd ed. Boca Raton, FL: CRC Press; 2005:177-230.
10. O'Malley B. General anatomy and physiology of reptiles. In: O'Malley B, ed. *Clinical Anatomy and Physiology of Exotic Species.* Atlanta: Elsevier; 2005:17-39.
11. Cecil TR. Amphibian renal disease. *Vet Clin North Am Exot Anim Pract.* 2006;9:175-188.
12. Wright KM, Whitaker BR. *Amphibian Medicine and Captive Husbandry.* Malabar, FL: Krieger Publishing Company; 2001.
13. Davis LE, Schmidt-Nielsen B, Stolte H, et al. Anatomy and ultrastructure of the excretory system of the lizard, *Sceloporus cyanogenys. J Morphol.* 1976;149:279-326.
14. Bentley PJ. Osmoregulation. In: Gans C, Huey RB, eds. *Biology of the Reptilia.* London: Academic Press; 1976.
15. Minnich J. Water procurement and conservation by desert reptiles in their natural environment. *Isr J Med Sci.* 1976;12:740.
16. Gibbons PM. Advances in reptile clinical therapeutics. *J Exot Pet Med.* 2014;23:21-38.
17. Holz P, Barker IK, Burger JP, et al. The effect of the renal portal system on pharmacokinetic parameters in the red-eared lider (*Trachemys scripta elegans*). *J Zoo Wildl Med.* 1997;28:386-393.
18. Tully TN. Birds. In: Mitchell MA, Tully TN, eds. *Manual of Exotic Pet Practice.* Philadelphia: Saunders; 2008.
19. Lumeij JT. Nephrology. In: Ritchie BW, Harrison GJ, Harrison LR, eds. *Avian Medicine: Principles and Application.* Lake Worth, FL: Wingers Pub.; 1994:538-555.

20. Rommel SA, Lowenstine LJ. Gross and microscopic anatomy. In: Dierauf LA, Gulland FMD, eds. *CRC Handbook of Marine Mammal Medicine*. 2nd ed. New York: CRC Press; 2001:129-158.

21. Emerson H, Norris C. "Red-Leg"—An infectious disease of frogs. *J Exp Med*. 1905;7:32-58.

22. Urbain A. La paratyphose des grenouilles *(Rana esculenta)*. *J Soc Biol*. 1944;183:458-549.

23. Temple R, Fowler M. Amphibians. In: Fowler M, ed. *Zoo and Wild Animal Medicine*. 1st ed. Philadelphia: W.B. Saunders; 1978:79-88.

24. Reichenbach-Klinke H, Elkin E. Bacterial diseases. In: *Diseases of Amphibians*. New York: Academic Press; 1965:221-246.

25. Cranshaw G. Amphibian medicine. In: Fowler M, ed. *Zoo and Wild Animal Medicine: Current Therapy*. 3rd ed. Philadelphia: W.B. Saunders; 1993:131-139.

26. Wright K. Taxonomy of amphibians kept in captivity. In: Wright K, Whitaker BR, eds. *Amphibian Medicine and Captive Husbandry*. Malabar, FL: Krieger Publishing; 2001:3-6.

27. Green DE. Pathology of amphibia. In: Wright K, Whitaker BR, eds. *Amphibian Medicine and Captive Husbandry*. Malabar, FL: Krieger Publishing; 2001:401-485.

28. Cranshaw G. Anurans (Anura, Salienta): Frogs, toads. In: Fowler M, ed. *Zoo and Wild Animal Medicine*. 5th ed. Philadelphia: W.B. Saunders; 1999:20-33.

29. Brayton C. Wasting disease associated with cutaneous and renal nematodes, in commercially obtained *Xenopus laevis*. *Ann NY Acad Sci*. 1992;653:197-201.

30. Kudo R. On the protozoa parasitic in frogs. *Trans Am Microscop Soc*. 1922;41:59-76.

31. McKinnell RG. Incidence and histology of renal tumors of leopard frogs from the North Central States. *Ann N Y Acad Sci*. 1965;126:85-98.

32. Duncan AE, Garner MM, Bartholomew JL, et al. Renal myxosporidiasis in Asian horned frogs *(Megophrys nasuta)*. *J Zoo Wildl Med*. 2004;35:381-386.

33. Mutschmann F. Pathological changes in African hyperoliid frogs due to a myxosporidian infection with a new species of *Hoferellus* (Myxozoa). *Dis Aquat Organ*. 2004;60:215-222.

34. McKinnell RG, Cunningham WP. Herpesviruses in metastatic Lucke renal adenocarcinoma. *Differentiation*. 1982;22:41-46.

35. Meyer-Rochow V, Asashima M, Moro S. Nephroblastoma in the clawed frog *Xenopus laevis*. *J Exp Anim Sci*. 1990;34:225-228.

36. Stacy BA, Parker JM. Amphibian oncology. *Vet Clin North Am Exot Anim Pract*. 2004;7:673-695.

37. Wright K, Whitaker BR. Nutritional disorders. In: Wright K, Whitaker BR, eds. *Amphibian Medicine and Captive Husbandry*. Malabar, FL: Krieger Publishing; 2001:73-84.

38. Frye FL. *Biomedical and Surgical Aspects of Captive Reptile Husbandry*. 2nd English ed. Malabar, FL: Krieger Publishing Company; 1991.

39. Frye F. Diagnosis and surgical treatment of reptilian neoplasms with a compilation of cases 1966-1993. *In Vivo*. 1993;8:885-892.

40. Done LB. Neoplasia. In: Mader D, ed. *Reptile Medicine and Surgery*. St. Louis, MO: Saunders; 1996:125-141.

41. Kölle P, Hoffman R, Wolters M, et al. Cystic calculi in reptiles. *Proceedings of the Association of Amphibian and Reptile Veterinarians*. 2001;190-192.

42. Dalbeth N. Management of gout in primary care: challenges and potential solutions. *Rheumatology (Oxford)*. 2013;52:1549-1550.

43. Mader DR. Gout. In: Mader DR, ed. *Reptile Medicine and Surgery*. 2nd ed. St. Louis, MO: Elsevier/W.B. Saunders; 2006.

44. Neogi T. Gout. *N Engl J Med*. 2011;364:443-452.

45. Harrold L. New developments in gout. *Curr Opin Rheumatol*. 2013;25:304-309.

46. Schumacher J, Toal RL. Advanced radiography and ultrasonography in reptiles. *Sem Avian Exot Pet Med*. 2001;10:162-168.

47. Jones YL, Fitzgerald SD. Articular gout and suspected pseudogout in a basilisk lizard *(Basilicus plumifrons)*. *J Zoo Wildl Med*. 2009;40:576-578.

48. Carpenter JW, Marion CJ. *Exotic Animal Formulary*. 4th ed. St. Louis, MO: Elsevier Saunders; 2013.

49. Burgos-Rodriguez AG. Avian renal system: clinical implications. *Vet Clin North Am Exot Anim Pract*. 2010;13:393-411.

50. Marshall KL, Craig LE, Jones MP, et al. Quantitative renal scintigraphy in domestic pigeons *(Columba livia domestica)* exposed to toxic doses of gentamicin. *Am J Vet Res*. 2003;64:453-462.

51. Schmidt RE. Types of renal disease in avian species. *Vet Clin North Am Exot Anim Pract*. 2006;9:97-106.

52. Speer BL. Diseases of the urogenital system. In: Altman RB, Clubb SL, Dorrestein GM, et al., eds. *Avian Medicine and Surgery*. Philadelphia: W.B. Saunders; 1997:625-644.

53. King AS, McLelland J. *Birds: Their Structure and Function*. Eastbourne: Bailliere Tindall; 1984.

54. Bounous DI, Schaeffer DO, Roy A. Coagulase-negative *Staphylococcus* sp. septicemia in a lovebird. *J Am Vet Med Assoc*. 1989;195:1120-1122.

55. Bhaiyat MI, Hariharan H, Chikweto A, et al. Isolation of Coagulase-Negative *Staphylococcus* Spp. and *Kocuria varians* in Pure Culture from Tissues of Cases of Mortalities in Parrots in Grenada, West Indies. 2013. International Journal of Veterinary Medicine: Research & Case Reports. http://www.ibimapublishing.com/journals/IJVMR/2013/149634/a149634.html.

56. Gevaert D, Nelis J, Verhaeghe B. Plasma chemistry and urine analysis in *Salmonella*-induced polyuria in racing pigeons *(Columba livia)*. *Avian Pathol*. 1991;20:379-386.

57. Naldo JL, Samour JH. Causes of morbidity and mortality in falcons in Saudi Arabia. *J Avian Med Surg*. 2004;18:229-241.

58. Pollock C. Diagnosis and treatment of avian renal disease. *Vet Clin North Am Exot Anim Pract*. 2006;9:107-128.

59. Lierz M. Avian renal disease: pathogenesis, diagnosis, and therapy. *Vet Clin North Am Exot Anim Pract*. 2003;6:29-55, v.

60. Mushi E, Binta M, Isa J. Biochemical composition of urine from farmed ostriches *(Struthio camelus)* in Botswana: short communication. *J S Afr Vet Assoc*. 2001;72:46-48.

61. Deem SL. Fungal diseases of birds of prey. *Vet Clin North Am Exot Anim Pract*. 2003;6:363-376.

62. Greenacre CB, Latimer KS, Ritchie BW. leg paresis in a black palm cockatoo *(Probosciger aterrimus)* caused by aspergillosis. *J Zoo Wildl Med*. 1992;23:122-126.

63. Tham V, Purcell D, Schultz D. Fungal nephritis in a grey-headed albatross. *J Wildl Dis*. 1974;10:306-309.

64. Martin MP, Bouck KP, Helm J, et al. Disseminated *Aspergillus flavus* infection in broiler breeder pullets. *Avian Dis*. 2007;51:626-631.

65. Sak B, Kasickova D, Kvac M, et al. Microsporidia in exotic birds: intermittent spore excretion of *Encephalitozoon* spp. in naturally infected budgerigars *(Melopsittacus undulatus)*. *Vet Parasitol*. 2010;168:196-200.

66. Lee SC, Corradi N, Byrnes EJ 3rd, et al. Microsporidia evolved from ancestral sexual fungi. *Curr Biol*. 2008;18:1675-1679.

67. Snowden K, Phalen DN. *Encephalitozoon* infection in birds. *Sem Avian Exot Pet Med*. 2004;13:94-99.

68. Malcekova B, Valencakova A, Luptakova L, et al. First detection and genotyping of *Encephalitozoon cuniculi* in a new host species, gyrfalcon *(Falco rusticolus)*. *Parasitol Res*. 2011;108:1479-1482.

69. Lobo ML, Xiao L, Cama V, et al. Identification of potentially human-pathogenic *Enterocytozoon bieneusi* genotypes in various birds. *Appl Environ Microbiol*. 2006;72:7380-7382.

70. Kašičková D, Sak B, Kváč M, et al. Sources of potentially infectious human microsporidia: molecular characterisation of microsporidia isolates from exotic birds in the Czech Republic, prevalence study and importance of birds in epidemiology of the human microsporidial infections. *Vet Parasitol*. 2009;165:125-130.

71. Haro M, Izquierdo F, Henriques-Gil N, et al. First detection and genotyping of human-associated microsporidia in pigeons from urban parks. *Appl Environ Microbiol*. 2005;71:3153-3157.

72. Lee S-Y, Lee S-S, Lyoo YS, et al. DNA detection and genotypic identification of potentially human-pathogenic microsporidia from asymptomatic pet parrots in South Korea as a risk factor for zoonotic emergence. *Appl Environ Microbiol.* 2011;77:8442-8444.

73. Malcekova B, Valencakova A, Molnar L, et al. First detection and genotyping of human-associated microsporidia in wild waterfowl of Slovakia. *Acta Parasitol.* 2013;58:13-17.

74. Pulparampli N, Graham D, Phalen D, et al. *Encephalitozoon hellem* in two eclectus parrots *(Eclectus roratus):* identification from archival tissues. *J Eukaryot Microbiol.* 1998;45:651-655.

75. Reetz J. Natural transmission of microsporidia *(Encephalitozoon cuniculi)* by way of the chicken egg. *Tierarztl Prax.* 1994;22:147-150.

76. Reetz J, Rinder H, Thomschke A, et al. First detection of the microsporidium *Enterocytozoon bieneusi* in non-mammalian hosts (chickens). *Int J Parasitol.* 2002;32:785-787.

77. Santin M, Fayer R. Microsporidiosis: *Enterocytozoon bieneusi* in domesticated and wild animals. *Res Vet Sci.* 2011;90:363-371.

78. Slodkowicz-Kowalska A, Graczyk TK, Tamang L, et al. Microsporidian species known to infect humans are present in aquatic birds: implications for transmission via water? *Appl Environ Microbiol.* 2006;72:4540-4544.

79. Lallo MA, Calabria P, Milanelo L. *Encephalitozoon* and *Enterocytozoon* (Microsporidia) spores in stool from pigeons and exotic birds: microsporidia spores in birds. *Vet Parasitol.* 2012;190:418-422.

80. Pirestani M, Sadraei J, Forouzandeh M. Molecular characterization and genotyping of human related microsporidia in free-ranging and captive pigeons of Tehran, Iran. *Infect Genet Evol.* 2013;20:495-499.

81. Reetz J. Naturally-acquired microsporidia *(Encephalitozoon cuniculi)* infections in hens. *Tierarztl Prax.* 1993;21:429-435.

82. Kašičková D, Sak B, Kváč M, et al. Detection of *Encephalitozoon cuniculi* in a new host—cockatiel *(Nymphicus hollandicus)* using molecular methods. *Parasitol Res.* 2007;101:1685-1688.

83. Snowden K, Logan K, Phalen D. Isolation and characterization of an avian isolate of *Encephalitozoon hellem. Parasitology.* 2000;121:9-14.

84. Snowden K, Logan K. Molecular identification of *Encephalitozoon hellem* in an ostrich. *Avian Dis.* 1999;43:779-782.

85. Snowden K, Daft B, Nordhausen RW. Morphological and molecular characterization of *Encephalitozoon hellem* in hummingbirds. *Avian Pathol.* 2001;30:251-255.

86. Carlisle MS, Snowden K, Gill J, et al. Microsporidiosis in a Gouldian finch *(Erythrura* [Chloebia] *gouldiae). Aust Vet J.* 2002;80:41-44.

87. Nakamura A, Homem C, Garcia S, et al. Keratoconjunctivitis by *Encephalitozoon hellem* in lovebirds *(Agapornis* spp.) in Brazil: case report. *Arq Bras Med Vet Zootec* 2010;62:816-820.

88. Barton CE, Phalen DN, Snowden KF. Prevalence of microsporidian spores shed by asymptomatic lovebirds: evidence for a potential emerging zoonosis. *J Avian Med Surg.* 2003;17:197-202.

89. Gelis S, Raidal SR. Microsporidiosis in a flock of tricolor parrot finches *(Erythrura tricolor). Vet Clin North Am Exot Anim Pract.* 2006;9:481-486.

90. Muller MG, Kinne J, Schuster RK, et al. Outbreak of microsporidiosis caused by *Enterocytozoon bieneusi* in falcons. *Vet Parasitol.* 2008;152:67-78.

91. Graczyk TK, Sunderland D, Rule AM, et al. Urban feral pigeons *(Columba livia)* as a source for air-and waterborne contamination with *Enterocytozoon bieneusi* spores. *Appl Environ Microbiol.* 2007;73:4357-4358.

92. Bart A, Wentink-Bonnema EM, Heddema ER, et al. Frequent occurrence of human-associated microsporidia in fecal droppings of urban pigeons in Amsterdam, The Netherlands. *Appl Environ Microbiol.* 2008;74:7056-7058.

93. Haro M, Henriques-Gil N, Fenoy S, et al. Detection and genotyping of *Enterocytozoon bieneusi* in pigeons. *J Eukaryot Microbiol.* 2006;53(suppl 1):S58-S60.

94. Friend M, Franson JC. Field manual of wildlife diseases. General Field Procedures and Diseases of Birds: Information and Technology Report 1999-001. Washington, DC: U.S. Geological Survey, Biological Resources Division, 1999.

95. Yabsley MJ. *Eimeria.* In: Atkinson CT, Thomas NJ, Hunter DB, eds. *Parasitic Diseases of Wild Birds.* Ames, IA: Wiley-Blackwell; 2008:162-180.

96. Schmidt RE, Reavill DR, Phalen DN. Urinary system. In: Schmidt RE, Reavill DR, Phalen DN, eds. *Pathology of Pet and Aviary Birds.* Ames, IA: Iowa State Press; 2008:95-107.

97. Lindsay DS, Blagburn BL, Hoerr FJ, et al. Cryptosporidiosis in zoo and pet birds. *J Protozool.* 1991;38:180S-181S.

98. Gardiner C, Imes G Jr. *Cryptosporidium* sp. in the kidney of a black-throated finch. *J Am Vet Med Assoc.* 1984;185:1401-1402.

99. Randall CJ. Renal and nasal cryptosporidiosis in a junglefowl *(Gallus sonneratii). Vet Rec.* 1986;119:130-131.

100. Goodwin MA. Cryptosporidiosis in birds—a review. *Avian Pathol.* 1989;18:365-384.

101. Trampel DW, Pepper TM, Blagburn BL. Urinary tract cryptosporidiosis in commercial laying hens. *Avian Dis.* 2000;44:479-484.

102. Godoy SN, De Paula CD, Cubas ZS, et al. Occurrence of *Sarcocystis falcatula* in captive psittacine birds in Brazil. *J Avian Med Surg.* 2009;23:18-23.

103. Smith JH, Neill PJ, Box ED. Pathogenesis of *Sarcocystis falcatula* (Apicomplexa: Sarcocystidae) in the budgerigar *(Melopsittacus undulatus).* III. Pathologic and quantitative parasitologic analysis of extrapulmonary disease. *J Parasitol.* 1989;75:270-287.

104. Olias P, Gruber AD, Heydorn AO, et al. A novel *Sarcocystis*-associated encephalitis and myositis in racing pigeons. *Avian Pathol.* 2009;38:121-128.

105. Remple JD. Intracellular hematozoa of raptors: a review and update. *J Avian Med Surg.* 2004;18:75-88.

106. Goswami P, Swamy M. Avian malaria: Diagnosis and management. Jawaharlal Nehru Krishi Vishwa Vidyalaya Jabalpur 482004 (Madhya Pradesh) India:19.

107. Donovan TA, Schrenzel M, Tucker TA, et al. Hepatic hemorrhage, hemocoelom, and sudden death due to *Haemoproteus* infection in passerine birds: eleven cases. *J Vet Diagn Invest.* 2008;20:304-313.

108. Rotstein DS, Flowers JR, Wolfe BA, et al. Renal trematodiasis in captive double-toothed barbets *(Lybius bidentatus). J Zoo Wildl Med.* 2005;36:124-126.

109. Rubio-Godoy M, de León GP-P, Mendoza-Garfias B, et al. Helminth parasites of the blue-footed booby on Isla Isabel, México. *J Parasitol.* 2011;97:636-641.

110. Luppi MM, de Melo AL, Motta RO, et al. Granulomatous nephritis in psittacines associated with parasitism by the trematode *Paratanaisia* spp. *Vet Parasitol.* 2007;146:363-366.

111. Borah MK, Rahman T, Goswami S, et al. On the incidence and pathology of *Paratanaisia bragai* dos Santos, 1934 (Freitas, 1959) infection in domestic pigeon *(Columba livia). J Vet Parasitol.* 2009;23:159-161.

112. Sahara A, Prastowo J, PriyoWidodo D, et al. Identifikasi cacing trematoda dan gambaran patologi ginjal burung merpati yang terinfeksi (Identification and pathological features of trematodes in pigeon's kidney). *Jurnal Veteriner.* 2013;14.

113. Brener B, Tortelly R, Menezes RC, et al. Prevalence and pathology of the nematode *Heterakis gallinarum*, the trematode *Paratanaisia bragai*, and the protozoan *Histomonas meleagridis* in the turkey, *Meleagris gallopavo. Mem Inst Oswaldo Cruz.* 2006;101:677-681.

114. Abdo W, Sultan K. Histopathological findings of the kidney *Trematoda paratanaisia* spp. (Digenea: Eucotylidae) in cattle egret *(Bubulcus ibis). Rev Bras Parasitol Vet.* 2013;22:312-313.

115. Arnizaut AB, Hayes L, Olsen GH, et al. An epizootic of *Tanaisia bragai* in a captive population of Puerto Rican plain pigeon *(Columba inornata wetmorei). Ann N Y Acad Sci.* 1992;653:202-205.

116. Santos V. Monostomose renal das aves domésticas. *Rev Dep Nac Prod Animal.* 1934;1:203-211.

117. Unwin S, Chantrey J, Chatterton J, et al. Renal trematode infection due to *Paratanaisia bragai* in zoo housed Columbiformes and a red bird-of-paradise *(Paradisaea rubra). Int J Parasitol Parasites Wildl* 2013;2:32-41.

118. Mahdy OA, Shaheed I. Histopathological study on the effect of *Renicola heroni* on the kidneys of giant heron Ardea goliath. *Helminthologia.* 2001;38:81-83.

119. Woodall P. *Cloacotaenia megalops* (Cestoda, Hymenolepididae) in the redbilled teal. *Ostrich.* 1977;48:1-4.

120. Green AJ, Georgiev BB, Brochet A-L, et al. Determinants of the prevalence of the cloacal cestode *Cloacotaenia megalops* in teal wintering in the French Camargue. *Eur J Wildl Res.* 2011;57:275-281.

121. Meyerholz DK, Vanloubbeeck YE, Hostetter SJ, et al. Surveillance of amyloidosis and other diseases at necropsy in captive trumpeter swans *(Cygnus buccinator). J Vet Diagn Invest.* 2005;17:295-298.

122. Huffman JE, Friedm B. Schistosomes. In: Atkinson CT, Thomas NJ, Hunter DB, eds. *Parasitic Diseases of Wild Birds.* Ames, IA: Wiley-Blackwell; 2008:246-261.

123. Franson JC, Derksen DV. Renal coccidiosis in oldsquaws *(Clangula hyemalis)* from Alaska. *J Wildl Dis.* 1981;17:237-239.

124. Wobeser G. Renal coccidiosis in mallard and pintail ducks. *J Wildl Dis.* 1974;10:249-255.

125. Skírnisson K. Mortality associated with renal and intestinal coccidiosis in juvenile eiders in Iceland. *Parasitologia.* 1997;39:325-330.

126. Sercy O, Nie K, Pascalon A, et al. Receptivity and susceptibility of the domestic duck *(Anas platyrhynchos)*, the Muscovy duck *(Cairina moschata)*, and their hybrid, the mule duck, to an experimental infection by *Eimeria mulardi. Avian Dis.* 1996;40:23-27.

127. Oksanen A. Mortality associated with renal coccidiosis in juvenile wild greylag geese *(Anser anser anser). J Wildl Dis.* 1994;30:554-556.

128. Gomis S, Didiuk AB, Neufeld J, et al. Renal coccidiosis and other parasitologic conditions in lesser snow goose goslings at Tha-anne River, west coast Hudson Bay. *J Wildl Dis.* 1996;32:498-504.

129. Tuggle BN, Crites JL. Renal coccidiosis in interior Canada geese, *Branta canadensis interior* Todd, of the Mississippi Valley population. *J Wildl Dis.* 1984;20:272-278.

130. Gajadhar AA, Leighton FA. *Eimeria wobeseri* sp. n. and *Eimeria goelandi* sp. n. (Protozoa: Apicomplexa) in the kidneys of herring gulls *(Larus argentatus). Journal of Wildlife Dis.* 1988;24:538-546.

131. Yabsley MJ, Gibbs SE. Description and phylogeny of a new species of *Eimeria* from double-crested cormorants *(Phalacrocorax auritus)* near Fort Gaines, Georgia. *J Parasitol.* 2006;92:385-388.

132. Yabsley MJ, Gottdenker NL, Fischer JR. Description of a new *Eimeria* sp. and associated lesions in the kidneys of double-crested cormorants *(Phalocrocorax auritus). J Parasitol.* 2002;88:1230-1233.

133. Montgomery RD, Novilla MN, Shillinger RB. Renal coccidiosis caused by *Eimeria gaviae* n. sp. in a common loon *(Gavia immer). Avian Dis.* 1978;22(4):809-814.

134. Leighton FA, Gajadhar AA. *Eimeria fraterculae* sp. n. in the kidneys of Atlantic puffins *(Fratercula arctica)* from Newfoundland, Canada: species description and lesions. *J Wildl Dis.* 1986;22:520-526.

135. Morgan KJ, Alley MR, Pomroy WE, et al. Extra-intestinal coccidiosis in the kiwi *(Apteryx* spp.). *Avian Pathol.* 2013;42:137-146.

136. Echols SM. Evaluating and treating the kidneys. In: Harrison GJ, Lightfoot TL, eds. *Clinical Avian Medicine.* Palm Beach, FL: Spix Publishing, Inc.; 2006:451-492.

137. Johne R, Muller H. Polyomaviruses of birds: etiologic agents of inflammatory diseases in a tumor virus family. *J Virol.* 2007;81:11554-11559.

138. Lafferty SL, Fudge AM, Schmidt RE, et al. Avian polyomavirus infection and disease in a green aracaris *(Pteroglossus viridis). Avian Dis.* 1999;43:577-585.

139. Tomasek O, Kubicek O, Tukac V. Unusual fatal avian polyomavirus infection in nestling cockatiels *(Nymphicus hollandicus)* detected by nested polymerase chain reaction. *Vet Med (Praha).* 2007;52:193.

140. Phalen DN. Papillomaviruses and polyomaviruses. In: Thomas NJ, Bruce Hunter D, Atkinson CT, eds. *Infectious Diseases of Wild Birds.* Ames, IA: John Wiley & Sons; 2008:206-215.

141. Ladds P. Viral diseases in birds. In: Ladds P, eds. *Pathology of Australian Native Wildlife.* Collingwood, Victoria (Australia): Csiro Publishing; 2009:29-52.

142. Alley MR, Rasiah I, Lee EA, et al. Avian polyomavirus identified in a nestling Gouldian finch *(Erythrura gouldiae)* in New Zealand. *NZ Vet J.* 2013;61:359-361.

143. Guerin JL, Gelfi J, Dubois L, et al. A novel polyomavirus (goose hemorrhagic polyomavirus) is the agent of hemorrhagic nephritis enteritis of geese. *J Virol.* 2000;74:4523-4529.

144. Cattoli G, Susta L, Terregino C, et al. Newcastle disease: a review of field recognition and current methods of laboratory detection. *J Vet Diagn Invest.* 2011;23:637-656.

145. Leighton FA, Heckert RA. Newcastle disease and related avian paramyxoviruses. In: Thomas NJ, Hunter DB, Atkinson CT, eds. *Infectious Diseases of Wild Birds.* Ames, IA: Blackwell Pub.; 2007:3-16.

146. Wakamatsu N, King DJ, Kapczynski DR, et al. Experimental pathogenesis for chickens, turkeys, and pigeons of exotic Newcastle disease virus from an outbreak in California during 2002-2003. *Vet Pathol.* 2006;43:925-933.

147. Kaleta EF, Baldauf C. Newcastle disease in free-living and pet birds. In: *Newcastle Disease.* Boston MA: Kluwer Academic Publishers; 1988:197-246.

148. Ritchie BW. *Avian Viruses: Function and Control.* Lake Worth, FL: Wingers Pub.; 1995.

149. Cox W. Avian pox infection in a Canada goose *(Branta canadensis). J Wildl Dis.* 1980;16:623-626.

150. Maeda M, Imada T, Taniguchi T, et al. Pathological changes in chicks inoculated with the picornavirus "avian nephritis virus." *Avian Dis.* 1979;23:589-596.

151. Styles DK, Phalen DN. Clinical avian urology. *Sem Avian Exot Pet Med.* 1998;7(2):104-113.

152. Brandão J, Beaufrère H. Clinical update and treatment of selected infectious gastrointestinal diseases in avian species. *J Exot Pet Med.* 2013;22:101-117.

153. Neumann U, Kummerfeld N. Neoplasms in budgerigars *(Melopsittacus undulatus)*: clinical, pathomorphological and serological findings with special consideration of kidney tumours. *Avian Pathol.* 1983;12:353-362.

154. Reece RL. Observations on naturally occurring neoplasms in birds in the state of Victoria, Australia. *Avian Pathol.* 1992;21:3-32.

155. Garner M. Overview of tumors, Section II: A retrospective study of case submissions to a specialty diagnostic service. In: Harrison GJ, Lightfoot TL, eds. *Clinical Avian Medicine.* Palm Beach, FL: Spix Publishing, Inc.; 2006:566-572.

156. Gould WJ, O'Connell PH, Shivaprasad HL, et al. Detection of retrovirus sequences in budgerigars with tumours. *Avian Pathol.* 1993;22:33-45.

157. Simova-Curd SA, Huder JB, Boeni J, et al. Investigations on the diagnosis and retroviral aetiology of renal neoplasia in budgerigars *(Melopsittacus undulatus). Avian Pathol.* 2010;39:161-167.

158. Sanchez C, Bush M, Montali R. Polycystic kidney disease associated with unilateral lameness in a northern pintail *(Anas acuta). J Avian Med Surg.* 2004;18:257-262.

159. Latimer KS, Ritchie BW, Campagnoli RP, et al. Metastatic renal carcinoma in an African grey parrot *(Psittacus erithacus erithacus). J Vet Diagn Invest.* 1996;8:261-264.

160. Rosen LB. Avian reproductive disorders. *J Exot Pet Med.* 2012;21:124-131.

161. Leach S, Heatley JJ, Pool RR Jr, et al. Bilateral testicular germ cell-sex cord-stromal tumor in a pekin duck *(Anas platyrhynchos domesticus).* *J Avian Med Surg.* 2008;22:315-319.

162. Sonnenfield JM, Carpenter JW, Garner MM, et al. Pheochromocytoma in a Nicobar pigeon *(Caloenas nicobarica).* *J Avian Med Surg.* 2002;16:306-308.

163. Campbell JG. *Tumours of the Fowl.* London, UK: William Heinemann Medical Books Ltd.; 1969.

164. Hahn KA, Jones MP, Petersen MG, et al. Metastatic pheochromocytoma in a parakeet. *Avian Dis.* 1997;41:751-754.

165. Filippich LJ. Tumor control in birds. *Semin Avian Exotic Pet Med.* 2004;13:25-43.

166. Macwhirter P, Pyke D, Wayne J. Use of carboplatin in the treatment of a renal adenocarcinoma in a budgerigar. *Exotic DVM.* 2002;4: 11-12.

167. Steinohrt LA. Avian fluid therapy. *J Avian Med Surg.* 1999;83-91.

168. DiBartola SP. Disorders of sodium and water: hypernatremia and hyponatremia. In: DiBartola SP, ed. *Fluid, Electrolyte, and Acid-Base Disorders in Small Animal Practice.* St. Louis, MO: Saunders/Elsevier; 2012:45-79.

169. Bartholomew GA, Cade TJ. The water economy of land birds. *Auk.* 1963;80:504-539.

170. Goldstein DL, Braun EJ. Contributions of the kidneys and intestines to water conservation, and plasma levels of antidiuretic hormone, during dehydration in house sparrows *(Passer domesticus).* *J Comp Physiol [B].* 1988;158:353-361.

171. Machado C, Mihm F, Buckley D, et al. Disintegration of kidney stones by extracorporeal shockwave lithotripsy in a penguin. *Proc First Inter Conf Zool Avian Med Oahu (Hawaii).* 1987;1987: 343-349.

172. Dennis PM, Bennett RA. Ureterotomy for removal of two ureteroliths in a parrot. *J Am Vet Med Assoc.* 2000;217:844-865, 865-868.

173. Gonçalves GAM, Salgado BS. Post-mortem lesions of urolithiasis in a lesser seed finch *(Sporophila angolensis).* *Acta Veterinaria Brasilica.* 2012;6:52-55.

174. Hicham S, Fettah A, Lounas A. Descriptive study of an outbreak of avian urolithiasis in a large commercial egg complex in Algeria. *Notulae Scientia Biologicae.* 2011;3:22-25.

175. Herbert JD, Coulson JO, Coulson TD. Quantification of tissue uric acid levels in a Harris's hawk with visceral gout. *Avian Dis.* 2011;55: 513-515.

176. Carro MD, Falkenstein E, Radke WJ, et al. Effects of allopurinol on uric acid concentrations, xanthine oxidoreductase activity and oxidative stress in broiler chickens. *Comp Biochem Physiol C Toxicol Pharmacol.* 2010;151:12-17.

177. Lumeij J, Sprang E, Redig P. Further studies on allopurinol-induced hyperuricaemia and visceral gout in red-tailed hawks *(Buteo jamaicensis).* *Avian Pathol.* 1998;27:390-393.

178. Dallwig R. Allopurinol. *J Exot Pet Med.* 2010;19:255-257.

179. Czarnecki CM, Olivero DK, McVey AS. Plasma uric acid levels in ethanol-fed turkey poults treated with allopurinol. *Comp Biochem Physiol C.* 1987;86:63-65.

180. Settle T, Carro M, Falkenstein E, et al. The effects of allopurinol, uric acid, and inosine administration on xanthine oxidoreductase activity and uric acid concentrations in broilers. *Poult Sci.* 2012;91:2895-2903.

181. Poffers J, Lumeij J, Timmermans-Sprang E, et al. Further studies on the use of allopurinol to reduce plasma uric acid concentrations in the red-tailed hawk *(Buteo jamaicensis)* hyperuricaemic model. *Avian Pathol.* 2002;31:567-572.

182. Poffers J, Lumeij J, Redig P. Investigations into the uricolytic properties of urate oxidase in a granivorous *(Columba livia domestica)* and in a carnivorous *(Buteo jamaicensis)* avian species. *Avian Pathol.* 2002;31:573-579.

183. Snoeyenbos G, Reynolds I, Tzianabos T. Articular gout in turkeys: a case report. *Avian Dis.* 1962;6:32-36.

184. Guzman D. Renal disease. In: Mayer J, Donnelly TM, eds. *Clinical Veterinary Advisor, Birds and Exotic Pets, 1: Clinical Veterinary Advisor.* Philadelphia: Elsevier Health Sciences; 2013:228-229.

185. Georgiades CS, Neyman EG, Barish MA, et al. Amyloidosis: review and CT manifestations. *Radiographics.* 2004;24:405-416.

186. Merlini G, Bellotti V. Molecular mechanisms of amyloidosis. *N Engl J Med.* 2003;349:583-596.

187. Chiti F, Dobson CM. Protein misfolding, functional amyloid, and human disease. *Annu Rev Biochem.* 2006;75:333-366.

188. Obici L, Perfetti V, Palladini G, et al. Clinical aspects of systemic amyloid diseases. *Biochim Biophys Acta.* 2005;1753:11-22.

189. Tanaka S, Dan C, Kawano H, et al. Pathological study on amyloidosis in *Cygnus olor* (mute swan) and other waterfowl. *Med Mol Morphol.* 2008;41:99-108.

190. Sato A, Koga T, Inoue M, et al. Pathological observations of amyloidosis in swans and other Anatidae. *Nihon Juigaku Zasshi.* 1981;43:509-519.

191. Cowan DF. Avian amyloidosis. I. General incidence in zoo birds. *Pathol Vet.* 1968;5:51-58.

192. Cowan DF. Avian amyloidosis. II. Incidence and contributing factors in the family Anatidae. *Pathol Vet.* 1968;5:59-66.

193. Karstad L, Sileo L. Causes of death in captive wild waterfowl in the Kortright Waterfowl Park, 1967-1970. *Wildl Dis.* 1971;7:236-241.

194. Landman WJ, Gruys E, Gielkens AL. Avian amyloidosis. *Avian Pathol.* 1998;27:437-449.

195. Schneider RR, Hunter DB, Waltner-Toews D, et al. A descriptive study of mortality at the Kortright Waterfowl Park: 1982-1986. *Can Vet J.* 1988;29:911-914.

196. Carpenter JW, Andrews GA, Beyer NW. Zinc Toxicosis in a free-flying trumpeter swan *(Cygnus buccinator).* *J Wildl Dis.* 2004;40:769-774.

197. Stepanets V, Vernerova Z, Vilhelmova M, et al. Amyloid A amyloidosis in non-infected and avian leukosis virus-C persistently infected inbred ducks. *Avian Pathol.* 2001;30:33-42.

198. Blagburn BL, Lindsay DS, Hoerr FJ, et al. *Cryptosporidium* sp. infection in the proventriculus of an Australian diamond firetail finch *(Staganoplura bella:* Passeriformes, Estrildidae). *Avian Dis.* 1990;34: 1027-1030.

199. Nakamura K, Tanaka H, Kodama Y, et al. Systemic amyloidosis in laying Japanese quail. *Avian Dis.* 1998;42:209-214.

200. Brayton C. Amyloidosis, hemochromatosis, and atherosclerosis in a roseate flamingo *(Phoenicopterus ruber).* *Ann NY Acad Sci.* 1992;653: 184-190.

201. Sato Y, Aoyagi T, Matsuura S, et al. An occurrence of avian tuberculosis in hooded merganser *(Lophodytes cucullatus).* *Avian Dis.* 1996; 40(4):941-944.

202. Kapakin KAT, Gursan N, Kutsal O. Generalized amyloidosis in a partridge *(Alectoris chukar).* *J Fac Vet Med, Univ Kafkas, Kars (Turkey).* 2010;16:143-146.

203. Beyer WN, Spann JW, Sileo L, et al. Lead poisoning in six captive avian species. *Arch Environ Contam Toxicol.* 1988;17:121-130.

204. Pascucci S, Maestrini N, Govoni S, et al. *Mycoplasma synoviae* in the guinea-fowl. *Avian Pathol.* 1976;5:291-297.

205. Cassone LM, Phalen DN. Avian pathology challenge. *J Avian Med Surg.* 2002;16(1):65-68.

206. Mayahi M, Esmaeilzadeh S, Mosavari N. Histopathological study of avian tuberculosis in naturally infected domestic pigeons with *Mycobacterium avium* subsp. avium. *Iranian J Vet Sci Technol.* 2013;5: 45-56.

207. Hampel MR, Kinne J, Wernery U, et al. Increasing fatal AA amyloidosis in hunting falcons and how to identify the risk: a report from the United Arab Emirates. *Amyloid.* 2009;16:122-132.

208. Forbes NA, Cooper JE. Fatty liver-kidney syndrome of merlins. In: Redig PT, Cooper JE, Remple D, et al., eds. *Raptor Biomedicine.* Minneapolis, MN: University of Minnesota Press; 1993:45-48.

209. Wadsworth P, Jones D, Pugsley S. Fatty liver in birds at the zoological society of London. *Avian Pathol.* 1984;13:231-239.
210. Siller WG. Renal pathology of the fowl—a review. *Avian Pathol.* 1981;10:187-262.
211. Marthedal H, Vellinge G. Lever-og nyrelidelse hos Kyllinger. *Nordisk Veterinärmötet, Helsinki.* 1958;8:250-255.
212. Cooper J, Forbes N. A fatty liver-kidney syndrome of merlins. *Vet Rec.* 1983;112:182-183.
213. Nicholls P, Bailey T, Samour J. Fatty liver syndrome in captive bustards: clinical, pathological and epidemiological findings. *Avian Pathol.* 1997;26:19-31.
214. Davies RR. Avian liver disease: etiology and pathogenesis. *Semin Avian Exotic Pet Med.* 2000;9(3):115-125.
215. Van Alstine W, Trampel D. Polycystic kidneys in a pigeon. *Avian Dis.* 1984;28(3):758-764.
216. Lightfoot TL, Yeager JM. Pet bird toxicity and related environmental concerns. *Vet Clin North Am Exot Anim Pract.* 2008;11:vi, 229-259.
217. Crespo R, Chin RP. Effect of feeding green onions (*Allium ascalonicum*) to white Chinese geese (*Threskiornis spinicollis*). *J Vet Diagn Invest.* 2004;16:321-325.
218. Wade LL, Newman SJ. Hemoglobinuric nephrosis and hepatosplenic erythrophagocytosis in a dusky-headed conure (*Aratinga weddelli*) after ingestion of garlic (*Allium sativum*). *J Avian Med Surg.* 2004;18:155-161.
219. Gartrell BD, Roe WD. The Effects of Chocolate and Chocolate By-Product Consumption on Wild and Domestic Animals. In: Watson RR, Preedy VR, Zibadi S, eds. *Chocolate in Health and Nutrition.* London, UK: Humana Press; 2013:135-141.
220. Gartrell B, Reid C. Death by chocolate: a fatal problem for an inquisitive wild parrot. *N Z Vet J.* 2007;55:149-151.
221. Cole G, Murray M. Suspected chocolate toxicosis in an African Grey parrot (*Psittacus erithacus*). *Proc Ann Conf Assoc Avian Vet.* 2005;2005:339-340.
222. Sara MG. Treatment of chocolate toxicosis in a Mynah bird (a case report). Fourth Inter Vet Poult Congress, Tehran, Iran; 2014.
223. Kinde H. A fatal case of oak poisoning in a double-wattled cassowary (*Casuarius casuarius*). *Avian Dis.* 1988;32:849-851.
224. Ozcan K, Ozen H, Karaman M. Nitrosative tissue damage and apoptotic cell death in kidneys and livers of naturally ethylene glycol (antifreeze)-poisoned geese. *Avian Pathol.* 2007;36:325-329.
225. Orosz SE. Clinical avian nutrition. *Vet Clin North Am Exot Anim Pract.* 2014;17:397-413.
226. Koutsos EA, Matson KD, Klasing KC. Nutrition of birds in the order Psittaciformes: a review. *J Avian Med Surg.* 2001;15:257-275.
227. de Matos R. Calcium metabolism in birds. *Vet Clin North Am Exot Anim Pract.* 2008;11:vi, 59-82.
228. Swenson J, Bradley GA. Suspected cholecalciferol rodenticide toxicosis in avian species at a zoological institution. *J Avian Med Surg.* 2013;27:136-147.
229. Eason CT, Wickstrom M, Henderson R, et al. Non-target and secondary poisoning risk associated with cholecalciferol. *NZ Plant Protection.* 2000;53:299-304.
230. Huff W, Kubena L, Harvey R, et al. Mycotoxin interactions in poultry and swine. *J Anim Sci.* 1988;66:2351-2355.
231. Peraica M, Radic B, Lucic A, et al. Toxic effects of mycotoxins in humans. *Bull World Health Organ.* 1999;77:754-766.
232. Glahn RP. Mycotoxins and the avian kidney: assessment of physiological function. *World's Poultry Science J.* 1993;49:242-250.
233. Singh VK, Meena M, Zehra A, et al. Fungal Toxins and Their Impact on Living Systems. In: Kharwar RN, Upadhyay RS, Dubey NK, Raghuwanshi R, eds. *Microbial Diversity and Biotechnology in Food Security.* New Delhi: Springer; 2014:513-530.
234. Oberheu DT, Dabbert CB. Exposure of game birds to ochratoxin A through supplemental feeds. *J Zoo Wildl Med.* 2001;32:136-138.
235. Dhanasekaran D, Shanmugapriya S, Thajuddin N. Aflatoxins and aflatoxicosis in human and animals. In: Guevara-González RG, ed. *Aflatoxins—Biochemistry and Molecular Biology Croatia.* Croatia: InTech; 2011:221-254.
236. Oberheu DG, Dabbert CB. Aflatoxin production in supplemental feeders provided for northern bobwhite in Texas and Oklahoma. *J Wildl Dis.* 2001;37:475-480.
237. Henke SE, Gallardo VC, Martinez B, et al. Survey of aflatoxin concentrations in wild bird seed purchased in Texas. *J Wildl Dis.* 2001;37:831-835.
238. Boermans HJ, Leung MC. Mycotoxins and the pet food industry: toxicological evidence and risk assessment. *Int J Food Microbiol.* 2007;119:95-102.
239. Scudamore K, Hetmanski M, Nawaz S, et al. Determination of mycotoxins in pet foods sold for domestic pets and wild birds using linked-column immunoassay clean-up and HPLC. *Food Addit Contam.* 1997;14:175-186.
240. Redig PT, Arent LR. Raptor toxicology. *Vet Clin North Am Exot Anim Pract.* 2008;11:261-282, vi.
241. Degernes LA. Waterfowl toxicology: a review. *Vet Clin North Am Exot Anim Pract.* 2008;11:283-300, vi.
242. Scheuhammer A. The chronic toxicity of aluminium, cadmium, mercury, and lead in birds: a review. *Environ Pollut.* 1987;46:263-295.
243. Wolfe MF, Schwarzbach S, Sulaiman RA. Effects of mercury on wildlife: a comprehensive review. *Environ Toxicol Chem.* 1998;17:146-160.
244. Dorrestein Gv, Van Gogh H, Rinzema J. Pharmacokinetic aspects of penicillins, aminoglycosides and chloramphenicol in birds compared to mammals. A review. *Vet Q.* 1984;6:216-224.
245. Goetting V, Lee KA, Tell LA. Pharmacokinetics of veterinary drugs in laying hens and residues in eggs: a review of the literature. *J Vet Pharmacol Ther.* 2011;34:521-556.
246. Schroeder EC, Frazier DL, Morris PJ, et al. Pharmacokinetics of ticarcillin and amikacin in blue-fronted Amazon parrots (*Amazona aestiva aestiva*). *J Avian Med Surg.* 1997;260-267.
247. Ramsay EC, Vulliet R. Pharmacokinetic properties of gentamicin and amikacin in the cockatiel. *Avian Dis.* 1993;37(2):628-634.
248. El-Gammal AA, Ravist WR, Krista LM, et al. Pharmacokinetics and intramuscular bioavailability of amikacin in chickens following single and multiple dosing. *J Vet Pharmacol Ther.* 1992;15:133-142.
249. Bird JE, Miller KW, Larson AA, et al. Pharmacokinetics of gentamicin in birds of prey. *Am J Vet Res.* 1983;44:1245-1247.
250. Dinev TG. Comparison of the pharmacokinetics of five aminoglycoside and aminocyclitol antibiotics using allometric analysis in mammal and bird species. *Res Vet Sci.* 2008;84:107-118.
251. Itoh N, Okada H. Pharmacokinetics and potential use of gentamicin in budgerigars (*Melopsittacus undulatus*). *Zentralbl Veterinarmed A.* 1993;40:194-199.
252. Pedersoli WM, Ravis WR, Askins DR, et al. Pharmacokinetics of single doses of gentamicin given intravenously and intramuscularly to turkeys. *J Vet Pharmacol Ther.* 1989;12:124-132.
253. Pedersoli WM, Ravis WR, Askins DR, et al. Pharmacokinetics of single-dose intravenous or intramuscular administration of gentamicin in roosters. *Am J Vet Res.* 1990;51:286-289.
254. Dimitrova D, Lashev L, Nikiforov I. Pharmacokinetics of tobramycin following intravenous and intramuscular administration in homing pigeons (*Columba livia*). *Folia Medica A.* 1998;2:32-33.
255. Bloomfield RB, Brooks D, Vulliet R. The pharmacokinetics of a single intramuscular dose of amikacin in red-tailed hawks (*Buteo jamaicensis*). *J Zoo Wildl Med.* 1997;55-61.
256. Lashev L, Mihailov R. Pharmacokinetics of apramycin in Japanese quails. *J Vet Pharmacol Ther.* 1994;17:394-395.
257. Haritova A, Djeneva H, Lashev L, et al. Pharmacokinetics of gentamicin and apramycin in turkeys roosters and hens in the context

of pharmacokinetic–pharmacodynamic relationships. *J Vet Pharmacol Ther*. 2004;27:381-384.

258. Hawkins MG, Paul-Murphy J. Avian analgesia. *Vet Clin North Am Exot Anim Pract*. 2011;14:61-80.

259. Green RE, Newton I, Shultz S, et al. Diclofenac poisoning as a cause of vulture population declines across the Indian subcontinent. *J Appl Ecol*. 2004;41:793-800.

260. Watson RT, Gilbert M, Oaks JL, et al. The collapse of vulture populations in South Asia. *Biodivers*. 2004;5:3-7.

261. Oaks JL, Meteyer CU, Rideout BA, et al. *Diagnostic investigation of vulture mortality: the anti-inflammatory drug diclofenac is associated with visceral gout. Raptors worldwide World Working Group on Birds of Prey and Owls, Berlin, Germany*. Blaine, WA: Hancock House Publishers; 2004:241-243.

262. Cuthbert RJ, Taggart MA, Prakash V, et al. Avian scavengers and the threat from veterinary pharmaceuticals. *Philos Trans R Soc Lond B*. 2014;369:20130574.

263. Swan GE, Cuthbert R, Quevedo M, et al. Toxicity of diclofenac to *Gyps* vultures. *Biol Lett*. 2006;2:279-282.

264. Green RE, Taggart MA, Das D, et al. Collapse of Asian vulture populations: risk of mortality from residues of the veterinary drug diclofenac in carcasses of treated cattle. *J Appl Ecol*. 2006;43:949-956.

265. Gilbert M, Watson RT, Ahmed S, et al. Vulture restaurants and their role in reducing diclofenac exposure in Asian vultures. *Bird Conserv Int*. 2007;17:63-77.

266. Prakash V. Status of vultures in Keoladeo National Park, Bharatpur, Rajasthan, with special reference to population crash in *Gyps* species. *J Bombay Nat Hist Soc*. 1999;96:365-378.

267. Prakash V, Bishwakarma MC, Chaudhary A, et al. The population decline of *Gyps* vultures in India and Nepal has slowed since veterinary use of diclofenac was banned. *PLoS ONE*. 2012;7:e49118.

268. Oaks JL, Gilbert M, Virani MZ, et al. Diclofenac residues as the cause of vulture population decline in Pakistan. *Nature*. 2004;427:630-633.

269. Sharma P. Aceclofenac as a potential threat to critically endangered vultures in India: a review. *J Rapt Res*. 2012;46:314-318.

270. Naidoo V, Swan GE. Diclofenac toxicity in *Gyps* vulture is associated with decreased uric acid excretion and not renal portal vasoconstriction. *Comp Biochem Physiol C Toxicol Pharmacol*. 2009;149:269-274.

271. Cuthbert R, Taggart MA, Prakash V, et al. Effectiveness of action in India to reduce exposure of *Gyps* vultures to the toxic veterinary drug diclofenac. *PLoS ONE*. 2011;6:e19069.

272. Chaudhry MJI, Ogada DL, Malik RN, et al. First evidence that populations of the critically endangered long-billed vulture *Gyps indicus* in Pakistan have increased following the ban of the toxic veterinary drug diclofenac in South Asia. *Bird Conserv Int*. 2012;22:389-397.

273. Mahapatro G, Arunkumar K. The case for banning diclofenac and the vanishing vultures. *Biodivers*. 2014;15:265-268.

274. Cuthbert RJ, Dave R, Chakraborty SS, et al. Assessing the ongoing threat from veterinary non-steroidal anti-inflammatory drugs to critically endangered *Gyps* vultures in India. *Oryx*. 2011;45:420-426.

275. Galligan TH, Amano T, Prakash VM, et al. Have population declines in Egyptian vulture and red-headed vulture in India slowed since the 2006 ban on veterinary diclofenac? *Bird Conserv Int*. 2014;24:1-10.

276. Cuthbert R, Green R, Ranade S, et al. Rapid population declines of Egyptian vulture *(Neophron percnopterus)* and red-headed vulture *(Sarcogyps calvus)* in India. *Anim Conserv*. 2006;9:349-354.

277. Zorrilla I, Martinez R, Taggart MA, et al. Suspected flunixin poisoning of a wild Eurasian Griffon Vulture from Spain. *Conserv Biol*. 2014;29(2):587-592.

278. Dama M. The diclofenac ban is helping vulture conservation; what further pharmaceutical threats loom ahead? *Curr Sci*. 2014;107:564-565.

279. Naidoo V, Wolter K, Cromarty D, et al. Toxicity of non-steroidal anti-inflammatory drugs to *Gyps* vultures: a new threat from ketoprofen. *Biol Lett*. 2010;6:339-341.

280. Naidoo V, Venter L, Wolter K, et al. The toxicokinetics of ketoprofen in *Gyps coprotheres*: toxicity due to zero-order metabolism. *Arch Toxicol*. 2010;84:761-766.

281. Cuthbert R, Parry-Jones J, Green RE, et al. NSAIDs and scavenging birds: potential impacts beyond Asia's critically endangered vultures. *Biol Lett*. 2007;3:91-94.

282. Pereira ME, Werther K. Evaluation of the renal effects of flunixin meglumine, ketoprofen and meloxicam in budgerigars *(Melopsittacus undulatus)*. *Vet Rec*. 2007;160:844-846.

283. Sharma AK, Saini M, Singh SD, et al. Diclofenac is toxic to the steppe eagle *Aquila nipalensis*: widening the diversity of raptors threatened by NSAID misuse in South Asia. *Bird Conserv Int*. 2014;24:282-286.

284. Acharya R, Cuthbert R, Baral HS, et al. Rapid decline of the bearded vulture *Gypaetus barbatus* in Upper Mustang, Nepal. *Forktail*. 2010;26:117-120.

285. Rattner BA, Whitehead MA, Gasper G, et al. Apparent tolerance of turkey vultures *(Cathartes aura)* to the non-steroidal anti-inflammatory drug diclofenac. *Envir Toxicol Chem*. 2008;27:2341-2345.

286. Naidoo V, Mompati KF, Duncan N, et al. The pied crow *(Corvus albus)* is insensitive to diclofenac at concentrations present in carrion. *J Wildl Dis*. 2011;47:936-944.

287. Naidoo V, Duncan N, Bekker L, et al. Validating the domestic fowl as a model to investigate the pathophysiology of diclofenac in *Gyps* vultures. *Env Toxicol Pharm*. 2007;24:260-266.

288. Swarup D, Patra R, Prakash V, et al. Safety of meloxicam to critically endangered *Gyps* vultures and other scavenging birds in India. *Anim Conserv*. 2007;10:192-198.

289. Naidoo V, Wolter K, Cromarty AD, et al. The pharmacokinetics of meloxicam in vultures. *J Vet Pharmacol Ther*. 2008;31:128-134.

290. Santos T, de Oliveira JB, Vaughan C, et al. Health of an ex situ population of raptors (Falconiformes and Strigiformes) in Mexico: diagnosis of internal parasites. *Rev Biol Trop*. 2011;59:1265-1274.

291. Baker DG, Morishita TY, Bartlett JL, et al. Coprologic survey of internal parasites of northern California raptors. *J Zoo Wildl Med*. 1996;27:358-363.

292. Ferrer D, Molina R, Adelantado C, et al. Helminths isolated from the digestive tract of diurnal raptors in Catalonia, Spain. *Vet Rec*. 2004;154:17-20.

293. Joseph V. Infectious and parasitic diseases of captive passerines. *Sem Avian Exot Pet Med*. 2003;12:21-28.

294. Helmboldt CF, Eckerlin RP, Penner LR, et al. The pathology of capillariasis in the blue jay. *J Wildl Dis*. 1971;7:157-161.

295. Miller AD, Townsend AK, McGowan KJ, et al. Non-West Nile virus-associated mortality in a population of American crows *(Corvus brachyrhynchos)*: a gross and histopathologic study. *J Vet Diagn Invest*. 2010;22:289-295.

296. Ford S. Raptor gastroenterology. *J Exot Pet Med*. 2010;19:140-150.

297. Howard LL, Papendick R, Stalis IH, et al. Fenbendazole and albendazole toxicity in pigeons andd. *J Avian Med Surg*. 2002;16:203-210.

298. Gozalo AS, Schwiebert RS, Lawson GW. Mortality associated with fenbendazole administration in pigeons *(Columba livia)*. *J Am Assoc Lab Anim Sci*. 2006;45:63-66.

299. Lewandowski AH, Campbell TW, Harrison GJ. Clinical chemistries. In: Harrison GJ, Harrison LR, eds. *Clinical Avian Medicine and Surgery*. Philadelphia: W.B. Saunders; 1986:192-200.

300. Weber MA, Terrell SP, Neiffer DL, et al. Bone marrow hypoplasia and intestinal crypt cell necrosis associated with fenbendazole

administration in five painted storks. *J Am Vet Med Assoc.* 2002;221:417-419, 369.

301. Acierno MJ, Mitchell MA, Freeman DM, et al. Determinination of plasma osmolality and agreement between measured and calculated values in healthy adult Hispaniolan Amazon parrots (*Amazona ventralis*). *Am J Vet Res.* 2009;70:1151-1154.

302. Beaufrère H, Acierno M, Mitchell M, et al. Plasma osmolality reference values in African Grey parrots (*Psittacus erithacus erithacus*), Hispaniolan Amazon parrots (*Amazona ventralis*), and red-fronted macaws (*Ara rubrogenys*). *J Avian Med Surg.* 2011;25:91-96.

303. Langston C. Managing fluid and electrolyte disorders in renal failure. *Vet Clin North Am Small Anim Pract.* 2008;38:xiii, 677-697.

304. Olanrewaju HA, Thaxton JP, Dozier WA 3rd, et al. Electrolyte diets, stress, and acid-base balance in broiler chickens. *Poult Sci.* 2007;86:1363-1371.

305. Verbalis JG. Diabetes insipidus. *Rev Endocr Metab Disord.* 2003;4: 177-185.

306. Starkey SR, Wood C, de Matos R, et al. Central diabetes insipidus in an African Grey parrot. *J Am Vet Med Assoc.* 2010;237:415-419.

307. Davis H, Jensen T, Johnson A, et al. 2013 AAHA/AAFP fluid therapy guidelines for dogs and cats. *J Am Anim Hosp Assoc.* 2013;49:149-159.

308. Rinaldi M, Brandao J, Nevarez J, et al. Hypernatremia in an umbrella cockatoo (*Cacatua alba*). *Exot Con 2015 Main Conf Proc.* 2015;2005:123.

309. Lamberski N, Daniel GB. Fluid dynamics of intraosseous fluid administration in birds. *J Zoo Wildl Med.* 1992;23(1):47-54.

310. Goudas P, Lusis P. Case report. Oxalate nephrosis in chinchilla (*Chinchilla laniger*). *Can Vet J.* 1970;11:256.

311. Jackson CN, Rogers AB, Maurer KJ, et al. Cystic renal disease in the domestic ferret. *Comp Med.* 2008;58:161.

312. Nelson W. Hydronephrosis in a ferret. *Vet Med Small Anim Clin.* 1984;79:516-521.

313. Hernandez-Divers SJ, Stahl SJ, Stedman NL, et al. Renal evaluation in the healthy green iguana (*Iguana iguana*): assessment of plasma biochemistry, glomerular filtration rate, and endoscopic biopsy. *J Zoo Wildl Med.* 2005;36:155-168.

314. Kolle P. Urinalysis in tortoises. *Proc Assoc Amphib Reptile Vet.* 2000; 2000:111-113.

315. Hernandez-Divers S, Hernandez-Divers S. Diagnostic imaging of reptiles. *In Pract.* 2001;23:370.

316. Donsbough A, Powell S, Waguespack A, et al. Uric acid, urea, and ammonia concentrations in serum and uric acid concentration in excreta as indicators of amino acid utilization in diets for broilers. *Poult Sci.* 2010;89:287-294.

317. Kolmstetter CM, Ramsay EC. Effects of feeding on plasma uric acid and urea concentrations in blackfooted penguins (*Spheniscus demersus*). *J Avian Med Surg.* 2000;14:177-179.

318. Harr KE. Clinical chemistry of companion avian species: a review. *Vet Clin Pathol.* 2002;31:140-151.

319. Capitelli R, Crosta L. Overview of psittacine blood analysis and comparative retrospective study of clinical diagnosis, hematology and blood chemistry in selected psittacine species. *Vet Clin North Am Exot Anim Pract.* 2013;16:71-120.

320. Wimsatt J, Canon N, Pearce RD, et al. Assessment of novel avian renal disease markers for the detection of experimental nephrotoxicosis in pigeons (*Columba livia*). *J Zoo Wildl Med.* 2009;40:487-494.

321. Stoev SD, Daskalov H, Radic B, et al. Spontaneous mycotoxic nephropathy in Bulgarian chickens with unclarified mycotoxin aetiology. *Vet Res.* 2002;33:83-93.

322. Radin M, Swayne D, Gigliotti A, et al. Renal function and organic anion and cation transport during dehydration and/or food restriction in chickens. *J Comp Physiol [B].* 1996;166:138-143.

323. Pegram RA, Wyatt R. Avian gout caused by oosporein, a mycotoxin produced by *Chaetomium trilaterale*. *Poult Sci.* 1981;60:2429-2440.

324. Pegram R, Wyatt R, Smith T. Oosporein-toxicosis in the turkey poult. *Avian Dis.* 1982;26(1):47-59.

325. Bird JE, Walser MM, Duke GE. Toxicity of gentamicin in red-tailed hawks. *Am J Vet Res.* 1983;44:1289-1293.

326. Lumeij JT, Remple JD. Plasma urea, creatinine and uric acid concentrations in relation to feeding in peregrine falcons (*Falco peregrinus*). *Avian Pathol.* 1991;20:79-83.

327. Lumeij JT. Pathophysiology, diagnosis and treatment of renal disorders in birds of prey. In: Lumeij JT, Remple JD, Redig PT, et al., eds. *Raptor Biomedicine III.* Lake Worth, FL: Zoological Education Network, Inc.; 2000:169-178.

328. Koutsos EA, Smith J, Woods LW, et al. Adult cockatiels (*Nymphicus hollandicus*) metabolically adapt to high protein diets. *J Nutr.* 2001;131:2014-2020.

329. Muriel R, Schmidt D, Calabuig CP, et al. Factors affecting plasma biochemistry parameters and physical condition of osprey (*Pandion haliaetus*) nestlings. *J Ornithol.* 2013;154:619-632.

330. Casado E, Balbontin J, Ferrer M. Plasma chemistry in booted eagle (*Hieraaetus pennatus*) during breeding season. *Comp Biochem Physiol A Mol Integr Physiol.* 2002;131:233-241.

331. Chan FT, Lin PI, Chang GR, et al. Hematocrit and plasma chemistry values in adult collared scops owls (*Otus lettia*) and crested serpent eagles (*Spilornis cheela hoya*). *J Vet Med Sci.* 2012;74: 893-898.

332. Scholtz N, Halle I, Flachowsky G, et al. Serum chemistry reference values in adult Japanese quail (*Coturnix coturnix japonica*) including sex-related differences. *Poult Sci.* 2009;88:1186-1190.

333. Hanauska-Brown LA, Dufty AM Jr, Roloff GJ. Blood chemistry, cytology, and body condition in adult northern goshawks (*Accipiter gentilis*). *J Raptor Res.* 2003;37:299-306.

334. Scope A, Filip T, Gabler C, et al. The influence of stress from transport and handling on hematologic and clinical chemistry blood parameters of racing pigeons (*Columba livia domestica*). *Avian Dis.* 2002;46:224-229.

335. Halliday WG, Ross JG, Christie G, et al. Effect of transportation on blood metabolites in broilers. *Br Poult Sci.* 1977;18:657-659.

336. Bowles H, Lichtenberger M, Lennox A. Emergency and critical care of pet birds. *Vet Clin North Am Exot Anim Pract.* 2007;10: 345-394.

337. Lumeij J. Plasma urea, creatinine and uric acid concentrations in response to dehydration in racing pigeons (*Columba livia domestica*). *Avian Pathol.* 1987;16:377-382.

338. Levy A, Perelman B, Grevenbroek MV, et al. Effect of water restriction on renal function in ostriches (*Struthio camelus*). *Avian Pathol.* 1990;19:385-393.

339. Chandra M, Singh B, Soni GL, et al. Renal and biochemical changes produced in broilers by high-protein, high-calcium, urea-containing, and vitamin-A-deficient diets. *Avian Dis.* 1984;28:1-11.

340. Woods R, Jones H, Watts J, et al. Diseases of Antarctic seabirds. In: Kerry KR, Riddle MJ, eds. *Health of Antarctic Wildlife.* Berlin, London, New York: Springer; 2009:35-55.

341. Scope A, Schwendenwein I, Schauberger G. Plasma exogenous creatinine excretion for the assessment of renal function in avian medicine-pharmacokinetic modeling in racing pigeons (*Columba livia*). *J Avian Med Surg.* 2013;27:173-179.

342. Vanderhasselt R, Buijs S, Sprenger M, et al. Dehydration indicators for broiler chickens at slaughter. *Poult Sci.* 2013;92: 612-619.

343. Williams JB, Pacelli MM, Braun EJ. The effect of water deprivation on renal function in conscious unrestrained Gambel's quail (*Callipepla gambelii*). *Physiol Zool.* 1991;64(5):1200-1216.

344. Martin HD, Kollias GV. Evaluation of water deprivation and fluid therapy in pigeons. *J Zoo Wildl Med.* 1989;20:173-177.

345. Fair J, Whitaker S, Pearson B. Sources of variation in haematocrit in birds. *Ibis.* 2007;149:535-552.

346. Quezada T, Cuellar H, Jaramillo-Juarez F, et al. Effects of aflatoxin B₁ on the liver and kidney of broiler chickens during development. *Comp Biochem Physiol C Toxicol Pharmacol.* 2000;125:265-272.

347. Cray C, Tatum LM. Applications of protein electrophoresis in avian diagnostics. *J Avian Med Surg.* 1998;12(1):4-10.

348. Melillo A. Applications of serum protein electrophoresis in exotic pet medicine. *Vet Clin North Am Exot Anim Pract.* 2013;16:211-225.

349. Kummrow MS. Ratites or struthioniformes: Struthiones, rheae, cassuarii, apteryges (ostriches, rheas, emus, cassowaries, and kiwis), and tinamiformes (tinamous). In: Miller RE, Fowler ME, eds. *Fowler's Zoo and Wild Animal Medicine.* St. Louis, MO: Elsevier/Saunders; 2015:75-82.

350. Duke GE, Degen AA, Reynhout JK. Movement of urine in the lower colon and cloaca of ostriches. *Condor.* 1995;97(1):165-173.

351. Skadhauge E, Erlwanger K, Ruziwa S, et al. Does the ostrich *(Struthio camelus)* coprodeum have the electrophysiological properties and microstructure of other birds? *Comp Biochem Physiol A Mol Integr Physiol.* 2003;134:749-755.

352. Skadhauge E, Warui CN, Kamau JM, et al. Function of the lower intestine and osmoregulation in the ostrich: preliminary anatomical and physiological observations. *Q J Exp Physiol.* 1984;69:809-818.

353. Yang Y, Jiang Y. Anatomy and histology of cloaca in African ostrich *(Struthio camelus).* *Remote Sens Env Transport Eng.* 2011;2011:8058-8060.

354. Warui C, Erlwanger K, Skadhauge E. Gross anatomical and histomorphological observations on the terminal rectum and the cloaca in the ostrich *Struthio camelus.* *Ostrich.* 2009;80:185-191.

355. Fowler ME. Comparative clinical anatomy of ratites. *J Zoo Wildl Med.* 1991;22(2):204-227.

356. Halsema WB, Alberts H, de Bruijne JJ, et al. Collection and analysis of urine from racing pigeons *(Columba livia domestica).* *Avian Pathol.* 1988;17:221-225.

357. Heatley JJ, Villalobos A. Avian bornavirus in the urine of infected birds. *Vet Med.* 2012;3:19-23.

358. Goldstein DL, Braun EJ. Structure and concentrating ability in the avian kidney. *Am J Physiol Reg Int Comp Phys.* 1989;256:R501-R509.

359. Bolton W, Tucker F, Sturgill B. Experimental autoimmune glomerulonephritis in chickens. *J Clin Lab Immunol.* 1980;3:179-184.

360. Casotti G, Braun EJ. Renal anatomy in sparrows from different environments. *J Morphol.* 2000;243:283-291.

361. Goecke CS, Goldstein DL. Renal glomerular and tubular effects of antidiuretic hormone and two antidiuretic hormone analogues in house sparrows *(Passer domesticus).* *Physiol Zool.* 1997;70(3):283-291.

362. Roberts J. The effect of acute or chronic administration of prolactin on renal function in feral chickens. *J Comp Physiol [B].* 1998;168:25-31.

363. Forman MF, Wideman RF. Renal responses of normal and preascitic broilers to systemic hypotension induced by unilateral pulmonary artery occlusion. *Poult Sci.* 1999;78:1773-1785.

364. Jones KH, Turner B, Brandão J, et al. Pilot study: colostomy and urine collection protocol for investigating potential inciting causes of hen diuresis syndrome. *Avian Dis.* 2015;59(2):227-234.

365. Manangi MK, Clark FD, Coon CN. Improved colostomy technique and excrement (urine) collection device for broilers and broiler breeder hens. *Poult Sci.* 2007;86:698-704.

366. Belay T, Bartels KE, Wiernusz CJ, et al. A detailed colostomy procedure and its application to quantify water and nitrogen balance and urine contribution to thermobalance in broilers exposed to thermoneutral and heat-distressed environments. *Poult Sci.* 1993;72:106-115.

367. Forman M, Beck M, Kachman S. N-Acetyl-β-D-glucosaminidase as a marker of renal damage in hens. *Poult Sci.* 1996;75:1563-1568.

368. Tschopp R, Bailey T, Di Somma A, et al. Urinalysis as a noninvasive health screening procedure in Falconidae. *J Avian Med Surg.* 2007;21:8-12.

369. Kurtenkov A. Effect of different drinking regimes on water economy in domestic ostriches *(Struthio camelus domesticus)* at different ages. *Agricult Agricult Pract Sci J.* 2009;71(3–4):209.

370. Brock AP, Grunkemeyer VL, Fry MM, et al. Comparison of osmolality and refractometric readings of Hispaniolan Amazon parrot *(Amazona ventralis)* urine. *J Avian Med Surg.* 2013;27:264-268.

371. Vereecken M, De Herdt P, Vanrobaeys M, et al. Plasma biochemistry in pigeons experimentally infected with *Salmonella. Avian Dis.* 2001;45:467-472.

372. Layton HE, Davies JM, Casotti G, et al. Mathematical model of an avian urine concentrating mechanism. *Am J Physiol Renal Physiol.* 2000;279:F1139-F1160.

373. Calder W, Bentley P. Urine concentrations of two carnivorous birds, the white pelican and the roadrunner. *Comp Biochem Physiol.* 1967;22:607-609.

374. Janes DN. Osmoregulation by Adelie penguin chicks on the Antarctic peninsula. *Auk.* 1997;114(3):488-495.

375. Lyons ME, Goldstein DL, Karasov W. Osmoregulation by nestling and adult American kestrels *(Falco sparverius).* *Auk.* 2002;119:426-436.

376. Jones JS, Thomas JS, Bahr A, et al. Presumed immune-mediated hemolytic anemia in a blue-crowned conure *(Aratinga acuticaudata).* *J Avian Med Surg.* 2002;16:223-229.

377. Johnston MS, Son TT, Rosenthal KL. Immune-mediated hemolytic anemia in an eclectus parrot. *J Am Vet Med Assoc.* 2007;230:1028-1031.

378. Hanley CS, Thomas NJ, Paul-Murphy J, et al. Exertional myopathy in whooping cranes *(Grus americana)* with prognostic guidelines. *J Zoo Wildl Med.* 2005;36:489-497.

379. Tully TN Jr, Hodgin C, Morris JM, et al. Exertional myopathy in an emu *(Dromaius novaehollandiae).* *J Avian Med Surg.* 1996;96-100.

380. Candeletta SC, Homer BL, Garner MM, et al. Diabetes mellitus associated with chronic lymphocytic pancreatitis in an African grey parrot *(Psittacus erithacus erithacus).* *J Assoc Avian Vet.* 1993;7:39-43.

381. Wallner-Pendleton EA, Rogers D, Epple A. Diabetes mellitus in a red-tailed hawk *(Buteo jamaicensis).* *Avian Pathol.* 1993;22:631-635.

382. Pilny AA, Luong R. Diabetes mellitus in a chestnut-fronted macaw *(Ara severa).* *J Avian Med Surg.* 2005;19:297-302.

383. Desmarchelier M, Langlois I. Diabetes mellitus in a nanday conure *(Nandayus nenday).* *J Avian Med Surg.* 2008;22:246-254.

384. Harr KE. Diagnostic value of biochemistry. In: Harrison GJ, Lightfoot TL, eds. *Clinical Avian Medicine.* Palm Beach, FL: Spix Publishing, Inc.; 2006:611-629.

385. McMillan MC. Imaging of avian urogenital disorders. *AAV Today.* 1988;2(2):74-82.

386. Daniel GB, Mitchell SK, Mawby D, et al. Renal nuclear medicine: a review. *Vet Radiol Ultrasound.* 1999;40:572-587.

387. Freeman KP, Hahn KA, Jones MP, et al. Right leg muscle atrophy and osteopenia caused by renal adenocarcinoma in a cockatiel *(Melopsittacus undulatus).* *Vet Radiol Ultrasound.* 1999;40:144-147.

388. Sanchez-Migallon Guzman D. Renal disease. In: Mayer J, Donnelly T, eds. *Clinical Veterinary Advisor, Birds and Exotic Pets. 1. Clinical Veterinary Advisor.* Philadelphia, Pennsylvania: Elsevier Health Sciences; 2013:228-229.

389. Ngo TC, Assimos DG. Uric acid nephrolithiasis: recent progress and future directions. *Rev Urol.* 2007;9:17.

390. McNeel SV, Zenoble RD. Avian urography. *J Am Vet Med Assoc.* 1981;178:366-368.

391. Krautwald-Junghanns ME, Schloemer J, Pees M. Iodine-based contrast media in avian medicine. *J Exotic Pet Med.* 2008;17:189-197.

392. Forbes N. Avian radiology and endoscopy. *Vet Q*. 1998;20:S66-S67.

393. Rivers BJ, Johnston GR. Diagnostic imaging strategies in small animal nephrology. *Vet Clin North Am Small Anim Pract*. 1996;26:1505-1517.

394. Hofbauer H, Krautwald-Junghanns ME. Transcutaneous ultrasonography of the avian urogenital tract. *Vet Radiol Ultrasound*. 1999;40:58-64.

395. Simova-Curd S, Nitzl D, Mayer J, et al. Clinical approach to renal neoplasia in budgerigars *(Melopsittacus undulatus)*. *J Small Anim Pract*. 2006;47:504-511.

396. Bang-asan PE, Acorda JA. Ultrasonographic features of the kidneys in apparently healthy ostriches *(Struthio camelus)* raised in captivity. *Philippine J Vet Anim Sci*. 2013;39(2):259-268.

397. Canny C. Gross anatomy and imaging of the avian and reptilian urinary system. *Sem Avian Exotic Pet Med*. 1998;7(2):72-80.

398. Krautwald-Junghanns M-E, Pees M. Urogenital tract. In: Krautwald-Junghanns M-E, Pees M, Reese S, et al., eds. *Diagnostic Imaging of Exotic Pets: Birds, Small Mammals, Reptiles*. Hannover, Germany: Schlütersche Verlagsgesellschaft mbH & Co.; 2011:122-135.

399. Tyson R, Daniel GB. Renal scintigraphy in veterinary medicine. *Semin Nucl Med*. 2014;44:35-46.

400. Orosz SE, Toal RL. Tomographic anatomy of the golden eagle *(Aquila chrysaetos)*. *J Zoo Wildl Med*. 1992;23(1):39-46.

401. Mackey EB, Hernandez-Divers SJ, Holland M, et al. Clinical technique: application of computed tomography in zoological medicine. *J Exotic Pet Med*. 2008;17:198-209.

402. Petnehazy O, Benczik J, Takacs I, et al. Computed tomographical (CT) anatomy of the thoracoabdominal cavity of the male turkey *(Meleagris gallopavo)*. *Anat Histol Embryol*. 2012;41:12-20.

403. Kusmierczyk J, Wall CR, Hoppes S, et al. Comparison of computed tomographic images of birds obtained with sedation vs general anesthesia. *J Exotic Pet Med*. 2013;22:251-257.

404. Romagnano A, Shiroma JT, Heard DJ, et al. Magnetic resonance imaging of the brain and coelomic cavity of the domestic pigeon *(Columba livia domestica)*. *Vet Radiol Ultrasound*. 1996;37:431-440.

405. Grando AP. Utilização de tomografia por ressonância magnética nuclear para sexagem de aves silvestres sem dimorfismo sexual. Master's thesis. Universidade de São Paulo, 2002.

406. Grunkemeyer VL. Advanced diagnostic approaches and current management of avian hepatic disorders. *Vet Clin North Am Exot Anim Pract*. 2010;13:413-427.

407. Kerl ME, Cook CR. Glomerular filtration rate and renal scintigraphy. *Clin Tech Small Anim Pract*. 2005;20:31-38.

408. Radin MJ, Hoepf TM, Swayne DE. Use of a single injection solute-clearance method for determination of glomerular filtration rate and effective renal plasma flow in chickens. *Lab Anim Sci*. 1993;43:594-596.

409. Divers SJ. Avian diagnostic endoscopy. *Vet Clin North Am Exot Anim Pract*. 2010;13:187-202.

410. Müller K, Göbel T, Müller S, et al. Use of endoscopy and renal biopsy for the diagnosis of kidney disease in free-living birds of prey and owls. *Vet Rec*. 2004;155:326-329.

411. Murray MJ, Taylor M. Avian renal disease: endoscopic applications. *Sem Avian Exotic Pet Med*. 1999;8(3):115-121.

412. Pizzi R. Spiders. In: Lewbart GA, ed. *Invertebrate Medicine*. 2nd ed. Ames, IA: Wiley-Blackwell Publishing; 2012:187-221.

413. Gore SR, Harms CA, Kukanich B, et al. Enrofloxacin pharmacokinetics in the European cuttlefish, *Sepia officinalis*, after a single i.v. injection and bath administration. *J Vet Pharmacol Ther*. 2005;28:433-439.

414. Scimeca J. Cephalopods. In: Lewbart GA, ed. *Invertebrate Medicine*. 2nd ed. Ames, IA: Wiley-Blackwell Publishing; 2012:113-125.

415. Roberts HE, Palmeiro B, Weber ES 3rd. Bacterial and parasitic diseases of pet fish. *Vet Clin North Am Exot Anim Pract*. 2009;12:609-638, table of contents.

416. Nouws JF, Grondel JL, Schutte AR, et al. Pharmacokinetics of ciprofloxacin in carp, African catfish and rainbow trout. *Vet Q*. 1988;10:211-216.

417. Treves-Brown KM. *Applied Fish Pharmacology*. Dordrecht, Boston: Kluwer Academic Publishers; 2000.

418. Kim MS, Lim JH, Park BK, et al. Pharmacokinetics of enrofloxacin in Korean catfish *(Silurus asotus)*. *J Vet Pharmacol Ther*. 2006;29:397-402.

419. Stoskopf MK. Fish pharmacotherapeutics. In: Fowler ME, Miller RE, eds. *Zoo and Wild Animal Medicine Current Therapy 4*. 4th ed. Philadelphia: W.B. Saunders; 1999:182-189.

420. Wright KM, Whitaker BR. Pharmacotherapeutics. In: Wright KM, Whitaker BR, eds. *Amphibian Medicine and Captive Husbandry*. Malabar, FL: Krieger Publishing Company; 2001:309-330.

421. Letcher J, Papich M. Pharmacokinetics of intramuscular administration of three antibiotics in bullfrogs *(Rana catesbeiana)*. *Proc Am Assoc Zoo Vets*. 1994;1994:79-93.

422. Gibbons PM, Klaphake E, Carpenter JW. Reptiles. In: Carpenter JW, Marion CJ, eds. *Exotic Animal Formulary*. 4th ed. St. Louis, MO: Elsevier/Saunders; 2013:83-182.

423. Frye FL. *Reptile Care. An Atlas of Diseases and Treatments*. Neptune City, NJ: TFH Publications; 1991.

424. Funk RS. A formulary for lizards, snakes, and crocodilians. *Vet Clin North Am Exot Anim Pract*. 2000;3:viii, 333-358.

425. Stahl SJ. Pet lizard conditions and syndromes. *Sem Avian Exotic Pet Med*. 2003;12(3):162-182.

426. White SD, Bourdeau P, Bruet V, et al. Reptiles with dermatological lesions: a retrospective study of 301 cases at two university veterinary teaching hospitals (1992-2008). *Vet Dermatol*. 2011;22:150-161.

427. Marin P, Bayon A, Fernandez-Varon E, et al. Pharmacokinetics of danofloxacin after single dose intravenous, intramuscular and subcutaneous administration to loggerhead turtles *Caretta caretta*. *Dis Aquat Organ*. 2008;82:231-236.

428. Stein G. Reptile and amphibian formulary. In: Mader DR, ed. *Reptile Medicine and Surgery*. Philadelphia: W.B. Saunders; 1996:465-472.

429. Divers S. Clinician's approach to renal disease in lizards. *Proc Assoc Rep Amphib Vet*. 1997;1997:5-11.

430. Mautino M, Page CD. Biology and medicine of turtles and tortoises. *Vet Clin North Am Small Anim Pract*. 1993;23:1251-1270.

431. Raiti P. Veterinary care of the common kingsnake, *Lampropeltis getula*. *Bull Assoc Rept Amph Vet*. 1995;5:11-18.

432. Mader DR. Gout. In: Mader DR, ed. *Reptile Medicine and Surgery*. 1st ed. Philadelphia: W.B. Saunders; 1996:374-379.

433. Frye FL. *Reptile Clinician's Handbook: A Compact Clinical and Surgical Reference*. Malabar, FL: Krieger Publishing Company; 1994.

434. Bennett R. Management of common reptile emergencies. *Proc Assoc Reptil Amphib Vet Kansas City*. 1998;1998:67-72.

435. Funk RS, Diethelm G. Reptile formulary. In: Mader DR, ed. *Reptile Medicine and Surgery*. 2nd ed. St. Louis, MO: Saunders/Elsevier; 2006:1119-1139.

436. Boyer T. *Essentials of Reptiles: A Guide for Practitioners*. Lakewood, CO: American Animal Hospital Association; 1998:1-253.

437. Gauvin J. Drug therapy in reptiles. *Sem Avian Exotic Pet Med*. 1993;2:48-59.

438. Jenkins J. Medical management of reptile patients. In: *The Compendium on Continuing Education for the Practicing Veterinarian*. 1991;13:980-988.

439. Plumb DC. Probenecid. In: Plumb DC, ed. *Plumb's Veterinary Drug Handbook*. 6th ed. Ames, IA: Blackwell Publishing; 2008:1028-1030.

440. Perry SM, Mader DM. Clinical use of Epogen (Epoetin Alfa) in green sea turtles *(Chelonia mydas)* and loggerhead sea turtles *(Caretta caretta)*. Exotics Con. 2015;531.

441. Forbes NA. Birds of prey. In: Beynon PH, Cooper JE, eds. *BSAVA Manual of Exotic Pets*. Cheltenham, UK: British Small Animal Veterinary Association; 1991:212-220.

442. Phalen DN. Common bacterial and fungal infectious diseases in pet birds. *Comp Contin Ed Pract Vet*. 2003;25:43.

443. Flammer K. Treatment of bacterial and mycotic diseases of the avian gastrointestinal tract. *Proc North Am Vet Conf*. 2002;2002:851-852.

444. Rupley AE. Critical care of pet birds. Procedures, therapeutics, and patient support. *Vet Clin North Am Exot Anim Pract*. 1998;1:v, 11-41.

445. El-Gendi A, El-Banna H, Abo NM, et al. Disposition kinetics of danofloxacin and ciprofloxacin in broiler chickens. *Dtsch Tierarztl Wochenschr*. 2001;108:429-434.

446. Flammer K, Aucoin DP, Whitt DA. Intramuscular and oral disposition of enrofloxacin in African grey parrots following single and multiple doses. *J Vet Pharmacol Ther*. 1991;14:359-366.

447. Byrne RF, Davis C, Lister SA. Prescribing for birds. In: Bishop Y, ed. *The Veterinary Formulary*. 5th ed. London: Pharmaceutical Press; 2001:43-56.

448. Ritchie BW, Harrison GJ. Formulary. In: Ritchie BW, Harrison GJ, Harrison LR, eds. *Avian Medicine: Principles and Application*. Lake Worth, FL: Wingers Pub.; 1994:457-478.

449. Joyner K. Pediatric therapeutics. *Proc Annu Conf Assoc Avian Vet*. 1991;1991:188-189.

450. Tully TN Jr. Psittacine therapeutics. *Vet Clin North Am Exot Anim Pract*. 2000;3:vi, 59-90.

451. Krautwald-Junghanns M, Straub J. Avian cardiology: part 1. *Proc Annu Conf Assoc Avian Vet*. 2001;2001:330.

452. Johnson-Delaney CA. Therapeutics of companion exotic marsupials. *Vet Clin North Am Exot Anim Pract*. 2000;3:vii, 173-181.

453. Morrisey JK, Carpenter JW. Formulary. In: Quesenberry KE, Carpenter JW, eds. *Ferrets, Rabbits, and Rodents: Clinical Medicine and Surgery*. 2nd ed. St. Louis, MO: Saunders/Elsevier; 2004:436-444.

454. Isenbügel E, Baumgartner RA. Diseases of the hedgehog. In: Fowler ME, ed. *Zoo and Wild Animal Medicine: Current Therapy 3*. 3rd ed. Philadelphia: W.B. Saunders; 1993:294-302.

455. Smith AJ. General husbandry and medical care of hedgehogs. In: Bonagura JD, ed. *Kirk's Current Veterinary Therapy XIII: Small Animal Practice*. 13th ed. Philadelphia: W.B. Saunders; 2000:1128-1133.

456. Hillyer EV, Brown SA. Ferrets. In: Birchard SJ, Sherding RG, eds. *Saunders Manual of Small Animal Practice*. Philadelphia: W.B. Saunders; 1994:1317-1344.

457. Pye G, Carpenter J. Guide to medicine and surgery in sugar gliders. *Vet Med*. 1999;94:891-905.

458. Stocker L. *Medication for Use in the Treatment of Hedgehogs*. UK: The Wildlife Hospital Trust; 1992.

459. Brown SA. Ferret drug dosages. In: Antinoff N, Bauck L, Boyer TH, eds. *Exotic Formulary*. 2nd ed. Lakewood, CO: American Animal Hospital Association; 1999:43-61.

460. Johnson-Delaney CA. *Exotic Companion Medicine Handbook for Veterinarians*. Lake Worth, FL: Wingers Publishing; 1996.

461. Bistner SI, Ford RB, Kirk RW. *Kirk and Bistner's Handbook of Veterinary Procedures and Emergency Treatment*. 6th ed. Philadelphia: W.B. Saunders; 1995.

462. Nelson CL, McLaren SG, Skinner RA, et al. The treatment of experimental osteomyelitis by surgical debridement and the implantation of calcium sulfate tobramycin pellets. *J Orthop Res*. 2002;20:643-647.

463. Harkness JE. *A Practitioner's Guide to Domestic Rodents*. Lakewood, CO: American Animal Hospital Association; 1993.

464. Hillyer EV. Pet rabbits. *Vet Clin North Am Small Anim Pract*. 1994;24:25-65.

465. Collins BR. Antimicrobial drug use in rabbits, rodents, and other small mammals. In: Collins BR, Dorrestein G, Jacobson E, et al., eds. *Antimicrobial Therapy in Caged Birds and Exotic Pets*. Trenton, NJ: Veterinary Learning Systems; 1995:3-10.

466. Ness RD, Johnson-Delaney C. Sugar gliders. In: Quesenberry KE, Carpenter JW, eds. *Ferrets, Rabbits, and Rodents: Clinical Medicine and Surgery*. 3rd ed. St. Louis, MO: Saunders/Elsevier; 2012:393-410.

467. Smith A. Husbandry and medicine of African hedgehogs *(Atelerix albiventris)*. *Small Exp Anim Med*. 1992;2:21-28.

468. Hoefer HL. Clinical approach to the African hedgehog. *Proc North Am Vet Conf*. 1999;1999:836-838.

469. Carpenter JW, Mashima TY, Gentz EJ, et al. Caring for rabbits: an overview and formulary. *Vet Med*. 1995;April:340-364.

470. Adamcak A, Otten B. Rodent therapeutics. *Vet Clin North Am Exot Anim Pract*. 2000;3:viii, 221-237.

471. Bishop CR. Reproductive medicine of rabbits and rodents. *Vet Clin North Am Exot Anim Pract*. 2002;5:vi, 507-535.

472. Powers L. Subcutaneous implantable catheter for fluid administration in an African pygmy hedgehog. *Exotic DVM*. 2002;4:16-17.

473. Schweigart G. *Arzneimittelanwendung bei Nagetieren und Kaninchen Handbücher für die Heimtierpraxis*. 2nd ed. Berlin: Veterinärmedizinischer Fachverlag; 2009.

474. Brown SA. Rabbit urinary tract disease. *Proc North Am Vet Conf*. 1997;1997:785-787.

475. Ness R. Sugar glider *(Petaurus breviceps)*: general husbandry and medicine. *Proc of Assoc Avian Vet*. 2000;2000:99-107.

476. Brust DM. What every veterinarian needs to know about sugar gliders. *Exotic DVM*. 2009;11:32-41.

477. Lightfoot TL. Therapeutics of African pygmy hedgehogs and prairie dogs. *Vet Clin North Am Exot Anim Pract*. 2000;3:vii, 155-172.

478. Hoefer H. Common problems in guinea pigs. *Proc North Am Vet Conf*. 1999;1999:831-832.

479. Johnson-Delaney CA. Other small mammals. In: Meredith A, Redrobe S, eds. *BSAVA Manual of Exotic Pets*. 4th ed. Quedgeley, UK: British Small Animal Veterinary Association; 2002:102-115.

480. Harcourt-Brown F, Harcourt-Brown NH. *Textbook of Rabbit Medicine*. Oxford, UK: Butterworth-Heinemann; 2002.

481. Harrenstien L. Critical care of ferrets, rabbits, and rodents. *Semin Avian Exotic Pet Med*. 1994;3:217-228.

482. Antinoff N. Musculoskeletal and neurologic diseases. In: Quesenberry KE, Carpenter JW, eds. *Ferrets, Rabbits, and Rodents: Clinical Medicine and Surgery*. 2nd ed. St. Louis, MO: W.B. Saunders; 2004:115-120.

483. Allen DG, Pringle JK, Smith DA. *Handbook of Veterinary Drugs*. Philadelphia: Lippincott; 1993.

484. Jepson L. *Exotic Animal Medicine: A Quick Reference Guide*. Philadelphia, PA: Saunders/Elsevier Health Sciences; 2009.

485. Wixson SK. Anesthesia and analgesia. In: Manning PJ, Ringler DH, Newcomer CE, eds. *The Biology of the Laboratory Rabbit*. 2nd ed. San Diego: Academic Press; 1994.

486. Dombrowski D, De Voe R. Emergency care of invertebrates. *Vet Clin North Am Exot Anim Pract*. 2007;10:621-645.

487. Hadfield CA, Whitaker BR, Clayton LA. Emergency and critical care of fish. *Vet Clin North Am Exot Anim Pract*. 2007;10:647-675.

488. Kirchgessner M, Mitchell MA. Chelonians. In: Mitchell MA, Tully TN, eds. *Manual of Exotic Pet Practice*. St. Louis, MO: Saunders/Elsevier; 2009:207-249.

489. Macwhirter P. Passeriformes. In: Ritchie RW, Harrison GJ, Harrison LR, eds. *Avian Medicine: Principles and Application*. Lake Worth, FL: Wingers Pub.; 1994:1172-1199.

490. Lichtenberger M, Orcutt C, DeBehnke D. Mortality and response to fluid resuscitation after acute blood loss in mallard ducks. *Proc Assoc Avian Vet*. 2003;2003:7-10.

491. Harkness JE, Wagner JE. *The Biology and Medicine of Rabbits and Rodents*. 4th ed. Baltimore: Williams & Wilkins; 1995.

492. Stamper MA, Miller SM, Berzins IK. Pharmacology in elasmo-branchs. In: Smith M, War-molts D, Thoney D, eds. *The Elasmo-branch Husbandry Manual: Captive Care of Sharks, Rays and Their Relatives.* Columbus Zoo, Columbus (OH): Biological Survey; 2004: 447-466.

493. Lewbart GA. Emergency pet fish medicine. In: Bonagura JD, ed. *Kirk's Current Veterinary Therapy XII Small Animal Practice.* Phila-delphia: W.B. Saunders; 1995:1369-1374.

494. Crawshaw GJ. Amphibian emergency and critical care. *Vet Clin North Am Exot Anim Pract.* 1998;1:207-231, vii.

495. Jarchow JL. Hospital care of the reptile patient. In: Jacobson ER, Kollias GV, eds. *Exotic Animals.* New York: Churchill Livingstone; 1988:19-34.

496. Gibbons PM. Critical care nutrition and fluid therapy in reptiles. *Proc 15th Annu Intl Vet Emerg Crtit Care Symp.* 2009:91-94.

497. Mader DR, Rudloff E. Emergency and critical care. In: Mader DR, ed. *Reptile Medicine and Surgery.* 2nd ed. St. Louis, MO: Saunders/ Elsevier; 2006:533-548.

498. Lichtenberger M. Shock and cardiopulmonary-cerebral resuscita-tion in small mammals and birds. *Vet Clin North Am Exot Anim Pract.* 2007;10:275-291.

499. Chew DJ, DiBartola SP. *Manual of Small Animal Nephrology and Urology.* New York: Churchill Livingstone; 1986.

Index

Page numbers followed by "*f*" indicate figures and by "*t*" indicate tables.

long ascending and long descending
pathways of, 398*t*
metabolic bone disease (MBD) in, 359-360
miscellaneous fluids in, 536*t*
musculoskeletal diseases in
neoplastic, 366-367
nutritional, 362
musculoskeletal system of, 354
diagnostic imaging of, 355
myopathies in, 363-364, 364*f*
normal heart rates of, 195*t*
ocular diseases in, diagnostics and
treatment of, 446-448
osteomyelitis in, 373
physical examination of, 9, 13*f*
pituitary of, neoplasia in, 282
reproductive cycle of, 464
reproductive diseases in, 471-473, 472*f*
treatment of, 486-487
reproductive system of, 463-464, 463*f*
diagnostics for, 482-483
respiratory diseases in, 105-110
extrarespiratory diseases, 109-110
in lungs and air sacs, 107-109, 109*f*
nasal and sinusal diseases, 105-106
noninfectious lower, medical therapy for,
135
surgical therapy for, 135-138
tracheal diseases, 106-107
upper, medical therapy for, 134
respiratory mechanics and regulation in,
92-93
respiratory system of, 88-93
clinical implications of, 88*t*
larynx, trachea, and syrinx, 89-90
lung-air sac system, 90-92, 91*f*
mammals *vs.*, 88*t*
upper, 88-89, 89*f*
skin diseases in, 54-56, 55*f*
treatment of, 64*t*-65*t*
specific diagnostics for, 119-125
advanced imaging, 124-125
clinical pathology and laboratory tests,
120-121, 121*f*
endoscopy, 123, 123*f*
physical examination, 119-120, 120*f*
pulmonary and air sac biopsy, 123-124
radiology, 121-123, 122*f*
respiratory monitoring, 121
ultrasound, 124
thyroid glands of, 287-288
tracheoscopy in, 106*f*
urinary system diseases in, 505-520
advanced imaging for, 533
bacterial, 505-506
diagnostics for, 527-534
fungal, 506-507
iatrogenic, 518-520
imaging for, 531-534
neoplasia, 513
nutritional diseases in, 516-518
parasitic, 507-510
treatment for, 535*t*
viral, 510-513, 511*t*-512*t*
valvular diseases in, 178
vascular diseases in, 178
ventilatory muscles in, 92*t*

Bite wounds, in reptiles, 31
Blanding's turtle, endoscopic sexing, 8*f*
Blepharitis, 448-449, 449*f*
"Blister disease," 34
Blood pressure measurement
in birds, 194-195, 195*t*
in mammals, 190, 190*t*
in reptiles, 186
Blood uric acid quantification, limitation of,
527-528
BMR. *see* Basal metabolic rate (BMR)
Body-condition scoring, 9
Bohle iridovirus, 501
Bone
composition of, 374-375
healing, 375
Bone plates, 378*f*
Bordetella bronchiseptica, 102-103
Bornavirus, avian, 238
Botflies, in rabbits, 44-45
Bradycardia, in ferrets, 190
Branchial sieve, 222
Brinzolamide, 453
Bromocriptine, for prolactinomas, 282
Bronchodilators, 127
Bronopol, 129*t*
Brooklynella hostilis, in fish, 26, 26*f*
Buccopharyngeal cavity, 81
Bufolucilia bufonivora, 97
Bufolucilia silvarum, 97
Bullfrogs (*Rana catesbeiana*), 3-7
Bumblefoot, in birds, 38-39, 39*f*
Buphthalmos, 441

C

Cabergoline
for mammary tumors, in mammals, 489
for prolactinomas, 282
Caecilian, musculoskeletal system of, 353
Calcidiol, 290
Calciferol, 290
Calcitonin, 283, 290, 292-293, 358, 534*t*-535*t*
Calcitriol, 289-290, 357
Calcium, 289
in extracellular fluid, 356
metabolic bone disease and, 292, 357
for nutritional secondary
hyperparathyroidism (NSHP), 358
Calcium ethylenediaminetetraacetic acid
therapy, for heavy metal toxicity, 409
Calcium glubionate, 358, 534*t*-535*t*
Calcium gluconate, 534*t*-535*t*
Calcium homeostasis, 289-294
in birds, 292-293
in reptiles, 290-292
in small mammals, 293-294
Calcium metabolism hormones and related
molecules
in birds, 332*t*
in reptiles, 324*t*-326*t*
in small mammals, 341*t*-345*t*
Calcium-phosphorus ratio, in birds, 359-360
Calcium supplementation, for metabolic bone
disease, 403-404
Californian desert tortoise (*Gopherus agassizii*),
pericardial diseases in, 170
Campylobacter spp., in birds, 241

Cancellous bone, 374
Candida albicans, 39, 242
Candidiasis, in birds, 242
Canine distemper virus (CDV), in ferrets, 41,
103, 422, 422*f*, 454
Cannibalism, in rodents, 474
Capnometry, 121
Carbon dioxide (CO_2) laser, for castrating
sugar glider, 490, 490*f*
Carboplatin, 513
Cardiac lung, 83
Cardiac tamponade, 202
Cardiomegaly
in ball python, 185*f*
secondary to DCM, in mammals, 173*f*
Cardiovascular system, 151-220
anatomy and physiology of, 152-166
diseases in, 166-182
general therapeutics of, 202-203
function of, 151
thyroid gland and, 283
Cataracts
in birds, 448, 448*f*
in ferrets, 454
in fish, 440
in guinea pigs, 456
in reptiles, 446
Catfish, enteric septicemia of, 228
Caudata, respiratory system of, 81
Caudo-ventral approach, for avian urogenital
tract, 533
Cavum nasi proprium, of reptiles, 82
C-cell carcinoma, in ferrets, 288-289
CDV. *see* Canine distemper virus (CDV)
Cecoliths, in rabbits, 256
Cecotroph staining, in rabbits, 256
Cecotrophs, 227
Cecum, in rabbits, 227
Cefazolin 5% solution, 451
Cefotaxime, 127*t*
Ceftazidime, 130*t*-131*t*, 534*t*-535*t*
Ceftiofur sodium, 131*t*
Celioscopy, 201-202
Central nervous system, 392-434
anatomy and physiology of, 392-399
diseases in, 399-427
specific diagnostics for, 427-431
Cephalic lateral line system, in fish, 394-395,
394*f*
Cephalopods, 78
central nervous system of, anatomy and
physiology in, 393
closed circulatory system of, 153-154, 154*f*
Cerclage wire, for fractures, 377
Cervicocephalic diverticulum rupture, 106,
106*f*
in birds, surgical therapy for, 136-137
Cestodes, in fish, 230
Chandlerella quiscali, 415, 415*f*
Cheilitis, in guinea pigs, 46
Chelonians
endoscopy for, 117
musculoskeletal system of, 354
respiratory system of, 83
shell abscess in, 373
Chemical bioregulation, 277, 278*f*
Chemosis, 443, 443*f*